MEDICAL LIBRARY
WATFORD POSTGRADUATE
MEDICAL CENTRE
WATFORD GENERAL HOSPITAL
VICARAGE ROAD
WATFORD WD1 8HB

FUNDAMENTALS OF ANAESTHESIA

Second Edition

FUNDAMENTALS OF ANAESTHESIA

Second Edition

Edited by

Colin Pinnock

Ted Lin

Tim Smith

Associate Editor

Robert Jones

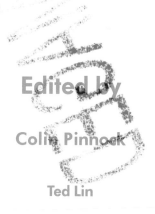

\\G\M\M/

© 2003
Greenwich Medical Media Ltd.
137 Euston Road
London
NW1 2AA

ISBN 1 900151 618

First Published 1999

Reprinted 2000

Second Edition 2003

While the advice and information in this book is believed to be true and accurate, neither the authors nor the publisher can accept any legal responsibility or liability for any loss or damage arising from actions or decisions based in this book. The ultimate responsibility for the treatment of patients and the interpretation lies with the medical practitioner. The opinions expressed are those of the authors and the inclusion in this book relating to a particular product, method or technique does not amount to an endorsement of its value or quality, or of the claims made of it by its manufacture. Every effort has been made to check drug dosages; however, it is still possible that errors have occurred. Furthermore, dosage schedules are constantly being revised and new side effects recognised. For these reasons, the medical practitioner is strongly urged to consult the drug companies' printed instructions before administering any of the drugs recommended in this book.

Apart from any fair dealing for the purposes of research or private study, or criticism or review, as permitted under the UK Copyright Designs and Patents Act, 1988, this publication may not be reproduced, stored, or transmitted, in any form or by any means, without the prior permission in writing of the publishers, or in the case of reprographic reproduction only in accordance with the terms of the licences issued by the Copyright Licensing Agency in the UK, or in accordance with the terms of the licences issued by the appropriate Reproduction Rights Organization outside the UK. Enquiries concerning reproduction outside the terms stated here should be sent to the publishers at the London address printed above.

The right of Colin Pinnock, Ted Lin and Tim Smith to be identified as editors of this work has been asserted by them in accordance with the Copyright, Designs and Patents Act 1988.

The publisher makes no representation, express or implied, with regard to the accuracy of the information contained in this book and cannot accept any legal responsibility or liability for any errors or omissions that may be made.

A catalogue record for this book is available from the British Library

Project Manager
Gavin Smith

Production and Design by
Saxon Graphics Limited, Derby

Printed in Great Britain by
William Clowes, Beccles, Suffolk

CONTENTS

Preface   vii

Section Editors   xi

Contributors   xi

Acknowledgements   xiii

List of abbreviations   xv

SECTION 1: CLINICAL ANAESTHESIA

Chapter 1:   Pre-operative Management   1
Chapter 2:   Induction of Anaesthesia   25
Chapter 3:   Intra-operative Management   43
Chapter 4:   Postoperative Management   59
Chapter 5:   Special Patient Circumstances   81
Chapter 6:   The Surgical Insult   109
Chapter 7:   Regional Anaesthesia &
             Analgesia   123
Chapter 8:   Principles of Resuscitation   147
Chapter 9:   Major Trauma   171
Chapter 10: Clinical Anatomy   189

SECTION 2: PHYSIOLOGY

Chapter 1:   Cellular Physiology   219
Chapter 2:   Body Fluids   241
Chapter 3:   Haematology and Immunology   257
Chapter 4:   Muscle Physiology   283
Chapter 5:   Cardiac Physiology   299
Chapter 6:   Physiology of the Circulation 331
Chapter 7:   Renal Physiology   361
Chapter 8:   Respiratory Physiology   395
Chapter 9:   Physiology of the Nervous
             System   425
Chapter 10: Gastro-intestinal Physiology   453
Chapter 11: Metabolism and Temperature
             Regulation   473
Chapter 12: Endocrinology   495

Chapter 13: Physiology of Pregnancy   511
Chapter 14: Foetal and Newborn Physiology 529

SECTION 3: PHARMACOLOGY

Chapter 1:   Physical Chemistry   537
Chapter 2:   Mechanisms of Drug Action   549
Chapter 3:   Pharmacodynamics   559
Chapter 4:   Pharmacokinetics   571
Chapter 5:   Anaesthetic Gases and Vapours 587
Chapter 6:   Hypnotics and Intravenous
             Anaesthetic Agents   601
Chapter 7:   Analgesic Drugs   619
Chapter 8:   Neuromuscular Blocking
             Agents   639
Chapter 9:   Local Anaesthetic Agents   653
Chapter 10: Central Nervous System
             Pharmacology   667
Chapter 11: Autonomic Nervous System
             Pharmacology   681
Chapter 12: Cardiovascular Pharmacology   699
Chapter 13: Respiratory Pharmacology   713
Chapter 14: Endocrine Pharmacology   721
Chapter 15: Gastro-intestinal Pharmacology 729
Chapter 16: Intravenous Fluids   737
Chapter 17: Pharmacology of Haemostasis   745
Chapter 18: Antimicrobial Therapy   753
Chapter 19: Clinical Trials – Design and
             Evaluation   767

SECTION 4: PHYSICS, CLINICAL MEASUREMENT AND STATISTICS

Chapter 1:   Applied Physics   773
Chapter 2:   Clinical Measurement   831
Chapter 3:   Anaesthetic Equipment   875
Chapter 4:   Basic Statistics   913

Index   927

This book is dedicated to Samuel and Edd

I am delighted that the success of 'Fundamentals' has enabled us to proceed to an early second edition. It will be apparent to the familiar reader that this edition has undergone rather more than a simple facelift. A great deal of feedback from both examiners and candidates has been used to modify and shape this current volume. New authors have been brought in to Section 1 to revise and modify the clinical chapters where necessary, (incorporating several important and new areas of emerging knowledge) whilst resuscitation and trauma chapters have been updated by their original writers. Anatomy has been extended in scope to reflect subjects that are currently popular in the Primary FRCA.

In Section 2, there are new chapters on neurology and endocrinology and an extra chapter on neonatal physiology has been incorporated to satisfy the demands of the examination syllabus.

Section 3 has been updated comprehensively with the removal of some drugs now lapsed and the incorporation of newer agents that have become available. By popular demand a new chapter on clinical trial design rounds off the pharmacology section.

It is, however, Section 4 that has undergone the most radical changes. I am very grateful to Ted Lin for the completely new physics and equipment chapters, which provide excellent core revision in these important areas. A greater number of diagrams (and many revised graphics) throughout the book and a completely new index complete the modifications over the first edition.

I thus believe that the second edition of 'Fundamentals' is an even better revision aid to the Primary FRCA examination and will build on the reputation of its forerunner. Once again my thanks go to my three co-editors for their hard work and determination.

Colin Pinnock
Redditch
October 2002

The advent of a syllabus for the FRCA examination, itself a requirement of the STA, seemed to me to provide an ideal opportunity for a dedicated revision textbook. It will therefore be of no surprise to readers that this volume mirrors closely the syllabus for the primary FRCA in both structure and content.

Having enlisted the willing help of my two co-editors, Tim Smith and Ted Lin, we set about recruiting authors to contribute. Chapter authors have been chosen for their ability and known prowess as teachers and a deliberate policy of not inviting 'usual' contributions from frequently seen names was taken. Having said that, several primary examiners appear as contributors and within each chapter coverage of revision topics has been kept as appropriate to the examination as possible.

To reduce the variability that is the bane of multi author texts I have personally edited every chapter to ensure consistency of style and it is a reflection of the workload involved that it has taken three years to complete this project. I am grateful to all contributing authors for their tolerance and good humour during alteration of their golden prose.

Whilst no single book can cover the entire syllabus as a 'one stop' aid, the majority of material covered in the examination is detailed within these pages. Some items lately included in the syllabus, after completion of the manuscript, will be added in future editions (such as the anatomy pertaining to ankle block). Candidates will, however, be well served if this book is used as a general basis for revision.

I am extremely grateful to Rob Jones who has been responsible for generating virtually all the artwork within this text, the few other diagrams being credited to their sources.

Thanks are also due to both my co-editors for their extensive work and dedication. If this volume enables any candidate to pass the primary examination, who would not have done so otherwise, then our job will have been well done.

C A Pinnock
July 1999

SECTION EDITORS

Section 1: Clinical Anaesthesia
C A Pinnock and R P Jones

Section 2: Physiology
E S Lin and C A Pinnock

Section 3: Pharmacology
C A Pinnock and T C Smith

Section 4: Physics and Clinical Measurement
E S Lin and C A Pinnock

CONTRIBUTORS

Dr B L Appadu
Consultant Anaesthetist
Peterborough General Hospital
Peterborough

Dr I T Campbell
Reader in Anaesthesia
University of Manchester

Dr G Cavill
Consultant Anaesthetist
Wansbeck General Hospital
Northumberland

Dr H B J Fischer
Consultant Anaesthetist
Alexandra Hospital
Redditch

Dr A K Gupta
Director of Neurocritical Care and Consultant Anaesthetist
Addenbrooke's Hospital
Cambridge

Dr R M Haden
Consultant Anaesthetist
Alexandra Hospital
Redditch

Dr C D Hanning
Consultant Anaesthetist
Leicester Royal Infirmary
Leicester

Dr R P Jones
Associate Specialist in Anaesthesia
Alexandra Hospital
Redditch

Dr K Kerr
Consultant Anaesthetist
Alexandra Hospital
Redditch

Dr T Leach
Consultant Anaesthetist
Alexandra Hospital
Redditch

Dr K E Lewis
Consultant Anaesthetist
Princess of Wales Hospital
Bridgend
West Glamorgan

Dr E S Lin
Consultant Anaesthetist
Glenfield Hospital
Leicester

Dr C J Lote
Senior Lecturer
University of Birmingham
Birmingham

Dr T McLeod
Consultant Anaesthetist
Birmingham Heartlands Hospital
Birmingham

Dr M C Mushambi
Consultant Anaesthetist
Leicester Royal Infirmary
Leicester

Dr J R Neilson
Consultant in Haematology
Russells Hall Hospital
Dudley

Dr J P Nolan
Consultant Anaesthetist
Royal United Hospital
Bath

Dr A Ogilvy
Consultant Anaesthetist
Leicester General Hospital
Leicester

Dr S M Parr
Consultant Anaesthetist
Solihull Hospital
Solihull

Dr F J Pickford
Consultant Anaesthetist
Prince Charles Hospital
Merthyr Tydfil

Dr C A Pinnock
Consultant Anaesthetist
Alexandra Hospital
Redditch

Professor D Rowbotham
Professor of Anaesthesia
Leicester Royal Infirmary
Leicester

Dr A M Sardesai
Specialist Registrar in Anaesthesia
Addenbrooke's Hospital
Cambridge

Dr J Stone
Consultant Microbiologist
Alexandra Hospital
Redditch

Dr J L C Swanevelder
Consultant Anaesthetist
Glenfield Hospital
Leicester

Dr T C Smith
Consultant Anaesthetist
Alexandra Hospital
Redditch

Dr M Tidmarsh
Consultant Anaesthetist
City General & Maternity Hospitals
Carlisle

Dr L Vries
Consultant Anaesthetist
Alexandra Hospital
Redditch

Professor A Wolf
Professor of Anaesthesia
Bristol Children's Hospital
Bristol

Dr J K Wood
Consultant Haematologist
Leicester Royal Infirmary
Leicester

ACKNOWLEDGEMENTS

The Association of Anaesthetists of Great Britain and Ireland
9 Bedford Square, London WC1B 3RA

Section 1

Chapter 2
PR.12   Pre-operative assessment of the pacemaker patient

Chapter 3
I.4   Clinical features of anaphylaxis
I.5   The first observed clinical features of anaphylaxis
I.6   Management of a patient with suspected anaphylaxis

Chapter 4
IN.6   Recommendations for standards of monitoring during anaesthesia and recovery

Chapter 5
PO.1   Criteria to be met before transfer from recovery room to general ward

Chapter 6
SC.9   Indications for intubation and ventilation after head injury
SC.10   Transfer checklist for neurosurgical patients

Section 4

Chapter 3
EQ.10   Association of Anaesthetists checklist

British Journal of Anaesthesia
BMJ Publishing Group, BMA House, Tavistock Square, London WC1H 9JR

Section 1

Chapter 1
EQ.4   Mapleson classification of breathing systems

Chapter 5
PO.10   DVT risk group classification

European Resuscitation Council
PO Box 13, B-2610 Antwerpen, Belgium
Resuscitation Council (UK)

Section 1

Chapter 9
RS.1   Adult basic life support   ERC 1997

RS.2   Assessment of the airway   ERC 1996
RS.3   Guidelines for treatment of an unconscious victim   ERC 2000
RS.4   The ALS algorithm for the management of cardiac arrest in adults   ERC 2000
RS.5   Differential diagnosis of SVT & VT by treatment   ERC 2000
RS.6   Algorithm for treatment of broad complex tachycardia   ERC 2000
RS.7   Algorithm for treatment of narrow complex tachycardia and high risk atrial fibrillation   ERC 1996
RS.8   Algorithm for bradycardia and heart blocks   ERC 1996
RS.9   Drugs used in life threatening peri-arrest arrythmias
RS.11   Management of upper airway obstruction by a foreign body in the infant or child   Resuscitation Council (UK) 2000
RS.12   Summary of assessment of circulation and compression techniques in infants and children   Resuscitation Council (UK) 2000
RS.13   Paediatric advanced life support   Resuscitation Council (UK) 2000

Penlon Ltd
Radley Road, Abingdon, Oxon, OX14 3PH

Section 1

Chapter 3
I.8   Laryngoscope blades

Pharmacokinetics of Anaesthesia
Ed. Prys-Roberts C, Hug C. Blackwell Scientific Publications, Oxford 1984

Section 3

Chapter 4
PK.9   Mapleson's water analogue models

Proctor & Gamble Pharmaceuticals UK Ltd
Staines, TW18 3AZ

Section 1

Chapter 4
IN.10   Features of MH
IN.11   Treatment of MH

**The Sourcebook of Medical Illustration
Ed. Cull P. The Parthenon Publishing Group,
Carnforth, UK, 1989**

Section 1

Chapter 8

RA.7	Patient positions for spinal anaesthesia
RA.21	Patient position for caudal anaesthesia
RA.22	Needle angulation for caudal anaesthesia

Chapter 11

A.1	The mouth
A.2	Nerve supply of the tongue
A.3	Lateral view of the nasal cavity
A.4	Coronal section of the nose and maxillary sinus
A.6	Larynx, direct laryngoscopic view
A.7	Larynx, anterior view
A.8	Larynx, posterior view

A.9	Larynx, lateral view
A.10	Larynx, sectional view
A.11	The respiratory tree
A.19	Cervical plexus
A.20	The brachial plexus
A.22	Nerves of the lumbar plexus
A.23	Nerves of the sacral plexus
A.24	Cervical vertebra, superior and leteral views
A.25	Thoracic vertebra, superior and lateral views
A.26	Lumbar vertebra, superior and leteral views

Section 2

Chapter 9

| NE.9 | Structure of the eye |
| NE.23 | Distribution of the autonomic nervous system |

Chapter 11

| MT.20 | Structure of the liver |

The editors gratefully acknowledge the help given by the above parties in granting permission to use the material cited.

α	alpha
β	beta
2,3-DPG	2,3-diphosphoglycerate
5-HT	5-hydroxytryptamine
A	adenine
A	ampere
A&E	accident and emergency
ABC	airway, breathing, circulation
ABV	arterial blood volume
AC	alternating current
ACE	angiotensin converting enzyme
Ach	acetyl choline
ACT	activated clotting time
ACTH	adrenocorticotrophic hormone
ADCC	antibody dependent cell mediated cytotoxicity
ADH	anti diuretic hormone
ADP	adenosine diphosphate
AED	automated external defibrillator
AER	audio evoked response
AF	atrial fibrillation
AID	autoimmune deficiency disease
ALS	advanced life support
AMP	adenosine monophosphate
ANF	atrial natriuretic factor
Ang I	angiotensin I
Ang II	angiotensin II
ANOVA	analysis of variance
ANP	atrial natiuretic peptide
ANSI	American National Standards Institute
AP	action potential (in cardiac physiology)
AP	antero posterior
AP	anaesthetic proof
APC	antigen presenting cell
APCR	activated protein C resistance
APG	anaesthetic proof category
APL	adjustable pressure limiting
APTT	activated partial thromboplastin time
AQP	aquaporins
ARDS	adult respiratory distress syndrome
ASA	American Society of Anaesthesiology
ASIS	anterior superior iliac spine
ATLS	advanced trauma life support
ATP	adenosine triphosphate
ATPS	ambient temperature and pressure saturated
AUC	area under curve
AV block	atrio ventricular block
AV	atrioventricular
bd	twice a day
Bl/G	blood/gas
BLS	basic life support
B_M	B memory cell
BMI	body mass index
BMR	basal metabolic rate
$BMRO_2$	basal metabolic rate of oxygen consumption
BNP	brain natiuretic peptide
BP	blood pressure
bpm	beats per minute
Br/Bl	brain/blood
BSA	body surface area
BSER	brain stem evoked responses
BTPS	body temperature and pressure saturated
c	centi
C	coulomb
Ca	arterial compliance
CAM	cell adhesion molecules
cAMP	cyclic adenosine monophosphate
CAO_2	alveolar oxygen content
CaO_2	arterial oxygen content
CAPD	continuous ambulatory peritoneal dialysis
CB	cannabinoid
CBF	cerebral blood flow
CBG	corticosteroid binding globulin
CC	closing capacity
CcO_2	capillary oxygen content
cd	candela
CFAM	cerebral function analysing monitor
CGRP	calcitonin gene related peptide
CI	cardiac index
CI	confidence interval (statistics)
CK	creatinine kinase
Cl	clearance
C_L	lung compliance
$CMRO_2$	cerebral metabolic rate of oxygen consumption
CNS	central nervous system
CO	cardiac output
CO_2	carbon dioxide
CoA	co-enzyme A
COAD	chronic obstructive airways disease
COMT	catechol-o-methyl transferase
COP	colloid oncotic pressure
COPA	cuffed oropharyngeal airway
cos	cosine
COSHH	control of substances hazardous to health
COX	cyclo-oxygenase
CP	creatine phosphate
CPAP	continuous positive airway pressure
CPD-A	citrate phosphate dextrose adenine

CPK MB	creatinine phosphokinase (cardiac iso-enzyme)
CPP	coronary perfusion pressure
CPR	cardiopulmonary resuscitation
C_R	respiratory system compliance
CRH	corticotrophin releasing hormone
CSE	combined spinal epidural
CSF	cerebrospinal fluid
CSM	Committee for Safety of Medicines
CT	computerised tomography
CTZ	chemo receptor trigger zone
$C\bar{v}O_2$	mixed venous oxygen content
CVP	central venous pressure
CVS	cardiovascular system
CW	chest wall compliance
d	deci
D	dopaminergic
da	deca
DC	direct current
DCR	dacrocystorhinostomy
DDAVP	1-deamino-8-arginine vasopressin
DIC	disseminated intravascular coagulation
DIT	di-iodothyronine
DLCO	diffusing capacity of the lungs for carbon monoxide
DNA	deoxyribonucleic acid
DNR	do not resuscitate
DNAR	do not attempt resuscitation
$\dot{D}O_2$	oxygen delivery
DVT	deep vein thrombosis
Ea	arterial elastance
EAR	expired air respiration
EBC	effective blood concentration
EC	effective concentration
ECA	electrical control activity
ECF	extra cellular fluid
ECF-A	eosinophil chemotactic factor of anaphylaxis
ECFV	extra cellular fluid volume
ECG	electrocardiogram
ECV	effective circulating volume
ED_{50}	effective dose in 50% of population
ED_{95}	effective dose in 95% of population
EDP	end diastolic point
EDPVR	end diastolic pressure volume relationship
EDRF	endothelium derived relaxing factor
EDTA	ethylenediaminetetra-acetate
EDV	end diastolic volume
EEG	electroencephalogram
Ees	ventricular systolic elastance
EF	ejection fraction
EM	electromagnetic
EMD	electromechanical dissociation
EMF	electro motive force
EMG	electromyogram

EMLA	eutectic mixture of local anaesthetic
EMS	emergency medical service
ENT	ear nose and throat
EPO	erythropoietin
EPSP	excitatory post synaptic potential
ER	endoplasmic reticulum
ERC	European Resuscitation Council
ERV	expiratory reserve volume
ESP	end systolic point
ESPVR	end systolic pressure volume relationship
ESR	erythrocyte sedimentation rate
ESRA	European Society of Regional Anaesthesia
ESV	end systolic volume
ET	endothelium
ETC	oesophageal tracheal combitube
$ETCO_2$	end tidal carbon dioxide
f	femto
f	frequency of breaths
F	gas flow
F/M	foeto maternal ratio
FA	fatty acid
FAC	fractional area change
$FACO_2$	fractional alveolar carbon dioxide concentration
$FADH_2$	flavine adenine dinucleotide
FBC	full blood count
FDC	F-decalin
FDP	fibrin degradation products
Fe^{2+}	ferrous iron state
$F\bar{E}CO_2$	fractional mixed expired carbon dioxide concentration
FEMG	frontalis electromyogram
FEV%	ratio of FEV_1 to FVC
FEV_1	forced expiratory volume in one second
FFA	free fatty acids
FFP	fresh frozen plasma
FFT	fast Fourier transform
FG	fat group
FGF	fresh gas flow
FiO_2	fractional inspired oxygen concentration
FNHTR	febrile non haemolytic transfusion reactions
FRC	functional residual capacity
FSH	follicle stimulating hormone
FTPA	F-tripropylamine
FVC	forced vital capacity
G	giga
G	guanine
GCS	Glasgow coma scale
GDP	guanine diphosphate
GFR	glomerular filtration rate
GH	growth hormone
GI	gastro-intestinal
GIT	gastro-intestinal tract
GMP	guanine monophosphate

GP	glycolytic phosphorylation		ISI	international sensitivity index
GTN	glyceryl trinitrate		IT	implant tested
GTP	guanosine triphosphate		ITP	idiopathic thrombocytopaenia purpura
h	hecto		ITU	intensive therapy unit
H	hour		IU	International units
H_2	histamine receptor 2		IV	intravenous
HAFOE	high air flow oxygen entrainment		IVC	inferior vena cava
HAS	human albumin solution		IVIg	intravenous immunoglobulin
Hb	haemoglobin		IVRA	intravenous regional anaesthesia
HbA	adult haemoglobin		J	joule
HbCO	carboxyhaemoglobin		JVP	jugular venous pressure
HbF	foetal haemoglobin		K	Kelvin
Hbmet	methaemoglobin		k	kilo
HbS	haemoglobin sickle		KCCT	kaolin clotting time
Hbsulph	sulphaemoglobin		KE	kinetic energy
HCG	human chorionic gonadotrophin		LAK	lymphokine activated killer
HCO_3^-	bicarbonate		LAP	left atrial pressure
Hct	haematocrit		Laser	light amplification by stimulated emission of radiation
HD	haemodialysis			
HDL	high density lipoprotein		LBP	lipopolysaccharide binding protein
HDN	haemolytic disease of the newborn		LD_{50}	lethal dose 50%
HDU	high dependency unit		LDL	low density lipoprotein
HELLP	hemolytic anaemia elevated liver enzymes low platelets		LED	light emitting diode
			LH	luteinising hormone
HFJV	high frequency jet ventilation		LIS	lateral intracellular spaces
HIV	human immunodeficiency virus		LMA	laryngeal mask airway
HME	heat and moisturiser exchanger		LMW	low molecular weight
HMWK	high molecular weight kininogen		LOH	loop of Henle
HPL	human placental lactogen		LOR	loss of resistance
HPV	hypoxic pulmonary vasoconstriction		LOS	lower oesophageal pressure
HR	heart rate		LT	leukotriene
Hz	hertz		LV	left ventricle
I	current		LVEDP	left ventricular end diastolic pressure
I:E	inspiratory:expiratory ratio		LVEDV	left ventricular end diastolic volume
ICAM	intercellular adhesion molecule		LVF	left ventricular failure
ICF	intracellular fluid		LVH	left ventricular hypertrophy
ICP	intracranial pressure		LVSW	left ventricular stroke work
IDDM	insulin dependant diabetes mellitus		LVSWI	left ventricular stroke work index
IgA	immunoglobulin A		M	mega
IgE	immunoglobulin E		M	metre
IgG	immunoglobulin G		m	milli
IGF	insulin like growth factor		M	muscarinic
iGluR	ionotropic glutamine receptor		mA	milliamps
IgM	immunoglobulin M		MAC	minimum alveolar concentration
IHD	ischaemic heart disease		MAO	monoamine oxidase
IL	interleukin		MAOI	monoamine oxidase inhibitor
ILCOR	International Liaison Committee on Resuscitation		MAP	mean arterial pressure
			MCH	mean cell haemoglobin
IM	intramuscular		MCV	mean cell volume
IML	intermediolateral		MDA	manual dilatation of anus
INR	international normalised ratio		MDP	maximum diastolic potential
IOP	intra-ocular pressure		MEFR	mid expiratory flow rate
IPPV	intermittent positive pressure ventilation		MEP	miniature end plate potential
IR	infra red		MET	medical emergency teams
IRV	inspiratory reserve volume		MFR	mannosyl-fucosyl receptor

MG	muscle group
MH	malignant hyperthermia
MHC	major histocompatability
MI	myocardial infarction
MIC	minimum inhibitory concentration
μ	micro
MILS	manual in line stabilisation
MIR	minimum infusion rate
MIRL	membrane inhibitor of reactive lysis
MIT	mono-iodothyronine
MMC	migratory motor complex
mmHg	millimetres of mercury (pressure)
MODS	multiple organ dysfunction syndrome
mol	mole
MONA	morphine, oxygen, nitrates, aspirin
MPAP	mean pulmonary arterial pressure
mRNA	messenger RNA
MRSA	methicillin resistant *Staphyloccocus aureus*
MSH	melanocyte stimulating hormone
MUGA	multigated scan
MV	minute volume
MW	molecular weight
n	nano
N	newton
nAChR	nicotinic acetylcholine receptors
NADH	nicotinamide adenine dinucleotide
NADPH	nicotinamide adenine dinucleotide phosphate
$NaHCO_3$	sodium bicarbonate
NANC	non adrenergic non cholinergic
Nd-YAG	neodymium yttrium-aluminium garnet
NIBP	non invasive blood pressure
NIST	non interchangeable screw thread
NK	natural killer
NMDA	N-methyl-D-aspartate
NMJ	neuro muscular junction
NO	nitric oxide
NSAID	non steroidal anti-inflammatory drug
NTS	nucleus tractus solitarius
NV	nausea and vomiting
NWC	number of words counted
O/G	oil/gas
O/W	oil/water
OCI	oesophageal contractility index
ODC	oxyhaemoglobin dissociation curve
Ω	ohm
OP	oxidative phosporylation
OPAC	oximetric pulmonary artery catheter
Osm	Osmoles/litre
π	osmotic pressure
p	pico
P	probability
Pa	pascal
PABA	para-amino benzoic acid
PAC	pulmonary artery catheter

$PACO_2$	alveolar carbon dioxide partial pressure
$PaCO_2$	arterial carbon dioxide partial pressure
PAF	platelet activating factor
PAH	para-aminohippuric acid
PAO_2	alveolar oxygen partial pressure
PaO_2	arterial oxygen partial pressure
PART	patient at risk team
Paw	airway pressure
PBP	penicillin binding proteins
PCA	patient controlled analgesia
PCC	prothrombinase complex concentrates
PCEA	patient controlled epidural analgesia
PCWP	pulmonary capillary wedge pressure
PD	photodiode
PDE	phosphodiesterase enzyme
PDGF	platelet derived growth factor
PDPH	post dural puncture headache
PE	potential energy
PE	pulmonary embolus
$PE'CO_2$	partial pressure end tidal carbon dioxide
PEA	pulseless electrical activity
PEEP	positive end expiratory pressure
PEFR	peak expiratory flow rate
PF4	platelet factor 4
PFC	perfluorocarbon
PGE	prostaglandin E
PGI	prostaglandin I
Pi	inorganic phosphate
PIH	prolactin inhibiting hormone
PK	prekallikrein
PLOC	provoked lower oesophageal contractions
PMN	polymorphonuclear neutrophils
PONV	post operative nausea and vomiting
PPF	plasma protein fraction
PPHN	persistent pulmonary hypertension of the newborn
ppm	parts per million
PPP	pentose phosphate pathway
PRI	pain rating index
PRST	pressure, rate, sweating, tears
PSI	pounds per square inch
PT	prothrombin time
PTC	post tetanic count
PTH	parathormone
PTT	partial thromboplastin time
PTTK	partial thromboplastin time with kaolin
PV	pressure volume
PVC	poly vinyl chloride
PVD	peripheral vascular disease
PVR	pulmonary vascular resistance
$\dot{Q}$	cardiac output
Q	charge
$\dot{Q}$	flow
$\dot{Q}s$	shunt flow
R	resistance (electrical)

R	universal gas constant		SVWI	stroke volume work index
RAP	right atrial pressure		SW	stroke work
RAST	radioallergosorbent test		T	absolute temperature
RBC	red blood cell		T	tera
RBF	renal blood flow		T	thiamine
Re	Reynold's number		$t_{\frac{1}{2}}$	half life
REM	rapid eye movement		T_3	tri-iodothyronine
RH	relative humidity		T_4	thyroxine
RIMA	reversible inhibitor of monoamine oxidase A		tan	tangent
			TBG	thyroxine binding globulin
RMP	resting membrane potential		TBV	total body volume
RNA	ribonucleic acid		TBW	total body water
RNU	regional neurosurgical unit		TCR	T cell receptor
ROC	receptor operated ion channels		TCRE	trans cervical resection of the endometrium
RPF	renal plasma flow			
RQ	respiratory quotient		TENS	transcutaneous electrical nerve stimulation
rRNA	ribosomal RNA			
RS	respiratory system		T_H	T helper cell
RSI	rapid sequence induction		THR	total hip replacement
RT_3	reverse tri-iodthyronine		TIVA	total intravenous anaesthesia
RV	residual volume		TKR	total knee replacement
RV	right ventricle		TLC	total lung capacity
RVSWI	right ventricular stroke work index		TLV	total lung volume
s	second		T_m	tubular maximum
S/N	signal to noise ratio		TNF	tumour necrosis factor
SA	sino atrial		TNF-α	tumour necrosis factor α
SAGM	saline adenine glucose mannitol		TOE	transoesophageal echocardiography
SaO_2	arterial oxygen saturation		TOF	train of four
SD	standard deviation		TP	threshold potential
SEM	standard error of the mean		t-PA	tissue type plasminogen activator
SFH	stroma free haemoglobin		TPP	thiamine pyrophosphate
SI	stroke index		TRALI	transfusion related acute lung injury
SI	System of International units		TRH	thyrotrophin releasing hormone
SIADH	syndrome of inappropriate ADH secretion		tRNA	transfer RNA
			TSH	thyroid stimulating hormone
sin	sine		TT	thrombin time
SIRS	systemic inflammatory response syndrome		TTN	transient tachypnoea of the newborn
			TUR	trans urethral resection
SL	semilunar		TURBT	trans urethral resection of bladder tumour
SLE	systemic lupus erythematosis		TURP	trans urethral resection of the prostate
SLOC	spontaneous lower oesophageal contractions		TXA_2	thromboxane A_2
			U&E	urea and electrolytes
SNGFR	single nephron glomerular filtration rate		UBF	uterine blood flow
SpO_2	pulse oximeter oxygen saturation		UK	United Kingdom
SR	sarcoplasmic reticulum		UOS	upper oesophageal sphincter
SRS-A	slow reacting substance of anaphylaxis		URT	upper respiratory tract
SSRI	selective serotonin re-uptake inhibitors		URTI	upper respiratory tract infection
STOP	suction termination of pregnancy		UTP	uridine triphosphate
Σ	sum of		UV	ultra violet
SV	stroke volume		v	velocity
SVC	superior vena cava		V	volt
SVI	systemic vascular index		V/Q	ventilation/perfusion
$S\bar{v}O_2$	mixed venous oxygen saturation		VA	alveolar volume
SVP	saturated vapour pressure		V_{BL}	blood volume
SVR	systemic vascular resistance		VC	vital capacity

$\dot{V}CO_2$	carbon dioxide flux	V_{PL}	plasma volume
VD	anatomical dead space	V_{RBC}	red blood cell volume
Vd	volume of distribution	VRE	vancomycin resistant enterococci
VER	visual evoked response	VRG	vessel rich group
VF	ventricular fibrillation	V_T	tidal volume
VIC	vaporiser inside circle	VT	ventricular tachycardia
VIE	vacuum insulated evaporator	V_TCO_2	volume of carbon dioxide per breath
V_{INT}	interstitial fluid volume	vWF	von Willebrand's factor
VIP	vasoactive intestinal polypeptide	W	watt
VLDL	very low density lipoprotein	WBC	white blood cell
VMA	vannilyl mandelic acid	WCC	white cell count
$\dot{V}O_2$	oxygen uptake in the lungs	WHO	World Health Organisation
VOC	vaporiser outside circle		
VPC	ventricular premature contractions		

SECTION 1: 1
PRE-OPERATIVE MANAGEMENT

G. Cavill and K. Kerr

ASSESSMENT
The Airway
ASA Status

PREPARATION FOR ANAESTHESIA
Premedication
Pre-operative factors
    starvation
    fluid status
    electrolyte disturbances
    smoking

CONCURRENT MEDICAL DISEASE
Respiratory disease
    infection
    asthma
    chronic obstructive pulmonary disease
Cardiovascular disease
    hypertension
    ischaemic heart disease
    pacemakers
    valvular disease
Haematological disease
    anaemia
    sickle cell
    clotting abnormalities
Musculoskeletal disease
    rheumatoid arthritis
Renal disease
    renal failure
Endocrine disease
    diabetes mellitus

CONCURRENT MEDICATION

CONCURRENT SURGICAL DISEASE
Intestinal obstruction
Acute abdomen

ASSESSMENT

The safe conduct of anaesthesia requires meticulous pre-operative assessment and planning, the primary objectives of a pre-operative visit. Such a visit provides the opportunity for the anaesthetist to introduce himself and provide a brief explanation of his role. This in itself will do much to allay patient anxiety, arguably more effectively than premedication. Effective pre-operative assessment requires accurate identification of pre-existing problems and anticipation of difficulties that might result during or after anaesthesia. Through appropriate planning the patient's pre-operative condition can then be optimised.

A history should be taken of previous anaesthetic experiences and of any family history of problems connected with anaesthesia. The patient's general health should be assessed and drug treatment, allergies, history of reflux and smoking and alcohol habits noted. An examination of the patient's dentition and airway must be made. The results of relevant investigations should be noted. The pre-operative visit also allows the anaesthetist to explain what will happen during anaesthesia and to discuss post operative analgesia and any other concerns the patient may have. Premedication may also be prescribed at this time.

THE AIRWAY

Ease of intubation has been graded according to the best possible view obtained on laryngoscopy (Cormack 1984). Grades 3 and 4 are difficult intubations.

- Grade 1 Whole of glottis visible
- Grade 2 Glottis incompletely visible
- Grade 3 Epiglottis but not glottis visible
- Grade 4 Epiglottis not visible

The reported incidence of difficult intubation varies, but is around 1 in 65 intubations. Despite careful history and examination, 20% of difficult intubations are not predicted. The consequences may be disastrous. A history of previous difficult intubation is important but a history of straightforward intubation several years earlier may be falsely reassuring as the patient's weight, cervical spine movement and disease process may all have changed. Some congenital conditions may predict a difficult intubation e.g. Pierre Robin syndrome, Marfan's syndrome or cystic hygroma. Pathological conditions can make intubation difficult e.g. tumour, infection or scarring of the upper airway tissues. There is no one test that is able to predict all difficult intubations. Clinical assessment of the airway is therefore essential. In the Mallampati scoring system the patient sits opposite the anaesthetist with mouth open and tongue protruded. The structures visible at the back of the mouth are noted (Mallampati 1985) as described below.

- Class 1 Faucial pillars, soft palate and uvula visible
- Class 2 Faucial pillars and soft palate visible, uvula masked by base of tongue
- Class 3 Only soft palate visible
- Class 4 Soft palate not visible

The modified Mallampati classification produces a high incidence of false positives. If the thyromental distance with the neck extended is less than 6.5 cm or the width of three fingers, difficult intubation is predicted. A thyromental distance of less than 6.5 cm and Mallampati class 3 or 4 predicts 80% of difficult intubations.

The Wilson risk factors may provide additional predictive information on the airway. The Wilson risk factors each score 0–2 points, to give a maximum of 10 points. A score > 2 predicts 75% of difficult intubations, also with a high incidence of false positives. The Wilson risk factors are:

- Obesity
- Restricted head and neck movements
- Restricted jaw movement
- Receding mandible
- Buck teeth

Inability to flex the chin onto the chest indicates poor neck movement. Once the neck is fully flexed, a patient should be able to move their head more than 15° to demonstrate normal occipito-axial movement. Reduced jaw movements are demonstrated by poor mouth opening (particularly if of less than two fingers' width) and by inability to protrude the lower teeth beyond the upper.

Radiological features may aid prediction of a difficult intubation but are not routinely performed. They include:

- Reduced distance between occiput and spine of C1 and between spines of C1 and C2
- Ratio of mandibular length to posterior mandibular depth > 3.6
- Increased depth of mandible

AMERICAN SOCIETY OF ANESTHESIOLOGISTS (ASA) SCORING SYSTEM

The ASA scoring system describes the pre-operative condition of a patient (Sacklad 1941) and is used routinely for every patient in the UK. It makes no allowances for the patient's age, smoking history, any obesity or pregnancy. Anticipated difficulties in intubation are not relevant. Addition of the postscript E indicates emergency surgery. There is some correlation between ASA score and peri-operative mortality. Definitions applied in the ASA system are given below in Figure PR.1.

THE ASA SCORING SYSTEM
(PERI-OPERATIVE MORTALITY GIVEN IN BRACKETS)

I	Healthy patient (0.1%)
II	Mild systemic disease, no functional limitation (0.2%)
III	Moderate systemic disease, definite functional limitation (1.8%)
IV	Severe systemic disease that is a constant threat to life (7.8%)
V	Moribund patient, unlikely to survive 24 hours with or without operation (9.4%)

In 1983 a sixth category was introduced to describe "a declared brain-dead patient whose organs are being removed for donor purposes"

Figure PR.1

PREPARATION FOR ANAESTHESIA

PREMEDICATION

As more day surgery is performed and more patients are admitted to hospital close to the scheduled time of surgery, premedication has become less common. The main indication for premedication remains anxiety, for which a benzodiazepine is usually prescribed, sometimes with metoclopramide to promote absorption. Premedication serves several purposes: anxiolysis; smoother induction of anaesthesia; reduced requirement for intravenous induction agents and possibly reduced likelihood of awareness.

Intramuscular opioids are now rarely prescribed as premedication. The prevention of aspiration pneumonitis in patients with reflux requires premedication with an H_2-antagonist, the evening before and morning of surgery, and sodium citrate administration immediately prior to induction of anaesthesia. Topical local anaesthetic cream over two potential sites for venous cannulation is usually prescribed for children. Anticholinergic agents may be prescribed to dry secretions or to prevent bradycardia e.g. during squint surgery. Usual medication should be continued up to the time of anaesthesia.

PRE-OPERATIVE FACTORS

Starvation

It is routine practice to starve patients prior to surgery in attempt to minimise the volume of stomach contents and hence decrease the incidence of their aspiration. Aspiration of solid food particles may cause asphyxiation and aspiration of gastric acid may cause pneumonitis (Mendelson's Syndrome). Guidelines for pre-operative starvation are becoming less restrictive as more information becomes available. Currently many centres forbid their patients to eat for five hours or to drink for three hours prior to theatre. Milky drinks are not allowed because their high fat content increases gastric transit time. Pre-operative chewing of gum does not increase intragastric volumes.

Prolonged periods of starvation give rise to problems. Dehydration may occur, particularly in children and in patients who are pyrexial or who have received bowel preparation. Infants may become hypoglycaemic. In patients with cyanotic heart disease, sickle cell disease or polycythaemia dehydration may precipitate thrombosis. In jaundiced patients the hepato-renal syndrome may be precipitated. It is thus essential that these patients receive intravenous therapy while they are being starved.

Fluid status

Healthy patients can balance daily fluid intake and output. Adults exchange approximately 5% of body water each day, while infants exchange about 15% and so are at greater risk of dehydration. A patient's fluid status may be affected by the underlying disease process or by its treatment (Figure PR.2) and there may be associated electrolyte disturbances. In certain conditions such as trauma, infection or ileus, fluid is redistributed rather than lost from the body, but will nonetheless still require replacing to maintain fluid

Disturbances of fluid balance		
	Increased	**Decreased**
Input	Excessive IV fluids	Nausea
		Dysphagia
		Nil by mouth orders
		Coma
		Severe respiratory disease
Output	Sweating	Syndrome of inappropriate
	Diarrhoea (including	ADH secretion (SIADH)
	bowel preparation)	
	Vomiting	Renal impairment
	Polyuria	
	Haemorrrhage	
	Burns	

Figure PR.2

balance. If patients have been ill for longer periods malnutrition may also be a problem.

Fluid balance should be assessed pre-operatively in all patients who are at risk of disturbances which is most likely in emergencies. A history of any of the above will direct clinical examination. Postural hypotension, tachycardia and hypotension may be found in volume depletion, while a raised jugular venous pressure (JVP) and peripheral oedema may be found in volume overload. Skin turgor, or fontanelle tension in infants, is a useful guide and assessment of urine output is very important. Oliguria is defined as a urine output of less than 0.5 ml/kg/H. Relevant investigations include serum electrolytes, urea and creatinine. A urea raised proportionally more than the creatinine value indicates dehydration.

Correction of fluid balance

Therapy should be guided by central venous pressure (CVP), urine output, blood pressure, heart rate and electrolyte balance. Where fluid overload is diagnosed, fluid restriction and possibly diuretic therapy are required. If fluid depletion is diagnosed, replacement of the lost fluid, plus maintenance fluids, is required. Hypovolaemia resulting from blood loss, necessitates red cell transfusion. If plasma has been lost, as in burns patients, plasma protein fraction (PPF) will be required. Maintenance fluid requirements are 40 ml/kg/day in adults (greater for children). Excessive administration of 5% dextrose to correct dehydration may lead to hyperglycaemia and hyponatraemia, while

excessive administration of 0.9% saline may cause hypernatraemia and peripheral and pulmonary oedema.

Electrolyte disturbances

Disturbances of electroytes may be due to the underlying disease process, to drugs, particularly diuretics, or to iatrogenic causes. It is rare for a patient to exhibit overt clinical signs but electrolyte disturbances present several potential problems for the anaesthetist (Figure PR.3). It is particularly important to assess the volume status of the patient who has an electrolyte disturbance. Electrolyte disturbances are more likely to be acute and hence more serious in patients presenting for emergency surgery.

Pre-operatively, hyponatraemia may be long standing, commonly due to diuretics and this situation rarely requires treatment. More acutely, pre-operative hyponatraemia is often due to inappropriate intravenous therapy on the ward. Treatment should comprise the administration of intravenous normal saline and, if there are signs of fluid overload, diuretics. Severe symptomatic hyponatraemia has a high mortality and is seen most commonly as part of the TUR syndrome. Hyponatraemia should be treated promptly with diuretics and only rarely with hypertonic saline. Too rapid correction of severe acute hyponatraemia may result in subdural haemorrhage, pontine lesions and cardiac failure. Hypernatraemia is mainly a problem when associated with volume

PROBLEMS AND CAUSES OF ELECTROLYTE DISTURBANCES

Problems	Causes
Hyponatraemia	
Confusion, fits and coma possible	Excess water intake (particularly intravenously)
If water excess: hypertension, cardiac failure, anorexia and nausea	Diuretics
	TUR syndrome
	Impaired water excretion (SIADH, hypothyroidism cardiac failure, nephrotic syndrome)
Hypernatraemia	
Rarely symptons if simple water loss	Reduced intake (impaired consciousness, unable to swallow, no water)
If severe, there may be muscle weakness, signs of volume depletion and coma	Increased insensible loss (fever, hot environment hyperventilation)
	Impairment of urinary concentrating mechanism (diabetes insipidus, hyperosmolar non ketotic coma or diabetic ketoacidosis)
Hypokalaemia	
Muscular weakness .	Diuretics
Potentiates non depolarising muscle relaxants	Gastro-intestinal loss (diarrhoea, vomiting, fistula, ileus, villous adenoma of large bowel)
Cardiac arrhythmias	Recovery phase of diabetic ketoacidosis and acute tubular necrosis
Rhythm problems if on digoxin	Post relief of urinary tract obstruction
	Reduced intake
	Cushing's syndrome
	Hyperaldosteronism
Hyperkalaemia	
Spurious if blood sample haemolysed	Acute or chronic renal disease
Cardiac arrest may occur if plasma K^+ > 7 mmol/l	Shift of K^+ out of cells (tissue damage)
	Acidosis (particularly diabetic ketoacidosis)
	Increased intake
	Drugs impairing secretion (K^+ retaining diuretics)
	Addison's disease
	Tissue breakdown (rhabdomyolysis)

Figure PR.3

depletion and it should be corrected by administration of 5% dextrose intravenously taking care not to fluid overload the patient.

Chronic changes in plasma potassium are well tolerated but acute changes are associated with electrocardiogram (ECG) changes and cardiac dysrhythmias (Figure PR.4). It is the ratio of intracellular to extracellular potassium that is relevant to myocardial excitability. Where the disturbance is chronic, this ratio will be nearly normal. Hypokalaemia may be treated by giving potassium either orally or intravenously. Care must be taken in the presence of renal insufficiency or low cardiac output states as hyperkalaemia may result. A flow controlled pump should be used to control the intravenous infusion rate if the concentration of potassium exceeds 40 mmol/L and ECG monitoring will be required as ventricular fibrillation may occur if hypokalaemia is corrected too quickly. Hyperkalaemia should be treated over several days by the administration of calcium resonium. If

ECG changes are noted or more rapid correction of acute changes is required pre-operatively insulin, 20 units in 100 ml 20% dextrose over 30–60 minutes, may be given. This may be repeated depending on the next serum potassium. Intravenous calcium, 10 ml 10% calcium gluconate, immediately (but temporarily) improves automaticity, conduction and contractility.

Smoking

A heavy smoker is anyone who smokes 20 or more cigarettes per day. Smoking causes several peri-operative problems: increased airway reactivity; increased sputum production and retention; bronchospasm; coughing and atelectasis associated with an increased risk of postoperative chest infection. Associated diseases include ischaemic heart disease and chronic obstructive pulmonary disease. Up to 15% of the haemoglobin in smokers combines with carbon monoxide to form carboxyhaemoglobin, reducing the oxygen carrying capacity of blood. After 12–24 hours of stopping smoking the effects of carbon monoxide and nicotine are significantly reduced and after 6–8 weeks ciliary and immunological activity are restored. All smokers should be encouraged to abstain prior to theatre.

CONCURRENT MEDICAL DISEASE

It is important to be aware of any medical condition affecting a patient and to ensure that its management prior to surgery is optimal. Emergency cases present particular problems as nausea or vomiting may have caused the patient to omit usual medication. An understanding of the pharmacology and possible interactions of concurrent medication with anaesthetic drugs is also essential.

RESPIRATORY DISEASE

Viral infection

The commonest respiratory problem of relevance to anaesthesia is viral upper respiratory tract infection (URTI) which causes increased bronchial reactivity, particularly in asthmatics, persisting for 3–4 weeks following resolution of the URTI. Current or recent URTI is also associated with an increased incidence of post-operative chest infection. Hence, unless surgery is urgent, such patients should be postponed for 4 weeks.

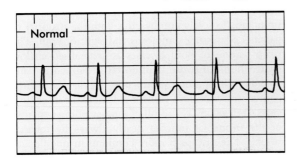

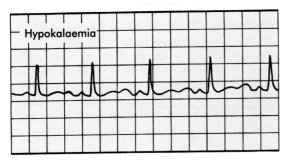

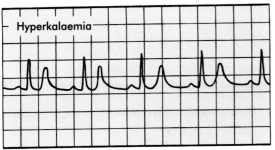

Figure PR.4 ECG changes associated with hypo- and hyperkalaemia

Asthma

Asthma is common, affecting 10–20% of the population. In many patients the condition is mild and requires only occasional treatment, but in others there may be frequent and severe attacks requiring hospital admission and, in a few patients, ventilation on the Intensive Care Unit. There are two main groups although there is some overlap: **early onset** asthma (atopic or extrinsic) and **late onset** asthma (non-atopic or intrinsic). The symptoms of asthma are wheeze, cough, chest tightness and dyspnoea. They are caused by an inflammatory reaction within the bronchial wall which results in bronchospasm, mucosal swelling and viscid secretions. In atopic asthma exposure to allergens results in the formation of IgE which causes a Type 1 or anaphylactic antigen-antibody hypersensitivity reaction.

The treatment of mild asthma is the occasional or regular use of inhaled selective beta$_2$-adrenoreceptor agonists such as salbutamol or terbutaline. Some patients may be using prophylactic inhaled sodium chromoglycate. In moderate cases regular inhaled corticosteroids are required. More severely affected patients may also be taking oral theophylline or regular oral steroids. Acute exacerbations of asthma may be treated with short courses of high dose oral steroids. Regular steroids may cause adrenocortical suppression and prevent the normal stress response to surgery and thus peri-operative hydrocortisone cover may be required. Usual bronchodilator therapy should be continued pre-operatively. It is common practice to prescribe a pre-operative dose of inhaled beta$_2$-adrenoreceptor agonist immediately prior to the patient going to theatre and to ensure that the patient brings their inhaler to theatre in case it is required post operatively. As bronchospasm may be precipitated by anxiety, benzodiazepine premedication is often prescribed. Sedative drugs are contraindicated in anyone experiencing an acute exacerbation of their asthma.

Assessment of the severity of a patient's asthma may be made from the history; frequency of attacks, whether the patient has ever been admitted to hospital with an attack or has ever required ventilation, whether oral steroids are ever necessary and if so how frequently. Nocturnal cough and frequent waking with symptoms indicate poor control of asthma. A chest radiograph in an asthmatic patient who is currently well, is often normal and not necessary pre-operatively. In long standing cases there may be hyperinflation of the lungs. Pulmonary function tests provide a useful indication of the degree of airflow obstruction, in particular, the forced expiratory volume in one second (FEV$_1$) and the peak expiratory flow rate (PEFR) are used. If a patient's normal PEFR is known, the current state of their asthma may be ascertained from measurement of PEFR pre-operatively. If the patient has experienced a recent exacerbation of their asthma, with an increase in symptoms and medication required and reduced PEFR, it is appropriate to postpone elective surgery until their condition has returned to normal which may take several weeks. Where surgery is urgent, steps should be taken to optimise the patient's condition in the time available by the use of a nebulised beta$_2$-adrenoreceptor agonist and, if severe, the commencement of enteral or parenteral steroids.

Chronic obstructive pulmonary disease

Chronic bronchitis and emphysema are different pathologically but frequently co-exist as chronic obstructive pulmonary disease. A patient's condition may fall anywhere in a spectrum from solely chronic bronchitis to solely emphysema, with the majority of patients possessing symptoms and signs of both. The main feature of both diseases is generalised airflow obstruction. **Chronic bronchitis** is defined as daily cough with sputum production for at least three consecutive months a year for at least two consecutive years. It develops as a result of long-standing irritation of the bronchial mucosa nearly always by tobacco smoke. The disease is more common in middle and later life, in smokers than in non smokers and in urban than in rural dwellers. Pathologically there is hypertrophy of mucus secreting glands and mucosal oedema, leading to irreversible airflow obstruction. Air becomes 'trapped' in the alveoli on expiration causing alveolar distension which may result in associated emphysema. Chronic bronchitis is a progressive disease, worsening with each acute exacerbation. Eventually respiratory failure develops characterised by hypoxia, polycythaemia, pulmonary hypertension and cor pulmonale. Rarely, chronic hypercapnia may lead to loss of the central response to carbon dioxide, resulting in a 'blue bloater' whose hypoxia is the only stimulus to ventilation. If these patients undergo general anaesthesia they are extremely difficult to wean and to extubate. Symptoms of chronic bronchitis are cough with sputum, dyspnoea and wheeze. Clinical signs include hyperinflation of the chest, variable inspiratory and expiratory wheeze and often basal crackles which may disappear after coughing. Peripheral oedema and raised jugular venous pressure are found with cor pulmonale and there may be cyanosis.

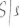

Emphysema is defined as enlargement of the air spaces distal to the terminal bronchioles with destructive changes in the alveolar wall. The main cause of emphysema is smoking although the rare genetic deficiency of alpha$_1$-antitrypsin may cause severe emphysema in young adults. The complications of emphysema include rupture of a pulmonary bulla leading to pneumothorax and later respiratory failure and cor pulmonale may occur. Classically emphysematous patients are described as 'pink puffers'. The only symptom of emphysema is exertional dyspnoea or dyspnoea at rest as the condition worsens. The main clinical sign of emphysema is a hyperinflated chest.

The treatment of chronic obstructive pulmonary disease is mostly symptomatic once the patient has stopped smoking. Bronchodilators are useful if there is an element of reversible airways obstruction. Patients may be prescribed inhaled beta$_2$-agonists, ipratropium bromide and theophylline. Diuretic therapy may be used to control right sided heart failure. Patients who are hypoxic with pulmonary hypertension may be on domiciliary oxygen therapy, a bad prognostic indicator.

There are no characteristic radiological abnormalities due to chronic bronchitis, but co-existing emphysema may result in the appearance of hyperinflation with low flat diaphragms, loss of peripheral vascular markings and prominent hilar vessels (bat winging) and bullae. The heart is narrow until cor pulmonale develops. The presence of bullae supports the diagnosis of emphysema and occasionally a giant emphysematous bulla will be seen when surgical ablation may improve symptoms and lung function. Pre-operative pulmonary function tests may help determine which of the two pathological conditions predominates. Arterial blood gas analysis is indicated to assess gas exchange if a patient has severe dyspnoea on mild or moderate exertion.

If there is a history of recent onset of green sputum production rather than white, and clinical signs support a diagnosis of chest infection, surgery should if possible be postponed and a course of antibiotics and physiotherapy commenced.

PULMONARY FUNCTION TESTS

Peak expiratory flow rate (PEFR) is the rate of flow of exhaled air at the start of a forced expiration and is measured using a simple flowmeter. Reduced values compared to predicted values for age, height and sex indicate airflow obstruction. Serial measurements are useful for monitoring disease progress and for demonstrating a response to bronchodilator therapy.

Spirometric tests of lung function are easy to perform. If a subject exhales as hard and as long as possible from a maximal inspiration, the volume expired in the first second is the forced expiratory volume in one second (FEV$_1$) and the total volume expired is the forced vital capacity (FVC). The measured values are compared to predicted values for age, height and sex. The ratio of FEV$_1$ to FVC (FEV%) is most useful (normal range 65–80%). Obstructive airways disease e.g. asthma, reduces the FEV$_1$ more than the FVC, so the FEV% is low. Restrictive airways disease e.g. pulmonary fibrosis, reduces the FVC and, to a lesser degree, the FEV$_1$, so the FEV% is normal or high (Figure PR.5).

Arterial blood gas analysis may be useful and interpretation should be systematic. Look first at the pH value (acidosis or alkalosis) to determine the direction of the primary change. Although there may be partial compensation for the underlying abnormality, there is never full or over-compensation. Then look at the PCO$_2$, which is determined by alveolar ventilation. A low PCO$_2$ (hyperventilation) indicates a respiratory alkalosis or respiratory compensation for a metabolic acidosis. Conversely a raised PCO$_2$ (hypoventilation) indicates a respiratory acidosis. The PCO$_2$ does not increase above normal to compensate for a metabolic alkalosis. Next, consider the standard bicarbonate value (HCO$_3^-$). This is defined as the extracellular fluid (ECF) bicarbonate concentration the patient would have if the PCO$_2$ were normal. If standard bicarbonate is raised, there is either a metabolic alkalosis or metabolic compensation for a respiratory acidosis. If the standard bicarbonate is low, there is a metabolic acidosis or metabolic compensation for a respiratory alkalosis. The base excess is defined as the number of mmol of HCO$_3^-$ which must be added to (or removed from) each litre of ECF to return the ECF pH to 7.4, if the PCO$_2$ were normal. A negative base excess (a base deficit) indicates metabolic acidosis, so is found with a low standard bicarbonate, and a positive base excess, which is found with a raised standard bicarbonate, indicates metabolic alkalosis. Finally, the PO$_2$ should be examined. A low PO$_2$ indicates hypoxaemia and a raised PO$_2$ indicates that the patient is receiving additional oxygen.

CARDIOVASCULAR DISEASE

Hypertension

Hypertension occurs in 15% of the UK population. Although mean systemic diastolic and systolic arterial pressure rise with increasing age, hypertension is defined by arbitrarily set levels (Figure PR.6). In 97%

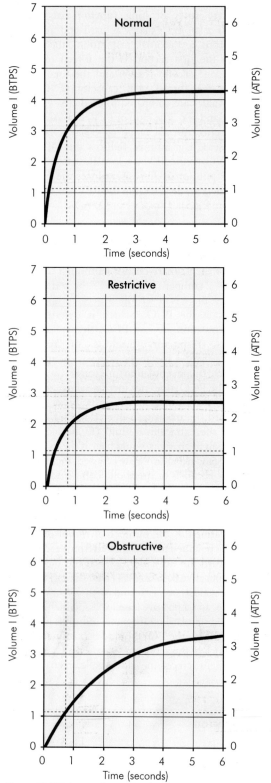

Figure PR.5 Spirometric tests in obstructive and restrictive pulmonary disease

of these patients the cause is unknown and they are said to have "essential" or primary hypertension. In the remaining 3% hypertension is secondary to renal or endocrine disease, coarctation of the aorta, drugs or pregnancy. It is important that hypertension is adequately controlled pre-operatively.

Whilst degree of hypertension is traditionally defined in terms of diastolic blood pressure the problem of isolated systolic hypertension is a topic currently receiving much interest. Isolated systolic hypertension is most prevalent in the elderly population and is a significant risk factor for stroke as well as cardiovascular morbidity in this group.

The pathogenesis of primary hypertension is not understood, but it is known that systemic vascular resistance is increased leading to a possible decrease in cardiac output by 15–20%. Additionally, the level of sympathetic nervous system activity is high resulting in a greater than normal response to any stimulus. In a hypertensive patient there is a much greater fall than normal in systemic arterial pressure on induction of anaesthesia due to a fall in cardiac output resulting from decreases in both heart rate and stroke volume. This exaggerated fall is lessened in controlled hypertension. Importantly, there is an increased risk of post-operative myocardial infarction in hypertensive patients. Hypertension is associated with other diseases of relevance to the anaesthetist such as ischaemic heart disease, peripheral vascular disease (PVD), renal disease, cerebrovascular disease and diabetes mellitus. At pre-operative assessment the anaesthetist should look for evidence of any of these conditions and for end organ damage due to hypertension. An ECG may reveal left ventricular hypertrophy (LVH) or ischaemic heart disease. Serum urea, electrolytes and creatinine may reveal renal impairment and serum glucose may show diabetes. Chest X-ray may reveal left ventricular enlargement and distended upper pulmonary lobe veins indicate left ventricular failure. In advanced failure there is generalised hazy opacification spreading out from the hilum and possibly Kerley 'B' lines or pleural effusions.

DRUG TREATMENT

Usual anti-hypertensive therapy should be continued on the day of surgery. Anti-hypertensive agents tend to potentiate the hypotensive effects of general anaesthesia. Thiazide diuretics are a common first line treatment for hypertension, particularly in the elderly. Thiazide treatment can often result in hypokalaemia or hypovolaemia. Beta-adrenergic antagonists are frequently employed in conjunction with a thiazide. Despite their advantages during anaesthesia

RELEVANCE OF DEGREE OF HYPERTENSION TO ANAESTHESIA		
Degree of hypertension	Diastolic pressure (mmHg)	Prognosis with anaesthesia
Mild	90–104	No evidence that treatment makes any difference to outcome
Moderate	105–114	Not really looked at but presumably increased risk, particularly if evidence of end organ damage
Severe	> 114	Probably increased risk of ischaemia, arrhythmia and poor outcome therefore cancel and treat

Figure PR.6

(depression of the cardiovascular response to laryngoscopy and to surgical stimulation) beta-blockers may cause problems: bradycardia, atrioventricular block, decreased myocardial contractility, bronchoconstriction and altered response to inotropes. If beta-blockers are stopped pre-operatively, hypertension, arrhythmias and myocardial ischaemia are increased intra-operatively, as is postoperative myocardial ischaemia. Calcium channel antagonists are also prescribed for hypertension. Diltiazem and verapamil may cause bradycardia. Angiotensin converting enzyme (ACE) inhibitors are also used for the treatment of cardiac failure and these agents are associated with hypotension and hyperkalaemia. Drugs more recently introduced for the treatment of hypertension include angiotensin II type 1 receptor antagonists and imidazoline receptor antagonists.

Sedative premedication is often prescribed for hypertensive patients to reduce endogenous catecholamine levels which may exacerbate the hypertension.

Ischaemic heart disease (IHD)

In the UK 12–20% of patients undergoing surgery have pre-operative evidence of myocardial disease. This is almost always due to atheroma although rarely other disease processes may be responsible. With increasing age atheromatous plaques form in the intima of arteries. These plaques grow and evolve with time, decreasing blood flow through a vessel and possibly occluding it. The rate of progression of individual plaques within any patient is variable and explains why although peripheral vascular and cerebrovascular disease will often co-exist with coronary artery disease, the patient may be asymptomatic of these other conditions.

IHD may be diagnosed from a history of angina or myocardial infarction (MI). It may also be the underlying cause of a conduction defect or arrhythmia. A guide to the severity of angina is the exertion necessary to precipitate an attack. The distance that is regularly walked on the flat before an attack occurs should be elicited in the history. It may be that angina is only occasional, such as when climbing more than one flight of stairs or in very cold weather. If angina is

TIME ELAPSED FROM MYOCARDIAL INFARCTION AND RISK OF PERI-OPERATIVE MYOCARDIAL INFARCTION	
Time elapsed	Risk
< 3 months	High
3–6 months	Medium
> 6 months	Low

Figure PR.7

precipitated by minimal exertion or is even occurring at rest (unstable angina), the patient has severe myocardial insufficiency and anaesthesia may present problems. If elective surgery is proposed, this should be cancelled and the patient further investigated with a view to cardiac surgery. It is important to establish the timing of any previous MI. Peri-operative MI has a mortality of up to 70%. The risk of peri-operative MI is O.1–0.2% if there is no history of previous MI. If there is such a history then the overall reinfarction rate is 6–7% and can be related to the time from previous infarct. The actual level of risk is however uncertain particularly since the introduction of thrombolysis.

The progressive, episodic nature of IHD has led many workers to attempt to make predictions about the postoperative risk of cardiac complications following major, non-cardiac surgery.

The Goldman cardiac risk index was one of the earlier multifactorial scoring systems designed to predict clinical risk. Although there have since been a number of modifications, notably by Detsky 1986, it still forms the basis of a system in use currently. (Goldman 1977, Figure PR.8). Each risk factor is awarded points and the total out of a possible 53 points calculated. If the total is <5 points, the predicted cardiac mortality (serious cardiac morbidity) is 0.2%(0.7%), if the total is 6–25 points, 2%(17%) and if the total is >25 points, 56%(22%). Evidence of cardiac failure is the most important factor, closely followed by recent MI.

Despite modifications of this scoring system and the introduction of alternatives, overall predictive accuracy has remained disappointingly limited. The modified cardiac risk index has however proven useful in the development of guidelines for the pre-operative assessment of patients with IHD. Those published by the American College of Physicians in 1997 provide guidance for the level of investigation required for patients with IHD. Thus, more sophisticated investigations such as echocardiography and radionuclide scanning can be carried out where appropriate. Different scoring systems have produced conflicting and thus confusing data regarding peri-operative cardiac risk. However much of the work supports the likelihood that certain factors consistently reduce peri-operative cardiac morbidity and mortality. These include pre-operative optimization of cardiac status, aggressive invasive monitoring and prompt treatment of intra-operative haemodynamic disturbance.

THE ELECTROCARDIOGRAM

A 12 lead ECG is essential in males aged >45 years, females aged > 55 years, diabetics aged > 40 years and

GOLDMAN RISK INDEX

Pre-operative 3rd heart sound or jugular venous distension (11 points)

MI in previous 6 months (10 points)

More than 5 premature ventricular contractions per minute documented at any time before operation (7 points)

Rhythm other than sinus or presence of premature atrial contractions on last pre-operative ECG (7 points)

Age over 70 years (5 points)

Emergency operations (4 points)

Intraperitoneal, intrathoracic or aortic operations (3 points)

Significant aortic stenosis (3 points)

Poor general medical conditions (3 points), defined by any one of the following:
PaO_2 < 8 kPa or $PaCO_2$ >6.5 kPa
K^+ < 3.0 mmol/l or $HCO3^-$ < 20 mmol/l
Urea > 7.5 mmol/l or Creatinine > 270 mmol/l
Chronic liver disease
Patient bedridden from non cardiac causes

Figure PR.8

in all patients with a history suggestive of IHD (Figure PR.9). Left axis deviation indicates IHD while right axis deviation may be normal. Only 50% of old MIs will be seen. An exercise ECG may be indicated in patients in at risk groups e.g. undergoing peripheral vascular surgery, if the resting ECG is normal, there is no LVH and no previous MI. Continuous ambulatory ECG may be useful if the patient's ability to exercise is limited. Although abnormal rhythms may be detected clinically an ECG is needed to confirm diagnosis. Rate and rhythm should be noted (Figure PR.10) and a 24 hour ECG may be useful.

Sinus tachycardia has several common causes such as anxiety, pyrexia, cardiac failure and anaemia. Supraventricular tachyacardia may be due to a congenital conduction abnormality. IHD is the main cause of the other arrhythmias, although thyroid

ECG ABNORMALITIES ASSOCIATED WITH MYOCARDIAL ISCHAEMIA

Conduction abnormalities	Degrees of heart block Bundle branch block
Arrhythmias	Multifocal ventricular Ectopics Episodes of VT or VF
QRS	Presences of Q waves Poor R wave progression
ST segment	>1 mm depression > 2 mm depression
T wave	Isoelectric Inverted Reverted

Figure PR.9

disease should not be forgotten. Atrial tachyarrhythmias should be controlled pre-operatively with digoxin or amiodarone therapy. Complete heart block, any form of bifascicular block and sick sinus syndrome require pre-operative pacing. Multifocal ventricular ectopics are more significant than uni-focal ectopics, indicating IHD. Atrial ectopics are not usually significant.

OTHER CARDIAC INVESTIGATIONS

Echocardiography uses ultrasound to study blood flow, the structure of the heart and the movement of valves and cardiac muscle. Ventricular volumes, ejection fraction and gradients across valves can be estimated. The ejection fraction is particularly useful. It is normally > 60% and if < 40 % serious problems associated with anaesthesia should be anticipated.

Chest X-ray may show cardiomegaly, with a cardiothoracic ratio of > 0.5. 70% of patients with cardiomegaly have an ejection fraction of less than 50%.

Radionucleotide scanning provides a relatively non-invasive means of accurately assessing myocardial function. In blood pool scanning ^{99}Technetium-labelled red blood cells are injected intravenously and then both the amount of blood in the heart at each stage of the cardiac cycle and the shape of the cardiac chambers can be determined. The scanning camera may be linked to ECG and pictures collected over multiple cardiac cycles (multigated or MUGA scans). In perfusion scintigraphy, acute MI may be detected by "hot spot" scanning. This technique also uses ^{99}Technetium which is taken up into the acutely infarcted myocardial tissue thus revealing the position and extent of the damage. Conversely "Cold spot" scanning uses ^{201}Thallium to demonstrate areas of myocardial ischaemia and scarring. ^{201}Thallium behaves like a potassium ion and is distributed throughout the heart muscle depending on coronary blood flow. It is taken up by normal myocardium so areas that are not being perfused show on the scan as perfusion defects. A coronary vasodilator, such as dipyridamole, may then be given. A fixed perfusion defect indicates scar tissue while a reperfusion defect indicates ischaemia. Reperfusion defects are more significant because ischaemia may develop peri-operatively whereas a fixed perfusion defect cannot deteriorate.

DIAGNOSIS OF ARRHYTHMIAS

Rate	Rhythm	Diagnosis
Normal	Irregular	Multiple ectopics
Fast	Regular	Sinus tachycardia Atrial flutter Supraventricular tachycardia
Fast	Irregular	Atrial fibrillation Atrial flutter with variable block
Slow	Regular	Complete heart block
Fast and slow	Irregular	Sick sinus syndrome

Figure PR.10

Pacemakers

The need for cardiac pacing results from disease of the conducting system of the heart which may or may not be associated with general ischaemic heart disease. The most common scenario is that of an elderly patient without associated cardiac conditions.

A variety of pacemakers may be encountered depending on the age of the unit. Modern pacemakers operate through a lead in the atrium, ventricle or both. Depolarisation arising endogenously may either inhibit or trigger a paced beat. Pacemakers are classified using a five letter code as in Figure PR.11

As an illustration an AAI unit paces atrially and will be inhibited by sensing an endogenous depolarisation in the atrium. In contrast a VVT unit paces ventically and is triggered if an endogenous depolarisation is sensed in the ventricle.

Most modern units are dual units which work in DDD mode, providing atrial pacing in the presence of atrial bradycardia and ventricular pacing after an atrial depolarisation (endogenous or paced) if a spontaneous ventricular beat is absent.

The characteristics of an implanted pacemaker can sometimes be changed externally, either by application of magnets or radio-frequency generators. The most usual indication for this being a change of demand to fixed rate. The most modern units require a cautious approach to the use of magnets which may expose a programmable unit to the risk of being re-set in a variable fashion. All patients who have an implanted pacemaker have a registration card with details of the device (see Figure PR.12)

Pre-operative assessment should be directed to determining the type of unit and its characteristics. Examination of the cardiovascular system should be undertaken in detail. Chest X-ray will help identify the pulse generator siting and lead placement and number. The use of surgical diathermy is associated with various hazards. These are detailed below.

SURGICAL DIATHERMY AND PACEMAKERS

Use of surgical diathermy in the presence of an indwelling pacemaker may produce the following problems:

- Ventricular fibrillation. Most common when the pacemaker unit is an older type
- Inhibition of demand function
- Unpredictable setting of programmable types
- Asystole
- Unit failure

Recommendations for the use of surgical diathermy in the presence of an indwelling pacemaker unit are as follows:

- Place the indifferent electrode on the same side as the operation and as far from the pacemaker unit as possible
- Limit the use of diathermy as much as possible
- Use the lowest current setting possible
- Use bipolar diathermy (but power of coagulation is less)

GENERIC PACEMAKER CODE

1st Code Letter Paced Chamber	2nd Code Letter Sensed Chamber	3rd Code Letter Response to Endogenous Depolarisation	4th Code Letter Programmable Functions	5th Code Letter Antiarrhythmic Function
I	II	III	IV	V
V (ventricle)	V (ventricle)	T (trigger)	P (rate)	S (scanning)
A (atrium)	A (atrium)	I (inhibited)	M (multiprogrammable)	E (externally activated)
D (double)	D (double)	D (double)	C (communicating)	
	O (none)	O (none)	R (rate responsive)	
			B (impulse burst)	
			N (normal rate competition)	
			O (none)	

Figure PR.11

PRE-OPERATIVE ASSESSMENT OF THE PACEMAKER PATIENT

Coded information recorded at implantation on European Pacemaker Registration Card			
	Symptom	01-02	unspecified
		03-04	dizziness or syncope
		05	bradycardia
		06	tachycardia
		07-09	miscellaneous conditions
	ECG	01-04	sinus or unspecified
	Rhythm	05-07	second degree AV block
		08-10	complete heart block
		11-21	bundle branch or bifascicular block
	Aetiology	01-03	unspecified
		04-05	idiopathic or ischaemic
		06	post infarction
		07-11	miscellaneous conditions

ECG rhythm
1. All beats preceded by a pacemaker spike: assume patient is pacemaker-dependent
2. If native rhythm predominates patient is unlikely to be pacemaker-dependent
3. No evidence of pacemaker activity; magnet may be applied over pulse generator to switch to fixed rate pacing
4. If pacemaker spike is not followed by P or QRS wave suspect pacemaker malfunction (note if pacemaker is activated by a magnet to pace at a fixed rate, the spike may fall in the refractory period and fail to stimulate the ventricle)

Chest X-ray
1. Location of pulse generator
2. Location of leads in atrium, ventricle or both
3. If necessary pulse generator model can be identified

Ref: Bloomfield and Bowler (1989)

Figure PR.12

- Monitor patient ECG constantly
- Keep the pacemaker programmer available, where appropriate

Valvular heart disease

The availability of echocardiography today means that any patient with suspected valve disease should be properly investigated and a diagnosis made prior to anaesthesia. Valve angioplasty or replacement is sometimes indicated before elective surgery. Unfortunately, patients with significant valve disease may still present for emergency surgery. Any patient with a heart valve lesion, including replacement valves, requires prophylactic antibiotics for dental, genito-urinary, obstetric, gynaecological and gastro-intestinal procedures. The current recommended regimes are

found in the British National Formulary. The main causes of valvular heart disease are shown in Figure PR.13. Note that multiple valve lesions may co-exist.

AORTIC STENOSIS

The symptoms of aortic stenosis occur late and include angina, syncope, dyspnoea and sudden death. Clinical signs are difficult to assess but generally include plateau pulse, LVH and an aortic ejection systolic murmur which is similar in character to that of aortic sclerosis. The ECG may show LVH with strain. On chest X-ray left ventricular enlargement may not be evident and the aortic valve may be calcified. Echocardiography determines the gradient across the valve and will provide information on ventricular function. If the valve gradient is greater than 50 mmHg, angioplasty or valve replacement should be considered. The main anaesthesia related problems are fixed cardiac output, ventricular arrhythmias and incipient cardiac failure.

AORTIC REGURGITATION

Aortic regurgitation gives rise to few symptoms until the LV fails, when dyspnoea occurs. Clinical signs include a collapsing pulse, LV enlargement and an early diastolic murmur. The ECG shows changes of LVH and on chest X-ray the heart will be enlarged. Echocardiography shows a dilated left ventricle and aortic root. Problems with respect to anaesthesia are poor myocardial reserve and cardiac failure.

MITRAL STENOSIS

Symptoms of mitral stenosis are dyspnoea, tiredness and haemoptysis. Clinical signs include malar flush and a mid-diastolic murmur. Mitral stenosis may be complicated by systemic embolism or pulmonary hypertension. The ECG will often demonstrate atrial fibrillation (AF), P mitrale and right ventricular hypertrophy. On chest X-ray there may be left atrial enlargement and pulmonary venous congestion. Patients with a small valve area on echocardiography or moderate symptoms need surgery. Anaesthesia related problems include AF, anti-coagulant therapy, fixed cardiac output and pulmonary oedema.

MITRAL REGURGITATION

Progressive dyspnoea and tiredness are common symptoms of mitral regurgitation. Left ventricular enlargement and a pansystolic murmur are the predominant clinical signs. The ECG shows LVH, P mitrale and atrial fibrillation. Chest X-ray demonstrates left sided enlargement of the heart, particularly atrial enlargement, and indications of pulmonary oedema may be seen. Echocardiography is useful to assess left ventricular function. Specific problems with respect to anaesthesia include pulmonary oedema, AF and anticoagulant therapy.

TRICUSPID VALVE LESIONS

Tricuspid stenosis is usually associated with mitral and aortic valve disease. Tricuspid regurgitation is usually due to right ventricular enlargement. Anaesthesia related problems are usually due to the accompanying other valve disease rather than to the tricuspid lesion itself.

PULMONARY VALVE LESIONS

Pulmoary stenosis is usually congenital and may be part of Fallot's tetralogy. Pulmonary regurgitation is rare and most often secondary to pulmonary hypertension.

HAEMATOLOGICAL DISEASE

Anaemia

A patient is considered anaemic if the haemoglobin is below the normal range and polycythaemic if above the normal range. For adult females this is 12–16 g/dl and for adult males 13–17 g/dl. In children the range varies and a child is considered to be anaemic if the haemoglobin value is less than 18 g/dl at birth, less than 9 g/dl at 3 months, less than 11 g/dl from 6 months to 6 years and less than 12 g/dl from 6–12 years.

The causes of anaemia are blood loss, inadequate production of erythrocytes and excessive destruction of erythrocytes. Anaemia may be classified by the mean cell volume of the erythrocyte (MCV) (Figure PR.14).

CAUSES OF VALVULAR DISEASE

Valve regurgitation	Valve stenosis
Congenital	Congenital
Rheumatic fever	Rheumatic fever
Infective endocarditis	Senile degeneration
Syphilitic aortitis	
Valve ring dilation, e.g. dilated cardiomyopathy	
Traumatic valve rupture	
Senile degeneration	
Damage to chordae and papillary muscles, e.g. MI	

Figure PR.13

The mean cell haemoglobin (MCH) is also useful and defines hypo- and normo-chromic types of anaemia.

Iron deficiency is the most common cause of anaemia but the cause is often multifactorial. Those patients in whom anaemia should be suspected include all females of child-bearing age (due to menstrual loss), the elderly (due to poor diet and other diseases) and all patients who are undergoing gastro-intestinal or gynaecological surgery (due to blood loss). Most patients suffering from anaemia are completely asymptomatic. If severely anaemic, symptoms may include tiredness and dyspnoea on exertion and in the elderly angina, heart failure and confusion may be precipitated.

A full blood count also provides the platelet count (raised in acute blood loss and acute inflammation) and the white cell count (raised in infection). A differential white cell count distinguishes between neutrophilia (bacterial infection, inflammation) and lymphocytosis (viral infection). If the platelet count, white cell count and haemoglobin are all low, this indicates marrow aplasia or infiltration. Abnormalities which may be detected on examination of the blood film include a raised reticulocyte count (haemolytic anaemia, continued bleeding), sickle cells or malarial parasites. Further investigation may be indicated prior to blood transfusion e.g. additional blood tests (ferritin, vitamin B_{12}, folate, reticulocyte count, direct Coombs test) or bone marrow aspiration.

Of most relevance to anaesthesia is a decrease in oxygen carrying capacity of the blood. Although anaemia decreases blood viscosity and hence improves blood flow with a consequent increase in oxygen delivery to the tissues, once the haemoglobin is less than 10 g/dl the increase in blood flow no longer compensates for the decreased oxygen-carrying capacity. Some authorities consider a haemoglobin value of greater than 8 g/dl, rather than 10 g/dl acceptable for anaesthesia. A secondary anaemia related problem is the fact that cardiac output increases in order to maintain oxygen flux. In some patients this leads to cardiac failure and in all cardiac reserve is decreased, reducing the ability to compensate for the myocardial depressant effects of anaesthesia. It is important to remember that cyanosis is only evident clinically when the level of deoxyhaemoglobin equals or exceeds 5 g/dl. Hence in severely anemic patients cyanosis is rarely seen.

In patients with chronic anaemia, there is an increase in 2,3-diphosphoglycerate (2,3-DPG) concentration in the reticulocytes which causes the oxygen dissociation curve to shift to the right, improving the off-loading of oxygen in the tissues. Stored blood contains decreased levels of 2,3-DPG which take 24 hours to reach normal levels following transfusion. Hence blood transfusion in an anaemic patient immediately prior to anaesthesia confers minimal advantage and may lead to fluid overload. For elective surgery, transfusion should be completed at least 24 hours earlier.

In patients who are acutely anaemic (for example due to recent blood loss), heart rate, arterial pressure, CVP and urine output should be closely monitored during fluid replacement to ensure normovolaemia is restored prior to anaesthesia. Blood should be transfused to

A CLASSIFICATION OF ANAEMIA	
MCV	**Cause**
Microcytic	Iron deficiency (hypochromic)
	Thalassaemia (hypochromic)
	Chronic disease
Normocytic	Chronic disease (normochromic or hypochromic)
	Mixed deficiency
	Acute blood loss (normochromic)
Macrocytic	Alcohol (normochromic)
	B_{12} or folate deficiency (normochromic)
	Pregnancy
	Hypothyroidism (normochromic)
	Low-grade haemolytic anaemia with high reticulocyte count

Figure PR.14

achieve a haemoglobin of greater than 10 g/dl and a haematocrit of greater than 0. 3. Administration of oxygen therapy will increase oxygen delivery by ensuring maximal saturation of the available haemoglobin and an increase in the dissolved oxygen in blood. Urgent surgery may be indicated to stop the bleeding, so resuscitation may need to be continued during anaesthesia and surgery.

Sickle cell disease

Sickle cell disease is due to a haemoglobinopathy which is inherited autosomally resulting in the formation of Haemoglobin S instead of Haemoglobin A. The S variant consists of 2 normal alpha chains and 2 abnormal beta chains in which glutamic acid has been substituted by valine in the sixth amino acid from the N-terminal. Small decreases in oxygen tension cause HbS to polymerise and form pseudo-crystalline structures which distort the red blood cell membrane to produce the characteristic sickle-shaped cells. Sickled cells increase blood viscosity and obstruct blood flow in the microvasculature leading to thrombosis and infarction. These sickled cells are also subject to abnormal sequestration. Patients homozygous for another haemoglobinopathy, HbC, suffer minimal morbidity but patients heterozygous for HbS and HbC (Haemoglobin SC disease) suffer from a mild form of sickle-cell anaemia as the presence of HbC causes the HbS to sickle more easily.

Sickle cell anaemia results from a patient being homozygous for haemoglobin S. Sickle cell trait results from a patient being heterozygous for haemoglobin S. Patients with sickle cell trait are resistant to falciparum malaria and it is in those areas of the world where falciparum malaria is endemic that the gene is particularly common i.e. tropical Africa, north-east Saudi Arabia, east central India and around the Mediterranean. The prevalence of HbSS in the UK black population is around 0.25% and the prevalence of HbAS in the same population is around 10%.

The main clinical problems for patients suffering from sickle cell anaemia are chronic haemolytic anaemia and infarction crises. Infarction crises may be precipitated by dehydration, infection, hypoxia, acidosis or cold, although they may also occur spontaneously. Crises are very painful, often involving bones or the spleen, and may also cause cerebrovascular accidents, haematuria due to renal papillary necrosis and chest pain due to pulmonary infarction. Patients with sickle cell trait have a normal haemoglobin and are clinically well. Most of their red blood cells contain less than 50% HbS and sickling only occurs when the oxygen tension is very low.

Pre-operatively all patients in the at-risk population for HbS should be screened. A Sickledex test detects the presence of HbS by precipitating sickling of the red blood cells on exposure to sodium metabisulphite. If this test is positive then electrophoresis is necessary to distinguish between the heterozygote and the homozygote. In an emergency situation, if the Sickledex test is positive but there is no history to suggest sickle cell anaemia and the haemoglobin, the reticulocyte count and the blood film are normal, then it is safe to assume that the patient has the trait only. Haematological advice should always be sought for patients with sickle cell anaemia. Evidence of renal, pulmonary or cerebrovascular complications should be assessed pre-operatively. Blood transfusion prior to elective surgery may be indicated if the anaemia is particularly severe and exchange transfusion will be necessary prior to major surgery to reduce the concentration of HbS to around 40%. An intravenous infusion should always be set up pre-operatively to avoid dehydration and heavy premedication should be avoided. Depending on the type of surgery planned, the proposed surgeon should be sufficiently experienced to proceed without the use of a tourniquet, as its use is contraindicated in both the homozygote and the heterozygote.

Clotting abnormalities

If a patient has a history of liver disease, bleeding problems or is taking anticoagulants a clotting screen is indicated. Clotting may also be abnormal after massive blood transfusion or in pregnancy-induced hypertension. The activated partial thromboplastin time (APPT) measures factors VIII, IX, XI and XII in the intrinsic system. It is prolonged by warfarin therapy and liver disease. In contrast the prothrombin time (PT) measures factors I, II, VII and X in the extrinsic system and is prolonged by heparin therapy and in dilutional coagulopathy. The International Normalised Ratio (INR) is the ratio of the PT sample time to control time, a widely used indicator of clotting function. A ratio of < 2.0 is considered safe for most surgery.

Coagulation abnormalities due to liver disease should be corrected by Vitamin K administration. The effects of warfarin should be temporarily reversed by fresh frozen plasma (FFP), not by Vitamin K which will prevent the recommencement of warfarin therapy. Heparin coagulopathy is corrected by stopping the heparin or, more urgently, by protamine. FFP is required to correct a dilutional coagulopathy, as may occur with massive blood transfusion.

Disseminated intravascular coagulation (DIC) is indicated by decreased platelets, increased fibrin degradation products, decreased fibrinogen and prolonged APPT and PT. The underlying cause should be identified and treated and clotting corrected with FFP (or cryoprecipitate) and platelet tranfusion.

Thrombocytopenia may be asymptomatic, but haematological advice should be sought and platelets are usually given to ensure a platelet count above 50×10^9. For specific factor deficiencies, such as Haemophilia, the purified factor or FFP should be given immediately pre-operatively.

MUSCULO-SKELETAL DISEASE

Although many musculoskeletal conditions may be encountered prior to anaesthesia and surgery, by far the most common of these is rheumatoid arthritis.

Rheumatoid arthritis

Rheumatoid arthritis is an autoimmune connective tissue disease. The dominant pathological feature is a chronic, destructive synovitis, which causes an inflammatory, typically symmetrical, deforming polyarthritis. Rheumatoid arthritis has many extra-articular features which greatly influence the morbidity and mortality of the disease (Figure PR.15). Approximately 70% of patients are positive for

rheumatoid factor, which is a circulating IgM antibody to the patient's own IgG. The overall prevalence is approximately 1% with a male to female ratio of 1: 3. Over the age of 55 years 5% of females and 2% of men are affected.

Rheumatoid arthritis is necesarily associated with a large number of drug-induced complications. Non-steroidal anti-inflammatory drugs (NSAIDs) are commonly used to treat pain and stiffness and may cause gastric erosions. The disease-modifying drugs used in the management of rheumatoid arthritis can similarly be associated with serious side effects. **Chloroquine** may cause haemolytic anaemia and ocular problems. **Sulphasalazine** rarely causes megaloblastic anaemia or hepatitis. **Oral gold** is less likely to cause marrow suppression or proteinuria than intramuscular gold. **Methotrexate** may cause marrow suppression or abnormal liver function. Although **Penicillamine** may cause the nephrotic syndrome, it is also associated (rarely) with generalised marrow suppression and conditions which mimic myasthenia gravis or systemic lupus erythematosus. Some patients will be receiving systemic steroids for their disease and others may be taking immunosuppressant drugs.

Rheumatoid arthritis most commonly affects the joints of the hands and feet, but the larger joints of the hips, knees and elbows may also be involved. 25% of patients with rheumatoid arthritis have cervical instability. Not all will have long-standing disease and a quarter will

EXTRA-ARTICULAR FEATURES OF RHEUMATOID ARTHRITIS	
Respiratory	Fibrosing alveolitis, pleural effusion, rheumatoid nodules, bronchiolitis, Caplan's syndrome
Cardiovascular	Pericarditis, pericardial effusion, vasculitis, heart block, cardiomyopathy, aortic regurgitation
Renal	Amyloidosis (may affect other systems), drug induced
Neurological	Cervical cord compression, peripheral neuropathy, entrapment neuropathy, mononeuritis multiplex
Haematological	Anaemia of chronic disease, iron deficiency anaemia (NSAIDs), marrow suppression (gold), thrombocytosis, Felty's syndrome
Ocular	Keratoconjunctivitis sicca, scleritis, episcleritis, scleromalacia perforans

Figure PR.15

have no clinical signs of cervical cord compression. The most common cervical problem is atlanto-axial subluxation, although subaxial subluxation may also occur. The atlanto-axial ligaments become lax and the odontoid peg is eroded making neck flexion dangerous by risking cord compression. Also of interest to the anaesthetist are limited mouth opening due to temporomandibular joint involvement and rarely, airway obstruction due to dislocation of the cricoarytenoid joints. A hoarse voice suggests cricoarytenoid arthritis. Respiratory function may be additionally impaired by costo-chondrial joint disease which can add to any restrictive defect.

It is therefore important pre-operatively to carefully assess the rheumatoid patient for evidence of extra-articular involvement. A full blood count is essential and if the patient is taking any disease-modifying drugs, serum electrolytes, urea and creatinine and liver function tests will also be necessary. Chest X-ray and pulmonary function tests may be indicated. Neck mobility and mouth opening should be assessed clinically. A lateral X-ray of the cervical spine in flexion and extension must be performed. If the gap between the odontoid peg and the posterior border of the anterior arch of the atlas is > 3 mm (or > 4 mm if aged over 40 years), subluxation is present. Care should be taken when asking the patient to attempt maximal flexion of the cervical spine. Awake intubation may be indicated if a difficult intubation is anticipated and if there is cervical spine involvement it will be necessary for the patient to wear a semi-rigid collar during anaesthesia to ensure peri-operative cervical stability. If there is evidence of severe cervical spine instability, it is appropriate to refer the patient for surgical stabilisation.

RENAL DISEASE

Renal failure

Renal disease covers a wide spectrum of clinical pictures from decreased renal reserve, through varying degrees of renal impairment to end-stage renal failure. Up to 80% of excretory function may be lost before a rise in serum urea or creatinine is seen. The creatinine value gives a useful indication of the degree of renal failure. The corresponding urea value is more readily affected by dietary protein, tissue breakdown and hydration and is therefore less useful. The cause of renal impairment or failure is very relevant to anaesthesia because the underlying disease process may have other manifestations. Renal failure may be acute or chronic (Figure PR.16).

The majority of renal patients presenting for anaesthesia will have chronic renal failure and most

will be on a dialysis programme, involving either intermittent haemodialysis (HD) or continuous ambulatory peritoneal dialysis (CAPD). At pre-operative assessment, the anaesthetist should establish the cause of renal failure and look for evidence of other systems affected by the same disease process. Renal failure affects all systems of the body (Figure PR.17).

Necessary investigations include urea and electrolytes, creatinine, full blood count, clotting screen, liver function tests and hepatitis B surface antigen. Chest X-ray and ECG are also required. In evaluating the renal failure patient for anaesthesia, particular reference should be made to the fluid status. 24 hours post-haemodialysis is the optimal time for elective surgery. Immediately following HD a patient may be volume depleted. CAPD has far less effect on circulating volume and may be continued until surgery. Most patients will be chronically anaemic but if asymptomatic and with no evidence of cardiovascular disease blood transfusion will probably not be necessary. Transfusion may precipitate fluid overload and should be undertaken prior to or during the last HD before anaesthesia. Hypertension should be controlled and fluid balance optimised. Acidosis and hyperkalaemia must be corrected by dialysis. The site of any arterio-venous fistula should be noted and arrangements made for it to be protected peri-operatively by wrapping in gamgee. The limb with the fistula should **never** be used for intravenous access.

ENDOCRINE DISEASE

Patients suffering from endocrine disease should have their condition stabilised by consultation (where time allows) with the responsible physician. The most frequently encountered endocrine disease in surgical practice is diabetes mellitus which is considered in more detail below and in Chapter 5.

Diabetes mellitus

Diabetes mellitus is characterised by a persisting state of hyperglycaemia due to lack or diminished effectiveness of endogenous insulin. It presents problems to the anaesthetist both in respect of the need to ensure adequate peri-operative control of blood glucose and in respect of the known long term complications of the condition. Diabetes mellitus may be classified as primary or secondary (Figure PR.18). There are two types of primary diabetes mellitus: insulin dependent diabetes mellitus (IDDM or type I) and non-insulin dependent diabetes mellitus (NIDDM or type II). The

CAUSES OF CHRONIC AND ACUTE RENAL FAILURE

Chronic renal failure

Diabetic nephropathy
Hypertensive nephropathy
Chronic urinary tract obstruction
Chronic glomerulonephritis
Polycystic kidney disease
Chronic bilateral pyelonephritis
Collagen diseases
Persisting acute renal failure

Acute renal failure

Pre-renal

Severe hypotension (hypovolaemia, cardiac failure, septic shock, drug overdose)
Major vessel disease (thrombosis, aortic aneurysm)
Intravascular haemolysis
Rhabdomyolysis

Renal

Acute tubular necrosis (acute ischaemia, drugs, bacterial endotoxins)
Vasculitis
Acute glomerulonephritis
Acute interstitial nephritis
Coagulophathies
Eclampsia

Post renal

Urinary tract obstruction (prostatic hypertrophy, renal or ureteric stones, surgical mishap)

Figure PR.16

SYSTEMIC EFFECTS OF RENAL FAILURE

Cardiovascular

Premature atheroma
Hypertension
Left ventricular failure
Pericardial effusions

Respiratory

Pulmonary venous congestion or oedema
Pneumonia

Haematological

Normochromic normocytic anaemia
Prolonged bleeding time due to platelet dysfunction
Increased incidence hepatitis B carriage

Gastro-intestinal

Delayed gastric emptying
Increased gastric acidity
Peptic ulceration
Impaired liver function

Neurological

Peripheral and autonomic neuropathies
Encephalopathy

Biochemical

Metabolic acidosis with compensatory respiratory alkalosis
Hyperkalaemia
Hypocalcaemia
Hypoalbuminaemia

Figure PR.17

prevalence in the UK is 2% with a ratio of NIDDM: IDDM of 7: 3. The aetiology of diabetes mellitus remains unclear but it is known to be the result of environmental factors interacting with genetic factors. IDDM usually presents before the age of 40 years and NIDDM usually presents after the age of 50 years.

Glycosuria which has been detected on routine urine testing performed pre-operatively may often be the first indication that a patient has diabetes. As there is individual variation in the renal threshold for glucose, diagnosis should be confirmed by examining blood glucose. The diagnosis of diabetes mellitus may be made from a random blood glucose of >11.1 mmol/l or a fasting blood glucose of >7.8 mmol/l. If the patient is a known diabetic, control may be assessed from the patient's diary of the results of home testing of blood glucose. Single random blood glucose estimations are of little value, although measurement of glycosylated haemoglobin is more useful and reflects blood glucose control over the previous 6–8 weeks.

The long-term complications of diabetes are equally likely in both IDDM and NIDDM and are related to the duration of the disease and the effectiveness of blood sugar control. Complications are due to disease of both large blood vessels (atheroma) and small blood vessels (microangiopathy). Atheroma causes the same pathological changes as in non-diabetic patients, but the disease occurs earlier, is more extensive and more severe. Atheroma is the cause of the increased incidence in diabetics of IHD and PVD. Diabetic microangiopathy is the cause of diabetic nephropathy, retinopathy and neuropathy. Diabetes is a common cause of autonomic neuropathy, which can be detected at the bedside by demonstrating postural hypotension. Diabetic patients frequently present for surgery for the complications of their disease and pre-operative assessment must include screening for evidence of other complications. An ECG and other cardiac investigations may be indicated. Serum urea, electrolytes and creatinine should be performed to assess renal function.

The management of approximately 50% of diabetics is by diet alone. 20–30% require diet and an oral hypoglycaemic drug and 20–30% require diet and insulin. Oral hypoglycaemic agents fall into two groups, both of which depend on the presence of some endogenous insulin. **Sulphonylureas** act by augmenting insulin secretion and may also alter peripheral insulin receptor number and sensitivity. The commonly used sulphonylureas include glibenclamide, gliclazide and tolazamide. These drugs should be omitted on the day of surgery because of the risk of peri-operative hypoglycaemia. Glibenclamide should be stopped 24 hours prior to surgery and chlorpropamide 48 hours, because of their prolonged durations of action. In all cases blood sugar should be carefully monitored peri-operatively.

The second group of oral hypoglycaemic agents are the **biguanides**. Metformin is the only available biguanide and is often used in conjunction with a sulphonylurea. It enhances the peripheral action of insulin. Hypoglycaemia is very unusual with metformin although it may cause lactic acidosis. Biguanide therapy should be stopped on the morning of surgery and blood glucose concentration monitored. Surgery itself is a cause of stress resulting in increased secretion of

CLASSIFICATION OF DIABETES MELLITUS

	Primary	Secondary
Type I	Insulin-dependent diabetes mellitus	Pancreatic disease, e.g. pancreatitis, pancreatectomy, neoplastic disease, cystic fibrosis
Type II	Non insulin-dependent diabetes mellitus	Excess production of insulin antagonists, e.g. growth hormone (acromegaly), glucocorticoids (Cushing's syndrome), thyroid hormones, catecholamines (phaeochromocytoma)
		Drugs, e.g. corticosteroids, thiazides
		Liver disease

Figure PR.18

the catabolic hormones (cortisol, growth hormone and glucagon) which results in increased catabolism and may lead to diabetic ketoacidosis in both NIDDM and IDDM. Thus, NIDDM patients who are undergoing major surgery will require insulin in the peri-operative period and IDDM patient will experience an increase in their insulin requirements.

The two main types of insulin preparation are unmodified, rapid onset, short-acting (soluble) insulin and modified, delayed onset, intermediate- or long-acting insulin. The insulin regime used varies from patient to patient but involves a combination of short- and longer-acting insulins injected before meals and at bedtime. It is important to remember that IDDM patients need insulin even when they are being starved. Soluble insulin is the only form which can be given intravenously as well as subcutaneously and is used for peri-operative control of blood glucose. The management of diabetic patients presenting for surgery is given in Chapter 5.

CONCURRENT MEDICATION

Concurrent medication may interact with drugs administered during anaesthesia.

Furthermore the surgical procedure itself may be affected by, or indeed affect, such medication. For this reason it is important that careful consideration is given to pre-operative drug management. Medication may have to be continued, stopped or modified. Alternatively, anaesthetic technique may have to be modified to minimise the risk of adverse interaction. A change in mode of administration or formulation is sometimes required. Examples of drugs that should be continued are; anticonvulsants, most cardiovascular drugs (antihypertensives, anti-anginals, anti-arrythmics), bronchodilators, corticosteroids and antiparkinsonian drugs. All are important in terms of providing optimal control of underlying conditions. It is seldom necessary to stop drugs pre-operatively however a number of possible exceptions are worthy of discussion. Warfarin should be stopped several days pre-operatively and the patient heparinised. In certain circumstances, usually when there is a risk of excessive bleeding, NSAIDs and aspirin may be stopped although the risks of stopping aspirin may outweigh the benefits. To minimise the risk of thromboembolism oral contraceptives and hormone replacement therapy are often stopped several weeks before surgery. Lithium therapy should be stopped 24 hours before surgery. Most drugs that have been stopped pre-operatively can be restarted when oral intake resumes. Should this be delayed alternative routes of administration may have to be sought.

It is occasionally necessary to modify dose and formulation of a drug peri-operatively as is the case with corticosteroid therapy. Adrenal suppression has not been reported with prednisolone doses below 5 mg daily. Patients on higher doses undergoing major surgery will require additional corticosteroid support administered as intravenous hydrocortisone.

Monoamine oxidase inhibitors (MAOIs) irreversibly inhibit monoamine oxidase. Stopping these drugs three weeks prior to anaesthesia, to allow resynthesis of the enzyme, is no longer considered necessary, but anaesthetic technique may need to modified. MAOIs interact with opioids, particularly pethidine, to cause cardiovascular and cerebrovascular excitation (hypertension, tachyacardia, convulsions) or depression (hypotension, hypoventilation, coma). Hypertensive crises may be precipitated by sympathomimetic agents.

Tricyclic antidepressants competitively block norepinephrine re-uptake by postganglionic sympathetic nerve endings. Patients taking these drugs are hence more sensitive to catecholamines so sympathomimetics may cause hypertension and arrhythmias. Under the influence of anesthesia arrythmias and hypotension may be seen.

Herbal preparations are more frequently encountered as alternative medicine gains popularity. Certain preparations do require consideration in the preoperative period. St. John's Wort for example, used to treat depression, may have MAOI effects. Feverfew, a migraine treatment has anticoagulant effects.

The use of low molecular weight heparins (LMWH) in thromboprophylaxis must be considered when central nerve blockade is planned during anaesthesia. To minimise the risk of vertebral canal haematoma a period of at least 12 hours should elapse between administration of a LMWH and epidural or spinal anaesthesia.

CONCURRENT SURGICAL DISEASE

INTESTINAL OBSTRUCTION

Patients with intestinal obstruction often have electrolyte disturbances due to vomiting or, if incomplete obstruction, diarrohoea. They may have been ill at home for several days and not been able to take their usual medication for any concurrent medical condition. These patients may be dehydrated and possibly hypovolaemic due to gastro-intestinal losses or to third space losses into their gut. Inappropriate intravenous fluid therapy on a surgical ward may have exacerbated the problems. Abdominal distension splints the diaphragm and decreases respiratory reserves. If long standing, a chest infection may have developed. Fluid and electrolyte disturbances should be corrected prior to theatre and pre-operative chest physiotherapy may be useful. A nasogastric tube should be inserted before induction of anaesthesia in attempt to empty the stomach and decrease the risk of peri-operative regurgitation and aspiration.

ACUTE ABDOMINAL EMERGENCIES

All patients with an acute abdomen from whatever cause are at increased risk of regurgitation of stomach contents and so a nasogastric tube should be inserted prior to theatre. Patients with testicular problems e.g. torsion, should be included in this category because of the abdominal origin of the nerve supply of the testis.

References and further reading

American College of Physicians. Guidelines for assessing and managing the peri-operative risk from coronary artery disease associated with major non-cardiac surgery. Annals of Internal Medicine 1997;**127:** 309–328.

Bloomfield P, Bowler GMR. Anaesthetic management of the patent with a permanent pacemaker. Anaesthesia 1989;**44:** 42–46.

Cormack RS, Lehane J. Difficult tracheal intubation in obstetrics. Anaesthesia 1984;**39:** 1105–1111.

Detsky AS, Abrams HB, Forbath N, Scott JG, Hilliard JR. Cardiac assessment for patients undergoing noncardiac surgery-multifactorial clinical risk index. Arch Intern Med 1986; 146(11):2131-4.

Goldman L, Caldera DL, Nussbaum SR, Southwick FS, Krogstad D, Murray B. Multifactorial index of cardiac risk in noncardiac surgical procedures. N Engl J Med 1977;**287:** 45–850.

Hopkins P.M, Hunter J.M. (ed.), Endocrine and Metabolic Disorders in Anaesthesia and Intensive Care. British Journal of Anaesthesia 2000;**85:** 1.

Mallampati SR, Gatt SP, Gugino LD, Desai SP, Waraksa B, Freiberger D. A clinical sign to predict difficult tracheal intubation: a prospective study. Can Anaesth Soc J 1985;**32:** 429–434.

Mason R, Anaesthesia Databook A Peri-operative and Peripartum Manual, 3rd Edition. Greenwich Medical Media, London 2001.

Prys-Roberts C. Isolated systolic hypertension: pressure on the anaesthetist. Anaesthesia 2001;**56:** 505–510

Sacklad M. Grading of patients for surgical procedures. Anesthesiology 1941;**2:** 281–284.

Drug and Therapeutics Bulletin. Drugs in the peri-operative period:
1 – Stopping or continuing drugs around surgery. Vol.37 No.8 1999.

2 – Corticosteroids and therapy for diabetes mellitus. Vol.37 No.9 1999.

4 – Cardiovascular drugs. Vol.37 No.12 1999.

SECTION 1: 2
INDUCTION OF ANAESTHESIA

S. M. Parr

METHODS OF INDUCTION
Intravenous induction
Inhalational induction

ANAPHYLAXIS
Recognition
Treatment
Follow up

TRACHEAL INTUBATION
Indications
Management of a difficult intubation
Management of failed intubation
Confirmation of correct placement
 of endotracheal tube

**REGURGITATION AND VOMITING
DURING INDUCTION**
Causes
Prevention
Pulmonary aspiration

SPECIAL CIRCUMSTANCES
Full stomach
Head injury
Upper airway obstruction

METHODS OF INDUCTION

The objective of modern anaesthesia is to rapidly obtain a state of unconsciousness, to maintain this state and then achieve a rapid recovery. For any anaesthetic agent to be effective, whether administered intravenously or by inhalation, it must achieve a sufficient concentration within the central nervous system. Inhalational anaesthetic agents are administered by concentration rather than dose and as the concentration delivered rapidly equilibrates between alveoli, blood and brain, this allows a way of quantifying the anaesthetic effect for each agent. The minimum alveolar concentration (MAC) is defined as that concentration of anaesthetic agent that will prevent reflex response to a skin incision in 50% of a population. MAC is, therefore, an easily defined measure of depth of anaesthesia. Intravenous induction agents are, in contrast, administered by dose rather than concentration. To administer a 'sleep dose' of an induction agent requires an assessment of the likely response from an individual and knowledge of the pharmacokinetics and pharmacodynamics of the particular agent used. Figures I.1 and 2 summarise the main advantages and disadvantages of each route of administration.

INTRAVENOUS INDUCTION

The intravenous route of induction is the most common method of induction, allowing delivery of a bolus of drug to the brain, which results in rapid loss of consciousness. This is generally more acceptable to the patient than inhalational induction and has the advantage of minimising any excitement phase. The rapid intravenous administration of a drug sufficient to achieve a plasma concentration which results in central nervous system depression will necessarily be associated with effects on other organ systems, in particular the cardiovascular system. The rapid smooth induction of anaesthesia by the intravenous route, therefore, co-exists with an equally rapid onset of side effects. Hypotension, respiratory depression and rapid loss of airway control may provide cause for concern. Some of these potential problems can be minimised. Choosing an induction agent that demonstrates cardiovascular stability (such as etomidate) may be beneficial. The required dose may be reduced by premedication with benzodiazepines or pre treatment with intravenous opioids. Most importantly whatever induction agent is chosen it should be administered at an appropriate dosage and suitable rate for the individual patient. This will depend on consideration of all relevant factors taking special account of pre existing morbidity.

INHALATIONAL INDUCTION

Venepuncture, especially for children, still remains a great fear and many would see the avoidance of needles as the major advantage of inhalational induction. The slow speed of induction remains the major problem with this route. To achieve a sufficient concentration of inhalational agent in the central

---

INTRAVENOUS INDUCTION OF ANAESTHESIA

Advantages

Rapid onset
Dose titratable
Depression of pharyngeal reflexes allows early insertion of LMA
Anti-emetic and anti-convulsive properties

Disadvantages

Venous access required
Risk of hypotension
Apnoea common
Loss of airway control
Anaphylaxis

Figure I.1

INHALATION INDUCTION OF ANAESTHESIA

Advantages

Avoids venepuncture
Respiration is maintained
Slow loss of protective reflexes
End tidal concentration can be measured
Rapid recovery if induction is abandoned
Upper oesophageal sphincter tone maintained

Disadvantages

Slow process
Potential excitement phase
Irritant and unpleasant, may induce coughing
Pollution
May cause a rise in ICP/IOP

Figure I.2

nervous system to produce unconsciousness requires adequate uptake by the lungs and sufficient distribution to the brain. The uptake of an inhaled agent is dependent on a number of factors: the inspired concentration, the alveolar ventilation, the blood gas partition coefficient and the rate at which the agent is removed by the pulmonary circulation. Agents that are pleasant and non irritant (regardless of concentration), and which have a low blood gas partition coefficient allowing rapid equilibration between inspired and alveolar concentrations allow rapid induction and recovery.

An important advantage of the inhalational route over the intravenous route is the maintenance of airway control. If ventilation ceases either because of profound respiratory depression or airway obstruction the induction process will be reversed. This may be particularly important in patients with a compromised airway where a gradual loss of consciousness with the preservation of ventilation maintains a degree of safety. The technique of an inhalational induction requires practice. Co-operative patients can sometimes be persuaded to take a vital capacity breath of isoflurane or sevoflurane in an attempt to speed up induction but for the majority of cases volatile agents need to be introduced gradually. This is especially true with young children who may be disturbed by anaesthetic masks and pungent volatile agents. In this situation the gradual introduction of the volatile agent and use of a cupped hand rather than a face mask is likely to meet with greater approval.

ANAPHYLAXIS

Modern anaesthesia requires the use of several drugs to provide hypnosis, analgesia and muscular relaxation and thus, in view of the large number of patients receiving anaesthesia annually it is not surprising that untoward reactions occasionally occur. An adverse reaction to drugs administered by the intravenous route, rather than by inhalation, is likely to be more severe because the absorption of drugs across mucous membranes is relatively slow and may offer a degree of immunological protection.

Anaphylactic reactions are immediate type hyper-sensitivity reactions resulting from the interaction of antigens with specific IgE antibodies bound to mast cells and basophils. The mast cells and basophils respond by releasing vasoactive and bronchoconstrictive substances, which include histamine, leukotrienes (see Section 3, Chapter 13)

and eosinophil chemotactic factor of anaphylaxis (ECF-A). Anaphylactic reactions occur in individuals who have become sensitised to an allergen. Anaphylactoid reactions are clinically indistinguishable from anaphylaxis but do not result from prior exposure to a triggering agent. They are often mediated via IgG causing activation of complement and the liberation of anaphylatoxins C3a, C4a and C5a. The frequency of allergic reactions to individual drugs is difficult to quantify. Approximate figures for the incidence of IgE-dependent anaphylaxis under anaesthesia are given in Figure I.3. For details on latex allergy see page 107–108.

RECOGNITION

Irrespective of the mode of triggering, all the clinical manifestations of an allergic reaction occur as a result of the liberation of vasoactive substances. The typical clinical features of anaphylaxis are hypotension, bronchospasm, oedema and the development of a rash (Figure I.4). Cardiovascular collapse is one of the most common early signs (Figure I.5). This is usually the result of vasodilatation and may be compounded by arrhythmias (usually supraventricular tachycardia), hypovolaemia and a reduction in venous return, which will be exacerbated if high inflation pressures are necessary to facilitate ventilation of the lungs. Bronchospasm is variable in its severity from a

SUBSTANCES IDENTIFIED IN IgE DEPENDENT ANAPHYLAXIS (INCIDENCE IN %)

Muscle relaxants

comprising 70% of total of which

–	suxamethonium	43%
–	vecuronium	37%
–	pancuronium	13%
–	atracurium	7%

Others

comprising 30% of total of which

–	latex	15%
–	colloids	5%
–	hypnotics	4%
–	antibiotics	2%
–	benzodiazepines	2%
–	opioids	2%

Figure I.3

CLINICAL FEATURES OF ANAPHYLAXIS

Cardiovascular collapse		88%
Bronchospasm		36%
Swelling of the face		24%
Generalised swelling		7%
Cutaneous signs	rash	3%
	erythema	45%
	urticaria	8.5%

Association of Anaesthetists of Great Britain and Ireland 1995

Figure I.4

THE FIRST OBSERVED CLINICAL FEATURES OF ANAPHYLAXIS

No pulse/fall in arterial pressure	28%
Difficulty inflating lungs	26%
Flushing	21%
Coughing	6%
Rash	4%
Desaturation	3%
Cyanosis	3%
Others (ECG changes, swelling, urticaria)	9%

Association of Anaesthetists of Great Britain and Ireland 1995

Figure I.5

transient degree of difficulty with ventilation to the situation where gas exchange is impossible despite the use of high airway pressures and slow inspiratory and expiratory times. The presence of wheals and erythema near the point of venous access is usually a sign of localised histamine release which usually does not require any treatment and resolves spontaneously within an hour. Generalised erythema, wheals and oedema are signs of systemic histamine release which may herald the onset of a major reaction.

TREATMENT

The prompt and aggressive treatment of a patient with a severe anaphylactic reaction is life saving. 100% oxygen should be administered and consideration given to early intubation before the onset of angio-oedema. The administration of epinephrine is a priority, and if there is circulatory collapse 1 ml of 1 in 10 000 epinephrine should be administered IV at 1 minute intervals. Intravenous colloids are the most effective treatment to restore intravascular volume, up to two litres may be infused rapidly (note that allergic reaction to colloids administered at this time is virtually unknown). Arrhythmias should be treated symptomatically. Bronchospasm can be difficult to overcome and although epinephrine is often effective aminophylline and nebulised salbutamol may be useful for persistent bronchospasm. Intratracheal injections of local anaesthetic agents (such as lidocaine 100 mg) have also been advocated. Although such reactions are rare all anaesthetists should rehearse a simulated 'anaphylaxis drill' at regular intervals (Figure I.6).

FOLLOW UP

After a suspected drug reaction associated with anaesthesia the patient should be counselled and investigated. This is the responsibility of the anaesthetist who administered the drug and should be conducted in consultation with a clinical immunologist. No tests or investigations of any kind should be performed until the resuscitation period is completed. Approximately one hour after the reaction occurred 10 ml venous blood should be taken into a plain glass tube, the serum separated and stored at –20°C for estimation of serum tryptase concentration. Elevation of this enzyme indicates that the reaction was associated with mast cell de-granulation. Blood samples in EDTA containing tubes are useful for complement assays and haematology; the disappearance of basophils being indicative of a Type I anaphylactic reaction. When more than one drug has been administered skin prick tests are useful to establish the agent involved. These should be carried out by specialised departments with full resuscitation facilities.

RAST testing

The radio-allergosorbent test (RAST) is an in vitro method of measuring circulating allergen specific IgE antibodies. The allergen is first attached to a paper disc and is then incubated with serum from the patient. Circulating antibody will become bound and a second incubation is carried out with radiolabelled allergen-specific anti-IgE. The amount of bound radioactivity is related to the amount of specific IgE in the original serum. RAST capable of measuring IgE antibodies to thiopentone, muscle relaxants and latex are available, among others.

MANAGEMENT OF A PATIENT WITH SUSPECTED ANAPHYLAXIS

Initial therapy

1. Stop administration of drug(s) likely to be responsible
2. Maintain airway, give 100% oxygen
3. Lay patient flat with feet elevated
4. Give adrenaline
    IM   0.5 mg to 1.0 mg and repeated every 10 minutes as required
    IV   50 to 100 mcg over 1 minute and repeated as required
    For cardiovascular collapse 0.5 to 1.0 mg (5 to 10 ml of 1 in 10 000) may be required intravenously in divided doses by titration. This should be given at a rate of 0.1 mg (1 ml of 1 in 10 000) per minute until a response is obtained
5. Start intravascular volume expansion with crystalloid or colloid

Secondary therapy

1. Antihistamines (chlorpheniramine 10–20 mg by slow intravenous infusion)
2. Corticosteroids (100–300 mg hydrocortisone IV)
3. Catecholamine infusions consider   epinephrine   4–8 mcg/min
                                          norepinephrine   4–8 mcg/min
4. Consider bicarbonate 0.5–1.0 mg/kg IV for acidosis
5. Airway evaluation (before extubation)
6. Bronchodilators may be required for persistent bronchospasm

Association of Anaesthetists of Great Britain and Ireland 1995

Figure I.6

Detailed written records should be kept of all events especially the timing of administration of all drugs. The anaesthetist is responsible for submitting a report using the 'yellow card' system to the Committee on Safety of Medicines and advising the patient about future anaesthesia. This must include an explanation to the patient and a full and detailed record in the case notes with a copy to the general practitioner. The patient should also be given a written record of the reaction and be advised to wear a 'Medic alert' bracelet.

TRACHEAL INTUBATION

INDICATIONS

There are two major indications for tracheal intubation in the anaesthetised patient. Firstly to ensure airway patency and, second, to protect the airway from aspiration.

Airway patency

Assuming that the tracheal tube is kept clear of obstructions and free of kinks, tracheal intubation affords the anaesthetist the guarantee of a patent airway. This is particularly useful in the following situations:

*   Prolonged operations such as neurosurgical, cardiac and extensive abdominal surgery.

*   Operations where access to the airway is difficult such as head and neck surgery and patients in the prone position.

*   Operations involving excessive movement of the head and neck, where other forms of airway control may become dislodged.

- Situations where it is difficult to achieve a clear airway with a laryngeal mask airway or face mask.

- Situations where a major intra-operative complication develops (severe haemorrhage, anaphylaxis or malignant hyperpyrexia).

Protection from aspiration

A cuffed endotracheal tube forms an air tight seal at the level of the cuff and greatly reduces the risk of contamination of the lower respiratory tract. This is particularly useful in patients with an increased risk of regurgitation and during surgery when there may be extensive bleeding from the mouth, nose or oropharynx. Other indications for tracheal intubation include thoracic operations that require isolation of one lung and those patients in whom the aspiration of secretions from the lower respiratory tract is necessary.

MANAGEMENT OF A DIFFICULT INTUBATION

Clinical examination of the patient and bedside assessments of the airway are useful in identifying those patients posing the risk of a potentially difficult intubation but it is not unusual to be confronted with a patient of normal appearance in whom the glottis cannot be visualised on direct laryngoscopy. The latest Triennial report into maternal mortality in the UK (HMSO 1993) describes eight cases of death directly attributable to anaesthesia. In five of these cases there was difficulty with the airway.

When faced with a potentially difficult airway it is important to remain calm. The degree of difficulty should be assessed and senior assistance sought if available. It is essential to ensure that the patient is adequately ventilated, oxygenated and anaesthetised at all times, and it may be necessary to wake the patient up. The drama of a difficult intubation can easily be turned into a crisis when there are multiple attempts at laryngoscopy in a hypoxic patient with a mouth full of blood and secretions. The use of rapidly redistributed intravenous induction agents such as propofol will allow rapid return of consciousness unless the patient receives adequate amounts of volatile agent or further incremental doses of induction agent.

If ventilation by mask is easy and gas exchange can be maintained there are a number of manoeuvres and aids available to improve the chances of correct endotracheal tube placement. These are detailed below.

1. Positioning

The 'sniffing the morning air' position is the most important manoeuvre that can improve intubating conditions. The neck is flexed on the chest to about 35 degrees, this can usually be achieved with one pillow under the head. The head is then extended on the neck so that the face is tilted back 15 degrees from the horizontal plane. In this position the oral, pharyngeal and tracheal axes are aligned. The practice of placing one hand on the chin and the other on the back of the head to force the head into severe extension will not only push the larynx into an anterior position and make intubation more difficult, but also in patients with osteoporosis or rheumatoid arthritis it runs the risk of fracturing the odontoid peg against the body of C1. In very obese patients it may be necessary to place pillows under the shoulders and neck as well as the head to allow the head to be extended on the neck.

2. Laryngoscopy technique

The Macintosh laryngoscope blade has a flange on its left side to keep the tongue out of the line of sight. The blade should be inserted into the right side of the mouth and advanced centrally towards the base of the tongue. The blade is then lifted to expose the epiglottis and advanced into the vallecula with continued lifting to expose the laryngeal opening. There is a natural tendency amongst inexperienced anaesthetists to advance the blade insufficiently and then lever the laryngoscope to try and achieve visualisation of the glottis which will cause the proximal end of the blade to act as a lever on the upper incisors or gums resulting in dental damage or bleeding. Other causes of difficulty include inserting the blade past the epiglottis and elevating the entire larynx so that the oesophagus is visualised or allowing the tongue to slip over the right side of the laryngoscope blade impairing the view. Difficulty may be encountered in inserting the laryngoscope correctly in obese patients and large breasted women and it may occasionally be necessary to insert an unattached blade into the mouth and then reattach the handle. The use of external laryngeal pressure applied to the thyroid cartilage in a posterior direction can improve the view obtained at laryngoscopy. With respect to the grading of the view at laryngoscopy described by Cormack and Lehane (Cormack 1984) a grade 3 may be changed into a grade 2 See Figure I.7.

THE VIEW OBTAINED AT LARYNGOSCOPY

Grade 1	Visualisation of the vocal cords
Grade 2	Visualisation of the posterior portion of the laryngeal aperture
Grade 3	Visualisation of the epiglottis
Grade 4	Visualisation of the soft palate only

Figure I.7

3. Gum elastic bougie

This simple device is probably the single most important aid to help difficult intubation available to the anaesthetist. It is a 60 cm long introducer, 5 mm in diameter with a smooth angled tip at the end. The bougie is made from braided polyester with a resin coat, which provides both the necessary stiffness and flexibility to enable it to be passed into the larynx. It may be bent before insertion to aid placement. The device is especially useful in cases where the glottic opening cannot be visualised. In this situation correct placement may be confirmed by the detection of clicks as the introducer is gently passed down into the trachea. The tracheal tube can then be slid over the bougie into the trachea with a 90 degree anti-clockwise rotation to facilitate passage through the laryngeal inlet.

4. Stylet

A pre curved malleable stylet when placed within an endotracheal tube will enable the tube to be curved and thus aid placement of the tube especially when the larynx is anteriorly situated. The stylet should on no account be allowed to protrude beyond the tip of the endotracheal tube, as this may cause trauma to the larynx.

5. Lightwand

A lightwand (trachlight) uses the principle of transillumination of the neck when a light is passed into the trachea. In this situation a distinct glow can be seen below the thyroid cartilage which is not apparent when the light is placed in the oesophagus. The light emitted by the wand should project laterally as well as forward and there should be little associated heat production. The lightwand is usually advanced without the aid of a laryngoscope and once in the trachea the internal stylet that gives the wand its stiffness can be retracted to allow the pliable wand to be advanced into the trachea and used as a guide for the placement of the endotracheal tube.

6. Alternative laryngoscope blades (Figure I.8)

The standard Macintosh laryngoscope was introduced in 1943. It has a relatively short curved blade designed to rest in the vallecula and lift the epiglottis. Several alternative laryngoscope blades are available, some of which are described below.

Miller. Straight bladed laryngoscope with a slight curve at the tip. The blade is longer, narrower and smaller at the tip and is designed to trap and lift the epiglottis

McCoy. The McCoy levering laryngoscope (McCoy 1993) has a 25 mm hinged blade tip controlled by a spring loaded lever on the handle of the laryngoscope which allows elevation of the epiglottis without the use of excessive forces on the pharyngeal tissues

Bullard. The Bullard laryngoscope is a rigid bladed indirect fibre-optic laryngoscope with a shape designed to match the airway. The fibre-optic bundle passes along the posterior aspect of the blade and ends 26 mm from the distal tip of the blade allowing excellent visualisation of the larynx. Intubation can be achieved using an attached intubating stylet with pre loaded endotracheal tube. Although this device requires a considerable amount of practice it is particularly useful in those patients with upper airway pathology, limited mouth opening or an immobile or unstable cervical spine

Prism. The Huffman prism is an example of a laryngoscope using refraction to aid visualisation of the larynx. It employs a modification of the Macintosh blade whereby a block of transparent plastic in a prism shape is attached to the proximal end of the blade. The ends of the prism are polished to provide optically flat surfaces, the nearest to the eye being cut at 90 degrees to the line of vision and the distal surface at 30 degrees. The net result to the view obtained is a refraction of approximately 30 degrees.

Polio. The Polio blade was originally designed to enable patients in an iron lung to be intubated. In the UK the 'polio blade' is actually a 90 degree adaptor located between the handle and blade of a standard Macintosh laryngoscope. It allows the easier introduction of the blade in situations where the chest gets in the way of the handle.

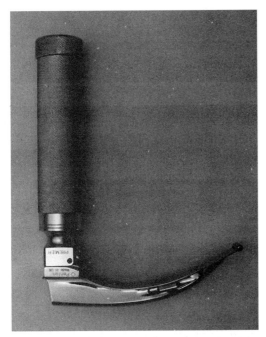

Macintosh

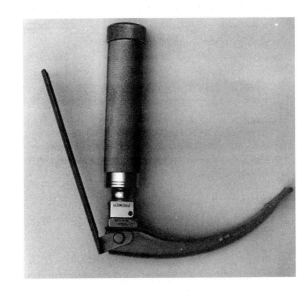

McCoy

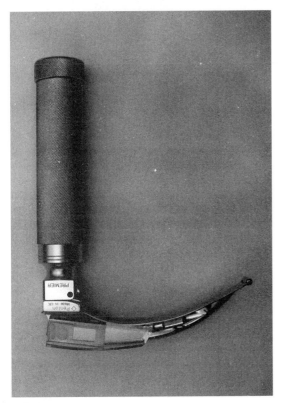

Huffman

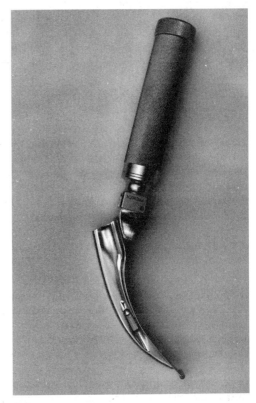

Polio

Figure 1.8 Laryngoscope blades

Flexiblade. A flexible bladed laryngoscope based on the Macintosh shape is now available. This takes the principle of the McCoy one step further in that the blade is muti-segmented and able to change its radius of curvature. This device may be manipulated to optimise the view of the cords during laryngoscopy.

7. Laryngeal mask airway (LMA)

The laryngeal mask airway is a useful means of airway control in difficult and failed intubations. Note that the LMA has been shown to be life saving in cases of failed intubation in obstetric anaesthesia (Gataure and Hughes 1995). A number of insertion methods have been advocated and in the case of difficulty it seems wise to use a familiar technique. Anterior displacement of the mandible often prevents down folding of the epiglottis and in cases of difficulty is recommended. If intubation is difficult and the airway can be secured with a laryngeal mask there are then several choices available to the anaesthetist.

- Use the LMA to oxygenate the patient whilst allowing to wake up. Consider regional anaesthesia or securing the airway by alternative means

- Use the LMA to maintain anaesthesia. The laryngeal mask can be used for both spontaneous and controlled ventilation. The laryngeal mask is in popular use for gynaecological surgery (such as laparoscopy) and there have been reports of its use in patients normally requiring intubation (such as coronary artery bypass grafting)

- Use the LMA to intubate the trachea. In adults a well lubricated uncut cuffed 6 mm internal diameter endotracheal tube can be passed through the lumen of a size 3 or 4 laryngeal mask. The patient needs to be correctly positioned 'sniffing the morning air' and the laryngeal mask needs to be correctly sited with no down folding of the epiglottis. The patient should be deeply anaesthetised with or without muscle relaxation to prevent coughing or laryngospasm. Rotation of the tube through 90 degrees will prevent the bevel of the tube catching on the bars of the laryngeal mask aperture, and the tube can then be passed into the trachea. If cricoid pressure has been applied this tends not to be compromised by the presence of a laryngeal mask and should be continued at least until the moment of

intubation when it may need to be momentarily released. If difficulty is encountered the position of the head and neck can be altered, firstly by extension at the atlanto-occipital joint and then with varying degrees of flexion of the neck. If an endotracheal tube larger than a size 6.0 is required a gum elastic bougie can be passed through the laryngeal mask into the trachea and an endotracheal tube railroaded over the bougie into place. A development of the LMA specifically designed for secondary intubation is now available.

The intubating laryngeal mask is a shortened version of the usual device with a forwardly directed metal handle. The aperture has a single wider bar which is designed to elevate the epiglottis as a narrow endotracheal tube is advanced through the laryngeal mask lumen. The intubating laryngeal mask therefore has a role in the temporary establishment of the airway prior to securing it with a cuffed ET tube. The usual risks of aspiration during the process are, however, present.

8. Other airway management devices

Several other devices are available for the management of the airway. These include:

- The combitube airway. This is a double lumen device designed for blind placement in the pharynx. Its role is to allow ventilation of the lungs whether the tube enters the trachea or oesophagus. There are eight supraglottic apertures and a single distal lumen. Two cuffs, a large volume pharyngeal one and a small volume distal cuff create a seal and both are fitted with pilot tubes. In practice it is most common that the combitube enters the oesophagus. Ventilation may not always be possible and there have been instances of trauma and oesophageal damage.

- The cuffed oropharyngeal airway. This device is a modification of the standard Guedel airway, mainly differing in having a distal inflatable cuff.

- The airway management device (AMD). The AMD is a single lumen device designed for blind placement. It has a double cuff each with pilot balloon. There is limited experience with the AMD in practice.

- The laryngeal tube. This device is similar to the AMD but has two cuffs (a small distal and large proximal) and a single pilot balloon. Early experience suggests that this device has a limited role in airway management. It has however been successfully used to aid nasotracheal intubation in difficult circumstances.

9. Blind nasal intubation

In blind nasal intubation a nasotracheal tube is passed through the nose with the head extended at the atlanto-axial joint. The tip of the tube, if kept in the midline, will usually impact anteriorly and flexion of the head will allow advancement of the tube into the larynx. If the tube is not in the midline it will tend to lodge in the pyriform fossa and this usually shows as a bulge on the anterior aspect of the neck. If the tube enters the oesophagus it can often be relocated in the trachea by first withdrawing and then advancing again. This technique requires a great deal of practice and is not recommended for the novice. A topical vasoconstrictor solution (such as xylometazoline spray) should be used to minimise the risk of bleeding from the nasal mucosa.

10. Retrograde intubation

Retrograde intubation involves the passage of a catheter through a cricothyroid incision upwards so as to protrude at the mouth. It is then possible to use the catheter to railroad an endotracheal tube into the larynx. The technique may be carried out under local or general anaesthesia but it has complications (Figure I.9) and is not recommended for inexperienced hands. For detail of the practical method see Figure I.10.

COMPLICATIONS OF RETROGRADE INTUBATION

Bleeding

Perforation of posterior wall of trachea with needle

Subcutaneous emphysema of neck

Pneumothorax

Infection at puncture site

Figure I.9

MANAGEMENT OF FAILED INTUBATION

Failed intubation may be the result of an anticipated degree of difficulty with the airway or a totally unexpected event.

Unexpected

A suitable failed intubation drill is mandatory. Generally patients do not come to harm because they

TECHNIQUE OF RETROGRADE INTUBATION

Pass a Tuohy needle attached to a saline filled syringe through a cricothyrotomy puncture. Verify penetration of the larynx by aspiration of air. Angulate the needle 45 degrees cephalad with the bevel pointing anteriorly. Push an epidural catheter through the needle until it appears at the mouth. Anchor the catheter at its entry point in the neck. Keeping the catheter tensioned pass a lubricated endotracheal tube over the catheter, advancing until passage through the vocal cords is indicated by a 'click'. If there is any obstruction to passage at this point, rotate the tube through 90 degrees and if this fails try a smaller tube size.

Figure I.10

cannot be intubated, they come to harm because of inadequate oxygenation, inadequate anaesthesia, trauma to the airway and aspiration. Persistent and prolonged attempts at intubation using conventional laryngoscopy cause oedema and bleeding in the airway with progressive difficulty in ventilation. Over vigorous mask ventilation fills the stomach with gas leading to an increasing likelihood of regurgitation.

A major problem relating to the use of a failed intubation drill is the timing of the decision as to when it should be implemented. Although there must be an early acceptance of failure it is probably reasonable to have three or four attempts at endotracheal intubation using some of the manoeuvres designed to aid success such as proper positioning of the patient, anterior laryngeal pressure and use of the gum elastic bougie. The use of totally unfamiliar equipment such as alternative laryngoscope blades is unlikely to be of help. If the patient cannot be intubated, Figure I.11 describes appropriate management.

Anticipated

When a potentially difficult airway is recognised careful steps should be taken to assess the patient pre-operatively. The previous medical history should be sought and past anaesthetic records scrutinised. The presence of respiratory or cardiac disease may require special attention during intubation or induction. The assessment of the airway should be particularly thorough and include mouth opening, neck extension, thyro-mental distance, nostril patency, Mallampatti score and state of dentition.

Possible options in anticipated difficult intubation are:

Call for help. If cricoid pressure has been applied it should not be released. Tilt the table head down. Suction pharynx as required. Insert oral airway and institute bag and mask ventilation with 100% oxygen. If this is difficult a two person effort may be required, one to maintain the airway, the other to squeeze the reservoir bag. If ventilation is satisfactory consider waking the patient up. In an emergency (Caesarean section for foetal distress, for example) maintain cricoid pressure and allow spontaneous respiration to return. Continue anaesthesia via a face mask.

If ventilation is difficult try inserting a laryngeal mask airway. If ventilation is impossible both with a conventional mask and through a laryngeal mask airway, consider severe laryngeal spasm as a cause. If this has been excluded perform an emergency cricothyroid puncture with a 16 or 14 G cannula. Once in the trachea remove the needle and connect the catheter to a 2 ml syringe. Discard the plunger and insert a size 7.0 mm endotracheal tube (Portex) connector inside the syringe, attach this to a catheter mount and anaesthetic circuit.

Figure I.11

- Awake intubation
- Intubation attempts after induction of anaesthesia
- Elective surgical tracheostomy under local anaesthesia
- Cricothyroid puncture and HFJV

Awake intubation is indicated in the following patients. Those with congenital airway anomalies, those with trauma to the face, airway or cervical spine and those with a history of previous difficult intubation. The practical technique of awake intubation is described in Figure I.12. Although awake intubation is an unpleasant experience for the patient it provides a number of advantages:

- The airway is preserved
- There is no loss of muscle tone (facilitating fibre-optic visualisation)
- Consciousness and respiration are unaffected

CONFIRMATION OF CORRECT PLACEMENT OF ENDOTRACHEAL TUBE

After intubation of the trachea the tip of the endotracheal tube will ideally lie above the carina but below the vocal cords. The two major malplacements

Use sedative premedication cautiously and not at all in the presence of severe airway compromise. Anticholinergic premedication may be given to reduce secretions. Prescribe aspiration prophylaxis (such as ranitidine and sodium citrate) pre-operatively. Check all equipment in the anaesthetic room, attach monitoring and secure intravenous access. Prepare the airway by achieving local anaesthesia as described on p 158. Spray the nasal mucosa with a vasoconstrictor if this is the chosen route. Having loaded the chosen endotracheal tube onto the fibreoptic scope proceed via mouth or nose until the larynx is visualised. Pass the tube off the scope into the trachea and check for correct placement.

Figure I.12

are accidental endobronchial intubation and accidental oesophageal intubation. Endobronchial intubation is generally the result of an endotracheal tube being cut to a length greater than necessary. It is more usual for the right main bronchus to become intubated due to its more vertical nature. The signs of accidental endobronchial intubation are an unexplained drop in oxygen saturation, higher than expected airway pressure (and a feel of poor compliance in the reservoir bag) and asymmetrical chest movement. If ausculation confirms endobronchial intubation, withdraw the tube until bilateral ventilation returns then re-inflate the cuff.

Unrecognised oesophageal intubation is still a major cause of anaesthetic morbidity and mortality. Fortunately most oesophageal intubations are easily recognised but there are still occasions where failure to recognise misplacement of the tube has serious, often fatal consequences. The oft quoted maxim 'When in doubt take it out' is still valid. The methods used to verify the position of the endotracheal tube can be divided into clinical indications of correct tube placement and objective signs such as tests based on the detection of CO_2 from expired-gas (Figure I.13).

Clinical signs

Direct visualisation of the tracheal tube passing between the vocal cords
This simple method is one of the most reliable means of confirming correct intubation. Unfortunately, in grade 3 intubations and patients with an anterior larynx a satisfactory view may be impossible to obtain. Excessive movement of the head and neck, alterations in patient position, traction on the trachea or

CONFIRMATION OF CORRECT ENDOTRACHEAL TUBE PLACEMENT

Clinical signs

Direct visualisation of the tube through the cords
Auscultation for breath sounds
Chest movement with positive pressure ventilation
"Feel" of the reservoir bag
(Absence of cyanosis)

Objective signs

Carbon dioxide detectors
Oesophageal detectors

Figure I.13

ERRORS IN CONFIRMATION OF CORRECT INTUBATION

False negative results

Equipment failure
Disconnection or apnoea
Kinked or obstructed gas sampling tube
Kinked or obstructed tracheal tube
Dilution of expired gas by high fresh gas flow
    with sidestream sampling
Severe airway obstruction
Poor pulmonary perfusion (severe hypotension,
    pulmonary/air embolism)

False positive results

Tube in oesophagus after exhaled gases have
    been forced into stomach
Tube in oesophagus after drinking carbonated
    beverages
Distal end of endotracheal tube in pharynx

Figure I.14

oesophagus and poor fixing of the tracheal tube are all potential causes of tube displacement.

Auscultation of breath sounds

This can and should be done repeatedly to ensure that the tube is still within the trachea whenever there has been movement of the tube or movement of the patient. Auscultation in both axillae to confirm symmetrical breath sounds will usually verify correct tube placement although there have been occasions where transmitted sounds from oesophageal intubations have caused confusion. This is often the case in infants where the presence of bilateral abnormal breath sounds should alert the anaesthetist to the possibility of oesophageal intubation. For this reason in both adults and children it is wise to auscultate in both axillae and in the epigastrium as the gurgling sound of air entering the stomach is quite characteristic.

Observation of chest movement

This cannot be relied upon to distinguish oesophageal from tracheal intubation.

The 'feel' of the reservoir bag

The characteristic feel of the reservoir bag on manual ventilation is a good guide to the location of the tracheal tube and in particular the rapid refilling of the bag during expiration is unlikely to occur in cases of oesophageal intubation. Unfortunately, there have been occasions where confusion has arisen particularly in patients with poor compliance or high airway resistance. Oesophageal pressures tend to reflect intrapleural pressures and the movement of the reservoir bag with spontaneous respiration cannot be regarded as an indication of tracheal intubation.

The appearance of cyanosis

Although oesophageal intubation will eventually cause severe decreases in oxygen saturation there may be a delay of some minutes before cyanosis occurs. Cyanosis usually becomes apparent when there is 5 g of reduced haemoglobin per 100 ml blood (in cases of severe anaemia this may reflect oxygen saturations of 60%). Pre-oxygenation followed by a period of apnoea may delay the fall in oxygen saturation for up to 3 minutes and normal oxygen saturations detected by a pulse oximeter should not be regarded as a sign of successful tracheal intubation. If a patient is making respiratory efforts through an unintubated trachea recovery of consciousness may well occur before a significant reduction in oxygen saturation.

Objective signs

Identification of carbon dioxide in expired gas

Alveolar gas normally contains about 5% carbon dioxide. If the lungs are being perfused and effective alveolar ventilation is occurring then identification of carbon dioxide in exhaled gas by capnography should confirm correct tube placement. There are however a number of causes of false-negative results where the tube is correctly placed but the capnograph waveform is absent (Figure I.14). There is also potential for false-positive results where there is carbon dioxide passing out of a misplaced tube. This can occur after a period of vigorous mask ventilation with inflation of the stomach with gas containing carbon dioxide. The CO_2 waveform in this situation may initially appear normal but rapidly diminishes to zero after a few breaths. Carbon dioxide in expired gas can also be detected chemically. pH-sensitive chemical indicator devices that reversibly change colour on exposure to CO_2 are available. These are often disposable devices that do not require a power source, are simple and safe in operation with a quick response time but may be relatively costly. In areas where sophisticated equipment is not available bubbling expired gases through a diluted solution of bromothymol blue will cause a rapid colour change from a reddish-blue to a greenish yellow on exposure to CO_2.

Oesophageal detector devices

The oesphageal detector device consists of a 60 ml syringe that can be attached to an endotracheal tube connector. A negative pressure applied to the lumen of the oesophagus will cause it to collapse whereas the adult trachea contains cartilaginous rings and will not collapse under the same conditions. Aspiration of the plunger will therefore freely withdraw gas if the tube is in the trachea but will encounter resistance if the tube is located in the oesophagus. If the syringe is replaced by a self inflating bulb then the principle of use remains the same; compression of the bulb is followed by immediate refill if the tracheal tube is correctly placed whereas if the tube is in the oesophagus the bulb will remain collapsed. Although these devices are simple and sensitive they may fail to confirm tracheal tube placement if the tube is partially obstructed or if the patient has bronchospasm or is morbidly obese.

REGURGITATION AND VOMITING DURING INDUCTION

CAUSES

There are multiple factors which may pre dispose to regurgitation and vomiting. The major causes are detailed in Figure I.15.

CAUSES OF REGURGITATION AND VOMITING

Factors that increase gastric volume	Full stomach
	Intestinal or pyloric obstruction
	Air inflation during mask ventilation
Factors that delay gastric emptying	Pregnancy
	Head injury
	Diabetic autonomic neuropathy
	Opioids
	Sympathetic stimulation; pain or anxiety
Incompetence of the gastro-oesophageal junction	Hiatus hernia
	Nasogastric tube *in situ*
	Scleroderma
Raised intra-abdominal pressure	Obesity
	Steep head down position
	Pregnancy
Other causes	Peritonitis
	Pancreatitis
	Hypotension in the awake patient
	Drugs; opioids, ergometrine, magnesium, volatile agents
	Vagal stimulation (for example pressure on the epiglottis from a polio blade)

Figure I.15

PREVENTION

The aims in prevention of pulmonary aspiration are threefold; to render the gastric contents as innocuous as possible, to prevent gastric contents reaching the pharynx and to prevent contamination of the lower respiratory tract (Figure I.16).

GUIDELINES FOR PREVENTING PULMONARY ASPIRATION

Avoid oversedation

Starve patient (elective procedure)

Aspirate nasogastric tube

Reduce gastric acidity

Employ rapid sequence induction

Figure I.16

Gastric volume

The concept that a critical volume of 25 ml and pH of 2.5 is necessary to produce aspiration pneumonitis has been around since the time of Mendelson's original study (Mendelson 1946) and although these values maybe somewhat arbitrary it is true that any mechanism that reduces gastric volume or acidity will tend to minimise the severity of aspiration pneumonitis. Ensure that the patient is starved. In recent years the value of conventional fasting regimes (6 H for solids and 4 H for liquids) has been challenged and from these studies a few general conclusions can be drawn. Clear fluids are rapidly removed from the stomach and in healthy adults and children clear fluid intake within 2–3 H of induction does not affect gastric contents. Solid, semi-solid food and milk products are not cleared from the stomach as rapidly. The application of suction to an orogastric or nasogastric tube allows liquid gastric contents to be removed from the stomach before the induction of anaesthesia. It cannot be relied upon, however, to completely empty the stomach. It has been argued that the presence of a gastric tube will interfere with the mechanics of the lower oesophageal sphincter allowing reflux of gastric contents and should, therefore, be removed before a rapid sequence induction. In the authors' opinion the tube should be aspirated immediately before induction and left in situ open to allow the free passage of fluid and gas out of the stomach. Vomiting can be induced by the slow intravenous injection of up to 5 mg apomorphine. Not surprisingly this is rather unpleasant for the patient and cannot ever be recommended.

Gastric acidity

Gastric acidity may be reduced by the administration of an alkali or a deliberate inhibition of gastric acid production. Sodium citrate, magnesium trisilicate, H_2 blocking agents and proton pump inhibitors are the most commonly used agents.

Sodium citrate is a clear, soluble, non particulate alkali. 30 ml of 0.3 M sodium citrate is particularly effective at raising gastric pH, but may cause an increase in gastric volume. Failure to neutralise gastric acidity in some patients may be related to inadequate mixing with stomach contents. Unfortunately, the duration of action of sodium citrate is dependent on the rate of gastric emptying and may be as short as 20 minutes thereby not providing adequate prophylaxis at the time of recovery.

Magnesium trisilicate mixture contains magnesium trisilicate, magnesium carbonate and sodium carbonate made up with peppermint emulsion and chloroform water. Although an effective antacid, the solution is particulate in nature and studies have suggested a link between the aspiration of gastric fluid containing particulate antacids and severe pulmonary reactions.

H_2 receptor blockade by cimetidine or ranitidine will suppress acid secretion by gastric parietal cells. Cimetidine 400 mg administered orally or intravenously will reduce gastric volume and raise pH in most patients after 1–2 hours. Unfortunately, cimetidine has a range of side effects when used long term including mental confusion, dizziness and headaches as well as hypotension and arrhythmias following bolus administration. Cimetidine reduces hepatic blood flow and inhibits cytochrome P_{450} and will prolong the duration of action of drugs cleared by the liver such as warfarin, propanolol, phenytoin, diazepam and bupivacaine. Rantidine 150 mg orally is more rapid in onset, more effective and has a longer duration of action than cimetidine. Furthermore it is relatively free of side effects. For these reasons it is generally preferred to cimetidine for pre-operative use.

Omeprazole is a non competitive proton pump inhibitor effectively suppressing the final step of gastric acid secretion. A single dose of omeprazole 40 mg will reduce gastric acidity for up to 48 hours. It has been used as a prophylactic agent for acid aspiration and although a single dose will reduce gastric volume and acidity, better results have been obtained with two doses, the first given the evening before surgery.

Gastric emptying

Gastric emptying may be encouraged pharmacologically by drugs such as metoclopramide. Metoclopramide possesses central and peripheral anti-dopaminergic activity and will raise the lower oesophageal barrier pressure and accelerate gastric emptying within 10–20 minutes of an intravenous dose. Metoclopramide exhibits an inconsistent anti-emetic action secondary to inhibition of the chemoreceptor trigger zone. Extrapyramidal reactions are the commonest serious side effect and can occur following a single dose of 10 mg.

Lower oesophageal sphincter tone

The lower oesophageal sphincter maintains closure of the distal oesophagus through tonic contraction of smooth muscle. The resulting pressure gradient between the distal oesophagus and the stomach is known as the lower oesophageal barrier pressure and in healthy adults is normally 30 mmHg. The sphincter cannot be relied upon to prevent reflux in a patient with gastric distension, obesity and pregnancy and is affected by various drugs. Dopaminergic and adrenergic stimulation decrease the lower oesophageal barrier pressure whereas cholinergic stimulation increases the lower oesophageal barrier pressure. Anticholinergic drugs such as atropine and glycopyrrolate will, therefore, decrease the contractility of the lower oesophageal sphincter and may encourage reflux.

Cricoid pressure

The application of cricoid pressure to prevent passive regurgitation at induction of anaesthesia was proposed by Sellick (1961). The cricoid cartilage is a ring shaped cartilage which when pressed backwards onto the vertebral column will occlude the upper end of the oesophagus. Sellick described having the head and neck extended, stabilising the cricoid cartilage between the thumb and second finger and applying pressure on the cricoid cartilage with the index finger. Firm pressure should be applied, sufficient to cause mild discomfort but not so severe as to cause breathing difficulties. The usual method of applying cricoid pressure is a modification of the original technique with the patient in the 'sniffing the morning air position' and pressure applied with the thumb and index finger. If flexion of the neck occurs hindering insertion of the laryngoscope this can be prevented by the assistant placing the other hand behind the neck and applying gentle support. Lower oesophageal sphincter pressure decreases as anaesthesia is induced and cricoid pressure should, therefore, be applied whilst the patient is still awake and increased immediately consciousness is lost. Cricoid pressure should be maintained until the trachea has been intubated, the cuff inflated and the correct position of the tube confirmed. It should then be the responsibility of the anaesthetist to determine the moment at which cricoid pressure is released. Cricoid pressure should still be maintained if active vomiting occurs as the risk of aspiration outweighs the potential risk of oesophageal rupture from high intra-oesophageal pressures. The application of cricoid pressure may prove difficult in patients with short, thick necks and if pressure has been applied incorrectly the larynx may be pushed away from the midline making the process of intubation more difficult.

PULMONARY ASPIRATION

If regurgitation or vomiting occurs during induction, the upper airway should be cleared by immediately sucking out the pharynx and turning the patient head down. If the patient is paralysed tracheal intubation should be performed and the airway protected. If gastric contents are thought to have entered the trachea these should be aspirated before ventilation is commenced as positive pressure will force the acidic contents further into the lungs. Attempted neutralisation of acid at this stage is ineffective but the injection of 10 ml boluses of saline into the trachea followed by immediate suction is a useful form of bronchial lavage. Large volumes of saline will be absorbed and should, therefore, be avoided.

Early clinical signs of acid aspiration in the anaesthetised patient include a fall in arterial oxygen saturation and the presence of wheezing and ronchi which may be localised to one lung. Aspiration of solid material causes plugging of the large airways and is often fatal. Bronchospasm, pulmonary oedema and ventilation perfusion mismatch all contribute to worsening arterial hypoxaemia and often the only way to maintain adequate oxygenation is to institute a period of mechanical ventilation with 100% oxygen and the addition of positive end expiratory pressure (PEEP). Bronchodilators and physiotherapy are often helpful and prophylactic antibiotics should be administered, particularly in the case of gross soiling of the airways. Systemic steroids are of no benefit and may increase the risk of secondary bacterial infection.

SPECIAL CIRCUMSTANCES

THE FULL STOMACH

A patient with a full stomach requires a rapid sequence induction (RSI) to minimise the time from loss of consciousness to intubation with a cuffed

RAPID SEQUENCE INDUCTION

Place patient on tilting table. Check all equipment. Keep active suction readily to hand. Attach monitoring and secure intravenous access. Pre-oxygenate with 100% oxygen administered from a close fitting facemask for two minutes. Apply cricoid pressure (the role of a trained assistant). Administer a sleep dose of an appropriate induction agent intravenously. Once consciousness has been lost administer suxamethonium 1 mg/kg intravenously. When the patient is relaxed perform laryngoscopy and intubate the trachea. Inflate the cuff and check position of the tube before releasing cricoid pressure. Secure the tube.

Figure I.17

endotracheal tube. Before beginning the induction it is necessary to minimise the pH and volume of gastric contents. This can be achieved by pharmacological methods if time allows and physical methods such as the aspiration via a nasogastric tube (see above).

The term 'Rapid sequence induction' is preferable to 'crash induction', which implies an element of panic which is clearly undesirable! Skilled assistance is mandatory and the procedure should be explained to the patient in advance. Practical detail of RSI is given in Figure I.17.

HEAD INJURY

A patient with a head injury may require intubation and ventilation for a number of reasons; to protect the airway from aspiration, to maintain adequate oxygenation, to allow controlled hyperventilation as a means of reducing intracranial pressure and to facilitate the management of convulsions. Intubation is often performed in emergency departments before transfer for CT scanning or neurosurgery and it is important that anaesthetists are aware that a protected airway and adequate oxygenation take priority over the wishes of neurosurgeons to be able to make a clinical examination of an unconscious patient. Great care should be taken to minimise rises in intracranial pressure in patients with a head injury. A slight (15 degree) head up tilt is, therefore, beneficial. Patients with a head injury should be assumed to have a full stomach and, therefore, require a rapid sequence induction. Head injured patients must also be assumed to have suffered a cervical spine injury and if this cannot be excluded the neck should be immobilised in the neutral position. The use of an induction agent such as thiopentone or propofol will attenuate the rise in intracranial pressure associated with laryngoscopy and should be used even in unconscious patients. Coughing on the tracheal tube and turning of the head cause an increase in intracranial pressure and should, therefore, be avoided.

UPPER AIRWAY OBSTRUCTION

Upper airway obstruction is always a matter of concern to the anaesthetist. Patients often require anaesthesia in order to assess the cause of the obstruction and may require a period of endotracheal intubation or a formal tracheostomy. Inhalational induction is the preferred route in a patient with respiratory obstruction. This should be performed under controlled conditions by a senior anaesthetist in an operating theatre environment using full monitoring. Equipment for a difficult intubation must be available, and if necessary a surgeon should be standing by to perform an emergency tracheostomy. The conduct of the induction will depend on the age and fitness of the patient and the severity of the obstruction. Venous access should be secured before induction unless the patient is a child when crying can precipitate complete obstruction. Patients often prefer to sit up and should be induced in this position. Halothane in 100% oxygen is a suitable agent being potent and relatively non irritant and should be introduced gradually and built up to an inspired concentration of 4–5%. Helium–oxygen mixtures have been advocated in airway obstruction due to the low density of helium which results in greater flow under conditions of turbulence. It is doubtful that any significant advantage results over the use of 100% oxygen as carrier for the volatile agent. The newly introduced vapour, sevoflurane shows promise as an agent for gaseous induction and is currently under evaluation. With any form of airway obstruction the uptake of a volatile agent will be reduced and it may take up to 15 minutes to achieve a sufficient depth of anaesthesia. Once the patient is deeply anaesthetised and breathing spontaneously then laryngoscopy may be performed. Alternatively, if the degree of obstruction is not too severe it may be possible to gently assist ventilation by hand and if this is easy a dose of suxamethonium can be given and direct laryngoscopy performed. It is essential that the ability to ventilate the patient be confirmed before giving muscle relaxant drugs.

References and further reading

Cormack RS, Lehane J. Difficult tracheal intubation in obstetrics. *Anaesthesia* 1984; **39:** 1105–1111.

Gataure PS, Hughes JA. The laryngeal mask airway in obstetrical anaesthesia. *Can J Anaes* 1995; **42:** 130–133.

McCoy EP, Mirakhur RK. The levering laryngoscope. *Anaesthesia* 1993; **48:** 516–519.

Mendelson CL. Aspiration of stomach contents into lungs during obstetric anaesthesia. *Am J Obstet Gynecol* 1946: **52:** 191–205.

Report on Confidential Enquiries into Maternal Deaths in the UK – The Series, London, HMSO.

Sellick BA. Cricoid pressure to control regurgitation of gastric contents during induction of anaesthesia. *Lancet* 1961; **2:** 404–405.

SECTION 1: 3

INTRA-OPERATIVE MANAGEMENT

C. A. Pinnock

POSITIONING THE SURGICAL PATIENT

MAINTENANCE OF ANAESTHESIA

Techniques of maintenance
Prevention of awareness
Analgesia
Airway control
IPPV
Monitoring
Fluid therapy

CRITICAL INCIDENTS

Cyanosis
Hypertension and hypotension
Arrhythmias
Bronchospasm
Respiratory obstruction
Massive haemorrhage
Emboli
Malignant hyperthermia
Pneumothorax

FAILURE TO BREATHE

Causes of failure to reverse

The intra-operative period follows induction of anaesthesia and is terminated by discharge of the patient from the operating theatre into the recovery area. After leaving the confines of the anaesthetic room the first task is the safe positioning of the patient for surgery and the re-establishment of monitoring and the anaesthesia delivery system as soon as possible.

POSITIONING THE SURGICAL PATIENT

Manipulation of a patient into the desired position for surgery carries its own problems. The main hazards are related to the effects of pressure and the physiological changes associated with a change in posture.

The anaesthetised patient is at risk of developing pressure sores in those areas where perfusion may be compromised. Likely sites are the occiput, the sacrum and the heel, all of which must be padded. External pneumatic compression devices applied to the lower limbs both confer a degree of protection from pressure effects and also improve circulation which helps to prevent deep vein thrombosis. No patient should ever be allowed to lie with the legs crossed and where possible an evacuable mattress should be used. Compartment syndrome, usually related to trauma or arterial surgery, and for which immediate fasciotomy is essential to save life or limb, can be a rare complication of prolonged lower limb compression in the lithotomy position.

The physiological effects which result from positioning are posture related. In the respiratory system a reduction in functional residual capacity (FRC) and total lung volume (TLV) is usually seen, accompanied by ventilation and perfusion imbalance and a degree of mechanical embarrassment to the respiratory process.

Cardiovascular effects are generally the result of gravitationally dictated venous pooling which leads to a fall in pre load and reduced cardiac output. Embarrassment of venous return due to abdominal compression is a specific complication of the prone position, but one that may be overcome by correct support so that the abdomen is unrestricted.

Steep head down (Trendelenburg) positioning may increase intra-ocular pressure. Air embolism is a risk if the operative site lies above the right atrium.

The potential damage to nerves from the common positions is detailed in Figure IN.1.

MAINTENANCE OF ANAESTHESIA

TECHNIQUES FOR MAINTENANCE OF ANAESTHESIA AND ANALGESIA

The maintenance of anaesthesia may be conveniently divided into those techniques applied to patients who are self ventilating and those techniques applied to patients who are receiving artificial ventilation of their lungs. Techniques suitable for self ventilating patients are summarised in Figure IN.2.

ANAESTHETIC TECHNIQUES FOR SELF VENTILATING PATIENTS

Local anaesthesia by tissue infiltration, central or peripheral neural blockade

General anaesthesia by inhalation of anaesthetic vapours with or without nitrous oxide

General anaesthesia by intermittent manual or by target controlled intravenous administration of anaesthetic agents, with or without inhalation of nitrous oxide

General anaesthesia by intramuscular injection (ketamine)

Hypnosis

Acupuncture

Figure IN.2

Local anaesthesia

Maintenance of anaesthesia by local anaesthetic techniques is covered on pages 125–126.

General anaesthesia by inhalation of volatile agents

The ideal is to keep the patient safely asleep, pain free, and appropriately relaxed. This ideal cannot always be met. Unawareness (sometimes referred to as hypnosis) is an absolute priority. To an extent, hypnosis is related to the minimum alveolar concentration (MAC) of any specified volatile agent.

In unpremedicated subjects MAC (sometimes referred to as 1 MAC) is the alveolar concentration of a volatile anaesthetic (in oxygen) which will prevent

Position	Nerve injury	Cause

SUPINE	supra-orbital
	nerves innervating the eyeball
	cranial nerve VII
	brachial plexus
	
	radial nerve
	ulnar nerve
		pressure from an endotracheal tube connector
		pressure by a face mask
		pressure by a tight face mask harness
		traction injury due to incorrect positioning or from
		   shoulder retainers in the Trendelenberg position
		pressure by screen supports
		pressure by the edge of the operating table
		   mattress

Position	Nerve injury	Cause

LITHOTOMY
as above plus
	cervical spine
	sciatic nerve
	
	femoral nerve
	
	posterior tibial nerve
	common peroneal nerve
	saphenous nerve
	obturator nerve
		movement up or down the operating table
		stretching of nerve between sciatic notch and
		   neck of fibula
		flexion of thigh may stretch nerve against ingunal
		   ligament
		pressure from stirrups
		compression against head of fibula
		compression against the medial tibial condyle
		flexion at the obturator foramen

Position	Nerve injury	Cause
PRONE	cervical spinal cord brachial plexus radial nerve ulnar nerve LCNT	over extension of the cervical spine overdistension direct compression compression at the elbow against a mattress pressure on the anterior superior iliac spine

Figure IN.1 Nerve damage related to positioning

movement in response to a standard surgical stimulus in one half of the population. MAC is, thus, the ED_{50} (the effective dose in 50% of patients). MAC may be higher or lower in the other 50% of the population. MAC may, therefore, be considered to equal the median of a normal distribution of alveolar concentrations. It is important to consider where in the distribution an individual patient lies. The issue can only be resolved by clinical observation and monitoring. During anaesthesia (assuming normal respiratory function) the alveolar concentration of a volatile agent, or its MAC, is close to the concentration of the agent measured at the end of exhalation, the end tidal concentration.

MAC is the standard way to compare the potencies of volatile agents, and is also useful because it is additive. Thus, if the patient inhales 0.5 MAC of one agent and inhales 0.5 MAC of another agent, the MAC value is $0.5 + 0.5 = 1.0$. MAC does not always relate to the 'depth' of anaesthesia. Various reasons apply and these are listed in Figure IN.3.

CHARACTERISTICS OF MAC VALUES

Normally distributed

Relate to movement and not to awareness (MAC for awareness is less than MAC for movement)

Vary with age and well being

Inferred from end tidal concentration (may not correlate with arterial blood concentration)

Reduced by concurrent administration of sedatives, hypnotics and analgesics

Increased by fear and by drug abuse (including alcohol)

Figure IN.3

General anaesthesia by using IV agents via bolus or infusion

Various agents have been employed for intravenous techniques. **Thiopentone** was widely used in the 1950s and 1960s for continuous IV anaesthesia but its accumulation in the tissues and hence prolonged recovery phase proved disadvantageous. **Ketamine** has proved useful in the Third World. **Propofol** is currently popular in the UK and is in common use for total intravenous anaesthesia (TIVA). There are three popular techniques:

1. An induction dose of propofol is followed by smaller bolus doses on an empirical basis. This technique is adequate for short procedures (< 15 min).

2. Manually controlled infusion

   In this system blood concentrations of propofol are achieved by the use of a syringe pump which delivers the induction dose at a fixed rate (about 600 ml/H) until verbal contact with the patient is lost. Maintenance of anaesthesia is continued at 6 mg/kg/H and the rate adjusted manually if the patient moves. The patient is allowed to breathe spontaneously a mixture of nitrous oxide in oxygen or oxygen in air. A 'stepdown' regimen is described, based on pharmacokinetic principles (e.g. after induction 10 mg/kg/H for 10 min, 8 mg/kg/H for 10 min and 6 mg/kg/H thereafter). Supplementary boluses of propofol may be needed to ensure adequate depth of anaesthesia.

3. Target controlled infusion

   Target controlled infusion techniques are computer controlled. The aim is to reach the effective blood concentration (EC) of propofol in mcg/ml needed to prevent response to a surgical incision; and to keep it there. Minimum infusion rate (MIR), the infusion rate necessary to maintain EC, is the intravenous equivalent of MAC. The syringe pump, controlled by computer, is the equivalent of a vaporiser. If the target EC (say, 6 mcg/ml) is set too low or too high the 'vaporiser concentration' can be adjusted as for an inhalational anaesthetic technique. Systems usually require programming for individual patient characteristics (age, weight, ASA status, concomitant opioid administration). Success depends on the software (a three compartment pharmacokinetic model, a set of specific pharmacokinetic variables for propofol, and special instructions, or algorithms, to vary the rate of infusion).

PREVENTION OF AWARENESS DURING SURGERY

The primary purpose of maintenance of anaesthesia is to ensure the adequacy of anaesthesia so as to prevent awareness during surgery. Awareness may be defined as follows:

• Awareness (explicit memory)

  Conscious awareness with recall but without pain. The patient recalls conversations in the operating theatre. The incidence is thought to be about 4/1000 in obstetrics and 2/1000 in non obstetric surgery.

Conscious awareness with recall and pain. The incidence is thought to be about 1/10 000 in elective surgery and 2/1000 in the 'shocked' patient.

- Awareness (implicit memory)

   Perception without conscious awareness or recall. The patient denies recall, but may remember 'something' under hypnosis. Psychologists are sceptical about the existence of this phenomenon.

- Awareness (deliberate)

   Surgery conducted under local anaesthesia is discussed on pages 125-145.

   Surgery for spinal deformities under general anaesthesia. The 'wake-up' test to see whether surgery has affected the integrity of the spinal cord has been replaced by observing motor evoked and (or) somato sensory evoked potentials.

Recall after surgery under general anaesthesia can be a psychological disaster from which the victim may take months to recover (post traumatic stress disorder). There remains no reliable means of measuring depth of anaesthesia or level of consciousness despite a large amount of research into automated real time analysis of the EEG.

Recall is almost always linked to a general anaesthetic technique which has employed muscle relaxation and artificial ventilation (IPPV). It may occur at any time: during induction (intubation of the trachea); during maintenance; and during emergence. Awareness may arise from several causes:

- Clinical fault (misjudged requirement)
- Technical fault (the anaesthesia system does not deliver the required mixture)
- Mixture of the above

Clinical observation remains the mainstay of the diagnosis of impending or actual awareness may be heralded by an increase in autonomic (sympathetic) activity, reflected by the following signs:

- Increase in pulse rate
- Increase in systemic arterial blood pressure
- Dilatation of the pupils
- Sweating
- Lacrimation
- Increase in metabolic rate

- Changes in the EEG (bispectral analysis, auditory evoked potentials)

It is important to note that there need not necessarily be an obvious sympathetic response. A significant change may not signify awareness (a 'false-positive') but merely imply an increase in ascending spinal cord traffic as reflected in the EEG. Effective maintenance of anaesthesia as described in Figure IN.4 minimises the risk of awareness.

RECOMMENDATIONS FOR AVOIDANCE OF AWARENESS

Constantly observe the patient

Administer a muscle relaxant only when necessary

Deliver 1 MAC of volatile agent, monitor and record MAC with an anaesthetic vapour analyser

Provide good analgesia, for example by combining a general anaesthetic technique with a local anaesthetic block

Monitor and record pulse rate, arterial blood pressure, pupil size, sweating, lacrimation, end-tidal carbon dioxide, core and skin temperature and the neuromuscular junction

---

Figure IN.4

ANALGESIA

With the exception of nitrous oxide (whose effect is limited) volatile anaesthetics are not analgesic agents but rather hypnotics and, to an extent, muscle relaxants. Thus, a specific form of analgesia needs to be provided. This might take the form of local or regional anaesthesia, augmented by opioids, with or without non steroidal anti-inflammatory drugs (NSAID) orally, parenterally or rectally. For cultural and medico-legal reasons it is best to seek a patient's consent for rectal administration of any drug and to write that consent on the anaesthetic record.

AIRWAY CONTROL

Airway control is a vital component of anaesthesia. Despite the best pre-operative assessment it is not always possible to foresee problems. Control of the airway is to some extent dictated by the technique used for the maintenance of anaesthesia.

Spontaneous breathing

While oropharyngeal (Guedel) or nasopharyngeal airways are satisfactory (and sometimes essential) the laryngeal mask airway has virtually replaced them. One reason is the ease with which it is possible to maintain the airway with no hands, freeing the anaesthetist to deal with other tasks. The LMA also provides, in most patients, a better and more secure airway. Provided the depth of anaesthesia and muscular relaxation is appropriate for the surgery regurgitation of gastric contents and their aspiration into the trachea should be no more common, and perhaps even less common, than with other airways. Should artificial ventilation become necessary it can be readily commenced and maintained.

Artificial ventilation

Endotracheal anaesthesia was developed by Magill and Rowbotham in 1920 and early tracheal tubes were not cuffed. Today, endotracheal intubation with a cuffed tube is generally thought of as the 'gold standard' for intermittent positive pressure ventilation (IPPV). In experienced hands, it is feasible and usually safe to ventilate the lungs artificially with an LMA. Although there are fears about the risk of tracheal aspiration, there have been no reported deaths or serious morbidity even when the LMA has been used for emergency obstetrical surgery or for resuscitation from cardiac arrest. The LMA has retrieved the situation when tracheal intubation was impossible. Recovery from anaesthesia and the establishment of spontaneous breathing have proved to be very smooth and in contrast with intubation post operative sore throats and transient cranial nerve palsies are uncommon.

At present the cuffed endotracheal tube is recommended in patients who are thought to have a full stomach, those with a radiologically proven hiatus hernia, severe oesophagitis or gross obesity, when airway access is difficult (prone position, intracranial surgery) and in prolonged surgery.

INTERMITTENT POSITIVE PRESSURE VENTILATION (IPPV)

Indications for IPPV

The decision to use IPPV, with or without a muscle relaxant, is often a personal one and depends upon the site, nature, extent and (to a degree) the likely duration of the operation. Posture and access to a secure airway are also important. Advice must be coloured by the introduction in the last decade of 'minimally invasive surgery' and by the increasing use of the laryngeal mask. Operations may be divided into 'surface' and 'non surface'. Surface procedures should not need muscle relaxation and IPPV. Consideration should be given about whether IPPV is more or less likely than spontaneous breathing to affect functional residual capacity (FRC) and, hence, oxygenation. If the surgical technique is likely to impair the mechanics of breathing or there is a need to secure the airway with a cuffed tracheal tube, IPPV should be employed. A patient who is already apnoeic from whatever cause (e.g. from drug overdose or head injury) will obviously require ventilation of their lungs.

The pattern of IPPV

IPPV may be considered by evaluating its respective components as detailed in Figure IN.5.

COMPONENTS OF IPPV
Minute volume ventilation (MV)
Tidal volume (V_T) and hence the respiratory frequency (f)
Ratio of inspiratory time to expiratory time (I:E ratio)
Fresh gas inflow (FGF) from the anaesthetic apparatus
Fractional inspired oxygen concentration (F_IO_2)
End tidal carbon dioxide tension ($P_E'CO_2$)
Airway pressure (consequent on the above)

Figure IN.5

The aim is to choose a pattern of IPPV which combines effective anaesthesia delivery with the best oxygen flux or 'oxygen availability' (oxygen delivery to the cell depends upon regional blood flow). The following factors are of importance: oxygen flux, cardiac output and saturation of haemoglobin with oxygen.

OXYGEN FLUX

The concept of oxygen flux relates to the delivery of oxygen to the tissues and is encapsulated in the following equation:

Oxygen flux = [cardiac output × Hb% × Sat% × k] + Z,

where k = Hüfner constant (1.39) and Z = the amount of oxygen dissolved in plasma

One of the main determinants of cardiac output is pre-load. Venous return to the heart depends not only upon posture and on the blood volume but on mean intrathoracic pressure. Increasing the mean intrathoracic pressure decreases venous return. During IPPV mean intrathoracic pressure relates to the pattern of ventilation. Any positive pressure (that is, any pressure above atmospheric) will reduce venous return; thus, lowest positive pressure compatible with an adequate oxygen saturation (> 96%) should be chosen.

SATURATION OF HAEMOGLOBIN WITH OXYGEN

Saturation may be measured invasively by an arterial blood sample (SaO_2) or, more commonly, by non invasive pulse oximetry (SpO_2). If the oxyhaemoglobin dissociation curve is shifted to the left (for example by hyperventilation or by hypothermia) the haemoglobin molecule will have a greater affinity for oxygen and will be less able to release oxygen to the tissues. In which case, no matter what the oxygen flux or availability, oxygen delivery to the tissues may be reduced. If on the other hand, the curve is shifted to the right (for example by hypoventilation) the haemoglobin molecule will have a lesser affinity for oxygen and oxygen delivery to the tissues may be increased. Note that the shape and position of the curve is affected by body temperature, pH, and to some degree by the concentration of 2,3-DPG in the red cell but these are far less easy to manipulate than end tidal carbon dioxide concentration. The choice of pattern of IPPV is, therefore, always a compromise. Normocapnia is desirable.

Choosing a pattern of IPPV-practical guidelines

MINUTE VOLUME VENTILATION (MV)

The simplest method is to use a calculation based on body weight (for example 70 ml/kg/min) which is unlikely to lead to underventilation of the lungs. The exhaled minute volume should be measured because, for various reasons (respiratory compliance, compliance of the anaesthesia system, leaks in the system, compression of the inspired gases), it may be less than both the inhaled and the prescribed volume.

TIDAL VOLUME (VT) AND FREQUENCY OF BREATHING (f)

The minute volume is divided into tidal volumes. A tidal volume of 10 ml/kg is reasonable for an adult. On this choice will depend the respiratory frequency (f) and, in combination with the minute volume and I:E ratio, the mean intrathoracic pressure. In the adult a respiratory frequency of 12–14 breaths per min is usually suitable.

RATIO OF INSPIRATORY TIME TO EXPIRATORY TIME (I:E RATIO)

In adult patients with healthy lungs choice is generally empirical. When the frequency of respiration is 10 breaths per min then inspiration of 2 s, and expiration 4 s, giving an I:E ratio of 1:2 is suitable. In obstructive airways disease, a longer time may be needed to allow full expiration.

FRESH GAS INFLOW (FGF)

Choice of FGF will depend on the selected breathing system and, if an automatic ventilator is used, upon its design.

FRACTIONAL INSPIRED OXYGEN CONCENTRATION (FiO_2)

The value depends on the measured SpO_2, which should be kept above 93% (a value at which oxyhaemoglobin is very close to the steep part of the dissociation curve) and preferably at 96–100%.

END TIDAL CO_2 CONCENTRATION ($Pe'CO_2$)

The desired $Pe'CO_2$ (as a reflection of the $PaCO_2$) may be achieved by manipulation of alveolar ventilation using the above characteristics.

AIRWAY PRESSURE (PAW)

Airway pressure will be consequent on the decisions made on the above characteristics. It is a measure of the energy needed to deliver a given tidal volume and minute volume ventilation at a prescribed I:E ratio.

MONITORING DURING ANAESTHESIA

In the UK the standards of monitoring are set out in Association of Anaesthetists of Great Britain and Ireland (2000) and they are summarised in Figure IN.6.

The devices necessary for minimal non invasive monitoring are listed in Figure IN.7.

MANAGEMENT OF INTRA-OPERATIVE FLUID THERAPY

Intra-operative fluid therapy is required for several different reasons. Pre-operative starvation leaves a residual deficit that should be made up, direct loss of blood requires replacement and the so-called third space creates an additional need for extracellular fluid replenishment.

Third space is a concept which was developed to explain the phenomenon of patients having undergone surgery whose fluid requirements were not explained by measurable loss. Experimentally, in such patients the extracellular fluid volume had become depleted in a degree related to the degree of

RECOMMENDATIONS FOR STANDARDS OF MONITORING DURING ANAESTHESIA AND RECOVERY

The Association of Anaesthetists of Great Britain and Ireland regards it as essential that certain core standards of monitoring must be used whenever a patient is anaesthetised. These standards should be uniform irrespective of duration or location of anaesthesia.

1. The anaesthetist must be present throughout the conduct of an anaesthetic.

2. Monitoring devices must be attached before induction of anaesthesia and their use continued until the patient has recovered from the effects of anaesthesia.

3. The same standards of monitoring apply when the anaesthetist is responsible for a local anaesthetic or sedative technique for an operative procedure.

4. All information provided by monitoring devices should be recorded in the patient's notes. Trend display and printing devices are recommended as they allow the anaesthetist to concentrate on managing the patient in emergency situations.

5. The anaesthetist must check all equipment before use. All alarm limits must be set appropriately. Infusion devices and their alarm settings must be checked before use. Audible alarms must be enabled when anaesthesia commences.

6. The recommendations state the monitoring devices which are essential and those which must be immediately available during anaesthesia. If a monitoring device deemed essential is not available and anaesthesia continues without it, the anaesthetist must clearly state in the notes the reasons for proceeding without the device.

7. Additional monitoring may be necessary as adjudged by the anaesthetist.

8. Only a brief interruption of monitoring is acceptable if the recovery area is immediately adjacent to the operating theatre. Otherwise monitoring should be continued during transfer to the same degree as any other intra or inter hospital transfer.

Association of Anaesthetists of Great Britain and Ireland 2000

Figure IN.6

MINIMAL MONITORING

Spontaneous breathing

ECG
Pulse oximeter
Indirect BP
Capnograph
Inspired gas O_2 analyser
Fresh gas O_2 analyser
Anaesthetic vapour analyser

Artificial ventilation – **All** the above plus

Airway pressure gauge
Ventilation disconnect device
Ventilation volume
Peripheral nerve stimulator
Temperature

Figure IN.7

surgery, but the patients body weight had not reduced. The fluid depletion of the extracellular space was said to have occurred due to the movement of fluid into a 'third space'. This concept is widely applied today. A useful formula for intra-operative fluid replacement is therefore: Input = basal requirements + deficit + losses + third space. Basal requirement of crystalloid for an adult is 2 ml/kg/H. Hartmann's is the usual solution of choice due to its ionic composition being close to that of plasma. Existing deficits from starvation are usually replaced in an empirical manner although CVP, if available, will give a useful guide. Direct loss of blood may be replaced by crystalloid at twice the estimated loss (up to 15% blood volume) or volume for volume with a colloid solution (gelatin or similar). Losses of greater than 15% blood volume should be replaced on a volume for volume basis with blood. If packed cells are used, additional plasma or colloid will be necessary. Whole blood is rarely supplied today. For the management of massive transfusion see later in this chapter.

CRITICAL INCIDENTS DURING ANAESTHESIA

CYANOSIS

Central cyanosis can usually be detected at an arterial oxygen saturation of about 80–85%, depending on whether the patient is anaemic. Note that 'Absence of cyanosis does not necessarily mean normal arterial oxygen levels' (Nunn, 1993). Even at an oxyhaemoglobin saturation of 93% the patient is very close to the steep part of the saturation curve. At 89% saturation the PaO_2 is only 7.5 kPa so that by the time central cyanosis is detectable the patient can be severely compromised. Cyanosis may be the result of failure to pre-oxygenate, airway obstruction, tracheal aspiration, drug overdose, a fall in cardiac output (haemorrhage, septicaemia, other surgical causes), inadequate ventilation and oxygenation (intubation of the right main bronchus, bronchospasm, laryngospasm), gross dehydration, and cardiac arrhythmias. Treatment depends upon the diagnosis but the first act must be to cut off all volatile and intravenous anaesthetics and administer 100% oxygen.

HYPERTENSION DURING ANAESTHESIA

Hypertension under anaesthesia may be defined as systolic arterial blood pressure > 20% above the preoperative value. This usually happens because the depth of anaesthesia is inappropriate to the intensity of the stimulus. Hypercarbia during the surgery is another possibility; and, in the supposedly paralysed patient, when the neuromuscular junction has not been continually monitored, there may be a need for another dose of a muscle relaxant. Techniques to complement general anaesthesia (such as central and peripheral neural blockade) are not always successful and inadequate depth may become revealed by a rise in arterial pressure.

HYPOTENSION DURING ANAESTHESIA

Hypotension under anaesthesia may be defined as a systolic arterial blood pressure < 20% pre-operative value. The most common causes of unwanted hypotension, apart from surgical consequences (of which haemorrhage is the most frequent) and central neural blockade, are bradycardias, hypovolaemia and drug overdose (which may be relative or absolute).

CARDIAC ARRHYTHMIAS

Cardiac arrhythmias are relatively common during general anaesthesia. Strangely, some pre-operative arrhythmias (e.g. ventricular ectopics) may disappear during or after induction of anaesthesia, only to reappear on recovery. Others, particularly atrial fibrillation, or temperature dependent sinus tachycardias, do not show this pattern.

Sinus bradycardia

This is a matter of definition, but an adult patient who arrives in the anaesthetic room with a heart rate of less than 60 beats per minute may, after induction and especially when an opioid is used, drop their heart rate to less than 40 beats per minute. The systemic arterial blood pressure may be adversely affected. In such patients, it may be wise to increase the heart rate before induction to 70 beats per minute or more by the judicious use of vagolytic agents. During maintenance of anaesthesia glycopyrrolate (0.2–0.6 mg) can be used.

Bradycardia

Bradycardia, proceeding to nodal rhythm, is typical of halothane anaesthesia: Other causes of bradycardia are consequent on vagal stimulation (traction on mesentery or extra-ocular muscles, for example).

Sinus tachycardia

The definition of sinus tachycardia is a matter of opinion. Adult heart rates above 100/min in the anaesthetic room usually mean inadequate pre-operative medication, and during surgery (unless secondary to haemorrhage) inadequate anaesthesia or muscle relaxation.

Ventricular bigeminy

Ventricular bigeminy is associated with endotracheal intubation (a sympathoadrenal response). Bigeminy is very often associated with halothane anaesthesia; given time the bigeminy will disappear, but if it does not intravenous lidocaine (50–100 mg) may be helpful.

The management of arrhythmias is shown in Figure IN.8.

MANAGEMENT OF INTRA-OPERATIVE ARRHYTHMIAS

Atrial fibrillation (AF)
Digoxin will reduce the ventricular response rate to atrial activity but takes too long to be effective in acute situations. Both amiodarone and verapamil can be employed to reduce ventricular rate. DC cardioversion is indicated for the acute onset of AF

Atrial flutter
Drug control of the ventricular rate is not often successful. DC cardioversion or atrial pacing may restore sinus rhythm

Atrial tachycardia with A-V block
After halting glycoside therapy (and ensuring normokalaemia), lidocaine 1 mg/kg IV is the drug of choice. Alternatively DC cardioversion or atrial pacing may be effective

Paroxysmal supraventricular tachycardia
Vagal tone should be increased by applying carotid sinus massage (or a Valsalva manoeuvre). Second line treatment is verapamil 5–10 mg IV (contra-indicated contemporaneously with beta blockers). Alternatively, give adenosine by rapid IV injection of 3 mg over 2 seconds, if necessary followed by 6 mg after 2 minutes, then by 12 mg after a further 2 minutes. Other potential pharmacological agents include propranolol, quinidine, procainamide, disopyramide and digoxin. DC cardioversion can also be used

Atrial ectopic beats
Treatment is not usually necessary

Ventricular ectopic beats
Treatment is unnecessary, unless the ectopic beats are frequent (one in four), or 'R on T' type in which situation an infusion of lidocaine or beta blocker therapy is indicated

Ventricular fibrillation
A single precordial thump should be administered followed by immediate DC defibrillation if unsuccessful. If the rhythm does not respond to defibrillation, prior treatment with IV bretylium tosylate may help

Ventricular tachycardia
In the acute situation when there is haemodynamic embarrassment DC cardioversion should be immediate. For brief episodes of VT suitable pharmacological agents include lidocaine (drug of choice), flecainide, disopyramide, amiodarone and mexiletine

Figure IN.8

BRONCHOSPASM

Bronchospasm during surgery may be detected clinically by listening to breath sounds in the anaesthesia system's expiratory limb or in the presence of IPPV, by observing an increase in ventilatory pressure or a decrease in tidal volume or both. Auscultation will confirm the finding. Capnography will show a rising end tidal CO_2 concentration and a typical trace showing a prolonged and flattened expiratory curve (and occasionally a slightly lengthened inspiratory time).

The smoker, the asthmatic, the patient with chronic obstructive airways disease and inadequate anaesthetised patients are susceptible to bronchospasm. Pre-operative physiotherapy and appropriate drug therapy should be arranged. Unexpected bronchospasm during anaesthesia in a patient with normal lungs is a matter for concern and may reflect tracheal aspiration, abutment of a tracheal tube on the carina, or an intra-operative drug hypersensitivity (e.g. hypersensitivity to an antibiotic). Bronchospasm may also be the first physical sign of impending pulmonary oedema.

Treatment of intra-operative bronchospasm should be instituted as follows. Stop the surgery and increase the inspired concentration of volatile agent. The vagus nerve should be blocked (with atropine or glycopyrrolate). Check the position of a tracheal tube. Give sympathomimetic agents (ephedrine, aminophylline). Aspirate the tracheo-bronchial tree. Stop the administration of any antibiotic; and with drug hypersensitivity in mind, re-evaluate the patient's history. Continue to monitor end tidal carbon dioxide and observe the ECG for evidence of a change in the S-T segment. Analysis of an arterial blood sample may be helpful.

RESPIRATORY OBSTRUCTION (INCREASED PEAK INSPIRATORY PRESSURE)

Respiratory obstruction should be very rare during maintenance of anaesthesia but demands instant relief. Inattention to detail (e.g. incorrect placement of Guedel or laryngeal mask airways or tracheal tubes, or their dislodgement) may be one cause and laryngeal spasm under too light anaesthesia another. The siting and patency of endotracheal tubes cannot always be relied upon; for example, the cuff may have been over inflated and herniated over the tracheal end. An increase in peak inspiratory pressure (during IPPV) will be inevitable if there is respiratory obstruction or bronchospasm. Other causes of raised airway pressure include the insufflation of carbon dioxide into the peritoneal cavity (minimally invasive surgery), strong surgical retraction (intra-abdominal, intrathoracic), and inadequate anaesthesia.

HYPERCARBIA AND HYPOCARBIA

Hyper- and hypocarbia refer to high or low carbon dioxide tensions in arterial blood. The reference range for the homeostatically 'normal' tension in a patient with normal lungs remains constant throughout life, unlike the arterial oxygen tension which tends to decrease, and varies from 4.8 to 5.3 kPa. Hyper- and hypocapnoea refer to carbon dioxide tensions in end-expired, or end tidal gas, which is taken to represent fairly closely the concentration of carbon dioxide in most, but not all, alveoli and to reflect arterial carbon dioxide. Simultaneous sampling of arterial blood and end tidal gas in the same patient should provide similar results, although arterial carbon dioxide is usually higher (by about 0.2–1 kPa), than end tidal carbon dioxide. Since arterial sampling is uncommon in everyday anaesthesia but end tidal sampling extremely common, the latter is usually equated with the former.

In spontaneously breathing patients end tidal carbon dioxide concentration is determined by the response of the patient to a surgical stimulus, to the respiratory depressant effects of the anaesthetic agents and on cardiac output. In artificially ventilated patients end tidal carbon dioxide concentration is open to manipulation. As a general consensus, the value should be kept within the reference range (normocapnia).

MANAGEMENT OF MASSIVE HAEMORRHAGE

Massive haemorrhage may be self evident (a traumatised patient in an accident and emergency department); anticipated (elective cardiac, vascular, neurosurgical and obstetrical operations); or unexpected.

A sudden reduction in end tidal carbon dioxide concentration may be a useful sign if the situation is not self evident, but once the diagnosis is made, the steps detailed in Figure IN.9 should be taken:

MANAGEMENT OF MASSIVE HAEMORRHAGE

Alert the surgeon to the problem. Summon help (pairs of hands). Alert the consultant haematologist and the blood bank. Request blood coagulation studies. Maintain systemic arterial blood pressure by warmed intravenous infusions of blood, if available, and colloid (or) crystalloid. Improve intravenous access. Begin invasive monitoring (CVP, intra-arterial line).

Figure IN.9

If greater than 50% of the patient's blood volume requires replacement the situation becomes one of massive transfusion. Transfusion of large amounts of stored blood results in several unphysiological effects mainly due its composition. Stored blood has a potassium concentration of 5–20 mmol/l, a pH of 6.5–7.2 and a temperature of 4–6°C. The initial acidosis that may be seen after transfusion is rapidly replaced by alkalosis as the citrate in the blood becomes metabolised. Transfused red cells rapidly take up the potassium and, thus, transient hyperkalaemia will become normokalaemia, or hypokalaemia. Filtration to remove debris of micro-aggregates and effete cells is desirable. A 20 μm filter is suitable. Fluid warming is essential and the device used should be able to cope with rapid rates of infusion. Due to dilutional effects a paucity of clotting factors and platelets will be seen. Treatment should be directed at the replacement of the relevant factors (using fresh frozen plasma or cryoprecipitates) and transfusion of platelet concentrates. Haematological advice as to how much of what is required is invaluable and will usually be based on the results of extensive testing of clotting function.

Mortality is related to the degree of embarrassment of organ oxygenation. High inspired oxygen concentrations are desirable and the maintenance of adequate circulating volume and cardiac output should be high priorities.

Choice of blood products

Haematological advice may recommend, on a descending scale, red cells, fresh frozen plasma and possibly, when the situation is desperate, cryoprecipitate and platelets, it is best to assume that all these blood products will be needed.

Incompatibility reactions

Incompatibility reactions are extraordinarily rare; but in the very often crucial situations described above the overextended anaesthetist may be tempted to transfuse blood products without rigorous checking, which should never occur. A stock of uncrossmatched blood is usually available for use in the direst emergencies. This 'universal recipient' blood is of blood group O negative, and transfusion of this will always carry a risk of incompatibility reaction.

EMBOLI

Intra-operative embolism most commonly results from thrombus, although other situations include gas, fat and rarely tumour or amniotic fluid.

Thrombus

The risk of developing intra-operative thrombosis is increased by various factors. These include:

- Smoking
- Immobility
- Malignancy
- Contraceptive pill
- Previous surgery
- Pelvic or lower limb surgery

Thrombus usually develops in the deep veins of the lower limb and pelvis and detachment of formed thrombus into the circulation results in venous thrombo-embolism which may result in the clinical condition of pulmonary embolism. Measures to reduce the risk of thrombus formation should be taken in all patients. These include:

- Good hydration
- Pre-operative low molecular weight heparin therapy
- Pneumatic leg compression
- Elastic stockings
- Spinal or epidural techniques (if appropriate)

Although rare, pulmonary embolism may occur during the intra-operative period. Diagnosis is usually made by a combination of signs such as unexplained tachyarrhythmias, hypoxia and an acute fall in end tidal carbon dioxide concentration. Management consists of increasing FiO_2, haemodynamic support and thrombolytic therapy. Transfer to ITU is usually needed. Embolisation of fat or tumour results in a similar, though generally more severe picture. Fat globules may be detectable in pulmonary secretions. Fat embolism is more common after long bone fractures and orthopaedic procedures where profound reaming of the intramedullary cavity is undertaken (such as femoral nailing). Amniotic fluid embolism is uncommon and results in a profound derangement of clotting function which leads to severe disseminated intravascular coagulation (DIC).

Gas

Embolisation of gas results from the ingress of gas into the circulation via the venous route. The usual cause of room air embolism is the site of surgery being above the level of the right atrium when air may enter an open vein. Air embolism via venous catheters must also be included. Laparoscopic procedures may result in embolisation of the insufflating gas (which is usually carbon dioxide).

The resulting clinical picture after gas embolism is dictated by the amount of gas which has entered the circulation (although in the case of carbon dioxide, little change will be seen). Embolisation of air at a rate exceeding 0.5 ml/kg/min will result in clinical signs, usually resulting from the air reaching the cardiac chambers. Features include:

- Millwheel murmur over the chest
- Fall in end tidal CO_2
- Hypoxia
- Tachyarrhythmias
- Raised pulmonary artery pressure

After diagnosing air embolism further entry of gas should be prevented by flooding the operative site with saline and a wet pack. Venous pressure at the operative site should be increased and ventilation of the lungs with 100% oxygen applied (nitrous oxide should be stopped immediately). Occasionally gas can be aspirated through an existing central line especially if the patient is turned laterally with right side uppermost. Post operative circulatory support and general supportive therapy on ITU may be required.

MALIGNANT HYPERTHERMIA (HYPERPYREXIA) (MH)

MH is exceedingly rare but of great importance. The mortality rate in the 1970s was > 70% and although today it is closer to 25% even that is a high price to pay for what is often minor surgery. The reduction in mortality probably reflects an increased awareness of the condition, more intensive patient monitoring for sensitive indicators, such as end tidal carbon dioxide tension, which assist early diagnosis; and the availability of an intravenous form of dantrolene sodium, a drug which has played an important role in the treatment of MH.

Pathophysiology

MH may represent a spectrum of conditions rather than a specific pharmacogenetic entity as the inheritance is complex. Presentation under anaesthesia is usually that of a marked increase in metabolic rate arising from accelerated muscle metabolism. At cellular level the exact defect remains unclear but dysfunction of the sarcoplasmic reticulum and abnormalities of intracellular ionic calcium transport occur, with a secondary effect of increased sympathetic nervous system activity. Agents known to induce MH cause an enhanced release of calcium from the sarcoplasmic reticulum and a generalised membrane permeability defect develops. Genetic studies indicate that the MH gene is on chromosome 19, in a position close to the ryanodine receptor gene. Features of MH are given in Figure IN.10.

FEATURES OF MH

Cardinal physical signs

Hyperthermia (core temperature rising by a minimum of 1–2°C/H)
Respiratory acidosis (hypercarbia)
Metabolic acidosis (with or without muscle rigidity)
Cardiac arrhythmias
Hypoxaemia
Cyanosis (from a large rise in oxygen consumption plus ventilation perfusion defects)

Signs of abnormal muscle activity

Failure of the jaw to relax after suxamethonium
Rigidity of certain, but not necessarily of all groups of muscles
Hyperkalaemia
Myoglobinuria and renal failure
Rise in creatinine kinase

Other signs

Disseminated intravascular coagulation (DIC)
Cerebral and pulmonary oedema

Triggering agents

ALL the inhalational agents including desflurane and sevoflurane
Suxamethonium (avoid if possible-phenothiazines, atropine)

Agents thought to be safe

Thiopentone
Propofol
Nitrous oxide
Opioids
Pancuronium
Vecuronium
Benzodiazepines
Amide local anaesthetics

Figure IN.10

TREATMENT OF MH

Stop the use of all MH trigger agents. Change the anaesthesia machine; and change from the circle system, if it is being used, to a non rebreathing system. Terminate surgery if possible. Monitor the ECG and capnograph. Alert the intensive care unit. Commence invasive monitoring. Delegate one person to prepare dantrolene sodium 1 mg/kg.

Record core temperature, pulse rate and blood pressure every 5 min. Estimate arterial pH and blood gases. Treat hypercarbia with vigorous hyperventilation, acidosis with sodium bicarbonate 2–4 mmol/kg. Maintain oxygenation. Save one venous sample for serum CK and send one for electrolytes and serum calcium estimations. Give IV dantrolene sodium 1 mg/kg. Repeat at 10 minute intervals if necessary, up to a maximum of 10 mg/kg.

Figure IN.11

Clinical management of a suspected fulminant case

CALL FOR HELP. Then treat as in Figure IN.11.

Secondary management

Cool the patient and keep the first urine sample for myoglobin estimation. Measure urine output. If obvious myoglobinuria occurs, give intravenous fluids, and mannitol or frusemide to promote urine flow. The use of steroids is controversial, but may be indicated for cerebral oedema in the severe case. Repeat the serum CK estimation at 24 H. Treat DIC if necessary. Dantrolene may need to be repeated for up to 24 H as re-triggering may occur.

ACCIDENTAL PNEUMOTHORAX

Accidental pneumothorax, uncommon in urgent, scheduled or elective surgery but to be expected during emergency surgery on patients admitted with trauma, may become more frequent with the use of interpleural anaesthesia and with today's emphasis on minimally invasive surgery, when it should more properly be renamed 'carbondioxidethorax'.

A patient with a pneumothorax without the presence of a chest drain with an underwater seal should not be anaesthetised. If, during anaesthesia, a pneumothorax is suspected, either unilateral or bilateral (e.g. by clinical observation, by percussion, by auscultation of the lungs, by hypoxia and hypercarbia, and by changes in the required ventilatory pressure accompanied by hypotension) surgery should be stopped and a chest drain with underwater seal promptly inserted. A tension pneumothorax is rapidly lethal and requires insertion of a large bore cannula into the affected side. A formal chest drain can be subsequently sited.

FAILURE TO BREATHE

Failure to breathe at the end of the procedure is commonly due to delayed recovery from the use of muscle relaxants. A full differential diagnosis is given on pages 62–67.

At the end of the surgical procedure the aim is to have the patient pain free, breathing spontaneously, cardiovascularly stable with reactive pupils, opening the eyes and mouth to command, and remembering nothing of the surgery. Delayed recovery from the use or abuse of muscle relaxants is less common than it used to be although there may be occasional problems secondary to the use of suxamethonium and mivacurium. Monitoring of the neuromuscular junction throughout anaesthesia with a peripheral nerve stimulator has become much more widespread reducing the empirical nature of relaxant dosage.

CAUSES OF FAILURE TO REVERSE

Suxamethonium apnoea

Suxamethonium is metabolised by plasma cholinesterase (pseudocholinesterase). A relative lack of pseudocholinesterase (some patients in the third trimester of pregnancy; severe malnutrition and genetic abnormality) will result in a prolongation of action of the drug.

The inheritance of abnormal cholinesterase is linked to several autosomal recessive genes, which are classified by their percentage inhibition of action when exposed to different substances (for example dibucaine or fluoride). Figure IN.12 describes the different situations.

The degree of prolongation of action is related to the genetic inheritance of the above enzymes.

PLASMA CHOLINESTERASE VARIANTS			
Enzyme	**Prevalence**	**Dibucaine number**	**Fluoride number**
Normal	94% (homozygous)	75–85	60
Atypical	0.03% (homozygous)	15–25	20
None (silent gene)	0.001% (homozygous)	N/A	N/A
Fluoride resistant	0.0001%	65–75	30

Figure IN.12

Heterozygotes for the normal enzyme will obviously have a normal response. Two to 4 H of paralysis after a 1 mg/kg dose of suxamethonium will be seen in homozygotes for the silent or atypical genes. Homozygotes for the fluoride resistant gene will show a prolongation of effect of 1–2 H. Most heterozygotes who have one normal and one abnormal gene will have a minor increase in duration of effect of about 20 minutes. Combinations of abnormal genes are rare with an unpredictable result. For details on inheritance see Section 3, Chapter 8.

Mivacurium apnoea

The action of mivacurium is mainly terminated by plasma cholinesterase and, thus, the defective forms of this enzyme will result in prolonged action of the drug. This is usually in the region of 2–4 H from a typical dose. Other elimination pathways include liver esterase metabolism and biliary and renal excretion.

Other reasons for greater than expected duration of muscle relaxant drugs include:

- Relative or absolute overdose of drug
- Electrolyte or acid base imbalance
- Incorrect prescription of reversal agent
- Relative or absolute overdose of a volatile anaesthetic

References and further reading

Anderton JM, Keen RI, Neave R. *Positioning the surgical patient*. London: Butterworths, 1988.

Association of Anaesthetists of Great Britain and Ireland. Recommendations for Standards of Monitoring during Anaesthesia and Recovery, 2000.

Buck N, Devlin HB, Lunn JN. *The report of a confidential enquiry into perioperative deaths*. London: The Nuffield Provincial Hospitals Trust and the King's Fund for London, 1987.

Lunn JN, Mushin WW. *Mortality associated with anaesthesia*. London: The Nuffield Provincial Hospitals Trust, 1982.

Mushin WW, Rendell-Baker L, Thompson PW, Mapleson WW. Automatic ventilation of the Lungs, 2nd edn. Oxford and Edinburgh: Blackwell Scientific Publications, 1969.

NCEPOD. Callum KG, Gray AJG, Hoile RW, Ingram GS, Martin IC, Sherry KM, Whimster F. Then and Now. The 2000 report of the National Confidential Enquiry into Perioperative Deaths. London.

Nunn JF. *Applied respiratory physiology*, 4th ed. London: Butterworth-Heinemann, 1993.

Rosen M, Lunn JN (eds). *Consciousness, awareness and pain in general anaesthesia*. London: Butterworths, 1987.

Servant C, Purkiss S. *Positioning Patients for Surgery*. London: Greenwich Medical Media, 2002.

SECTION 1: 4
POST OPERATIVE MANAGEMENT

T. McLeod

CARE OF THE UNCONSCIOUS PATIENT

POST OPERATIVE COMPLICATIONS

Respiratory
  Airway obstruction
  Hypoxaemia
  Inadequate pulmonary ventilation
Cardiovascular
  Hypertension
  Hypotension
  Cardiac arrhythmias
  Thromboembolism
CNS
  Shivering
  Failure to regain consciousness

OXYGEN THERAPY

Indications
Types of devices

POST OPERATIVE ANALGESIA

Treatment of pain
Pain assessment
Acute pain service

NAUSEA AND VOMITING

Prevention
Treatment

FLUID THERAPY

Physiology
Clinical assessment
Fluid replacement

SEQUELAE FOLLOWING ANAESTHESIA

Eye trauma
Airway trauma
Musculoskeletal trauma
Skin damage
Medico-legal issues

CARE OF THE UNCONSCIOUS PATIENT

Emergence from anaesthesia, although usually uneventful, can be associated with major morbidity. In the immediate post operative period, patients are at risk from respiratory and cardiovascular complications, which comprise approximately 70% and 20% of critical recovery room incidents respectively. The unconscious patient may develop upper airway obstruction or inadequate ventilation with subsequent hypoxaemia and hypercapnia and is at increased risk of aspiration due to the absence of the protective airway reflexes. Ongoing blood loss and residual drug effects may compound cardiovascular compromise. The importance of observation and early intervention during this period has been recognised for many years. Hazards may be reduced by the provision of adequate post operative recovery facilities along with fully trained staff that should ideally be available at all times.

The recovery room

Recommendations for the situation and design of the recovery room and equipment required have been made by a working party of the Association of Anaesthetists of Great Britain and Ireland (1993) and are summarised below.

Patient transfer from operating theatre

The design of trolleys should comply with the Association of Anaesthetists recommendations in that there is a need for oxygen cylinders, masks and tubing, airway support equipment, protective sides and a tilting mechanism. Portable monitoring equipment may be required. Care should be taken to avoid injury to eyes, dentition and peripheral nerves. Transfer to the recovery room should be undertaken by suitably trained staff under the supervision of the anaesthetist who is additionally responsible for handing over information about relevant medical conditions, the anaesthetic technique, intra-operative problems and post operative management to the recovery staff.

Management

Continuous observation must be made on a one-to-one basis by a nurse trained in recovery procedures until the patient is conscious and able to maintain their own airway. Respiratory and cardiovascular parameters, pain severity and conscious level should be documented at appropriate intervals.

Clinical observations should be supplemented by pulse oximetry and blood pressure measurement with an ECG, peripheral nerve stimulator, temperature monitor and capnography immediately available.

Patient discharge

Set criteria must be met before a patient is discharged to the ward (Figure PO.1). The patient being transferred to the high dependency or intensive care unit is an obvious exception to this.

CRITERIA TO BE MET BEFORE TRANSFER FROM RECOVERY ROOM TO GENERAL WARD

Level of consciousness
Obeys commands
Spontaneous eye opening

Respiratory System

| Upper airway | Able to maintain a clear airway |
| | Protective reflexes are present |

| Respiration | Satisfactory respiratory rate |
| | Satisfactory oxygenation |

Cardiovascular System

Haemodynamically stable
Pulse rate acceptable
Blood pressure acceptable
No persistent bleeding
Peripheral perfusion adequate

Pain Control

Adequate pain control
Adequate analgesic and anti-emetic provisions made

Temperature

No evidence of developing hypothermia or malignant hyperthermia

(Modified from Association of Anaesthetists of Great Britain and Ireland, 1993)

Figure PO.1

CAUSES OF UPPER AIRWAY OBSTRUCTION IN THE POST OPERATIVE PERIOD

	Oropharyngeal obstruction	Laryngeal obstruction
Common	Decreased muscle tone Secretions Sleep apnoea	Laryngospasm Secretions
Rare	Foreign body Oedema Wound haematoma Neuromuscular disease	Oedema Bilateral recurrent laryngeal nerve palsy Tracheal collapse

Figure PO.2

POST OPERATIVE COMPLICATIONS

Respiratory complications

UPPER AIRWAY OBSTRUCTION

The causes of oropharyngeal and laryngeal obstruction are shown in Figure PO.2.

In the unconscious patient, the tongue may fall backward and occlude the airway at the level of the oropharnyx. This occurs because of a decrease in oropharyngeal muscle tone, which is related to the residual effects of general anaesthesia and inadequate recovery from muscle relaxants. Rarely, oropharyngeal obstruction results from a foreign body e.g. failure to remove throat pack or post traumatic airway oedema. Wound haematoma can occur after neck surgery (e.g. carotid endarterectomy, thyroidectomy, radical neck dissection) and can rapidly produce upper airway obstruction. Oedema formation resulting from external compression of the venous and lymphatic drainage of the head and neck will make matters worse.

Laryngospasm is the commonest cause of laryngeal obstruction and is often associated with airway manipulation during emergence from anaesthesia e.g. airway insertion at light levels of anaesthesia, or the presence of secretions or blood. After thyroidectomy, bilateral recurrent laryngeal nerve palsies and tracheal collapse can occur although this is very rare. Laryngeal oedema secondary to prolonged or traumatic intubation can occasionally cause obstruction although this is more likely in the paediatric than adult patient because of the smaller size of the airway.

CLINICAL SIGNS

The clinical signs of upper airway obstruction include absence of air movement, "see-saw" motion of the chest and abdomen, and suprasternal and intercostal recession. Oxygen desaturation is a late sign. Incomplete laryngospasm typically produces stridor, an inspiratory "crowing" noise, although this is absent if the laryngospasm is complete.

MANAGEMENT

Initial measures are directed at preventing the tongue from falling backwards and obstructing the airway. The unconscious patient should be recovered in the lateral position with the jaw supported. Blood and secretions should be cleared by suction and supplemental oxygen given via a face mask. If upper airway obstruction develops the head should be tilted backwards and the jaw pushed forward by applying pressure behind the angle of the jaw. If this measure does not rapidly clear the airway then an oropharyngeal or nasopharyngeal airway should be inserted. Care should be taken on insertion of an oral airway as this may cause laryngospasm, coughing or vomiting in the waking patient and, if in doubt, a nasal airway should be passed. If this does not immediately rectify the situation then senior help should be sought and 100% oxygen administered via a tight fitting mask. Continuous positive airway pressure (CPAP) at this stage may help to open the airway or "break" the laryngospasm. However, in the presence of continued airway obstruction and falling oxygen saturation intravenous suxamethonium (1–2 mg/kg) should be given followed by manual ventilation with 100% oxygen and subsequent orotracheal intubation. In the rare event when this is not possible the failed intubation drill should be followed. Extubation of the trachea should occur when the patient has regained full muscle power and is awake. An algorithm for airway management is shown in Figure PO.3.

Upper airway obstruction secondary to wound haematoma must be immediately treated. The surgeon and an experienced anaesthetist should be called, the airway supported, 100% oxygen administered and the trachea intubated. The wound stitches should be removed and the haematoma evacuated. It is important to remember that the airway anatomy may be grossly distorted and it may be impossible to intubate the trachea. In this situation, a surgical airway will be required

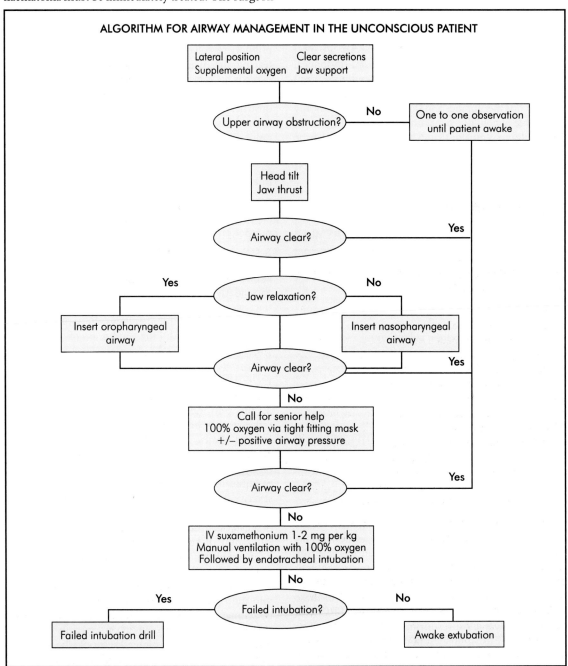

Figure PO.3

Hypoxaemia is defined as an oxygen saturation of less than 90%. In the post operative period it occurs due to a combination of factors which are listed in Figure PO.4 (Mangat 1993). Prevention, early recognition and treatment are important because of the increased morbidity and mortality associated with this condition.

Clinical features

Clinical signs associated with hypoxaemia are non specific and include central cyanosis, dyspnoea, tachycardia, arrhythmias, hyper or hypotension and agitation. Cyanosis is a dusky, blue discolouration of the mucous membranes and skin. It is usually clinically detectable when the concentration of deoxygenated haemoglobin is greater than 5 g/dl. However, it may be absent in the hypoxaemic anaemic patient and present in the polycythaemic patient with a normal PaO_2 and is therefore an unreliable indicator of hypoxaemia.

CAUSES OF POST OPERATIVE HYPOXAEMIA

Upper airway obstruction
Alveolar hypoventilation
Ventilation-perfusion mismatch
Diffusion hypoxia
Increased oxygen utilisation
Low cardiac output states

Figure PO.4

Upper airway obstruction and alveolar hypoventilation are important causes of hypoxaemia in the post operative period.

Ventilation-perfusion (V/Q) mismatch

There is about a 20% reduction in functional residual capacity (FRC) after induction of anaesthesia. This may lead to airway closure in dependent parts of the lung resulting in ventilation-perfusion mismatch with subsequent hypoxaemia. The very young, elderly, obese and smokers are particularly at risk, as in these groups, closing capacity may equal or exceed FRC with resultant airway closure during tidal breathing. The reduction in FRC is greatest in the supine position and oxygen saturation may be improved by sitting the patient up provided they are awake enough.

Causes of V/Q mismatch include: -

ATELECTASIS

Post operative pulmonary collapse or atelectasis is a common cause of hypoxaemia, particularly after upper abdominal and thoracic surgery. Onset is usually within 15 minutes of induction of anaesthesia, in both the spontaneously breathing and mechanically ventilated patient and lasts up to four days into the post operative period. Absorption atelectasis has been implicated in the development of post operative pulmonary collapse. It develops when the rate of gas leaving the alveolus due to uptake into the blood exceeds the rate of inspired gas entering it. This occurs when the airway to an area of lung is closed or obstructed, usually with secretions or blood. It is also found in areas of lung with a marked reduction in V/Q ratios. The rate of gas uptake is increased when insoluble gases such as nitrogen are replaced by soluble gases such as oxygen and nitrous oxide in an anaesthetic mixture (Joyce 1995).

Effective treatment includes adequate pain control, supplemental oxygen, chest physiotherapy and promotion of deep breathing exercises and coughing.

BRONCHOPNEUMONIA

Bronchopneumonia may occur after major surgery particularly if the patient is unable to clear respiratory tract secretions because of poor cough or inability to deep breathe. Treatment follows the same pattern as for atelectasis with the addition of appropriate antibiotic therapy.

ASPIRATION

There is a significant risk of aspirating gastric contents in the post operative period as protective airway reflexes may be absent or impaired. Patients with delayed gastric emptying (e.g. bowel obstruction, obesity, pregnancy or an incompetent gastro-oesophageal sphincter) are at increased risk. Aspiration of liquid material results in a pneumonitis of varying severity dependent on the volume and acidity of the fluid. Severe pneumonitis is associated with aspiration of greater than 25 ml of fluid with a pH of less than 2.5. Aspiration of solid material results in bronchial or laryngeal obstruction, and, if not immediately relieved, can be fatal. In the supine position, due to the anatomy of the bronchial tree, aspiration is most likely to occur into the right lung although, after a large aspiration, both lungs are often involved. The chance of aspiration may be reduced by recovering patients in the lateral position and those at high risk should be extubated after full recovery of protective reflexes. The treatment of aspiration is detailed on page 40.

PULMONARY OEDEMA

This is a relatively rare cause of V/Q mismatch in the recovery room which usually occurs within an hour of the end of surgery. Causes include fluid overload, cardiac failure or after relief of prolonged airway obstruction.

PNEUMOTHORAX

Pneumothorax may result from direct lung or airway trauma, rib fractures, central venous cannulation, brachial plexus block, intercostal nerve and inter pleural blocks and after thoracic, neck or renal surgery. A pneumothorax due to barotrauma associated with mechanical ventilation is unusual unless ventilation pressures are high. Patients with emphysematous bullae are particularly at risk

The characteristic features are pleuritic chest pain or breathlessness but these may not be detected if the pneumothorax is small or may be masked by the residual effects of anaesthesia. Spontaneously breathing patients with a pneumothorax of less than 20% of the lung field may be observed and the chest x-ray repeated. Any patient with a larger pneumothorax or who is mechanically ventilated should be treated with an intercostal drain. A tension pneumothorax is associated with marked shift of the trachea and mediastinum away from the affected side, hypoxaemia, hyper resonance to percussion and hypotension. It is a clinical diagnosis and a true medical emergency requiring immediate decompression by insertion of a chest drain at the fifth intercostal space in the anterior axillary line. A 14 gauge cannula should be inserted at the second intercostal space in the mid clavicular line if a chest drain is not immediately available.

DIFFUSION HYPOXIA

At the end of anaesthesia nitrous oxide leaves the blood and enters the alveoli diluting the gases already present. If the patient is breathing air, nitrogen will be absorbed into the blood at a slower rate than nitrous oxide enters the alveoli resulting in a decrease in alveolar oxygen concentration and a potentially hypoxic gas mixture. In practice, the effect of diffusional hypoxia is transient and is simply overcome by administering supplemental oxygen for approximately 10 minutes in the immediate post operative period.

OTHER CAUSES

Hypoxaemia may also occur as a result of increased oxygen consumption (e.g. shivering, pyrexia) or increased tissue oxygen extraction. These both result in a reduction in mixed venous oxygen concentration. A variable amount of mixed venous blood is shunted from the right to left side of the heart and mixes with oxygenated blood producing a fall in PaO_2. The extent of this fall is dependent on the mixed venous oxygen concentration and the degree of right to left shunt.

INADEQUATE PULMONARY VENTILATION

Reduced alveolar ventilation has many causes in the post operative period (see Figure PO.5). It results from a reduction in tidal volume, respiratory rate or a combination of both and, by definition, produces a raised arterial carbon dioxide tension ($PaCO_2$). Hypoxaemia and respiratory acidosis may be associated features.

**CAUSES OF ALVEOLAR HYPOVENTILATION
IN THE POST OPERATIVE PERIOD**

Upper airway obstruction

Decreased ventilatory drive
　Inhalational anaesthetics
　Opioids
　Benzodiazepines
　Central nervous system trauma

Inadequate respiratory muscle function
　Incomplete reversal of neuromuscular blockade
　Neuromuscular disease
　Diaphragmatic splinting (obesity, abdominal distension)
　Thoracic or upper abdominal surgery
　Acute or chronic lung disease

Figure PO.5

Decreased ventilatory drive

The commonest cause of central respiratory depression is the residual effect of inhalational anaesthetic agents or peri-operative opioid administration. The effect of volatile anaesthetic agents is compounded as they are predominantly excreted via the lungs.

An unconscious patient with low respiratory rate and pin-point pupils is typical of opioid overdosage. Supportive treatment includes the administration of oxygen, maintenance of the airway and manual ventilation by mask or tracheal tube if required. Opioid induced respiratory depression can be reversed by administration of naloxone, a competitive opioid antagonist. This agent should be given in small incremental doses of 50 to 100 mcg intravenously in order to prevent reversal of analgesia. Tachycardia and hypertension associated with sudden development of pain increases myocardial oxygen consumption and may lead to ischaemia in susceptible patients. The onset of action of naloxone is within 1 to 2 minutes but the duration of action is only 20 minutes, which is shorter than that of many opioids, hence a repeat dose may be required. The patient must not return to the ward until full recovery from the respiratory depressant effects of the opioid has occurred.

Benzodiazepines are often used as adjuncts to general anaesthesia. The elderly, sick and patients with liver disease are at risk of prolonged effects from these agents. Oversedation can be treated with flumazenil, a competitive benzodiazepine receptor antagonist. It is administered intravenously in 100 mcg increments titrated against clinical response. Onset of action is within 30 to 60 seconds and duration of effect varies from 15 to 120 minutes.

Decreased ventilatory drive may be related to a period of intra-operative hyperventilation with a resultant marked decrease in $PaCO_2$ which may continue into the immediate post operative phase. Neurosurgical and head injury patients may also develop hypoventilation in the post operative period as a direct result of central nervous system trauma.

Inadequate mechanical function of the respiratory muscles

INCOMPLETE REVERSAL OF NON-DEPOLARISING MUSCLE BLOCKADE

This is distressing and potentially dangerous to the patient. It is an important cause of both hypoventilation and upper airway obstruction. There are many factors that contribute to incomplete reversal (see Figure

FACTORS ASSOCIATED WITH PROLONGED NEUROMUSCULAR BLOCKADE

Hypothermia	
Respiratory acidosis	
Electrolyte abnormalities	Hypokalaemia Hypocalcaemia Hyponatraemia Hypermagnesaemia
Drug interactions	Volatile agents Calcium channel blockers Aminoglycosides Diuretics
Decreased excretion	Renal failure Liver failure

Figure PO.6

PO.6). The use of short acting non-depolarising muscle relaxants and neuromuscular monitoring to assess the degree of muscle blockade should, help to avoid this complication.

Typically the inadequately reversed patient can initiate movements but cannot complete them, as a result of which they appear twitchy with uncoordinated actions. Patients may exhibit extreme distress and in addition complain of difficulty or visual disturbance. Adequate muscle function may be confirmed clinically if the patient can lift their head off the pillow for five seconds; strength of hand grip is also assessed but is more subjective. A peripheral nerve stimulator may also be used, with a train of four ratio of greater than 70% and absence of fade after double burst stimulation indicating adequate recovery.

Treatment of inadequate reversal includes reassurance, along with sedation and ventilatory support if it is severe. All patients should receive supplemental oxygen and a further dose of neostigmine 1.25 to 2.5 mg intravenously (maximum of 5 mg total dose) may be given.

SUXAMETHONIUM APNOEA

Recovery from the effect of suxamethonium is dependent on the enzyme plasma cholinesterase which hydrolyses suxamethonium to succinyl monocholine and choline. Succinyl monocholine is further hydrolysed to succinic acid and choline. A prolonged neuromuscular block after suxamethonium administration is described as suxamethonium apnoea and can be due to both acquired (Figure PO.7) and genetic factors (Davis 1997).

The majority of acquired causes produce a minor prolongation of apnoea of only a few minutes. Decreased cholinesterase synthesis occurs in liver disease and to a lesser extent in pregnancy and hypothyroidism. Drugs decrease the activity of the enzyme by either competing with suxamethonium for it or binding with the enzyme, either reversibly or irreversibly, or inactivating it.

In cases of suxamethonium apnoea the type 1 block normally seen on using a nerve stimulator (absence of fade on train of four, no post tetanic facilitation) progresses through a transitional phase (development of tetanic fade and, later on, fade on train of four) or dual block and finally develops into a type 2 block (fade on train of four, post tetanic facilitation).

Treatment of suxamethonium apnoea includes on-going sedation and ventilation until there is spontaneous recovery of muscle function. Active measures such as administration of fresh frozen plasma have been used although risk of infection and cost have limited this practice. The patient may have to be managed in the intensive care unit if recovery is prolonged.

NEUROMUSCULAR DISEASE

Patients with neuromuscular disease may be particularly sensitive to the residual effects of general

anaesthesia and to neuromuscular blocking agents which, if possible, should be avoided or used at a reduced dose with monitoring of neuromuscular function.

DIAPHRAGMATIC SPLINTING

The obese, patients with gastric distension, and the post thoracotomy or upper abdominal surgical patient can develop diaphragmatic splinting. Good pain relief with thoracic epidural or patient controlled analgesia, chest physiotherapy, and nasogastric tube insertion where indicated can help prevent hypoventilation in these cases.

PRE-EXISTING LUNG DISEASE

Patients with chronic obstructive airways disease (COAD) are at increased risk of hypoventilation in the post operative period. They may not be able to further increase their work of breathing to maintain an adequate $PaCO_2$, particularly if bronchospasm or excessive airway secretions are present.

Bronchospasm may occur in asthma, COAD, smokers and in patients with acute respiratory infection. It is commonly precipitated by upper airway irritation either during airway manipulation or if secretions are present. Other causes of wheeze include aspiration, pulmonary oedema, and bronchospasm associated with anaphylaxis. Treatment of bronchospasm will depend on the underlying cause and the severity but should include supplemental oxygen and inhaled bronchodilator therapy.

Cardiovascular complications

Cardiovascular problems comprise approximately 20% of critical events in the recovery room. They present most commonly as hypertension, hypotension or cardiac arrhythmias.

HYPERTENSION

This is defined as a 20% or greater increase in pre-operative systolic blood pressure and is often short lived. It usually develops within 30 minutes of the end of surgery and may be precipitated by acute withdrawal of anti hypertensive medication. There are multiple causes (see Figure PO.8) of which pain, pre-operative hypertension and blood gas abnormalities are the commonest.

Management of high blood pressure is directed at establishing and treating the underlying cause, of which pain is the most common. Other causes include

---

ACQUIRED CAUSES OF SUXAMETHONIUM APNOEA

Decreased plasma cholinesterase concentration

Pregnancy
Liver disease
Chronic renal failure
Haemodialysis
Hypothyroidism

Decreased plasma cholinesterase activity

Induction agents (etomidate and ketamine)
Ester local anaesthetics
Anticholinesterases

Figure PO.7

FACTORS ASSOCIATED WITH HYPERTENSION IN THE IMMEDIATE POST OPERATIVE PERIOD

Patient factors	Agitation
	Pre-operative hypertension
	Pain
Inadequate ventilation	Hypoxaemia
	Hypercapnia
Drug interaction	Monoamine oxidase inhibitors
Bladder distension	
Malignant hyperpyrexia	
Endocrine (phaeochromocytoma)	

Figure PO.8

hypoxia, hypercapnia and intravascular fluid overload. Further measures at this stage are determined by the degree of hypertension and associated medical or surgical factors. In general, a moderate elevation in blood pressure of 30% of the pre-operative value is well tolerated.

Post operative hypertension is usually short lived and as such agents used to treat it should be short acting and may include the following:

Labetalol is a beta$_1$ adrenoceptor antagonist with some alpha$_1$ adrenoceptor antagonist activity. 5 mg bolus doses administered intravenously act within 5 minutes and last for up to an hour. Esmolol is a very short acting beta adrenoceptor antagonist with a rapid onset of action. It is given as a bolus of 500 mcg/kg over 60 seconds followed by an infusion at a rate of 50–300 mcg/kg per min dependent on clinical effect. Both of these drugs are contra-indicated in asthmatics. Nifedepine, a calcium antagonist, given sublingually at a dose of 5–20 mg is an effective means of reducing post operative hypertension. Hydralazine, a direct acting peripheral vasodilator, administered intravenously in 5 mg boluses has an onset of action within 10–20 minutes but may cause tachycardia. Glyceryl trinitrate, a direct acting arterial and venous dilator is usually used intra-operatively to control blood pressure but can be administered at a rate of 0.2–8 mcg/kg per min intravenously to rapidly reduce blood pressure in the post operative period.

HYPOTENSION

Hypotension occurs frequently in the recovery room and, in the majority of cases, is transient and benign. It is usually related to the residual effects of anaesthetic and analgesic drugs (Figure PO.9).

Whilst the causes of hypotension are manifold, hypovolaemia due to inadequate peri-operative fluid replacement or ongoing fluid loss is the most common. Sympathetic blockade associated with spinal anaesthesia or analgesia, with a resultant fall in systemic vascular resistance (SVR), is also an important cause of hypotension in the post operative period. The reduction in SVR related to rewarming of a hypothermic patient may also cause a decrease in blood pressure as may rarer causes such as anaphylaxis, cardiac arrhythmias, tension pneumothorax, and pulmonary embolus.

Once hypotension is evident the cause must be sought and treatment initiated to prevent ischaemia to vital organs. The patient should be laid flat or slightly head down and given supplemental oxygen whilst further assessment takes place

The hypovolaemic patient has a tachycardia, with a low JVP, decreased urine output, and poor peripheral perfusion, there may be obvious blood loss e.g. into drains. A rapid intravenous bolus of 250–500 ml of crystalloid or colloid should be given and the

CAUSES OF POST OPERATIVE HYPOTENSION

Frequent causes

Hypovolaemia	Blood loss or third space losses
Vasodilation	Subarachnoid and extradural block
	Residual effects of anaesthetic and analgesic agents
	Rewarming
	Sepsis
	Anaphylaxis

Infrequent causes

Arrhythmias

Myocardial ischaemia/infarction

Heart failure

Tension pneumothorax

Pulmonary embolism

Pericardial tamponade

Hypothyroidism

Figure PO.9

haemodynamic response assessed. Patients assumed to have normal left ventricular function who fail to respond to fluid therapy require central venous pressure monitoring. A pulmonary artery catheter may be required if left ventricular function is impaired. On-going blood loss may require further surgical intervention.

Patients with marked peripheral vasodilatation can be hypotensive despite adequate volume replacement. This is commonly seen after subarachnoid or extradural anaesthesia where administration of vasoconstricting drugs with or without further intravenous fluid should be given. Marked vasodilatation also occurs in sepsis and anaphylaxis where management is both supportive and guided at treating the specific underlying abnormality.

80% of hypotensive patients in recovery will respond to intravenous fluid therapy alone. It is potentially dangerous to use vasopressor drugs in the face of inadequate fluid replacement as they may cause ischaemia of the visceral organs such as the liver and kidneys, however, they may be useful in severe hypotension whilst a diagnosis is being sought and in the presence of vasodilatation. Vasopressor agents used include: Ephedrine, a sympathomimetic agent with alpha and beta adrenoceptor agonist activity, produces peripheral vasoconstriction, and an increase in heart rate and myocardial contractility. It has a rapid onset of action when given intravenously in 3 mg boluses. Metaraminol, an alpha-adrenoceptor agonist with some beta-adrenoceptor agonist activity, can also be used in the post operative period. It has a rapid onset of action and is given in incremental doses of 0.5 mg titrated against effect.

CARDIAC ARRHYTHMIAS

The majority of arrhythmias in the post operative period are benign. They may be related to hypercapnia, hypoxaemia, electrolyte and acid-base disturbance, pain, pre-existing cardiac disease, and myocardial ischaemia or infarction.

Sinus bradycardia (pulse <60 beats per minute) – this may be normal in the young, healthy patient or result from vagal stimulation, hypoxaemia, and drug effects e.g. beta-adrenoceptor antagonists, neostigmine. Treatment with intravenous glycopyrrolate 0.2–0.4 mg or atropine 0.2–0.6 mg will usually increase the heart rate.

Sinus tachycardia (pulse >100 beats per minute) – Pain, hypovolaemia, anaemia, pyrexia, and an increased metabolic rate can all produce a tachycardia. Tachycardia is usually harmless and treatment of the underlying cause is all that is warranted in the majority of cases. If it is associated with myocardial ischaemia, treatment with a beta blocker may be required.

Atrial or ventricular premature contractions – no specific treatment other than correction of hypercapnia and electrolyte abnormalities is usually required.

Supraventricular tachycardia – management of this arrhythmia depends on the degree of haemodynamic instability. Hypoxaemia, hypercapnia and electrolyte imbalance should be corrected. Carotid sinus massage may result in the return of sinus rhythm. Intravenous adenosine 6 mg over 5 seconds followed by a further dose, 2 minutes later, of 12 mg if required is often effective, although it should not be used in the asthmatic patient. Esmolol or verapamil can also be used. Synchronised direct current (DC) cardioversion is indicated if the patient is haemodynamically compromised.

Ventricular tachycardia – this is rare in the post operative period but can progress to ventricular fibrillation and must be treated immediately. If the blood pressure and cardiac output are not compromised, an intravenous bolus of lidocaine 50–100 mg should be given over a few minutes followed by a lidocaine infusion of 1–4 mg/min. DC cardioversion is indicated if hypotension is present.

Thrombo-embolism

Deep venous thrombosis (DVT) and pulmonary embolus (PE) are significant causes of morbidity and mortality in the post operative period. The incidence of DVT is difficult to accurately assess as many cases are not clinically detected. In the post operative period 10–80% of patients may, dependent on patient risk factors and type of surgery, develop DVT (Wheatley 1997). The risk of subsequent PE in this group of patients is unknown although up to 0.9% of all hospital admissions suffer fatal PE after DVT.

DEEP VENOUS THROMBOSIS

The commonest sites for venous thrombosis are in the leg and pelvis although any vein may be affected. The classic presentation of a painful calf which is red, swollen and warmer than the unaffected side is often not present and many cases are asymptomatic. The investigation of choice for below knee thrombosis is venography although iliofemoral thrombosis can usually be detected with Doppler ultrasound.

The main aim of treatment in established venous thrombosis is to minimise the risk of subsequent PE. All patients with above knee thrombosis must be formally anticoagulated for a period of three months. Treatment of below knee thrombosis is controversial because, although a PE can occur with any DVT, it is rare in cases confined to veins situated below the knee. For this reason, formal anticoagulation is not always carried out in this group.

PROPHYLAXIS

Effective prevention of DVT is an important aspect of peri-operative care and requires accurate identification of the at risk patient (see Figure PO.10). All moderate and high risk patients should be given prophylaxis. Prophylactic measures often vary from hospital to hospital and local guidelines should be followed.

Physical methods available include the application of graduated compression or thrombo-embolic deterrent stockings and intermittent compression devices that work by preventing venous stasis. Early ambulation and leg exercises should be encouraged in the post operative period.

Pharmacological methods include the subcutaneous administration of unfractionated and low molecular weight heparin. The main advantage of low molecular weight heparin is that it can be given as a once daily dose with a resultant improvement in patient acceptability.

Due to the increased risk of bleeding associated with pharmacological prophylaxis the mechanical methods are preferred in certain situations where the consequences of bleeding are severe as in major head and neck surgery or neurosurgery.

PULMONARY EMBOLUS

This usually results from dislodgement of thrombus in the systemic veins or, rarely, from the right atrium (atrial fibrillation may promote thrombus formation) or right ventricle (post-septal/right ventricular infarction). It has a mortality of approximately 10%.

Clinical features depend on the size of the PE, a small embolus may present with exertional dyspnoea and lassitude, a moderate sized embolus with pleuritic chest pain of sudden onset, haemoptysis and dyspnoea, and a massive embolus with severe chest pain, tachycardia, tachypnoea, and syncope. Physical signs may be absent after a small PE. Larger infarcts may produce a tachycardia, gallop rhythm, right ventricular heave, and a prominent *a* wave in the jugular venous wave form. A pleural rub may be present and signs and symptoms of DVT must be sought.

The investigation of choice is a ventilation-perfusion scan looking for ventilated but non-perfused areas of lung. The ECG usually only shows a sinus tachycardia although right ventricular hypertrophy, right axis deviation, and right bundle branch block may be present after large emboli. The classical S wave in lead I, Q wave and inverted T wave in lead III is usually absent. The chest X-ray is also often normal. Arterial blood gas sampling usually shows hypoxaemia and hypocapnia.

Anticoagulant therapy should be initiated, after confirmation of the diagnosis, to prevent further embolisation. In cases where a delay in ventilation-perfusion scan is expected anticoagulation should be started on clinical suspicion alone. The duration of anticoagulation depends on the risk of further venous emboli, with treatment continuing for up to six months. Thrombolysis with streptokinase is occasionally used after large emboli.

CNS complications

SHIVERING

Post-anaesthetic shivering occurs in up to 65% of cases (Crossley 1993) and is related to age, gender, duration of anaesthesia and anaesthetic technique. The consequences of shivering include marked increases in minute ventilation and cardiac output secondary to greater oxygen demand and carbon dioxide production. This may have a detrimental effect particularly in the patient with cardiorespiratory

---

DVT RISK GROUP CLASSIFICATION

Low risk patients:
  <40 yr old without additional risk factors
  Minor surgery (<30 min)

Moderate risk patients:
  >40 yr old
  Oral contraceptive medication
  Major surgery (>30 min)

High risk patients:
  Previous DVT/PE
  Major surgery for malignant disease
  Orthopaedic surgery to lower limbs

(adapted from Wheatley with permission)

Figure PO.10.

disease. Shivering can also interfere with post operative haemodynamic and oxygen saturation monitoring.

The incidence of post anaesthetic shivering is increased in hypothermic patients, however not all patients who shiver are hypothermic. Prolonged anaesthesia is associated post operative shivering. Methods to prevent a fall in core temperature such as raising ambient temperature in the operating theatre, warming intravenous fluids and using forced warm air blankets in the intra- and post operative period should be used in the at risk patient. Premedication with anticholinergic agents is associated with an increased incidence of shivering. The use of propofol as opposed to thiopentone as an induction agent or clonidine, an alpha$_2$ adrenergic agonist, given at induction reduces the incidence of shivering in the post operative period.

Treatment includes oxygen administration to prevent hypoxia, active warming and the use of specific drugs. Pethidine at a minimum dose of 0.35 mg per kg is the most effective opioid in the treatment of post-anaesthetic shivering with a 95% success rate. Fentanyl and alfentanil have some effect although this is less marked and shorter in duration than with pethidine. Doxapram, an agent usually used as a respiratory stimulant, is also effective at a dose of 0.2 mg/kg.

FAILURE TO REGAIN CONSCIOUSNESS

In most instances, failure to regain consciousness may be attributed to residual drug effects. Other causes include endocrine abnormalities such as hypoglycaemia or hypothyroidism, cerebral events including cerebrovascular accident or cerebral hypoxia or existing physiological derangements such as hypothermia, hypoxia, hypercapnia or hypotension.

Residual drug effects may be reversed with specific antagonists if unconsciousness is particularly prolonged. These may include naloxone for opioids and flumazenil, up to 1 mg intravenously, for benzodiazepines.

Diabetic patients should have their blood sugar levels checked both intra and post operatively. Hypoglycaemia should be treated with 50 mls of 50% dextrose intravenously.

OXYGEN THERAPY

INDICATIONS

Supplemental oxygen should be administered for at least 10 min to all patients during emergence from anaesthesia to prevent the development of tissue hypoxia.

The indications for oxygen therapy to continue after emergence from anaesthesia are listed in Figure PO.11 (Leach 1993). Any patient who is at risk of developing tissue hypoxia or is already hypoxaemic should be given supplemental oxygen.

TECHNIQUES OF ADMINISTRATION

Delivery systems used in the post operative period are listed in Figure PO.12. They may be subdivided into variable or fixed performance devices.

Variable performance devices are so called because the

INDICATIONS FOR OXYGEN THERAPY IN THE POST OPERATIVE PERIOD

Patient factors	Cardiorespiratory disease
	Obesity
	Elderly
	Shivering
Surgical factors	Upper abdominal procedures
	Thoracic surgery
Physiological factors	Hypovolaemia
	Hypotension
	Anaemia
Post operative analgesic technique	Patient controlled analgesia
	IV opioid infusion
	Epidural infusion (both local anaesthetic agents and opioids)

Figure PO.11

OXYGEN DELIVERY SYSTEMS IN THE POST OPERATIVE PERIOD

Variable performance	Fixed performance
Hudson Mask	Venturi masks
MC mask	Anaesthetic breathing
Nasal cannulae	circuits
Nasal catheter	
(nasopharyngeal catheter)	

Figure PO.12

inspired oxygen concentration (FIO_2) and degree of rebreathing vary from patient to patient and at different times in the same patient. This is dependent on the respiratory rate, inspiratory flow rate and length of expiratory pause. This type of device is most commonly used, as an accurate FIO_2 is not required in the majority of patients. The Hudson mask is a clear plastic facemask that is placed over the nose and mouth and, at a flow rate of four litres per minute, provides an FIO_2 of approximately 0.4. Addition of a reservoir bag to these masks increases the maximum obtainable FIO_2 to approximately 98%. Patient compliance is poor due to a claustrophobic feeling and the need to remove it during eating and drinking and for routine mouth care. The use of nasal cannulae provide a more comfortable and continuous method of oxygen delivery. At a flow rate of two to four l/min these devices provide an FIO_2 comparable with the face mask.

The fixed performance devices provide an accurate FIO_2 and avoid rebreathing. They may be further subdivided into high airflow oxygen enrichment (HAFOE) devices e.g. Venturi masks or lower flow devices such as anaesthetic breathing systems. Venturi masks use injectors of different sizes to deliver set oxygen concentrations varying from 24% to 60% by entraining air in oxygen using the venturi principle. The appropriate oxygen flow rate for each mask is printed on the injector which is also colour coded. For example, a 24% oxygen valve requires an oxygen flow of two litres per minute and entrains 38 litres of air per minute. Patients who require these masks include those at risk of respiratory failure if given high oxygen concentrations i.e. those who are reliant on a hypoxic drive for ventilation.

In patients who are taken to recovery with a laryngeal mask in situ, a T-piece may be connected to it to provide supplemental oxygen. These may also be varible performance – simply open ended tubing, or fixed performance.

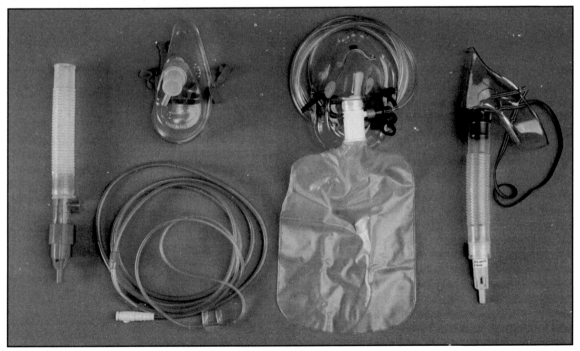

Figure PO.13 Left to right (clockwise): Venturi T piece, Hudson Facemask, mask with oxygen reservoir bag, Ventimask, nasal speculae.

The use of anaesthetic breathing systems is reserved for the immediate post operative period when 100% oxygen may need to be delivered via a tight fitting mask for example when there is airway obstruction or laryngeal spasm.

Humidification

Humidification is only required when oxygen is delivered at high flow rates or when the upper airway humidification processes are bypassed as occurs after tracheostomy or during prolonged tracheal intubation. It is therefore rarely required during the post operative period.

Duration

There is no consensus on how long supplemental oxygen therapy should be given. However, the incidence of hypoxaemia is greatest on the second or third post operative night after major surgery and the PaO_2 may not return to pre-operative levels until the fifth night. Supplemental oxygen should therefore be given, where indicated, for at least three days post operatively.

Complications

Supplemental oxygen administration is a safe technique. However, problems may occur when inappropriate methods are used. Two common problems are the occurrence of barotrauma and the risk of interference with hypoxic drive in certain patients.

BAROTRAUMA

Barotauma occurs when oxygen is directly delivered to the lower airway without free outflow of any excess gas. The practice of placing a variable performance facemask over the open end of a tracheal tube or laryngeal mask should be avoided as there have been reports of the oxygen inlet part of the facemask impacting on the male connector of the tracheal tube. This resulted in delivery of oxygen at a flow rate of 4 l/min minute and a pressure of 400 kPa with fatal consequences. The use of a T-piece system, where excess gas is vented to the atmosphere, is a much safer alternative.

LOSS OF HYPOXIC VENTILATORY DRIVE

Approximately 10% of patients with chronic respiratory failure depend on hypoxic ventilatory drive to maintain an adequate $PaCO_2$. In this group of patients administration of a high FIO_2 will cause hypoventilation with subsequent CO_2 retention and respiratory acidosis. However, the fear of causing CO_2 retention must not prevent the provision of appropriate oxygen therapy. A PaO_2 of 7 to 8 kPa must be attained. At this level of PaO_2 a slight increase will have a marked effect on oxygen content as this equates to the steepest part of the oxygen haemoglobin dissociation curve. In practice, 24–28% oxygen should be given in the first instance followed by blood gas analysis to assess clinical response. A higher FIO_2 should be administered if the PaO_2 is too low and, if required, ventilatory support should be instituted to control the $PaCO_2$.

POST OPERATIVE ANALGESIA

The provision of effective pain relief during the post operative period is dependent on anaesthetic technique, type and extent of surgery and the patient factors such as age and personality. In practice, a combination of opioid, non steroidal anti-inflammatory drugs (NSAID) and local anaesthetic techniques is often used.

Good pain control not only alleviates patient distress but also prevents or modifies many adverse effects (see Figure PO.14). The increase in sympathetic activity associated with pain results in tachycardia, hypertension, and increased myocardial oxygen demand, which, in patients with cardiac disease, may produce myocardial ischaemia. Post operative chest infection and basal atelectasis are more frequent in the patient who is unable to deep breathe or cough such as after upper abdominal or thoracic surgery. Patient immobility associated with poor pain control increases the risk of thrombo-embolic disease.

TREATMENT OF PAIN

Opioids

Opioids may be given via the following routes: Intramuscular, subcutaneous, intravenous, oral, intrathecal or extradural.

The dose of opioid required in the post operative period shows marked interpatient variability. This is due to both pharmacokinetic and pharmacodynamic factors with up to a five-fold difference in plasma concentrations after identical doses of intramuscular opioid. There are also differences in opioid receptor sensitivity between patients.

The conventional regime of on-demand intramuscular opioid often fails to provide adequate pain relief as

ADVERSE EFFECTS OF POST OPERATIVE PAIN

Cardiovascular

Tachycardia
Hypertension
Increased myocardial oxygen demand

Respiratory

Decreased vital capacity
Decreased functional residual capacity
Decreased tidal volume
Chest infections
Basal atelectasis

Gastro-intestinal

Nausea and vomiting
Ileus

Other effects

Urinary retention
Deep venous thrombosis
Pulmonary embolus

Figure PO.14

delays in administration, lack of patient awareness of availability and time taken for onset of action result in plasma levels falling below that required to produce analgesia. Usual dosage is 10–15 mg 2–4 hourly. There may be slow absorption in patients with poor peripheral perfusion. Subcutaneous opioid administration via indwelling cannulae is associated with similar limitations but avoids repeated needle insertion.

Intravenous opioids

Intravenous administration of opioid is generally more effective. A bolus dose can be followed by increments every few minutes until acceptable pain control is reached. This technique minimises the risk of serious side effects but is labour intensive and is only suitable in the recovery room or high dependency unit.

Continuous intravenous administration via an infusion will ensure maintenance of adequate plasma levels but may be associated with over sedation and respiratory depression mandating observation of the patient in a high dependency unit

Patient-controlled analgesia (PCA) was developed to further improve opioid analgesia by accounting for the variation in opioid requirement from patient to patient and the reduction in opioid required with time. The theoretical advantage of this technique is that the patient should maintain a plasma concentration at around the minimum effective analgesic plasma concentration with resultant good pain control and reduced side effects. It is safer than intravenous infusion techniques as the associated sedation when the patients are pain free results in reduced usage. In practice, patients may not alleviate their pain completely with this technique due to their worries about addiction and side effects. The success of PCA is dependent on patient education during the pre-operative visit, adequate pain control in the recovery room and regular review by nursing and anaesthetic staff. Morphine is the most commonly used opioid although other drugs such as alfentanil and pethidine have been used with good effect. A demand dose of morphine 1mg is used with a lock-out period of 5 minutes. The demand dose should be large enough to provide an analgesic effect but small enough to prevent unwanted side effects and may have to be altered depending on the clinical effect. The lock-out period must be long enough to prevent repeat administration before the initial bolus has had a maximal effect. A maximum dose per hour can also be set to prevent inadvertent overdose although, due to the large variation in opioid requirements between patients, this may prevent some patients from attaining adequate pain relief. A background infusion can also be used with a PCA device although there is no evidence to suggest that this is of benefit

The main side effects associated with parenteral opioid administration are nausea and vomiting, and cardiorespiratory depression. The incidence of severe respiratory depression during PCA is approximately 0.5%, which compares favourably with the intramuscular route. The risk of this is increased in patients receiving background opioid infusions or other sedative drugs. The elderly and patients with pre-existing sleep apnoea also have an increased risk of respiratory depression.

Oral opioids

Patients who are able to tolerate oral intake may benefit from opioids given by this route. It is a particularly useful technique in children due to the avoidance of needle or cannula insertion. A dose of morphine 0.2 mg/kg is adequate in most instances. First pass metabolism results in lower plasma concentrations after oral than after parenteral administration of the same dose.

Spinal opioids

Opioid administration via the intrathecal or extradural route can provide excellent post operative pain control. The commonest side effects associated with this technique are nausea, pruritus, sedation and urinary retention. Respiratory depression is an infrequent complication, however, it can occur up to 24 hours after administration of intrathecal opioids and therefore patients must be observed in the high dependency unit for a 24-hour period to monitor their respiratory status. Patients receiving extradural opioids are at a lower risk of developing respiratory depression but they must also be managed on a ward where this potentially fatal complication can be recognised and treated.

The conscious level of the patient is as important, if not more so, than the respiratory rate. A patient with a decreased conscious level with or without a low respiratory rate requires immediate treatment. Intravenous naloxone given in titrated doses is effective at reversing the opioid induced respiratory depression without reducing the analgesic effect.

Non-steroidal anti-inflammatory drugs

This group of drugs have both analgesic and anti-inflammatory properties. They are effective for treatment of mild to moderate post operative pain and, after the first 24 to 36 hours, may be used as the sole analgesic in major surgical patients. NSAIDs also have an opioid-sparing effect with a reduction of opioid requirement after major surgery of greater than 20% when given regularly.

NSAIDs have several advantages over opioid analgesics. Their use is not associated with respiratory depression or gastric stasis and as they are not controlled drugs, they are readily available. However, their use is associated with potentially serious side effects, which include gastro-intestinal haemorrhage, gastric ulceration, renal impairment and an increased risk of post operative bleeding due to impairment of platelet function. NSAIDs are contra-indicated in patients with a history of peptic ulcer disease, gastro-intestinal bleeding, renal impairment, previous hypersensitivity reactions to aspirin or NSAIDs, asthma, and bleeding diathesis. They should be avoided in the dehydrated or hypovolaemic patient and care should be taken when using NSAIDs in the elderly. The newer cyclo-oxygenase-2 selective agents have, as yet, no proven benefits over standard NSAIDs in the management of acute post operative pain and are considerably more expensive.

The salicylates are absolutely contra-indicated in children less than 12 years of age. Reye's syndrome, an acute encephalopathy with fatty infiltration of the liver, is associated with administration of these drugs in this age group.

Local anaesthetics

Local infiltration, peripheral nerve blocks, and epidural analgesia are often used to produce post operative pain relief both alone and in conjunction with other analgesic methods.

The advantage of local anaesthetic techniques is that profound analgesia can be produced without respiratory depression or nausea and vomiting. However, local anaesthetic toxicity may occur as a result of inadvertent intravenous administration or after large doses. In addition, although rare, peripheral nerve damage, haemorrhage, infection, accidental arterial or subarachnoid injection, and pneumothorax can all occur depending on the site of the block.

PAIN ASSESSMENT

Pain, by definition, is a subjective sensation and is difficult for an observer to accurately assess. The provision of a reliable and valid means of assessing pain is important because it allows the degree of improvement, after an analgesic intervention, to be documented in a reproducible way.

Two pain severity scoring systems, the verbal rating scale and visual analogue scale are frequently used in the post operative setting.

The verbal rating scale is simple and easy to use. The patient is asked to rate their pain as either "none", "mild", "moderate", or "severe" when at rest and on movement. The visual analogue scale consists of a 10 cm long line which represents a spectrum of pain intensity from "no pain at all" on the extreme left of the line through to "the worst pain imaginable" on the extreme right. The patient is asked to mark the point on this line that corresponds to the severity of their pain.

ACUTE PAIN SERVICE

The importance of effective post operative pain relief and increased complexity of analgesic techniques such as PCA and continuous epidural infusions has resulted in the formation of acute pain services in many hospitals. They provide a multidisciplinary approach to post operative pain control with the involvement of anaesthetists, specialist nurses, and clinical pharmacists. An acute pain service carries out regular patient assessment and provides back up for ward staff. It is also involved in "in-house" training of medical and nursing staff to improve understanding of analgesic methods and pain assessment.

POST OPERATIVE NAUSEA AND VOMITING

Post operative nausea and vomiting (PONV) is one of the commonest complications in the post operative period despite the use of modern day anaesthetic techniques. It occurs in 20 to 40% of cases and results in patient discomfort and anxiety and can produce significant morbidity in some cases. Sudden increases in intra-ocular and intra-cranial pressure associated with vomiting may be detrimental in the ophthalmic and neurosurgical patient. Fluid and electrolyte disturbances can occur if the period of vomiting is prolonged.

PONV exhibits a multifactorial aetiology and is influenced by patient, anaesthetic and surgical factors (See Figure PO.15).

Females are 2.5 times more likely to develop PONV than males. The incidence also varies with age, the lowest incidence is found in infants aged less than twelve months with a peak in the six to sixteen year old age group followed by a slight decrease during adult life. Inadequate starvation or delayed gastric emptying, from whatever cause, is associated with an increase in PONV and anxiety may have its effect via this mechanism. The increased incidence in obesity may be related to anaesthetic problems associated with these patients such as stomach insufflation, and the development of hypoxaemia or hypercapnia rather than obesity itself.

Intravenous induction agents are incriminated to varying degrees. Propofol is associated with less PONV than thiopentone and may have specific anti-emetic properties. Thiopentone is less emetogenic than etomidate. Nitrous oxide is thought to be associated with PONV possibly as a result of gut distension and raised pressure in the middle ear. Neuromuscular blocking agents are not implicated but reversal with neostigmine has been shown to increase emesis. This is despite concurrent administration of atropine which has anti-emetic properties. The development of hypotension after spinal anaesthesia is associated with almost twice the incidence of PONV when compared with those patients where hypotension did not occur.

PREVENTION OF PONV

Prevention of PONV is difficult due to its multifactorial aetiology. The mainstay of management is the avoidance of emetogenic drugs and use of anti-emetic agents.

A patient presenting for surgery at risk of PONV should receive anxiolytic and anti-emetic premedication. Anaesthesia should be induced using intravenous propofol in a controlled manner taking care to avoid gastric insufflation with anaesthetic gases. Opioid drugs should be used sparingly and, where appropriate, NSAIDs and local anaesthetic techniques used instead. An oxygen/air/volatile mix or total intravenous anaesthesia should be used for maintenance of anaesthesia. Further anti-emetic therapy should be

RISK FACTORS ASSOCIATED WITH PONV

Patient factors
  Gender
  Age
  Anxiety
  History of motion sickness
  Previous PONV
  Delayed gastric emptying
  Obesity

Anaesthetic factors

  Drugs   Opioids
                 Intravenous induction agents
                 Nitrous oxide
                 Neostigmine
  Technique   Gastric insufflation
                 Subarachnoid block

Surgical factors
  Emergency procedure
  Day case surgery
  ENT surgery
  Strabismus correction
  Gynaecological procedures
  Gastro-intestinal surgery
  Post operative pain
  Ileus, gastric distension

Figure PO.15

given intra-operatively and continued, on a regular basis, into the post operative period.

TREATMENT

Vomiting in a semi conscious patient requires immediate action; the patient should be placed in the lateral position, the pharynx cleared of any secretions and supplemental oxygen administered.

The conscious patient should be reassured and supplemental oxygen administered although this will only have a placebo effect unless hypoxaemia is the cause. Other underlying causes such as hypercapnia, hypotension or pain should be treated. The majority of patients, however, will require an anti-emetic (Rowbotham 1992).

There are several classes of drugs used for the treatment of PONV: Prochlorperazine, a Phenothiazine, is a dopamine antagonist acting on the chemoreceptor trigger zone whose use is limited by low efficacy, lack of an intravenous preparation and central nervous system side effects. Metoclopramide has antidopaminergic activity and a peripheral action on the gut, which increases gastric emptying, and small intestine transit time. The incidence of side effects is less than 10% but there is little evidence supporting its efficacy. 5-HT$_3$ antagonists such as ondansetron have been used much more frequently over the last few years with good effect, however they are often used as second line treatment due to their high cost. Cyclizine, a histamine receptor antagonist with mild anticholinergic activity is increasing in popularity as it is inexpensive and can be given orally, intramuscularly or intravenously.

POST OPERATIVE FLUID THERAPY

The aims of post operative fluid therapy are to maintain adequate hydration, blood volume, renal function and electrolyte balance. It is indicated in patients with pre-operative fluid abnormalities or ongoing fluid losses, and also in any patient undergoing a major surgical procedure.

PHYSIOLOGY

Total body water (TBW) accounts for 50–70% of body weight dependent on age, sex, body habitus and fat content. TBW is distributed between three fluid compartments: the intravascular space (8% TBW), the interstitial space (32% TBW) and the intracellular space (60% TBW). The intravascular and interstitial space together form the extracellular fluid (ECF) compartment and are separated by the endothelial cells of the capillary wall, which are freely permeable to water and small ions, but not to proteins. The intracellular fluid (ICF) compartment is separated from the ECF by the cell membrane which is selectively permeable to ions.

Surgical incision produces a neurohumoral or "stress" response with increasing levels of circulating catecholamines, ADH, aldosterone and cortisol and resultant sodium and water retention.

POST OPERATIVE FLUID LOSS

There are many causes of fluid loss in the surgical patient (See Figure PO.16). Insensible losses from the skin and lungs are approximately 0.5 ml/kg/H. This figure increases by 12% for each degree rise in body temperature above 37° C. "Third space" loss is due to tissue oedema and is directly related to the extent of the surgical incision, varying from 1 to 15 ml/kg/H. The amount of on-going loss is often difficult to quantify and it may be difficult to accurately measure blood loss.

CAUSES OF POST OPERATIVE FLUID LOSS IN THE SURGICAL PATIENT

Insensible losses	Sweating Respiration Faeces Urine output
'Third space' losses	
Ongoing losses	Haemorrhage Drains Nasogastric Vomiting Diarrhoea

Figure PO.16

CLINICAL ASSESSMENT

Regular clinical evaluation to detect any fluid deficit should be carried out in the post operative period. Adequacy of volume status is associated with normal pulse, blood pressure, and jugular venous pressure, a urine output of at least 0.5 ml/kg/H, moist mucous membranes and warm extremities and good peripheral perfusion. Trends in haemodynamic parameters can guide further fluid management and central venous or pulmonary artery occlusion pressure monitoring may be indicated in some cases. Assessment can be difficult in patients with residual effects of general or regional anaesthesia or on beta-blocker therapy where normal responses (peripheral vasoconstriction, tachycardia) may be masked. Laboratory investigations including haemoglobin concentration, haematocrit and urea may be abnormal in moderate to severe fluid deficit.

FLUID REPLACEMENT

It is difficult to predict fluid requirements in the post operative period, particularly after major surgery. The fluid regime in Figure PO.17 acts only as a guide to fluid therapy during this period and emphasis must be placed on repeated clinical assessment. Patients undergoing minor surgery who will start drinking within a few hours of the procedure do not usually require additional intravenous fluids.

The choice of fluid replacement depends on which fluid compartment is depleted. Crystalloids, which are solutions of electrolytes and sugars in water, are distributed throughout the three fluid compartments depending on their sodium concentration. Isotonic fluids such as 0.9% saline remain predominantly within the ECF compartment whereas hypotonic solutions such as 5% dextrose are distributed throughout the ECF and ICF. Colloids, which are solutions of high molecular weight proteins (blood and blood products), gelatins, starches or dextrans are mainly confined to the intravascular compartment.

Insensible losses are replaced with 5% dextrose if there is no ECF loss. However, the majority of post operative patients has a degree of ECF loss and require additional sodium. 4% dextrose/0.18% saline is then the fluid of choice. Potassium should be added to maintenance fluids after the first post operative day at 1 mmol/kg/day. Estimated 'third space' loss is replaced with normal (0.9%) saline or a balanced salt solution such as Hartmann's solution. Blood loss is replaced with colloid on a one-to-one basis and, if the loss exceeds apporoximately 15% of

POST OPERATIVE INTRAVENOUS FLUID REGIME

Cause	Replacement fluid	Volume (ml/kg/H)	Comment
Insensible loss	5% Dextrose or 4% Dextrose/0.18% saline	1	
"Third" space loss	0.9% Saline or	1 – 3	Minor surgery e.g. Hernia repair
	Hartmann's solution	3 – 5	Intermediate e.g. Mastectomy
		5 – 10	Major surgery e.g. THR
		10 – 15	Major plus surgery e.g. Aortic aneurysm repair
Blood loss	0.9% Saline (3x blood loss) or Colloid (1x blood loss) or Packed red blood cells (1x blood loss)		Aim for Hb of 10 g/dl

Figure PO.17

the patients blood volume, packed red blood cells to maintain the haemoglobin concentration at about 10 g/dl. Normal saline or Hartmann's solution can also be used to maintain intravascular volume although a volume three times the estimated blood loss has to be infused.

Post operative fluid therapy should continue until there is adequate oral intake, fluid deficits have been corrected and there are no major ongoing fluid losses.

SEQUELAE OF ANAESTHESIA

Complications occurring after surgery result from a combination of patient, surgical, and anaesthetic factors. Morbidity directly attributable to anaesthetic practice is often relatively minor e.g. post operative sore throat, but can result in permanent disability e.g. hypoxic brain damage. An increasing number of medicolegal claims are made against anaesthetists each year which highlight the virtues of diligence, accurate record keeping, attention to detail and continued observation throughout the administration of anaesthesia and into the post operative period.

The sequelae of anaesthesia are related to anaesthetic technique and patient positioning:

EYE TRAUMA

Corneal abrasions can occur if the eyelids remain open during anaesthesia and the cornea is allowed to dry out. This is easily preventable by applying adhesive tape, which should be removed with care, to ensure that the eyelids remain closed. Corneal abrasion may also occur if the eye comes into direct contact with equipment such as laryngoscope blades or anaesthetic masks. Retinal ischaemia has been reported after prolonged eyeball compression with resultant transient blindness. Eye pads should be used if the prone or lateral position is adopted.

AIRWAY TRAUMA

Instrumentation of the oropharynx with a laryngoscope blade, a laryngeal mask, or oral airway can result in lip, tongue, and gum abrasions. Care should be taken to prevent the lips or tongue from being caught on the teeth.

Broken teeth and damaged dental work not only put the patient at risk of aspiration but are also a cause of

significant inconvenience after recovery. For this reason, dental damage is a major cause of litigation. Poor dentition, loose teeth and the presence of caps, crowns and bridges should be documented at the pre-operative visit. Methods employed to decrease the risk of dental trauma include the use of nasal airways, mouth guards, and fibre-optic intubation.

Up to 50% of patients complain of post operative sore throat. This may be related to tracheal intubation although it is often associated with airway or laryngeal mask insertion, nasogastric tube placement, and administration of dry gases.

MUSCULOSKELETAL TRAUMA

Muscle pains can occur in the post operative period and are usually related to suxamethonium administration. Suxamethonium pains are more common in the young, ambulant patient with large muscle bulk. During pregnancy and childhood the muscle pains are less intense. The onset is typically delayed by 24 hours and may mimic influenza-like symptoms. Administration of low dose non-depolarising muscle relaxants, benzodiazepines, or lidocaine before anaesthetic induction have all been used in an attempt to reduce the muscle pains with variable effect. Patients should be informed of the possibility of this complication.

Backache and neck pain can occur from poor patient positioning and as a result of stretched ligaments and relaxed skeletal muscle. Arms and legs can slip off operating tables or trolleys, if inadequately secured, with the potential for ligament and bony injuries.

Nerve injuries have been extensively reported and are a result of direct compression or stretching of the nerve. Correct patient positioning and extensive padding of exposed sites are mandatory. The brachial plexus can be damaged if there is excessive abduction of the arm (>90 degrees) with the humeral head impinging on the axillary neurovascular bundle. The radial nerve, as it runs down the lateral border of the arm 3–5 cm above the lateral epicondyle, is at risk of being damaged by a blood pressure cuff. The ulnar nerve is exposed at the elbow and can be damaged by direct trauma or the blood pressure cuff. The common peroneal nerve can be damaged, when the patient is placed in the lithotomy position, as it passes laterally around the neck of the fibula resulting in foot drop and loss of sensation on the dorsum of the foot. The saphenous nerve is also at risk in the lithotomy position when there is compression of the medial aspect of the leg against the leg support and results in loss of sensation along the medial aspect of the calf. Facial and supraorbital nerve palsies due to direct nerve compression have also been reported.

SKIN DAMAGE

Bruising and skin breakdown over pressure areas can occur after prolonged procedures and in the elderly. The occiput, elbows, and heels should be padded and the undersheet smoothed out. Skin contact with metal must be prevented because of the risk of electrical burns if diathermy is used. Excessively frequent blood pressure cuff inflation is associated with localised bruising and should be avoided. In the post operative period, patients with residual local anaesthetic blocks or epidural analgesia are at increased risk of skin breakdown due to immobility and loss of sensation.

MEDICO-LEGAL ISSUES

After receiving a verbal or written complaint from a patient a copy of all the relevant clinical information should be made. A senior member of the anaesthetic department should be informed and, if in any doubt, advice should be sought from the relevant medical defence institution. Under no account must any documented information be altered. The importance of completing an accurate and legible anaesthetic form for every patient undergoing anaesthesia can not be stressed enough.

References and further reading

Association of Anaesthetists of Great Britain and Ireland. Post-anaesthetic recovery facilities. Recommendations of a working party, (Chairman Marks RL). Association of Anaesthetists of Great Britain and Ireland, 1993.

Crossley AW. Post operative shivering. *British Journal of Hospital Medicine* 1993; **49:** 204–208.

Davis L, Britten JJ, Morgan M. Cholinesterase: its significance in anaesthetic practice. *Anaesthesia* 1997; **52:** 244–260.

Joyce CJ, Baker AB. What is the role of absorption atelectasis in the genesis of peri-operative pulmonary collapse? *Anaesthesia and Intensive Care* 1995; **23:** (6); 691–696.

Leach RM, Bateman NT. Acute oxygen therapy. *British Journal of Hospital Medicine* 1993; **49:** 637–644.

Mangat PS, Jones JG. *Anaesthesia Review 10* (ed. Kaufman L). Churchill Livingstone; Edinburgh; 1993: 95–102.

Rowbotham DJ. Current management of post operative nausea and vomiting. *British Journal of Anaesthesia* 1992; **69** (Suppl. 1): 46S–59S.

The Royal College of Surgeons of England and The College of Anaesthetists. Pain after Surgery. Report of a Working Party (Chairman AA Spence) of the Commission on the Provision of Surgical Services, 1990.

Wheatley T, Veitch PS. Recent advances in prophylaxis against deep vein thrombosis. *British Journal of Anaesthesia* 1997; **78:** 118–120.

SECTION 1: 5
SPECIAL PATIENT CIRCUMSTANCES

C. A. Pinnock
R. M. Haden

THE PREGNANT PATIENT
    Analgesia in labour
    Operative anaesthesia

THE PAEDIATRIC PATIENT
    Assessment
    Equipment
    Fluid therapy
    Analgesia
    Specialist surgery

THE HEAD INJURED PATIENT
    Applied physiology
    Management of head injury

THE DAY CASE PATIENT
    Social circumstances
    Category of surgery
    Medical fitness
    Anaesthetic technique

THE OBESE PATIENT
    Applied physiology
    Anaesthesia

THE METABOLICALLY COMPROMISED PATIENT
    Liver disease
    Renal disease
    Diabetes mellitus

INFECTIVE RISK GROUPS
    Hepatitis
    HIV
    Precautions
    Needlestick Injury
    Prion Disease

LATEX ALLERGY

THE PREGNANT PATIENT

Obstetric anaesthesia requires detailed knowledge of the physiological changes associated with pregnancy. Whilst these are covered thoroughly in Section 2, Chapter 13, the salient points are outlined below to aid the reader.

As pregnancy progresses, the maternal blood volume increases and, although total haemoglobin increases, the haemoglobin concentration falls by dilution. The concentration of clotting factors increases causing a tendency to deep vein thrombosis exacerbated by pressure on the pelvic veins from the increasingly bulky uterus. Cardiac output increases throughout pregnancy due to increases in stroke volume and heart rate. Thoracic volume rises so that although tidal volume remains comparable to pre-pregnancy values, there becomes an impression of hyperinflation. At the end of pregnancy $PaCO_2$ is reduced to 4 kPa. The hormonal changes of pregnancy cause relaxation of smooth muscle and ligaments, resulting in a reduction in lower oesophageal sphincter tone which, combined with increasing intra-abdominal pressure, leads both to functional hiatus herniae and oesophageal reflux. Gastric contents are more voluminous than usual and gastric emptying is slowed. In labour, gastric emptying virtually ceases.

Patients in the third trimester of pregnancy should not be allowed to lie in the supine position for any reason without left lateral tilt to displace the uterus because the weight of the uterus compresses the inferior vena cava. The substantial reduction in venous return to the heart that follows may produce fainting. If compensatory vasoconstriction is abolished by epidural blockade, serious falls in cardiac output may result.

ANALGESIA IN LABOUR

Pain in labour is the result of a hollow organ, the uterus, contracting against an obstruction, the foetus, in an attempt to expel it. The pain is the result of tension in the uterine wall. The patient's response to the pain of contractions is a psychological response that depends on culture, history and preparation; therefore, each patient must be taken on her own merits. The pain of labour is transmitted to the spinal cord via two routes, depending on the stage of labour. The impulses from the body and fundus of the uterus pass via the lower thoracic spinal roots, T10 to L1, while those from the cervix and birth canal pass via the sacral roots. The net result is that pain in the first stage of labour is perceived to be lower abdominal while in the second stage it changes focus to pelvis and perineum

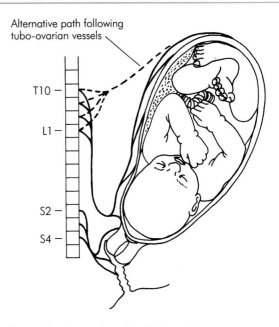

Figure SC.1 Innervation of the birth canal

(see Figure SC.1). Nocioceptive impulses pass up the spinal cord and are interpreted in the brain. The various methods of providing analgesia in labour are detailed in Figure SC.2.

METHODS OF PAIN RELIEF IN LABOUR	
Psychological	
Complementary	TENS
	Acupuncture
Systemic analgesia	Nitrous oxide
	Inhalational agents
	IM opioids
	PCA
Epidural analgesia	Bolus
	Infusion

Figure SC.2

Psychological methods

There is no doubt that adequate psychological preparation for labour significantly reduces pain. Breathing and relaxation techniques are taught routinely in antenatal classes. Self hypnosis can also be successful in the suitably motivated patient.

Complementary methods

Transcutaneous electrical nerve stimulation (TENS) can work well if introduced early enough in labour. The technique depends on the gate theory of pain transmission (as described by Melzack and Wall 1965). Stimulation must be applied to the dorsal columns of the spinal cord in the mid-thoracic region, above the level of the affected nerve roots, i.e. T10. TENS is effective early in labour but begins to lose its effect after 5 cm cervical dilatation is reached. Acupuncture has been advocated for use in labour but it is not in common use in the UK.

Systemic analgesia

Systemic administration of analgesic drugs remains the mainstay of labour analgesia. Administration is usually by inhalation of nitrous oxide or anaesthetic vapours or alternatively by intravenous or intramuscular administration of opioids.

Nitrous oxide is usually administered as a 50% mixture with oxygen (Entonox®). Effective use of nitrous oxide depends on beginning the inhalation before the painful part of the contraction so that an analgesic concentration is reached by the time that a contraction becomes painful, which is difficult to achieve. Anaesthetic vapours have been advocated in sub-anaesthetic concentrations (such as isoflurane 0.2%) but have not achieved large scale use.

Opioid analgesia may be given either by the intramuscular or intravenous routes. Local rules and preferences dictate the choice of opioid. Midwives may administer intramuscular opioids on their own responsibility, subject to local protocols relating to which drug, number of doses and accountability. Agents in widespread use include the agonists pethidine and diamorphine while some units favour partial agonists such as meptazinol. All opioids have a reputation for causing foetal respiratory depression.

The intravenous route, via a patient controlled analgesia device (PCA) has not yet become popular, despite the advantages of patient control and lower total dose. PCA devices may be simple 'elastic recoil' systems with a reservoir refilled at a fixed rate or complex computer controlled devices with adjustable background infusions and lockout times. Pethidine remains the most popular drug for obstetric PCA.

Epidural analgesia

Epidural analgesia is the most effective form of labour analgesia, but has disadvantages in that it requires the availability of a trained anaesthetist and is accompanied by rare but potentially major complica-

---

CONTRA-INDICATIONS TO EPIDURAL ANAESTHESIA

Maternal refusal
Bleeding diathesis
Anatomical abnormalities
Hypovolaemia
Cardiac disease
Neurological disease
Sepsis

Figure SC.3

tions. Epidural analgesia comes into its own in long or complicated labours, malpresentations (such as occipito-posterior position or breech) and pre eclampsia where control of the blood pressure and improvements in placental blood flow are vital to the well being of both mother and foetus. Indications for epidural analgesia are numerous, contra-indications are listed in Figure SC.3.

CONTRA-INDICATIONS TO EPIDURAL ANALGESIA

1) Maternal refusal

   The only absolute contra-indication to the technique. If after, reasonable explanation of the risks and benefits, the patient refuses then to continue constitutes assault. On this basis there is no need for written consent to epidurals in labour; first, a woman in labour is in pain and distressed and cannot, under those circumstances, be expected to make a balanced judgement and, second, if the basis of the service is **request**, then the fact that the patient, via her midwife, asks for this method of analgesia can be taken as verbal consent. This has not been tested in court. The available methods of analgesia should have been explained in antenatal classes and the patient should, therefore, be able to make an informed choice without lengthy explanation during labour.

2) Bleeding diathesis

   There is controversy about the provision of epidural and spinal blockade in patients with a bleeding tendency, whether this is congenital, such as haemophilia, or acquired, such as warfarinisation. It is generally accepted that any patient whose clotting times are more than 50% extended should probably not have an epidural (in practice this means an INR > 1.5). The potential problem is the vulnerability of the epidural venous plexus and concern that if an epidural vein is punctured there will be an uncontrolled bleed from it, causing an haematoma, which could compress the spinal cord. While this sequence of events is certainly possible, it is also exceptionally rare and occurs with the same incidence as spontaneous epidural haematoma.

The suitability of epidural analgesia for patients taking low dose heparin or aspirin is also controversial. Aspirin causes a permanent block of platelet thromboxane A2 which affects any platelets in the circulation at the time the aspirin is administered. This continues for the life of any individual platelet, roughly 10 days from new. While this may appear to be a contra-indication to epidural puncture with its attendant risk of haemorrhage, the effect is quite limited because new, unaffected platelets are being produced continually. The best indicator of platelet function is the bleeding time, which suffers from poor reproducibility and a wide normal range. The ESRA guidelines on epidural use and anticoagulation are given on page 134.

In obstetric anaesthesia there are a number of other causes of acquired clotting failure which may contra-indicate epidural puncture. Pre-eclampsia is associated with deranged clotting function particularly if severe or late in pregnancy. The platelet count will give an indication of the severity of the problem before it becomes clinically important. The **HELLP** syndrome is a variant of pre eclampsia (**H**aemolytic anaemia, **E**levated **L**iver enzymes and **L**ow **P**latelets). This condition is highly dangerous and causes extreme physiological upsets which can only be restored using the full facilities of an intensive care unit and haematological support. The pronounced coagulopathy that occurs in HELLP syndrome is a contra-indication to epidural analgesia.

Intra-uterine foetal death causes a failure of clotting as the foetus begins to macerate and breakdown products enter the maternal circulation. The process does not become significant until the foetus has been dead for more than about 5 days but it is usual to measure clotting in this situation before an epidural is sited.

Placental abruption and other significant intra-uterine bleeds may cause clotting failure secondary to the consumption of clotting factors in a vain attempt to stop bleeding from the spiral arteries. The spiral arteries pass through the myometrium to the placental bed and are usually closed off by uterine contraction after delivery. If the uterus is kept open by the presence of a foetus, blood clots or placental remnants the bleeding will continue until the uterus is emptied or the patient exsanguinates. The blood loss may not be seen as vaginal bleeding because it can remain concealed entirely within the uterus.

Amniotic fluid embolus causes a syndrome similar to major fat embolism with clouding of consciousness, petechial haemorrhages, respiratory distress, hypotension and severe disseminated intravascular coagulation (DIC). This condition is rare but often fatal. Management consists of general supportive therapy and replacement of clotting factors and blood.

3) Anatomical abnormalities
Previous back surgery or spina bifida are relative contra-indications to epidural analgesia because of difficulty in identifying bony landmarks. If the patient has had a lumbar laminectomy or spinal fusion then it is wise to check the level of surgery from previous notes or X-rays so that a level can be chosen for the puncture which has bony landmarks and avoids scar tissue or implanted metal. In spina bifida occulta, the landmarks are missing congenitally but the epidural space is relatively normal. The ligamentum flavum may, however, be absent. In the more severe forms of neural tube defect the epidural space and dural tube may be abnormal and so the situation is more complicated. None of the above situations is an absolute contra-indication to epidural analgesia but the technique may be difficult or impossible, the spread of local anaesthetic in the epidural space may not be normal and the resulting pattern of block may be patchy or deficient.

4) Hypovolaemia
Hypovolaemia must be corrected before any form of anaesthesia or analgesia, unless the situation is so dire that immediate surgery is the only way to reduce massive blood loss, in which case general anaesthesia will be indicated. In this situation, as with any hypovolaemic patient, induction must be carried out with extreme care. Sympathetic blockade caused by epidural or spinal anaesthesia in a hypovolaemic patient can have catastrophic consequences.

5) Cardiac disease
Cardiac disease is often taken as a contra-indication to central neural blockade. In general, the effects of epidural anaesthesia are falls in both cardiac pre load and afterload, which can be controlled by the gentle administration of local anaesthetic agents and by judicious use of fluids and vasoconstrictors. Pregnancy itself carries such major vascular and cardiac changes that it is difficult to reach term unless there are reasonable cardiac reserves. Unfortunately, more and more patients with

congenital cardiac disease, whether corrected or not, are being brought to term. In addition, the age of onset of major coronary artery disease is now falling within the childbearing years. These patients may be on the verge of major cardiac decompensation by the time they reach term. Each woman must be considered on her merits.

6) Neurological disease

Chronic neurological disease is often quoted as a contra-indication to local or regional anaesthesia without evidence to confirm this view. Most of the chronic neurological disorders, such as multiple sclerosis follow a relapsing and remitting course, usually deteriorating at times of physical or mental stress and following a slow progression downward. If at the time of childbirth (one of the stressful times likely to cause relapse) central nerve block is provided for analgesia or anaesthesia then it is likely that the relapse will be blamed on the technique, regardless of whether it is in fact to blame. Provided that this is explained and accepted by the patient there is no reason why this form of analgesia should be withheld.

7) Sepsis

Sepsis at the proposed site of puncture is a contra-indication to epidural anaesthesia but there is usually a non infected space available close by which can be used. Maternal pyrexia, however, should be taken as a contra-indication because of the risk of blood-borne infection with a foreign body, the epidural catheter, in situ or a potential haematoma from epidural vein puncture providing an infective focus. Epidural analgesia limits maternal thermoregulation, and foetal death rate increases dramatically in maternal pyrexia, thus it may be preferable to avoid the use of epidural anaesthesia in this situation.

EPIDURAL TECHNIQUE

Detailed knowledge of the relevant anatomy is essential. See Figure SC.4 and Section 1, Chapter 7.

The epidural space is a potential space within the spinal canal. It is broadly triangular in shape with the apex posteriorly. The shape varies considerably from level to level, being more oval in the neck. Superiorly it is closed at the foramen magnum where the spinal dura mater and the periosteum of the spinal canal fuse to form the intracranial dura mater. It is, therefore, impossible for a true epidural injection to extend intracranially. Inferiorly, the epidural space is closed at the sacrococcygeal ligament. The anterior boundary lies within the spinal canal being formed by the posterior longitudinal ligaments of the spinal column, the vertebral bodies and the intervertebral discs. Posteriorly the space is bounded by the ligamenta flava (these may be paired at each level or one pair of continuous ligaments – opinion varies) and the vertebral laminae. There may be a plane of cleavage between the ligamenta flava that can give an impression that there is no ligament when a needle passes through it. Laterally the epidural space is bounded by the pedicles and laminae of the vertebrae and by the intervertebral foraminae, thus, it is not a closed space laterally. Interiorly the space contains the spinal dural sac and its contents; the spinal cord and nerve roots. The epidural space itself contains fat, arterioles, a complex of thin walled valveless veins which drain into the azygos system, lymphatics and the spinal nerve roots after they cross the dura and before they exit through the intervertebral foraminae. The nerve roots carry with them a cuff of dura that may extend out into the paravertebral space.

To reach the epidural space from the skin of the back, the tip of the needle must pass through successive layers of tissue. The bones over the lumbar area are palpated and the spaces between spinous processes

---

ANATOMY OF THE EPIDURAL SPACE

Boundaries	Superior	Closed at foramen magnum
	Inferior	Closed at sacrococcygeal membrane
	Anterior	Posterior longitudinal ligaments, vertebral bodies
	Posterior	Vertebral laminae, ligamenta flava
	Lateral	Open, pedicles and intervertebral foraminae
Shape		Broadly triangular, apex posteriorly
Contents		Veins, arteries, fat, lympathics, nerve roots and dural cuffs

Figure SC.4

identified. Once a suitable space has been identified (L2/3 is usually the easiest and most consistent to use) the needle is inserted through the skin staying strictly on the midline, although a deliberate paramedian approach is acceptable. The first ligament encountered is the supraspinous ligament. This has a 'crunchy' consistency and is up to 1 cm thick. The interspinous ligament feels 'spongy' and can be up to 6 cm thick. The ligamentum flavum is very variable in thickness up to 2 cm but is usually tough and difficult to penetrate. The essence of the technique is that with the needle tip in the ligamentum flavum, nothing can be injected through the needle whereas after careful advancement, the tip will emerge into the epidural space and there will be a sudden total loss of resistance to injection.

COMBINED SPINAL —EPIDURAL IN LABOUR

Combined spinal-epidural techniques may be used for analgesia in labour. An epidural needle is sited in the epidural space and a longer small-gauge spinal needle is then passed through it. A small dose of a mixture of bupivacaine and fentanyl is injected through the spinal needle which is then withdrawn and an epidural catheter passed through the epidural needle. The spinal solution establishes analgesia for the early part of the first stage of labour and, when this analgesia becomes inadequate, the epidural catheter is used for further doses. The patient is allowed some mobility while the spinal solution is effective but this may be limited by the need for continuous monitoring of the fetus. Each unit must have written policies to establish the limits to mobility in labour.

TEST DOSES

It is impossible to be absolutely sure of the correct placement of an epidural catheter until a dose of local anaesthetic agent has been injected. A test dose serves two purposes, first to identify vascular placement and, second, to identify intrathecal placement. To achieve this, a test dose must be small enough to do no harm if in the wrong place but large enough to show an effect. Most practitioners use a 3 ml dose of either 0.5% or 0.25% plain bupivacaine. There are advocates for both epinephrine containing and dextrose containing test-doses but neither is in popular use.

In practice, 3 ml plain isobaric bupivacaine, placed directly into the CSF, will produce total spinal anaesthesia within 5 min. Hyperbaric bupivacaine (Heavy Marcain®) will have a less extensive result and if placed intravenously there will be no noticeable effect. Larger volumes of local anaesthetic agent injected into the lumbar epidural venous plexus tend to pass backwards up the basilar vessels and cause a short-lived loss of consciousness or at least a period of light-headedness with lingual and circumoral paraesthesia. The rationale behind using an epinephrine containing solution is that, on intravenous injection, there will be a measurable increase in heart rate. While this may be so, the increase so caused will be within the pulse rate variation of any woman in labour and so may not be distinguished from normal.

Having given the test dose and waited an appropriate time for an effect to appear, usually 5 minutes, the main dose may to be given. Traditionally the choice is 0.25% or 0.5% plain bupivacaine by bolus top ups of between 6 and 10 ml as necessary to relieve the pain. The top ups may be given either all in one position, usually semi-reclining or half of the dose given in each lateral position with 5 minutes between. This method, while still in widespread use, is being superseded by a variety of low-dose infusion techniques that have the advantage of both reducing the drug load and reducing the unwanted effects of the traditional epidural such as high-density motor block and the increased incidence of instrumental delivery.

The majority of infusion epidurals begin with a single top up to rapidly establish the analgesia before commencing the infusion. Increasingly, the local anaesthetic agent in the top up is supplemented by small doses of an opioid (such as fentanyl). The combination appears to increase both the analgesia and the penetration of the block without any obvious drawbacks. Recent evidence suggests that there are no measurable foetal effects of the opioid at doses in current use. Infusion regimes vary considerably but most are based on either 0.1% bupivacaine or 0.2% ropivacaine, each with between 1 and 5 mcg per ml of fentanyl. Each unit should have a single standard mixture with which all anaesthetists and midwives should be familiar. This mixture is infused at a variable rate up to 15 ml per hour, though occasionally this mixture is given by bolus top-up rather than infusion.

Patient controlled epidural analgesia (PCEA) is gaining popularity slowly either as patient administered boluses alone or patient administered boluses to supplement a background infusion.

COMPLICATIONS

Epidural anaesthesia carries a risk of complications, the more major of which are listed below in Figure SC.5.

1) Dural tap
   Dural tap occurs in about 0.5% of obstetric

COMPLICATIONS OF EPIDURAL ANALGESIA

Dural tap
Intrathecal injection
Intravascular injection
Neurological
Backache
Pressure areas

Figure SC.5

epidurals. Once recognised, the management is straightforward. A working epidural must be established in another space. There should be no bearing down in the second stage of labour and there should be an elective forceps delivery. After delivery an epidural infusion should be set up with 0.9% saline or Hartmann's solution, and 1 litre infused over 24 hours. The patient should be reviewed daily by a senior member of staff. If the patient develops a postural occipito-frontal headache then this should initially be treated by encouraging oral fluids and by simple analgesia. Ibuprofen in regular doses is often effective. If the headache becomes incapacitating, an epidural blood patch should be offered. If accepted, this should be carried out with the minimum of delay. Infection or pyrexia will contra-indicate the technique. Under aseptic conditions a new epidural puncture is carried out and up to 20 ml of the patient's blood is injected into the epidural space. Further blood is sent for culture. To reduce the already small risk of epidural infection, some units advocate the systemic administration of a broad spectrum antibiotic before the blood is taken. Blood patch is usually successful in alleviating the headache.

2) Intravascular injection
While proper use of test doses will identify intrathecal and intravascular injections at that stage, epidural catheters can migrate into vessels or across the dura at any stage during the conduct of the technique and the full dose of local anaesthetic may be inadvertently injected into the circulation. For this reason full resuscitation facilities should be immediately available at all times and all staff involved, both anaesthetists and midwives, should be prepared for this eventuality.

Injection of local anaesthetic into the epidural veins may only cause paraesthesia of the tongue and lips but can also cause sudden loss of consciousness as the local anaesthetic agent affects the brain. The effect is usually temporary but in the case of bupivacaine, may be prolonged. The airway and respiration must be adequately maintained, tracheal intubation and controlled ventilation may be necessary. Once this has been achieved the circulation must be supported by fluids, vasopressors and cardiac massage if appropriate.

3) Intrathecal injection
The effects of intrathecal injection may be slower in onset but no less of a problem than intravascular injection. Progressive rising paralysis of the whole body, including the muscles of respiration, occurs accompanied by significant falls in blood pressure. The feature which distinguishes intrathecal injection from massive epidural is the onset of cranial nerve effects, particularly facial paralysis, trigeminal anaesthesia and rapid loss of consciousness. As with intravenous injection, the airway must be addressed first followed by the circulation, as detailed above.

These rare but major problems are the reason for direct observation of the patient for twenty minutes after an epidural injection or top up.

4) Neurological complications
Neurological complications of epidural analgesia are extremely rare and usually relate to cauda equina syndrome if there has been local neural toxicity by either too high a concentration of epinephrine in the injected drug or, more likely, the wrong drug administered. The majority of neurological complications following childbirth are related not to epidurals but to the management of labour, particularly where a large foetus has become obstructed in the second stage of labour for a prolonged time. This scenario results in compression of the roots and trunks of the lumbo-sacral plexus within the pelvis, especially L1 as it passes over the brim of the true pelvis. The most common defects subsequently are foot drop (lateral peroneal nerve), sciatic palsies or femoral nerve palsies.

5) Backache
Epidural analgesia in labour has developed a reputation for causing low grade but persistent backache after delivery which is probably related not to epidural analgesia itself but to the management of the back in labour. In the absence of pain sensation, proprioception and muscle tone to protect the joints and ligaments of the back there is a possibility of musculo-skeletal strain.

6) Pressure sores

Pressure sores are not usually associated with young women but the lack of sensation and motor block provided by epidural analgesia prevent the patient moving during labour. Patients should be encouraged to move regularly to prevent pressure sores developing, particularly over the sacrum.

OPERATIVE ANAESTHESIA

Anaesthesia for operative surgery in obstetrics falls into two main areas. First, operative delivery, for example Caesarean section (the most common) and forceps procedures. Second, post delivery procedures such as retained placenta. Both groups are amenable to being carried out under regional or general anaesthesia. In the case of retained placenta, it is essential before considering a regional technique (such as spinal anaesthesia) which removes sympathetic tone and causes profound vasodilatation, to accurately assess blood loss and restore circulating volume.

Regional anaesthesia

Central neural blockade for operative obstetric anaesthesia requires a different approach to the provision of analgesia in labour. In labour the only essential feature is analgesia – motor block is a distinct disadvantage. For obstetric surgery, including forceps delivery, removal of retained placenta and Caesarean section, complete anaesthesia of the relevant area is necessary. In labour, the highest dermatome required is T10 whereas for Caesarean section the upper limit needs to be a minimum of T6, though there is still some debate about whether it should be even higher than this to adequately cover the variable innervation of the peritoneum. The dose of local anaesthetic agent necessary to achieve this at term is only about two-thirds of that required in the non pregnant patient for a comparable result.

For obstetric surgery an epidural catheter is inserted in the usual way and, after a test dose, a main dose of local anaesthetic agent is given. This may be given as one dose or in divided doses. The local anaesthetic agent of choice should ensure rapid onset of an intense block with a duration of action in excess of 1 H. Bupivacaine 0.5% up to 30 ml (with or without adrenaline) or 20 ml 2% lidocaine with epinephrine usually produce satisfactory blockade.

Spinal anaesthesia for obstetrics offers advantages over epidural anaesthesia because of speed of onset and intensity of block but disadvantages because of severity and speed of onset of hypotension and the less adjustable nature of the technique. The major disadvantage of spinal anaesthesia in obstetric anaesthesia has always been the incidence of post dural puncture headache (PDPH). This has been significantly reduced by the use of solid-tipped needles with side holes such as the Sprotte and Whitacre point needles. The only spinal solutions with current product licences are 0.5% hyperbaric bupivacaine and 0.5% plain levobupivacaine. This latter solution is slightly hypobaric. Hyperbaric solutions of 0.5% ropivacaine are being investigated with a view to commercial availability.

The prevention and management of hypotension as a result of central neural blockade falls into two areas: volume loading and vasopressors. Volume loading before the administration of the block requires administration of 500–1000 ml of crystalloid solution or 500 ml colloid solution. Traditionally ephedrine has also been used in small intravenous doses (3 mg) to correct hypotension. Ephedrine crosses the placental barrier and may, thus, cause a foetal tachycardia.

In the pre-operative period the patient should be warned that regional anaesthesia may not give total loss of sensation but that general anaesthesia can be offered if necessary. This is an increasing field of complaint and litigation.

There is increasing use of combined spinal - epidural anaesthesia for operative delivery. This provides the speed of onset and intensity of spinal anaesthesia with the adjustability and duration of epidural anaesthesia.

General anaesthesia

Obstetric general anaesthesia is usually considered to be one of the higher risk specialities of anaesthesia because of the potential for urgency, uncontrolled bleeding and inhalation of gastric contents. In fact, as a cause of maternal mortality, anaesthesia ranks very low, on a par with amniotic fluid embolism and ruptured thoracic aneurysm. This low mortality is not a reason for complacency but a result of sustained work in eliminating the main causes of anaesthetic-related problems by intensive training in managing difficult intubation, and universal antacid prophylaxis.

As a rule of thumb, there is no such thing as a pregnant woman with an empty stomach. The gastric contents also tend to be more acid than in the non pregnant woman. Progesterone induced relaxation of the lower oesophageal sphincter, along with the higher intra-abdominal pressure in late pregnancy all tend to encourage the regurgitation and aspiration of gastric contents into the trachea. While Mendelson actually described obstruction to respiration by solid matter, the aspiration of liquid and the resulting chemical pneumonitis are usually called Mendelson's syndrome. Acid aspiration in pregnancy causes a gross chemical pneumonitis, which distinguishes it from the aspiration pneumonia of the non pregnant. Routine antacid prophylaxis in the delivery suite reduces both the volume and acidity of gastric contents. Common regimes involve administration of regular oral H_2 receptor antagonists to all admissions to the delivery suite and 0.3 molar sodium citrate solution when a decision is made to proceed to surgery. Variations on this theme include the administration of intravenous ranitidine and metoclopramide, this latter to encourage gastric emptying, although this effect is difficult to show and variable. Magnesium trisilicate mixture is little used now because it is particulate and does not mix well with gastric contents.

In the second and third trimesters of pregnancy tracheal intubation is considered mandatory because of the potential for acid aspiration. For the same reasons rapid sequence induction (RSI) with cricoid pressure is also necessary. The hormonal changes of pregnancy, as pertaining to intestinal function, remain for some 48 H post partum and so it is wise to apply RSI for up to a week after delivery. The standard general anaesthetic technique involves a wedge under the right buttock to displace the uterus from the inferior vena cava, rapid sequence induction with thiopentone and suxamethonium (propofol has no licence for use in late pregnancy). Tracheal intubation should be followed by controlled ventilation of the lungs with 50–70% nitrous oxide and a volatile agent of choice. Suitable muscle relaxants include atracurium and vecuronium. Mivacurium should be used with care due to the reduced activity of plasma cholinesterase in late pregnancy which may delay its offset. At the end of the procedure the tracheal tube should be removed with the patient in the lateral position, head down. Extubation should only be considered after the return of protective reflexes.

Tracheal intubation in the pregnant woman can be notoriously difficult. The anatomy of the chest changes in pregnancy with an increase in functional residual capacity (FRC) giving an impression of hyperinflation. This is combined with an increase in the size of the breasts and an apparent shortening of the neck (because of the increase in FRC). Note that the majority of pregnant women have a full set of natural teeth.

Pre-eclampsia may cause laryngeal oedema and it is now recognised that the Malampatti score may change as labour progresses, causing further difficulties. Endotracheal tube size should be reduced in expectation of difficulty. While the laryngeal mask does not provide sufficient barrier to gastric contents for routine use, in a case of difficult tracheal intubation, it may have a role (See Section 1 Chapter 2).

Equipment for the management of difficult intubation must be available at all times and within arms reach whenever obstetric anaesthesia is practised. Desirable equipment includes a range of laryngoscope blades and handles, including a polio blade, a variety of tube sizes down to 6.0 mm and stylets and bougies to aid intubation. Where death has occurred after difficult or failed intubation the cause has not been the failure to intubate but the failure to oxygenate the patient between attempts. **This point cannot be emphasised enough**.

Accidental awareness is more commonly encountered in obstetric general anaesthesia than any other specialty. The causes are usually failure to introduce sufficiently high concentrations of vapour sufficiently early, before the brain concentration of the induction agent begins to fall, or failure to maintain sufficiently high concentrations of vapour and nitrous oxide throughout the procedure.

WHEN TO CONSIDER A PATIENT PREGNANT

As a general rule, the risks of acid aspiration begin to outweigh the risks of tracheal intubation at about 16 weeks gestation and from this time onwards the patient should be considered as an obstetric problem. The hormonal changes of pregnancy fade rapidly after delivery, along with the effects on gastric function and so it is probably safe to revert to non pregnancy anaesthetic techniques at about 1 week post partum.

THE PAEDIATRIC PATIENT

For the purposes of this volume only those children of 20 kg in weight or greater will be considered. In practice, this will usually equate with an age of about five years.

ASSESSMENT

Pre-operative assessment in children should be as rigorous as in adults and questions should be addressed to the child even though the parents may answer for them. Most children are healthy but chronic conditions such as asthma, multiple allergies, congenital heart disease and systemic conditions (such as muscular dystrophy) may also be encountered. The presence of one congenital abnormality should stimulate the search for others. Chromosomal abnormalities may be linked particularly with congenital heart disease. Except for true emergency surgery, children with colds or upper respiratory tract infections should have their surgery cancelled and rescheduled to a later date. The inflamed airway is exquisitely sensitive to any kind of manipulation, resulting in laryngeal spasm. Laryngeal spasm in children is particularly dangerous because of the rapid onset of severe desaturation, made more marked by their higher metabolic rate.

There is no universally good premedicant for children, trimeprazine makes many children irritable and uncontrollable in an unpredictable way and the injectable premedicants are probably better avoided because of the distress caused by the injection. Day case admission can result in insufficient time for anxiolytic premedication to have effect (and the use of sedatives in day surgery may be undesirable). All children should have topical local anaesthetic cream or gel applied to the proposed venepuncture site at least 1 hour before anaesthesia. Drug doses in children should always be calculated on a weight-related basis, a calculation which will give an approximation of the required dose. If dilution of a drug is proposed then each syringe should be labelled with the drug name and concentration. Ambiguity must be avoided at all costs.

EQUIPMENT

Anaesthetic equipment for patients under 20 kg body weight is quite specialised and there is no gradation to adult equipment. For all paediatric patients the breathing system dead space and resistance should be kept to a minimum by avoiding catheter mounts, angle pieces and valves. Controlled ventilation may be preferable because of the inevitable increase in dead space after induction of anaesthesia and the increased work of breathing. The Mapleson E or F system is preferable for patients less than 20 kg but can also be used for heavier patients if the volume of the expiratory limb is more than the calculated tidal volume and the fresh gas flow for spontaneous ventilation is more than 2.5 times minute volume. Tidal volume approximates to 8 ml/kg in the child and a respiratory rate of about 20 per minute is usual. If ventilation is to be controlled then a minute volume divider type of ventilator should only be used for tidal volume settings greater than 300 ml. The reason for this is that below this the ventilator becomes inaccurate in delivery due to the higher proportion of compressible volume related to total tidal volume. For required tidal volumes less than 300 ml either a 'T piece occluder' type system

should be used or a Mapleson D with a ventilator such as the Nuffield Anaesthesia Ventilator Series 200.

If tracheal intubation is proposed then account should be taken of the increased resistance to breathing that this introduces. The resistance to flow in a tube is inversely related to the fourth power of the radius and so halving the diameter will increase resistance by 16 times. Any tracheal tube will have a smaller internal diameter than the natural airway, particularly if the tube is cuffed. Unless there is a risk of tracheal soiling uncuffed tubes are preferable because of the larger internal diameter that this allows. The anatomy of the child larynx is different from the adult (Figure SC.6). In consequence, the use of cuffed tubes in the < 10 age group renders the subglottic region vulnerable to oedema particularly if an overly large tube is introduced with force. Even small amounts of secretion in a tracheal tube will significantly increase the resistance to gas flow.

FLUID THERAPY

Intravenous fluids in children should be given via a burette giving set or a volume controlled pump and should always

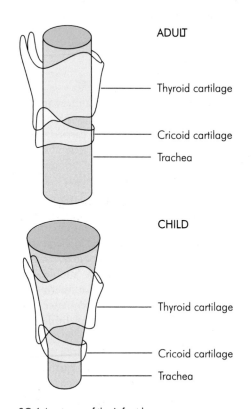

Figure SC.6 Anatomy of the infant larynx

be calculated on a weight related basis. A minimum of 2 ml/kg/H should be given to those not receiving oral fluids. Blood replacement can be very difficult to calculate and is based on replacing loss for loss when 10% blood volume has been spilt. Losses are assessed by swab weighing and accurate suction measurement. Blood volume may be estimated as 80 ml/kg in small children falling to 70 ml/kg in adults. Blood loss of 8 ml/kg will, therefore, need replacing during surgery.

ANALGESIA

Post operative analgesia should not be withheld because the dose calculations are inconvenient. Much of the surgery carried out on children lends itself very well to regional anaesthesia when used to supplement light general anaesthesia and this method provides very high quality early post operative analgesia. Although intramuscular opioids remain popular, there are many other routes of administration for analgesic drugs. Most children over six years of age can use PCA to advantage using skills learned at computer controls. Subcutaneous infusions of opioids may be useful and oral preparations (such as Oromorph®) should not be forgotten. Rectal administration of non steroidal agents (such as diclofenac) is rapidly gaining ground.

SPECIALIST SURGERY

General and urological surgery

Elective general and urological surgery in childhood tends to be restricted to herniotomy, orchidopexy and circumcision, all of which can be carried out on a day case basis with a combination of general and regional anaesthesia. Appendicectomy is another frequent operation in children and is always an inpatient (emergency or urgent) procedure. Groin incisions can be covered very well by inguinal field blockade while penile block is particularly good for circumcision. In contrast, the more widespread and bilateral anaesthesia of a caudal block may restrict mobility, particularly in larger children. Oral analgesia should be given before the effect of the local anaesthetic wears off. For appendicectomy, a rapid sequence induction technique should be used. Wound infiltration with local anaesthetic provides some post operative pain relief. While some of these children are relatively well, others are pyrexial and toxic, particularly if the diagnosis is made late. These latter need to be managed very carefully and their state of hydration properly assessed and corrected in the pre-operative period.

Orthopaedic surgery

Much of the orthopaedic surgery in this age group is the result of trauma. A full skeletal survey should be carried out so that other injuries are not missed, particularly head injuries and cervical spine injuries. Blood loss and analgesia requirements should receive particular attention before anaesthesia. After trauma, patients are usually assumed to have a full stomach and should be managed as such with pre-oxygenation and rapid sequence induction techniques. Post operative analgesia for fractures and soft tissue injuries is best provided by regional anaesthesia, although there is some debate about the development of compartment syndrome being masked if there are forearm or lower leg fractures. Elective orthopaedic procedures in children aged five years and over differ little in their anaesthesia requirements from adults.

ENT and dental surgery

The core of both ENT and dental anaesthesia is the problem of the shared airway. In both types of surgery the anaesthetist and the surgeon need good access to a clear airway kept free of debris and blood. This has resulted in the development of special equipment and techniques for this situation.

In the main, dental surgery in children is restricted to simple exodontia. Historically the main indication was caries but with improvements in dental hygiene and fluoridation of water the reason has changed but the procedure has not. Currently children lose teeth not because of caries but because of crowding within the mouth. Until the conclusions of the Poswillow report (Poswillow 1990) were applied, this procedure tended to be carried out in general dental surgeries with little or no monitoring equipment and minimal facilities. The report concluded that whenever and wherever dental anaesthesia were carried out the equipment and monitoring should be to the same standard as in the best equipped hospital operating theatres. Consequently, dental extraction under general anaesthesia is now carried out in very few practices, all of which are licensed and carry the full range of monitoring and resuscitation equipment.

Unless there are medical reasons for inpatient surgery, dental extraction is always carried out on a 'walk in, walk out' basis. The day case rules should be applied rigidly. Pre-operative assessment is carried out as usual, with particular reference to fasting and respiratory conditions (such as asthma). There is little opportunity for pre-operative investigation or correction of abnormalities. Induction of anaesthesia may be intravenous or inhalational, but venous access should be obtained in all cases. Care should be taken with intravenous drugs because of the risks of unrecognised fainting on induction, leading to hypotension and cerebral vascular insufficiency. Propofol has too great a potential for cardiovascular depression to be used regularly in the dental chair. Thiopentone is more appropriate. Inhalational induction is well tolerated in children, particularly if halothane (or the newer agent, sevoflurane) is used and a good rapport is obtained between anaesthetist and patient. The standard method involves 30–40% oxygen in nitrous oxide with up to 2% halothane introduced via a nasal mask. Once the mouth can be opened without resistance a pack is inserted by the surgeon which should separate the mouth from the pharynx. The teeth are then removed. The anaesthetist must maintain the airway, ensure oxygenation and anaesthesia and monitor the patient. Once the teeth have been removed and the mouth cleared of debris the inhaled anaesthetic agents are turned off and 100% oxygen administered until the child is awake. Recovery should be in the lateral position so that blood and debris are not inhaled. Debate has continued about whether the sitting or the supine position is better or safer. The supine position avoids unrecognised major falls in blood pressure but encourages regurgitation whereas the sitting position discourages regurgitation but increases the likelihood of unrecognised fainting on induction.

The majority of older children will accept dental extraction with local anaesthesia but if extractions are proposed in more than two quadrants of the mouth then it is unwise to do this all at one sitting because of the inevitable risk of total anaesthesia of the tongue and palate leading to obstruction or aspiration.

General anaesthesia may be necessary for conservative dentistry in those with severe learning difficulties. This may be a prolonged procedure involving multiple restorations and should be carried out with the airway protected by either an endotracheal tube or a laryngeal mask and an absorbent pack in place. Dental drills have an incorporated water spray, which can precipitate laryngeal spasm in the unprotected airway.

ENT surgery requires a shared airway, typical procedures being tonsillectomy and adenoidectomy, where the surgeon is both operating in the airway and causing bleeding from it! Adenoidectomy in isolation requires the airway to be maintained via the mouth, either by tracheal tube or laryngeal mask. Suction clearance of the mouth at the end of the procedure should be carried out under direct vision. Tonsillectomy in isolation may be carried out using either a naso-tracheal tube or, as suggested recently a laryngeal mask airway, although this remains contro-

versial against securing the airway with endotracheal intubation (oral or nasal). Suction at the end must again be carried out under direct vision but gently so as not to disturb the tonsillar bed. In both of these cases post operative analgesia should be provided parenterally before the recovery phase. There are advocates of both spontaneous and controlled ventilation for these procedures. Anaesthesia for myringotomy or suction clearance of the ears can be relatively simple, intravenous or inhalational induction with facemask or laryngeal mask for airway maintenance.

Ophthalmic surgery

Ophthalmic surgery in the over five's is usually for squint surgery or penetrating eye injury, probing and syringing of lachrymal ducts being confined to younger children.

Squint surgery is usually carried out as a day case, though the facility for overnight stay should always be available. Pre-operative assessment should be as rigorous as for any other form of surgery. Induction of anaesthesia should include a weight related dose of a vagolytic drug such as glycopyrrolate to prevent the severe bradycardia which results from even gentle traction on the extra-ocular muscles. Induction may be by the inhaled or intravenous route. Squint correction causes the same airway access problems for the anaesthetist as other head and neck surgery. The choice of tracheal intubation or laryngeal mask airway is largely a matter of personal preference, though tracheal tubes cause much more emergence laryngospasm than do laryngeal mask airways. Ventilation may be controlled or spontaneous. Post operative analgesia may be by provided by topical local anaesthetic agents, systemic opioids or NSAIDs.

THE HEAD INJURED PATIENT

APPLIED PHYSIOLOGY

The skull is a closed box containing brain tissue, extracellular fluid, CSF and blood. In the presence of space-occupying lesions, either tumour, blood clot or oedema, for example, the fixed volume of contents increases at the expense of the rest. Early in the disease process, when the incremental change in volume is still small, any sudden increase in pressure can be compensated for by changes in CSF or blood volume, cushioning the effect of the insult. Later, in the presence of a larger space-occupying lesion the compliance of the intracranial contents is reduced and so the pressure change is unbuffered and there may be

FACTORS AFFECTING CEREBRAL BLOOD FLOW

Arterial PCO_2
Arterial PO_2
Cerebral perfusion pressure
Intracranial pressure
Temperature
Drugs

Figure SC.7

damage to tissue either directly, by distortion of nerve tracts or by secondary reductions in blood flow.

In the normal (uninjured) brain cerebral blood flow (CBF) is affected by several factors. These are listed in Figure SC.7.

Arterial PCO_2

A relatively linear response exists between $PaCO_2$ values of 2.6 and 10.7 kPa. At the lower end of this range CBF will be half normal and correspondingly double at the higher end. Reduced $PaCO_2$ decreases both cerebral blood flow and intracranial pressure (ICP), mediated by CSF pH. After a step change in $PaCO_2$, the CSF bicarbonate concentration returns to normal over the next 24 H and the ICP and CBF return to normal even if the change in $PaCO_2$ is maintained. Hyperventilation can, therefore, only be used in the short term to reduce ICP.

Arterial PO_2

A small increase in CBF occurs with the administration of 100% oxygen. Hypoxia on the other hand, if severe, (PO_2 less than 6 kPa) will result in greatly increased CBF.

Cerebral perfusion pressure

Cerebral perfusion pressure (CPP) is calculated as the mean arterial pressure minus (ICP + CVP). Autoregulation maintains steady CBF between CPP values of 50–150 mmHg.

Intracranial pressure

Raised ICP will obviously reduce CBF and similarly raised venous pressure secondarily raises ICP with the same net result. Sudden rises in venous pressure during coughing or straining may cause serious falls in CBF, putting cerebral perfusion at risk in the compromised brain.

Temperature

Hypothermia reduces both CBF and the cerebral metabolic rate for oxygen. Similarly, rises in temperature increase CBF and oxygen consumption.

Drugs

The anaesthetic induction agents, with the exception of ketamine reduce CBF and cerebral metabolism. Ketamine and the inhalational agents cause rises in CBF via a vasodilator effect, with consequent increases in ICP. This can be mitigated to some extent by hyperventilation.

Management of head injury

Head injury should be considered significant if there has been certain loss of consciousness (however brief). Blood or CSF in the ear canal or nose imply skull fracture with the accompanying risk of meningitis due to the ingress of pathogens. In closed head injury, even of a relatively minor nature, there is a variable amount of oedema and cerebral contusion which increases the volume of the intracranial contents, displacing both CSF and blood volume and reducing compliance. Extra- and subdural haematomata also behave as large space-occupying lesions causing compression and distortion of the brain. Functional disabilities may be seen at an early stage. These include unsteadiness of gait, disorientation, irritability, nausea and vomiting. As the oedema or space occupation increases or becomes more widespread, the compliance is reduced further and cerebral blood flow is compromised causing hypoxic damage to brain tissue. Cerebral blood flow depends on the cerebral perfusion pressure, which in turn depends on the relationship between mean arterial blood pressure and intracranial pressure. As intracranial pressure increases so CBF falls. The standard international assessment of cerebral function is the Glasgow Coma Scale (GCS), see Figure SC.8. This is a very useful indicator but should not be taken in isolation. The best response in each category gives a maximum score of 14, indicating minimal injury while the minimum score is 3, indicating a very poor state with a very poor outcome. Trends in GCS are more valuable than single estimations.

The crux of immediate management in head injury is to avoid secondary injury. The primary injury has already occurred and any damage done will be largely irreversible. Oedema develops around the injury site and secondary injury must be avoided by reducing ICP (especially avoiding dramatic rises in ICP) and preventing hypoxic damage. The main decision to be made is whether the patient requires tracheal intubation, for control of ICP, surgery to other parts

GLASGOW COMA SCALE

Category	Score
Best performance	
Eye opening	
spontaneous	4
to speech	3
to pain	2
nil	1
Verbal response	
oriented	5
confused	4
inappropriate	3
incomprehensible	2
nil	1
Motor response	
obeying commands	5
localising	4
flexing	3
extending	2
nil	1

Figure SC.8

INDICATIONS FOR INTUBATION AND VENTILATION AFTER HEAD INJURY

Immediately:

- Coma – not obeying commands, not speaking no eye opening i.e. GCS ≤ 8
- Loss of protective laryngeal reflexes
- Ventilatory insufficiency as judged by blood gases hypoxaemia (PaO_2 < 9 kPa on air or < 13 kPa on oxygen) hypercarbia ($PaCO_2$ > 6 kPa)
- Spontaneous hyperventilation causing $PaCO_2$ < 3.5 kPa
- Respiratory arrhythmia

Before the start of a journey:

- Significantly deteriorating conscious level, even if not in coma
- Bilateral fractured mandible
- Copious bleeding into the mouth (e.g. from skull base fracture)
- Seizures

An intubated patient must be ventilated with muscle relaxation, and should receive sedation and analgesia
Aim for a PaO_2 > 13 kPa, $PaCO_2$ 4.0–4.5 kPa

Modified from Gentleman et al BMJ 1993; 307: 547–552

Association of Anaesthetists of Great Britain and Ireland 1996

Figure SC.9

of the body, investigation such as CT scanning or for transport to other facilities. In general, a GCS less than 8 indicates the need for major intervention and intensive care management. In addition to the GCS, the pattern of respiration, pulse and blood pressure should be taken into consideration. Spontaneous hyperventilation indicates significantly raised ICP, as does arterial hypertension accompanied by bradycardia. Control of ICP is of the utmost importance. Uncontrollable confusion and irritability may indicate significant brain injury and indicates the need for intervention. Indications for intubation after head injury are listed in Figure SC.9.

Practical technique

By and large secondary brain injury may be avoided by good oxygenation and airway management and by avoiding rises in ICP, particularly as a result of an unmodified pressor response to intubation. Although it might appear that unconscious patients do not need to be anaesthetised before intubation, this is not so. In this particular situation induction agents are used not primarily for the abolition of consciousness but to reduce ICP before intubation. Intubation without previous pharmacological reduction of ICP or without modification of the pressor response may cause more

damage than the original injury and should be avoided at all costs. The sympatho-adrenal response to intubation may be minimised by the administration of an adequate dose of induction agent accompanied by an opioid agent such as alfentanil. The appropriate muscle relaxant to use for intubation is potentially controversial. Rapid intubation is desirable but suxamethonium can cause a significant rise in ICP. This is certainly the case in the normal brain but recent work suggests that it may not be the case in the injured (and, therefore, less compliant) brain. The rise in ICP may be an effect of the drug itself rather than the fasciculations it causes. The non depolarising relaxants are, therefore, preferable in terms of ICP management but this ignores the fact that many head-injured patients have full stomachs, a soiled airway or are vomiting because of their raised ICP. A possible solution lies in the administration of a large dose of a non depolarising relaxant such as vecuronium, given after careful pre-oxygenation and the application of cricoid pressure. The fasciculations of suxamethonium may be modified or abolished by pre curarization with a small dose of a non depolarising relaxant (such as 20 mg Gallamine) or by pre treatment with 0.1 mg/kg suxamethonium, both of which may inhibit intubating conditions. The risk of aspiration must be carefully weighed against any minor advantage in ICP control.

Subsequently, ventilation of the lungs must be maintained by facemask or laryngeal mask airway until the relaxant reaches maximum clinical effect so as to avoid coughing and movement which will increase the intracranial pressure even more than intubation itself. Once intubation has been safely achieved the pressor response to the presence of the tube must also be modified to control ICP. This can be achieved by adequate sedation or general anaesthesia with controlled ventilation and moderate hyperventilation. Inhalational agents should be avoided because of their cerebral vasodilator effect and anaesthesia maintained by repeated bolus or infusions of intravenous agents. If possible, fluid loading should be restricted or avoided. Excessive crystalloid resuscitation may increase cerebral oedema. Intravenous mannitol (as 10 or 20 g boluses) may reduce cerebral oedema to some extent but should not be given unless a urinary catheter is in situ because the stimulation from a full bladder may increase ICP and also anaesthetic dose requirements.

Monitoring should conform to the accepted minimum monitoring standards and should include non invasive blood pressure, pulse oximetry and end tidal CO_2 analysis. Blood loss from scalp wounds may be significant in itself and should not be forgotten.

Transfer of the head injured patient

Head injured patients and those with suspected intracranial haemorrhage may require transfer between hospitals for either CT scanning or definitive management of their injuries. This can be a difficult and dangerous enterprise and should be carried out with the greatest of care. Facilities in ambulances, helicopters and scanning rooms are limited, as is space, but nevertheless the management of the airway and ICP must take precedence over speed or convenience. The patient must be stabilised before transfer. The escort must be capable of managing the predictable eventualities; re-intubation, hypertension, hypotension and, thus, must take with them sufficient equipment, drugs and fluids to maintain anaesthesia and relaxation. Ambulances should be able to travel quickly but

TRANSFER CHECKLIST FOR NEUROSURGICAL PATIENTS

System	Checklist
Respiration	$PaO_2 > 13$ kPa? $PaCO_2 < 4.5$ kPa? Airway clear? Airway protected adequately? Intubation and ventilation required?
Circulation	BP systolic > 120 mmHg? Pulse < 100/min? Peripheral perfusion? Reliable large IV cannula *in situ*? Estimated blood loss already replaced?
Head injury	GCS? GCS trend? (improving/deteriorating) Focal signs? Skull fracture?
Other injuries	Cervical spine injury, chest injury, fractured ribs, pneumothorax excluded? Intrathoracic, intra-abdominal bleed? Pelvic, long bone fracture? Extracranial injuries splinted?
Escort	Doctor and nurse adequately experienced? Instructed about **this** case? Adequate equipment and drugs? Can use equipment and drugs? Case notes and X-rays? Where to go in the neuro-unit? Telephone numbers programmed into portable phone? Portable phone battery fully charged? Name and bleep number of receiving doctor? Money in case of emergencies?

Modified from Gentleman *et al Lancet* 1990; **335**: 330–334

Association of Anaesthetists of Great Britain and Ireland 1996

Figure SC.10

smoothly without the severe shocks of fast travel. Monitoring should include automatic blood pressure, pulse oximetry and preferably end tidal CO_2 measurement. For CT scanning, there must be appropriate equipment in the scanning room. An anaesthetic machine with automatic ventilator, piped gases and full monitoring are essential. Figure SC.10 gives a useful checklist for transfer of a head injured patient.

THE DAY CASE PATIENT

Day stay surgery implies that the patient's admission to the hospital is scheduled and that admission and discharge are planned for the same day. In practice this usually means that admissions in the morning are discharged at mid day while mid day admissions are discharged in the early evening and the facility then closed overnight.

For the patient, this means that they are away from their work or home environment for the shortest possible time and their social circumstances are disrupted as little as possible.

Anaesthesia and surgery are major insults to the patient's physiology, however minor they may appear, thus there must be rigorous policies and protocols for the day surgery unit with patients carefully selected with regard to fitness and type of surgery.

The criteria to be applied fall into several categories:

SOCIAL CIRCUMSTANCES

The patient's social circumstances must provide a safe environment for the post operative care of a recently anaesthetised patient, even if the procedure was carried out with local anaesthetic or sedation only. For the first 24 H after anaesthesia, there must be a responsible adult present on the premises to care for the patient and to manage untoward events. The patient must be brought to, and taken from, hospital by a responsible adult. They must live within easy travelling distance of the hospital in case of urgent re-admission (this is usually taken as within 30 min travelling time). Patients must not go home by public transport and preferably not by taxi. If these criteria cannot be fulfilled then the surgery must be carried out on an inpatient basis. If the patient arrives for day surgery without these criteria being satisfied then the operation should be cancelled and their admission re-organised. Part of the admission process must be to check that these criteria have been satisfied.

Specific advice should be given to each patient concerning their post operative welfare. The patient

OPERATIONS SUITABLE FOR DAY STAY

General surgery	Unilateral hernia repair
	Unilateral varicose veins (not prone)
	Sebaceous cysts
	Small benign breast lumps
	Child circumcision
Urology	Cystoscopy ($\pm$ biopsy)
	Diathermy to small bladder tumours
	Hydrocoele
	Varicocoele
	Vasectomy
Gynaecology	Diagnostic laparoscopy
	Laparoscopic test of tubal patency
	Termination of pregnancy
Ophthalmology	Probing of tear ducts
	Cataract surgery (rigid application of other criteria)
	Squint surgery (single eye)
Orthopaedics	Arthroscopy (minor arthroscopic surgery)
	Joint/back manipulation
Oral surgery	Removal of third molars
ENT	Myringotomy
	Antral washout
	Septal vessel diathermy
Haematology	Blood sampling and chemotherapy

Figure SC.11

must be told to avoid alcohol for 24 hours post operatively because the depressant effect of alcohol acts synergistically with the residual anaesthetic drugs and, especially if barbiturate anaesthetics are used, may cause unconsciousness. The patient must be told not to drive vehicles or operate machinery because their physical and mental reactions may not be good enough to keep them out of danger. Car insurance may be invalidated by driving under the residual influence of anaesthetics and the police may charge the driver with driving under the influence of drugs. Similarly they must not cook or be involved in baby care. Lifetime or important decisions should not be made in the post operative period, because patients may be residually disinhibited.

Pre-operatively the day case patient must be told these rules in front of witnesses, or sign a form to say that they have read them at a time when they are not under the influence of anaesthetic drugs. The responsible escorting adult must also understand these rules.

CATEGORY OF SURGERY

The types of surgery suitable for day case work include those with only minor disturbances of nutrition, which last only a short time (usually taken to be less than 45 minutes of anaesthesia) and which do not usually require opioid analgesia afterward. Surgery, where significant blood loss is predicted or where the abdomen is electively opened, is not suitable (except for minor laparoscopic surgery). Surgery where there will be major limitation of mobility is not suitable. Unilateral inguinal hernia repair may be suitable (especially if local anaesthesia is employed), bilateral repair is not. Surgery should only be carried out by surgeons experienced in the procedure in question. Figure SC.11 indicates some procedures that may be suitable for day case work, other factors being satisfied.

MEDICAL FITNESS

Patients must be ASA I or II and between the ages of 16 and 65. Patients outside this age range may be acceptable subject to special arrangements between the anaesthetist and the surgeon. If it is planned to carry out surgery on small children (3 years old or more in a district general hospital) organisationally it is better to arrange a full list of children with a paediatric trained nurse in attendance rather than to have children interspersed within an adult list (Welfare of Children in Hospital 1991). Patients over 65 may be acceptable if they are otherwise healthy. Drug-controlled diabetic patients are never suitable for day case surgery. Essential hypertension is not necessarily a contra-indication provided control is good. Cardiovascular diseases such as angina, cardiac failure or arrhythmias are unacceptable. Controlled atrial fibrillation may be an exception to this if stable and treated.

Obesity is not acceptable (criteria differ but 100 kg or body mass index greater than 30 may be taken as exclusion guidelines). These rules apply to regional anaesthesia and general anaesthesia equally.

ANAESTHETIC TECHNIQUE

Intra-operative: Anaesthesia should be restricted to simple techniques with proven good recovery characteristics, particularly in terms of post operative nausea and vomiting and analgesia. Techniques that employ regional analgesia are particularly suitable provided that mobility is not restricted by the local block. Spinal anaesthesia and femoral nerve blockade are considered unsuitable because of the major inhibition of mobility that results. Caudal analgesia is acceptable in small children but for circumcision a penile block provides good post operative analgesia without motor effects. Spinal anaesthesia in ambulatory young people is notorious for post dural puncture headache and for postural hypotension and should be avoided. Elective tracheal intubation should be avoided because of the risk of laryngeal oedema (and major nasal haemorrhage if nasal intubation is employed) but, having said that, it has been in routine use for day-stay removal of third molar teeth for many years. This latter situation is changing with the increasing use of the laryngeal mask airway. Elective-controlled ventilation used to be considered as a contra-indication to day surgery until the advent of mivacurium, which is short acting and does not need reversal. The use of reversal drugs may reduce the likelihood of patient discharge because of their autonomic and central nervous effects. The laryngeal mask makes day case controlled ventilation feasible where it would not otherwise be so. Thiopentone is not a suitable induction agent for day case general anaesthesia whereas propofol is indicated because of the relatively rapid recovery without significant hangover.

Post operative: Pain should be controlled by the use of regional anaesthetic techniques with the addition of non steroidal anti-inflammatory drugs (NSAIDs) if suitable. Rectal diclofenac is in widespread use but should be discussed with the patient pre-operatively. Account must be taken of the fact that local anaesthesia will wear off after several hours. The patient should be encouraged to take moderate analgesics before the effect of the local anaesthetic wears off and discharged with a suitable supply to take home.

ADMISSION FACILITIES

Wherever surgery is carried out on a day stay basis there must always be the facility to admit the patient overnight. If that facility does not exist either because there are no inpatient beds available or because the day unit is a remote site then surgery should not proceed. Day units should always be within the confines of a general hospital.

The usual anaesthetic reasons for overnight admission following day surgery are nausea and vomiting or pain requiring opioid analgesia. Complications of surgery are a common reason for admission, as is prolonged surgery with consequent slow post operative recovery, usually because the criteria for day surgery have been breached, either by unsuitable surgery or unsuitable surgeon. Records should be kept of the reasons for refusal of day case surgery and the incidence and reasons for unplanned post operative admission.

THE OBESE PATIENT

Obesity can be defined as a body mass index (BMI) of more than 30. The BMI is calculated by dividing the weight (kg) by the square of the height (m^2).

In obesity physiology is altered in several ways as detailed below.

APPLIED PHYSIOLOGY

Oxygen consumption and the work of breathing are increased while chest compliance and functional residual capacity are reduced. Tidal volume and closing volume may overlap while conscious, resulting in poor aeration and a tendency to hypoxia even at rest. These factors increase shunting and the incidence of hypoxia and, when FRC is reduced by anaesthesia or positional changes on the operating table, shunting is further increased. Hypoxia is commonly seen because of these changes and the tendency for the diaphragm to be elevated by pressure from abdominal wall fat. Post operative hypoxia is particularly frequently encountered and, because of the failure to adequately expand the chest, the incidence of atelectasis and hypostatic infection increases.

Blood volume and cardiac output are increased, increasing cardiac work. There is also a tendency to coronary artery disease that is exacerbated by lack of exercise. The increase in both intra-abdominal and abdominal wall fat increases the intra-abdominal pressure, raising the incidence of functional and anatomical hiatus hernia. The resting volume of gastric juice is also increased, as is its acidity. The increase in intra-abdominal pressure also reduces venous return from the legs, predisposing to DVT and pulmonary embolism. There is a higher incidence of wound infection and wound dehiscence. Surgical access can be difficult because of the distribution of fat.

ANAESTHESIA

For the anaesthetist there are often anatomical problems in establishing venous access, particularly if central venous access is needed. Airway maintenance may be difficult because of the tendency to short fat neck and, in females, protruding breasts. Intubation may also be difficult and pre-oxygenation is recommended. Chest compliance is reduced and so the work of ventilation increases, sometimes to the extent

that mechanical ventilators may be unable to generate the inflation pressure necessary to achieve adequate tidal volumes. This can also be a problem if a laryngeal mask airway is used because the inflation pressure may exceed the LMA leak pressure. The high inflation pressures necessary will further reduce venous return and falls in cardiac output may be significant.

Non invasive blood pressure measurements may give erroneous readings if the cuff size is not chosen correctly. A cuff that is relatively too small will give falsely high readings. Regional anaesthetic techniques may be more difficult because of difficult nerve location and loss of landmarks and extra long needles may be necessary. There is more fat in the epidural space and so **smaller** doses of local anaesthetic agents may produce the same effect as in the normal patient. Placing epidural and spinal needles can be particularly difficult because of the increased distance between skin and landmarks. The sitting position may help because the skin and bone midlines may come into opposition whereas in the lateral position these may be some distance apart, making the technique impossible. Finding bony landmarks with a standard hypodermic needle before inserting the epidural needle will improve the chances of success.

All induction agents and vapours are fat soluble and a significant proportion of the cardiac output supplies fat, therefore these drugs are diverted from the brain and into fat stores, increasing the requirement for induction agents and slowing the rise in brain concentration, tending to increase the incidence of awareness. Similarly, emergence may be slower because of the slower leaching of agents from the fat stores. This latter causes obese patients to be exposed to volatile agents for longer so increasing their biotransformation. This can be a particular problem with halothane where the incidence of halothane related liver dysfunction is increased in obesity. Halothane should, therefore, be avoided in the obese patient.

THE METABOLICALLY COMPROMISED PATIENT

LIVER DISEASE

Applied physiology

The liver is the largest organ in the body receiving 30% of cardiac output. The majority of nutritional, haematological and detoxification metabolism occurs in the liver, including the breakdown or excretion of many anaesthetic drugs. Other physiological roles of the liver include the manufacture of proteins, lipoproteins and carbohydrates which includes the clotting factors and the proteins to which most anaesthetic drugs are bound. Globulins are not produced in the liver. The liver also acts as a store for vitamins, minerals and carbohydrates. In the presence of significant liver disease, all these processes become disturbed.

Different conditions cause differing patterns of dysfunction. Excessive red cell turnover causes jaundice by overloading the pathways of haem breakdown even though other liver functions may remain relatively normal. Obstructive and cholestatic jaundice causes major disruption to metabolic pathways and to the absorption of fats and fat soluble vitamins, causing further problems. Hepatocellular dysfunction may be toxic or infective in origin but will result in the same picture of unconjugated bilirubinaemia, fat malabsorption and metabolic disturbance. In the end stage of hepatic failure, virtually all the body's metabolic processes are disturbed. Clinical features include clotting failure, coma from ammonia toxicity because of disturbed protein metabolism, hypoglycaemia because of poor glycogen metabolism, water overload and major electrolyte imbalance. There is usually portal hypertension that causes the formation of collateral circulation including oesophageal varices. If these bleed then the sudden high protein meal provided by enteral haemoglobin may precipitate hepatic coma in an otherwise compensated patient, a desperate situation which may be irretrievable. Anaesthesia in liver failure is, therefore, not for the inexperienced.

Assessment of patients with liver disease

Full haematological and biochemical screening results should be available to supplement clinical evaluation of the patient. Absorption of vitamin K from the gut depends entirely on the presence of bile salts and so the synthesis of prothrombin and other clotting factors, which depend on vitamin K are sensitive barometers of liver function. Albumin has a long plasma half-life and so is an indicator of more chronic disease when its value will be lowered. Transaminases are released from damaged hepatocytes but as these enzymes are also present in other tissues, this cannot be taken as specific to liver function (which also applies to alkaline phosphatase). Conjugated bilirubinaemia suggests obstructive jaundice whereas unconjugated bilirubinaemia suggests a pre hepatic or hepatic cause. In the presence of established liver disease anaesthetic agents and techniques must be chosen with care and with due consideration for disturbed metabolism, pharmacokinetics, and water and electrolyte balance.

DRUGS

Benzodiazepines have a prolonged and more intense effect than usual and, thus, should be avoided as pre medicants and induction agents. Opioids have a greatly prolonged effect. The metabolism of the barbiturate induction agents is prolonged, but as their effect as induction agents is not terminated by metabolism but by redistribution this is relatively academic except in severe disease where minimum doses should be used. Etomidate behaves similarly. While suxamethonium is not specifically contra-indicated, its effect may be prolonged by reduced plasma cholinesterase activity (which also applies to mivacurium). The behaviour of the other non depolarising muscle relaxants is largely dependent on protein binding and excretion. All these agents are highly bound to plasma proteins and so in the hypoproteinaemia of liver disease they will have a higher unbound fraction and a greater effect for the same dose. The exception to this is d-tubocurarine, which is bound to globulins rather than albumin and so, because plasma globulins are often normal or raised in liver disease, the effect of this drug may be reduced. Although the majority of excretion of both curare and pancuronium is by the renal route, reduced biliary excretion may prolong their effect. In the case of atracurium or cisatracurium, much of the breakdown is via non specific plasma esterases and so subject to prolonged effect in liver disease. In severe hepatic dysfunction the spontaneous degradation which these drugs also undergo may be disturbed by acid base changes. Patients with severe liver disease tend to be water overloaded because of secondary hyperaldosteronism and the volumes of distribution of all drugs will be affected. Liver function has little effect on the choice of anaesthetic vapours. The use of halothane is not contra-indicated unless by other considerations although sevoflurane is the more popular choice.

Local anaesthetic agents may have delayed excretion though not a prolonged anaesthetic effect. Regional anaesthetic techniques may be contra-indicated by abnormal clotting.

FLUIDS

Fluid and electrolyte balance must be scrupulous and blood glucose monitored frequently because of disturbed glycogen metabolism in the later stages of the disease.

TECHNIQUES

Standard general anaesthetic techniques may be used

with care in liver disease. Peripheral and central regional anaesthesia, including epidural and spinal techniques are acceptable unless the INR is greater than 1.5. Renal function is often disturbed in obstructive jaundice and is always affected in hepatic failure. Urine output must be encouraged to avoid the onset of renal failure in the post operative period. Pre-operative infusion of mannitol in the jaundiced patient may help to avoid hepato-renal syndrome, 500 ml 20% mannitol is appropriate.

REPEAT ANAESTHESIA

Patients may require repeat anaesthesia either fortuitously or during a planned course of treatment and over a short or longer time scale.

The main considerations at pre-operative assessment for repeat anaesthesia are to identify if possible the anaesthetic technique used, the drugs involved and any related problems. Problems of particular interest are nausea and vomiting, difficult airway management, difficult intubation, drug reactions and the use of halothane.

Derangement of liver function following halothane exposure shows two clinical pictures. In the first instance a mild and transient disturbance in liver function is seen and this may be accompanied by mild pyrexia. Resolution is seen within a few days without permanent sequelae. It is suggested that the mechanism underlying this mild picture is the result of the phase 1 transformation products of halothane reacting directly with hepatic macromolecules to cause tissue necrosis. In the second instance massive and fulminant hepatic necrosis occurs. Although rare, mortality is in the region of 40–70%. It is thought that the underlying mechanism of this process is the formation of a hapten–protein complex resulting in immune mediated destruction of liver tissue. The hapten is likely to be a halothane metabolite, tri-fluroacetyl halide is the most likely culprit.

The Committee on Safety of Medicines (CSM) recommendations for repeated use of halothane are that it should not be used within three months of a previous administration unless there is an overwhelming clinical reason for the second use, and that it should not be used if there was unexplained pyrexia or jaundice within 1 week after a previous exposure.

As there are alternative vapours and techniques easily available, and halothane is falling into disuse, many anaesthetists avoid it within a three month period unless there is a good clinical reason for second exposure, such as the need for inhalational induction.

Even this is being overtaken with the introduction of sevoflurane, which is almost as good as halothane when used for inhalational induction. Many anaesthetists believe that halothane should only ever be used once per patient.

Even though a patient may be a regular patient it is important to go through a full pre-operative assessment each time because there is always the possibility of new intercurrent disease, particularly in the elderly. Notice should be taken of any problems encountered by previous anaesthetists and the patient should be asked when their last anaesthetic was. The vapour used should be noted and avoided in repeat if necessary.

RENAL DISEASE

APPLIED PHYSIOLOGY

The kidneys excrete water, electrolytes, water-soluble drugs and water-soluble products of metabolism. Plasma electrolytes, urea and creatinine provide an indication of renal function. While the plasma urea also depends on liver function, the creatinine concentration also depends on the level of protein metabolism in the body. For the plasma creatinine to rise, renal function must be < 30% of normal. As renal function is reduced below this the creatinine and urea will rise, as will the plasma potassium concentration. Water is retained and the production of new red cells is depressed by reductions in erythropoietin secretion. Acidosis develops, compensated by respiratory alkalosis and cardiac output increases. In established chronic renal failure the haemoglobin may fall to 5–6 g/dl with a creatinine concentration > 700 mmol/l and potassium > 6 mmol/l. In the early stages of the disease some improvement may be possible by correction of the precipitating cause and by careful attention to fluid and electrolyte balance. One of the more common causes of chronic renal impairment is obstructive uropathy and the simple expedient of indwelling urinary catheterisation may return the patient to a relatively normal biochemical state.

Patients in renal failure (even if mild) should not be transfused to correct their anaemia unless there is a situation of acute blood loss. To do so will precipitate cardiac failure by volume overload and will suppress the production of normal red cells. Owing to changes in 2,3-DPG concentration, stored red cells do not carry oxygen at their full capacity for some 24 H post transfusion and so the effect of transfusion can be a reduction of oxygen delivery to the tissues.

Drugs and techniques

In choosing anaesthetic drugs and techniques, care should be taken to avoid those drugs that are excreted solely through the kidney. Fortunately, all of the induction agents undergo redistribution and biotransformation to inactive products before excretion. Renal impairment may delay the excretion of the opioids and prolong their action. Suxamethonium should be avoided as it causes the release of potassium from muscle cells and may precipitate cardiac arrhythmias in an already hyperkalaemic patient. The volume of distribution of the non depolarising relaxants may be increased, reducing their effect while their breakdown and excretion are reduced. Mivacurium, atracurium and cisatracurium may have a relatively normal duration of action, altered only by acidosis. Pancuronium and vecuronium should be used with great care because they are largely excreted unchanged in the urine. Renal impairment has little bearing on the choice of anaesthetic vapours though there is a theoretical risk of additional renal toxicity if enflurane or isoflurane are used in high concentration for prolonged periods as fluoride ion is released during their metabolism and high concentrations of fluoride are known to be nephrotoxic. Aminoglycoside antibiotics should be used with extreme care in renal impairment as they are renally excreted and both nephrotoxic and ototoxic at the high and sustained levels which are found if normal doses are given to patients with impaired excretion. Attention to fluid and electrolyte balance must be rigorous, replacing only that which has been lost and avoiding potassium containing fluids. Occasionally a patient may present who maintains their renal function only if they have a high urine output or with a high output type of renal failure. These patients must not be fluid restricted in the pre-operative period. Venous access must be considered very carefully in patients likely to need dialysis as chronic fistula or shunt formation may be necessary. It is better to preserve the vessels in one arm if possible. If a fistula is already present then this limb should be avoided at all costs and the limb protected from pressure during surgery. Regional anaesthesia is useful in the renally impaired patient provided that there are no other contra-indications. The choice of airway maintenance technique will depend on the proposed surgery.

DIABETES MELLITUS

Diabetes mellitus is the most common endocrine disorder and one of the more common co-existing conditions in patients presenting for surgery.

COMPLICATIONS OF DIABETES

Nephropathy
Peripheral neuropathy
Autonomic neuropathy
Cerebral vascular disease
Coronary artery disease
Peripheral vascular disease
Retinopathy
Lipo-atrophy
Fetal macrosomia
Hypoglycaemia
Hyperglycaemia
Ketoacidosis
Lactic acidosis
Obesity
Infection
Wound infection
Delayed healing

Figure SC.12

Complications

The complications of diabetes are listed in Figure SC.12.

Patients with diabetes may present for incidental surgery or for surgery related to their diabetes, particularly abscesses, wound debridement, amputation of toes, feet or limbs, and cataract surgery, although diabetic patients do not have a higher incidence of cataracts, simply an earlier presentation of the condition. Whether the surgery is incidental or not, and whether the diabetes is insulin or non insulin dependent, there is an interaction between the surgical insult and the diabetes that needs to be properly managed to maintain stability and avoid further complications of both the diabetes and the surgery. Inadequately managed diabetes can result in hyper- or hypoglycaemia, ketoacidosis, wound infection and delayed healing. Occasionally the surgical condition can result in instability and toxic confusion, which will, of course, make the diabetes more unstable and worsen the surgical condition. Patients should not be presented for anaesthesia unless their diabetes is under reasonable control with blood glucose between 3 and 10 mmol/l during the pre-operative fasting period. Any patient whose blood glucose is outside this range should have their surgery postponed until the situation has been corrected, unless the surgical condition is a

MANAGEMENT OF DIABETES

ELECTIVE SURGERY

Ideally all diabetic patients will have been assessed by a physician before admission and brought into adequate control.

Diet controlled

Minor disturbance
May be suitable for day case admission. No specific treatment regimen. Blood glucose result available one hour pre-operatively. Return to usual diet same day.

Major disturbance
No specific treatment regimen. Blood glucose result available one hour pre-operatively. Return to usual diet as soon as surgery allows.

Tablet controlled

Minor disturbance
Not suitable for day case surgery. Admit at least the day prior to surgery. No diabetic tablets the day prior to or the day of surgery. Blood glucose and electrolyte results available one hour prior to surgery. Test glucose four hourly until discharge. Return to normal tablet regimen the day after surgery. Dextrose infusion necessary only if glucose result less than 4 mmol/l.

Major disturbance
Admit 48 hours pre-operatively for stabilisation on insulin infusion regimen (for 24 hours prior to surgery). No oral hypoglycaemics the day prior to or the day of surgery. Two hourly glucose estimation

until stable. Infusion regimen to continue until normal oral intake resumes, then return to oral diabetic therapy for at least 48 hours before discharge. Monitor glucose four hourly thereafter.

Insulin controlled

Minor disturbance
Not suitable for day case surgery. Admit the day before surgery. Half usual dose of short acting insulin the evening before surgery.

Morning operation:
Fast from midnight for a morning list. No insulin in the morning. Blood glucose result one hour pre-operatively. The evening after surgery give one third dose of short acting insulin with supper. Check blood glucose three hours after supper. Return to usual treatment the day after surgery.

Afternoon operation:
Fast from 08-00 for an afternoon list. Half dose of short acting insulin with light breakfast. Start slow infusion of 5% Dextrose (four hours per half litre). Check blood glucose two hourly after breakfast. Half dose of short acting insulin with supper. Check glucose three hours after this. Return to usual treatment the day after surgery.

Major disturbance
Admit 48 hours pre-operatively for stabilisation on insulin infusion regimen. Monitor glucose two hourly in the first 24 hours of the regimen. Continue insulin infusion regimen until full oral intake is resumed. Return to normal treatment for at least 36 hours before discharge. Monitor glucose four hourly.

Figure SC.13

---

true emergency. Similarly, any tendency to acidosis or ketosis and any co-existing electrolyte disturbance must be fully corrected before anaesthesia. Unfortunately, there are many patients with gangrene or infection of ischaemic tissue whose diabetes will not come into adequate control until debridement has been carried out. This should not prevent the attempt being made. Patients presented for elective surgery should be seen by a physician with a special interest in diabetes before the day of operation so that their diabetes is under optimal control.

Effect of complications on anaesthesia

Nephropathy causes hypertension and electrolyte disturbances, particularly of potassium and creatinine. These disturbances are a reflection of renal function and give some indication of the adequacy of fluid and electrolyte homeostasis and drug excretion.

Neuropathy. Diabetic peripheral neuropathy is unpredictable in both distribution and effect. This may make the testing of peripheral nerve blocks more difficult. Autonomic neuropathy is not usually formally sought, the test being a formal Valsalva

MANAGEMENT OF DIABETES

EMERGENCY SURGERY

Diet controlled

Minor disturbance
Check blood glucose. Return to usual diet same day if possible.

Major disturbance
Check blood glucose prior to operation. Check fasting glucose daily until return to full oral intake. Insulin intervention may be necessary depending on result. Return to usual diet before discharge.

Tablet controlled

Minor disturbance
Dextrose infusion from time of admission. Check blood glucose prior to operation. Check fasting glucose daily until return to full oral intake. Insulin intervention may be necessary depending on result. Return to usual diet before discharge.

Major disturbance
Commence on insulin infusion regimen after admission and continue until full oral intake re-established, then return to tablets. Check blood glucose two hourly until on full oral intake. Discharge 48 hours after tablets recommenced, if stable.

Insulin controlled

Minor disturbance
Insulin infusion regimen from admission. Check blood glucose two hourly. Return to usual insulin doses only when on full oral intake. Stabilise before discharge.

Major disturbance
Insulin infusion regimen from admission. Continue infusion until re-established on full oral intake then return to usual doses. Stabilise on usual doses for 48 hours before discharge.

INSULIN INFUSION REGIMEN

Laboratory blood sugar and electrolytes before starting regimen. Dextrose 5% 1000 ml eight hourly by pump (125 ml/hr). Soluble insulin 60 units in 60 ml saline via syringe pump at a rate determined by sliding scale. Two hourly glucose evaluation.

Blood glucose	Insulin rate
<5 mmol/l	zero
5–10 mmol/l	1 unit/hour
10–15 mmol/l	2 units/hour
15–20 mmol/l	3 units/hour
>20 mmol/l	5 units/hour

Note: Potassium should be added to the infusion bag according to pre-infusion value and twice daily electrolyte results.

Figure SC.13 (continued)

manoeuvre, but is probably present in a large number of diabetics. The heart may be partly de-nervated and so variations in heart rate may not follow the expected patterns. Similarly the peripheral autonomic responses may not be adequate to prevent variations in blood pressure. Gastro-intestinal autonomic neuropathy may delay gastric emptying, increasing the likelihood of regurgitation.

Vascular disease. Diabetic vascular disease tends to involve small vessels rather than large vessels and though there may be no obvious major coronary or cerebral vessel disease, as a general rule it should be assumed that anyone who has peripheral vascular disease also has central and coronary vascular disease. As it is mostly small vessels that are affected the fall in blood pressure associated with regional or central nerve blockade tends not to be so manifest.

Pregnancy. Diabetic management in pregnancy can be very difficult with significant increases in insulin requirement during the pregnancy and major, sudden falls in requirement in the puerperium. Diabetics tend to have large immature babies that may need forceps delivery or Caesarean section for delivery. All pregnant diabetics should be managed by a competent physician in addition to their obstetrician. Gestational diabetes may also need careful management to prevent complications.

Management

Diabetes may be controlled by diet, oral therapy or insulin, depending on severity. Both oral therapy and some of the insulins may last more than 24 hours from the last dose. This must be borne in mind when preparing patients for surgery. The metabolic disturbances of diabetes may take the form of hypo- or hyperglycaemia, keto-acidosis or lactic acidosis. Surgery tends to produce a slight hyperglycaemia as a normal 'stress' response.

Whichever diabetic management protocol is followed, it must be a straightforward regimen so that problems are avoided while being flexible enough to cope with major and minor surgery and both elective and emergency surgery. A suitable regimen is detailed above. Minor disturbance may be considered surgery with no significant disturbance of physiology, lifestyle or nutrition, the disturbances lasting less than 24 hours. Major disturbance involves substantial disturbance of physiology, lifestyle or nutrition for more than 24 hours. Figure SC.13 shows a suggested management plan for various situations.

INFECTIVE RISK GROUPS

The major risk to healthcare workers is represented by the blood borne viruses, a group which contains hepatitis A, B and C as well as human immunodeficiency virus (HIV).

HEPATITIS A

The hepatitis A virus is a common infection acquired by close contact with infected persons or by food contamination, particularly sewage contaminated water and shellfish. The incubation period is 2–7 weeks. Carriers have not been reported.

There is a prodromal 'flu-like' illness with marked myalgia proceeding to hepatocellular jaundice which resolves spontaneously without chronic damage.

HEPATITIS B

Infection with the hepatitis B virus is much more serious than hepatitis A in that hepatic failure is more common, chronic damage is frequent, the disease is endemic in many parts of the world and some 10% of all those infected will become chronic carriers. The infection may be acquired by vertical transmission from mother to child in utero or in childhood or by heterosexual or homosexual contact or direct inoculation of body fluids. The virus is highly infective in small inoculates, unlike HIV. In countries with adequate blood transfusion services this route of transmission is now rare. The prodromal illness may be severe with arthralgia and urticaria followed by hepatocellular jaundice. The illness is not usually severe and the majority of patients clear the virus within a few weeks. All healthcare workers should be immunised against this condition, though occasionally the immunisation may have to be repeated several times.

HEPATITIS C

Hepatitis C is indistinguishable from the other viral hepatitides except on serological testing. The usual route of transmission is parenteral inoculation with large inoculates required to stimulate the infection. Until recently, transfusion of blood and blood products was the major route of infection, which suggests that there must be a pool of chronic carriers in the community. Blood products can now be screened for this infection but there must be a large number of previously transfused patients who carry the disease. Up to 40% of those infected will develop progressive chronic liver disease.

HIV/AIDS

Infection with the human immunodeficiency virus was only recognised in 1983 but there must have been numerous unrecognised cases before that. The virus is delicate, easily destroyed and has low infectivity. The main routes of transmission are by promiscuous sexual activity (both heterosexual and homosexual) and by the sharing of injection equipment. Many haemophiliacs have been infected by pooled blood transfusion products which were drawn from an infected community before the problem was recognised. Needle stick injury is not a major route of infection except in the case of a large innoculate or frequent small innoculation from an infected population, such as when performing surgery in sub-Saharan Africa. HIV and Hepatitis B frequently occur together, particularly in prostitutes and in the homosexual and drug abusing communities.

Infection with HIV may be asymptomatic for many years but usually progresses towards AIDS or one of the related conditions. Drug treatments in use at present may slow this progress and extend the patient's life but there is currently no treatment which will prevent or reverse the inevitable downhill course. Infected persons remain infectious even when asymptomatic.

CLINICAL PICTURES IN HIV INFECTION

No symptoms
Generalised lymphadenopathy
Chronic fatigue
Weight loss
Night sweats
Recurrent fever
Chronic skin infections
Intermittent/continuous diarrhoea
Myalgia
Low grade encephalopathy
Immune deficiency with opportunistic infections
Kaposi's sarcoma

Figure SC.14

The main presentations are in terms of related opportunistic infections such as tuberculosis, Pneumocystis carinii, Candida oesophagitis or Cryptosporidium colitis. Kaposi's sarcoma is diagnostic.

HIV/AIDS is a spectrum of conditions rather than presenting as one or more specific syndromes. (Figure SC.14)

Persistent generalised lymphadenopathy is characterised by the presence of extra-inguinal lymph nodes for more than 3 months, and may be painful. Histology generally shows reactive change. One third progress to AIDS within 5 years.

AIDS encephalopathy is a psychomotor and psychoneurological condition with poor memory, apathy, poor concentration and behavioural changes.

AIDS. A diagnosis of full AIDS depends on the demonstration of immunodeficiency-related opportunistic infections or related cancers such as Kaposi's sarcoma.

PRECAUTIONS

Hepatitis B and C may cause chronic liver damage and due account should be taken of liver function in those patients known to be carriers or known to have had B or C hepatitis. Hepatitis A does not produce chronic sequelae but may present for surgery during the active or prodromal phases of the disease and again, liver function should be tested and the anaesthetic managed accordingly. The AIDS-related conditions may be of interest to the anaesthetist when the patient presents for surgery but the possibilities are so broad that each must be taken on its merits. Patients may present for lymph node biopsy. Unfortunately, the majority of people infected with hepatitis B, C and HIV are asymptomatic and not known to the medical community. While precautions against cross infection are usually taken in those patients known, to be infected, it is more logical to take precautions in all patients and assume that every patient is potentially infectious. It is thus, wise for anaesthetists to develop the habit of wearing gloves and eye protection in all cases. Contaminated needles should **never** be re-sheathed but disposed of immediately in sharps disposal containers. Syringes should not be transferred from one patient to another and the person using sharps should dispose of them to reduce the number of staff potentially exposed. All cuts and abrasions on both staff and patients should be covered with waterproof dressings and all spillages of body fluids should be cleaned immediately with a viricidal solution.

In anaesthetising patients known to have one of the HIV related syndromes, extreme care should be taken to avoid introducing infections into the patient, who has a life threatening immune deficiency akin to immunosuppressed leukaemics or transplant recipients. This involves effective skin disinfection before venepuncture and full aseptic technique for other invasive procedures. All other equipment used should be either disposable single use or have been autoclaved and be re-autoclaved as soon as possible after the event. Figure SC.15 details recommended precautions to prevent occupational transmission of HIV from patients to healthcare workers.

NEEDLESTICK INJURY

Although great care is taken to avoid needlestick injury, inevitably occasional accidental inoculation can occur. Following injury the puncture site should be encouraged to bleed vigorously and thoroughly washed with soap and water. Eye splashes should be rinsed with sterile eye-wash or water.

PREVENTION OF OCCUPATIONAL TRANSMISSION OF HIV

Risk	Precaution
Hand contact with body fluids	Wear gloves
Blood splashes	Wear apron/mask/goggles
Needle stick injury	Dispose of sharps into safe container Do not pass to another person
Exposed skin lesion	Cover with waterproof dressing
Salivary contact	Minimise handling of used airway equipment; sterilise after use
Contaminated equipment	Sterilise as per local policy

Figure SC.15

Occupational exposure must be reported and recorded in an accident book. Each unit may have a different protocol for this, most require attendance at A and E. Blood should be taken from the victim, and in high risk scenarios from the patient (after appropriate consent). If after consideration of the relative risk (taking into account HIV and hepatitis status) prophylaxis is considered desirable this should be instistued. Triple therapy is usual and this comprises three antiviral drugs, a combination of protease inhibitors and nucleoside analogue reverse transcriptase inhibitors. Counselling should be made available through the occupational health department.

PRION DISEASE

Alterations in the native prion proteins by gene mutation may give rise to infective particles which cause the transmissible spongiform encephalopathies. Although there are various forms of these conditions, most attention has focused on Creutzfeld-Jakob disease in its variant (non spontaneous) form. Dementia, loss of memory and personality changes comprise the clinical presentation and death occurs within months of diagnosis.

Prion particles are resistant to destruction by most normal sterilisation procedures and are small enough to 'hide' in crypts within stainless steel.

Patients at risk are those with a presumptive diagnosis of CJD and those who have received hormone treatment from human pituitary glands or human dura mater grafts. Prion particles are found in lympho-reticular tissue and it has now been recommended that cases for adeno-tonsillectomy be regarded as potentially infective. Single use equipment, both surgical and anaesthetic must be used in such cases. Advice on the management of patients with known CJD may be obtained from a specific CJD incidents panel at the Department of Health.

Latex Allergy

Allergy to natural rubber latex is an increasing problem for health care workers who may have to carry out procedures on patients who react to latex or who may themselves develop reactions to latex. The reactions tend to fall into two groups, either skin contact or anaphylactic in type. Both are serious problems and no distinction should be made between them. Natural latex contains a variety of highly allergenic proteins, which cause reaction by repeated exposure and hypersensitivity. Continued exposure increases the severity of the reaction. It is interesting that there are reports of cross-reactions to similar proteins in fruits such as banana, avocado and kiwi fruit as well as nuts.

If a patient reports possible latex allergy then, while skin testing by dermatologists is possible, it is time consuming and potentially dangerous so it may be wise to accept the patient at face value and treat them as if they are positive.

PERI-OPERATIVE CARE

For planned surgery the patient should be first on a morning operating list to avoid the possibility of latex particles being in the operating theatre atmosphere. All staff should be familiar with the local latex allergy policy and aware of their responsibilities. Traffic in the room should be kept to a minimum.

All staff should wear non-latex gloves.

If possible all anaesthetic breathing system tubing should be made of plastics or man-made rubbers such as neoprene. If it is not possible to replace this tubing then it should be covered with stockinet gauze to prevent transfer of particles from the rubber to the patient by staff handling the exposed rubber. Similarly blood pressure cuff bladders and tubing should be covered so that there is no contact with the patient. All breathing systems should have a bacterial filter at the patient end to prevent latex particles entering the patient's airway. For airway maintenance PVC tracheal tubes and laryngeal mask airways are acceptable, as they do not contain latex. Facemasks should be made of plastic. IV cannulae are usually latex-free though it is always wise to check beforehand.

Syringes should be checked for latex, though most modern syringes are latex-free and labeled as such. Standard blood giving sets contain latex in the injection port at the cannula connection. These should be avoided. Even supposedly latex-free fluid giving sets may contain latex in injection ports. These should be removed but if this is not possible, should not be used as injection ports because of the possibility of coring and embolising particles of latex. A three-way tap is preferable.

Equipment for local and regional anaesthesia does not usually contain latex but each anaesthetic department should identify which products are latex-free and keep a stock of these products. There are lists of latex-free and latex-containing products on the internet at **www.immune.com/rubber/ukdatabase**

Note that the rubber seals on drug ampoules do not contain latex.

An anaphylaxis pack should be available in the operating theatre while a latex-allergic patient is present. The patient should be anaesthetised in the operating theatre and recover in the same room rather than being transferred to a recovery room where the atmosphere is less well controlled.

Each anaesthetic and operating theatre department should develop a policy on the management of latex allergy and a box containing latex-free equipment. All staff should familiarise themselves with both of these.

References and further reading

Day case surgery. Association of Anaesthetists of Great Britain and Ireland. 1994.

HIV and other blood borne viruses. Association of Anaesthetists of Great Britain and Ireland. 1992.

Melzack R, Wall PD. Pain mechanism: a new theory. *Science* 1965; **150:** 971–979.

Michenfelder JD. *Anaesthesia and the brain.* Edinburgh: Churchill Livingstone, 1988.

Poswillow DE (Chairman). *General anaesthesia, sedation and resuscitation in dentistry.* Report of an Expert Working Party. 1990.

Recommendations for the transfer of patients with acute head injuries to neurosurgical units. Association of Anaesthetists of Great Britain and Ireland. 1996.

Report on Confidential Enquiries into Maternal Deaths in the United Kingdom – The Series. London, HMSO.

Steward DJ. *Manual of paediatric anaesthesia,* 5th Edition. Edinburgh: Churchill Livingstone, 2001.

Welfare of children in hospital. London, HMSO, 1991.

SECTION 1: 6
THE SURGICAL INSULT

C. A. Pinnock
R. M. Haden

GENERAL SURGERY

Laparotomy
Head and neck
Rectum and anus
Laparoscopic surgery

UROLOGY

Trans urethral procedures
Nephrectomy
PCNL
TVT

ORTHOPAEDICS

Arthroplasty
Laminectomy
Fractured neck of femur

GYNAECOLOGY

Hysterectomy and TCRE
Laparoscopy
Ectopic pregnancy
Termination and evacuation

ENT

Laryngoscopy
Tonsils and adenoids
Middle ear
Tracheostomy

OPHTHALMOLOGY

Cataract
Squint
Retinal surgery
Penetrating injury
DCR

ORAL SURGERY

Dental extraction
Fractured mandible
Fractured zygoma
Fractured maxilla

Surgery of any kind represents a genuine traumatic insult to the body and is accompanied by a verifiable stress response dependent on the magnitude of the insult. While the general principles of broad based anaesthesia have been covered in Chapters 2, 3 and 4, the purpose of this chapter is to alert the reader to operative procedures that have specific problems or caveats associated with them. For reasons of space, only the more frequently encountered operations have been included.

GENERAL SURGERY

LAPAROTOMY

The majority of patients requiring laparotomy will present an aspiration risk and, therefore, require rapid sequence induction and subsequent muscular relaxation with intermittent positive pressure ventilation (IPPV). In the case of a perforated viscus (duodenal ulcer, for example) electrolyte imbalance, dehydration and cardiovascular instability make for a high risk procedure. The presence of faecal soiling of the peritoneum is a particularly bad prognostic indicator. Anastomosis of the bowel requires special consideration. Survival of anastomoses is maximised if the blood supply to the joined section is not compromised in any way. In practice, this requires the avoidance of reversal drugs (and, therefore, atracurium is indicated) and the use of epidural anaesthesia, usually combined with general anaesthesia if there are no contra-indicating factors to the technique (such as poor haemodynamic resuscitation). Epidural anaesthesia provides better post operative pain relief than patient controlled analgesia (PCA) which is important in the avoidance of pneumonia in upper abdominal incisions. Extubation of patients following a surgical procedure which has involved handling of the bowel should be left until the protective reflexes have returned, as the risk of regurgitation is ever present.

HEAD AND NECK SURGERY

Surgery to the head and neck, whether thyroid, parathyroid or salivary glands is the target, encompasses the same basic principles. Airway security is of paramount importance and the likely situation is one of obscuration of the patient and breathing circuitry with head towels making intubation and subsequent IPPV preferable to the use of the laryngeal mask airway although this device is in use. Avoidance of coughing is important and

adequate muscular relaxation and depth of anaesthesia will ensure that this complication does not arise. Spontaneous respiration is not recommended. In the case of thyroid surgery adequate assessment of the airway is necessary if there is any degree of goitre. Parathyroidectomy can be a prolonged procedure in which case warming precautions (mattress and fluids) should be used. Patients covered with head towels require suitable eye protection to avoid corneal damage.

RECTUM AND ANUS

Surgery to the rectum and anus (e.g. manual dilatation of the anus and haemorrhoidectomy) is highly stimulating and requires adequate depth of anaesthesia to prevent the development of hypertension, tachycardia and laryngeal spasm. Caudal anaesthesia is appropriate in this situation but may be technically difficult in adults. Pilonidal sinus deserves special mention. Many of these patients are obese and for reasons of surgical access require placing in the prone position. Airway security is best achieved by endotracheal intubation followed by IPPV (although some practitioners use the reinforced laryngeal mask airway) and eye protection should be employed. Caudal anaesthesia is contra-indicated in the presence of active infection close to the site of injection.

LAPAROSCOPIC CHOLECYSTECTOMY

While the recovery from laparoscopic cholecystectomy is both quicker and less problematic than from the traditional open operation, the procedure itself carries a considerably greater physiological insult and greater morbidity. Patients who are fit for the open procedure may not be fit for a laparoscopic procedure. The abdomen is filled to high pressure with carbon dioxide and the patient is required to be positioned in a steep head-up position with left rotation. The diaphragm therefore becomes splinted and the lungs compressed, widening the carina and moving it to a higher position in the chest. A properly placed tracheal tube may enter a main bronchus once the abdomen is inflated. The heart may be rotated from its usual position, distorting the great vessels. The venous return from the lower half of the body is compromised by the intra-abdominal pressure and position. Hypertension is induced by the absorption of carbon dioxide. These factors combine to produce a patient with poor venous return, low cardiac output and high systemic resistance, a recipe for significant cardiac strain even in the absence of coronary artery disease. The increased intragastric pressure encourages regurgitation. Peritoneal stretching can also induce severe vagal bradycardia. The standard anaesthetic technique for this procedure is a controlled ventilation technique via a tracheal tube. A dose of a vagolytic drug may be given before the start of surgery in order to avoid the vagal bradycardia of peritoneal stretching. Post operative analgesia with systemic opioids and NSAIDs is usually sufficient though the pneumoperitoneum causes shoulder pain which may be resistant to opioids until the carbon dioxide has been absorbed. There is a risk that laparoscopic procedures may be converted to open procedures if the anatomy is difficult or if bleeding becomes a problem.

Laparoscopic hernia repair is becoming popular. The physiological insult is less than for cholecystectomy, but the procedure may be accompanied by significant post operative pain.

UROLOGICAL SURGERY

TRANSURETHRAL RESECTION OF THE PROSTATE (TURP)

Open prostatectomy has become a very infrequent procedure, the majority being undertaken as transurethral resection of the prostate (TURP). Prostatic hypertrophy, whether benign or malignant is one of the conditions of the ageing population and tends to coincide with other conditions of the ageing population; ischaemic heart disease, hypertension, diabetes and respiratory disease which must all be taken into account in planning anaesthesia. Patients requiring prostatectomy may have disturbed plasma electrolytes because of chronic back pressure on the kidneys. This situation may improve with good pre-operative drainage by urethral or suprapubic catheterisation, but the electrolyte results rarely return to normal, thus mild elevations of urea or creatinine values are common. Urethral instrumentation is notorious for causing gram negative septicaemia and so patients with indwelling catheters or those known to have pre-existing infection should have their operations covered by a renal function related dose of a suitable antibiotic, such as gentamicin. Blood loss in prostatectomy is related to resection time rather than size of the prostate and is generally accepted to be less if spinal anaesthesia is used rather than general anaesthesia. This also has the advantage that any catheter manipulations or bladder washouts necessary in the immediate post operative period will be covered by the residual effects of the anaesthetic.

Spinal anaesthesia has advantages in those with pre-existing respiratory disease, though its use in the presence of ischaemic heart disease is more contentious. Prolonged surgery with continuous irrigation can cause dramatic falls in the patient's temperature, which can only be partly corrected by warming the irrigation and intravenous fluids. Blankets covering the upper body may also help but the majority of re-warming must be done in the post operative period. Blood loss at prostatectomy can be difficult to assess though a variety of methods are available. The lithotomy position tends to increase peripheral resistance until the patient is returned to the supine position when there is a major fall in peripheral resistance often accompanied by a fall in arterial pressure which should, therefore, be measured and corrected before transfer from the operating theatre into recovery.

TRANSURETHRAL RESECTION OF BLADDER TUMOUR (TURBT)

Bladder tumours are not usually large and rarely result in major blood loss. Occasionally patients will be anaemic at presentation from frank blood loss over a period of time. Anaemia should be corrected. Use of diathermy in the bladder can stimulate the obturator nerve, which is close by in the pelvis, lateral to the bladder. This causes mass movement of the patient's legs which can result in perforation of the bladder and vascular or bowel damage by the resectoscope. This situation can only be prevented by using muscular relaxation and IPPV. Good relaxation is also necessary for adequate bi-manual surgical assessment of the tumour and the bladder, anaesthesia should not be terminated until this is complete. Patients with bladder tumours become regular attenders and so at each attendance the anaesthetist must establish the time since the last general anaesthetic, which agents were used and the patient's response to them. As time passes new medical conditions may appear or pre-existing conditions deteriorate and so a full pre-operative assessment should be carried out at each admission.

Transurethral syndrome

Endoscopic surgery requires continuous irrigation with a solution of glycine (1.5% in water). This solution is deliberately non electrolytic so that the diathermy current is applied to the tissue rather than being dissipated in the fluid. If significant volumes of this solution get into either the general circulation or the tissues, from where it is absorbed, then there may be serious fluid and electrolyte disturbances. The most obvious are water excess and hyponatraemia. Cerebral oedema develops leading to confusion, hypertension and bradycardia, though loss of consciousness or convulsions is not uncommon. Respiratory distress accompanied by hypoxia (because of interstitial pulmonary oedema) and cardiac effects such as rhythm and contractility changes may also be seen. The plasma sodium concentration may fall to extreme levels, below 100 mmol/l is not unknown. If the irrigation fluid is in the tissues or free in the peritoneal cavity then laparotomy for drainage may be the only possible method of treatment. Emergency anaesthesia in this situation is fraught with difficulties but is one of those occasions when the patient must be accepted as they are without any attempt to improve the situation in the pre-operative period. General anaesthesia employing intubation and IPPV is the first choice.

A glycine solution containing 1% ethanol is now available. The use of breath alcohol estimations can give an estimate of fluid absorption during the procedure and this technique is gaining popularity for resectoscopic surgery.

NEPHRECTOMY

Nephrectomy for benign disease is usually carried out through a loin incision whereas if malignancy is involved (including ureteric disease) the operation is generally performed through a laparotomy. The essential difference is the position of the patient who is supine for laparotomy but in the lateral position for the loin approach. When in the lateral position the operating table may be arched to increase the distance between the rib cage and the pelvis to improve surgical access. This may cause kinking of the great vessels in the abdomen. In both positions there may be significant blood loss because of damage to renal vessels close to the aorta or inferior vena cava. In left-sided operations the diaphragm and pleura are in danger and the anaesthetist should be prepared to deal with pneumothorax.

The vessels of the dependent arm may be partly occluded in this position, therefore all monitoring and infusions should be on the upper arm. Loin incisions are particularly painful post operatively because of their proximity to the ribcage. Continuous epidural analgesia is particularly effective for both types of incision. Pyeloplasty is usually carried out in the lateral position through a loin incision and the above comments apply.

PCNL

Percutaneous nephrolithotomy (PCNL) is an endoscopic procedure to remove stones from the kidney without open surgery. The patient is placed prone. A large needle is passed under X-ray control into the relevant renal calyx and a large bore cannula passed along the track. The endoscope is then passed through this cannula accompanied by continuous irrigation with glycine or saline, depending upon the method used to extract the stones. Saline is used with electrohydraulic lithotripsy whereas glycine or saline may be used with the lithoclast.

PCNL can take several hours and it therefore becomes difficult to maintain patient temperature throughout, particularly with the use of large volumes of irrigant. There can be considerable blood loss and significant absorption of irrigating solution causing facial and cerebral oedema. If glycine is used there may be features of the TUR syndrome. Severe pain is the norm in the immediate post operative period. Standard anaesthetic techniques for this involve tracheal intubation, controlled ventilation and epidural analgesia for post operative pain relief. The epidural dressing must be waterproof and be placed away from the operative puncture site. The usual precautions are necessary for the prone position, particularly eye protection and padding of pressure points. Care should be exercised in the tension of any bandage used to tie in the tracheal tube, as the facial oedema may cause this to cut into the patient, increasing the possibility of a restricted cerebral vascular supply. This procedure can be a major physiological strain on patients with ischaemic heart disease. It carries a significant mortality. The patients should be admitted to a high dependency unit for the immediate post operative period, though the less healthy patients may require the full facilities of an intensive care unit on a planned basis.

TVT

Transvaginal tension-free tape support of the bladder neck (TVT) is a relatively new procedure for stress incontinence. It is usually performed using spinal anaesthesia because of the surgeon's need to adjust the tension of the buttressing tape to the minimum (which prevents leakage). This involves the patient either coughing or straining part way through the procedure thus it is necessary to limit the level of block to no higher than the T 10 dermatome so that some power remains in the abdominal musculature. This is difficult to achieve in a predictable way.

ORTHOPAEDIC SURGERY

JOINT REPLACEMENT SURGERY

The most frequently performed operations in this category are hip and knee arthroplasty. Total hip replacement may be carried out under epidural, spinal or general anaesthesia. Peripheral nerve blockade may be useful for post operative analgesia (e.g. paravascular '3 in 1' and iliac crest block) but the hip joint is not easy to denervate in this manner due to its multiple nerve supply. Hip replacement may be carried out in the supine or lateral positions with the specific problems of these (see Chapter 3). Revision surgery and bone grafting to the acetabulum complicate the procedure greatly and add to the likelihood of extensive blood loss and the need for close haemodynamic monitoring. The most major incident to anticipate is cement reaction that generally occurs with cementing of the femoral, rather than acetabular prothesis. Various mechanisms have been suggested as implicated in cement reactions and these are listed in Figure SI.1. The clinical picture is one of hypotension accompanied by falling oxygen saturation which usually reverts over a 10–20 minute time course. Increase of inspired oxygen and circulatory support may become necessary. It is important that fluid balance is adequate before the cementing of the femoral component. Measures which have been used to reduce the likelihood of cement reaction include: distal bone plug in the shaft to limit the spread of cement, venting of the shaft to reduce pressure and air trapping, and waiting for the mixture to be relatively non viscous before insertion to reduce the likelihood of monomer absorption. Although less common a similar reaction may be seen after cemented humeral prostheses.

MECHANISMS OF CEMENT REACTION

Pulmonary embolisation	Marrow
	Fat
	Cement
	Air

Methylmethacrylate absorption

Pressurisation of femoral cavity

Heat from cement reaction within femoral cavity

Figure SI.1

Anaesthesia for total knee arthroplasty is broadly similar but does not show the same picture of cement reaction unless extra long femoral components are used after extensive reaming. Femoral and sciatic blockade may be used for analgesia or operation and in general techniques of anaesthesia are as for hip arthroplasty. The use of tourniquet restricts blood loss intra-operatively but post operative losses may be brisk. After release of the tourniquet metabolic products are released into the circulation representing an acid load which may cause temporary acidosis and a rise in end tidal carbon dioxide. Bilateral joint replacements are severe surgical insults that should not be undertaken lightly.

LAMINECTOMY

The primary requirement of back surgery is the prone position. Adequate eye care is important and there is no substitute for endotracheal intubation (possibly with an armoured tube) and IPPV using individual drugs of choice. The patient's arms must be carefully and symmetrically moved when turning into the prone position to avoid shoulder dislocation and pressure points should be padded. A suitable support should be employed to avoid abdominal compression, which will both embarrass ventilation and cause venous congestion in the epidural plexus. The Montreal mattress and Toronto frame are frequently used (Figure SI.2).

FRACTURED NECK OF FEMUR

There are several operations for the treatment of fractured neck of femur (dynamic hip screw, cannulated screws, etc.) depending on the precise site of the break. The majority of patients presenting for this procedure are elderly and frail, and maybe the victims of severe polypharmacy. A picture of dehydration and cardiac decompensation is frequently seen. As the operation is urgent rather than emergency attention should be paid to the correction of those features which can be improved (uncontrolled atrial fibrillation and electrolyte imbalance, to name but two).

Spinal anaesthesia is the most commonly employed technique for this procedure although care must be taken to ensure adequate fluid resuscitation otherwise severe hypotension may result from sympathetic blockade of the lower limbs. Turning the patient for spinal insertion may necessitate analgesia (particularly in the case of heavy solutions when the injured leg will be underneath) and small incremental

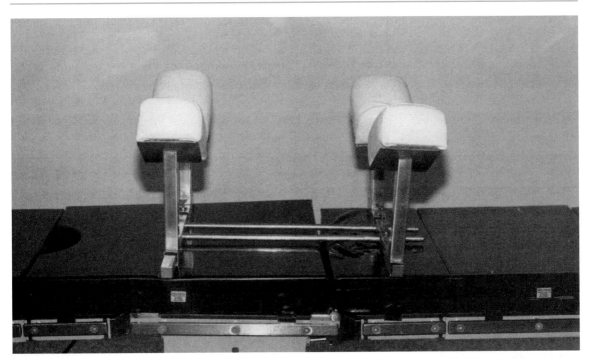

Toronto frame

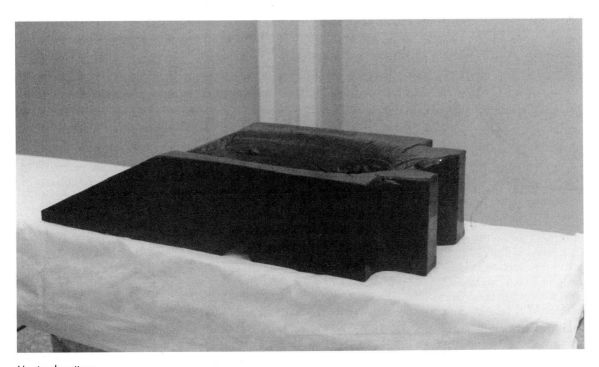

Montreal mattress

Figure SI.2 Supports for patients in the prone position

doses of IV ketamine with or without midazolam are frequently used. Epidural and general anaesthesia may also be used and although the mortality from general anaesthesia is higher in the short term, there is very little difference after three months or so have elapsed when death rates from all techniques approximate.

GYNAECOLOGICAL SURGERY

HYSTERECTOMY

Hysterectomy may be undertaken by abdominal or vaginal route. Abdominal hysterectomy equates to a laparotomy in its anaesthesia requirements although the use of a low transverse incision has encouraged the use of the laryngeal mask airway instead of endotracheal intubation (assuming no other contra-indications, such as morbid obesity). Muscular relaxation and IPPV are usually required with volatile agent and opioid of choice. Post operative pain relief may be delivered by the use of epidural infusions or PCA. The combination of PCA with a rectally administered non steroidal anti-inflammatory drug (such as diclofenac 100 mg) is widespread. Rectal administration of non steroidal anti-inflammatory agents in gynaecological surgery is especially indicated as the high concentrations of the drug which are found in the pelvic venous plexus after absorption ensure delivery to the surgical field. Vaginal hysterectomy is less of an insult than abdominal hysterectomy but has broadly similar anaesthesia requirements. Caudal injection of local anaesthetic agents provides a degree of post operative analgesia although it is unlikely that the level of block from this technique will reach sufficient height to be fully effective (T10); therefore, additional analgesia should be provided. If rectal drug administration after pelvic floor repair is desired, this is best administered by the operating surgeon after completion, when the suppository can be gently inserted without damage to the suture line.

Transcervical resection of endometrium (TCRE) is starting to replace hysterectomy as a treatment for uncomplicated menorrhagia. A resectoscope is inserted through the cervix after which endometrium is resected by laser or diathermy under direct vision. Fluid irrigation of the uterus is necessary in the same way as for TUR. The irrigating solution is isotonic glycine and the problems of absorption are identical to those of TUR syndrome (see above). The use of irrigating solutions containing 1% alcohol is recommended as absorption can be monitored by the measurement of breath alcohol using a suitable meter and normogram tables. TCRE is not accompanied by significant post operative discomfort.

LAPAROSCOPY

Laparoscopy involves the inflation of the abdomen with carbon dioxide before the insertion of a scope to examine the abdominal contents. The degree of inflation of the abdomen varies greatly between surgeons. Although the procedure is accomplishable with the patient breathing spontaneously, this is not recommended and IPPV with muscular relaxation is the norm (suitable agents being mivacurium and atracurium). Use of the laryngeal mask airway is common but not universal. The procedure is usually of short duration and not accompanied by great post operative discomfort except in the case of sterilisation where the presence of occluding clips on the Fallopian tubes may precipitate spasm. In this situation opioid drugs may be needed post operatively although non steroidal anti-inflammatory drugs are probably a better first line treatment (especially if a day case patient). The most alarming problem during laparoscopy is that of a severe bradycardia which may be precipitated on inflating the abdomen. Vagolytic drugs should be always at hand and if necessary the abdomen should be deflated until the heart rate stabilises. Asystolic arrest has been reported. Laparoscopy may be used to confirm the diagnosis of ectopic pregnancy. The patient must be carefully assessed to ensure that there is no great degree of concealed blood loss. The onset of muscle relaxation under anaesthesia in a patent with a bleeding ectopic pregnancy can result in sudden, massive haemorrhage in which case aggressive fluid replacement and urgent laparotomy are required. Large scale blood replacement should always be followed by haematological assessment of coagulation and appropriate remedial therapy.

EVACUATION AND TERMINATION (ERPC/STOP)

Evacuation of retained products of conception (ERPC) and suction termination of pregnancy (STOP) are similar in their anaesthesia requirements. As the volatile anaesthetic agents have a relaxant effect on the uterus, their use is associated with increased blood loss although this may not reach clinical significance. For this reason a technique of intermittent (or infused) induction agent is usual. Propofol with or without supplemental opioid agent is popular for what is a short, minimally disruptive procedure.

Patients requiring ERPC should be assessed for pre-operative blood loss and resuscitated as necessary. The use of oxytocics during anaesthesia for STOP is occasionally accompanied by untoward effects (peripheral vasoconstriction for example).

EAR, NOSE AND THROAT SURGERY

LARYNGOSCOPY

Direct laryngoscopy and its variants (which may include the use of lasers in the airway) demand special techniques of airway management because the surgeon works directly in the airway and needs access to the larynx. Specially designed small tracheal tubes, tubes with a cuff and an insufflation port or special laser-proof tubes are available and all have their uses. Because of the difficulties of maintaining spontaneous or controlled ventilation under these circumstances, the usual techniques involve a total intravenous technique with controlled ventilation using an insufflation device such as the Sanders injector or high frequency jet ventilator. If lasers are to be used in the airway then great care must be taken to isolate the trachea below the tube cuff from the airway above the cuff because any backwash of gas containing oxygen might result in an explosion or fire when the laser is next fired. Nitrous oxide is flammable.

TONSILLECTOMY

Anaesthesia for tonsillectomy with or without adenoidectomy requires defence of the shared airway from blood and debris. This necessarily involves endotracheal intubation after induction, which may be gaseous or IV. If an uncuffed tube is used in the child patient, a suitable pack (ribbon gauze, for example) should be placed around the laryngeal additus to protect the larynx from contamination of blood and saliva. Use of a Boyle–Davis gag (Figure SI.3) will prevent compression of the tube during surgical positioning. Having decided upon intubation, IPPV should be used and commonly a non depolarising relaxant, opioid, vapour combination is used for the maintenance of anaesthesia. Extubation should be undertaken in the head down lateral position after adequate pharyngeal suction. There are two choices for timing of this event, while the patient is still deep or after protective reflexes have returned. The latter is more common today. Blood loss should be particularly carefully assessed in young children. Because of the risk of Prion disease, disposable anaesthetic and surgical equipment is now mandatory.

Post tonsillectomy haemorrhage is a specific problem that requires mention. Following post tonsillectomy haemorrhage, the patient will usually be pale, tachycardic and sweaty. Intravenous

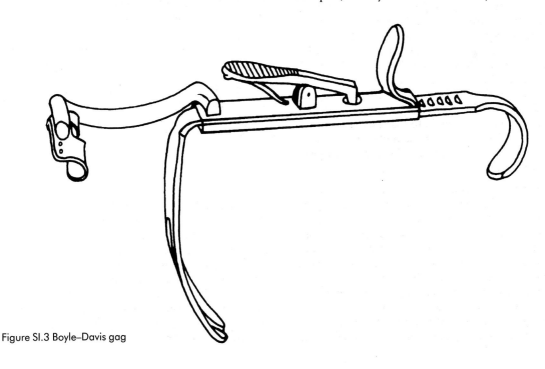

Figure SI.3 Boyle–Davis gag

resuscitation is essential before induction and two different techniques of anaesthesia have been recommended. In both situations the patient should be placed head down, in left lateral position with suction to hand. Following preparation of all equipment a choice may be made between intravenous or gaseous induction. In the first instance after the usual RSI precautions (pre-oxygenation, cricoid pressure) a cautious dose of induction agent is given, followed by suxamethonium and securement of the airway by endotracheal intubation. Alternatively, a gaseous induction of halothane and oxygen may be employed using suction as necessary and enough time to achieve a plane of anaesthesia deep enough to permit laryngoscopy and intubation. Maintenance and extubation are as described above. Some authorities recommend the emptying of swallowed blood from the stomach with a nasogastric tube before extubation which would appear a wise counsel.

MIDDLE EAR SURGERY

Middle ear surgery has one main requirement which differentiates it from other surgical procedures. This is the need for control of blood loss to achieve the surgeon the best possible view down the microscope. In practice, 'smooth' anaesthesia is desirable (for example no coughing or straining) and a relaxant, opioid, vapour technique is usually employed after intubation with an armoured endotracheal tube. Lidocaine spray to the larynx has been advocated before intubation to reduce the response to the presence of the tube as has the use of alfentanil with induction. Arterial hypotension is often requested, and provided there are no contra-indications this may be achieved by the use of sodium nitroprusside by controlled infusion or beta-blockade (esmolol is a suitable choice). Inspired oxygen concentration should be increased and a slight head up tilt will reduce bleeding by aiding venous drainage. It has been suggested that avoidance of nitrous oxide is beneficial to avoid pressure rises in the middle ear as it diffuses in. Oxygen air mixtures are, therefore, recommended in this situation. An anti-emetic agent should be administered during the procedure as nausea from disturbance of labyrinthine function is frequent and post operative vomiting is particularly undesirable.

TRACHEOSTOMY

The majority of elective tracheostomies are performed on intensive care patients following long term oral intubation. In this instance anaesthesia is usually maintained by the use of opioid agents with or without volatile supplementation and muscle relaxants as required to facilitate IPPV. The critical feature of the procedure is to avoid withdrawing the existing endotracheal tube before the surgeon gaining control of the airway by securing the tracheostomy tube in the correct position. If this is not achievable, the original tube can be re-advanced and oxygenation maintained. If the endotracheal tube has been removed without securing the trachostomy tube correctly a potentially dangerous situation develops which may be fatal. Transfer of connecting tubing from old to new tube should be as quick as possible to avoid desaturation. Emergency tracheostomy is a difficult and hazardous procedure best performed under local anaesthesia.

OPHTHALMIC SURGERY

CATARACT SURGERY

Cataracts may be congenital, traumatic, steroid- or radiation-induced, or degenerative. In degenerative cataracts there will also be other medical conditions of the ageing population. While diabetics have no more cataracts than the general population, they tend to present earlier and so there seems to be a preponderance of diabetic patients presenting for cataract surgery. Steroid induced cataracts present in patients taking long term steroids for other conditions, particularly eczema or asthma which should be taken into account. Cataract surgery demands a still eye with low intra-ocular pressure. This can usually be achieved by smooth anaesthesia with muscle relaxation and IPPV to achieve mild hypocapnia, whether via a tracheal tube or laryngeal mask, though the latter is preferable because of the lack of intubation pressor response or laryngeal spasm and coughing on extubation. There is a fashion for local anaesthesia for cataract surgery despite this having a higher failure rate, more complications and less predictable reduction of intra-ocular pressure. Patients who cannot lie flat without coughing or distress or cannot communicate because of language, deafness or dementia cannot safely have their cataract surgery under local anaesthesia. They may or may not be fit for general anaesthesia.

SQUINT SURGERY

The majority of patients for squint surgery are children, though occasional adults may present for cosmetic corrections. This operation is difficult to carry out with local anaesthesia because of the age of the patient and the manipulations necessary in the orbit. General anaesthesia should be carried out with the airway maintained by either a laryngeal mask or tracheal tube. There is little to choose between spontaneous or controlled ventilation. All patients having squint surgery should receive a weight related dose of a vagolytic such as glycopyrrolate to obtund the oculo-cardiac reflex, which can cause severe bradycardia on traction of the extra-ocular muscles. This is much easier to prevent than treat. Tracheal tubes in small children restrict the cross sectional area of the airway with a consequent increase in resistance to gas flow (resistance is inversely proportional to the 4th power of the radius). After extubation, the smallest amount of laryngeal or tracheal oedema can cause major falls in oxygen saturation. Laryngeal spasm at extubation causes sudden dramatic falls in saturation and the facilities for re-intubation with a muscle relaxant should be immediately to hand. Waiting for the spasm to break is a recipe for disaster. The tracheal tube used during the surgery should not be disposed of until the patient leaves the recovery room.

RETINAL SURGERY

Retinal detachments present sporadically but are not usually so urgent that they have to be done immediately on presentation. The patients are often hypertensive, though whether this is cause or effect is debatable. The surgery may be prolonged and is often carried out in semi-darkness. In this situation too soft an eye may be a disadvantage in that the low intra-ocular pressure may cause further tearing of the retina. Controlled ventilation is advantageous due to the duration of the surgery. A vagolytic agent should be given to prevent the oculo-cardiac reflex during surgical manipulation of the globe. The oculo-cardiac reflex also occurs during exenteration or enucleation. Occasionally the surgeon may wish to introduce a gas bubble between the vitreous and retina to tamponade the retina. If this is planned then nitrous oxide should be avoided or turned off as soon as the decision is made. Nitrous oxide diffuses into closed gas filled spaces and increases the volume of the bubble or, if the area has low compliance, the pressure will rise. While this may be acceptable during the procedure, it will diffuse out in the post operative period and the pressure or volume will reduce, reducing the tamponade effect.

PENETRATING EYE INJURY

Penetrating eye injuries may require induction of anaesthesia in the presence of a potentially full stomach. Unfortunately, suxamethonium causes a significant rise in intra-ocular pressure, which may cause further damage, especially if there is already vitreous loss or the lens is disrupted. An alternative is a rapid sequence induction using a generous dose of a rapid onset non depolarising relaxant instead of suxamethonium. Vecuronium or rocuronium are suitable choices. Rocuronium at 1.5 mg/kg gives equivalent intubating conditions to suxamethonium. It should be noted, however, that this dose ($3 \times ED_{95}$) may last up to 1 H. If the penetration of the globe has been with metallic fragments then the search for these may involve magnets or repeated X-rays which can require multiple changes of position or prolonged surgery.

DACROCYSTORHINOSTOMY (DCR)

Dacrocystorhinostomy is a potentially bloody procedure usually requiring an anaesthetic technique designed to reduce blood loss. The patient is usually placed with the table head up to improve venous drainage. A vasoconstrictor is introduced inside the nose to reduce mucosal bleeding. The blood pressure is often lowered to further reduce bleeding. Hypotension may be achieved by increasing the inspired concentration of anaesthetic vapour, particularly halothane (which depresses the myocardium) or isoflurane (which causes peripheral vasodilatation) or by introducing agents which cause peripheral vasodilatation such as trimetaphan or sodium nitroprusside. These agents must be used with extreme caution. Mild hyperventilation will also help to reduce the blood pressure. The airway is usually maintained with a tracheal tube, though the laryngeal mask will avoid the pressor response to the presence of the tube and so may avoid the need for active reduction of blood pressure. A pharyngeal pack is essential to absorb blood that trickles down from the nasopharynx.

ORAL AND MAXILLO FACIAL SURGERY

DENTAL EXTRACTION

Simple dental extraction demands good control of a shared airway and a degree of understanding between anaesthetist and dentist. Dental extraction should be carried out with the same standard of equipment and monitoring as in the best hospital operating theatres, including ECG, oximetry, NIBP and expired gas analysis. The majority of dental extractions are carried out on a day case basis unless there is significant co-existing disease. There is still some debate as to whether the sitting position or the supine position is better, both have advantages and disadvantages. The supine position provides some protection against fainting on induction of anaesthesia, a potentially dangerous event while encouraging regurgitation of stomach contents.

Induction of anaesthesia may be by inhalation or intravenous injection, but in both cases venous access should be obtained first. The sudden falls in blood pressure associated with propofol tend to limit its use in the dental chair, particularly in the sitting position. Methohexitone is less problematic in this regard while recovery is only marginally slower. There is no need for intravenous opioids and simple analgesics are adequate in the post operative period. Many children prefer inhalational induction that should be with halothane or sevoflurane in a nitrous oxide/oxygen mixture. Isoflurane has too pungent a smell and enflurane causes too much coughing and salivation to be useful. Inhalation induction and maintenance are carried out using a nasal mask. Once adequate anaesthesia has been established, the mouth is opened and a pack inserted between the mouth cavity and the pharynx, separating the nasal airway from the oral airway. In this way, the extraction can be carried out without dilution of the anaesthetic gases by mouth breathing and the airway can be maintained without contamination by blood and debris. Recovery should be in the lateral position, preferably head down.

Removal of wisdom teeth

Surgical removal of wisdom teeth demands that the surgeon has good access to the mouth cavity while the airway is protected from debris, water and blood. This is usually achieved by nasal intubation and use of a pharyngeal pack. The reinforced laryngeal mask is occasionally used but only by experienced anaesthetists. Nasal intubation can cause significant bleeding and pharyngeal tears. An accidental pharyngeal mucosal tear must be recognised and treated with a broad spectrum antibiotic to avoid major infective complications (including potential mediastinitis). The anaesthetist must choose between spontaneous and controlled ventilation. If spontaneous ventilation is used then there is a high incidence of cardiac arrhythmia, particularly with halothane. Most of the disturbances resolve with emergence from anaesthesia and require no intervention. Care must be taken to remove the pharyngeal pack at the end of the procedure. Recovery should be in the lateral position with observation of blood loss and post operative pain relief provided by NSAIDs.

FRACTURED MANDIBLE

Surgical treatment of fractured mandible involves stabilisation of the fracture against the mandible itself or against the maxilla via the upper teeth. The fracture may be plated, in which case the airway at the end of the procedure is clear, or the mandible may be wired to the upper teeth, in which case the mouth is closed at the end. It can be difficult to establish at the beginning of the procedure which situation will pertain at the end. Provided that the mouth can be opened before anaesthesia is induced, an IV induction may be used, followed by nasal intubation and a pharyngeal pack placed. Ventilation may be controlled or spontaneous but with due consideration for the duration of surgery and the recovery phase. An antiemetic should be given before the end of the procedure because vomiting in a semi-conscious patient with a closed mouth is disastrous. The pack must be removed before the end of the surgery. Spontaneous respiration must be re-established in the operating theatre following which the tube must not be removed until the patient is conscious and can maintain their own airway. The tracheal tube used must be retained until the patient leaves the recovery room. If the mouth is wired closed then a pair of wire cutters must go with the patient wherever they are while they are in hospital in case the wires need to be cut in an emergency. NSAID are suitable for post operative analgesia. The opioids are less suitable because of their sedative effects. There is a case to be made for patients with wired jaws to be nursed on an HDU or ITU overnight for airway observation.

FRACTURED ZYGOMA

Fracture of the zygoma indicates that severe trauma has taken place and the pre-operative assessment should take into account the possibility of closed head injury. The fracture is usually reduced via an incision above the temporal hair line and so the anaesthetist must be remote from the head. IV induction should be used, followed by controlled or spontaneous ventilation via an oral tracheal tube or a reinforced laryngeal mask airway. Whichever the airway device, it must be securely fixed because there may be significant head movement during the reduction. There is always the possibility of further open surgery if the initial manipulation fails.

FRACTURED MAXILLA

Anaesthesia for fractured maxilla is not for the inexperienced. The fracture indicates severe trauma and pre-operative assessment should take into account the possibility of closed head injury. The combination of significant head injury and maxillary fracture is an indication for tracheostomy as part of the surgical procedure, as is fracture of both maxilla and mandible together. The surgical procedure may involve stabilisation of the maxilla against the mandible or the skull, either of which will cause airway management problems. A compromised airway is an indication for inhalation induction followed by an 'exploratory' laryngoscopy before a muscle relaxant is given. An oral tracheal tube may be used unless the mouth is to be wired closed, in which case an oral tube will suffice while a tracheostomy is performed. Nasal tubes should not be used because of the displacement of the maxilla, usually backward. Ventilation should be controlled and the anaesthetic machine placed remotely. Access to the head is difficult, particularly at the end of the procedure if a 'halo' device is used to fix the maxilla to the skull. The patient should be nursed on an ITU/HDU after surgery.

Trismus

Fractures of the mandible and infection or haematoma in the mouth can cause significant swelling, inflammation of the tissues and spasm of the muscles of mastication, resulting in an inability to open the mouth adequately. The spasm may or may not relax after induction of anaesthesia. In this situation, intravenous induction can prove rapidly fatal because the patency of the airway is only maintained by muscle power, which is lost on induction of anaesthesia. If at this point it proves impossible to open the mouth or maintain the airway then the patient will die of hypoxia unless a cricothyrotomy is performed immediately. The presence of trismus, for whatever reason, demands inhalational induction. If, during the induction, the airway becomes compromised, then the anaesthetic may be terminated without risk to the patient and consciousness restored. Alternatives must then be considered with the patient awake, tracheostomy under local anaesthesia is one option. If the inhalational anaesthetic proceeds without difficulty then the degree of trismus can be assessed with the patient unconscious, with a view to tracheal intubation or laryngeal mask airway placement. Muscle relaxants should not be used unless a good view of the glottis has been obtained under anaesthesia. Blind nasal intubation has no place in this scenario because of the risk of torrential haemorrhage in an uncontrollable airway and because success is not guaranteed.

References and further reading

Atkinson R S, Rushman G, Lee J A. *Lee's Synopsis of Anaesthesia*, 11th ed. Oxford: Butterworth-Heinemann, 1993, Chapter 22.

Aitkenhead A, Smith G. *Textbook of Anaesthesia*, Churchill Livingstone 4th edition 2001. Chapters 55, 57, 58 and 61.

Williamson K M, and Mushambi M C. *Complications of hysteroscopic treatment of menorrhagia*. BJA 1996; **77**: 305–307.

SECTION 1: 7
REGIONAL ANAESTHESIA AND ANALGESIA

H. B. J. Fischer

GENERAL PRINCIPLES OF MANAGEMENT

Patient preparation
Performing the block
Peri-operative management

CENTRAL NEURAL BLOCKADE

Spinal anaesthesia
Epidural anaesthesia
Caudal anaesthesia

PERIPHERAL NERVE BLOCKADE

Brachial plexus block
Femoral nerve block
Ankle block
Inguinal field block
Penile block

LOCAL ANAESTHESIA OF THE UPPER AIRWAY

Topical
Superior laryngeal nerve block
Transtracheal block

INTRAVENOUS REGIONAL ANAESTHESIA

Regional anaesthesia has its origins in 1884, 38 years after the discovery of general anaesthesia, when Carl Koller instilled a solution of cocaine into a patient's eye and performed glaucoma surgery 'under local'. This landmark discovery led to an explosion of interest in blocking nerve conduction as surgeons looked for less dangerous alternatives to the general anaesthetic techniques then available.

GENERAL PRINCIPLES OF MANAGEMENT

Several important factors, common to all major regional anaesthesia techniques, require consideration to minimise risks and promote high standards of patient care.

PATIENT PREPARATION

Pre-operative preparation of the patient for regional anaesthesia should fulfil the same standards of care as for general anaesthesia because regional anaesthesia should not be regarded as a shortcut for high risk patients. A full explanation of the intended block should cover the conduct of the injection, patient management during surgery and recovery from the effects of the block. The advantages to patient, surgeon and anaesthetist may be discussed. The more common side effects that may be experienced should be outlined and the patient offered the choice of whether to remain fully conscious during surgery, have a sedative premedication or intravenous sedation during the procedure. Major complications of regional anaesthesia are rare (less than 1%). Contra-indications to regional anaesthesia are also relatively uncommon and are shown in Figure RA.1.

PERFORMING THE BLOCK

Major regional anaesthetic techniques require formal sterile procedures, especially central nerve blocks where meningitis and epidural abscess are rare but definite risks. All regional anaesthesia techniques have associated complications and local anaesthetic drugs have potentially toxic properties. Airway and resuscitation skills are, therefore, essential to the practice of regional anaesthesia. Figure RA.2 describes the general requirements for successful practice.

PERI-OPERATIVE MANAGEMENT

During performance of the block verbal contact with the patient should be maintained to offer reassurance and explanation of the unfolding events. Staff within the operating theatre must be aware of the impact of their noise and activity on the patient. Patients who have received premedication or intravenous

---

CONTRA-INDICATIONS TO REGIONAL ANAESTHESIA

Patient refusal despite adequate explanation

Unco-operative patient (obtunded conscious, for example)

Anticoagulation or coagulopathy

Untreated hypovolaemia (particularly applies to spinal anaesthesia)

Major infection

Trauma or burns over injection site

Raised intracranial pressure (particularly central blockade)

Figure RA.1

REQUIREMENTS FOR PERFORMING MAJOR REGIONAL ANAESTHESIA TECHNIQUES

Secure intravenous access

Full resuscitation apparatus

Adequate patient monitoring equipment

Ability to administer general anaesthesia rapidly

Fully trained anaesthetic assistance

Suitable sterile packs (re-usable or disposable)

A full range of sterile needles and other necessary equipment

Adequate space to maintain sterility

Surroundings that offer privacy, good lighting and warmth

Figure RA.2

sedation often sleep during surgery once the block is fully established and the initial surge of activity during preparation for surgery has subsided. Occasional verbal contact should still be maintained as part of the routine monitoring of the patient. Central neural blocks have the potential to cause hypotension due to peripheral vasodilatation and reduced venous return. Hypotension responds to changes in posture. Slight head down tilt with elevation of the legs will restore venous return and intravenous fluids may be required. Bradycardia should be treated with appropriate vagolytic therapy (for example glycopyrrolate 200–400 mcg IV) and vasopressors may be necessary if hypotension does not respond to the above measures. Ephedrine in 3 mg intravenous aliquots is most commonly used as it has both vasopressor and chronotropic effects without increasing myocardial oxygen requirements excessively.

The patient will be unable to protect anaesthetised limbs from pressure or extremes of posture and if the procedure is prolonged, may become distressed by being unable to change position. It is, therefore, important to protect the anaesthetised parts of the body and to maintain a comfortable posture for the patient. Post operatively, the affected limbs need protection from injury and pressure and patients should be mobilised with care to guard against postural hypotension until the effects of the block have worn off.

CENTRAL NEURAL BLOCKADE

There are three neuraxial techniques in common use and their terminology can confuse because terms are used interchangeably. **Spinal** (synonym: intrathecal or subarachnoid), **Epidural** (synonym: extradural or peridural) and **Caudal** (synonym: sacral epidural) are the preferred terms for anaesthesia and analgesia within the boundaries of the spinal column.

SPINAL ANAESTHESIA

Indications

Spinal anaesthesia is used for a wide variety of both elective and emergency surgical procedures below the level of the umbilicus. For surgery above the umbilicus, high spinals are now rarely used because of associated difficulties of maintaining spontaneous ventilation and abolishing the painful stimuli from traction on the peritoneum and pressure on the diaphragm.

Anatomy

Spinal anaesthesia requires the injection of a small volume of local anaesthetic agent directly into the cerebrospinal fluid (CSF) in the lumbar region, below the level of L1/2, where the spinal cord ends. Figure RA.3 shows the typical anatomy of the lumbar spine in cross section.

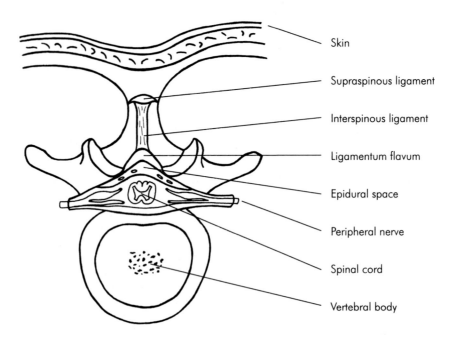

- Skin
- Supraspinous ligament
- Interspinous ligament
- Ligamentum flavum
- Epidural space
- Peripheral nerve
- Spinal cord
- Vertebral body

Figure RA.3 Cross section of the lumbar spine at L1

The meninges surround the spinal cord from the foramen magnum as far down as the second sacral segment (S 2). The **dura mater** is a tough fibro-elastic membrane, beneath that lies the delicate **arachnoid mater**. The dura mater invests the spinal cord and the spinal nerve roots forming the dural cuffs which extend laterally as far as the intervertebral foraminae. Although the arachnoid is attached to the dura there is a potential space between the layers (the sub dural space) and inadvertent injection into this space is a recognised complication of both spinal and epidural injections. The **pia mater** is a delicate vascular layer closely adherent to the spinal cord. Lateral projections of the pia form the dentate ligaments which attach to the dura and stabilise the spinal cord. The filum terminale is the caudal extension of the pia that anchors the spinal cord and dura to the peri-osteum of the coccyx. There are 31 pairs of spinal nerves (8 cervical, 12 thoracic, 5 lumbar, 5 sacral, one coccygeal) arising from the spinal cord which extends from the foramen magnum to the L 1/2 vertebral level. Below this level, the lumbar and sacral nerves form the **cauda equina** which offers a large surface area of nerve roots covered only by the pia mater and accounts for the sensitivity of these nerves to local anaesthetic agents administered centrally.

Physiology

CSF is a clear fluid with a mean specific gravity of 1.006 at 37°C, which is actively secreted by the choroid plexi in the lateral and fourth ventricles at a rate of up to 500 ml per day. There is no active flow, movement occurring by diffusion and changes in posture. Absorption occurs (at equilibrium with

---

FACTORS INFLUENCING INTRATHECAL SPREAD OF SOLUTIONS

Major influence

Baricity of solution
Posture of patient
Volume of solution
Mass of drug injected
Volume of CSF

Minor influence

Intervertebral level of injection
Height of patient
Age of patient
Weight of patient
Speed of injection
Induced turbulence (barbotage)
Posture

Figure RA.5

---

production) via the arachnoid villi of the major cerebral sinuses. The typical composition of CSF is shown in Figure RA.4. A number of factors affect the spread of local anaesthetic within the CSF these are listed in Figure RA. 5.

The maximal spread, duration and quality of the block is mostly influenced by the posture of the patient during and immediately after the injection and the density of the solution. The ratio of the density of the solution to that of CSF is expressed as baricity (where isobaricity = 1.0). If the injection is made at the L3/4 interspace with the patient in the left lateral position and the patient is then immediately turned supine, hypo- and hyperbaric solutions produce different effects due to their distribution patterns. **Hypobaric** solutions are not commonly available in the UK now but have been used traditionally for lower abdominal and lower extremity surgery as they tend to be restricted to the top of the lumbar lordosis when the patient lies supine. With the use of head up tilt, the height of the block can be encouraged in a cephalad direction but at the expense of a patchy quality of anaesthesia and an unpredictable height. Head down tilt will restrict the caudad limit of the block. **Isobaric** solutions are not influenced by posture and may be expected to produce a block influenced more by level of injection and volume. Commercially produced bupivacaine (normally described as isobaric) is slightly hypobaric (0.999) at

---

COMPOSITION OF CSF

Total volume (brain and spinal cord) approximately 130 ml

Volume around spinal cord approximately 35 ml

| CSF pressure in lumbar region | 60–100 mmH$_2$O (lateral position) |
| | 200–250 mmH$_2$O (sitting) |

Hydrogen ion concentration 40–45 nmol/l

Protein content 20–40 mg/l

Figure RA.4

body temperature and can produce unpredictable results with changing posture. **Hyperbaric** bupivacaine is the most commonly used drug for spinal anaesthesia in the UK at present. As hyperbaric solutions are hypertonic they remain affected by posture for up to 30 minutes after injection and so sensory levels may change within that time. This explains why so-called saddle blocks and unilateral spinals can rarely, if ever, be achieved with hyperbaric solutions.

The effects of a spinal anaesthetic on the physiology of the major organ systems are related primarily to the height of the block. Specific organ systems affected are detailed below.

NERVOUS SYSTEM

As a rule there is total neural blockade caudad to the injection site while cephalad to it the concentration of local anaesthetic decreases, producing a differential nerve block of the sensory, motor and autonomic fibres. Sympathetic fibres are most sensitive and may be blocked two to six segments higher than sensory fibres, which in turn may be a few segments higher than the associated motor block.

RESPIRATORY SYSTEM

Below the thoracic nerves, spinal anaesthesia has no clinical effect on respiratory function but as the intercostal nerves become progressively blocked, active expiratory mechanics are impaired producing a reduction in vital capacity and expiratory reserve volume. Tidal volume and other inspiratory mechanics remain normal due to increased diaphragm movement. Patients may complain of dyspnoea and may lose the ability to cough effectively. If there is exceptional cephalad spread and the cervical nerves become affected, apnoea due to phrenic nerve blockade can occur.

CARDIOVASCULAR SYSTEM

Progressive blockade of the thoraco-lumbar sympathetic outflow produces increasing vasodilatation of the resistance and capacitance vessels and a reduction of 15–18% in systemic vascular resistance. If the cardiac output is maintained, there will be a similar fall in mean arterial pressure. If, however, the cardiac output falls due to a reduction in pre load (for example due to hypovolaemia or a reduction in venous return due to postural changes) then hypotension may develop rapidly especially if the block reaches the cardioaccelerator fibres above the level of T4/5 when a reflex bradycardia may occur. Above the level of the block there is usually compensatory vasoconstriction but this is not sufficient to prevent significant falls in arterial pressure if the block is extensive.

GASTRO-INTESTINAL SYSTEM

Sympathetic blockade allows vagal, parasympathetic activity to predominate. Gastric emptying and peristalsis continue, sphincters relax and the bowel is generally contracted. This may preclude the use of central blockade in patients with obstructed bowel, at least until the obstruction has been relieved. However, the incidence of post operative ileus is reduced by spinal and epidural blockade and this is one of their main benefits. Nausea and vomiting can occur as a result of the unopposed vagal activity, if the peritoneal contents are stimulated in the awake patient.

Equipment

Spinal anaesthesia requires specialised needles and introducers in addition to the general equipment necessary for central nerve blocks (see Figure RA.6) There is an inevitable incidence of post dural puncture headache (PDPH) with spinal anaesthesia ranging from 0.2 to 24% and many designs of needle have been introduced to try and reduce this problem. Currently the lowest incidence of PDPH is associated with very narrow gauge, short bevel needles (26–29 G) and 24 G pencil point, Whitacre tip designs or the more specialised Sprotte designs with a large side opening hole. The narrow gauge and relatively blunt tips of these needles require insertion through a properly designed introducer, which should be closely matched to the type of spinal needle being used to avoid tip damage.

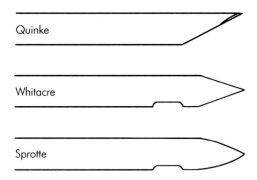

Figure RA.6 Tip design of spinal needles

Technique

Successful spinal anaesthesia depends on a reliable lumbar puncture technique. First establish venous access with a wide bore cannula and then position the patient either in the **lateral** position with the spine

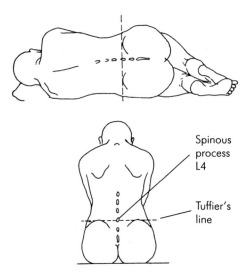

Figure RA.7 Patient positions for spinal anaesthesia

Sterilise the skin over the lumbar spine with a spirit based antiseptic and raise a skin wheal with 1% lidocaine over the appropriate interspace. Inject 2–3 ml more lidocaine into the subcutaneous tissue. Anchor the skin over the interspace by pressing the non dominant index finger on the spine of the cephalad vertebra and insert the needle or introducer in the midline at 90 degrees to the skin. Feedback from the needle tip will monitor the progress of the needle through the supraspinous and interspinous ligaments, the ligamentum flavum and sometimes the dura mater. If bone is contacted, withdraw the needle to the subcutaneous tissue and redirect slightly cephalad in the first instance. Puncture of the dura is usually obvious and when the stylet is removed CSF should flow freely.

Figure RA.8

flexed maximally to open up the gaps between the vertebral spines or in the **sitting** position with the feet placed on a low stool at the side of the bed and the elbows resting on the thighs (Figure RA.7). Each position has drawbacks and advantages and the choice is usually made on personal preference. In either case, a skilled assistant is necessary to position the patient correctly, maintain and support the posture and establish a rapport with them during the conduct of the block.

A line joining both iliac crests (Tuffier's line) passes across the spine of L 4 and is a reliable landmark for locating the L 3/4 interspace which is usually easily defined and is the one most often used. The technique for spinal anaesthesia is described in Figure RA.8.

Note that 22 G needles are robust enough to be used in patients with calcified ligaments or other anatomical difficulties and are recommended for elderly patients where these problems are more common and the risk of PDPH is very low. If an introducer is required, it should be inserted into the deep layers of the interspinous ligament, so that the needle has only a short distance to travel. Narrow gauge needles may deviate or be damaged by the ligamentum flavum, calcified ligaments or osteophytes and also will give little feedback. After performing the block the blood pressure, pulse rate and ECG should be monitored as the onset of sympathetic nerve blockade is quite rapid.

When using 3 ml 0.5% bupivacaine in 8% glucose (so called hyperbaric solution), motor and sensory loss will be apparent within a few minutes but the block may not be fully complete for up to 25 minutes. Sensory block can be tested using a blunt pinprick or loss of temperature sensation with an alcohol swab. Dermatomes should be tested bilaterally starting in the dermatome nearest to the level of injection. Motor loss is usually estimated using the Bromage scale (Figure RA.9).

THE BROMAGE MOTOR BLOCK SCALE (1965)

Degree of motor block	Bromage criterion	% Score
1. No block	Full flexion of knees and feet	0
2. Partial block	Just able to flex knees plus full flexion of feet	33
3. Almost complete	Unable to flex knees, some foot flexion still	66
4. Complete	Unable to move legs or feet	100

Figure RA.9

DRUG DOSES IN SPINAL ANAESTHESIA

Operation Site	Block level	Drug volume (hyperbaric bupivacaine 0.5%)
Peri-anal	L 4/5	2.5 ml
Urogenital	T 10	2.75–3.0 ml
Lower abdominal	T 6/7	3.0–3.25 ml

Figure RA.10

Normally, the whole procedure is conducted with the patient conscious or lightly premedicated, so as to maintain verbal contact and co-operation. If turning the patient is likely to be painful (for example those with fractured neck of femur) then intravenous ketamine 0.5 mg/kg may be administered to provide analgesia during insertion of the spinal.

Drugs, doses and volumes

Figure RA.10 gives a guide to drug administration for various operative sites.

Hyperbaric bupivacaine 0.5% gives a reliable surgical block for 2–3 hours. The above doses apply to a fit adult of normal stature (70 kg) and smaller volumes may be necessary for higher risk patients. Plain 'isobaric' bupivacaine 0.5% 3–4 ml is also commonly used but is less reliable above T 10. Lidocaine 5% in 8% glucose is sometimes indicated for short duration blocks; 2.5–3.0 ml lasts up to 1 hour at T 10 and up to 2 hours in the lower limbs.

Complications

Some complications (hypotension, urinary retention, bradycardia) are actually physiological consequences of central neural blockade and should not represent a clinical problem if correctly managed. If management is inappropriate, secondary effects such as nausea and vomiting, faintness or vasovagal loss of consciousness may follow.

HEADACHE

Loss of CSF through the dural puncture site will produce a low pressure headache due to traction on the cranial meninges. The main characteristics of a spinal headache are that it is minimal when lying flat, is severe when sat up or standing, occurs in the occipital and bi-frontal distribution and may be worsened by coughing or straining. In severe cases the traction may produce cranial nerve symptoms with alterations in vision and hearing. Onset is usually within 24 H of the injection and the majority of PDPH diminishes rapidly with rest, oral analgesia and adequate hydration and should resolve within 7 days. Occasionally more invasive treatment is required in high risk groups such as pregnant women and after puncture with large bore needles. **An epidural blood patch**, in which 20–30 ml of the patient's blood is withdrawn from a vein under the strictest sterile precautions and injected through an epidural needle placed as close to the level of the dural puncture as possible, is very effective at relieving a PDPH with > 90% success with the first injection. Other causes of headache should be considered before ascribing the cause to the spinal and a careful history of events should be elicited, as headaches are a very frequent complaint after surgery.

NEUROLOGICAL SEQUELAE

Temporary symptoms of paraesthesia, hypo-aesthesia and motor weakness may follow spinal anaesthesia but are not necessarily the result of trauma to a spinal nerve root. These symptoms occur from pressure, surgical trauma or stretching of the root or peripheral nerve and the great majority resolve spontaneously within a few weeks. Serious, permanent neurological damage is extremely rare (less than 1:10 000) but in view of the serious consequences of such an event, any neurological sequelae should be formally examined by a neurologist with experience of this type of damage as soon as the problem arises. Other rare causes of neurological damage include brain damage and anterior spinal artery syndrome due to excessive and prolonged hypotension, infection (meningitis and epidural abscess), arachnoiditis and cauda equina syndrome (both associated with the injection of incorrect solutions) and are usually the result of a failure of technique.

EPIDURAL ANAESTHESIA

Indications

Surgery can be undertaken within the abdomen and the lower limbs using an epidural as the sole anaesthetic technique but it is more usual to combine epidural anaesthesia and a light general anaesthetic. Epidural infusions are now extensively used for acute and chronic pain relief (Figure RA.11).

The salient significant differences between spinal and epidural approaches are summarised in Figure RA.12.

INDICATIONS FOR EPIDURAL ANAESTHESIA AND ANALGESIA

Surgery

Thoracic
Pulmonary
Cardiac
Vascular
Abdominal
Gastro-intestinal
Gynaecological
Urological
Orthopaedic and trauma

Acute pain relief

Post operative analgesia
Trauma
Miscellaneous (pancreatitis, ischaemic pain)

Chronic pain states

Chronic benign pain
Cancer pain

Figure RA.11

DIFFERENCES BETWEEN SPINAL AND EPIDURAL TECHNIQUES

	Spinal	Epidural
Onset	2–5 mins	20–30 mins
Duration	2–3 H (single shot)	3–5 H
Drug volume	2.5–4 ml	20–30 ml
Quality of block	rapid surgical anaesthesia	may be inadequate in some dermatomes

Figure RA.12

The differences in Figure RA.12 apply to single shot, local anaesthetic blocks and the addition of adjuvant drugs (such as opioids or alpha$_2$ agonists) can alter the characteristics of each technique. With regard to the epidural route it is customary to insert a catheter to allow top up doses or prolonged infusions whereas spinal catheters are not commonplace. Combined spinal and epidural (CSE) anaesthesia is increasingly used, especially for obstetric surgery to utilise the benefits of both techniques (Carrie 1990). Surgical block can be rapidly established with a small dose of spinal bupivacaine (2–2.5 ml hyperbaric solution) followed by the slower onset of a low dose epidural which can be used to extend operating time and post operative analgesia.

In summary, spinals provide rapid onset, short duration surgical anaesthesia below the umbilicus with small doses of drug. Epidurals have a slower onset time, require large doses of drug and produce less dense surgical anaesthesia but can be used more flexibly in the lumbar and thoracic regions and their duration may be extended to days or weeks for analgesia by the insertion of a catheter.

Anatomy

The anatomy of the epidural space is described on page 86. Refer also to Figure RA.3.

Physiology

The effects of epidural anaesthesia on the major organ systems are similar to those of spinal anaesthesia with the height of the block being the major determinant. In a patient with compromised cardiovascular or respiratory reserve, the slower onset of epidural blockade gives more time to manage the onset of hypotension and other side effects, although against this advantage must be weighed the risks of the need for a much larger dose of local anaesthetic drug. The spread of local anaesthetic solution within the epidural space and thus the ultimate height of block is determined by a number of factors (Figure RA.13).

Equipment

In addition to the equipment necessary for spinal anaesthesia (see previously) a suitable epidural pack will be required. There are several commercial packs readily available and most contain a loss of resistance syringe, Tuohy needle, catheter and bacterial filter.

Technique

The practical technique of lumbar midline approach to the epidural space is described in Figure RA.14 (overleaf).

FACTORS AFFECTING SPREAD OF EPIDURAL SOLUTIONS

Factors	Comment
Drug mass	Drug mass is critical and more important than either volume or concentration.
Drug volume	For a given drug mass, larger volume gives more spread than a small volume.
Site of injection	The epidural space increases in volume in a caudal direction. Thus a given volume will spread further in the cervical> thoracic> lumbar> sacral. Onset is fastest and the block most intense in the dermatomes nearest the site of injection.
Age	A given volume spreads further with increasing age over 40 years.
Raised abdominal pressure	Smaller volumes may be needed in pregnancy and morbid obesity.
Patient position	Prolonged sitting position may reduce upward spread. Earlier onset of block in dependant side.
Injection technique	Slow 'unfractionated' injection of dose through needle gives fewer incomplete blocks than 'fractionated' or incremental doses.

Figure RA.13

LOSS OF RESISTANCE (LOR) TO AIR OR SALINE

Air	Saline
Requires LOR syringe	Ordinary syringe
Intermittent testing and movement of needle	Continuous pressure on plunger and movement of needle
Easy to learn	More difficult to learn
One or two handed	One handed only control of needle
Air bubbles may form space and expand with N$_2$O	Saline may be confused with CSF

Figure RA.15

THE TECHNIQUE FOR EPIDURAL INSERTION

The Tuohy needle, the loss of resistance syringe, the catheter and filter must be examined and prepared for use. Connect the filter and catheter and fill with saline to ensure free passage of solution. Position the patient in either the lateral or sitting position as for a spinal injection and identify the appropriate vertebral interspace. Sterilise and drape the area, raise a skin wheal with 1% lidocaine and anchor the skin over the cephalad spine of the interspace with the non dominant index finger. Insert a 21G hypodermic needle at right angles to the skin exactly in the midline of the interspace to inject more local anaesthetic into the interspinous ligaments and identify the route of the Tuohy needle. Insert the Tuohy needle in the direction indicated by the hypodermic needle. The needle will pass easily through the superficial layers but as it passes through the supraspinous and interspinous ligaments, resistance will become more obvious. If the needle strikes bone withdraw it slightly and re-angle slightly cephalad but still in the midline. At this point remove the trochar and attach the loss of resistance syringe filled with air or saline as required. Carefully advance the needle and syringe combination through the deep layers of the interspinous ligament and into the ligamentum flavum. Constantly check for loss of resistance as the needle is advanced through the ligament which is 3–5 mm thick in the mid line. As the tip of the needle enters the epidural space, there will be a simultaneous loss of resistance in the syringe, an audible 'click' and a tactile feeling of the needle advancing more easily, which requires great control to prevent sudden advancement within the epidural space. Immobilise the Tuohy needle once the loss of resistance occurs, carefully remove the syringe and check that no blood or CSF drains from the needle. CSF will normally emerge from a Tuohy needle with sufficient volume and velocity to leave no doubt as to its identity.

Figure RA.14

The above description relates to loss of resistance to air. There are advocates for the use of saline and each technique has its own benefits and drawbacks. These are summarised in Figure RA.15.

Only 3 ml air or saline (or less) should be injected in order to minimise bubble formation, dilution of local anaesthetic and confusion with CSF. In distinguishing saline from CSF, saline should be cold on the skin compared with CSF and CSF will show positive for glucose on proprietary stick testing.

DRUG DOSES IN EPIDURAL ANAESTHESIA

Block height	Drug and volume			Duration
Lumbosacral (L1–S5 approx)	Lidocaine	2.0%	20–25 ml	2–3 H
	Bupivacaine	0.5%	18–20 ml	4–6 H
	Bupivacaine (racemic or levo)	0.75%	10–15 ml	4–6 H
	Ropivacaine	7.5 mg/ml	20–25 ml	4–6 H
Thoraco-lumbar (T5–L4/5 approx)	Lidocaine	2.0%	25–30 ml	2–3 H
	Bupivacaine	0.5%	20–25 ml	4–6 H
	Bupivacaine (racemic or levo)	0.75%	15–20 ml	4–6 H
	Ropivacaine	7.5 mg/ml	15–25 ml	4–6 H

Figure RA.16

Drugs, doses and volumes

INJECTION OF THE LOCAL ANAESTHETIC AGENT

Single shot technique. A test dose through the needle of 3 ml 2% lidocaine plus epinephrine 1:200 000 may detect inadvertent spinal or intravascular injection, denoted by the rapid onset of a spinal block or a sudden tachycardia (although there is an incidence of false negative test doses). The local anaesthetic agent may be injected slowly over 2 minutes in 5 ml aliquots to allow for detection of signs of impending toxicity.

Catheter techniques. The initial dose of local anaesthetic agent may be administered via the needle followed by insertion of a catheter for subsequent top up doses. This method dilates the epidural space, allows easier insertion of the catheter, and produces a more rapid onset of anaesthesia and fewer missed segments. Alternatively, the catheter is inserted immediately loss of resistance is confirmed, the test dose administered and the main dose given in incremental doses via the catheter. Figure RA.16 shows some indicative dosing requirements for a fit adult male with the injection made at L3/4. Lidocaine is usually used with 1:200 000 epinephrine to reduce absorption and prolong duration. Bupivacaine 0.75% offers the same duration as 0.5% solution but gives a better quality sensory and motor block.

Whichever method of epidural injection is used, the ECG, heart rate, oxygen saturation and blood pressure must be monitored frequently as the block develops over 15–20 minutes. The development of segmental sensory loss should be followed by testing of dermatomal levels as for a spinal block.

Complications

Complications of epidural block are similar to those of a spinal block but there is a difference of severity and incidence for each of the following complications.

POST DURAL PUNCTURE HEADACHE

This complication of accidental dural puncture carries a higher risk of headache developing and the headache is more severe due to the larger hole made in the dura. In non obstetric patients about half of the patients who have a dural puncture will develop a headache severe enough to require a blood patch but in the obstetric population over 90% of sufferers will require one.

BACK PAIN

Back pain is sometimes reported after epidural (and spinal) anaesthesia and may be related to several causes (Figure RA.17).

CAUSES OF BACK PAIN AFTER EPIDURAL OR SPINAL BLOCK

Cause	Notes
Needle track pain	Localised and temporary
Postural	Extremes of posture during surgery or labour
Drug or additive	2-Chloroprocaine and EDTA
Epidural abscess or haematoma	Rare but important to treat
Recurrence of previous low back pain	

Figure RA.17

EPIDURAL HAEMATOMA

Although reported after diagnostic lumbar puncture, haematoma formation is excessively rare after spinal and epidural anaesthesia. The majority of reported cases occurs in patients with a coagulopathy or anticoagulant treatment. Current knowledge suggests that it is safe to use spinal and epidural techniques in patients receiving prophylactic heparinisation for surgery. If there is doubt then the following limits (Figure RA.18) may help decide if it is safe to proceed with a central block. The same criteria apply to removing as well as inserting an epidural catheter.

RISK FACTORS FOR SPINAL HAEMATOMA AFTER CNB

Patient factors	Technique factors
Spinal abnormalities	Technical difficulty
Age over 70 years	Repeated attempts
Female	Traumatic puncture
Anticoagulant therapy	Catheter placement
Coagulopathy	Catheter removal

Figure RA.18

THROMBOPROPHYLAXIS AND CENTRAL NERVE BLOCKS

There are several million central nerve blocks (CNB) carried out in Europe each year. The majority of these patients receive either unfractionated heparin (UFH) or low molecular weight heparin (LMWH) pre-operatively. Despite such high numbers there has hitherto been a wide discrepancy between countries in guidelines for the use of thromboprophylaxis when central nerve blocks are desirable. The maximum probable incidence of spinal haematoma following CNB in patients without risk factors is 1/320 000 for spinals and 1/200 000 for epidurals. The maximum risk accompanies epidural catheterisation and the minimum single shot spinal techniques with fine gauge needles. Around 75% of significant spinal haematomas are associated with 'bloody taps' or bleeding diathesis. It is thought that 50% of significant haematomas are associated with catheter removal. Risk factors for spinal haematoma after CNB are summarised in Figure RA.18. Recently the European Society for Regional Anaesthesia (ESRA) has recommended good practice guidelines for thromboprophylaxis and CNB and these are given in Figure RA.19.

ESRA GOOD PRACTICE GUIDELINES FOR THROMBOPROPHYLAXIS AND CNB

UFH
Prophylactic doses.
Extensive experience within Europe. No appreciable risk if: interval of approximately 4 hours between a dose of 5000 units of UFH and insertion of CNB or removal of catheter or 1 hour interval after insertion of CNB (or removal of catheter) before next dose is given.

Therapeutic doses
For vascular or cardiac surgery. Start IV infusion 1 hour after CNB and maintain PTT at 1.5 times normal. Remove catheter 4 hours after stopping infusion and check for normal PTT, ACT and platelet count.

LMWH
For prophylaxis (up to 40 mg enoxaparin/day) no increase in risk compared to UFH provided there are no additional risk factors and there is a 10 – 12 hour interval between the last dose of LMWH and CNB (and removal of catheter).

There should then be 6–8 hour interval before next dose. Therefore a once daily dosage regimen is preferable.

Antiplatelet agents (aspirin, NSAIDs)
Very few case reports of problems in the absence of other risk factors.
Beware the use of concurrent therapy — dextrans, anticoagulants, heparin.
If time allows, stop therapy 1–3 days pre-op for NSAID's and 3 days or more for aspirin, ticlopidine and other antiplatelet drugs.
Otherwise, measure platelets, careful visual inspection and bleeding history. There are no universally accepted tests for adequate platelet function.

Oral anticoagulants
Therapeutic levels of coumarins are an absolute contraindication.
Stop agent, convert to heparin, monitor INR and prothrombin time (factor VII, but II and X also affected).
If INR exceeds 1.5, proceed with caution (spinal rather than epidural). Beware catheter removal.

Figure RA.19

CAUDAL ANAESTHESIA

INDICATIONS

The caudal route for injection of local anaesthetic agents provides a way of administering a sacral epidural. There are multiple indications for the use of caudal anaesthesia, which are listed in Figure RA.20.

Anatomy

The normal anatomy of the sacrum is subject to great variation in the extent to which the laminae of the five sacral vertebrae fuse in the midline to form the sacral canal. The sacral hiatus normally results from the failure of the lamina of S 4 and 5 to fuse but it can vary in size from complete absence (approximately 5% of the population) to complete bifida of the sacrum. The dural sac ends at the S 2 level in adults, a level which approximates to a line drawn between the posterior superior iliac spines. In pre-adolescent children, there is a predictable relationship between age, volume of injection and height of block (Schulte-Steinburg 1970) but pubertal growth changes the volume and shape of the sacral canal and this relationship is lost in adults.

Physiology

The effect of caudal anaesthesia is limited to the lumbar and sacral nerves and, therefore, there will be less effect on cardiovascular, respiratory and gastro-intestinal performance than other epidural techniques. Motor weakness is limited to the legs and sensory loss is usually subumbilical. Autonomic disturbance is limited to bladder and anorectal dysfunction as both sympathetic and pelvic parasympathetic outflow is blocked.

Equipment

A 22 G short bevel needle should be used for adults and larger children and a 23 G hypodermic needle for smaller children and babies. For prolonged anaesthesia and post operative analgesia in children, continuous caudal epidurals, employing a 20 G epidural catheter inserted through an 18 G Tuohy needle, are becoming popular.

Technique

It is most common to administer a caudal after inducing general anaesthesia. The practical technique is described in Figure RA.21.

THE TECHNIQUE OF CAUDAL ANAESTHESIA

Place the patient in the lateral position as for a spinal or lumbar epidural. Note that the posterior superior iliac spines and the sacral hiatus form an equilateral triangle (Figure RA.21). Use the index finger of the non dominant hand to palpate the sacral cornuae either side of the hiatus which normally feels like a small depression between the bony landmarks. With the hiatus located, sterilise and prepare the area and insert the needle at an angle of about 60 degrees to the skin through the subcutaneous tissues. The sacrococcygeal membrane is tough and offers obvious resistance to the needle; once through the membrane, re-angle the needle to 20–30 degrees (Figure RA.23) and carefully advance the needle a few millimetres, ensuring that it remains in free space. If it strikes bone or will not advance freely, withdraw slightly and reposition the needle or begin the whole procedure again. Do not advance the needle more than a few millimetres within the sacral canal, especially in children, because the dural sac extends beyond S2 in some individuals. Aspirate to check for blood and CSF and then slowly inject 3 ml of chosen solution to test for low resistance to injection. If this feels normal and there is no subcutaneous swelling denoting needle misplacement in the superficial tissues, slowly inject the main dose, with frequent aspiration checks.

INDICATIONS FOR CAUDAL ANAESTHESIA

Adult

Surgery
anorectal
gynaecology
orthopaedic surgery

Obstetric
episiotomy
removal of placenta

Chronic pain
coccydynia
spinal manipulation

Paediatric

Major abdominal and orthopaedic surgery
Inguinal hernia repair
Surgery to genitalia

Figure RA.20

Figure RA.21

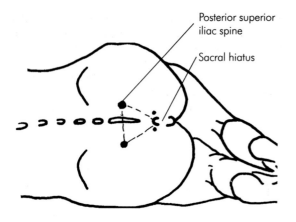

Figure RA.22 Patient position for caudal anaesthesia

DRUG DOSES FOR PAEDIATRIC CAUDAL BLOCK (0.25% BUPIVACAINE)

Block height	Volume in ml/kg
Lumbosacral	0.5
Thoracolumbar	1.0
Mid thoracic	1.25

Figure RA.24

DRUGS, DOSES AND VOLUMES

Paediatric: The linear relationship between age, volume and segmental spread is utilised in a number of formulae. The best known is that of Armitage (1979) and this is shown in Figure RA.24.

If the volume of bupivacaine used exceeds 20 ml, motor blockade can be minimised by using 0.19% bupivacaine (dilute 3 parts bupivacaine 0.25% with one part normal saline) and use the calculated volume as in Figure RA. 24. Lidocaine 1% in the same volumes gives analgesia for 3–4 hours compared with 6–8 hours for bupivacaine.

Adults: 25–30 ml 0.5% bupivacaine provides 6–8 hours of sub umbilical analgesia with a variable degree of segmental spread and motor blockade. If analgesia is necessary only within the sacral nerves, 20 ml is sufficient.

COMPLICATIONS

Incorrect needle placement is the commonest problem of the technique and is usually a matter of difficulty palpating landmarks. If the needle is too superficial, then the only adverse effect is a subcutaneous injection and a failed block. If the needle is inserted too deeply, it can pass through the sacrococcygeal joint into the pelvic cavity and thus the viscera, risking contamination of the epidural space. In pregnant patients there are reports of the needle entering the birth canal and damaging the foetal head. **Intravascular injection** is a risk due to the rich plexus of veins within the sacral canal. If the marrow of the sacral vertebra is cannulated and the dose injected, rapid systemic absorption can occur. **Infection** from a dirty technique in a potentially

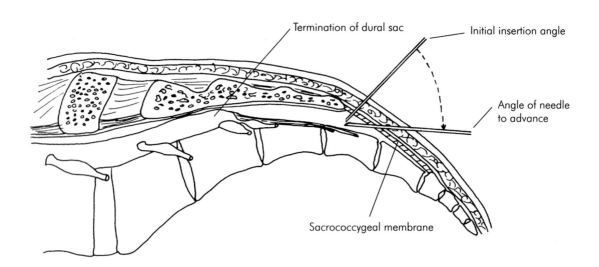

Figure RA.23 Needle angulation for caudal anaesthesia

unsterile area is a constant risk. **Dural puncture** is an uncommon but important complication because of the potentially large volume of local anaesthetic solution that can be inadvertently injected intrathecally.

PERIPHERAL NERVE BLOCKADE

There are several peripheral nerve blocks that have an important role in providing anaesthesia and post operative analgesia for surgery of the upper and lower extremities and the body surface (Pinnock 1996), a select few are detailed below.

BRACHIAL PLEXUS

INDICATIONS

Brachial plexus anaesthesia is indicated for a wide variety of surgical procedures and for the management of acute and chronic pain (Figure RA.25).

Anatomy

The anatomy of the brachial plexus is described on pages 205–207. The important, practical feature is the fascia that invests the plexus from its origins at the cervical roots between the middle and anterior scalene muscles to the five terminal nerves at the mid humeral level. Blockade of the brachial plexus is theoretically possible with entry into this fascia at any level, although the resulting block will vary according to the volume and subsequent spread of solution. There are

several techniques described in the literature but the three most common are the **Interscalene** (which blocks at the level of the five cervical roots), the **Supraclavicular** (which blocks at the level of the three trunks) and the **Axillary** (which blocks at the level of the five terminal nerves). Only the supraclavicular and the axillary are described below as the interscalene is technically more demanding.

Equipment

For single-shot injections, a short bevel 22 G, 3.5 cm regional block needle is ideal as it relays considerable information to the user about the tissue layers, particularly the sheath itself. The tactile response from the needle plus the frequent paraesthesiae when the needle is correctly placed should ensure a high success rate (> 85%). Experienced clinicians use a peripheral nerve stimulator to confirm accurate needle placement and this is a useful adjunct to teaching blocks or performing them in sedated or anaesthetised patients. To ensure that the needle is not displaced by manipulating or changing the syringes during injection, the 'immobile needle' concept (Winnie 1969) uses a short (10–15 cm) extension set from the needle to the syringe. This allows the operator to carefully control the needle while an assistant makes the injection or changes the syringes.

THE AXILLARY APPROACH

The axillary approach is the easiest technique to learn and carries the lowest risk of serious complications.

INDICATIONS FOR BRACHIAL PLEXUS BLOCKADE	
Indication	**Notes**

Trauma and orthopaedic surgery
    fracture manipulation or fixation
    joint replacement
    soft tissue trauma
	Possibility of compartment syndrome with
	    closed trauma

Vascular and reconstructive surgery
    shunt formation
    plastic reconstruction
    microvascular surgery
	Prolonged sympathetic blockade improves
	    blood flow to critical perfusion areas

Acute pain
    post operative analgesia
    continuous passive movement (after joint surgery)
	Up to 24 H analgesia with 0.75% bupivacaine

Chronic pain
    reflex sympathetic dystrophy
    terminal cancer pain
	Catheter insertion into sheath allows
	    prolonged infusions

Figure RA.25

The practical technique is described below in Figure RA.26.

Note: the needle may enter the axillary artery, in which case apply gentle aspiration and continue to slowly advance the needle through the posterior wall of the artery until blood can no longer be aspirated. At this point the patient may experience parasthesiae within the distribution of the radial nerve and after careful negative aspiration the injection can be completed – the **transarterial approach**. Firm digital pressure must be maintained for several minutes if the artery is punctured. In a fit adult, 40 ml local anaesthetic will usually produce an effective brachial plexus block but it may not uniformly block all five terminal nerves because of variable spread within the sheath. Thus a partial block may occur with a nerve territory being missed (usually the musculocutaneous) rather than a dermatomal pattern of failure as would be the case with an interscalene block, where the injection is made at the level of the roots. With a supraclavicular block, partial failure is manifested as both a dermatomal (C8/T1) and nerve territory (median or ulnar) failure, because the inferior trunk is the most likely to be missed.

Drugs, doses and volumes

Figure RA.28 illustrates the drugs, volume and average duration of block for surgical anaesthesia with respect to axillary and supraclavicular approaches to brachial plexus block. Although the relatively large volumes indicated may be above data sheet maxima, they are more effective than smaller volumes, widely used, and known to be safe due to the low rates of systemic absorption from the brachial plexus sheath. Regard should always be paid to maximum doses of local anaesthetic agent when calculated on a body weight basis. For axillary block, the technique will be most effective in the medial aspect of the upper arm, the forearm and hand; whereas for supraclavicular block, distribution is fairly uniform below the shoulder but may be less dense in the ulnar aspect of the hand.

THE SUPRACLAVICULAR APPROACH

There is a variety of techniques described but the subclavian perivascular approach (Winnie 1964) is very successful and deservedly popular. A line drawn from the cricoid cartilage laterally across the

---

THE TECHNIQUE OF AXILLARY APPROACH TO THE BRACHIAL PLEXUS

Position the patient supine with the shoulder abducted to 90 degrees and the elbow flexed to 90 degrees (Figure RA.27). Identify the lateral border of the pectoralis major and palpate the axillary arterial pulse at this level on the medial surface of the arm. Follow the pulsation proximal into the axilla to identify where the pulse is most obvious, and raise a skin weal with a 25 G needle and 1–2 ml of local anaesthetic over this point. Fix the artery with the non dominant index finger and insert a 22 G short bevel, 3.5 cm needle either above or below the index finger aiming towards the pulse; at a depth of 1–2 cm. In a normal adult arm there will be resistance from the fascial sheath followed by a distinct 'pop' and the patient may experience parasthesiae in the distribution of the ulnar nerve. The needle should be immobilised at this stage and the injection made after negative aspiration. Digital pressure applied distal to the needle during the injection and maintained while the needle is removed and the arm adducted after injection will encourage proximal spread of solution.

Figure RA.26

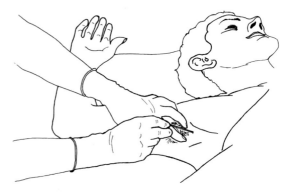

Figure RA.27 Patient position for axillary block

DRUG DOSES AND DURATION FOR BRACHIAL PLEXUS BLOCKADE

Drug	Volume	Duration
Lidocaine 1.5% + epinephrine	40–50 ml	3–4 H
Bupivacaine 0.5% (racemic or levo)	35–40 ml	9–11 H
Ropivacaine 0.5%	35–40 ml	9–11 H

Figure RA.28

sternomastoid muscle meets the posterior border of that muscle at the point where the interscalene groove emerges from under the sternomastoid, running caudally between the anterior and middle scalenus muscles laterally towards the midpoint of the posterior border of the clavicle providing useful landmarks. The practical technique is described in Figure RA.29, and patient position in Figure RA.30.

Complications

Some complications may be considered as inevitable side effects of a successful block whereas others are potentially dangerous (Figure RA.31).

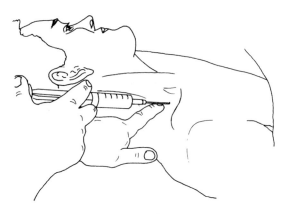

Figure RA.30 Patient position for subclavian brachial plexus block

THE TECHNIQUE OF SUBCLAVIAN PERIVASCULAR BRACHIAL PLEXUS BLOCK

Position the patient supine with the head supported by a single pillow and turned slightly away from the side to be blocked and the arm extended downwards, beside the thigh, to depress the clavicle (Figure RA.30). If the muscular landmarks are difficult to identify, ask the patient to lift their head slightly off the pillow to throw the muscle into relief; the interscalene groove can be highlighted by vigorous sniffing. Trace the interscalene groove distally with the non dominant index finger until the pulsation of the subclavian artery is palpable – usually about 1 cm behind the midpoint of the clavicle. Raise a skin wheal of local anaesthetic at this point and then insert a 22 G short bevel 3.5 cm needle parallel to the neck in the horizontal plane towards the pulse of the subclavian artery. It is not crucial to feel the arterial pulse, if the groove can be identified accurately. Advance the needle until the sheath is detected at a depth of about 1–2 cm as an increased resistance with a distinct 'pop' when the needle penetrates. The patient may experience parasthesiae in the distribution of the superior trunk (C 5/6, median, musculo-cutaneous or radial nerves). Aspirate to ensure that the needle has not entered the subclavian artery and slowly make the injection. If arterial blood is aspirated, carefully withdraw the needle a few millimetres until aspiration is negative; the needle will still be within the fascial sheath and the injection can be made as normal. Digital pressure proximal to the needle insertion will encourage distal spread; as the large volume is injected.

Figure RA.29

COMPLICATIONS OF BRACHIAL PLEXUS BLOCK

Axillary

Haematoma
Vascular damage

Supraclavicular

Phrenic nerve block
Horner's syndrome
Recurrent laryngeal nerve block
Pneumothorax

Figure RA.31

FEMORAL NERVE BLOCK

Indications

The femoral nerve is normally blocked in combination with the sciatic, obturator and lateral cutaneous nerves, as appropriate, to ensure an adequate block for the proposed site of surgery. The main indication is for major orthopaedic procedures of the lower limb, especially surgery to the femur and knee joint. Post operative analgesia following a total knee replacement or cruciate ligament reconstruction can be impressive as a single shot femoral nerve block may last up to 24 hours if 0.75% bupivacaine is used.

Anatomy

The femoral nerve is the largest branch of the lumbar plexus and enters the thigh lateral to the femoral artery in its own fascial sheath (Figure RA.32). It can be discretely blocked as a single nerve using 10 ml solution but a large volume (20–30 ml) produces, in effect, a distal approach to the lumbar plexus which also blocks the obturator nerve and lateral cutaneous nerve of thigh the so-called '3 in 1' block (Winnie 1973), although there is some uncertainty whether all three nerves are reliably blocked with this approach.

Technique

The practical technique of femoral nerve blockade is given in Figure RA.33.

Drugs, doses and volumes

Figure RA.34 shows the duration of a single shot femoral nerve block using a long acting local anaesthetic solution. Duration can be extended by the insertion of a catheter into the femoral nerve sheath for continuous infusion.

THE TECHNIQUE OF FEMORAL NERVE BLOCK

Position the patient supine and identify the inguinal ligament and the femoral arterial pulse immediately distal to it. The point of injection should be 1 cm lateral to the pulsation and 1–2 cm distal to the inguinal ligament. Having raised a skin weal of lidocaine, insert a 22 G short bevel regional block needle at about 45 degrees, aiming cephalad. A distinct pop as the needle pierces the fascia lata may be felt followed by a secondary pop as it enters the nerve sheath. Parasthesiae in the distribution of the femoral or saphenous nerves indicates close proximity to the nerve and after aspiration, slowly inject the chosen volume. In anaesthetised patients, a peripheral nerve stimulator will aid accurate location.

Figure RA.33

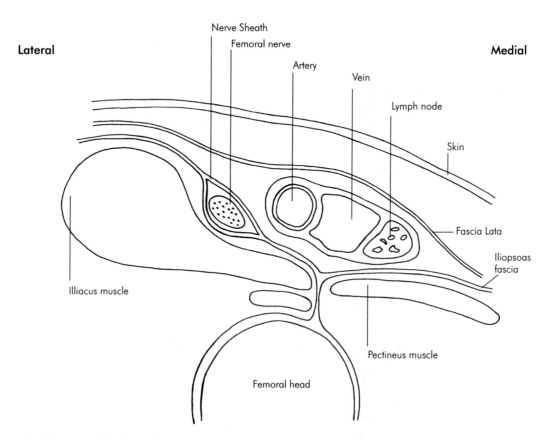

Figure RA.32 Anatomy of the femoral nerve in cross section

DRUG DOSES FOR FEMORAL NERVE BLOCK

Drug	Volume	Duration
Bupivacaine 0.5% (racemic or levo)	15 ml	12–18 H
Bupivacaine 0.75%	12 ml	18–24 H
Bupivacaine 0.5% (racemic or levo)	20–30 ml (for '3 in 1')	8–12 H

Figure RA.34

Complications

The only significant complication of femoral nerve block is the accidental injection of local anaesthetic into the femoral vessels, which are immediately adjacent to the nerve. Attention to detail when performing the block and careful aspiration prior to injection will prevent this avoidable complication. The limb will be anaesthetic for many hours and it must, therefore, be protected from pressure sores and prolonged immobility.

ANKLE BLOCK

Indications

The nerve supply to the foot can be blocked at the ankle to provide surgical anaesthesia and post operative pain relief for any operation performed distal to the malleoli. The main indications are orthopaedic and trauma surgery to the forefoot and digits. Surgery such as correction of hallux valgus is very painful and ankle blocks, using 0.5% bupivacaine, can provide 18 – 24 hours analgesia. Although it is usual to perform a combination of blocks at the ankle under light general anaesthesia, it is possible to use the technique in conscious patients. The practical techniques are described in Figure RA. 35.

Anatomy

The five nerves which supply the foot and the ankle are the terminal branches of the femoral and sciatic nerves. The saphenous nerve is the terminal branch of the femoral nerve and supplies the skin over the medial malleolus and a variable amount of the medial border of the foot. It passes anterior to the medial malleolus accompanied by the saphenous vein. The other nerves are branches of the sciatic nerve, which divides into the common peroneal and tibial nerves within the popliteal fossa. The deep and superficial peroneal nerves emerge onto the dorsum of the foot at the level of the extensor skin crease between the pulse of the dorsalis pedis and

the tendon of extensor hallucis longus. The deep peroneal nerve supplies the deep structures of the dorsum of the foot and the skin of the first webspace only; the superficial peroneal nerve supplies the skin of the dorsum of the foot and the lateral three webspaces. The tibial nerve runs in a sulcus behind the medial malleolus, deep to the medial collateral ligament of the ankle, accompanied by the corresponding tibial vessels and divides into medial and lateral plantar nerves which supply the sole of the foot and the deep plantar structures. The sural nerve runs subcutaneously between the lateral malleolus and the calcaneus to supply the lateral border of the foot.

Drugs, doses and volumes

Bupivacaine 0.5% will provide surgical anaesthesia for 3–4 hours and 12–18 hours analgesia, although up to 24 hours is possible. For minor surgery, especially in ambulant patients, 2% lidocaine will provide 1–2 hours surgical anaesthesia and 4–6 hours analgesia. Each nerve requires approximately 5–6 ml; thus the total volume used depends on the number of nerves blocked, although a maximum of 20 ml is recommended.

Complications

The main complications of these nerve blocks are the potential for intravascular injection or vascular trauma as all the injections are made into neurovascular bundles except the sural nerve. However, the volumes of local anaesthetic are small, the needle used should be no larger than 23 gauge and aspirating the needle before each injection will minimise the risk.

Many patients will be mobilised soon after surgery and they must be supervised and non-weight bearing whilst the blocks are still working because they will have no sensory or proprioceptive awareness in the sole of the foot if the tibial nerve has been blocked.

INGUINAL FIELD BLOCK

Indications

Inguinal field block in combination with light general anaesthesia is ideal suited to day case repair of a hernia. The technique offers rapid recovery from anaesthesia and post operative analgesia lasting for 6–8 H. If the surgery is to be performed using local anaesthesia as a sole technique, a larger volume of more dilute local anaesthetic is preferable and the surgeon may need to reinforce the anaesthesia by direct infiltration of the deeper structures within the inguinal canal. The technique of inguinal field block is detailed in Figure RA.36.

THE TECHNIQUE OF ANKLE BLOCK

Tibial nerve

Palpate the lower border of the medial malleolus and the medial surface of the calcaneal tuberosity. At the midpoint of a line between these two bony landmarks insert a 23 G needle at 90 degrees to the skin until it just touches the periosteum of the calcaneus just below the sustentaculum tali which can be felt as a crescent-shaped protuberance on the calcaneus. Withdraw the needle 1–2 mm, aspirate and slowly inject 5–6 ml. If the injection is in the correct plane, deep to the medical collateral ligament, the local anaesthetic will spread proximally and distally along the course of the tibial nerve.

Deep peroneal nerve

Position the foot at right angles to the tibia and palpate the pulse of dorsalis pedis. Identify the tendon of extensor hallucis longus by moving the great toe and insert a 23 G needle between these two landmarks at 45 degrees to the skin until contact is made with the distal end of the tibia. Withdraw the needle 1–2 mm, aspirate and slowly inject 4–5 ml of local anaesthetic.

Superficial peroneal nerve

Withdraw the needle into the subcutaneous tissue having completed the deep peroneal injection, and re-align it, aiming towards the lateral border of the foot. Advance the needle slowly and inject 4–5 ml of local anaesthetic, subcutaneously to produce a wheal of local anaesthetic extending laterally across the dorsum of the foot. This wheal can be gently massaged to spread it further laterally.

Sural nerve

Palpate the lower border of the lateral malleolus and the lateral aspect of the calcaneal tuberosity and make a subcutaneous injection of 5 ml of local anaesthetic between these two points.

Saphenous nerve

Identify the saphenous vein, if possible, anterior and proximal to the medial malleolus and inject a subcutaneous wheal of 3–4 ml of local anaesthetic around the vein, using a 23 G needle. Take care to avoid intravenous injection and trauma to the vein.

Figure RA.35

THE TECHNIQUE OF INGUINAL FIELD BLOCK

Lie the patient in the supine position and identify the anterior superior iliac spine (ASIS) and the pubic tubercle – the bony landmarks which define the two injection points. The top injection point will be 1 cm medial and 2 cm caudal to the ASIS. Make a skin wheal of lidocaine at this point and insert a 22 G short bevel regional block needle, at right angles to the skin, directly downwards through the skin and subcutaneous tissue. At a depth of 1–2 cm (more in obese patients), the needle will encounter the external oblique aponeurosis which will offer marked resistance to penetration. Move the needle from side to side in a horizontal plane and a distinct scratching over the surface of the aponeurosis will be felt. The iliohypogastric nerve (T 12/L 1) lies just deep to the aponeurosis, so once the needle penetrates it, immobilise the needle and inject 5 ml of local anaesthetic. Carefully advance the needle another 0.5–1 cm to penetrate the internal oblique muscle (there is often a slight loss of resistance as the needle leaves the inner surface of the muscle) and inject a further 5 ml of solution to block to ilioinguinal nerve (T 12/L 1), immediately deep to the muscle. Withdraw the needle to the subcutaneous tissues and infiltrate a subcutaneous, fan shaped area, using 10 ml of solution to block the terminal fibres of the subcostal nerve (T 12).

The second part of the injection should be made over the pubic tubercle. Insert the needle directly down to the tubercle and inject 5 ml of solution around the external inguinal ring to anaesthetise the genitofemoral nerve (L 1/2). Make a second fan shaped subcutaneous infiltration to block any fibres that may cross the midline.

Figure RA.36

Anatomy

The anatomy of the inguinal region is described in Chapter 10, page 215.

Drugs, doses and volumes

Bupivacaine 0.5% with epinephrine 1:200 000 to a total of 30 ml for supplementation of light general anaesthesia will provide up to 8 hours post operative analgesia. For local anaesthesia as a sole technique, 50 ml 1% prilocaine is suitable but only 2–3 hours post operative analgesia will result.

Complications

There are few important complications as the technique is mainly one of infiltration together with the discrete blockade of three small peripheral nerves. From the first point of injection, puncture of the peritoneum and viscera is possible if a long needle is used. Inadvertent intravascular injection is always a possibility with the second point of injection, especially the femoral vessels. It is also possible to block the femoral nerve from the same point and the patient may complain of pain in the hernia site and a numb, heavy leg!

PENILE BLOCK

Indications

The main indication for penile block is for post operative analgesia for adult and paediatric male circumcision, although any surgery on the shaft of the penis will benefit. Analgesia is comparable with that produced by a caudal block and avoids the motor and sensory effects on the legs and the autonomic dysfunction of bladder and bowel control. There are no major complications provided that epinephrine or other vasoconstrictors are not used and intravascular injection is avoided.

Anatomy

The shaft and glans of the penis are supplied by a pair of nerves (the dorsal penile nerves) which are terminal branches of the pudendal nerve (S2, 3, 4). The paired nerves emerge beneath the inferior surface of the pubic symphysis separated by the suspensory ligament and deep to Buck's fascia (the fascial sheath surrounding the corpora cavernosa). The perineal nerves (from the other branch of the pudendal nerve) which innervate the anterior part of the scrotum and the midline ventral surface of the penis need to be blocked for complete penile analgesia.

Technique

The technique of penile nerve block is given in Figure RA.37. It is customary to perform this block on anaesthetised or sedated patients.

Drugs, doses and volumes

Avoid epinephrine containing local anaesthetic solutions. Bupivacaine 0.5% will provide 6–8 hours post operative analgesia following circumcision. 10 ml is sufficient for an adult, children need 3–6 ml according to body weight and size. Limit total dose of bupivacaine to 2 mg/kg body weight.

THE TECHNIQUE OF PENILE BLOCK

Palpate the inferior edge of the pubic symphysis with the non dominant index finger and insert a 21 G (adult) or 23 G (paediatric) needle at about 45 degrees until it contacts the pubis or passes just caudad to it. If the needle contacts the pubis, re-angle it to walk it off the inferior edge and through Buck's fascia, which may be detectable as a slight resistance to the needle. After careful aspiration, make a single injection in the midline (both dorsal nerves may be reliably blocked by a single injection). In an adult, inject 7 ml and then inject a further 3 ml as a subcutaneous wheal across the midline of the ventral surface of the penis at its junction with the scrotum, starting approximately 1 cm lateral to the midline raphe and finishing 1 cm lateral on the other side. It is important to keep the needle subcutaneous while making this injection as the urethra is superficial at this point. In children the volume needs to be reduced *pro rata* according to body weight and penile size.

Figure RA.37

LOCAL ANAESTHESIA OF THE UPPER AIRWAY

The mucosal surfaces of the mouth, oropharynx, glottis and larynx may be anaesthetised by a combination of topical anaesthesia and discrete nerve blocks.

INDICATIONS

Intubation of trachea in patients with difficult airway due to trauma or disease.

Anatomy

The nerve supply of the airway comes from three sources. The trigeminal nerve supplies the nasopharynx, palate (V2), and anterior aspect of tongue (V3). The glossopharyngeal nerve supplies the oropharynx, posterior aspect of tongue and soft palate. The vagus nerve gives off two nerves – the superior laryngeal and recurrent laryngeal nerves which supply motor and sensory fibres to the airway below the epiglottis. The superior laryngeal nerve emerges beneath the inferior edge of the greater cornu of the hyoid before it divides into the internal and external branches.

Technique

The technique of local anaesthesia of the upper airway comprises three parts, topical anaesthesia, superior

THE TECHNIQUE OF LOCAL ANAESTHESIA OF THE AIRWAY

To topically anaesthetise the mouth and oropharynx, sit the patient up with their mouth open maximally and spray four metered puffs of lidocaine (10 mg per spray) onto the tongue and wait a few minutes for it to take effect. Depress the tongue and spray a further 4 puffs onto the posterior part of the tongue and pharynx. Although the superior laryngeal nerve can be topically anaesthetised by placing a pledget soaked in 2% lidocaine into each pyriform fossa with Krause forceps, once the mouth and tongue are blocked, it is more usually blocked discretely as follows: Place the patient supine with the head extended and palpate the hyoid bone just cephalad to the thyroid cartilage. Displace the hyoid slightly towards the side to be blocked and insert a 25 G, 2.5 cm needle just under the inferior border of the hyoid and inject 2–3 ml of 1% lidocaine, moving the needle gently in and out through the thyrohyoid membrane (Figure RA.39). Repeat on the other side. To complete the airway anaesthesia, with the patient in the same position as above, palpate the inferior border of the thyroid cartilage and having anaesthetised the skin first, insert a 21 G, 2.5 cm needle through the cricothyroid membrane into the lumen of the trachea. Ensure that air is freely aspirable and then rapidly inject 3–4 ml of 2% lidocaine. This will precipitate brisk coughing which spreads the local anaesthetic throughout the trachea and up into the larynx and vocal cords (Figure RA.40). Total dose of lidocaine in an average 70 kg adult should not exceed 200 mg.

Figure RA.38

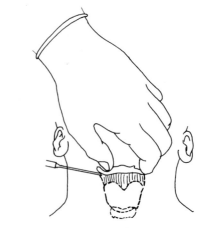

Figure RA.39 Superior laryngeal nerve block

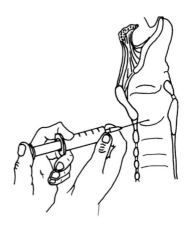

Figure RA.40 Transtracheal block

laryngeal nerve block and transtracheal anaesthesia. Practical details are given in Figure RA.36.

INTRAVENOUS REGIONAL ANAESTHESIA (IVRA)

The technique in current use differs from the original description of August Bier in 1908, although it is often called 'Bier's block'. Bier placed two tourniquets on the forearm and injected procaine directly into a vein isolated by surgical cut-down. Although a two tourniquet technique has been re-evaluated recently, one tourniquet is used in modern practice.

Indications

Any surgery lasting less than 1 hour below the level of the elbow in the arm or the ankle in the leg.

Equipment

The tourniquet used must be properly maintained with regular calibration of the pressure gauge and must be of an approved design. Sphygmomanometer cuffs should never be used. Specially designed double cuff tourniquets are available which allow the proximal cuff to be blown up while the block is established and then the distal cuff is inflated over anaesthetised skin for use during surgery and the proximal one deflated. This improves comfort during prolonged procedures but the patient may still experience deep pain from ischaemic muscle.

Technique

The practical technique for performing IVRA is shown in Figure RA.41.

Analgesia will be complete within 15 minutes using 0.5% prilocaine. The cuff should remain inflated for at least 20 minutes after which time deflation of the cuff and systemic release of the local anaesthetic drug should not cause untoward reactions, although occasionally some transient minor systemic symptoms such as light headedness or tinnitus are reported. IVRA in the leg is not practical if the cuff has to be placed around the thigh as inflation pressures of 300–400 mmHg above systolic and very large volumes of local anaesthetic are required. If the surgery is limited to below the ankle, however, then a cuff around the calf is possible using similar pressures and drug volumes to the arm, although exsanguination may not be ideal as the lower leg has a two-bone compartment and vessels between the tibia and fibula will not be compressed. There is also a risk of damage to the peroneal nerve in the region of the head of the fibula if a high tourniquet is applied.

Drugs, doses and volumes

The local anaesthetic agent currently licensed for IVRA is prilocaine 0.5%. For an adult male, 60 ml 0.5% (300 mg) produces good sensory and motor block and is well within the maximum recommended dose of 600 mg.

References and further reading

Armitage EN. Caudal block in children. *Anaesthesia* 1979; **34:** 396.

Bromage PR. A comparison of the hydrochloride and carbon dioxide salts of lidocaine and prilocaine in epidural analgesia. *Acta Anaesthsiol Scand Suppl* 1965; **16:** 55–69.

Brown DL. *Regional Anesthesia and Analgesia.* Philadelphia: Saunders, 1996.

Carrie LES. Extradural, spinal or combined block for obstetric surgical anaesthesia. *British Journal of Anaesthesia* 1990; **65:** 225–233.

Green NM. Distribution of local anaesthetic solutions within the subarachnoid space. *Anesth Analg* 1985; **64:** 715–730.

Pinnock CA, Fischer HBJ, Jones RP. *Peripheral Nerve Blockade.* Edinburgh: Churchill Livingstone, 1996.

Schulte-Steinburg O, Ralhfs VW. Spread of extradural analgesia following caudal injection in children. A statistical study. *British Journal of Anaesthesia* 1977; **49:** 1027–1034.

Winnie AP. An 'Immobile Needle' for nerve blocks. Anesthesiology 1969; 31: 577–578.

Winnie AP, Collins V. The subclavian perivascular technique of brachial plexus anesthesia. *Anesthesiology* 1964; **25:** 353–363.

Winnie AP, Rammamurthy S, Durrani A. The inguinal paravascular technic of lumbar plexus anesthesia; the '3 in 1' block. *Anesth Analg* 1973; **52:** 989–996.

THE TECHNIQUE OF PERFORMING IVRA

Place an intravenous cannula in the dorsum of both hands, one for injection of the local anaesthetic and the other to allow for drug and fluid requirements during surgery. Wrap a layer of wool padding around the upper arm and place the tourniquet over the padding, ensuring that it is of the correct dimensions for the limb and properly secured. Elevate the limb and use a compression bandage to exsanguinate it or simply compress the axillary artery and keep the arm elevated for three minutes. Inflate the tourniquet to 100 mmHg above the patient's systolic blood pressure, remove the compression bandage and observe the arm for one minute to ensure that the veins remain empty. If blood begins to flow under the tourniquet the procedure should be repeated, using a pressure 150 mmHg above systolic or an alternative anaesthetic technique considered. Inject the local anaesthetic solution slowly (20 ml per min) to avoid high intravenous pressures which could force it under the tourniquet.

Figure RA.41

SECTION 1: 8
PRINCIPLES OF RESUSCITATION

F. J. Pickford

CARDIORESPIRATORY ARREST

Causes
Recognition

CARDIOPULMONARY RESUSCITATION

Basic life support
Advanced life support
Drug usage
Complications of CPR
Management of life threatening peri-arrest
  arrhythmias

RESUSCITATION OF THE PREGNANT PATIENT

Causes of arrest
Basic life support
Advanced life support

RESUSCITATION OF INFANTS AND CHILDREN

Causes of arrest
Basic life support
Advanced life support
Drug usage

ETHICAL CONSIDERATIONS IN CPR

When not to start resuscitation
When to resuscitate
When to stop resuscitation
Witnessing the resuscitation

CARDIORESPIRATORY ARREST

This chapter is firmly linked to the algorithms taught by the Resuscitation Council (UK) which in turn are condensed from the evidence-based "International Guidelines 2000 for CPR and ECC – A Consensus on Science".

CAUSES

The commonest cause of cardiac arrest is heart disease and although ischaemic heart disease is usually the precipitating cause, other cardiac conditions, such as valvular heart disease or cardiomyopathy may lead to cardiac arrest, as may several non-cardiac conditions. Thus cardiac arrest may be precipitated by:

● gross electrolyte and metabolic disturbances

● drugs and poisons

● mechanical interference

— with cardiac filling (e.g. hypovolaemia)

— or cardiac ejection (e.g. pulmonary embolism)

● hypothermia

● anaphylaxis (see Section 1 Chapter 2)

Respiratory causes of cardiac arrest must also be considered. Hypoxia and hypercarbia leading to secondary cardiac arrest may occur due to:

● intracerebral causes (e.g. haemorrhage)

● acute upper airway obstruction (e.g. choking)

● lower airway obstruction (e.g. asthma)

● pulmonary disease

Early aggressive treatment of the problems listed above can prevent cardiac arrest.

Since new guidelines for resuscitation were introduced in 1997 there has been some improvement in survival rate following arrest with a shockable rhythm but not with other rhythms (Gwinnutt 1997). It has been established that lives can be saved if risk can be ascertained and treatment started **before** cardio-respiratory arrest occurs. Such measures include morphine, oxygen, nitrates and aspirin (MONA) and early thrombolysis and beta blockade for patients with myocardial infarction (Verheugt 1999). Similarly secondary cardiac arrest may be avoided if patients with deteriorating respiratory, circulatory or neurological function can be attended early by hospital medical emergency teams (METs) (McQuillan 1998) or patients at risk teams (PARTs) (Goldhill 1999). At

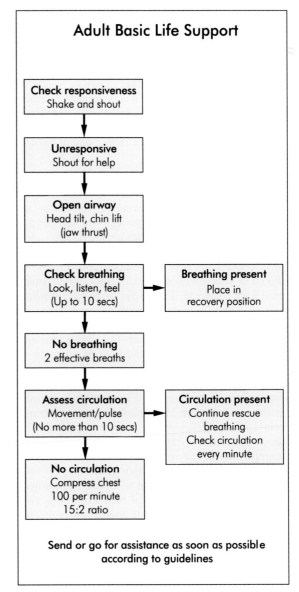

Figure RS.1 Adult basic life support ©RCUK 97

Ref. Single rescuer Adult Basic Life Support. An advisory statement from the Basic Life Support Working Group of the International Liaison Committee on Resuscitation (ILCOR) Resuscitation 34 (1977) 101-108

present however it is often the junior anaesthetist who is first called to these patients and it must be stressed that senior help should be sought early.

A primary cardiac arrest will rapidly be followed by cessation of respiration. Alternatively, if a respiratory arrest is the primary event, then without effective intervention, bradycardia will occur and secondary cardiac arrest, usually asystolic, will supervene.

RECOGNITION

For the healthcare professional, the diagnosis of cardiorespiratory arrest is made on the clinical findings of unresponsiveness with absent pulsations in major vessels. A carotid artery pulsation should be sought for no more than ten seconds; if it is thought to be absent and the patient is apnoeic and not moving, a diagnosis of cardiorespiratory arrest should be made. The victim may still be gasping if effective cardiac output has only recently ceased.

It is equally important to recognise the patient who has 'collapsed' but has **not** deteriorated to the point of cardiorespiratory arrest. Having assessed that the surroundings are safe and using basic life support assessment techniques (see under BLS), the patient should be categorised as shown in Figure RS.1. A conscious patient who is breathing and has a pulse should be checked for injuries and monitored visually until fully recovered. The unconscious patient who is breathing and has a pulse should be turned into the recovery position (unless there is evidence of cervical spine injury) and monitored for airway patency, breathing and adequate circulation. If there is no breathing (assessment for this may take up to ten seconds) help should be sought. However, if the likely cause of unconsciousness and apnoea is trauma, near drowning, alcohol or drug intoxication or the victim is a child, a lone rescuer should perform resuscitation for about one minute before going for help. Up to five attempts should be made to achieve two effective breaths. The patient should then be assessed for signs of a circulation and the carotid artery palpated for up to ten seconds, remembering that even within this time, diagnostic accuracy is poor. If circulation is present, rescue breathing should continue with pulse checks every minute. If it is deemed that there is no circulation, full cardiopulmonary resuscitation must ensue.

CARDIOPULMONARY RESUSCITATION (CPR)

Effective CPR combines the following two elements: Basic Life Support (BLS) techniques that ensure adequate delivery of blood to vital organs and maintain physiological normality at cell level, so that: Advanced Life Support (ALS) interventions can then provide the rapid return of a spontaneous circulation. However, because of the proven efficacy of early defibrillation, if the equipment is available, this intervention should ideally take precedence over institution of basic life support.

BASIC LIFE SUPPORT

Traditionally, and still in the community, techniques are taught as the 'ABCs' (airway, breathing, circulation) of BLS. Before any approach to a casualty, a check must be made for patient and rescuer safety. Conscious level must then be ascertained by calling and by gentle shaking of the shoulders.

AIRWAY

In the unconscious patient, who is not breathing and has no pulse, there can be several mechanisms of airway obstruction resulting from a variety of causes, including tongue displacement, tongue swelling from anaphylaxis, laryngeal spasm, oedema or trauma, foreign body obstruction at laryngeal, tracheal, or bronchial level, bronchospasm or pulmonary oedema. The commonest of these is backward displacement of the tongue and epiglottis in the unconscious supine patient. Three manoeuvres can be used to create a clear upper airway (ERC 1996). **Head tilt** achieves lower cervical spine flexion and extension of the head at the atlanto-occipital joint, and **chin lift** is then added to improve the airway. **Jaw thrust** can further displace the tongue and in addition the thumbs can be used to open the mouth. This technique can be useful if a cervical spine fracture is suspected. It should be used in conjunction with in-line stabilisation of the head and neck by another helper and if the base of the thumbs are placed over the maxilla during jaw thrust, some further control of head stability can be assured. With the airway presumed to be clear from tongue obstruction, assessment should be made by looking, listening and feeling for breathing. (Figure RS. 2). If the patient is breathing spontaneously and there is evidence of expired air, obstruction is not present. It must be emphasised that if the patient is apnoeic, then it is not until an applied ventilatory volume is given and is seen to produce rise and fall of the chest, that the airway can be confirmed as being clear.

ASSESSMENT OF THE AIRWAY	
Look	in the mouth for a foreign body for cyanosis for rise and fall of the chest
Listen	for breath sounds (normal or abnormal)
Feel	for air flow at the mouth for chest movements for tracheal position for chest abnormalities, e.g. surgical emphysema

Figure RS.2

UPPER AIRWAY OBSTRUCTION BY A FOREIGN BODY

Obstruction of the airway by a foreign body is an important diagnosis, which needs to be made swiftly in the patient who has not deteriorated to the point of cardiorespiratory arrest. Whether or not consciousness has been lost, if the patient is still making efforts to breathe, then the degree of obstruction can be assessed. Noisy, stridulous breathing with respiratory distress indicates partial obstruction. The conscious patient will also be coughing and indicating choking by clutching their neck. If there is cyanosis and distress, intervention is needed urgently. Complete obstruction is not accompanied by any airflow and is, therefore, silent. Treatment of the choking patient depends upon whether they are conscious or unconscious. The best treatment for the conscious patient is encouragement to cough. If this fails, up to five back blows (hitting with the heel of the hand between the patient's scapulae) may dislodge an impacted foreign body. The Heimlich manoeuvre of subdiaphragmatic or abdominal thrusts can cause visceral damage and should only be used in adults. The fist should be placed well below the xiphisternum and five firm inward and upward thrusts should be given.

If the victim is unconscious and is an adult, guidelines for treatment are given in Figure RS. 3. After tilting the head, finger sweep may be performed in adults if a foreign body is seen in the mouth. After lifting the chin, a check should be made for breathing and if this is absent, five rescue breaths should be attempted; the aim is to deliver two effective breaths. If these have not been achieved, fifteen chest compressions should be performed without assessing circulation as these may relieve foreign body obstruction. These compressions will also serve to circulate blood if there is no cardiac output.

Failure to clear the airway will lead to cardiac arrest and therefore in the unconscious patient, the anaesthetist should rapidly opt for advanced methods for the relief of obstruction e.g. direct visualisation and endotracheal intubation.

RESCUE BREATHING

Expired air respiration (EAR) practiced in the community, is used to supply rescue breathing. Whilst performing a manoeuvre to keep the airway open, the nose of the patient should be pinched and two gentle breaths given by the rescuer, observing for rise and fall of the chest. It is obvious that maintenance of a clear airway helps to avoid gastric inflation but EAR always poses the risk of aspiration. However, without supplemental oxygen, it is recommended that a tidal volume of 10 ml/Kg should be given over 2 seconds, watching for rise and fall of the chest.

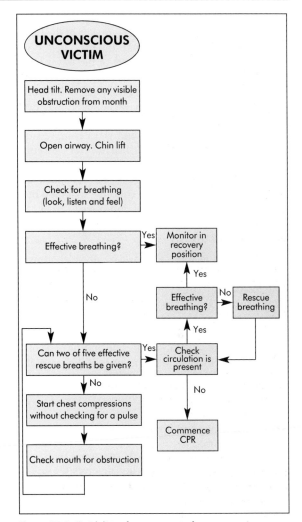

Figure RS.3. Guidelines for treatment of an unconscious victim. From International Guidelines 2000 for CPR and ECC

Disadvantages of EAR include:

- low inspired oxygen concentration

- aesthetic considerations

- risk of cross infection

CIRCULATION

The presence of a spontaneous circulation must be sought before initiating CPR. The carotid artery should be palpated for up to 10 seconds. If there is no pulse and if evidence of circulation is absent, i.e. there is no movement or coughing and the patient is not breathing normally, help should be summoned and chest compressions started with the patient on a firm flat surface. The hand position should be over the sternum, two finger breadths up from the xiphisternum, in the midline. The fingers of the upper hand should be interlocked with the hand below and pressure exerted through the heel of the lower hand. Chest compression using direct downward pressure with the arms straight, should be applied to a depth of 4–5 cm at a rate of 100/min (Handley 1997). Even following these guidelines accurately, the artificial circulation produced is poor and chest compressions should be stopped only briefly for essential interventions, or for palpation of the pulse if the clinical condition improves. It is recommended that ventilation and compressions continue in a ratio of 2: 15 whilst the patient remains unintubated.

EARLY DEFIBRILLATION

In adults the commonest cardiac arrest rhythm is ventricular fibrillation. Therefore in the community, solo rescuers are taught to phone **first** in unresponsive adults so that the nearest EMS (Emergency Medical Service) can provide early defibrillation which is cost effective and saves lives. If the single rescuer is dealing with a child or if trauma, submersion or drug or alcohol intoxication is thought to be the cause of the arrest, it is recommended that a minute of CPR is performed and then the EMS is called.

ADVANCED LIFE SUPPORT

Advanced life support (ALS) continues with the provision of BLS techniques but involves the use of extra equipment, which will be dealt with subsequently in the sequence ABC. ALS is specifically directed towards restoring a spontaneous circulation. As ventricular fibrillation is the most common rhythm of cardiac arrest, and since it offers the best opportunity for successful resuscitation if defibrillation occurs early (within 90 seconds) then there must be no delay in delivering up to three DC shocks.

ADVANCED AIRWAY MANAGEMENT

Simple adjuncts are often used to aid BLS techniques, but in practice, the use of any mechanical aid, however simple, may reduce efficacy and introduce complications.

PROTECTING THE AIRWAY

There are several devices available to aid the management of the airway:

1) **Pharyngeal airways** may be used via the oral or nasal routes. Neither type of airway should be used if there is evidence of pharyngeal trauma. The oropharyngeal airway is suitable for the unconscious patient; it should be removed if there is any evidence of gagging or retching. The cuffed oropharyngeal airway (COPA) may also be used effectively by non-anaesthetists. The nasopharyngeal airway, made of a soft material, can be used in situations where the mouth cannot be opened or the teeth are insecure. It may also be better tolerated by the semi-conscious patient.

2) **The laryngeal mask airway (LMA)**. The LMA partially protects the airway and is said to offer the best current alternative to endotracheal intubation by inexperienced personnel (ERC 1996). The basic principle that rise and fall of the chest during ventilation equates with a clear airway must be emphasised if relatively inexperienced staff are to be taught the techniques of LMA insertion. The practicalities of insertion may be relatively simple; the assessment of correct positioning is not so easy. Although endotracheal intubation is preferable to the LMA, the device may be useful if there is an unstable cervical spine fracture and where intubation is not deemed to be essential. In a difficult intubation a modified intubating LMA can be used to establish a clear airway and then a bougie and/or a small endotracheal tube inserted through it.

3) **The oesophageal tracheal combitube (ETC)** has been used as a device for airway maintenance during CPR. It has the advantage that once placed it does not matter whether it is in the trachea or oesophagus and ventilation is possible via one or other lumen. The airway has not gained popularity in this country and it may not be safe because EMS personnel may inadvertently ventilate the oesophagus.

4) **Endotracheal intubation**.
Endotracheal intubation is still the airway management of choice to achieve a protected airway. The technique may be more difficult in the emergency situation with unskilled help, poor head positioning, vomit in the mouth and endotracheal tubes of varying lengths. If the patient has already been intubated, it is the anaesthetist's duty to check for correct placement of the tube and to re-intubate if there is any doubt about oesophageal intubation or malplacement of the tube. The tube should then be firmly secured.

Once endotracheal intubation is achieved, chest compressions and ventilations should be asynchronous. This allows continuous chest compressions, which have been shown to improve perfusion pressures during CPR (Kern 1998).

5) **The surgical airway**
If an airway cannot be obtained by any other means,

then surgical access to the trachea must be obtained, preferably by a skilled operator. Two techniques have been advocated for use during CPR; they provide access through the cricothyroid membrane and both carry risk of misplacement and haemorrhage. **Needle cricothyroidotomy** is the technique of choice as it is least difficult to perform. In this technique, a specific tracheal needle or a 14G intravenous cannula is directed caudally through the cricothyroid membrane. If equipment is available, percutaneous transtracheal jet ventilation can be used. In an emergency a length of oxygen tubing with a side hole which can be intermittently occluded, can be used to provide temporary ventilation. **Surgical cricothyroidotomy is** more difficult but may be used. **Percutaneous dilatational tracheostomy** or **emergency tracheostomy** are both too time consuming in a situation where there is life-threatening hypoxia. Whichever technique is used to access the trachea, correct placement of the cannula or tube must be confirmed.

CONFIRMATION OF CORRECT TUBE PLACEMENT

During emergency airway management, as in the theatre setting, it is now recommended that end tidal carbon dioxide monitoring is used. It will be reliable where there is a perfusing rhythm; during cardiac arrest, where there is no CO_2 output, a second method for confirming correct tube placement, an oesophageal detector device, should be employed. (International Guidelines 2000 for CPR and ECC).

VENTILATION

Two methods of ventilation may be employed, simple adjuncts to EAR and self-inflating bags.

Disadvantages of EAR have been described. Mouth-to-barrier techniques, which incorporate a plastic sheet with a central filter with or without a bite block, remove the need for direct contact with the patient.

The problems of EAR can be overcome by use of a pocket mask with a one way valve and a port for the addition of oxygen; the tidal volume can then be reduced to approximately 500 ml or 6–7 ml/Kg.

Self inflating bag and valve devices should be of robust construction with reliable valves and standard diameter fittings. They should be used with a reservoir and 15 l/min of added oxygen to ensure an inspired oxygen concentration of up to 100%. Inexperienced personnel may find that they are difficult to use in conjunction with a face mask, and it is recommended that two hands are used to maintain a patent airway and an effective seal, while a second operator squeezes the bag.

If used with a device that does not isolate the trachea, care should be taken not to inflate the stomach with excessive inflation pressures. An oxygen powered resuscitator or a portable ventilator can be used instead of a self-inflating bag, once the patient has been intubated.

CIRCULATION

If the arrest is witnessed or monitored and no defibrillator is available a single precordial thump should be given as rapidly as possible. This may terminate VT and very occasionally, VF. If this is unsuccessful or has not been appropriate, then a diagnosis of cardiac arrest should be confirmed by the absence of any response, no evidence of normal breathing, and the inability to detect a major pulse, but a maximum of ten seconds should be spent doing this. A diagnosis of the underlying rhythm should also be made via the defibrillator paddles or from a formal lead II trace; there will be one of four patterns; ventricular fibrillation (VF), ventricular tachycardia (VT), asystole or pulseless electrical activity (PEA). However, for the purposes of treatment, there is now only one algorithm for advanced life support (See Figure RS. 4) divided into two limbs, one for VF/VT and one for non-VF/VT. In all cases of cardiac arrest, but particularly in asystole and PEA, potentially reversible causes must be considered and treated. Treatment aimed at alleviating hypoxia (including relief of tension pneumothorax) and correcting hypovolaemia, may restore a cardiac output.

VF / VT

VF is the commonest primary rhythm, especially in patients with ischaemic heart disease and is associated with a better prognosis than the other rhythms, particularly if DC defibrillation occurs as early as possible. Three shocks should be delivered sequentially; with a modern defibrillator this is possible within 45 seconds. The selected energy levels for a monophasic defibrillator should be 200 J, 200 J and 360 J. If VF persists and there is still no evidence of any output, basic life support should be provided for one minute (4 cycles of 15: 2 or 12 breaths with asynchronous chest compressions) (RC (UK) 2000). Intravenous access should be established and epinephrine should be given within this cycle. If not already in situ, the patient may be intubated after pre-oxygenation and chest compressions and ventilation may be interrupted temporarily to achieve this. During a one minute cycle of CPR, lead and paddle positions should be checked and thought should be given to potentially reversible causes of VF. If there is still no evidence of an output then three further 360 J shocks should be given. During a prolonged arrest, epinephrine 1 mg may be given at least every three minutes, and an anti-arrhythmic agent (amiodarone (Kudenchuk 1999) or if this is unavailable, lidocaine) or an alkalising agent (sodium bicarbonate, NaHCO₃) may be considered. Prolonged resuscitation attempts may be required in hypothermia or near drowning and specific treatment may be needed for gross electrolyte imbalance. Although resuscitation attempts should not usually be abandoned if the rhythm is still VF, persistent VF may indicate myocardial failure; more usually, however, an agonal rhythm will develop, which carries a poor prognosis.

NON VF / VT (ASYSTOLE AND PEA)

For these rhythms, basic CPR cycles should be three minutes (12 cycles of 15: 2 or 36 breaths with asynchronous chest compressions) (RC (UK) 2000), with rhythm and circulation checks at the end of each cycle.

However, if non-VF/VT rhythm follows successful defibrillation, it should be noted that this may represent myocardial stunning and sinus rhythm may return spontaneously. For this reason, the algorithm recommends one minute of CPR and then a check for an output.

ASYSTOLE

Asystole is characterised by ventricular standstill on the ECG but a mistaken diagnosis must be avoided since fibrillation can be more successfully treated. Causes of asytole include:

- acute hypoxia and hypovolaemia (both treatable)
- myocardial ischaemia (usually severe and terminal)
- electrolyte imbalance
- drug overdosage

If asystole is diagnosed, monitor gain should be increased and all lead connections checked to ensure accurate diagnosis. The ECG monitor should be switched to lead II, and then another lead considered in case the directional vector of the fibrillation waveform happens to be perpendicular to the sensing electrode therefore being hidden. If there is any doubt that the rhythm may be fine VF, a precordial thump may be given or the initial three shock sequence followed as in the VF algorithm. After these shocks or if asystole is definitely the presenting rhythm, the airway should be secured and IV access established early. Epinephrine should be given to support adequate cerebral and coronary perfusion. Strong cholinergic activity may depress the function of the sino-atrial and atrioventricular nodes, especially when sympathetic stimulation is reduced, for instance by infarction or beta blockade. Atropine may increase the chance of successful resuscitation therefore a full dose of atropine (3 mg IV) should be given. Pacing should be considered if there has been any evidence of electrical activity such as p waves or occasional QRS complexes. Sodium bicarbonate may be given but only if there is evidence of a severe acidosis.

PULSELESS ELECTRICAL ACTIVITY (PEA)

PEA describes mechanical asystole with an undetectable pulse, but accompanied by the presence of an ECG trace which can vary from being near normal to a bizarre agonal pattern. Primary PEA carries a very poor prognosis and reflects profound myocardial pump failure. Secondary PEA carries a better prognosis if potentially reversible causes are considered and treated early. If specific treatment of any of these causes fails to produce an immediate output, or the PEA is deemed to be a primary event, the algorithm (Figure RS. 4) should be followed, including three minute CPR cycles, with intubation and IV cannulation performed early, and epinephrine given as an adjunct to basic life support. If the QRS complexes in PEA occur at a rate slower than 60/min full atropinisation is recommended.

TECHNIQUES APPLIED IN ADVANCED LIFE SUPPORT

ELECTRICAL DEFIBRILLATION

Manual direct current (DC) defibrillators are usually powered by a rechargeable battery and have an on/off switch, an AC/DC converter, a charge selector, a capacitor and hand held electrodes each with a discharge button. Charging can be initiated by a button on the machine or one of the electrodes and energy levels are measured in joules. The waveform is usually sinusoidal, but newer lighter defibrillators deliver shocks with biphasic waveforms. An electrical current of sufficient size to depolarise a critical mass of the myocardium is passed through the chest wall between the electrodes; discharge should be unsynchronised. The current magnitude depends on the energy of the shock and the transthoracic impedance. Impedance is lessened by having large electrodes applied with good pressure and contact, by using self-adhesive conducting pads, and by the passage of previous shocks. One electrode should be placed below the right clavicle and the other over the apex of the heart. Safety is of paramount importance. The operator needs to

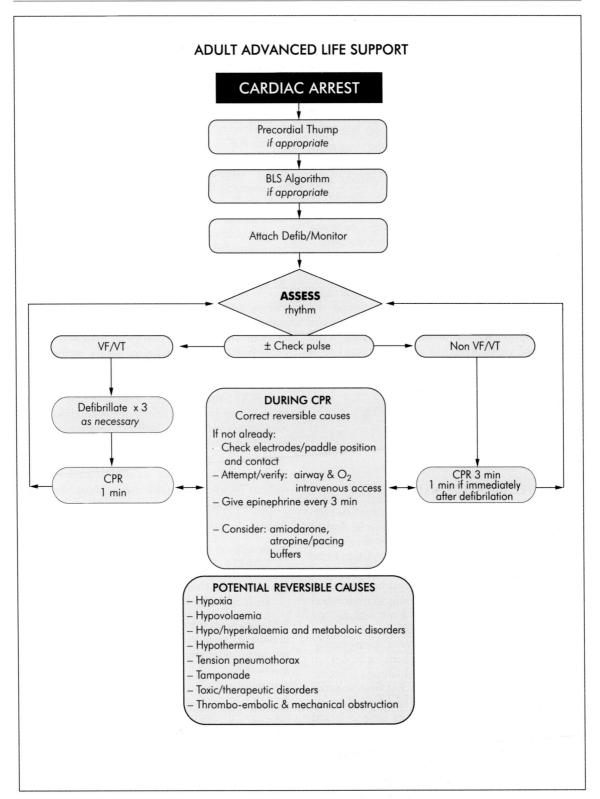

Figure RS.4 The ALS algorithm for the management of cardiac arrest in adults © ERC 96 and RC (UK) 2000 from Resuscitation 46 (2000) 169-184

issue a 'stand clear' command before discharge and to know how to dump any unused charge. The risk of explosion and arcing of the shock across the chest wall can be avoided by temporary removal of the oxygen source and glyceryl trinitrate transdermal patches before defibrillation.

Automated external defibrillators (AEDs) are available for non-medical personnel. The energy levels are preset but otherwise the principles are the same as for manual defibrillation, though fine VF may not be recognised.

All defibrillators, whatever their type, should be checked regularly and all users should be fully trained in the techniques of manual and automatic defibrillation and practice these techniques regularly.

PACING

Current recommendations state that non-invasive transcutaneous pacing should be used during the course of the asystole algorithm if any electrical activity occurs. The adhesive electrodes can be placed in the anterolateral configuration to allow continuation of chest compressions. Defibrillation can also be given through these electrodes.

DRUG USAGE IN ALS

During cardiac arrest, drug administration is always secondary to other interventions.

ACCESS FOR DRUGS AND FLUIDS

Peripheral intravenous access may not always be easy. All drugs given via a peripheral route must be flushed into the vein and it may take up to five minutes for boluses to become effective. The central venous route may, therefore, be a better option in the hands of an experienced anaesthetist. The internal jugular vein is the route of choice. Intratracheal drug administration has been used when venous access is not available and absorption of epinephrine via this route has been shown to be reliable if administered appropriately. Intra-osseous access has now been accepted in paediatric practice and is considered safe and effective; this route is also possible in adults but large volumes and drugs such as amiodarone and bicarbonate cannot be given. The intracardiac route is, unreliable and unsafe, and it is not recommended.

EPINEPHRINE

Epinephrine remains the recommended vasopressor in all forms of cardiac arrest, despite the fact that circulating catecholamine levels are already very high during cardiac arrest. It appears that exogenous epinephrine produces an increase in cerebral and coronary perfusion due to its alpha-adrenergic activity. Coronary blood flow occurs during the relaxation phase of CPR and is determined by the difference between aortic diastolic and right atrial diastolic pressure; epinephrine increases this difference. The beta-adrenergic activity of epinephrine increases myocardial oxygen consumption following resumption of cardiac output and, therefore, other drugs without beta-adrenergic activity have been investigated including vasopressin. However, epinephrine remains the recommended drug of choice (in a dosage of 1 mg at least every 3 minutes) and at present vasopressin, though promising, is not actively recommended as a substitute for epinephrine.

ALKALISING AGENTS

During cardiac arrest there is a rapid accumulation of carbon dioxide within tissues accompanied by build up of lactic acid, due to poor tissue perfusion. This is exacerbated by the inability of poorly perfused liver cells to metabolise lactic acid. In arrested patients the net result is a marked arteriovenous difference in pH and PCO_2, thus, a mixed venous sample of blood provides the best indicator of tissue conditions. The most appropriate treatment for the deleterious effects of acidosis is restoration of a spontaneous output and improved tissue perfusion. If this is not achievable it has been traditional to use an alkalising agent, usually sodium bicarbonate. Sodium bicarbonate has many known adverse effects such as:

- hypernatraemia and increased osmolarity

- generation of CO_2 and reduced intracellular and CSF pH

- increased affinity of haemoglobin for oxygen (reducing oxygen delivery)

Additionally, in the cardiac arrest situation and in the peri-arrest period bicarbonate can cause negative inotropy, reduction of cerebral blood flow and the inactivation of simultaneously administered epinephrine.

Sodium bicarbonate will precipitate if given with calcium salts. The European Resuscitation Council Guidelines (Koster 1992) recommend that sodium bicarbonate is used in doses of 50 mmol, either during prolonged resuscitation attempts or when the venous pH is 7.1 or less (or the base deficit exceeds −10). It is also specifically indicated in hypercalcaemia and tricyclic antidepressant overdose.

ANTI-ARRHYTHMIC AGENTS

No effective and safe anti-arrhythmic has been identified as successful adjunct therapy for the treatment of VF. Most anti-arrhythmic agents increase defibrillation thresholds. Lidocaine probably has more detrimental than beneficial effects but has traditionally been given (as a bolus of 100 mg). All anti-arrhythmic agents are also pro-arrhythmic. Amiodarone probably has a lower incidence of these side effects and following a study showing that this drug improved the rate of survival from community to hospital admission, it has now been recommended as the anti-arrhythmic of choice during cardiac arrest in refractory VF/VT (Kudenchuk 1999).

Amiodarone may be given as a bolus of 300 mg diluted to 20 mls with 5% Dextrose via a peripheral or ideally via a central vein. It can be given after the third shock but should not delay further shocks. Multiple anti-arrhythmic drugs should not be used. For anti-arrhythmic agents to be fully effective, blood gas and electrolyte disturbances must have been considered and treated.

COMPLICATIONS OF CPR

Iatrogenic complications of CPR are relatively common and may pose post resuscitation problems. Rib and sternal fractures occur frequently. Other complications of chest compressions may include visceral trauma (usually liver) and cardiac trauma. Complications related to poor airway and ventilatory management are inhalation of gastric contents, inadvertent oesophageal intubation and rarely gastric rupture. Other post arrest problems (not necessarily caused by CPR) are pulmonary oedema, recurrent cardiac arrest, cardiogenic shock, multiple organ dysfunction and adverse neurological outcome.

RECOGNITION AND MANAGEMENT OF LIFE THREATENING PERI-ARREST ARRHYTHMIAS

Life threatening peri-arrest arrhythmias include tachycardias (either broad complex or narrow complex) and bradycardias. Arrhythmias are common after myocardial infarction and in association with cardiac failure, hypotension and anti-arrhythmic drugs; if promptly treated, cardiac arrest can be averted. These arrhythmias can also be caused or potentiated by increased catecholamine levels (endogenous or exogenous), hypoxia, hypercarbia, severe acidosis, gross electrolyte disturbances, and pain or anxiety. These problems should be addressed. Arrhythmias

may compromise cardiac output because of loss of co-ordinated atrial and ventricular activity and rate problems; the resultant decreased cardiac output together with increase in myocardial oxygen consumption may rapidly lead to life threatening heart failure, hypotension, poor perfusion, acidosis and end organ dysfunction. Treatment must be instituted immediately. All patients with these life threatening arrhythmias should have reliable IV access established and high flow oxygen should be given.

TACHYCARDIAS

BROAD COMPLEX TACHYCARDIA

The normal upper width limit for a QRS complex is 0.11 second. In a tachycardia with a wide QRS complex, the diagnosis is usually that of a ventricular tachycardia (VT) but supraventricular tachycardia (SVT) with bundle branch block or accessory or aberrant conduction should also be considered. If a diagnosis cannot be made and there is a pulse the guidelines given in Figure RS. 5 should be followed.

DIFFERENTIAL DIAGNOSIS OF SVT & VT BY TREATMENT

- Consider previous history
- Study previous ECGs. If similar broad complex QRS morphology is seen in association with sinus rhythm this indicates a supraventricular rhythm
- Obtain a current ECG to exclude VT
- **The default position however is that broad complex tachycardias should be treated as if they were VT (see algorithm Figure RS.6)**

Figure RS.5

It may be very difficult to distinguish between the diagnoses of SVT and VT. The following guidelines have been suggested (Wellens 1978):

- give adenosine, which will be effective in abolishing SVT but not VT

- seek cardiological help

- use synchronised DC cardioversion (indicated in SVT and VT)

- only use verapamil, which is a myocardial depressant and potent vasodilator, when a diagnosis of SVT has been made with confidence

Current guidelines stress that adenosine should not be overused in a prolonged attempt to prove a diagnosis of SVT; in any life threatening, fast (more than 150 beats/min), wide complex tachycardia where the exact origin of the rhythm cannot be established, cardioversion is the common treatment of choice. Similarly, a common adjunctive drug choice is amiodarone.

In broad complex tachycardia, which is diagnosed as sustained ventricular tachycardia, oxygen should be administered and IV access secured. If the pulse is absent and there are no signs of a circulation, the protocol for VF should be followed. If a pulse is palpable but haemodynamic stability is poor or deteriorating rapidly or the rate is high (more than 150 beats/min), help should be sought and synchronised DC cardioversion should be performed. If cardioversion is not successful, hypokalaemia (K < 3.6 mmol/l) should be treated with intravenous potassium and magnesium, amiodarone should be given and DC cardioversion can then be repeated. Other anti-arrhythmics (lidocaine, procainamide or sotalol) can be given if amiodarone is not available, but never in combination, and overdrive pacing can be considered.

Polymorphic VT with prolonged baseline QT interval (Torsades-de-pointes) is treated differently with cessation of any causative drugs, magnesium infusion and overdrive pacing.

The algorithm for broad complex tachycardia is shown in Figure RS.6.

NARROW COMPLEX TACHYCARDIA

Narrow complex tachycardia is almost always supraventricular in origin and includes atrial flutter and fibrillation, atrioventricular junctional tachycardia, multifocal atrial tachycardia and paroxysmal re-entrant tachycardia. In the context of the peri-arrest situation, paroxysmal supraventricular tachycardia and atrial fibrillation with a fast ventricular rate are the commonest problems. Supraventricular tachycardia can be relatively benign but may be life threatening. The algorithm for narrow complex tachycardia is shown in Figure RS. 7.

If the rate is so high (more than 250 beats/min) that the pulse is absent and consciousness impaired, immediate cardioversion should be used (Resuscitation Council (UK) 2000).

If the rate is more than 200 beats/min, unilateral carotid sinus massage can be used to slow a paroxysmal supraventricular tachycardia but care must be taken as an increase in vagal tone in those with acute ischaemia or possible digoxin toxicity, may precipitate ventricular

fibrillation. Adenosine is now established as the preferred treatment for terminating the rhythm of supraventricular tachycardia but starting cautiously with a dose of 6 mg (Resuscitation Council (UK) 2000).

Adenosine should be avoided in the presence of known Wolff-Parkinson-White syndrome when a dangerously fast ventricular response can be precipitated.

Fast atrial fibrillation (more than 150 beats/min) may also cause haemodynamic compromise and underlying causes such as heart failure, mitral valve disease and thyrotoxicosis should be considered. As with the other tachyarrhythmias, urgent treatment is required in the form of synchronised DC cardioversion after prior general anaesthesia. Caution is required if digoxin toxicity is suspected, as there may be a risk of inducing a malignant arrhythmia. The 'universal' anti-arrhythmic, amiodarone, is recommended prior to repetition of cardioversion; in addition heparin must be given if the atrial fibrillation might have been present for more than twenty four hours and there is a risk of possible embolisation. DC cardioversion is also the treatment of choice in atrial flutter (whether or not there is haemodynamic compromise) and low energy shocks may be sufficient.

BRADYCARDIAS AND HEART BLOCKS

Although a bradycardia is classically defined as a heart rate of less than 60 beats/min, intervention is usually required only if the rate is less than 40 beats/min. However, in the context of a failing left ventricle, a pulse rate of more than 40 beats/min may require treatment. Bradycardias are usually manifestations of increased vagal tone, though Mobitz type I block may be associated with inferior myocardial infarction and is often temporary. They may however have an underlying cause such as hypoxia, hypothermia, severe head injury or poisoning. All patients who are symptomatic or have multiple escape beats, should be given oxygen and IV access is needed (Figure RS.8). For the purposes of treatment, sinus and junctional bradycardias (this includes first degree AV block) and Mobitz type I second degree AV block (Wenckebach phenomenon) are considered together and if there is a satisfactory response to atropine (0.5 mg IV), the patient can be observed. If there is no response or if the block is second degree AV block (Mobitz type II) or complete heart block when there is a risk of asystole, further measures are required whilst help is called for transvenous pacing. These measures include further atropine to a total dose of 3 mg, transcutaneous pacing, and epinephrine infusion. Isoprenaline is no longer used as this drug can compromise an ischaemic left

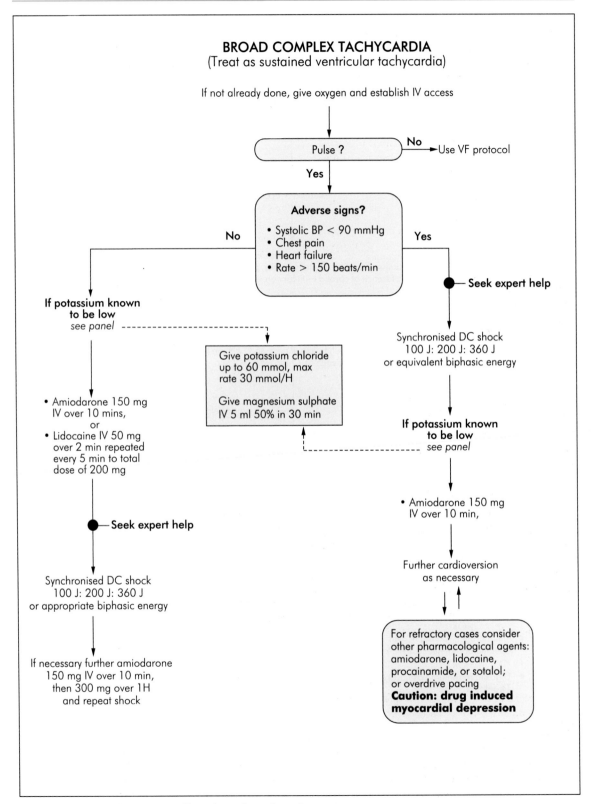

Figure RS.6 Algorithm for treatment of broad complex tachycardia © ERC 96 and RC (UK) 2000

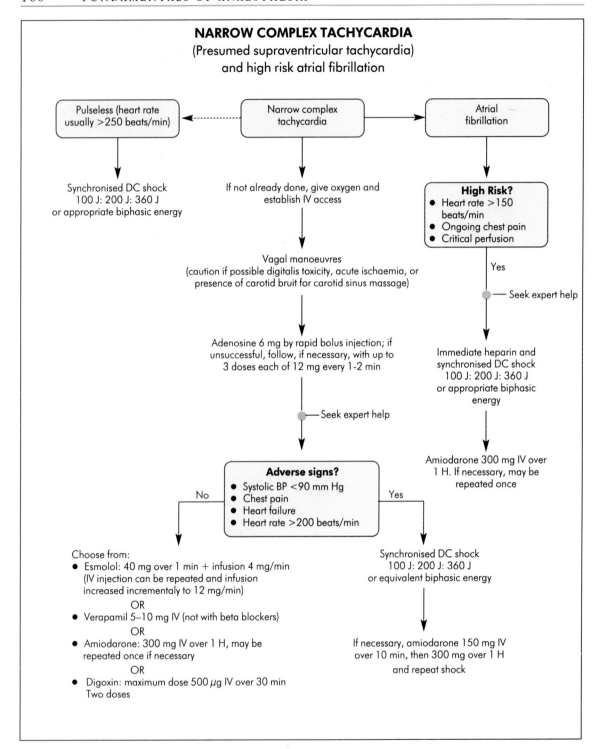

NARROW COMPLEX TACHYCARDIA
(Presumed supraventricular tachycardia)
and high risk atrial fibrillation

Pulseless (heart rate usually >250 beats/min)

Narrow complex tachycardia

Atrial fibrillation

Synchronised DC shock
100 J: 200 J: 360 J
or appropriate biphasic energy

If not already done, give oxygen and establish IV access

High Risk?
- Heart rate >150 beats/min
- Ongoing chest pain
- Critical perfusion

Vagal manoeuvres
(caution if possible digitalis toxicity, acute ischaemia, or presence of carotid bruit for carotid sinus massage)

Yes

Seek expert help

Adenosine 6 mg by rapid bolus injection; if unsuccessful, follow, if necessary, with up to 3 doses each of 12 mg every 1-2 min

Immediate heparin and synchronised DC shock
100 J: 200 J: 360 J
or appropriate biphasic energy

Seek expert help

Amiodarone 300 mg IV over 1 H. If necessary, may be repeated once

Adverse signs?
- Systolic BP <90 mm Hg
- Chest pain
- Heart failure
- Heart rate >200 beats/min

No

Yes

Choose from:
- Esmolol: 40 mg over 1 min + infusion 4 mg/min (IV injection can be repeated and infusion increased incrementaly to 12 mg/min)
  OR
- Verapamil 5–10 mg IV (not with beta blockers)
  OR
- Amiodarone: 300 mg IV over 1 H, may be repeated once if necessary
  OR
- Digoxin: maximum dose 500 μg IV over 30 min Two doses

Synchronised DC shock
100 J: 200 J: 360 J
or equivalent biphasic energy

If necessary, amiodarone 150 mg IV over 10 min, then 300 mg over 1 H and repeat shock

Figure RS.7 Algorithm for treatment of narrow complex tachycardia and high risk atrial fibrillation   © ERC 96 and RC (UK) 2000

ventricle and increase infarct size because of its effect in increasing myocardial oxygen demand.

MANAGEMENT OF LIFE THREATENING PERI-ARREST ARRHYTHMIAS

SYNCHRONISED CARDIOVERSION

This must be performed on anaesthetised patients only. A standard defibrillator is suitable but lower starting energies may be effective (100 J or even 50 J in atrial flutter). The shock should be synchronised to the R wave on the ECG trace; a dot will appear on each R wave when the mode is selected. Since there is usually some delay between pressing the discharge buttons and delivery of the shock, the paddles should be held on the chest until they are safely discharged.

TRANSCUTANEOUS PACING

The pacing electrodes should be placed in the antero-posterior or antero lateral position on the chest. The fixed or demand mode is selected at a rate of 60–90 beats/min. The pacing is started with the pacing current set at the lowest level, and then gradually increased until capture occurs. Skeletal muscle

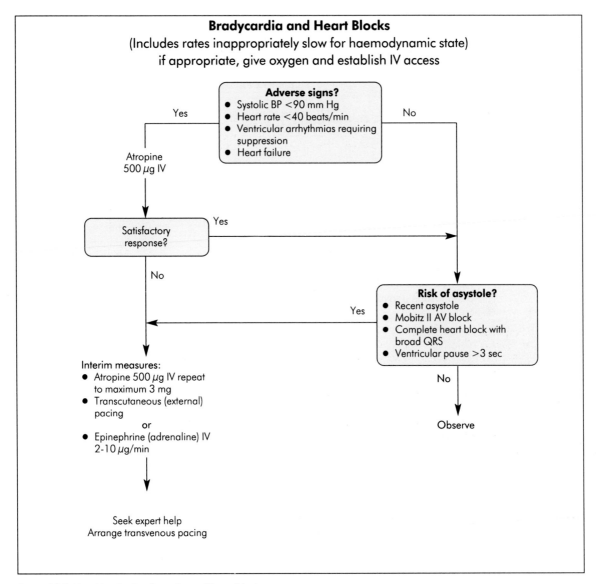

Figure RS.8 Algorithm for bradycardia and heart blocks © ERC 96 and RC (UK) 2000

contractions will also increase with gain and the patient may require analgesia. Failure to capture can be rectified by changing the electrode position.

DRUG ADMINISTRATION

The administration of drugs, their doses and their adverse side effects are summarised in Figure RS.9. Figure RS.10 shows examples of ECG tracings relating to the rhythms discussed.

RESUSCITATION OF THE PREGNANT PATIENT

CAUSES OF ARREST

The causes can be the same as in the non pregnant population (such as trauma or pre-existing heart disease) but other specific obstetric factors must be considered. These include severe haemorrhage, revealed or concealed, pulmonary embolism, toxaemia, amniotic fluid embolism, placental abruption and spinal and epidural mishaps. Resuscitation in early

DRUGS USED IN LIFE THREATENING PERI-ARREST ARRYTHMIAS

Drug	See algorithm	Dose and administration (all drugs given IV)	Comments (CI = Contraindications)
Adenosine	Narrow complex tachycardia	6 mg then 12 mg up to 3 times Very fast injection Flush with Saline	Transient asystole Chest pain CI Asthma CI with dipyrimadole CI with carbamazepine CI if heart is denervated CI in WPW syndrome
Amiodarone	All tachycardias	150 mg in 5% Dextrose over 10 mins	Hypotension Arrhythmogenesis CI with other anti-arrhythmics
Lidocaine	Refractory broad complex tachycardia if amiodarone unavailable	50 mg repeated every 10 mins to total 200 mg	Hypotension Arrhythmogenesis CI with other anti-arrhythmics CI in myocardial failure CI in AV block
Magnesium	Broad complex tachycardia if potassium low and hypo-magnesaemia suspected Torsades-de-pointes	Magnesium sulphate 5 mls of 50% solution over 30 min	
Potassium	Broad complex tachycardia if potassium low	KCl maximum 60 mmol at 30 mmol/H	Control infusion rate
Atropine	Bradycardia	0.5mg repeated to a maximum of 3 mg	
Epinephrine	Bradycardia unresponsive to atropine, while awaiting pacing	2-10μg/min (1mg in 100ml at 0.2 to 1ml/min)	Control infusion rate

Figure RS.9

pregnancy should be conducted as recommended for other adults and directed towards maternal considerations, ultimately both mother and foetus will die if a maternal circulation cannot be restored.

After the 24th gestational week when the foetus is potentially viable, there are two lives to save; obstetric and paediatric help should be sought early and after five minutes of unsuccessful resuscitation, Caesarean section should be considered while advanced life support continues (Lanoix 1995).

Differences between maternal resuscitation and that of the non pregnant patient are outlined overleaf.

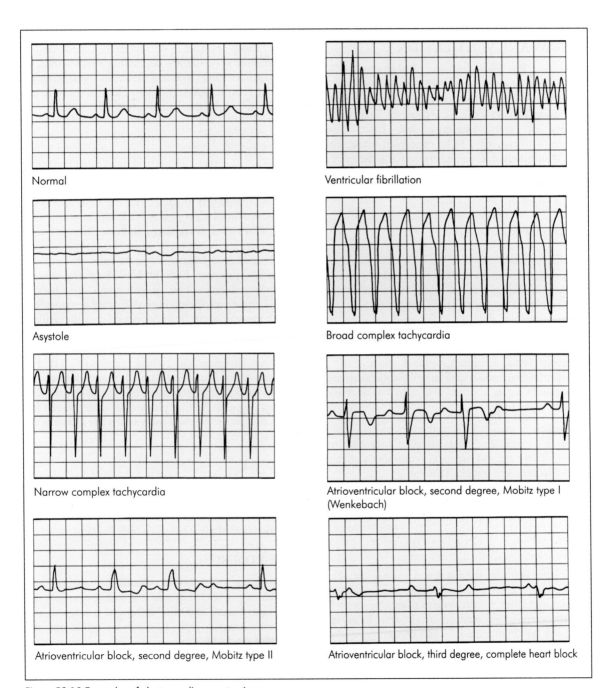

Figure RS.10 Examples of electrocardiogram tracings

To avoid venacaval compression by the gravid uterus, the patient must be placed with a wedge or sandbag under the right hip. Chest compression is feasible in this position but the compression point should be slightly higher up the sternum than otherwise.

AIRWAY AND VENTILATION

Owing to the increased risk of regurgitation and pulmonary aspiration, cricoid pressure should be applied and the airway secured as early as possible. Intubation may be difficult because of large breasts, obesity or glottic oedema and basic airway management may have to be continued while senior help is summoned. Once intubation is achieved, care must be taken to ensure adequate bilateral lung inflation and higher than normal inflation pressures will be required.

ARREST PROTOCOLS

In pulseless electrical activity, if occult haemorrhage is suspected, insertion of wide bore cannulae is essential but may be difficult; blood should be taken for cross matching and a rapid fluid challenge given.

Arrest protocols should be followed as usual and epinephrine is indicated every three minutes to support maternal and therefore foetal perfusion. It has been suggested that because repeated doses of IV epinephrine can cause uteroplacental vasoconstriction, then this factor is another reason to consider early delivery of the baby.

If lidocaine is used in VF and the patient has received epidural bupivacaine, local anaesthetic toxicity may occur. There is no specific contraindication to defibrillation in the pregnant patient.

RESUSCITATION OF INFANTS AND CHILDREN

Adult cardiac arrest usually has a cardiac aetiology; children more often arrest secondary to respiratory or circulatory failure. Adults present most often with VF but the commonest rhythm in children is asystole preceded by bradycardia. It is becoming evident, however, that if a child has known cardiac disease, the arrest rhythm will be more likely to be VF and early defibrillation is required.

The outcome from primary respiratory arrest with some cardiac output, is better than when prolonged hypoxia has progressed to full cardiopulmonary arrest, so early intervention with particular attention to the airway and breathing is extremely important in the sick child. The circulation must not be forgotten since circulatory failure due to hypovolaemia (secondary to haemorrhage, fluid losses or maldistribution in sepsis), is probably the second commonest cause of arrest. Repeated assessments of capillary refill must be made and fluid boluses administered. Resuscitation techniques vary slightly depending on whether the paediatric victim is an infant (less than 1 year of age) or a child (1 to 8 years). An older child of more than 8 years can be treated as a small adult.

In the collapsed child who has not progressed to a cardiac arrest, the principles of treatment are the same as those employed in adults, but the techniques vary. Conscious level is assessed as in adults, but gently and it should be remembered that an infant cannot talk and a scared child may not reply. If the child is unconscious but breathing and the airway is partially obstructed in the supine position, the child should be placed in a safe, lateral recovery position, given oxygen and observed until help arrives. If choking is suspected in a conscious child, coughing can be encouraged as in the adult; if this fails or the child is unconscious, then the algorithm for choking should be followed noting the difference between an infant and a child (Figure RS. 11). It is recommended that the Heimlich manoeuvre should not be used in infants because of the risk of iatrogenic visceral trauma. A blind pharyngeal finger sweep in a partially obstructed child can worsen the situation and should never be used.

AIRWAY

Airway patency is checked and maintained as in adults but smaller children will not need a pillow. Chin lift and jaw thrust must be applied gently without compression of the soft tissues of the neck.

BREATHING

Expired air resuscitation should be applied with inspiration over 1–1.5 seconds and for infants the mouth to 'mouth and nose' technique is taught. Up to 5 breaths may be given to achieve a minimum of 2 effective rescue breaths.

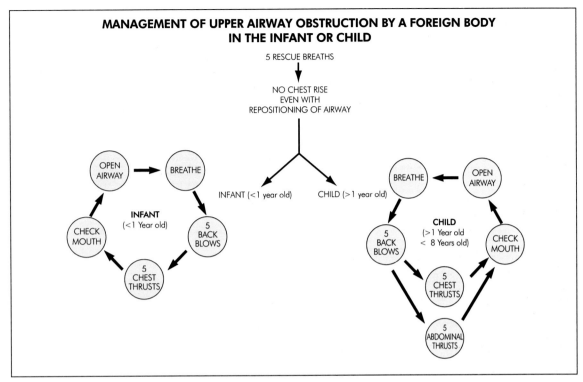

MANAGEMENT OF UPPER AIRWAY OBSTRUCTION BY A FOREIGN BODY IN THE INFANT OR CHILD

Figure RS.11 © ERC 94

SUMMARY OF ASSESSMENT OF CIRCULATION AND COMPRESSION TECHNIQUES IN INFANTS AND CHILDREN

	Infant less than 1 yr	Child 1-8 yrs	Child more than 8 yrs
Circulation Pulse check (taken while looking for signs of a circulation)	Brachial	Carotid	Carotid
Compressions Site	One finger breadth below nipple line	Lower half of sternum	As in adult
Technique	Two fingers (for single healthcare provider) Both thumbs with hands encircling chest (two healthcare providers)	Heel of one hand	1 or 2 hands
Rate/minute	100	100	100
Ratio (regardless of rescuer numbers)	5:1	5:1	15:2 (continuous chest compressions with protected airway)

Figure RS.12 From Resuscitation 46. 1-3. Pg 333

CIRCULATION

Circulation is best assessed in infants by palpation of the brachial pulse. If there are no signs of a circulation in a child or an infant or if there is a bradycardia of less then 60 beats/min with evidence of poor perfusion then chest compressions should be started. The techniques of chest compression are different in children of different ages (See Figure RS. 12). In particular, it is now recommended that the two thumb –encircling hand technique (rather than the two finger method) is used in infants when there are two rescuers (Dorfsman 2000).

ADVANCED LIFE SUPPORT

In paediatric resuscitation, endotracheal tube sizes, defibrillator settings and drug dosages must all be carefully calculated, but often the child's weight is unknown. An updated standard reference chart (Oakley 1993) allows an approximation of weight to be derived from the age, but care must be taken using this chart because drug volumes are quoted and relate to drug concentrations that may not be standardised throughout hospitals. The use of the Broselow tape is an alternative method. The tape is colour coded and lists drug dosages, defibrillator settings, fluid volumes and tube sizes in separate sections according to height and removes the need for guesswork.

AIRWAY AND VENTILATION

High concentrations of oxygen must be given prior to advanced airway management. Use of the LMA in paediatric resuscitation cannot yet be confidently recommended; however, intubation though desirable is often difficult if the operator is inexperienced and if the child is small. The epiglottis is long and leaf like and the larynx anteriorly placed. In the absence of any chart, a useful guideline suggests that the endotracheal tube should be the diameter of the child's own little finger; if the child's age is known the size and length of the tube can be calculated as follows:

Size = Age/4 + 4 mm internal diameter

Length = size X 3 cms

Care must be taken not to intubate a main bronchus. In unrelieved obstruction, senior help must be sought and needle cricothyroidotomy must be considered as a life saving procedure.

CIRCULATION

The Paediatric Advanced Life Support Algorithm should be followed, as in adults (See Figure RS. 13).

NON VF / VT

Asystole, often preceded by bradycardia, is the commonest cardiac arrest rhythm in children. As in adults, the possibility of VF must be excluded and treated. Confirmed asystole may be secondary to hypoxia and therefore the airway and ventilation must be the first priorities before any drug is administered. As in adults, causes of pulseless electrical activity must be looked for and treated. Hypovolaemia is a particularly likely diagnosis in the sick child and therefore an initial fluid challenge of 20 ml/kg should be given rapidly with the first dose of epinephrine. For both these rhythms, the protocols for cycles of epinephrine administration followed by three minutes of basic life support should be followed.

VF OR PULSELESS VT

These rhythms will not often be seen in children unless there is known heart disease. If they are encountered in a previously normal child, hypothermia, drug effects and electrolyte disturbances must be considered. Early defibrillation is essential; the recommended defibrillation energy levels are 2 J/kg for the first two shocks and thereafter 4 J/kg. Paediatric paddles should be used if the estimated weight is < 10 kg; however, transthoracic impedance is greater with these, and therefore, in an older child with a broader chest, adult paddles are preferred. Standard and alternative paddle positions are used as in adults; for infants the front and back paddle positions may be used. Automatic defibrillators may now be used in older children (more than 8 years) and this may be particularly useful in the out of hospital setting. Shocks should be repeated after a minute of CPR, and epinephrine given at least every three minutes.

DRUG USAGE

ADMINISTRATION

Peripheral venous access is notoriously difficult in small children. Central venous cannula insertion can be dangerous as well as difficult. Intra-osseous access may be life saving. If neither IV nor endotracheal access is available it is recommended that early intra-osseous access is secured. This route, using a bone marrow needle in the proximal tibia is safe, simple and rapid to acquire and drugs, fluids and blood can be given by this route. Endotracheal drug administration has been advocated and epinephrine can be given in doses ten times greater than the initial IV dose by this route. Endotracheal drugs should be injected into the endotracheal tube and then flushed with normal saline.

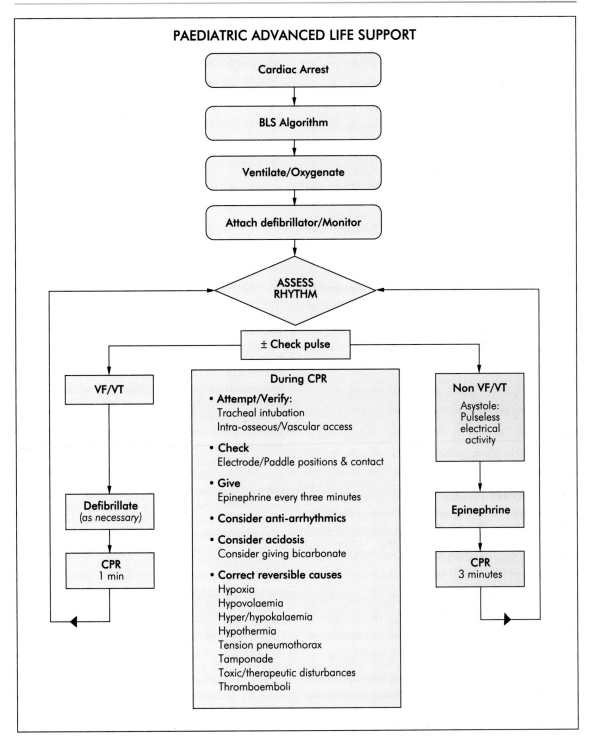

Figure RS.13 Paediatric Advanced Life Support © Resuscitation Council (UK) 2000

Atropine, lidocaine, naloxone and diazepam can also be given via the endotracheal tube, but there are no recommended doses. Bicarbonate should not be given intratracheally.

EPINEPHRINE (ADRENALINE)

Epinephrine should be given in doses of 0.01 mg/kg of 1: 10,000 solution (0.1 ml/kg) via the IV or intra-osseous route and 0.1 mg/kg of the 1: 1,000 solution (0.1 ml/kg) via the endotracheal tube. It should be repeated at least every three minutes. Although the outcome for children in refractory asystole is dismal, and there may be an increased chance of a return of spontaneous circulation after high dose epinephrine (0.1 mg/kg), concerns about coronary vasoconstriction and post arrest hypertension in adults has resulted in recommendations that the second and subsequent doses should be the same i.e. 0.01mg/kg. A dose larger than this can be considered only if severe vasodilatation was the cause of the cardiac arrest (Resuscitation Council (UK) Paediatric Advanced Life Support 2000).

ALKALISING AGENTS

As with adults, sodium bicarbonate should, where possible, be avoided. However, since cardiac arrest in children may be the terminal event following a prolonged episode of hypoxia or hypovolaemia, bicarbonate may need to be given for a proven severe metabolic acidosis. The recommended dose is 1 mmol/kg by slow intravenous injection or via the intra-osseous route.

ANTI-ARRHYTHMICS

Amiodarone is now the anti-arrhythmic of choice in persistent ventricular fibrillation as well as for peri-arrest supraventricular and ventricular tachycardias. The dose is 5mg/kg IV as a bolus.

ATROPINE

Since bradycardia and asystole in children is often secondary to hypoxia, ventilation with 100% oxygen is the recommended treatment followed by epinephrine. Atropine is not included in the asystole algorithm, it may however be given if vagal overactivity is evident in the peri-arrest situation particularly in association with intubation: the dose is 0.02 mg/kg IV with a minimum dose of 0.1 mg to avoid paradoxical bradycardia.

FLUIDS

In suspected hypovolaemia with severe circulatory failure or PEA, 20 ml/kg of a crystalloid or colloid solution should be infused rapidly, capillary refill and peripheral perfusion rechecked and the bolus repeated.

Glucose administration should be avoided during cardiac arrest but is indicated for infants with proven hypoglycaemia. In the child with known cardiac disease the volumes of all drugs should be counted in the total volumes given.

ETHICAL CONSIDERATIONS

All ethical decisions relating to CPR should be compatible with the European Convention on Human Rights Act, which has recently been implemented in the UK.

WHEN NOT TO START RESUSCITATION

It is obvious that in cases of mortal injury (decapitation, incineration) or longstanding death, resuscitation attempts will be futile. However, there are also other medical and ethical indications where resuscitation should not be started and there are now guidelines for the issue of hospital policies for the withholding and withdrawal of resuscitation. (BMA, RC (UK) and RCN 2001). Competent and fully informed patients who expressly and usually appropriately request not to be resuscitated should be respected and their wishes should be recorded clearly in writing in the presence of a witness (Doyal 1995) or communicated via their GP. Where the patient's condition indicates that resuscitation would be unsuccessful and futile or might cause unnecessary pain and suffering, and not be in the patient's best interest, then even without their explicit consent, the consultant could, in discussion with the relatives, consider such a policy. However, it should be noted that the relative's views have no legal status. The final decision of withholding resuscitation should be made by the consultant caring for the patient, in conjunction with other health professionals, acting in the patient's best interest. However the decision is reached, the 'do not attempt resuscitation' (DNAR) statement should be clearly written in both the medical and nursing notes. It should be reviewed regularly (BMA, RC (UK) and RCN 2001). All other treatment, however, should be given; the DNAR order relates to resuscitation alone.

WHEN TO RESUSCITATE

Outside the hospital setting, medical practitioners have an ethical, though not legal, obligation to provide appropriate and prompt action according to their skills and circumstances. In an emergency unit, if the arrested patient has only just reached the hospital, their previous history is unknown and they are attended by junior staff, then resuscitation should proceed and be instituted in full. The relatives can be questioned, old notes retrieved and senior help sought while resuscitative measures continue.

WHEN TO STOP RESUSCITATION

A lay person is taught to continue BLS until help arrives or exhaustion supervenes. In the hospital setting, decisions have to be made whether to continue or to abandon resuscitation. If the arrest has been caused by severe hypothermia, near drowning or drug overdose, particularly in children, then all possible measures should be continued, if necessary, for several hours. The decision to abandon resuscitation should not be solely influenced by the time spent resuscitating. However, persistence of asystole for more than twenty minutes with unresponsiveness to drug and fluid therapy and despite elimination of treatable conditions, should lead to a discussion between team members; the team leader should then make the final decision to stop. If resuscitation is proceeding unsuccessfully in a patient whose history is not initially known, and evidence of a recent valid DNAR decision is then found, the attempt should be abandoned. Equally, review of the futility and inappropriateness of resuscitative measures should lead to a decision by a senior doctor, in consultation with the team, to abandon the attempt.

WITNESSING THE RESUSCITATION

Increasingly, relatives are requesting to be present during the resuscitation procedures and although there is ambivalence in the medical profession about the effect that this may have on efficacy of treatment, the practice is becoming more common. Certainly the relative's wishes must be considered and their accompanied presence during resuscitation may positively influence their subsequent grieving process.

References and further reading

Decisions Relating to CPR. A Joint Statement from the BMA, the RC(UK) and the RCN, Feb. 2000.

Dorfsman ML, Menegazzi JJ, Wadas RJ, Auble TE. Two-thumb vs two-finger chest compression in an infant model of prolonged cardiopulmonary resuscitation. *Acad Emerg Med* 2000; **7(10):** 1077–82.

Doyal L. Editorial. Advance directives. *BMJ* 1995; **310:** 612–613.

European Resuscitation Council. Guidelines for Resuscitation. Antwerp, ERC, 1996.

Goldhill DR, Worthington L, Mulcahy A, Tarling M, Sumner A. The patient-at-risk team: identifying and managing seriously ill ward patients. *Anaesthesia* 1999; **54:** 853–860.

Gwinnutt CL, Columb M, Harris R. Outcome after cardiac arrest in adults in UK hospitals: effect of the 1997 guidelines. *Resuscitation* 2000; **47:** 125–135.

Handley AJ, Becker LB, Allen M, van Drenth A, Montgomery WH. Single rescuer basic life support. An Advisory Statement by the Basic Life Support Working Group of the International Liason Committee on Resuscitation. *Resuscitation* 1997; **34:** 101–107.

International Guidelines 2000 for CPR and ECC – A Consensus on Science. *Resuscitation* 2000; **46 (1–3):** 1–448.

Kern KB, Hilwig RW, Berg RA, Ewy GA. Efficacy of chest compression-only BLS CPR in the presence of an occluded airway. *Resuscitation* 1998; **39:** 179–188.

Koster R, Carli P. Acid-base management: a statement for the ALS Working Party of the ERC. *Resuscitation* 1992; **24:** 143–146.

Kudenchuk, PJ, Cobb LA, Copass MK, Cummins RO, Doherty,AM, Fahrenbruch CE et al. Amiodarone for resuscitation after out-of-hospital cardiac arrest due to ventricular fibrillation. *New England Journal of Medicine* 1999: **341:** 871–878.

Lanoix R, Akkapeddi V, Goldfeder B. Perimortem cesarean section: case reports and recommendations. *Acad Emerg Med* 1995; **2(12):** 1063–7.

McQuillan P, Pilkington S, Allan A, Taylor B, Short A, Morgan Get al. Confidential inquiry into quality of care before admission to intensive care. *BMJ* 1998; **317:** 631.

Oakley P, Phillips B, Molyneux E, Mackway-Jones K. Paediatric resuscitation. Updated standard reference chart. *BMJ* 1993; **306:** 1613.

Valenzuela TD, Roe DJ, Cretin S, Spaite DW, Larsen MP. Estimating effectiveness of cardiac arrest interventions: a logistic regression survival model. *Circulation* 1997; **96:** 3308–3313.

Verheugt FWA. Acute Coronary Syndromes: Drug Treatments. *Lancet* 1999; **353** (Suppl.II): 16–19.

Wellens HJ, Bar FW, Lie KI. The value of the electrocardiogram in the differential diagnosis of a tachycardia with a widened QRS complex. *The American Journal of Medicine* 1978; **64:** 27–33.

SECTION 1: 9
MAJOR TRAUMA

J. P. Nolan

PATHOPHYSIOLOGY OF TRAUMA
  Physiological response to haemorrhage
  Systemic inflammatory response syndrome

ASSESSMENT AND MANAGEMENT OF THE TRAUMA PATIENT
  Pre hospital phase
  Preparation for resuscitation
  Primary survey
  Secondary survey

MEDICAL HISTORY

ANALGESIA
  Systemic analgesia
  Regional anaesthesia

MANAGEMENT OF BURNS

CONTINUING MANAGEMENT

ANAESTHESIA IN THE TRAUMA PATIENT
  Induction
  Intra-operative phase

PRACTICAL TECHNIQUES
  Cut-down
  Femoral cannulation
  Subclavian vein cannulation
  Chest drainage

In the United Kingdom trauma kills 14,500 people annually and is the commonest cause of death in those aged under 40 years. The advanced trauma life support (ATLS) course (American College of Surgeons, 1997) provides a basic framework on to which hospital specialists can build their individual skills. The ATLS course focuses on the initial management of patients with major injuries during the so-called "golden hour". The golden hour reflects the importance of timely treatment. A severely injured patient who is in haemorrhagic shock, is hypoxic, or who has an expanding intracranial haematoma, for example, will need rapid, effective resuscitation. The aim is to restore cellular oxygenation before the onset of irreversible shock. This time critical period is better emphasised by the term "platinum 10 minutes".

PATHOPHYSIOLOGY OF TRAUMA AND HYPOVOLAEMIA

Several mechanisms are involved in the development of cellular injury after severe trauma. The commonest is haemorrhage resulting in circulatory failure with poor tissue perfusion and generalised hypoxia (hypovolaemic shock). Myocardial trauma may result in cardiogenic shock while spinal cord trauma may cause neurogenic shock. Severe trauma is a potent cause of the systemic inflammatory response syndrome (SIRS) and this may progress to the multiple organ dysfunction syndrome (MODS) and multiple organ failure.

PHYSIOLOGICAL RESPONSES TO HAEMORRHAGE

A reduction in blood volume immediately activates low pressure receptors in the atria, walls of the ventricles, pulmonary arteries and great veins. High pressure baroreceptors in the aortic arch and carotid sinus are stimulated by hypotension. Chemoreceptors in the carotid body are stimulated by severe hypotension (mean arterial pressure < 60 mmHg). Signals from these receptors are transmitted to the vasomotor centre in the medulla and pons. Autonomic efferents from the vasomotor centre increase peripheral arteriolar and venous tone, heart rate and myocardial contractility. In severe hypotension, large quantities of epinephrine are secreted by the adrenal medulla, and circulating norepinephrine is increased substantially by overspill from synaptic clefts. Adrenocorticotrophic hormone (ACTH), growth hormone (GH), antidiuretic hormone (ADH), and β-endorphins are released from

the pituitary in response to shock and plasma cortisol levels are also increased markedly. Reduced perfusion to the renal cortex stimulates the juxtaglomerular apparatus to release renin, which activates the angiotensin system. Angiotensin II stimulates secretion of aldosterone by the adrenal cortex causing sodium and water retention. The reduction in urine output contributes to restoration of circulating volume. In response to haemorrhage, interstitial fluid will move into the vascular compartment. This translocation of fluid may occur quite rapidly at first (perhaps 1 litre in the first hour), and may total 2 litres by 24 hours.

The goal of the compensatory mechanisms described above is to preserve vital organ perfusion. Perfusion to other tissues, such as skin and gut, may be sacrificed. Cells rendered hypoxic by decreased tissue perfusion will switch to anaerobic metabolism. In comparison with aerobic metabolism, considerably less adenosine triphosphate (ATP) is produced and lactate accumulates rapidly. The ensuing lactic acidosis represents an "oxygen debt", which is "repaid" after effective fluid resuscitation. Depletion of ATP will result in membrane ion-pump failure, cellular swelling, uncoupling of oxidative phosphorylation and, eventually, cell death. Uncoupling of oxidative phosphorylation and permanent loss of intracellular phosphate is the cellular representation of "irreversible shock". Cellular oxygenation must be restored quickly if the patient is to survive.

SYSTEMIC INFLAMMATORY RESPONSE SYNDROME

Crushed and wounded tissues activate complement which in turn triggers a cascade of inflammatory mediators [C3a, C5a, tumour necrosis factor-α (TNF-α), interleukin (IL) 1, IL-6, and IL-8] Thus, severe trauma is a potent cause of the systemic inflammatory response syndrome. The diagnostic features of SIRS (American College of Chest Physicians, 1992) and are summarised in Figure TT.1.

In response to trauma, large numbers of polymorphonuclear neutrophils (PMNs) are released from human bone marrow. Depending on the presence of various modulators, the PMNs adhere tightly to endothelium and migrate into the surrounding parenchyma where they are activated to release superoxide anion (O_2^-) and elastase (Roumen, 1995). This inflammatory response plays a key role in the development of acute respiratory distress syndrome (ARDS) and MODS (Saadia, 1996; Goris, 1996; Sauaia, 1996). Although infection may also play a

THE SYSTEMIC INFLAMMATORY RESPONSE SYNDROME (SIRS)

Manifested by two or more of the following conditions:

- Temperature > 38°C or < 36°C
- Heart rate > 90 beats/min
- Respiratory rate > 20 breaths/min or $PaCO_2$ < 4.3 kPa
- WBC > 12 000 cells/mm³, < 4000 cells/mm³, or > 10% immature (band) forms.

Figure TT.1

role subsequently, up to 50% of the patients developing organ failure early after trauma, do so in the absence of bacterial infection.

ASSESSMENT AND MANAGEMENT OF THE TRAUMA PATIENT

PREHOSPITAL PHASE

In the United Kingdom, prehospital management of severely injured patients is performed mainly by paramedics (Carney, 1999). These personnel are trained in tracheal intubation, intravenous cannulation, fluid resuscitation, the provision of analgesia, and spinal immobilisation. Paramedics are trained to minimise on-scene time; a prolonged time to definitive care will increase mortality. Unless the patient is trapped, on scene interventions should be restricted to control of the airway and ventilation, and stabilisation of the spine. The receiving hospital should be given advanced warning of the impending admission of a severely injured patient. The ambulance officer at the scene should be able to communicate directly with accident department staff via a talk-through link. Concise and essential information on the patient's condition and estimated time of arrival must be given. Accident department staff can then decide whether to alert the trauma team.

PREPARATION FOR RESUSCITATION

With advance warning, medical and nursing staff can prepare a resuscitation bay in readiness for the patient's arrival. This will include running through drip sets, turning on fluid warmers, and drawing up anaesthetic drugs. Members of the resuscitation team should put on protective clothing comprising gloves, plastic aprons, and eye protection. The relevant nurses and doctors should be assigned tasks before the patient arrives. In hospitals with formal trauma teams, the roles of individual team members are usually well established (Figure T.2). The team leader should be a suitably experienced doctor from one of the relevant specialties e.g., emergency medicine, anaesthesia, general surgery, or orthopaedic surgery.

PRIMARY SURVEY AND RESUSCITATION

The initial management of the trauma patient is considered in 4 phases:

- Primary survey
- Resuscitation
- Secondary survey
- Definitive care

COMPOSITION AND ROLE OF A TYPICAL TRAUMA TEAM

Team leader –	Primary and Secondary surveys, co-ordination of team, overall responsibility for the patient while in the A&E department
Anaesthetist –	Airway, ventilation, central venous access, difficult peripheral access, fluid balance, analgesia
Surgeon –	All other procedures, chest drain, fracture splintage, urethral catheter
Nurses × 2 –	Measure vital signs, record data, remove clothes, assist doctors
Radiographer –	Cervical spine, chest, and abdominal X-rays, other X-rays as requested by team leader
Porter –	To take samples to pathology labs, to retrieve urgent blood from blood bank

Figure TT.2

Although the first two phases are listed consecutively, they are performed simultaneously. The secondary survey, or head-to-toe examination of the patient, is not started until the patient has been adequately resuscitated. The aim of the primary survey is to look sequentially for immediately life-threatening injuries, in the order that they are most likely to kill the patient. The correct sequence is:

1. Airway with cervical spine control

2. Breathing

3. Circulation and haemorrhage control

4. Disability – a rapid assessment of neurological function

5. Exposure – while considering the environment, and preventing hypothermia

If life-threatening problems are detected they should be treated immediately, before proceeding to the next step of the primary survey.

Airway and cervical spine

The priority during the resuscitation of any severely injured patient is to ensure a clear airway and maintain adequate oxygenation. Apply a pulse oximeter probe to the patient as soon as possible but remember that peripheral vasoconstriction may make it difficult to obtain a reliable reading. If the airway is obstructed, immediate basic manoeuvres such as suction, chin lift, and jaw thrust may temporarily clear it. A soft nasopharyngeal airway (size 7.0 – 7.5 mm) is useful in the semi conscious patient who will not tolerate a Guedel airway. Every patient with multiple injuries should receive high concentration oxygen. In the unintubated, spontaneously breathing patient give this with a mask and reservoir bag ($FiO_2 = 0.85$) (Figure TT.3).

It should be assumed that every patient sustaining significant blunt trauma has a cervical spine injury, until proven otherwise. Paramedics should have applied cervical spine immobilisation at the accident scene (Figure TT.3). The most effective method comprises a combination of a correctly sized semi rigid cervical collar and lateral blocks joined with tape or straps across the forehead. A long spine board will minimise movement at the thoraco-cervical junction. This combination will minimise neck flexion, although 30% of normal extension is still possible. If the patient has an unstable cervical spine injury, further movement may result in permanent injury to the cord (McLeod, 2000). Minimise neck movement during any airway manoeuvres. Mask ventilation can produce at least as much displacement of the cervical spine as that produced by oral intubation. Manual in-line stabilisation (MILS) of the neck will minimise movement of the cervical spine during oral intubation (Nolan, 1997). The cervical spine cannot be deemed undamaged until the patient has been examined by an

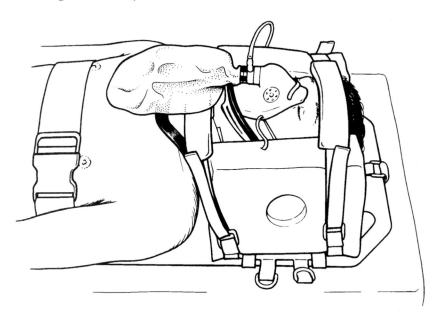

Figure TT.3 Cervical spine immobilisation with semi-rigid collar, lateral blocks and spine board

experienced clinician **and** adequate radiological views obtained (see secondary survey). A reliable clinical examination cannot be obtained if the patient has sustained a significant closed head injury, is intoxicated, or has a reduced conscious level from any other cause.

In the unconscious patient, or in the presence of haemorrhage (from maxillofacial injuries for example) secure the airway by placing a cuffed tube in the trachea. Other reasons for intubating the trauma patient are to optimise oxygen delivery, control ventilation, and to enable procedures to be performed on unco-operative patients.

The technique of choice for emergency intubation of a severely-injured patient is direct laryngoscopy and oral intubation with manual in-line stabilisation of the cervical spine, following a period of pre-oxygenation, intravenous induction of anaesthesia, paralysis with suxamethonium, and application of cricoid pressure. If performed with care, tracheal intubation of a patient with a cervical spine injury carries relatively little risk (McLeod, 2000). An assistant applies manual in-line stabilisation (MILS) to the patient's neck by grasping the patient's mastoid processes and holding the head firmly down on the trolley. This enables the intubator to use the laryngoscope without flexing the cervical spine. Placing the patient's head and neck in neutral alignment in this way impairs the view at laryngoscopy; in this position the view of the larynx is grade 3 or worse in approximately 20% of patients (Nolan, 1993). Intubation is helped by a gum elastic bougie and a McCoy levering laryngoscope. If intubation of the patient proves impossible, secure the airway by surgical cricothyroidotomy. A laryngeal mask can be inserted to provide oxygenation while a surgical airway is obtained. The LMA does not guarantee protection against aspiration and can be regarded as a temporary airway only. A new modification of the LMA, the ProSeal, provides a better seal with the larynx and has a gastric drainage tube to enable passage of a tube into the stomach (Brain, 2000). Needle cricothyroidotomy, with a 14 G cannula followed by jet insufflation of oxygen from a high pressure source (400 KPa), is an alternative method of providing temporary oxygenation but as with the LMA, will not protect against aspiration. Standard cannulae may kink and become obstructed so try to use a device manufactured specifically for needle cricothyroidotomy.

Breathing

Look and listen to the chest to confirm that both sides are being ventilated adequately and measure the respiratory rate. The following chest injuries are immediately life threatening and must be diagnosed and treated in the primary survey:

- Tension pneumothorax
- Open pneumothorax
- Flail chest
- Massive haemothorax
- Cardiac tamponade

TENSION PNEUMOTHORAX

Reduced chest movement, reduced breath sounds, and a resonant percussion note on the affected side, along with respiratory distress, hypotension and tachycardia, indicate a tension pneumothorax. Deviation of the trachea to the opposite side is a late sign, and neck veins may not be distended in the presence of hypovolaemia. Treatment is immediate decompression with a large cannula placed in the 2nd intercostal space, in the mid-clavicular line on the affected side. Once intravenous access has been obtained, insert a large chest drain (36 F) in the 5th intercostal space in the anterior axillary line, and connect to an under water seal drain.

OPEN PNEUMOTHORAX

Cover an open pneumothorax with an occlusive dressing and seal on three sides; the unsealed side should act as a flutter valve. Insert a chest drain away from the wound in the same hemithorax.

FLAIL CHEST

Multiple fractures in adjacent ribs will cause a segment of the chest wall to lose bony continuity with the thoracic cage. This flail segment will move paradoxically with inspiration. The immediately life-threatening problem is the underlying lung contusion, which can cause severe hypoxia. The patient must be given effective analgesia and a thoracic epidural is ideal (see below). Assisted ventilation, via a tracheal tube or by a non-invasive technique, is required if hypoxia persists despite supplemental oxygen.

MASSIVE HAEMOTHORAX

A massive haemothorax is defined as more than 1500 ml blood in a hemithorax and will cause reduced chest movement, a dull percussion note, and hypoxaemia. Start fluid resuscitation and insert a chest drain. The patient is likely to require a thoracotomy if blood loss from the chest drain exceeds 200 ml per hour but this decision will depend also on the patient's general physiological state.

CARDIAC TAMPONADE

Although not primarily a disorder of breathing, it is logical to consider the possibility of cardiac tamponade while examining the chest, particularly if the patient has sustained a penetrating injury to the chest or upper abdomen. Distended neck veins in the presence of hypotension are suggestive of cardiac tamponade, although after rapid volume resuscitation myocardial contusion will also present in this way. A classically described sign of cardiac tamponade is muffled heart sounds, but in the midst of a noisy resuscitation room this cannot be assessed. If cardiac tamponade is suspected, and the patient is deteriorating despite all resuscitative efforts, a resuscitative thoracotomy and open pericardiotomy is indicated. In the absence of someone skilled in thoracotomy, a pericardiocentesis may restore cardiac output temporarily.

Circulation

Control major external haemorrhage with direct pressure. Rapidly assess the patient's haemodynamic state and attach ECG leads. Until proven otherwise, assume hypotension to be caused by hypovolaemia. Less common causes include myocardial contusion, cardiac tamponade, tension pneumothorax, neurogenic shock, and sepsis. Hypovolaemic shock is divided into four classes according to the percentage of the total blood volume lost, and the associated symptoms and signs (Figure TT.4). Blood loss of 15–30% of the total blood volume is associated typically with a tachycardia > 100 beats per minute (bpm) and reduced pulse pressure; the rise in diastolic pressure reflects peripheral vasoconstriction. A fall in systolic

pressure implies a loss of > 30% of total blood volume (approximately 1500 ml in a 70 kg adult).

Insert two short, large-bore, peripheral intravenous cannulae (14 gauge or larger) and take blood samples for FBC, U&E's, and cross match. The easiest site is usually the ante-cubital fossa, but anywhere on the upper limb is acceptable. The femoral vein or the long saphenous vein at the ankle can be used, but are not ideal if the patient has pelvic or intra-abdominal injuries. If percutaneous, peripheral access is impossible, other options are cut down on to a peripheral vein, or central venous cannulation. Cut downs have few complications and can be performed quickly with minimal training (see below). Standard large-bore cannula can be inserted by cut down and possible sites are the antecubital fossa, the saphenous vein at the ankle, and the proximal saphenous vein. Central venous cannulation may not be easy in the hypovolaemic patient and there is a risk of creating a pneumothorax. Use a short, large bore catheter, such as a 8.5 F pulmonary artery introducer sheath, for rapid fluid resuscitation via central veins. After fluid challenging the hypovolaemic patient, monitor the central venous pressure continuously. The intra-osseous route (usually via the proximal tibia) is useful in children, but in adults will not enable adequate flow for effective fluid resuscitation. Take a sample for arterial blood gas analysis. Severely injured patients will have a marked base deficit, indicating lactic acidosis, and its correction will help to confirm adequate resuscitation. Insert an arterial cannula (radial, brachial, or femoral) for continuous direct blood pressure monitoring. A critically ill trauma patient warrants invasive monitoring at the earliest opportunity.

A CLASSIFICATION OF HAEMORRHAGIC SHOCK

	Class 1	Class 2	Class 3	Class 4
Blood loss (% of TBV)	< 15%	15–30%	30–40%	> 40%
Blood loss/70 kg (ml)	750	750–1500	1500–2000	> 2000
Systolic BP	Normal	Normal	Reduced	Very low
Diastolic BP	Normal	Raised	Reduced	Very low
Heart rate	< 100	> 100	> 120	> 140
Respiratory rate	14–20	20–30	30–40	30–40
Urine output (ml/H)	> 30	20–30	10–20	0
Mental state	Alert	Anxious or aggressive	Confused	Drowsy or unconscious

Figure TT.4

Give two litres of a crystalloid solution (e.g. Hartmanns solution) for the initial fluid challenge. The response to this will help to determine the patient's intravascular volume. Failure to improve the vital signs (the non-responder) suggests exsanguinating haemorrhage, and the need for immediate surgical intervention and transfusion of blood. A full cross match will take 45 minutes, but group confirmed blood can be issued in 10 minutes, and group O blood obtained immediately. A transient response to this fluid challenge implies that the patient has lost 20–40% of circulating blood volume and has ongoing bleeding. This requires immediate surgical assessment and probably blood transfusion. A sustained reduction in heart rate and increase in blood pressure implies only moderate blood loss (< 20% blood volume).

In the absence of obvious external haemorrhage, the likely source of severe haemorrhage is: the chest, abdomen, or pelvis. Explore these possibilities and treat them during the primary survey. Careful examination of the chest should exclude massive haemothorax. Obvious abdominal distension mandates a laparotomy, while an equivocal abdominal examination is an indication for computerised tomography (CT) or ultrasound (see under secondary survey). A severely disrupted pelvis may be detected by springing the iliac crests. This assessment should be made only once; repeated attempts will exacerbate bleeding from large pelvic vessels. The pelvis should be "closed" immediately by the application of an external fixator, which will reduce the bleeding.

Warm all intravenous fluids. A high capacity fluid warmer will be required to cope with the rapid infusion rates used during trauma patient resuscitation. Hypothermia, defined by a core temperature less than 35°C, is a serious complication of severe trauma and haemorrhage. The aetiology of hypothermia in the patient requiring massive transfusion is multifactorial and includes exposure, tissue hypoperfusion, and infusion of cold fluids. Hypothermia correlates with survival; those trauma patients with a core temperature below 34°C have a 40% mortality compared with a 7% mortality for those whose lowest recorded core temperature is 34°C or above. Hypothermia has a several adverse effects (Sessler, 2001):

- Gradual decline in heart rate and cardiac output while increasing the propensity for myocardial arrhythmias

- Shift of the oxyhaemoglobin curve to the left, thus impairing peripheral oxygen delivery

- Shivering which may compound the lactic acidosis which typically accompanies hypovolaemia

- Decreased metabolic clearance of lactic acid by the liver

- Hypothermia which contributes to the coagulopathy accompanying massive transfusion

Disability

Record the size of the pupils and their reaction to light, and rapidly assess the Glasgow Coma Scale (GCS) score, which is described in Chapter 5. If the patient requires urgent induction of anaesthesia and intubation, a quick neurological assessment should be performed first.

Exposure and environmental control

It is likely that the patient's clothes will have been removed by this stage. If not, completely undress the patient and apply a forced-air warming blanket to prevent the patient cooling.

Tubes

Insert a urinary catheter; urine output is an excellent indicator of the adequacy of resuscitation. Before inserting the catheter, check for indications of a ruptured urethra such as scrotal haematoma, blood at the meatus, or a high prostate. If any of these signs are present, get a urologist to assess the patient – the specialist may make one attempt to gently insert a urethral catheter before using the suprapubic route. Insert a gastric tube to drain the stomach contents and reduce the risk of aspiration. If there is any suspicion of a basal skull fracture, use the orogastric route, which eliminates the possibility of passing a nasogastric tube through a basal skull fracture and into the brain. Once the location of the gastric tube is confirmed, instil 300 ml of contrast – this will help to exclude a gastro-intestinal perforation if the patient has an abdominal CT scan.

Radiography

All patients who have sustained significant blunt trauma require radiographs of the chest and pelvis. Defer radiographs of the cervical spine to the secondary survey. Obtain the chest and pelvic radiographs in the resuscitation room as soon as possible, but without interrupting resuscitation. This is achieved best if the X-ray equipment is mounted on overhead gantry and members of the trauma team are wearing lead coats.

The secondary survey

Do not undertake the detailed head-to-toe survey until resuscitation is well underway and the patient's vital signs are stable. Re-evaluate the patient continually, so that ongoing bleeding is detected early. Patients with exsanguinating haemorrhage may need a laparotomy as part of the resuscitation phase. They should be transferred directly to the operating theatre; the secondary survey is postponed until the completion of life-saving surgery. Alert staff in the operating theatre and ITU as soon as any severely-injured patient is admitted to the resuscitation room. The objectives of the secondary survey are: to examine the patient from head to toe and front to back; to take a complete medical history; to gather all clinical, laboratory and radiological information; and to devise a management plan.

Head

Inspect and feel the scalp for lacerations, haematomas or depressed fractures. Look for evidence of a basal skull fracture:

- Racoon eyes

- Battle's sign (bruising over the mastoid process)

- Subhyaloid haemorrhage

- Scleral haemorrhage without a posterior margin

- Haemotympanum

- Cerebrospinal fluid rhinorrhoea and otorrhoea

Brain injury is divided into primary and secondary groups. Primary injury (concussion, contusion, and laceration) occurs at the moment of impact and, other than preventative strategies, there is nothing that can be done about it. Secondary brain injury is compounded by hypoxia, hypercarbia, and hypotension. The presence of hypotension and hypoxia doubles the mortality for head injury and they should be prevented or rapidly treated. Guidelines for the management of severe head injury are well described elsewhere (Gentleman, 1993; Maas, 1997; Bullock, 1996). Goals include a mean blood pressure of at least 90 mmHg, $SaO_2 > 95\%$ and, if mechanically ventilated, a $PaCO_2$ of approximately 4.5 kPa.

The conscious level is assessed using the GCS, which is reliable and reproducible. As the GCS is a dynamic measurement, the trend of conscious level change is more important than one static reading. Record the pupillary response and the presence of any lateralising signs. A dilated pupil in a patient in coma can be due to pressure on the occulomotor nerve from a displaced medial temporal lobe, and is a sign of ipsilateral haematoma or brain injury. A haematoma pressing on the motor cortex usually causes contralateral motor weakness. However, it may be of such a size that the whole hemisphere is shifted, pressing the opposite cerebral peduncle against the edge of tentorium. This will cause ipsilateral weakness, although its clinical detection is masked because the patient will be deeply comatose.

Indications for intubation and ventilation after head injury are listed in Figure TT.5. Patients requiring a CT scan will usually need to be intubated and ventilated for at least the duration of the scan.

Unless they are conscious and co-operative, trauma patients requiring a CT scan are normally intubated and ventilated for at least the duration of the scan. Depending on the results of CT scan, these patients are often sedated and mechanically ventilated for at least 24 hours even if their pre-induction GCS was greater than 9.

INDICATIONS FOR INTUBATION AND VENTILATION AFTER HEAD INJURY

Immediately:

GCS < 9

Loss of protective laryngeal reflexes

Ventilatory insufficiency (PaO_2 < 13 kPa on oxygen, $PaCO_2$ > 6 kPa)

Spontaneous hyperventilation causing $PaCO_2$ < 3.5 kPa

Respiratory arrhythmia

Before transfer of the patient to the regional Neurosurgical Unit:

Significantly deteriorating conscious level, even if not in coma

Bilaterally fractured mandible

Copious bleeding into mouth

Seizures

Figure TT.5

Indications for an urgent CT scan (Jennett, 1990) include:

- Coma after resuscitation

- Deteriorating conscious level

- Confusion and focal signs

- Skull fracture and GCS < 15, or neurological signs

- Multiply injured patients not fully orientated, and requiring ventilation and/or extracranial surgery

- Any head injury with previously known intracranial pathology

Referral to the regional neurosurgical unit is indicated for:

- All patients with an intracranial mass

- Primary brain injury requiring ventilation

- Compound depressed skull fracture

- Persistent CSF leak

- Penetrating skull injury

- Patients deteriorating rapidly with signs of an intracranial mass lesion

Mannitol 0.5 – 1.0 g/kg may be given after discussion with the neurosurgeon. This can reduce intracranial pressure and will buy time before surgery.

Face and neck

Careful examination of the face may reveal steps around the orbital margins and along the zygoma and mobile segments in the mid-face or mandible. With an assistant maintaining the head and neck in neutral alignment, inspect the neck for swelling or lacerations, and feel the cervical spinous processes to detect deformity and elicit tenderness.

Obtain lateral, anteroposterior (AP) and odontoid peg radiographs of the cervical spine. If the cervical spine cannot be seen clearly, down to the junction of the 7th cervical (C 7) and 1st thoracic (T 1) vertebrae, obtain a swimmers view (lateral oblique with one arm raised) or a CT scan of C 7-T 1. Interpretation of cervical spine radiographs is difficult. Check alignment of the four lordotic curves on the lateral radiograph: the anterior vertebral line, the anterior spinal canal, the posterior spinal canal, and the spinous process tips. Widening of the prevertebral space is an indication of cervical spine injury. Normal cervical radiographs alone do not "clear" the cervical spine – they must be supplemented by a reliable clinical examination. Treat all trauma

patients with unknown mechanisms of injury as having an unstable cervical spine injury, until the spine has been "cleared" formally by an experienced clinician.

Thorax

There are six potentially life threatening injuries (two contusions and four "ruptures") that can be identified by careful examination of the chest during the secondary survey:

- Pulmonary contusion

- Cardiac contusion

- Aortic rupture

- Diaphragmatic rupture

- Oesophageal rupture

- Rupture of the tracheobronchial tree

PULMONARY CONTUSION

Inspect the chest for signs of considerable decelerating forces, such as seat belt bruising. Even in the absence of rib fractures, pulmonary contusion is the commonest potentially lethal chest injury. Young adults and children have compliant ribs and considerable energy can be transmitted to the lungs in the absence of rib fractures. The earliest indication of pulmonary contusion is hypoxaemia (reduced PaO_2 / FiO_2 ratio). The chest radiograph will show patchy infiltrates over the affected area but it may be normal initially. Increasing the FiO_2 alone may provide sufficient oxygenation but failing that the patient may require continuous positive airway pressure (CPAP) by facemask, or tracheal intubation and positive pressure ventilation. Check the ventilator parameters continually. Use a small tidal volume (5–7 ml/kg) and keep the peak inspiratory pressure below 35 cmH_2O to minimise volutrauma and barotrauma. While avoiding hypoxaemia, try to keep the FiO_2 less than 0.5. These ventilation strategies have probably contributed to the recent reduction in trauma-associated acute respiratory distress syndrome (ARDS) (Navarrete-Navarro, 2001). The patient with chest trauma requires appropriate fluid resuscitation but fluid overload will worsen lung contusion.

CARDIAC CONTUSION

Consider the possibility of cardiac contusion in any patient with severe blunt chest trauma, particularly if there is a sternal fracture. Cardiac arrhythmias and ST changes on the ECG may indicate contusion but these signs are very non-specific. The right ventricle is most frequently injured because it is predominantly an anterior structure, but it is not well evaluated by a 12-lead ECG. An elevated CK-MB isoenzyme is equally insensitive for diagnosing myocardial contusion, but measurement of serum troponin I is better (Orliaguet, 2001). An elevated CVP, in the presence of hypotension, may be the earliest indication of myocardial dysfunction secondary to severe cardiac contusion, but cardiac tamponade must be excluded. Echocardiography will help to confirm the diagnosis of cardiac contusion. Patients with severe cardiac contusion tend to have other serious injuries that mandate their admission to an intensive care unit, thus, the decision to admit a patient to ITU rarely depends on the diagnosis of cardiac contusion alone. The severely contused myocardium is likely to require inotropic support.

TRAUMATIC AORTIC RUPTURE

The thoracic aorta is at risk in any patient subjected to a significant decelerating force, e.g., a fall from a height or high-speed road traffic accident. Only 10 – 15% of these patients will reach hospital alive and of these survivors, untreated, two thirds will die of delayed rupture within 2 weeks. The commonest site for aortic injury is at the aortic isthmus, just distal to the origin of the left subclavian artery at the level of the ligamentum arteriosum. Deceleration produces huge shear forces at this site because the relatively mobile aortic arch travels forward relative to the fixed descending aorta. The tear in the intima and media may involve either part of or all the circumference of the aorta, and in survivors the haematoma is contained by an intact aortic adventitia and mediastinal pleura. Patients sustaining traumatic aortic rupture usually have multiple injuries and may be hypotensive at presentation. However, upper extremity hypertension is present in 40% of cases as the haematoma compresses the true lumen causing a "pseudo-coarctation". The supine chest radiograph will show a widened mediastinum in the vast majority of cases. Although this is a sensitive sign of aortic rupture, it is not very specific. An erect chest radiograph provides a clearer view of the thoracic aorta (Figure TT.6). Other signs suggesting possible rupture of the aorta are listed in Figure TT.7.

If the chest radiograph is equivocal further investigation will be required. Helical CT scan is as good as arteriography for delineating aortic injury and a number of centres are now using transoesophageal echocardiography to diagnose traumatic aortic

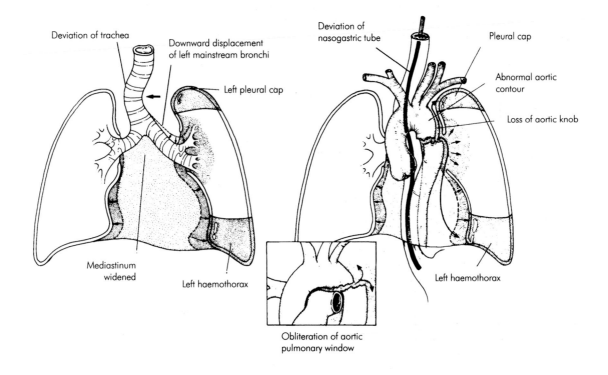

Figure TT.6 Radiological features of traumatic aortic rupture

SIGNS ASSOCIATED WITH TRAUMATIC RUPTURE OF THE AORTA

Widening of the mediastinum

Pleural capping

Left haemothorax

Deviation of the trachea to the right

Depression of the left mainstem bronchus

Loss of the aortic knob

Deviation of the nasogastric tube to the right

Fractures of the upper 3 ribs

Fracture of the thoracic spine

Figure TT.7

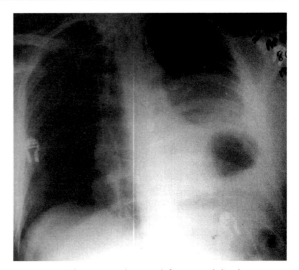

Figure TT.8 Chest X-ray showing left ruptured diaphragm

ruptures. If a rupture of the thoracic aorta is suspected, maintain the blood pressure at 80 – 100 mmHg systolic (using a beta-blocker such as esmolol), to reduce the risk of further dissection or rupture. Pure vasodilators, such as SNP, increase the pulse pressure and will not reduce the shear forces on the aortic wall. When bleeding from other injuries has been controlled, transfer the patient to the nearest cardiothoracic unit,.

RUPTURE OF THE DIAPHRAGM

Rupture of the diaphragm occurs in about 5% of patients sustaining severe blunt trauma to the trunk. It can be difficult to diagnose initially, particularly when other severe injuries dominate the patient's management, and consequently, the diagnosis is often made late. Approximately 75% of ruptures occur on the left side. The stomach or colon commonly herniates into the chest and strangulation of these organs is a significant complication. Signs and symptoms detected during the secondary survey may include: diminished breath sounds on the ipsilateral side, pain in the chest and abdomen, and respiratory distress. Diagnosis can be made on a plain radiograph (elevated hemidiaphragm, gas bubbles above the diaphragm, shift of the mediastinum to the opposite side, nasogastric tube in the chest). The definitive diagnosis is made by instilling contrast media through the nasogastric tube and repeating the radiographic examination (See Figure TT.8 and 9). Once the patient has been stabilised, the diaphragm will require surgical repair.

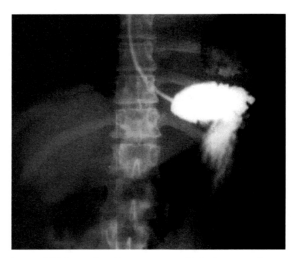

Figure TT.9 X-ray showing contrast media in the stomach (intrathoracic)

OESOPHAGEAL RUPTURE

A severe blow to the upper abdomen may result in a torn lower oesophagus, as gastric contents are forcefully ejected. The conscious patient will complain of severe chest and abdominal pain and mediastinal air may be visible on the chest X-ray. Gastric contents may appear in the chest drain. The diagnosis is confirmed by contrast study of the oesophagus or endoscopy. Urgent surgery is essential since accompanying mediastinitis carries a high mortality.

TRACHEOBRONCHIAL INJURY

Laryngeal fractures are, fortunately, rare. Signs of laryngeal injury include hoarseness, subcutaneous emphysema, and palpable fracture crepitus. Total airway obstruction or severe respiratory distress will have been managed by intubation or surgical airway during the primary survey and resuscitation phases. This is the one situation where tracheostomy, rather than cricothyroidotomy, is indicated. Less severe laryngeal injuries may be assessed by CT before any appropriate surgery. Transections of the trachea or bronchi proximal to the pleural reflection cause massive mediastinal and cervical emphysema. Injuries distal to the pleural sheath lead to pneumothoraces. Typically, these will not resolve after chest drainage, since the bronchopleural fistula causes a large air leak. Most bronchial injuries occur within 2.5 cm of the carina and the diagnosis is confirmed by bronchoscopy. Tracheobronchial injuries require urgent repair through a thoracotomy.

Abdomen

Examine the whole abdomen thoroughly. Quickly determine the need for laparotomy – at this stage, do not spend time trying to define precisely which viscus is injured. Inspect the abdomen for bruising, lacerations and distension, and feel carefully to elicit tenderness. Undertake a rectal examination to assess sphincter tone and to exclude the presence of pelvic fracture or a high prostate. Further diagnostic studies, such as CT, ultrasound, or diagnostic peritoneal lavage (DPL), are indicated whenever abdominal examination is unreliable, for example:

- In patients with a depressed level of consciousness, e.g., head injury, drugs, or alcohol

- In the presence of lower rib or pelvic fractures

- When the examination is equivocal, particularly if prolonged general anaesthesia for other injuries will make reassessment impossible.

Diagnostic peritoneal lavage should be performed by the surgeon who will be responsible for any subsequent laparotomy. Indications of a positive peritoneal lavage include:

- > 5 ml free blood aspirated from the peritoneal cavity

- Enteric contents aspirated from the peritoneal cavity

- Lavage fluid leaking into the chest drains or urinary catheter

- > 100, 000 red blood cells $\times$ 10^9 /l, bile, food, or bacteria in the lavage fluid

Computerised tomography and ultrasound are increasingly used in preference to DPL. In experienced hands, ultrasound has a sensitivity, specificity, and accuracy comparable to DPL and it can be done at the bedside. In the United Kingdom, 24 hour access to an experienced ultrasonographer is rare. In the other parts of the world, particular the United States, trauma surgeons and emergency physicians undertake ultrasound examinations to evaluate trauma patients rapidly. Focused assessment with sonography for trauma (FAST) involves scanning four distinct regions identified as the fours P's: pericardial, perihepatic, perisplenic and pelvic. While ultrasound and DPL are good for detecting blood, CT will provide information on specific organ injury. However, CT is time consuming and can miss some gastro-intestinal, diaphragmatic, and pancreatic injuries.

Major pelvic trauma resulting in exsanguinating haemorrhage should be treated during the resuscitative phase (see above).

Extremities

Inspect all limbs for bruising, wounds, and deformities, and examine for vascular and neurological defects. Correct any neurovascular impairment by re-alignment of any deformity and splintage of the limb.

Spinal column

If the patient is conscious, a detailed neurological examination should detect any motor or sensory deficits. Log roll the patient to enable a thorough inspection and palpation of the whole length of the spine. A safe log roll requires a total of five people: three to control and turn the patient's body, one to maintain the cervical spine in neutral alignment with the rest of the body, and one to examine the spine. The person controlling the cervical spine must command the team.

Unconscious trauma patients require AP and lateral radiographs of the thoracolumbar spine, as well as the three views of the cervical spine.

MEDICAL HISTORY

Obtain a medical history from the patient, relatives, and/or the ambulance crew. A useful mnemonic is:

A = Allergies

M = Medications

P = Past medical history

L = Last meal

E = Event leading to the injury and the environment

It is possible that a patient's pre-existing medical problem contributed to, or precipitated an accident, e.g., myocardial infarction while driving a car.

The paramedics will be able to give invaluable information about the mechanism of injury. The speed of a road traffic accident and the direction of impact will dictate the likely injury patterns.

ANALGESIA

SYSTEMIC ANALGESIA

Give effective analgesia as soon as practically possible. If the patient needs surgery imminently, then immediate induction of general anaesthesia is a logical and very effective solution to the patient's pain. If not, titrate intravenous opioid (e.g., fentanyl or morphine) to the desired affect. Head injured patients need adequate pain relief for any other injuries. **Careful** titration of intravenous morphine or fentanyl provides effective pain relief without serious respiratory depression. The popular use of intramuscular codeine in head injured patients is illogical. It is a weak opioid, and in equianalgesic doses it is a more potent histamine releaser than morphine. It has the same other side effects as morphine, including the ability to induce respiratory depression and miosis. This is hardly surprising since its effects are brought about by the 10–20% that is metabolised to morphine. The proportion of codeine converted to morphine varies considerably due to the genetic polymorphism that governs the enzymatic process, thus its effects are unpredictable. Although still licensed for intravenous use, codeine by this route is never clinically indicated and bolus injection may be associated with a significant risk of severe hypotension.

Non-steroidal anti-inflammatory drugs (NSAIDs) provide moderate analgesia but are relatively contraindicated in patients with hypovolaemia; these patients depend on renal prostaglandins to maintain renal blood flow. In normovolaemic trauma patients, use of NSAIDs may reduce the need for opioids.

LOCAL AND REGIONAL ANALGESIA

Local anaesthetic blocks are ideal in the acute trauma patient but there are relatively few blocks that are both simple and effective. A good example is the femoral nerve block for a fracture of the femoral shaft.

Regional analgesia has a useful role in some acute trauma patients but hypovolaemia and coagulopathy must be excluded before epidural or spinal analgesia is attempted. In patients with multiple ribs fractures, including flail segments, an appropriately placed thoracic epidural will provide excellent analgesia. This will help the patient to tolerate aggressive physiotherapy and to maintain adequate ventilation. All these factors help to reduce the requirement for intubation and mechanical ventilation. A lumbar epidural will benefit patients with lower limb injuries.

MANAGEMENT OF BURNS

The standard "ABC" principles apply to managing patients with severe burns. Patients with severe burns should be stabilised and transferred to the nearest burns centre. The patient with a thermal injury to the respiratory tract may rapidly develop airway obstruction from the oedema. Give humidified high concentration oxygen to all patients suspected of having thermal or smoke injury to the respiratory tract. Undertake arterial blood gas analysis and measure the carboxyhaemoglobin concentration. Consider the need for early intubation in the presence of any of the following:

- Altered consciousness

- Direct burns to the face or oropharynx

- Hoarseness or stridor

- Soot in the nostrils or sputum

- Expiratory rhonchi

- Dysphagia

- Drooling and dribbling saliva

Having established intravenous access, start fluid resuscitation and cover burnt areas with cling film. The simple "rule of nines" (Figure TT.10) allows an approximate calculation of the surface area of the burn, which is determined more precisely later using a Lund

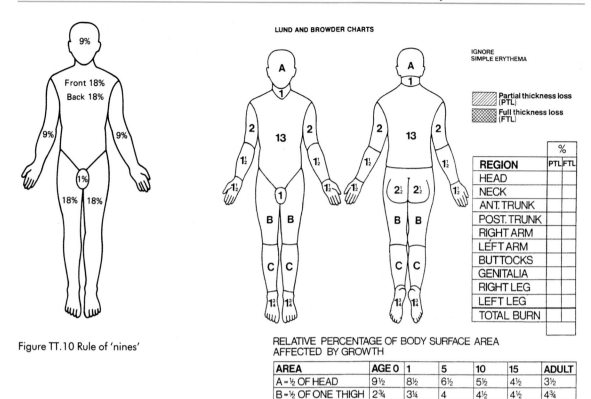

LUND AND BROWDER CHARTS

IGNORE
SIMPLE ERYTHEMA

Partial thickness loss (PTL)
Full thickness loss (FTL)

REGION	%	
	PTL	FTL
HEAD		
NECK		
ANT. TRUNK		
POST. TRUNK		
RIGHT ARM		
LEFT ARM		
BUTTOCKS		
GENITALIA		
RIGHT LEG		
LEFT LEG		
TOTAL BURN		

Figure TT.10 Rule of 'nines'

RELATIVE PERCENTAGE OF BODY SURFACE AREA AFFECTED BY GROWTH

AREA	AGE 0	1	5	10	15	ADULT
A = ½ OF HEAD	9½	8½	6½	5½	4½	3½
B = ½ OF ONE THIGH	2¾	3¼	4	4½	4½	4¾
C = ½ OF ONE LEG	2½	2½	2¾	3	3¼	3½

Figure TT.11 Lund and Browder chart

and Browder chart (Figure TT.11). Most burns centres are now using crystalloid for initial fluid resuscitation. Give 2–4 ml of crystalloid per kilogram body weight per percent burn area in the first 24 hours. Give one half of this fluid in the first eight hours, and the remainder over the next 16 hours. The exact volume of fluid given depends on vital signs, central venous pressure, and urine output. Patients with full thickness burns of > 10% of the body surface area will probably require blood. Patients with severe burns need potent analgesia, which is best given by carefully titrating intravenous opioids.

ANAESTHESIA FOR PATIENTS WITH SEVERE TRAUMA

INDUCTION OF ANAESTHESIA

Trauma patients can present the anaesthetist with a number of problems in the peri-operative period. A smooth induction of anaesthesia and neuromuscular blockade provides optimal conditions for intubation in high-risk trauma patients. The technique for intubation and stabilisation of the cervical spine is

described above. Continuous monitoring of central venous and arterial pressure is invaluable at this stage. Pressurise intravenous fluid bags to enable rapid infusion. Assume that the patient has a full stomach and take appropriate precautions when inducing anaesthesia. Too much induction drug can cause profound hypotension while, in the head injured patient, too little may result in serious intracranial hypertension. There is no evidence that the choice of induction agent alters survival in major trauma patients. In theory, etomidate is the most cardiovascularly stable of the intravenous induction drugs, but an inappropriate dose given by someone who does not use it regularly will cause significant hypotension. Thiopentone and propofol in appropriate doses are perfectly acceptable in the acute trauma patient. Use the induction drug with which you are most familiar – the trauma resuscitation room is not the place for experimentation.

Severely injured patients requiring intubation generally fall into three groups:

(a) Patients who are stable and adequately resuscitated – give a standard or slightly reduced dose of induction drug.

(b) Patients who are unstable or inadequately resuscitated but require immediate intubation – give a reduced, titrated dose of induction drug.

(c) Patients who are in extremis, and are severely obtunded and hypotensive – here induction agents are inappropriate but give a muscle relaxant to facilitate intubation. As soon as adequate cerebral perfusion is achieved, give anaesthetic and analgesic drugs.

Suxamethonium remains the neuromuscular blocker with the fastest onset of action, and is the first choice relaxant for intubation of the acute trauma patient. Provided adequate anaesthesia is provided, suxamethonium does not cause a rise in intracranial pressure in head-injured patients. Rocuronium is almost as fast in onset and is favoured by some experienced trauma anaesthetists.

INTRA-OPERATIVE MANAGEMENT

The following considerations are of relevance to the anaesthetist during surgery for the severely injured patient:

- Prolonged surgery – the patient is at risk from pressure areas and from heat loss. Anaesthetists and surgeons should rotate to avoid exhaustion. Avoid nitrous oxide in those cases expected to last more than six hours.

- Fluid loss – there may be heavy blood and "third space" losses. The combination of hypothermia and massive transfusion will cause profound coagulopathy. A significant metabolic acidosis will occur in patients with major injuries. This will need frequent monitoring (arterial blood gases) and correction with fluids and inotropes, as appropriate.

- Multiple surgical teams – it is more efficient if surgical teams from different specialties are able to work simultaneously, but this may severely restrict the space available to the anaesthetist.

- Acute lung injury – trauma patients are at significant risk of hypoxia caused by acute lung injury. This may be primary, from pulmonary contusion, or secondary, due to SIRS or fat embolism from orthopaedic injuries. Advanced ventilatory modes will be required to maintain appropriate oxygenation.

TECHNIQUES

CANNULATION OF MAJOR VESSELS FOR RESUSCITATION AND MONITORING

Peripheral cut down

If percutaneous cannulation is impossible, a short, large-bore cannula can be inserted via surgical cut-down. With minimal practice, this procedure can be accomplished very rapidly. The best site is the long saphenous vein at the ankle, although some surgeons prefer to use the proximal saphenous vein in the groin. The technique is given below in Figure TT.12.

Cannulation of the femoral vein

In hypovolaemic patients in whom percutaneous access to arm veins is impossible, a useful alternative is the femoral vein. This large vein is consistently located directly medial to the femoral artery in the groin and as long as the artery is palpable, the vein is normally easily cannulated using a Seldinger technique. A pulmonary artery introducer sheath (8.5 F internal diameter) will enable very high fluid flows.

Cannulation of the subclavian vein

The ATLS course manual does not recommend the central veins for rapid fluid resuscitation because, in their opinion, in the hypovolaemic patient, the complication rate is high and the time taken to achieve access is slower than that for peripheral cut down. In reality, many anaesthetists are more competent with central venous cannulation than peripheral cut-down

TECHNIQUE OF PERIPHERAL CUT DOWN

Having cleaned the skin and inserted local anaesthetic if appropriate, make a 2.5 cm horizontal incision 2 cm superior and anterior to the medial malleolus. Expose the vein using blunt dissection with haemostatic forceps. Pass a silk tie around the distal part of the vein and tie it off. Apply gentle traction on this to stabilise the vein. Pass a second tie around the proximal end of the vein but do not tie it. Make a small transverse venotomy and insert a large bore cannula (at least 14 G), using the proximal tie to control bleeding. Tie the proximal suture around the vein and cannula, attach the fluid infusion set and suture the skin wound.

Figure TT.12

and the choice must lie with the individual. The major complications are pneumothorax and accidental arterial puncture. Significant air emboli are very rare. In the blunt trauma patient, internal jugular venous cannulation is not recommended because most approaches to this vein require turning of the patient's head; this cannot be done unless the cervical spine has been cleared. Subclavian cannulation can be performed while the patient's cervical collar is on and with the head and neck in neutral alignment. If a pulmonary artery introducer sheath is used it will allow rapid flow and the ability to monitor central venous pressure. If a chest drain has been inserted, use the same side for subclavian access, unless a major vascular injury is suspected. Practical technique is given below in Figure TT.13

Chest drainage

A tension pneumothorax should be immediately decompressed by insertion of a cannula through the second intercostal space in the mid clavicular line. A chest drain is then inserted. Other indications for chest drainage in the trauma patient are: simple pneumothorax, haemothorax, and rib fractures in a patient requiring positive pressure ventilation. Do not use a trochar for chest drain insertion; it can cause serious lacerations of the lung and pulmonary vessels. Practical technique is given in Figure TT.14.

SUBCLAVIAN VEIN CANNULATION

Position the patient slightly head down (keeping the head and neck in neutral alignment) and clean the skin overlying the chosen site. Infiltrate with local anaesthetic if appropriate. Using a thin walled needle attached to a 10 ml syringe puncture the skin just below the midpoint of the clavicle and, keeping the needle very close to the underside of the clavicle, advance toward the suprasternal notch while aspirating on the syringe. Once blood can be aspirated freely, detach the syringe and feed in the guidewire for about 15 cm. Remove the needle, taking care not to displace the wire. Make a small incision in the skin, adjacent to the wire and insert the dilator over the wire. Remove the dilator, leaving the wire *in situ* and finally, insert the introducer sheath over the wire. Remove the wire and attach the intravenous giving set to the introducer sheath. Suture the sheath in position and cover with a sterile dressing.

Figure TT.13

INSERTION OF CHEST DRAIN

Place the patient supine with the ipsilateral arm at right angles to the chest. The insertion point is in the 5th intercostal space (nipple level) in the anterior axillary line. Infiltrate down to the upper border of the rib with 1% lidocaine. Make a 3 cm incision along the upper border of the 5th rib. Using Kelly's forceps, bluntly dissect down into the pleural cavity. Insert a finger into the pleural cavity and sweep around to ensure that the lung is clear of the chest wall. Select a large chest drain (32–36 F), remove the trochar, and insert the Kelly's forceps through the distal side hole. Insert the chest drain into the pleural cavity using the forceps as a guide. Suture the chest drain securely to the skin and connect it to a underwater drainage system. Obtain a chest X-ray to check for lung expansion and tube position. Leave the drain in situ until the lung is re-expanded and drainage of fluid and/or air has stopped. The chest drains of a patient receiving positive pressure ventilation should not be clamped – the intrapleural pressure is always positive and the patient can be transported safely as long the drains are not moved above the level of the chest.

Figure TT.14

References and further reading

American College of Chest Physicians/Society of Critical care Medicine Consensus Conference: Definitions for sepsis and organ failure and guidelines for the use of innovative therapies in sepsis. *Crit Care Med* 1992; **20**: 864–874.

The American College of Surgeons Committee on Trauma: *Advanced Trauma Life Support Program For Physicians: Instructor Manual*. Chicago: American College of Surgeons, 1997.

Brain AIJ, Verghese C, Strube PJ. The LMA 'Pro-Seal' – a laryngeal mask with an oesophageal vent. *Br J Anaesth* 2000; **84**: 650–4.

Bullock R, Chesnut RM, Clifton G et al. Guidelines for the management of severe head injury. *Eur J Emerg Med* 1996; **2**: 109–127.

Carney CJ. Prehospital care – a UK perspective. *Brit Med Bull* 1999; **55**: 757–766.

Gentleman D, Dearden M, Midgley S, Maclean D. Guidelines for resuscitation and transfer of patients with serious head injury. *Br Med J* 1993; **307**: 547–52.

Goris RJA. MODS/SIRS: result of an overwhelming inflammatory response? *World J Surg* 1996; **20**: 418–421.

Jennett B, Macpherson P. Implications of scanning recently head injured patients in general hospitals. *Clinical Radiology* 1990; **42**: 88–90.

Maas AIR, Dearden M, Teasdale GM et al. EBIC – Guidelines for management of severe head injury in adults. *Acta Neurochir* (Wien) 1997; **139**: 286–294.

McLeod ADM, Calder I. Spinal cord injury and direct laryngoscopy – the legend lives on. *Br J Anaesth* 2000; **84**: 705–708.

Navarrete-Navarro P, Rodriguez A, Reynolds N, West R, Habashi N, Rivera R, Chiu WC, Scalea T. Acute respiratory distress syndrome among trauma patients: trends in ICU mortality, risk factors, complications and resource utilization. *Intensive Care Med* 2001; **27**: 1133–40.

Nolan JP, Wilson ME. Orotracheal intubation in patients with potential cervical spine injuries. An indication for the gum elastic bougie. *Anaesthesia* 1993; **48**: 630–633.

Nolan JP, Parr MJA. Aspects of Resuscitation in Trauma. *Br J Anaesth* 1997; **79**: 226–240.

Orliaguet G, Ferjani M, Riou B. The heart in blunt trauma. *Anesthesiology* 2001; **95**: 544–8.

Roumen RMH, Redl H, Schlag G, et al. Inflammatory mediators in relation to the development of multiple organ failure in patients after severe blunt trauma. *Crit Care Med* 1995; **23**: 474–480.

Saadia R, Lipman J. Multiple organ failure after trauma. *Br Med J* 1996; **313**: 573–574.

Sauaia A, Moore FA, Moore EE, Lezotte DC. Early risk factors for postinjury multiple organ failure. *World J Surg* 1996; **20**: 392–400.

Sessler DI. Complications and treatment of mild hypothermia. *Anesthesiology* 2001; **95**: 531–43.

SECTION 1: 10
CLINICAL ANATOMY

C. A. Pinnock
R. P. Jones

RESPIRATORY SYSTEM
   Mouth
   Nose
   Pharynx
   Larynx
   Trachea
   Bronchial tree
   Lungs

PLEURA AND MEDIASTINUM
   Pleura
   Mediastinum
   Diaphragm
   Heart

NERVOUS SYSTEM
   Spinal cord
   Meninges
   Major plexi
   Autonomic nervous system
   Cranial nerves

VERTEBRAL COLUMN
   Cervical, thoracic and lumbar vertebrae
   Sacrum

SPECIAL ZONES
   Thoracic inlet
   First rib
   Intercostal space
   Abdominal wall
   Inguinal canal
   Antecubital fossa
   Great vessels of the head and neck
   Orbit
   Base of skull
   Coeliac plexus

RESPIRATORY SYSTEM

THE MOUTH

STRUCTURE (see Figure CA.1)

The mouth extends from the lips to the isthmus of the fauces. It contains the tongue, alveolar arches that comprise the gums and teeth and the openings of the salivary glands. The mouth may be divided into two sections, the vestibule and the cavity proper.

The vestibule is a slit like cavity bounded externally by cheeks and lips. The gingivae and teeth provide the boundary to the mouth cavity proper. The mucous membrane is stratified squamous epithelium and the opening of the parotid duct lies just above the second molar crown. **The oral cavity** proper is limited by the maxilla anteriorly and laterally. It is roofed by the hard and soft palates. The floor of the cavity mainly consists of the tongue. Posteriorly the oropharyngeal isthmus separates the oral cavity from the oropharynx. The lining consists of mucous membrane, which is stratified squamous epithelium with mucous glands beneath.

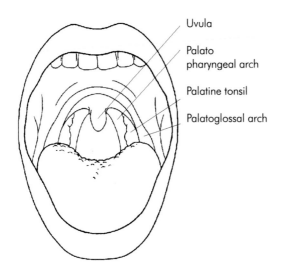

Uvula

Palato
pharyngeal arch

Palatine tonsil

Palatoglossal arch

Figure CA.1 The mouth

The Teeth

STRUCTURE

Each tooth has a crown, a neck and roots that penetrate the alveolar bone. The central cavity of the tooth is filled with pulp and surrounded by dentine. At the crown the dentine is covered by enamel whereas the dentine of the root is covered by cementum. Within the alveolar socket the peri-odontal membrane fixes the tooth in position.

NERVE SUPPLY

The teeth of the upper jaw are supplied by the anterior and posterior superior alveolar nerves whereas the teeth of the lower jaw are supplied by the inferior alveolar nerve.

The nerve supply of the gums is different for labial and lingual surfaces. The gums of the upper jaw receive supply to the labial surface via the infra-orbital and posterior superior alveolar nerves and supply to the lingual surface via the nasopalatine and greater palatine nerves. The gums of the lower jaw receive supply to the labial surface via the mental and buccal surfaces. The lingual nerve supplies the lingual surface of the gums of the lower jaw.

The Tongue

STRUCTURE

The tongue is a muscular structure occupying most of the mouth. It is attached to the mandible and the hyoid bone and rests on the geniohyoid and mylohyoid muscles. A 'V'-shaped groove separates the tongue into an anterior two thirds and a posterior one third.

MUSCLES

The tongue has both intrinsic and extrinsic muscles. The intrinsic muscles are arranged in vertical, horizontal and transverse bundles and mainly act to change the shape of the tongue. The extrinsic muscles are genioglossus, hyoglossus, styloglossus and palatoglossus. The extrinsic muscles move the tongue. Palatoglossus is supplied by the pharyngeal plexus (vagus) whereas all the other muscles are supplied by cranial nerve IX.

NERVE SUPPLY (see Figure CA.2)

The lingual nerve supplies the mucous membrane of the anterior two thirds. Taste fibres leave the lingual nerve in the chorda tympani and pass via the facial nerve to the nucleus of the tractus solitarius.

The glossopharyngeal nerve transmits taste and general sensation from the posterior third of the tongue. The salivary glands receive efferent parasympathetic supply from the superior salivary nucleus in the pons.

BLOOD SUPPLY

The tongue is supplied by the lingual artery and drains via the deep lingual vein into the internal jugular vein.

LYMPHATIC DRAINAGE

The tip of the tongue drains into the submental nodes, the sides into the submandibular glands and the posterior third drains into the retropharyngeal and jugulodigastric nodes.

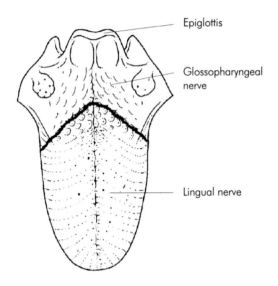

Figure CA.2 Nerve supply of the tongue

THE NOSE

STRUCTURE

The nose may be divided into the external nose, which is made up of bone and cartilage and the nasal cavities. The nasal septum divides the nasal cavity into two separate areas which open anteriorly through the nares and posteriorly through the choanae. The dilated area just within the external nose is termed the vestibule. Each nasal cavity has a roof, floor and two walls.

The roof — The roof is made of the nasal cartilages, nasal bones and frontal bones, the cribriform plate of the ethmoid and the body of the sphenoid. It is arched antero-posteriorly.

The floor — is concave and consists of the horizontal plate of the palatine bone and the palatine process of the maxilla.

The medial wall — is the nasal septum made of septal cartilage with a contribution from the ethmoid and vomer.

The lateral wall — has a bony framework which mainly comprises the ethmoidal labyrinth, the maxilla and the perpendicular plate of the palatine bone. The surface area is increased by the presence of three conchae: superior, inferior and middle each, of which overlies a meatus (Figure CA.3).

The paranasal sinuses and the nasolacrimal duct open onto the lateral wall through orifices. The sphenoid sinus opens into the spheno-ethmoidal recess. The middle ethmoidal cells cause a bulge in the middle meatus onto which they open. This is the bulla ethmoidalis. Below the bulla a semicircular groove, the hiatus semilunaris has the openings of the frontal, ethmoidal and maxillary sinuses (see Figure CA.4).

The nose is lined by vascular mucoperiosteum. Apart from the superior concha and its immediate surrounding area, which is covered by yellow olfactory epithelium, the nose is surfaced by respiratory epithelium.

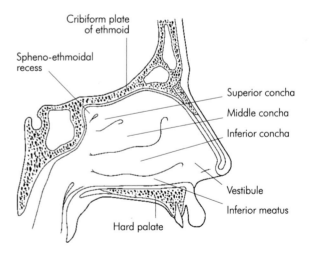

Figure CA.3 The lateral wall of the left nasal cavity

BLOOD SUPPLY

The ophthalmic and maxillary arteries supply the nose. Venous drainage is provided by the facial vein and pterygoid venous plexus.

NERVE SUPPLY

The specialised olfactory zone is supplied by the olfactory nerve. The first and second divisions of the trigeminal nerve provide general sensation.

The septum is mainly supplied by the nasopalatine branch of the maxillary nerve.

The lateral wall is supplied by the lateral posterior superior nasal nerve, the anterior superior alveolar nerve and the nasociliary nerve. All are branches of the maxillary nerve.

The floor is supplied by the anterior superior alveolar nerve and the greater palatine nerve.

LYMPHATIC DRAINAGE

The anterior nasal cavity drains into the submandibular nodes and the posterior into the retropharyngeal lymph nodes.

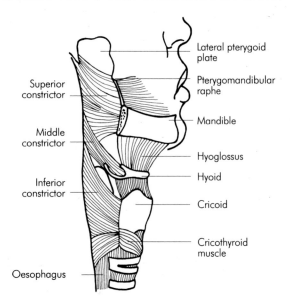

Figure CA.5 The pharynx

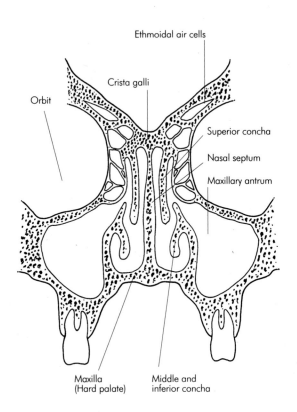

Figure CA.4 Coronal section of the nose and maxillary sinus

THE PHARYNX

STRUCTURE (see Figure CA.5)

The pharynx is basically a wide muscular tube forming the common upper pathway of alimentary and respiratory tracts. It extends from the base of the skull to the level of C 6. The pharynx lies posterior to, and communicates with, the nose, mouth and larynx. This relationship divides the pharynx into three sections – naso, oro- and laryngo-pharynx. The posterior surface of the pharynx lies on the pre vertebral fascia and cervical vertebrae. The pharynx has four coats:

1) Mucous coat. The mucosa is stratified squamous epithelium excepting the nasopharynx where the lining is ciliated, columnar epithelium.

2) Fibrous coat. This is generally thin, but becomes condensed to form the capsule of the tonsil.

3) Muscular coat. This comprises the three constrictor muscles superior, middle and inferior plus stylopharyngeus salpingopharyngeus and palatopharyngeus. The constrictor muscles have an extensive bilateral origin from mandible, hyoid and larynx. Each constrictor spreads out from its anterior attachment to pass posteriorly joining in the mid-line raphe. The superior constrictor arises from the pterygoid plate, the pterygoid hamulus, the pterygomandibular raphe and the inner aspect

of the mandible. The middle constrictor arises from the stylohyoid ligament, and the greater and lesser horns of the hyoid. The inferior constrictor is the largest muscle of the three, arising from the thyroid cartilage, cricoid cartilage and the tendinous arch of cricothyroid. Functionally the muscle has two parts with different muscle fibre orientation. It is between the two that the formation of a pharyngeal pouch may occur.

4) Fascial coat – buccopharyngeal fascia forms the thin fibrous coat of the pharynx.

Nasopharynx

The nasopharynx communicates with the oropharynx through the pharyngeal isthmus. The Eustachian tube opens into the nasopharynx just below the inferior nasal concha. The adenoids (nasopharyngeal tonsil) lie on the roof and posterior wall of the nasopharynx. The adenoid is a collection of lymphoid tissue covered by ciliated epithelium positioned against the superior constrictor. The sphenoid sinus lies posterior and slightly above the nasopharynx separating it from the sella turcica.

Oropharynx

Anteriorly the oropharynx communicates with the oral cavity via the faucial isthmus. It extends to the level of the upper border of the epiglottis where it becomes continuous with the laryngopharynx. The lateral wall of the faucial isthmus contains palatopharyngeus and palatoglossus lying within folds of mucous membrane, these are the arches of the fauces. The palatine tonsils are collections of lymphoid tissue lying on the pillars of the fauces.

Laryngopharynx

The laryngopharynx extends between the tip of the epiglottis and the lower border of the cricoid cartilage (C 6). Anteriorly the opening of the larynx presents together with the posterior surfaces of the arytenoid and cricoid cartilages. The recesses on each side of the larynx formed by its posterior bulging into the laryngopharynx are the piriform fossae. These are famous as the resting place of stray fish bones and other similar.

BLOOD SUPPLY

The pharynx receives arterial supply from the ascending pharyngeal, superior thyroid, lingual, facial and maxillary vessels. Venous drainage is provided by the internal jugular vein via the pharyngeal plexus.

NERVE SUPPLY

This is mainly from the pharyngeal plexus, which lies on the surface of the middle constrictor muscle. The plexus is formed by three main components:

1) Sensory fibres in the pharyngeal branches of the glossopharyngeal (CN IX) and vagus (CN X) nerves.

2) Motor fibres from the nucleus ambiguous travelling in the pharyngeal branch of the vagus supply all muscles except stylopharyngeus (which has its motor supply via the glossopharyngeal).

3) Branches from the cervical sympathetic chain.

An additional sensory supply to the nasopharynx is provided by the pharyngeal branch of the maxillary nerve. The laryngopharynx receives sensory branches from the internal and recurrent laryngeal nerves. Note that the tonsil has a three fold nerve supply: glossopharyngeal nerve via the pharyngeal plexus, posterior palatine branch of the maxillary nerve, fibres from the lingual branch of the mandibular nerve.

LYMPHATIC DRAINAGE

The nasopharynx drains into the retropharyngeal lymph nodes and the remainder of the pharynx into the deep cervical chain.

THE LARYNX

STRUCTURE

The larynx is a functional sphincter at the beginning of the respiratory tree to protect the trachea from foreign bodies. It is lined by ciliated columnar epithelium and consists of a framework of cartilages linked together by ligaments which are moved by a series of muscles.

CARTILAGES OF THE LARYNX

There are four cartilages of importance:

1) The **thyroid cartilage** is said to be shaped like a shield. It consists of two plates that join in the mid-line inferiorly to form the thyroid notch (Adam's apple). Each plate has a superior and inferior horn or cornua at the upper and lower limit of its posterior border, respectively. The inferior horn articulates with the cricoid cartilage.

2) The **cricoid cartilage** is shaped like a signet ring with the large laminal portion being posterior. Each lateral surface features a facet that articulates with the inferior horn of the thyroid cartilage. The upper border of the lamina has an articular facet for the arytenoid cartilage.

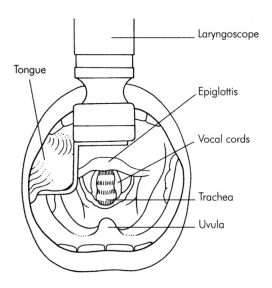

Figure CA.6 Larynx, direct laryngoscopic view

The crico-tracheal ligament joins the first ring of the trachea to the cricoid cartilage.

The crico-thyroid ligament joins the cricoid cartilage to the thyroid cartilage.

The hyo-epiglottic ligament joins the epiglottis to the body of the hyoid.

The intrinsic ligaments of the larynx are of minor importance being the capsules of the small synovial joints between cricoid and arytenoids. The larynx possesses a fibrous internal framework which is composed of the quadrangular membrane, the crico-vocal membrane and the vocal ligament (which is strictly a thickened upper border of the crico-vocal membrane) providing the framework of the true vocal cord.

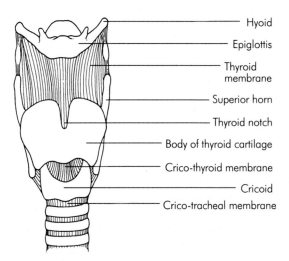

Figure CA.7 Larynx, anterior, external view

3) There is a pair of **arytenoid cartilages**, each being shaped like a triple sided pyramid possessing medial, posterior and antero-lateral surfaces. Each arytenoid cartilage projects anteriorly as the vocal process and in a similar fashion laterally as the muscular process. The posterior and lateral crico-arytenoid muscles are inserted into the muscular process.

4) The **epiglottis** is a leaf shaped cartilage. It has a lower tapered end which is joined to the thyroid cartilage by the thyro-epiglottic ligament. The free upper end is broader and projects superiorly behind the tongue. The lowest part of the anterior surface of the epiglottis is attached to the hyoid by the hyo-epiglottic ligament. Two other minor cartilages are the corniculate and the cuneiform.

LIGAMENTS OF THE LARYNX

The ligaments of the larynx may be divided into extrinsic and intrinsic.

Extrinsic ligaments are the thyro-hyoid membrane, crico-tracheal, crico-thyroid, and hyo-epiglottic ligaments.

The thyro-hyoid membrane joins the upper border of the thyroid cartilage and the hyoid. The membrane is pierced by two important structures: the internal branch of the superior laryngeal nerve and the superior laryngeal artery.

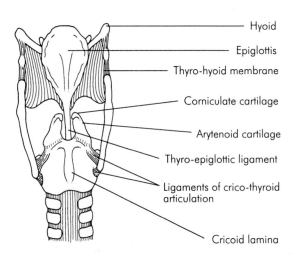

Figure CA.8 Larynx, posterior view

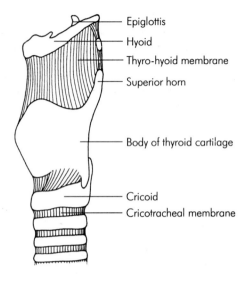

Epiglottis
Hyoid
Thyro-hyoid membrane
Superior horn

Body of thyroid cartilage

Cricoid
Cricotracheal membrane

Figure CA.9 Larynx, lateral view

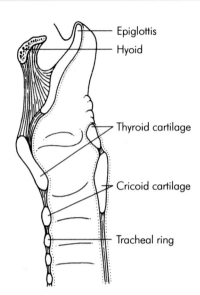

Epiglottis
Hyoid

Thyroid cartilage

Cricoid cartilage

Tracheal ring

Figure CA.10 Larynx, sectional view

MUSCLES OF THE LARYNX

There are three extrinsic muscles of the larynx and six intrinsic ones.

Extrinsic group

1) Sterno-thyroid arises from the manubrium to insert into the lamina of the thyroid cartilage. It is a depressor of the larynx.

2) Thyro-hyoid arises from the oblique line of the thyroid lamina to insert onto the greater horn of the hyoid. It is an elevator of the larynx.

3) The inferior constrictor is a constrictor of the pharynx (see above).

Intrinsic group

These are paired with the exception of the transverse (or inter) arytenoid:

1) Crico-thyroid arises from the anterior surface of the arch of the cricoid cartilage to insert on the inferior horn and adjacent lower border of the thyroid cartilage. Contraction of the muscle approximates the cricoid and thyroid cartilages causing tilting of the cricoid. The antero-posterior diameter of the glottis is thus increased. The net result is an increase in the tension of the vocal cords.

2) Posterior crico-arytenoid arises from the posterior surface of the lamina of the cricoid cartilage to

insert on the muscular surface of the arytenoid. Contraction of the muscle externally rotates the arytenoid and by doing so abducts the vocal cord.

3) Lateral crico-arytenoid arises from the outer lateral arch of the cricoid cartilage to insert into the muscular process of the arytenoid. Contraction of the muscle internally rotates the arytenoid which results in vocal cord adduction and closure, therefore, of the glottis.

4) The transverse arytenoid is attached to the posterior surfaces of both arytenoids. Contraction of the muscle increases tension between the two arytenoids and causes constriction of the glottis by narrowing of its posterior section.

5) Aryepiglottic muscle is a continuation of the oblique fibres of transverse arytenoid lying within the aryepiglottic fold. The only action of the muscle is to cause a minor constriction of the laryngeal inlet.

6) Thyro-arytenoid arises from the junction of the two laminae of the thyroid cartilage and is inserted into the antero-lateral surface of the arytenoid. Contraction of the muscle pulls the arytenoid anteriorly which results in vocal cord relaxation. Some fibres of thyro-arytenoid are inserted into the vocal cord to make the vocalis muscle. This may have a role in adjusting cord tension.

BLOOD SUPPLY

The larynx receives arterial supply from the laryngeal branches of the superior and inferior thyroid arteries. The respective veins provide venous drainage.

NERVE SUPPLY

The mucous membrane of the larynx above the vocal cords is supplied by the internal laryngeal nerve, that below by the recurrent laryngeal nerve. All muscles of the larynx are supplied by the recurrent laryngeal nerve **excepting** cricothyroid which is supplied by the superior (also known as external) laryngeal nerve.

LYMPHATIC DRAINAGE

Most lymphatic drainage passes to the deep cervical chain. A small amount of lymph from the anterior and inferior areas of the larynx passes to the pre laryngeal and pre tracheal nodes.

TRACHEA

STRUCTURE

The trachea descends from the lower border of the cricoid cartilage (C 6) to terminate at its bifurcation into the two main bronchi at the sternal angle (T 4). The length of the adult trachea varies between 10 and 15 cm. The walls of the trachea are formed of fibrous tissue reinforced by 15–20 incomplete cartilaginous rings. Internally the trachea is lined by respiratory epithelium. The trachea may be divided into two portions, that in the neck and that in the thorax.

RELATIONS IN THE NECK

The trachea lies in the midline, anterior to the oesophagus with the recurrent laryngeal nerve residing in a lateral position in a groove between the two. In front of the trachea lie the cervical fascia, infrahyoid muscles, isthmus of the thyroid gland and the jugular venous arch. Laterally lie the lobes of the thyroid gland, carotid sheath and the inferior thyroid artery. The relationships of the trachea at level C 6 are shown in Figure CA.11.

RELATIONS IN THE THORAX

The trachea is traversed anteriorly by two major vascular structures, the brachiocephalic artery and the left brachiocephalic vein. To the left lie the common carotid and subclavian arteries and the aortic arch. To the right lie the right branch of the vagus, azygos vein and mediastinal pleura. The carina is situated anteriorly to the oesophagus behind the bifurcation of the pulmonary trunk.

BLOOD SUPPLY

Arterial supply from the inferior thyroid artery and venous drainage via the inferior thyroid veins.

NERVE SUPPLY

Recurrent laryngeal branch of the vagus with an additional sympathetic contribution from the middle cervical ganglion.

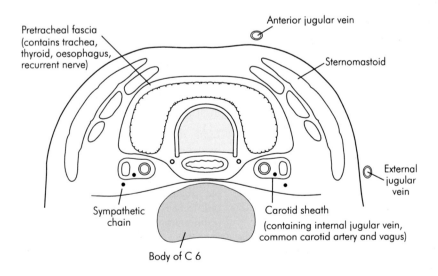

Figure CA.11 Cross section of the neck at level of C 6

LYMPHATIC DRAINAGE

Drainage flows to the deep cervical, pre tracheal and paratracheal lymph nodes.

BRONCHIAL TREE

The bronchial tree consists of extrapulmonary bronchi and intrapulmonary bronchi.

Extrapulmonary bronchi

At the carina, the two main bronchi arise. The right main bronchus is shorter, wider and more upright than the left. The right pulmonary artery and azygos vein are intimately related to the right main bronchus. The left main bronchus passes under the aortic arch anterior to the oesophagus, thoracic duct and descending aorta. The structure of the extrapulmonary bronchi is very similar to the trachea.

Intrapulmonary bronchi

Branching of the intrapulmonary bronchi gives rise to functional units – the bronchopleural segments. The right upper lobe bronchus arises from the right main bronchus just before the hilus and on entering the lung tissue it divides into apical, anterior and posterior segmental bronchi. The middle lobe bronchus arises from the right bronchus below the upper lobe bronchus and subsequently divides into the medial and lateral segmental bronchi. The continuing portion of the right bronchus runs to the lower lobe and divides into apical, anterior, medial, lateral and posterior basal segmental bronchi.

The left upper lobe bronchus arises from the left main bronchus within the lung and divides into five segmental bronchi, the superior and inferior of which supply the lingula. The continuing portion of the left bronchus runs to the lower lobe and then divides also into five segmental bronchi. Nomenclature is as for the right side – see Figure CA.12.

The successive divisions of the bronchial tree may be simplified as follows:

Main bronchus

Segmental bronchus

Bronchioli

Respiratory Bronchioli

Alveolar ducts

Atria

Alveolar sacs

Alveoli

MICROSTRUCTURE OF THE BRONCHIAL TREE

The epithelium of the large bronchi has several layers. The basal layer sits on a basal membrane, the intermediate layer consists of spindle cells and the superficial layer consists of ciliated columnar epithelium with occasional mucus secreting goblet cells. As the bronchi divide and become narrower the epithelium changes to ciliated cuboidal with few goblet cells. The epithelium in the alveoli is only 0.2 microns thick and the blood–air interface consists of: capillary wall, capillary basement membrane, alveolar basement membrane and alveolar epithelium. Interspersed with the flattened epithelial cells are larger cells with vacuoles. These are type II pneumocytes that secrete surfactant.

The submucous layer of the bronchial tree consists of an elastic layer of longitudinal fibres and a deeper unstriped muscle coat.

THE LUNGS

STRUCTURE

Each lung lies in its own pleural sac which is attached to the mediastinum at the hilus. The lung has an apex in the root of the neck and a base that rests on the diaphragm. The left lung has an indentation on its anterior surface, which is the cardiac notch. Deep fissures divide the lungs into lobes. The oblique fissure divides the left lung into upper and lower lobes. The right lung is divided into upper, middle and lower lobes by the oblique and horizontal fissures. The lingula represents the rudimentary middle lobe of the left lung. Each lung has a hilus containing a main bronchus, pulmonary artery, pulmonary veins, pulmonary nerve plexus and lymph nodes surrounded by a collar of pleura.

BLOOD SUPPLY

Lung tissue is directly supplied by the bronchial branches of the descending aorta. Venous drainage is by the bronchial veins that feed into the azygos vein. As regards oxygenation, poorly oxygenated blood travels to the alveoli via the pulmonary artery and returns ultimately to the pulmonary veins. See cardiac section for details.

NERVE SUPPLY

Direct parasympathetic supply via the vagus nerve. Sympathetic fibres from the thoracic sympathetic chain. Both travel in the pulmonary plexus. Sensory fibres arise from the vagus.

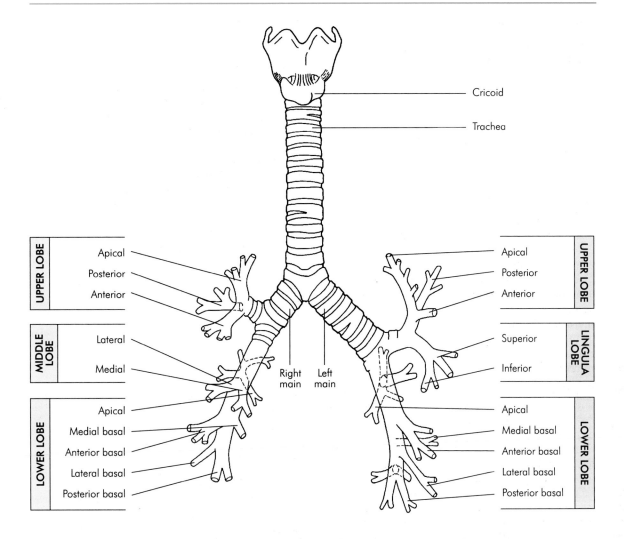

Figure CA.12 The bronchi of the respiratory tree

LYMPHATIC DRAINAGE

Most drainage is by way of the subpleural lymphatic plexus and the deep bronchial plexus both of which drain to the bronchopulmonary nodes and thence to the mediastinal lymph trunks

PLEURA AND MEDIASTINUM

THE PLEURA

STRUCTURE

The pleura is a twin walled serous lined sac. The two layers are termed visceral and parietal. The visceral pleura invests the lung tissue and the parietal pleura invests the diaphragm, chest wall, apex of the thorax and the mediastinum. The upper limit of the pleura is about 3 cm above the mid-point of the clavicle. From here the line of pleural reflections pass behind the sternoclavicular joints to meet in the midline at the level of the second costal cartilage. At the level of the fourth costal cartilage the lines deviate from each other. On the left the line of reflection deviates laterally descending along the lateral margin of the sternum as far as the sixth costal cartilage. On the right the line continues vertically downwards. At the level of the sixth costal cartilage both lines of reflection pass to the eighth rib in the mid clavicular line and then to the tenth rib in the mid axillary line and finally onto the twelfth rib in the paravertebral line.

BLOOD SUPPLY

The pleura receives a supply of arterial and venous vessels from the organs which it covers.

NERVE SUPPLY

The pulmonary pleura has no sensory supply but the parietal pleura is supplied by fibres from all subjacent tissue.

LYMPHATIC DRAINAGE

Visceral pleura initially drain to the superficial plexus of the lung and thence to the hilar nodes. The parietal pleura drains into parasternal, diaphragmatic and posterior mediastinal nodes.

THE MEDIASTINUM

The mediastinum is the area lying between the pleural sacs. The pericardium makes an artificial division into four regions: The middle mediastinum is the space occupied by the pericardium and its contents; the anterior mediastinum lies between the middle mediastinum and the sternum; the posterior mediastinum is that space between the pericardium and diaphragm and the superior mediastinum lies between pericardium below and thoracic inlet above.

THE DIAPHRAGM

A major muscle of respiration, the diaphragm is a musculotendinous septum between thorax and abdomen. It comprises a central tendinous portion and a peripheral muscular portion. The attachments of the diaphragm are **central** and **peripheral**. See Figures CA.13, CA.14.

CENTRAL ATTACHMENT

The fibres of the tendinous section are concentrated into a trilobed central tendon, which blends superiorly with the fibrous pericardium.

PERIPHERAL ATTACHMENT

A complex arrangement consisting of attachments to the crura, medial, median and lateral arcuate ligaments, costal margin and the xiphoid.

DIAPHRAGMATIC FORAMINAE

The inferior vena cava passes through the diaphragm within the central tendon to the right side at the level of T 8. This foramen also transmits the right phrenic nerve.

The oesophagus passes through the diaphragm to the left of the midline at the level of T 10. This foramen also transmits the vagi.

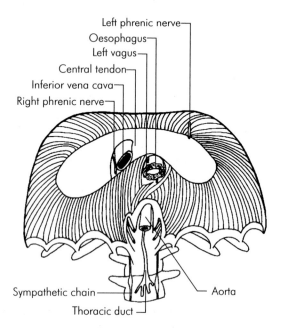

Figure CA.13 The diaphragm

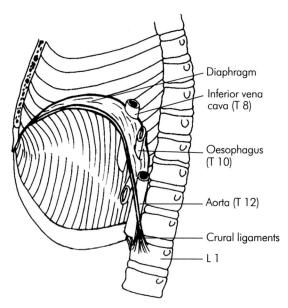

Figure CA.14 The diaphragmatic orifices

The aorta passes through the diaphragm behind the median arcuate ligament at T 12. The thoracic duct and azygos vein also pass through this foramina.

The left phrenic nerve pierces the left dome of the diaphragm.

RELATIONS

The heart and lungs within their respective sacs lie above. Inferiorly, on the right are the liver and right kidney and on the left the fundus of the stomach spleen and left kidney.

NERVE SUPPLY

The diaphragm is supplied by two phrenic nerves (C 3, 4, 5).

THE HEART

STRUCTURE

The heart is a muscular pump consisting of four chambers delineated by the coronary and interventricular sulci. The heart lies within the pericardial sac effectively suspended by the great vessels. Its shape is said to be that of an irregular cone with a base and an apex, lying obliquely across the middle mediastinum. The base is posterior facing and mainly consists of left atrium. The apex represents the tip of the left ventricle. The anterior surface is formed by the right ventricle (Figure CA. 15).

Chambers of the heart

1) Right atrium. The superior vena cava enters the right atrium in its supero-posterior part. The inferior vena cava and coronary sinus enter the right atrium inferiorly and the anterior cardiac vein enters the chamber anteriorly. A vertical ridge runs between the venae cavae and this is termed the crista terminalis. The openings of both inferior vena cava and coronary sinus are guarded by vestigial valves. An oval depression on the surface of the atrial septum, the fossa ovalis, marks the site of the foetal foramen ovale.

2) Right ventricle. The right ventricle communicates with the right atrium by way of the tricuspid valve that possesses three cusps medial, anterior and inferior. The pulmonary trunk communicates with the right ventricle by way of the pulmonary valve that also has three cusps, posterior, right anterior and left anterior. A division between inflow and outflow tracts is provided by the infundibulo-ventricular crest, a muscular ridge. Trabeculae on

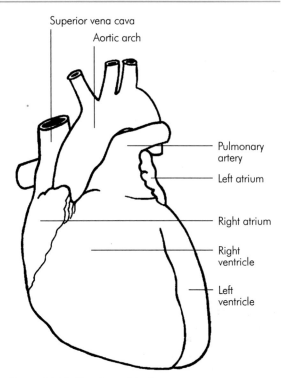

Figure CA.15 Chambers of the heart

the wall project papillary muscles which attach to the tricuspid valve by way of chordae tendinae.

3) Left atrium. The left atrium is a rectangular chamber behind the right atrium. Superiorly a small projection arises on the left of the pulmonary trunk, the left auricle. Four pulmonary veins enter the chamber posteriorly by way of valveless orifices. On the septal surface a shallow depression corresponds to the fossa ovalis of the right atrium.

4) Left ventricle. The left ventricle communicates with the left atrium via the mitral valve which has two cusps, anterior and posterior connected by chordae tendinae to papillary muscles. The origin of the aorta is defended by the aortic valve that has three cusps, right and left posterior and anterior above which lie the aortic sinuses. The right coronary artery arises from the anterior sinus and the left from the left posterior sinus. The wall of the left ventricle is ridged by thick trabeculae carnae.

CONDUCTING SYSTEM

The conducting system of the heart is provided by specialised cardiac muscle tissue within the sino-atrial, atrio-ventricular nodes and the bundle branch system of Purkinje fibres. The SA node consists of an area of conducting tissue in the wall of the right atrium at the upper end of the crista terminalis and to the right of the opening of the superior vena cava. The SA node transmits impulses through the atrial wall to the AV node, which is a similar structure in the septal wall of the right atrium above the opening of the coronary sinus.

The AV node gives rise to the AV bundle (the bundle of His) which descends across the interventricular septum to divide into right and left branches. The branches ramify into a subendocardial plexus in the ventricular wall.

NERVE SUPPLY

The nerve supply of the heart arises from the vagus, which provides cardio-inhibitory fibres, and the cervical and upper thoracic sympathetic ganglia that provide cardio-acceleratory fibres via the superficial and deep cardiac plexi.

BLOOD SUPPLY

The heart receives arterial blood from right and left coronary arteries (Figure CA.16).

The **right coronary artery** arises from the anterior aortic sinus passing forward between the right atrium and pulmonary trunk to then run in the right coronary sulcus to anastomose with the left coronary artery.

Branches: 1) Atrial branches
             2) Ventricular branches
             3) Marginal artery
             4) Posterior interventricular artery

The **left coronary artery** arises from the left posterior aortic sinus to pass between the left atrium and pulmonary trunk to run in the left coronary sulcus and then anastomose with the right coronary artery as described above.

Branches: 1) Atrial branches
             2) Ventricular branches
             3) Anterior interventricular artery
             4) Circumflex artery (sourcing marginal artery)

The sinuses of Valsalva are small outpocketings of the aortic wall in proximity to the coronary ostia. Their purpose is to produce small eddy currents which prevent the aortic valve cusps from obscuring the coronary ostia.

The venous drainage of the heart is complex (Figure CA.17). The majority of the venous drainage is provided by veins accompanying the coronary arteries, which then open directly into the right atrium. Some

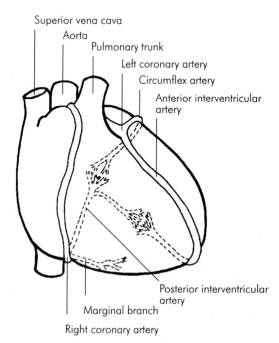

Figure CA.16 The coronary arteries

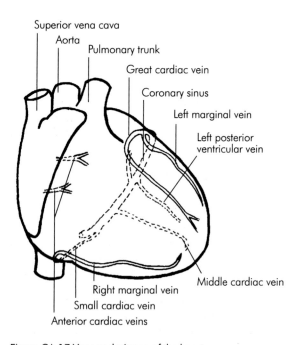

Figure CA.17 Venous drainage of the heart

venous blood drains directly into the cavity via the venae cordis minimae, very small veins. The anterior cardiac vein crosses the atrio ventricular groove and opens into the right atrium. The remainder of the venous drainage is provided by the coronary sinus, which has the following tributaries:

1) Great cardiac vein
2) Middle cardiac vein
3) Small cardiac vein
4) Oblique vein
5) Left posterior ventricular vein

LYMPHATIC DRAINAGE

Lymphatic drainage of the heart passes to the tracheobronchial lymph nodes.

Pericardium

The pericardium is a fibroserous membrane that surrounds the heart and great vessels. There are two layers, an outer fibrous pericardium and an inner serous pericardium.

The serous pericardium has the form of a closed sac in which the heart is invaginated. It has visceral and parietal layers. The fibrous pericardium exists as a strong sac containing the heart itself and the accompanying serous pericardium.

NERVOUS SYSTEM

THE SPINAL CORD

The spinal cord in the adult human is approximately 45 cm long. It is said to be cylindrical in shape, although flattened in the antero-posterior diameter. Above the spinal cord is continuous with the brain stem and below it tapers into the conus medullaris which is attached to the coccyx by the filum terminale. The cord usually ends at the level of L 1–2 although there is great variation in this.

Macroscopically the cord has slight grooves on its anterior and posterior surfaces, the anterior median fissure and posterior median sulcus respectively. In transverse section a central canal can be seen with an H shaped area of grey matter composed of nerve cells surrounded by white matter composed of nerve fibres. The grey matter is divided by virtue of its H shape into two anterior horns (carrying the anterior columns) and two posterior horns (carrying the posterior columns) the two being cross linked by the transverse comissure which corresponds to the cross bar of the H shape. The white matter is largely composed of medullated cells in a longitudinal orientation, which are classified according to their relationship to the grey matter into posterior, anterior and lateral white columns. See Figure CA.18.

Ascending tracts of the cord:

1) The posterior white column transmits fine touch sensation and proprioception. The two fasciculi (medial and lateral) connect to their respective cuneate and gracile nuclei in the medulla. The fibres then cross in the medullary decussation to reach the sensory cortex via the thalamus.

2) The lateral white column carries the lateral spino-thalamic tract, which conveys pain and temperature sensation. The cell bodies lie in the posterior horn of the opposite side and fibres then cross in the anterior white comissure to ascend to the thalamus.

3) The anterior and posterior spinocerebellar tracts ascend in the lateral column. Proprioception sensation is transmitted through these tracts, without crossing, to the cerebellum.

Descending tracts of the cord:

1) The pyramidal tract is the major motor pathway of the cord. It lies in the posterior part of the lateral white column. The tract arises from the pyramidal cells in the motor cortex to cross in the medulla and descend in the pyramidal tract of the contralateral side. At each segmental level fibres pass to the anterior horn of the same side to make the link between upper and lower motor neurones.

2) The direct pyramidal tract is a minor tract running close to the anterior median fissure. Fibres descend from the motor cortex without crossing, in contrast to the pyramidal tract. At each segmental level fibres cross to the opposite anterior horn.

BLOOD SUPPLY

The spinal cord receives arterial supply from the anterior and posterior spinal arteries with additional contributions from spinal branches of the vertebral, intercostal, lumbar and sacral arteries. Radicular arteries serve to reinforce the anterior spinal arterial supply and in the low thoracic or high lumbar level one of these is large and supplies most of the lower two-thirds of the cord, this is the arteria radicularis magna. Venous drainage is by way of a complex of anterior and posterior spinal veins which drain into segmental veins and thence to the azygos, lumbar and sacral veins according to level.

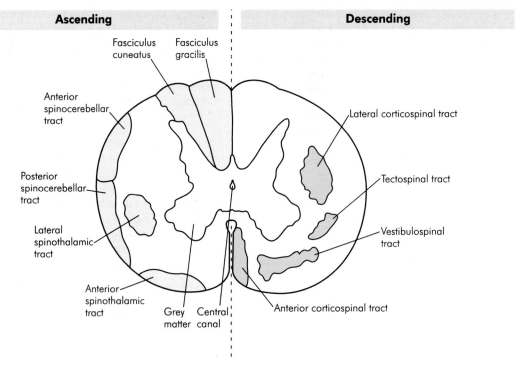

Figure CA.18 Tracts of the spinal cord

THE SPINAL MENINGES

There are three layers covering the spinal cord, the dura, arachnoid and pia mater.

Dura mater

The dura mater consists of two layers. On the surface of the brain the layers are separated by the cerebral venous sinuses. On the surface of the spinal cord the inner dural layer is densely fibrous and the outer layer less so. The outer or endosteal layer ends at the foramen magnum where it blends with the periosteum of the skull. Most commonly the dural sac ends within the sacrum at the level of S 2. It may however, terminate as high as L 5. The attachments of the dura are as follows:

1) Superiorly: the edges of the foramen magnum, bodies of C 2 and C 3 vertebrae

2) Anteriorly: posterior longitudinal ligament

3) Laterally: a sheath along the dorsal and ventral nerve roots

4) Inferiorly: the filum terminale

The anatomy of the epidural space is detailed on page 86.

Arachnoid mater

The arachnoid mater is a delicate membrane closely applied to the dura mater. In some areas the arachnoid herniates the dura mater to form the arachnoid villi which have a major role in the circulation of CSF. The cerebral layer of arachnoid loosely invests the brain and only dips into the main longitudinal fissure between the cerebral hemispheres.

Pia mater

The pia mater is the innermost layer of the three and is closely applied to the surface of the brain and spinal cord. The pia extends into all the sulci of the brain and invests both cranial and spinal nerves, their roots and the filum terminale. In the roof of the third and fourth ventricles and the medial wall of the lateral ventricles the two layers of the pia fuse and form the choroid plexuses. Anteriorly the spinal pia mater is thickened to form the linea splendens and on each side of the spinal cord a serrated fold of pia is termed the ligamentum denticulatum which pierces the arachnoid to attach to dura thus stabilising the cord within its dural sheath.

Spinal nerves

There are 31 pairs of spinal nerves (eight cervical, 12 thoracic, 5 lumbar, 5 sacral, 1 coccygeal) formed in the vertebral canal by the union of ventral and dorsal nerve roots. The ventral roots transmit efferent motor impulses from the cord and the dorsal roots transmit sensory information to the cord. The cell bodies of the sensory fibres are grouped in a ganglion on the dorsal root. When each nerve leaves the vertebral canal it divides into ventral and dorsal rami.

In most regions adjacent ventral rami connect to form major plexuses: cervical, brachial and lumbosacral. In the thoracic region the ventral rami become intercostal and subcostal nerves. Dorsal rami pass posteriorly to divide into medial and lateral branches to supply the muscles and skin of the posterior aspect of the body. See Figure CA.19.

There is a wide variation in the dermatomes corresponding to the spinal nerves, relatively consistent landmarks are nipple at T 4/5 and umbilicus at T 10. Important dermatomes are shown in Figure CA.20.

Peripheral nerves

The cervical plexus and its braches are shown in Figure CA. 21 The nerves of the upper limb derive from the brachial plexus. The branches and relationships of the brachial plexus are shown in Figures CA. 22–23. The nerves of the leg derive from the lumbosacral plexus (See Figures CA.24, 25). The sciatic nerve is the largest nerve in the body. It is derived from the roots of L 4,5 S 1,2,3 on the anterior surface of piriformis and descends through the greater sciatic foramen to run posteriorly within the thigh. On approaching the popliteal fossa it divides into tibial and common peroneal branches.
The tibial nerve is a terminal branch of the sciatic. it descends through the popliteal fossa through the flexor compartment to the level of the medial malleolus where it gives rise to medial and lateral plantar nerves.

The common peroneal nerve descends laterally in the popliteal fossa passing into peroneus longus where it divides into superficial and deep peroneal nerves. The sural nerve arises from the common peroneal high in the popliteal fossa before passing to lie behind the lateral malleolus.

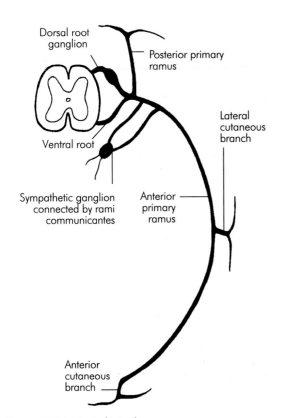

Figure CA.19 A typical spinal nerve

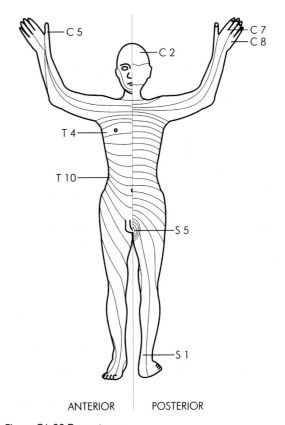

Figure CA.20 Dermatomes

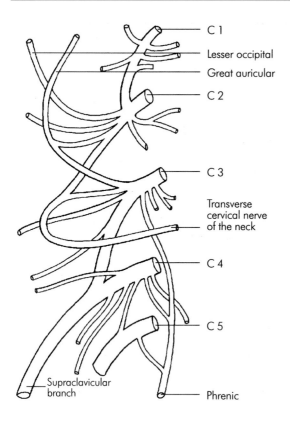

C 1

Lesser occipital

Great auricular

C 2

C 3

Transverse
cervical nerve
of the neck

C 4

C 5

Supraclavicular
branch

Phrenic

Figure CA.21 Cervical plexus

The obturator nerve is a branch of the lumbosacral plexus which descends medial to psoas and runs along the lateral pelvic wall after which it enters the thigh through the obturator foramen to divide into anterior and posterior branches.

The femoral nerve arises from the roots of L 2,3,4 and descends in the pelvis in the groove between psoas and iliacus to enter the thigh deep to the inguinal ligament. It divides into anterior, medial and muscular branches and also the important saphenous branch which emerges from sartorius to run medially in proximity with the saphenous nerve. For detail of the nerves of the foot see Section 1, Chapter 7.

AUTONOMIC NERVOUS SYSTEM

The autonomic nervous system consists of two complimentary components, the sympathetic and parasympathetic nervous systems whose fibres arise from the neurones of the visceral columns of the brain and spinal cord. Fibres synapse with peripheral ganglia before reaching their target organs.

Sympathetic nervous system

From T 1 to L 2 each ventral ramus gives a bundle of myelinated pre ganglionic fibres (rami communicantes) to form the sympathetic trunk. Each ventral ramus receives a bundle of unmyelinated post ganglionic fibres from the sympathetic trunk (rami communicans). The ganglia of the sympathetic system lie in two trunks either side of the vertebral column. There are 3 cervical, 12 thoracic, 5 lumbar and 5 sacral ganglia.

Parasympathetic nervous system

The system is formed by pre ganglionic fibres from the following cranial nerves: oculomotor, facial, glossopharyngeal and vagus and a sacral component comprising pre ganglionic fibres from S 2, 3 and 4. This is known as the cranio-sacral outflow. Although the ganglia of the parasympathetic system are usually ill defined and close to their target organs, the cranial nerves involved have anatomically discrete identifiable ganglia. Post ganglionic parasympathetic fibres are short and unmyelinated.

THE CRANIAL NERVES

Olfactory

The fibres of the olfactory nerve are actually the central processes of the olfactory cells rather than peripheral processes of a central group of ganglion cells.

The nerve fibres originate in the bipolar olfactory cells of the nasal mucosa and subsequently join to form approximately 20 bundles which pass through the cribriform plate of the ethmoid to terminate by synapsing with mitral cells in the olfactory bulb. Axons pass back from the mitral cells to the cortex of the uncus whereupon the final path becomes uncertain.

Optic II

Embryologically the optic nerve is part of the forebrain. Fibres originate in the ganglionic layer of the retina from which axons converge on the optic disc, piercing the sclera to form the optic nerve. The nerve runs posteriorly through the orbit and optic canal into the middle cranial fossa where it joins its partner from the contralateral side to form the optic chiasm. In the chiasm the fibres from the medial half of the retina cross to the opposite side while fibres from the lateral side of the retina pass in the optic tract of the same side. The optic tract passes backward to the lateral geniculate body of the thalamus and thence to the occipital visual cortex.

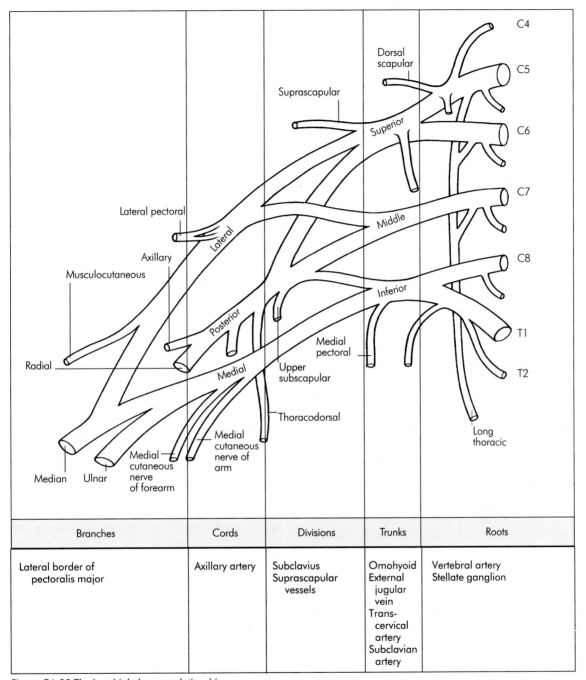

Branches	Cords	Divisions	Trunks	Roots
Lateral border of pectoralis major	Axillary artery	Subclavius Suprascapular vessels	Omohyoid External jugular vein Trans-cervical artery Subclavian artery	Vertebral artery Stellate ganglion

Figure CA.22 The brachial plexus – relationships

Oculomotor III

The oculomotor nerve has both somatic motor and parasympathetic motor fibres. The somatic fibres supply the muscles of the eye excepting superior oblique (VI) and lateral rectus (IV). The parasympathetic fibres synapse within the ciliary ganglion and supply the sphincter pupillae and ciliary muscles. The nerve arises in the upper midbrain where the nuclei lie within the peri-aqueductal grey matter. Fibres pass forwards through the midbrain exiting between the cerebral peduncles. Passing forwards the nerve pierces dura mater to run in the lateral wall of the

ANTERIOR

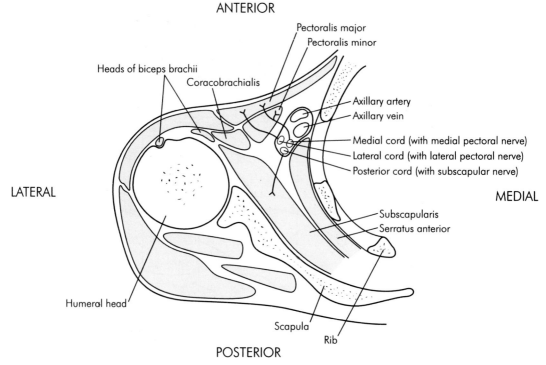

Figure CA.23 Relationships of the cords of the brachial plexus in the axilla

cavernous sinus after which it divides into superior and inferior branches. The superior branch passes through the superior orbital fissure to supply superior rectus and levator palpebrae superioris. The inferior division passes through the tendinous ring to supply medial rectus, inferior rectus and inferior oblique.

Trochlear IV

The trochlear nerve provides motor supply to the superior oblique muscle. It arises from a nucleus in the peri-aqueductal grey matter of the lower midbrain. Fibres pass dorsally around the cerebral aqueduct to decussate with the nerve of the opposite side then passing forward through posterior and middle cranial fossae to enter the orbit via the superior orbital fissure. In the middle cranial fossa the trochlear nerve pierces the dura and runs in the lateral wall of the cavernous sinus in a similar manner to the oculomotor nerve which is slightly more medially placed.

Trigeminal V

The trigeminal nerve is the principal sensory nerve of the face, nose and mouth. It also supplies motor fibres to the muscles of mastication. The nerve has three sensory nuclei: spinal, mesencephalic and superior (in the pons) and one motor also in the pons. The nerve

originates in the pons as a major sensory and more minor motor root. It passes forward to the trigeminal ganglion, which is situated on the petrous temporal bone. The three divisions, ophthalmic, maxillary and mandibular emerge from the anterior border of the ganglion. The motor root bypasses the ganglion to rejoin the mandibular nerve later.

Ophthalmic division: passes forward on the lateral wall of the cavernous sinus (below oculomotor and trochlear nerves) and divides into three branches, lacrimal, frontal and nasociliary. The branches of the nasociliary nerve are the anterior ethmoidal, posterior ethmoidal, infratrochlear and long ciliary nerves.

Maxillary division: runs along the inferior border of the cavernous sinus below the ophthalmic nerve and leaves the skull via the foramen rotundum. After traversing the pterygopalatine fossa the nerve is termed the infra orbital nerve and it emerges through the infra-orbital foramen to supply adjacent areas of the face. Fibres pass to the pterygopalatine ganglion and the maxillary nerve has the following branches: zygomatic, posterior superior alveolar and infra orbital which themselves branch into smaller nerves.

Mandibular division: sensory to the lower third of the face, the anterior two-thirds of the tongue and floor of the mouth. The mandibular nerve carries the motor

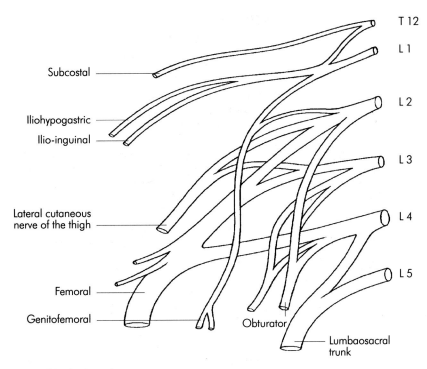

Subcostal

Iliohypogastric

Ilio-inguinal

Lateral cutaneous
nerve of the thigh

Femoral

Genitofemoral

T 12

L 1

L 2

L 3

L 4

L 5

Obturator

Lumbaosacral
trunk

Figure CA.24 Nerves of the lumbar plexus

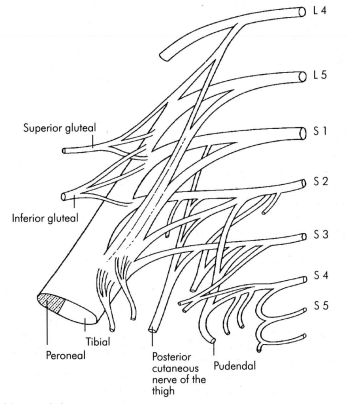

L 4

L 5

S 1

S 2

S 3

S 4

S 5

Superior gluteal

Inferior gluteal

Peroneal

Tibial

Posterior
cutaneous
nerve of the
thigh

Pudendal

Figure CA.25 Nerves of the sacral plexus

supply to the muscles of mastication tensor tympani, tensor palati, mylohyoid and the anterior belly of the digastric muscle.

The motor and sensory components pass separately through the foramen ovale and then join into a short trunk which lies on the tensor palati muscle. At this point the middle meningeal artery lies posterior to the nerve and the otic ganglion is medial to it. The sensory branches are as follows: meningeal, buccal, auriculotemporal, inferior alveolar and lingual.

Abducent VI

The nucleus of the abducent nerve resides in the lower pons. It leaves the inferior border of the pons to pass forward through the cavernous sinus, lying lateral to the internal carotid artery and medial to cranial nerves II, IV and V. The nerve enters the orbit to pierce lateral rectus which it supplies.

Facial VII

The facial nerve has a mixed function. It supplies motor fibres to the muscles of facial expression, parasympathtic secretomotor fibres to the sub-mandibular and sublingual salivary glands and taste sensation from the anterior two thirds of the tongue. There are three respective nuclei in the pons for these three functions. The fibres associated with taste pass to the geniculate ganglion and thence to the nucleus of the tractus solitarius from which they then cross to the opposite lateral nucleus of the thalamus ending in the sensory cortex. The secretomotor fibres arise in the superior salivary nucleus in the pons close to the motor nucleus. The motor nucleus lies within the reticular formation of the lower pons. The nerve leaves the pons to run laterally in conjunction with the vestibulocochlear nerve though the internal auditory meatus to the facial ganglion where the nerve takes a sharp posterior turn to pass downwards through the stylomastoid foramen just before which it gives off the chorda tympani which later joins the lingual nerve to supply taste sensation to the anterior two-thirds of the tongue. After emerging from the stylomastoid foramen the facial nerve is entirely motor and has the following branches: posterior auricular, digastric and stylohyoid.

Vestibulocochlear VIII

Within the auditory nerve are two types of fibre, vestibular and cochlear hence its alternative name. The nerve is formed in the internal meatus and then passes medially to join the brain stem at the cerebromedullary angle. Cochlear fibres arising from the bipolar spiral ganglion cells of the cochlea pass to the dorsal and ventral cochlear nuclei in the upper medulla. Efferent fibres cross to the opposite side to form the auditory striae in the floor of the fourth ventricle. Those from the ventral nucleus particularly forming the trapezoid body in the pons. Fibres ascend from the trapezoid body in the lateral lemniscus to reach the medial geniculate body and thence to the auditory cortex. Vestibular fibres arising from the semicircular ducts, saccule and utricle pass to the vestibular ganglion in the internal meatus and ultimately terminate in the vestibular nuclei in the floor of the fourth ventricle. Efferent fibres travel to the cerebellum in the inferior cerebellar peduncle and there are other vestibular connections to the nuclei of cranial nerves II, IV, VI and XI via the medial longitudinal bundle.

Glossopharyngeal IX

The glossopharyngeal nerve provides sensation to the pharynx, tonsil and posterior one-third of the tongue (including taste), motor supply to stylopharyngeus and secretomotor innervation to the parotid gland. The carotid branch of the glossopharyngeal supplies the carotid body and carotid sinus. Four nuclei correspond to the various roles of the nerve in the following way. The rostral part of the nucleus ambiguus (strictly vagus) is the nucleus of the motor path to stylopharyngeus. The inferior salivary nucleus supplies the secretomotor fibres to the parotid. The nucleus of the tractus solitarius (shared with fibres of VII and X) receives the taste fibres. General sensory fibres terminate in the dorsal sensory nucleus of the vagus. The roots of the glossopharyngeal leave the medulla just lateral to the olive. The nerve passes through the jugular foramen and pierces the pharyngeal wall between superior and middle constrictor muscles. There are two main branches, the tympanic branch and the carotid branch, which is of importance as it supplies the carotid sinus and carotid body.

Vagus X

The vagus nerve is the longest and most widely distributed of the cranial nerves. The vagus provides motor, sensory and secretomotor supply. It provides motor innervation to the larynx, bronchial muscles, gastro-intestinal tract and the heart (through cardio-inhibitory fibres). Sensory supply is distributed to the dura mater, respiratory tract, gastro-intestinal tract and heart. The vagus also provides secretomotor innervation to the bronchial mucus glands and gastro-intestinal tract. The vagus has three nuclei. The dorsal nucleus of the vagus is a mixed motor and sensory centre situated below the floor of the fourth ventricle. The nucleus ambiguus is a motor nucleus situated within the reticular formation of the medulla. The third nucleus is the nucleus of the tractus solitarius, which is concerned with taste sensation. It is situated in the central grey matter of the medulla. The vagus emerges from the medulla lateral to the olive as a group of rootlets, then leaving the skull through the jugular foramen as a single trunk. At the level of the base of skull the vagus has two ganglia, the superior and inferior sensory ganglia. Below the inferior ganglion the vagus receives a communication from the accessory nerve representing its cranial root. The nerve descends through the neck to reach the thorax where it is joined by its contralateral partner in the oesophageal plexus to form anterior and posterior vagal trunks that travel asymmetrically though the thorax and abdomen providing extensive visceral innervation en route.

Accessory XI

The accessory nerve provides the motor supply to sternomastoid and trapezius muscles. The nerve has two roots, a small cranial root travelling by way of the vagus and a larger spinal root from nuclei in the upper five cervical segments of the spinal cord. The nerve arises in the vertebral canal and ascends through the foramen magnum into the posterior cranial fossa. It leaves the skull by way of the jugular foramen and passes anterior to the internal jugular vein into the body of sternomastoid. Subsequently the nerve crosses the posterior triangle of the neck to pierce trapezius.

Hypoglossal XII

The hypoglossal nerve provides motor supply to all the intrinsic and extrinsic muscles of the tongue excepting palatoglossus. The nerve has its nucleus in the floor of the fourth ventricle and arises as a series of rootlets which leave the medulla between pyramid and olive. After uniting into one trunk the nerve leaves the skull by the hypoglossal canal. The nerve passes downwards between the internal carotid artery and jugular vein to the level of the angle of the jaw where it loops over the lingual artery before reaching hyoglossus and genioglossus and terminating in direct motor innervation of the muscles of the tongue. The hypoglossal nerve receives some fibres from the ventral ramus of C1 at the level of the base of skull. The majority of these fibres pass into the descendens hypoglossi which descends as a discrete branch being joined by the descendens cervicalis made of fibres from C2 and C3 to form the ansa hypoglossi which supplies omohyoid, sternothyroid and geniohyoid.

VERTEBRAL COLUMN

There are 7 cervical vertebrae, the atlas, axis and the similar C 3–6. There are 12 thoracic vertebrae and five lumbar vertebrae. Five fused sacral segments form the sacrum and the coccyx has four fused segments. Structures of typical vertebrae are shown below in Figures CA.26-CA.29.

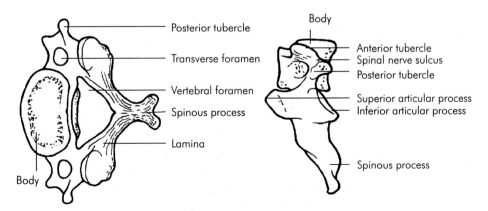

Figure CA.26 Cervical vertebra, superior and lateral views

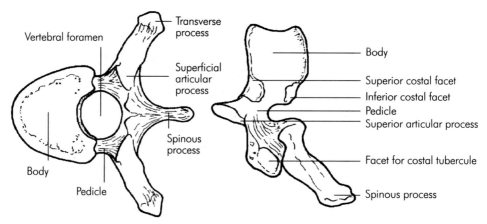

Figure CA.27 Thoracic vertebra, superior and lateral views

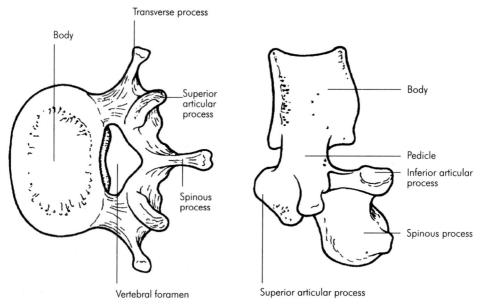

Figure CA.28 Lumbar vertebra, superior and lateral views

SPECIAL ZONES

THORACIC INLET

The thoracic inlet slopes downwards and forwards, making an angle of 60° to the horizontal. It is approximately 10 cm wide and 5 cm from front to back.

The thoracic inlet is bounded posteriorly by the first thoracic vertebra, anteriorly by the manubrium and first rib and laterally by the costal cartilage. The shape of the inlet is said to be kidney shaped due to the protrusion of the body of T 1 into what would otherwise be an oval. The thoracic inlet transmits the trachea, oesophagus, large vascular trunks (brachiocephalic, left carotid and left subclavian arteries and brachiocephalic vein), vagi, thoracic duct, phrenic nerves and cervical sympathetic chain. See Figure CA.30.

The first rib is short, wide and flattened. It lies in an oblique plane. The first rib has a rounded head with a facet that articulates with the body of T 1, a long neck and a tubercle that articulates with the transverse process of T 1. The inferior surface of the rib is smooth and lies on the pleura. The scalene tubercle on the medial border of the rib indicates the

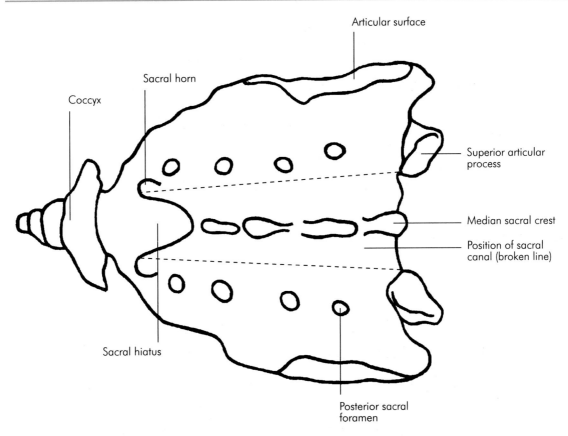

Figure CA.29 Sacrum, posterior view

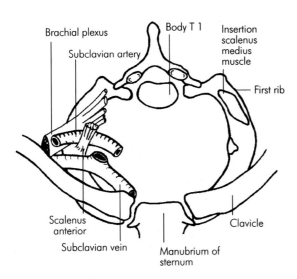

Figure CA.30 Thoracic inlet

attachment of the scalenus anterior muscle. Anteriorly the upper surface of the first rib gives attachment to the costoclavicular ligament and subclavius muscle. Between the pleura and the neck of the rib lie the sympathetic trunk, the large branch of the anterior primary ramus of T 1 passing to the brachial plexus and the superior intercostal vessels. The inner margin of the first rib gives attachment to the suprapleural membrane (Sibson's fascia) which joins the transverse process of C 7. See Figure CA.31.

INTERCOSTAL SPACES

The intercostal spaces are bounded by their related ribs and costal cartilages. They contain the intercostal muscles, vessels and nerves. Deep to the intercostal spaces lies the pleura. The intercostal muscles are arranged as follows: the external intercostal muscle descends in an oblique manner forwards from the lower border of the rib above to the upper border of the rib below. The internal intercostal muscle is an incomplete sheet between the ribs and the pleura which attaches to the sternum, costal cartilages and

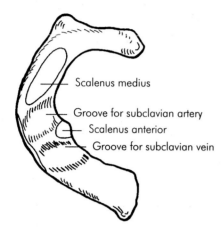

Figure CA.31 Surface markings of the first rib (superior view)

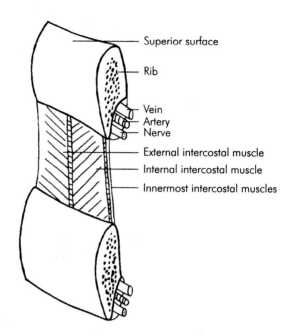

Figure CA.32 Intercostal space

ribs. Additionally, there is an innermost layer of muscles that is incomplete and consists of sternocostalis, the intracostals and subcostals. The contents of the intercostal space are the components of the neurovascular bundle. These are the posterior intercostal vein, the posterior intercostal artery and the intercostal nerve, from above downwards. The neurovascular bundle is protected by the costal groove of the upper rib as shown in Figure CA.32.

ABDOMINAL WALL
STRUCTURE

The most important muscle of the abdominal wall is the rectus abdominus. This is inserted into the pubic symphysis over a 3 cm wide area and inserts onto the 5th, 6th and 7th costal cartilages. The muscle generally is marked by three fibrous intersections on its anterior surface. Rectus abdominus lies within a sheath – the rectus sheath formed by a split in the aponeurosis of internal oblique. The rectus sheath is reinforced posteriorly by the aponeurosis of transversus abdominus and anteriorly by the aponeurosis of external oblique. At its uppermost extremity the rectus lies directly on the costal cartilages because neither internal oblique nor transversus abdominus extend superiorly to this level. Below the arcuate line of Douglas (half way between umbilicus and pubis) the aponeuroses of external oblique, internal oblique and transversus abdominus pass anterior to the rectus itself which therefore rests on transversalis fascia, fat and peritoneum. Fusion of the aponeuroses of the rectus sheath in the midline forms the linea alba which extends from the xiphoid to the pubis.

BLOOD SUPPLY

There is a substantial and varied blood supply to the abdominal wall. Of particular importance are the superior and inferior epigastric vessels. The surface marking of these vessels is represented by a line from the femoral pulse in the groin to a point just lateral to the umbilicus.

NERVE SUPPLY

The anterior primary rami of T 7–L 1 supply the anterior abdominal wall. The intercostal nerves (T 7–11) and the subcostal nerve (T 12) enter the abdominal wall between the interdigitations of the diaphragm eventually piercing the rectus abdominus to supply the skin. The first lumbar nerve, in contrast, divides anterior to quadratus lumborum muscle into the iliohypogastric and ilio-inguinal nerves. The iliohypogastric nerve pierces internal oblique close to the anterior superior iliac spine and then runs deep to external oblique to supply the skin of the suprapubic area. The ilio-inguinal nerve pierces internal oblique and traverses the inguinal canal. It emerges through the external ring (or occasionally through the aponeurosis of external oblique to supply a variable area of the genitalia and upper thigh). There is no deep fascia over the abdominal wall but the superficial fatty tissue may be termed Camper's and Scarpa's fascia (the latter being deeper) although there is no real distinction between the two.

Useful landmarks of the abdominal wall include the xiphoid-T 9, and the umbilicus-L 4.

INGUINAL CANAL

The inguinal canal is an obliquely angled path through the anterior abdominal wall. It extends from the deep ring, which is a weakness in the transversalis fascia at the midpoint of the inguinal ligament to the superficial ring, which is a deficiency in the aponeurosis of external oblique situated supero-medial to the pubic tubercle. The inguinal canal is approximately 5 cm long and has the following boundaries:

1) Anterior wall: external oblique aponeurosis reinforced laterally by internal oblique

2) Posterior wall: transversalis fascia reinforced medially by the conjoint tendon

3) Floor: edge of the inguinal ligament

4) Roof: internal oblique becoming conjoint tendon laterally

Contents: inferior epigastric artery, spermatic cord, round ligament and fat (see Figure CA.33).

ANTECUBITAL FOSSA

The antecubital fossa is a triangle bounded infero-medially by pronator teres, infero-laterally by brachio-radialis and superiorly by a line passing through the medial and lateral condyles of the humerus. The roof of the antecubital fossa consists of deep fascia, which is reinforced by the bicipital aponeurosis. On the deep fascia lie the median cubital vein and medial cutaneous nerve of the forearm. Lateral structures include the cephalic vein and lateral cutaneous nerve of the forearm and medially lies the basilic vein. Within the antecubital fossa from medial to lateral lie the median nerve, brachial artery, tendon of biceps and the radial nerve (see Figures CA.34 and CA.35).

VESSELS OF THE HEAD AND NECK

The major vessels of the head and neck are shown in Figures CA.36 and CA.37.

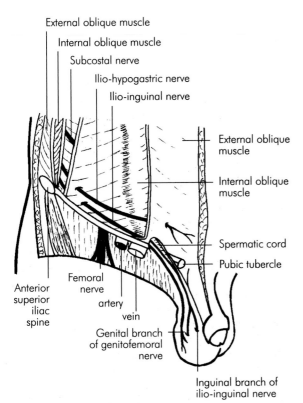

Figure CA.33 Inguinal canal

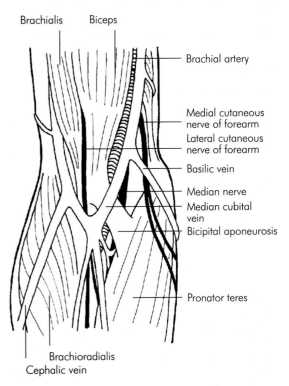

Figure CA.34 Antecubital fossa, superficial structures

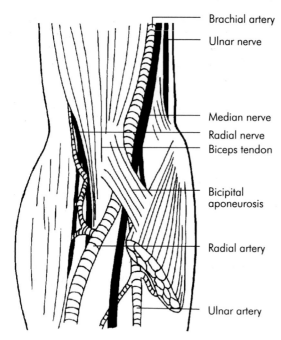

Brachial artery

Ulnar nerve

Median nerve

Radial nerve

Biceps tendon

Bicipital aponeurosis

Radial artery

Ulnar artery

Figure CA.35 Antecubital fossa, deep structures

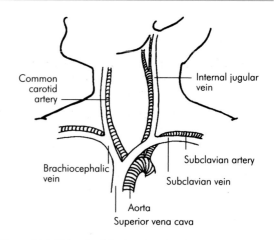

Common carotid artery

Internal jugular vein

Subclavian artery

Subclavian vein

Brachiocephalic vein

Aorta

Superior vena cava

Figure CA.36 Vessels of the head and neck

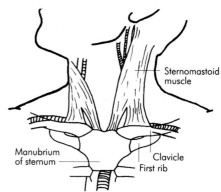

Sternomastoid muscle

Manubrium of sternum

Clavicle

First rib

Figure CA.37 Structures superficial to the vessels of the head and neck

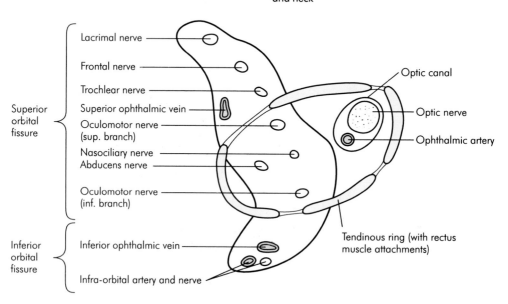

Lacrimal nerve

Frontal nerve

Trochlear nerve

Superior ophthalmic vein

Oculomotor nerve (sup. branch)

Nasociliary nerve

Abducens nerve

Oculomotor nerve (inf. branch)

Superior orbital fissure

Optic canal

Optic nerve

Ophthalmic artery

Tendinous ring (with rectus muscle attachments)

Inferior orbital fissure

Inferior ophthalmic vein

Infra-orbital artery and nerve

Figure CA.38 Structures passing through the orbital fissures

THE ORBIT

Orbital cavity

The orbital cavities lie within the facial skeleton. They are broadly pyramidal in shape and contain the globes, muscles, nerves, vessels and fat.

The **roof** of the orbit is mainly formed by the frontal bone but the posterior portion is derived from the greater wing of the sphenoid. It separates the orbit from the anterior cranial fossa. The **floor** is composed of the maxilla and zygoma with the maxillary air sinus lying beneath. The **lateral wall** is formed by the greater wing of the sphenoid and the zygomatic bone. The lateral wall separates the orbit from the temporal fossa. The **medial wall** has several components; from anterior to posterior these are the frontal process of the maxilla, the lacrimal bone, the orbital plate of the ethmoid and the sphenoid bone.

The orbit contains three posterior openings. The optic canal opens into the apex of the orbit and transmits the optic nerve together with its meninges and the ophthalmic artery. The superior orbital fissure lies between the greater and lesser wings of the sphenoid. The inferior orbital fissure lies between the floor and lateral wall. It opens into the pterygopalatine fossa medially and the infratemporal fossa laterally. The relationships of both fissures are shown in Figure CA.38

For the structure of the globe itself, see Section 2 Chapter 9.

Extra-ocular muscles

There are four **rectus** muscles; superior, inferior, medial and lateral. Anteriorly these muscles pass forward to attach to the sclera at the equator of the globe. Posteriorly they attach to a common tendinous ring around the optic canal and the medial end of the superior orbital fissure.

The **superior oblique** muscle is attached posteriorly to the common tendinous ring. The muscle passes forward around a cartilaginous 'pulley' (the trochlea) to travel backwards and laterally before inserting into the sclera behind the equator.

The **inferior oblique** is attached posteriorly to the floor of the orbit. It passes backwards and laterally below the inferior rectus muscle to attach to the sclera behind the equator. The lateral rectus muscle is supplied by the abducent nerve (VI), the superior oblique by the trochlear nerve (IV) and all the others by the oculomotor nerve (III). The relationships of the extraocular muscles are shown in Figure CA.39.

Blood supply

The ophthalmic artery is a branch of the internal carotid. It arises in the middle cranial fossa and enters the orbit through the optic canal lying inferior to the optic nerve. Branches include the central artery of the retina, ciliary branches, muscular branches and small branches which accompany the nerves within the orbit. The venous drainage of the orbit occurs via the superior and inferior ophthalmic veins which pass through the superior orbital fissure to empty into the cavernous sinus.

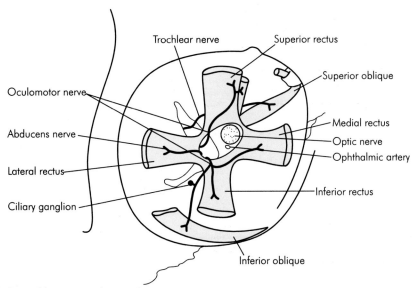

Figure CA.39 Relations of the extra-ocular muscles

BASE OF SKULL

The base of the skull contains various foramina which transmit contents of anatomical interest. These are illustrated in Figure CA.40.

COELIAC PLEXUS

The coeliac plexus is formed by the two interconnecting coeliac ganglia which lie either side of the coeliac artery. Each ganglion receives greater, lesser and renal (also called least) splanchnic nerves from the thoracic sympathetic trunk, branches pass anteriorly to the aorta to form the aortic sympathetic plexus. Post-synaptic fibres pass from the coeliac plexus to the alimentary tract, kidneys and testicles. Pre-synaptic sympathetic fibres pass through the coeliac plexus to end in the adrenal glands. The important relationships of the coeliac plexus are shown in Figure CA.41.

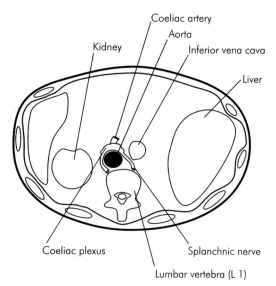

Figure CA.41 Relations of the coeliac plexus

Further reading

Ellis H, Feldman S. *Anatomy for Anaesthetists*, 7th ed. 1997 Blackwell Science, Oxford.

Erdmann A. *Concise Anatomy for Anaesthesia*. 2001 Greenwich Medical Media Ltd, London.

Lumley JS, Craven JL, Aitken JT. *Essential Anatomy*, 5th ed. 1995 Churchill Livingstone, Edinburgh.

Williams P, Warwick R, Dyson M, Bannister L. *Gray's Anatomy*, 37th ed. 1989 Churchill Livingstone, Edinburgh.

Greater palatine foramen
Greater palatine nerve and vessels

Lesser palatine foramen
Lesser palatine nerve and vessels

Foramen ovale
Mandibular division of V cranial nerve

Foramen spinosum
Middle meningeal artery

Carotid canal
Internal carotid artery and sympathetic fibres

Stylomastoid foramen
VII cranial nerve

Jugular foramen
Internal jugular vein
IX X XI cranial nerves

Hypoglossal canal
XII cranial nerve

Foramen magnum
Spinal cord
Medulla junction
Ascending spinal portion XI
    cranial nerve
Spinal and vertebral arteries
Branches of C 1-C 3 spinal nerves

Figure CA.40 Anatomy of the base of the skull

SECTION 2: 1
CELLULAR PHYSIOLOGY

E. S. Lin

ORGANISATION AND CONTROL
  Metabolism and metabolic control
  Cell function and cellular control
  Organ systems and homeostatic control

CELL STRUCTURE
  Basic cell morphology

CELL MEMBRANE
  Membrane functions
  Membrane structure
  Integral membrane proteins
  Membrane transport of substances
  Membrane transport mechanisms

CELL NUCLEUS
  Nucleus and nucleolus
  Nucleic acids
  Protein synthesis

CELL COMMUNICATION
  Chemical messengers
  Receptors
  Membrane signal transduction
  Second chemical messengers

AGEING
  Ageing and dyshomeostasis
  Theories of ageing

ORGANISATION AND CONTROL

The physiology of the body divides itself into different levels of functional organisation. Natural boundaries define three major levels, those of metabolism, cellular function and organ systems. The control mechanisms at each level form an essential part of the physiology, and direct function towards the ultimate goal of homeostasis. Homeostasis can be defined as maintenance of the composition and properties of extracellular fluid.

METABOLISM AND METABOLIC CONTROL

'Metabolism' is a global term encapsulating the mass of

HORMONE EFFECTS ON CELL METABOLISM

Hormone	Gland	Metabolic effects
Insulin	Beta cells in the islets of the Langerhans	↑ glycolysis ↑ glycogen synthesis ↑ protein synthesis ↑ triacylglycerol synthesis ↑ fatty acid synthesis ↓ glycogenolysis ↓ ketone formation ↓ breakdown of triglycerides
Glucagon	Alpha cells in the Islets of Langerhans	↑ glycogenolysis ↑ ketone formation ↑ gluconeogenesis
Epinephrine	Adrenal medulla	↑ glycogenolysis ↑ gluconegenesis ↑ lipolysis
Cortisol	Adrenal cortex	↑ gluconeogenesis ↑ lipolysis ↑ protein catabolism ↓ DNA synthesis
Growth hormone	Anterior pituitary	↑ gluconeogenesis ↑ lipolysis
Thyroid hormone	Thyroid	NORMAL CONCENTRATIONS ↑ RNA synthesis ↑ protein synthesis HIGH CONCENTRATIONS ↑ basal metabolic rate ↓ protein synthesis uncouples oxidative phosphorylation

Figure PG.1 Hormone effects on cell metabolism

biochemical pathways that form the chemical machine providing energy and materials for the maintenance of life. These pathways are controlled at biochemical level by various factors that determine the rate of metabolic reactions including:

- Chemical parameters affecting reaction rates, e.g. concentration of reactants, temperature, activation energy requirements, presence of catalysts
- Enzyme concentration and activity. Factors affecting the rate of enzyme-mediated reactions include substrate concentration, presence of co-factors or co-enzymes, and activation or inhibition by reaction products (see allosteric and covalent modulation)
- The law of mass action and feedback control

At a systemic level metabolism is controlled largely by the endocrine hormones. These substances produce broad physiological changes in the body by exerting multiple effects on cell biochemistry. Some examples of the cellular metabolic effects of hormones are given in Figure PG.1.

CELL FUNCTION AND CONTROL

Cell function involves both intra- and extracellular processes.

Intracellular functions

Intracellular functions include:

- Maintaining the internal milieu
- Reproducing DNA
- Production of RNA
- Repairing cell structures
- Synthesis of substances for export

- Metabolism of imported substances
- Production of chemical energy
- Cell motility

These functions are highly dependent on the intracellular milieu, which is in turn determined by the composition and properties of the extracellular fluid. Therefore intracellular control mechanisms are directed to maintaining these environments.

Intracellular control

Control of intracellular processes is achieved by various molecular mechanisms. All of the above intracellular functions are influenced by chemical messengers. Chemical signals are received at the extracellular membrane surface via molecular messengers. Often, second chemical messengers are activated at the inner surface of the cell membrane, which mediate intracellular changes. Intracellular control mechanisms include:

- Activation or inhibition of enzymes
- Regulation of gene expression
- Changes in membrane permeability
- Regulation of membrane receptor activity
- Changes in membrane potential

Extracellular function

Extracellular functions involve interaction and communication with other cells. This interaction may occur via mechanical, chemical or electrical mechanisms. The most common form of intercellular communication is via chemical messenger. Common groups of messengers are neurotransmitters, neurohormones, endocrine hormones and paracrine secretions.

Cell interactions can result in different types of response. Cells interacting with other cells in the immediate vicinity can produce local homeostatic responses such as an inflammatory response triggered by tissue injury. Co-ordinated functioning of masses of similar cells can result in specialised tissue or visceral activity such as myocardial contraction or gut peristalsis. Finally, interaction may occur with remote cells as occurs in the systemic effects of hormones or systemic responses of the immune system. Intercellular communication mechanisms are discussed in more detail below.

Local homeostatic responses

Local homeostatic responses involve the secretion of chemical messengers by cells in the immediate vicinity of the target cell (paracrine secretion). Alternatively, messengers may be secreted by a cell to act on itself (autocrine secretion). An example of such a local response is the inflammatory response in the case of injury, when local metabolites are released to increase blood flow to the injured tissues.

A group of paracrine agents commonly encountered is the eicosanoids, which are derivatives of arachidonic acid. These include prostaglandins, prostacyclin, leukotrienes and thromboxanes. These agents exert a wide spectrum of effects in many physiological processes including blood coagulation, smooth muscle contraction, pain mechanisms and local inflammatory responses.

ORGAN SYSTEMS AND HOMEOSTATIC CONTROL

Organ systems and their control mechanisms provide

the macroscopic means of controlling homeostasis and of interfacing the body with its external environment. The traditionally described systems such as the cardiovascular, respiratory and neurological systems all exert their control over the body's physiology by well-recognised mechanisms.

Negative feedback system

The most common homeostatic control mechanism is the negative feedback system. A negative feedback system operates to maintain a constant output parameter or steady-state, even if the output parameter is disturbed by an applied stimulus. When the steady-state is disturbed the system first detects the change in the output parameter. It then produces an opposite polarity signal (negative feedback signal) proportional to the output deviation, and feeds this signal back to the input of the system. This feedback signal changes the input and, thus, acts to correct the output deviation (Figure PG.2).

A simple physiological example of a negative feedback system is illustrated by the gamma efferent system controlling resting length in skeletal muscle to maintain posture. Here the output parameter is muscle

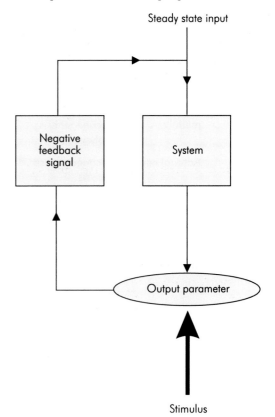

Figure PG.2 Negative feedback system

stretch and the input is the gamma efferent signal to the muscle. When stretch is increased, the displacement is detected by the muscle spindles, which feed back a signal to produce an increase in gamma efferent signal strength. This increases muscle tone thus acting to correct the original stretch or stimulus. Such a response is referred to as a reflex and describes the events in the simple 'knee jerk'.

The analogous homeostatic reflex is designed to maintain a given physiological parameter at a constant value or in a steady-state. The physiological parameter may be a variable such as mean arterial blood pressure, which rests normally at its operating point. When a change occurs in the blood pressure, the change is detected by a baroreceptor that relays a signal to an integrating centre (vasomotor centre of the medulla). The integrating centre then transmits a signal to an effector (vascular smooth muscle), which exerts a response to oppose the original change.

Positive feedback system

Positive feedback systems are also used for physiological control, although in these cases the system is not used to control a specific physiological parameter, but rather to produce a systemic response directed towards maintaining homeostasis. In such a system, there is no polarity change in the feedback signal and, thus, instead of opposing the detected physiological change the feedback signal acts to increase the deviation. This produces a cascade effect that can be identified in certain physiological responses, such as the coagulation cascade during blood clot formation.

CELL STRUCTURE

Cellular function is reflected by cell structure. In broad terms, a cell consists of the cell plasma membrane, the cytosol, intracellular organelles and the nucleus.

BASIC CELL MORPHOLOGY

A basic cell is illustrated in Figure PG.3. The outer cell membrane surrounds various functional structures or organelles, the largest of which is the nucleus. The medium surrounding the nucleus is the cytoplasm.

Cytoplasm

'Cytoplasm' is used to describe all intracellular contents outside the nucleus. It consists of the organelles and the cytosol.

Cytosol

Cytosol refers to the intracelluar fluid containing proteins and electrolytes. Intracellular fluid forms 40%

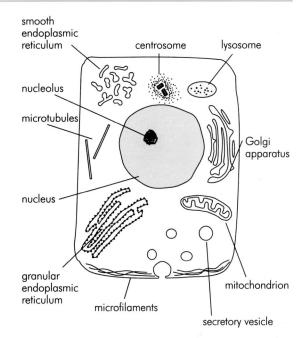

Figure PG.3 A basic cell

of body weight and possesses an electrolyte composition, which is discussed on pages 249–250.

Organelles

A summary of the organelles and their functions is shown in Figure PG.4.

Cytoskeleton

This system of microscopic fibres maintains the cell structure and enables cell movement to occur. Its main components are:

- Microtubules – 25 nm diameter structures with 5 nm-thick walls. Tubule length is a dynamic balance between assembly (at the +ve end) and disassembly (at the –ve end), of protein subunits
- Muscle thick filaments – composed of myosin 15 nm in diameter
- Intermediate filaments – solid fibres about 10 nm diameter
- Microfilaments – solid fibres about 5 nm in diameter made of polymerised actin

Cellular motion, shape changes and ciliary or flagellar movement all involve molecular motor mechanisms based on the action of ATPases. These form moving flexible cross bridges between cytoskeletal components and membranes or organelles. The actin–myosin mechanism responsible for muscle contraction is a molecular motor mechanism that occurs universally in

INTRACELLULAR ORGANELLES AND THEIR FUNCTIONS

Cytoskeleton	–	Maintans the structure of the cell
Membrane	–	Container for cell, nucleous and other organelles, Stuctural support and control of environment on either side
Mitochondria	–	Energy source for the cell generating ATP via oxidative phophorylation
Nucleus	–	Contains the genetic material in the form of chromosomes
		The central site of cell division or mitosis
		Nucleolus synthesises ribosomes
Centrosome	–	Formation of mitotic spindle in cell division
Endoplasmic reticulum (ER)	–	Rough (granular) ER has ribosomes attached and is responsible for protein synthesis
		Smooth (agranular ER is the site of steroid synthesis and detoxification
Ribosome	–	The actual site of protein synthesis in the ER or may occur free in cytoplasm
Golgi apparatus	–	Processes proteins for secretion from cell
Lyosomes	–	Breakdown and elimination of intracellular debris or exogenous substances
Peroxisomes	–	Catalyse various anabolic and catabolic reactions e.g. breakdown of long chain fatty acids
Cilia	–	Used by the cell to propel mucus or other substances over exposed mucosal surfaces

Figure PG.4 Intracellular organelles and their functions

other cells. Other examples of molecular motors include dynamin and kinesin, which act on microtubules.

Mitochondria

These are sausage-shaped structures with outer and inner membranes. Their main function is to produce chemical energy in the form of ATP by oxidative phosphorylation. The inner membrane is folded to form cristae, which are studded with units containing the oxidative phosphorylating and ATP-synthesising enzymes (Figure PG.5). The matrix contains enzymes required to drive the citric acid cycle, which in turn provides the substrate for oxidative phosphorylation.

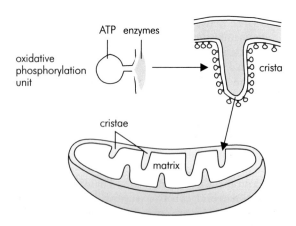

Figure PG.5 Mitochondrion structure

Mitochondria also contain a small amount of DNA, which is solely of maternal origin.

Endoplasmic reticulum (ER)

This membranous structure is composed of complex folds and tubules. In its granular form, ribosomes are attached to the cytoplasmic surfaces and are the primary site for protein synthesis in the cell. Agranular ER is free from ribosomes and is the site of steroid synthesis and detoxification.

Ribosomes

Ribosomes are about 32 nm diameter with large and small subunits. They are composed of 65% RNA and 35% protein and are the sites of protein synthesis. Free ribosomes exist in the cytoplasm and synthesise haemoglobin, peroxisomal and mitochondrial proteins.

Centrosome

This is composed of two centrioles at right angles to each other. The centrioles are cylindrical structures in which nine triplets of microtubules form the walls. A cylinder of pericentriolar material surrounds these structures. The whole structure is situated near the nucleus and is activated at the start of mitosis. Initially, the centrioles replicate and then the centriole pairs separate to form the mitotic spindle.

Golgi apparatus

This consists of flattened membranous sacs or cisterns that are stacked together to form a polarised structure

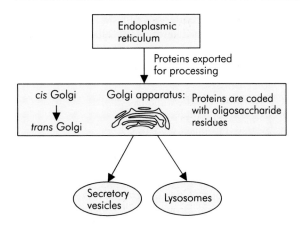

Figure PG.6 Golgi apparatus and protein processing

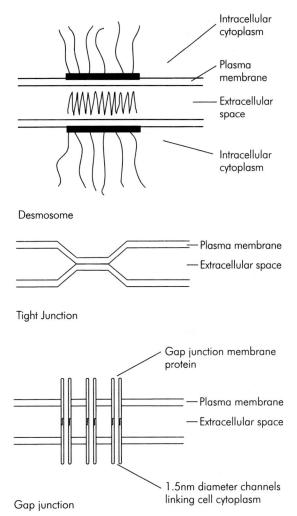

Desmosome

Tight Junction

Gap junction

Figure PG.7 Intercellular connections

with cis and trans ends, separated by a middle region. The Golgi apparatus prepares proteins for secretion (via exocytosis) by receiving the proteins from the ER at the cis side, coding them for destination and finally producing secretory granules or vesicles at the trans side (Figure PG.6).

Intercellular connections

The organisation of cells into tissues involves the formation of specialised junctions between the cells. Three basic types of junction are described (Figure PG.7).

- Desmosomes – disc-shaped junctions that provide mechanical bonding between cells subject to stress (e.g. epithelium, skin)
- Tight junctions – circumferential junctions that seal the extracellular space between epithelial cells, preventing the passage of molecules between cells
- Gap junctions – small channels (diameter 1.5 nm) that allow transfer of small ions and molecules between cells

Cilia

These projections on the luminal surface of epithelial cells are motile processes that move secretions and other substances across the surface of the cell. They are composed of nine pairs of microtubules arranged circumferentially around a central pair of microtubules. Each cilium is attached to a basal granule that has a structure similar to that of a centriole. Ciliary movement is produced by molecular motor mechanisms that cause the microtubules to slide relative to each other.

CELL MEMBRANE

MEMBRANE FUNCTIONS

Membranes surround all cells and the majority of intracellular organelles. The cell membrane has a primary function of controlling the passage of substances across it to maintain the intracellular environment, which is an essential requirement for cellular metabolism. Controlling the movement of ions across the membrane also establishes ion concentration gradients and electrical potential differences (membrane potential) across the membrane, which enable cells to perform specialised functions. A summary of cell membrane functions is outlined below:

- Regulation of the passage of substances across it for intracellular homeostasis
- Establishment of ion concentration gradients (K^+ and Na^+)
- Establishment of membrane potential
- Container for cell contents
- Anchorage for cytoskeleton
- Structural function for tissues acting as a site for intercellular connections
- Communication via chemical messengers
- Communication via action potentials

MEMBRANE STRUCTURE

Cell membranes are based on a double phospholipid layer structure. The phospholipid molecules are amphipathic, with one end charged and the other non polar. The membrane is formed by a double layer of these amphipathic molecules with the polar ends orientated outwards. This double layer is interrupted by integral membrane protein molecules, which often span the membrane completely and are referred to as transmembrane proteins. Membrane proteins and lipids may possess polysaccharide chains attached to their extracellular surface, which appears as a fuzzy coat visible on electron microscopy, known as the glycocalyx (Figure PG.8).

INTEGRAL MEMBRANE PROTEINS

Integral membrane proteins have various functions. Some form controllable channels for the passage of ions or water. Another group transmits chemical signals across the cell membrane by acting as active carriers. More recently, cell adhesion molecules have been identified that determine the cell's ability to attach to basal laminae and to other cells. Types of integral membrane proteins include:

- Ion channels
- Transport carriers
- Cell adhesion molecules
- Second messenger enzymes
- G proteins

Peripheral membrane proteins are located on the cytoplasmic membrane surface where they are attached to polar regions of the integral membrane proteins. These peripheral proteins are associated with cell motility and shape.

Cell adhesion molecules (CAM)

This is a large group of membrane proteins with several subdivisions and a wide range of functions. Their primary properties form the basis for cells to adhere either to other cells (to other CAMs) or to the extracellular matrix (i.e. collagen and glycoprotein elements in connective tissue). These adhesive properties are rapidly controllable and may also be linked to signal transduction by the same molecules. The scope of CAM function thus extends well beyond a simple structural role, and involves both normal and pathological processes. Some of the processes involving adhesion molecules are:

- Transduction of signals controlling differentiation, gene expression and motility
- Programmed assembly of cells to form the complex architecture of individual tissues
- Morphogenesis of embryological tissues and organs

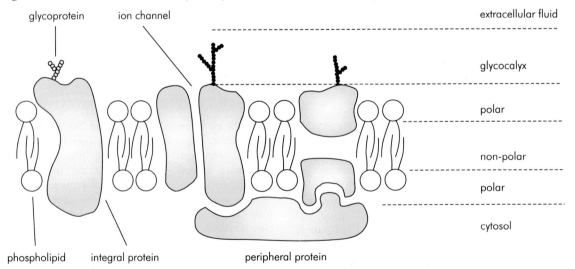

Figure PG.8 Cell plasma membrane

FAMILIES OF CELL ADHESION MOLECULES AND THEIR PROPERTIES

Adhesion molecule	Platelet adhesion
	Expressed on leukocytes and binds to IgSF (endothelium)
	Leukocyte motility
	Cell-matrix adhesion
Selectins	Expressed on circulating leukocytes
	Stored in endothelial cells and allow rolling of leukocytes
	Stored in platelets
	Leukocyte–endothelial adhesion
Cadherins	Morphogenesis of tissues
	Metastasis of tumours
	Embryological development
Immunoglobulin superfamily (IgSF)	Expressed on endothelium and binds to integrins (leukocytes)
	Expressed on gut mucosa binds integrins and selectins (lymphocytes)

Figure PG.9 Families of cell adhesion molecules and their properties

- Formation of intercellular connections in epithelial tissues
- Adhesion of leukocytes to vascular endothelium
- Enablement of leukocyte motility
- Directing of leukocyte migration in inflammation
- Platelet adhesion in blood coagulation
- Pathogenesis of airway inflammation in asthma
- Epithelial cell adhesion to basement membranes and the pathogenesis of bullous diseases

An outline of the different families of CAMs is summarised in Figure PG.9

G proteins

This group of membrane proteins has a high affinity for guanine nucleotides. Over 16 G proteins have been identified composed of alpha, beta and gamma subunits, suggesting the existence of many more. Activation of the G protein enables it to bind guanosine tri-phosphate (GTP) and interact with an effector protein. The activated G protein then de-activates itself by intrinsic GTPase activity (Figure PG.10). This reduces the GTP to GDP thus de-activating the G protein.

Activation of the G protein system can result in various effects. It can control the release of second messengers via Gs- and Gi-type proteins that have stimulatory or inhibitory effects on enzymes such as adenylyl cyclase. Some G proteins are directly coupled to ion channels and, thus, control membrane permeability to ions. Others can increase intracellular calcium concentrations and activate intracellular kinases. The heterogeneous nature of G proteins mean that a first

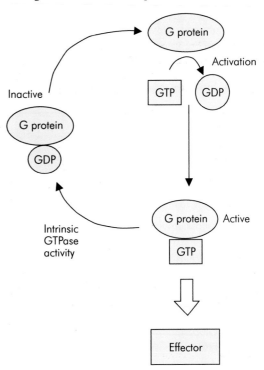

Figure PG.10 G protein activation and de-activation

messenger common to several tissues, can produce a spectrum of different cellular responses according to the tissue targeted. This variability is further increased by the fact that more than one G protein may be activated by a single receptor and several effector proteins can be coupled to a single G protein.

Second messenger enzymes

The production of second messengers; cyclic AMP, cyclic GMP, inositol triphosphate and diacylglycerol takes place at the cell membrane. The enzymes responsible for their production are adenylyl cyclase, guanylyl cyclase and tyrosine kinase. The activities of these enzymes are controlled by various pathways, which involve both activation and inhibition. Second messenger effects are multiple and widespread intracellularly.

MEMBRANE TRANSPORT OF SUBSTANCES

Cell membranes control the movement of a wide range of particles and substances between the intra- and extracellular spaces. These include gases, ions, water, proteins and intracellular granules or debris. Different components of the membrane are associated with different mechanisms of transport. The phospholipid bilayer areas of the membrane allow diffusion of water, small molecules and lipid soluble substances. Transmembrane proteins provide active mechanisms for transport and allow ion diffusion via channels.

Examples of substances transported across membranes are shown in Figure PG.11.

MEMBRANE TRANSPORT MECHANISMS

Various mechanisms exist for the transport of substances across the cell membrane. Mechanisms such as diffusion and osmosis are passive and do not require the expenditure of energy. Active transport is mediated by integral membrane proteins and uses energy often in the form of ATP. Membrane transport mechanisms include:

- Diffusion
- Ion channel diffusion
- Facilitated diffusion
- Primary active transport
- Secondary active transport
- Osmosis
- Exo- and endocytosis

Diffusion

This describes the resultant movement of solute molecules due to their random thermal motion. It is a passive process and net movement of the solute occurs when a concentration gradient is present (from a high to a low concentration). Certain molecules can diffuse across the phospholipid bilayer areas of a cell membrane.

EXAMPLES OF SUBSTANCES TRANSPORTED ACROSS MEMBRANES

Substance	Size nm	Site	Mechanism
Water	0.13	Lipid bilayer	Osmosis
Oxygen	0.12	Lipid bilayer	Diffusion
Nitrogen	0.12	Lipid bilayer	Diffusion
Carbon dioxide	0.12	Lipid bilayer	Diffusion
Sodium ions	0.19	Lipid bilayer	Ion diffusion
		ATPase pump	Active transport
Potassium ions	0.23	Ion channel	Ion diffusion
		ATPase pump	Active transport
Calcium ions	0.17	Ion channel	Ion diffusion
		ATPase pump	Active transport
Urea	0.23	Lipid bilayer	Diffusion
Steroids	<1.0	Lipid bilayer	Diffusion
Fatty acid	<1.0	Lipid bilayer	Diffusion
Glucose	0.38	Transport proteins	Facilitated diffusion
Proteins	>7.5	Vesicles	Exocytosis
			Endocytosis

Figure PG.11

In general, the rate of diffusion through a membrane, Q, is dependent on the concentration gradient ($C_1 - C_2$), the area of membrane exposed, A, the membrane thickness, D, and the permeability constant k_p:

$$Q = k_p A (C_1 - C_2)/D$$

The permeability constant, k_p depends on the local temperature and the characteristics of the membrane; molecular properties also affect it. The phospholipid bilayers are relatively impermeable to ions and large polar (hydrophilic) molecules, but permeable to small polar molecules and lipophilic substances. Thus, the rate of diffusion across the cell membrane:

- Increases with concentration gradient
- Increases with surface area
- Decreases with membrane thickness
- Increases with temperature
- Increases with lipid solubility
- Decreases with molecular weight
- Decreases with electrical charge of particle

A cell membrane acts as a diffusion barrier to solute molecules and can reduce their rates of diffusion by a factor of between 10^3 and 10^6, compared with free diffusion rates in water.

Osmosis

This term describes the net movement of water molecules due to diffusion between areas of different concentration. Pure water has a molar concentration of 55.5 M. In a solution, the addition of solute reduces the water concentration by replacing some water molecules with a solute molecule (or ion). Thus, a 1 M solution of glucose will have a reduced water concentration of 55.5 − 1 = 54.5 M. In the case of a solute that dissociates in solution, twice as many particles are formed. Thus, a 1 M solution of NaCl will reduce the water concentration by twice as much since each molecule of NaCl produces two particles, a sodium ion and a chloride ion. The 1 M solution of NaCl then has a water concentration of 55.5 − 2 = 53.5 M.

OSMOLARITY

The concentration of a solution can be expressed in terms of its osmolarity, reflecting the osmotic effect of the solute particles. The osmolarity of the 1 M glucose solution is, thus, 1 osm (osmol/l) while the 1 M NaCl solution has an osmolarity of 2 osm.

OSMOTIC PRESSURE

A concentration gradient of water can be produced between two compartments separated by a semipermeable membrane, such as a cell membrane, which is permeable to water but impermeable to solute. In this case, net diffusion of water molecules will occur from the compartment with the lower concentration of solute (higher concentration of water) across the membrane into the higher solute concentration (lower concentration of water). The movement of water into a compartment due to osmosis will have the physical effects of increasing the volume of the compartment and/or increasing the pressure in the compartment. This movement of water can be opposed by an increase in pressure in the compartment. The pressure required to oppose the net movement of water into a solution is the osmotic pressure. This is a property of the solution indirectly reflecting its osmolarity (Figure PG.12).

TONICITY

In a cell changes in volume can be produced according to the osmolarity of the intra- and extracellular fluids. Net movement of water into the cell occurs when the cell is placed in a solution of lower (hypotonic) osmolarity, giving rise to swelling and ultimately cell disruption or haemolysis. Placing a cell in a solution of higher osmolarity (hypertonic) than the intracellular contents causes shrinking. Normal extracellular fluid has an osmolarity of 300 mosm, which is equal to (isotonic) that of the intracellular fluid. Since intra- and extracellular solute concentrations are maintained due to the cell membrane permeability properties, no net movement of water occurs into or out of cells and they remain in equilibrium. Hyperosmotic, hypo-osmotic and iso-osmotic describe solution osmolarity irrespectively of the membrane permeability to the solute contained. Thus, the tonicity of such solutions may not correspond to their osmolarities.

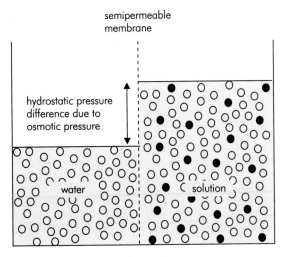

Figure PG.12 Osmosis and osmotic pressure

Ion diffusion

Although the phospholipid bilayer portions of the cell membrane are impermeable to ions, ion channels formed by transmembrane proteins render the cell membrane selectively permeable to Na^+, K^+, Ca^{2+} and Cl^-. The walls of these channels are formed by polypeptide subunits, which may number up to 12 per channel (Figure PG.13). Rapid changes in ion concentrations (such as in the production of action potentials) are produced by opening and closing the channels (gating) and consequently producing dramatic changes in permeability to a given ion. The gating of ion channels may be controlled by chemical messengers (ligand gating, e.g. acetyl choline receptors) binding to the subunits, changes in membrane potential (voltage gating, e.g. Na^+ channel) and stretching of the membrane (mechanical gating). Factors determining permeability of a cell membrane to a given ion are shown below:

• Chemical messenger concentration
• Membrane potential
• Membrane conformation
• Density of specific ion channels

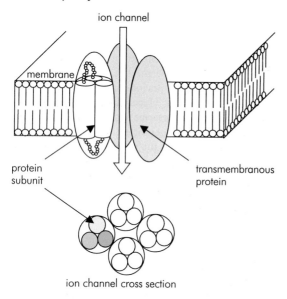

Figure PG.13 Ion channel

Active transport

Active transport is mediated by integral membrane proteins or carriers that bind a substance on one side of the membrane, undergo a conformational change and then release the substance on the opposite side of the membrane. Carriers may be specific for a given substance (uniport), alternatively they may transport a combination of substances (symport) and finally they can exchange one substance for another (anti-port). Factors affecting rate of active transport include:

• Degree of carrier saturation
• Density of carriers on membrane
• The speed of carrier conformational change

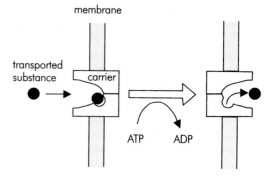

Figure PG.14 Primary active transport

PRIMARY ACTIVE TRANSPORT

Active transport requires the expenditure of energy since it usually moves substances against a concentration or electrical potential gradient (i.e. against an electrochemical gradient). In primary active transport, energy is obtained directly from the hydrolysis of ATP and then catalysed by the carrier, which binds the released phosphate (Figure PG.14). Phosphorylation of the carrier produces covalent

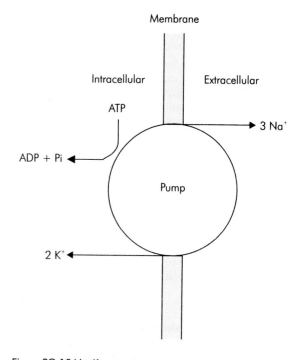

Figure PG.15 Na^+K^+ pump

modulation of its structure. Na⁺K⁺ATPase is an antiport carrier responsible for maintaining transmembrane ion gradients of Na^+ and K^+. This carrier 'pumps' three Na^+ ions out of the cell in exchange for two potassium ions (Figure PG.15), both against their respective concentration gradients. Other ion pumps (uniport systems) move calcium (Ca^{2+}ATPase) and hydrogen ions (H^+ATPase) across cell and organelle membranes against electrochemical gradients.

SECONDARY ACTIVE TRANSPORT

In this process a symport carrier transports a substance and an ion (usually Na^+) together. The carrier possesses two binding sites one for the substance and one for the ion. The substance binds to the first carrier site. The change in carrier conformation required to release the substance on the opposite side of the membrane is then powered by the ion binding to the second site, which produces allosteric modulation of the carrier structure. Since the ion always passes from high to low concentrations, there is no direct energy input required, and the energy for this secondary transport process is ultimately derived from the energy required to maintain the ion concentration gradient. The transported substance can travel in the same direction as the ion (co-transport) or in the opposite direction (counter transport). An example of such a system is the transport of glucose and Na^+ in the gut (Figure PG.16).

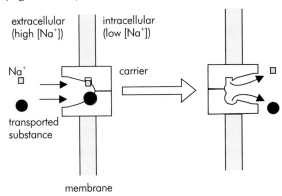

Figure PG.16 Secondary active transport

Facilitated diffusion

This is a misnomer since no diffusive process is involved. Facilitated diffusion describes the transport of a substance from a high to low concentration via a carrier. No energy coupling is required for this process since movement occurs down the concentration gradient. However, diffusion is not involved, thus the transport kinetics are characteristic of carrier-mediated

transport (Figure PG.17) and carrier saturation occurs. An example of this process is the transport of glucose intracellularly, which occurs via a set of four different carriers.

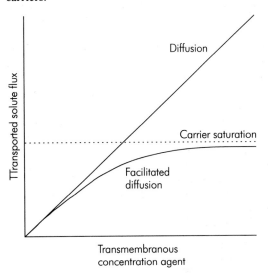

Figure PG.17 Facilitated diffusion and carrier kinetics

Endo- and exocytosis

This mode of transport does not require substances to pass through the membrane structure, but transports substances contained in membrane covered vesicles. In endocytosis, extracellular material is absorbed by being packaged into vesicles at the cell membrane. The vesicles are formed by invagination of the membrane. An equivalent process in reverse is exocytosis, which allows the cell to export intracellular substances or debris (Figure PG.18).

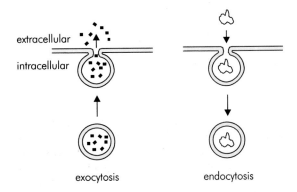

Figure PG.18 Endo- and exocytosis

CELL NUCLEUS

NUCLEUS AND NUCLEOLUS

Most cells in the body carry a single nucleus (exceptions are skeletal muscle cells which are multinucleate, and red blood cells which are anucleate). The nucleus is surrounded by a double membrane – the nuclear envelope. This envelope is interrupted at intervals by openings, the nuclear pores that allow the passage of specific proteins into and out of the nucleus.

The most important substances in the nucleus are the nucleic acids deoxyribonucleic acid (DNA) and ribonucleic acid (RNA).

Genetic material is contained as DNA–protein complex and forms the bulk of the nuclear contents. In addition, there is dense patch of granules visible under light microscopy known as the nucleolus. The nucleolus is rich in RNA and synthesises the ribosomal subunits for export to the cytoplasm. There the complete ribosomes are assembled and act as sites for protein synthesis.

NUCLEIC ACIDS

Nucleic acids are nucleotide polymers. Each nucleotide consists of a purine or pyrimidine base, a sugar (deoxyribose or ribose) and a phosphate group. The DNA molecule is a double helix, each component helix being a chain of nucleotides. DNA nucleotides contain deoxyribose sugar combined with one of the following bases: adenine (A), guanine (G), cytosine (C) and thymine (T). The deoxyribose molecules are linked by phosphate bonds to form the backbone of each spiral and the spirals are linked via the protruding bases to form the DNA double helix (Figure PG.19).

Genetic information is coded linearly along the double

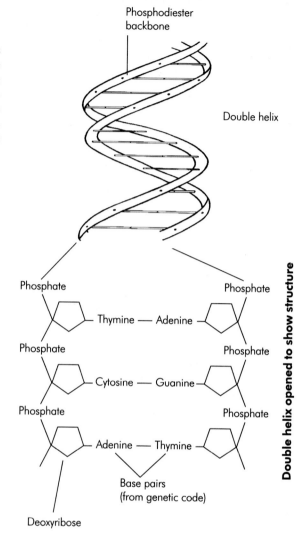

Figure PG.19 Double helix of DNA

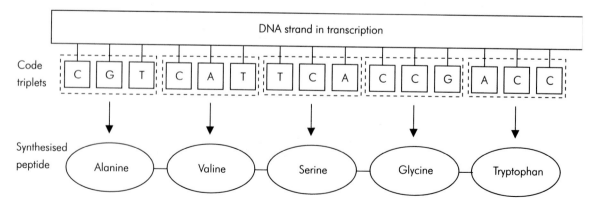

Figure PG.20 DNA coding for a peptide

helix structure by the sequence of the base pairs. The alphabet for this genetic code is formed by triplets of bases, each triplet coding for an amino acid, e.g. the triplet sequence cytosine–guanine–thymidine (CGT) codes for the amino acid alanine. Figure PG.20 shows the DNA coding for a small polypeptide.

RNA is a single-stranded nucleotide polymer that differs from DNA in function and structure (Figure PG.21). Three types of RNA are recognised: messenger (mRNA), transfer (tRNA) and ribosomal (rRNA). They are all synthesised in the nucleus using DNA as a template, but differ from each other in molecular size and function. The bulk of cellular RNA is rRNA, which together with specific proteins forms the ribosomal subunits; however, its function remains uncertain.

The human genome

The total genetic material in the nucleus forms a blueprint for the individual and is referred to as the genome. The genetic information is coded into giant molecules of deoxyribonucleic acid (i.e. DNA). These DNA molecules form large complexes with proteins, which appear as clumps of stained material, chromatin, under light microscopy. During cell division the chromatin forms paired bodies in the nucleus known as chromosomes. The human genome is contained in 46 chromosomes (23 pairs), each chromosome consisting of a single DNA molecule–protein complex. The genetic coding responsible for producing a single polypeptide is known as a gene, which represents a unit of hereditary information. There are between 50 000 and 100 000 genes in the human genome, which contain 3×10^9 base pairs.

PROTEIN SYNTHESIS

The process of synthesising proteins from the genetic information coded on DNA in the nucleus is outlined in Figure PG.22. Transcription describes the first stage in which mRNA is synthesised by RNA polymerase bound to the gene for the protein being synthesised. The mRNA then undergoes post transcriptional processing. The processed RNA passes from the nucleus into the cytoplasm, where one end binds to the surface of a ribosome. Free amino acids are concentrated around the ribosomal surface where they are loaded on to tRNA by aminoacyl-tRNA synthetase.

The surface-bound region of the mRNA is the site where the polypeptide is gradually elongated by the addition of amino acids in sequence. It provides two adjacent codons that recognise and bind tRNA by the corresponding anti-codon. The first codon binds tRNA carrying the incomplete peptide chain. The adjacent site binds tRNA carrying the next amino acid in the sequence, which is then added to the chain. The addition of each new amino acid is then completed by a shift of the active region along the mRNA strand by one codon. The cycle can then be repeated to add the next amino acid to the peptide.

PROPERTIES OF DNA AND RNA

	DNA	mRNA	tRNA
Structure	Double helix	Single strand	Single strand
Nucleotide sugar	Deoxyribose	Ribose	Ribose
Purines	Adenine Guanine	Adenine Guanine	Adenine Guanine
Pyrimidines	Cytosine Thymine	Cytosine Uracil	Cytosine Uracil
Number of bases in a molecule	$< 10^5$	$< 10^3$	80
Function	Stores amino acid sequences for protein synthesis	Transfers amino acid sequence as codons from DNA to ribosomes	Links amino acids to mRNA codons

Figure PG.21 Properties of DNA and RNA

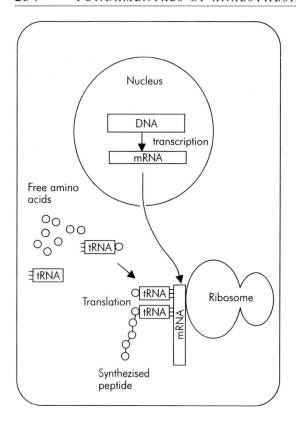

Figure PG.22 Protein synthesis

Control of protein synthesis

Genes possess different regions of which only the exons are transcribed to produce mRNA for protein synthesis (Figure PG.23). At any given time, only a fraction of the genes in a cell are being transcribed. Control of the transcription process in each gene is exerted via a promoter region to which RNA polymerase binds before commencing transcription. Control of protein synthesis is exerted via transcription factors that allow RNA polymerase to bind to the promoter site and to commence transcription. These controlling factors may originate from within the same cell, or originate from other cells via the extracellular fluid. A single transcription factor may control transcription for several genes.

Control of the rate of protein synthesis may also be exerted at the translation stage and by controlling the breakdown of mRNA in the cytoplasm.

CELL COMMUNICATION

Intercellular communication is the basic machinery through which homeostatic control is applied. Cells almost always use a chemical messenger to communicate with target cells, which may be local or remote in location. One group of chemical messengers is formed by the neurotransmitters, which are secreted by one neurone to target a neighbouring neurone just a synapse away. On the other hand, a hormone travels in the circulation to target multiple tissues remote from the secreting cells. In general terms, chemical messengers (ligands) are usually received by cell membrane proteins (receptors) and this interaction triggers the required cellular response by various mechanisms.

CHEMICAL MESSENGERS

Chemical messengers that reach a target cell in the extracellular fluid, whether via the circulation or through the interstitium, are referred to as first chemical messengers. The actions of a first chemical messenger often results in the intracellular release of an active ligand, which is termed a second messenger. Various groups of first messengers are recognised such as neurotransmitters, neuromuscular transmitters, hormones, paracrine agents and autocrine agents.

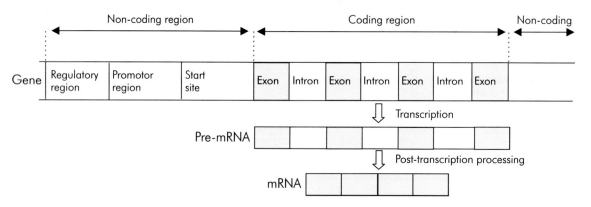

Figure PG.23 Gene regions

These are differentiated by their origin, the route travelled by the messengers and the cells targeted. Some examples are shown in Figure PG.24.

All chemical messengers or ligands interact with their target cells by binding to receptors and therefore have common properties that determine their performance.

Properties of a ligand

Ligands show the following properties:

- Affinity – strength of binding with the receptor
- Competition – ability of different ligands to bind to the same receptor
- Agonist activity – ability of a ligand to trigger the cell response
- Antagonist activity – ability of a ligand to bind to a receptor without triggering the cell response, i.e. to block the receptor
- half-life – time taken for ligand to be metabolized to half its concentration
- Lipid solubility – lipid-insoluble ligands activate receptors at the membrane surface. Lipid soluble ligands activate intracellular or intranuclear receptors.

RECEPTORS

'Receptor' refers to the region of a protein molecule that provides a binding site for a ligand. Receptors are usually situated on integral membrane proteins, and are activated by lipid-insoluble messengers at the membrane surface. Lipid-soluble messengers may cross the membrane to activate intracellular receptors. Receptors are not fixed components of the membrane, but are free to change position and to alter in population density.

Receptor properties

The properties of receptors are:

- Specificity – selectivity of a receptor determining how specifically it bind to a single ligand
- Saturation – percentage of receptors already occupied by ligand
- Down regulation – a decrease in the number of receptors available for a given ligand
- Up regulation – an increase in the number of available receptors for a given ligand
- Sensitivity – responsiveness of a target cell to a given ligand dependent on the density of receptors

TYPES OF FIRST CHEMICAL MESSENGER AND THEIR TARGET CELLS

Messenger	Origin	Route	Target cell

Neurotransmitters:
  norepinephrine
  acetylcholine
  serotonin
	Neurone	Synapse	Adjacent neurone

Hormones:
  thyroxine
  insulin
  cortisol
	Gland	Circulation	Multiple tissues

Neurohormones:
  vasopressin
  oxytocin
  ACTH
  TSH
	Neurone	Circulation	Multiple tissues
			Endocrine glands

Neuromuscular transmitter: acetylcholine	Neurone	Circulation	Muscle cell

Paracrine agents:
  eicosanoids
  cytokines
	Local cell	Extracellular fluid	Neighbouring cells

Autocrine agent:
  eicosanoids
  cytokines
	Local cell	Extracellular fluid	Cell of origin

Figure PG.24

- Supersensitivity – increased sensitivity of a cell as a result of up regulation

Binding site modulation

The first stage in transduction is the production of a change in shape or modulation of the binding site, when the ligand binds to the receptor. There are two main mechanisms by which this occurs, allosteric modulation and covalent modulation.

ALLOSTERIC MODULATION

In this case, the receptor possesses two binding sites one site, the functional site for the ligand and the other (regulatory site) for a modulator molecule. Binding of the modulator molecule enables ligand binding to occur at the functional site (Figure PG.25).

COVALENT MODULATION

This form of modulation requires the attachment of a phosphate group to the receptor (phosphorylation) to enable the functional site to bind the ligand (Figure PG.25).

MEMBRANE SIGNAL TRANSDUCTION

When a ligand binds to a receptor, modulation sets off a sequence of events into which can be thought of as transduction of a chemical signal received by the cell. Signal transduction ultimately results in alterations in cell function. These changes can affect:

- Membrane permeability
- Membrane potential
- Membrane transport
- Contractile activity

Allosteric modulation

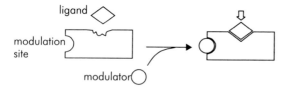

Covalent modulation

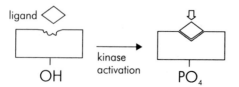

Figure PG.25 Allosteric and covalent modulation

- Secretory activity
- Protein synthesis

Different mechanisms are activated following modulation of the receptor protein.

Membrane signal transduction mechanisms

Receptors act as ion channels that are opened or closed by ligand binding (Figure PG.26).

Receptors function as protein kinases that are activated on ligand binding (Figure PG.26).

Receptors activate G proteins, which then mediate further actions. These include gating ion channels or releasing second messengers intracellularly (Figure PG.27).

Receptor ion channel

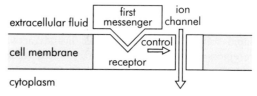

Receptor kinase

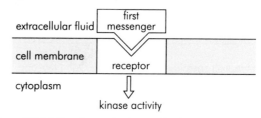

Figure PG.26 Signal transduction mechanisms

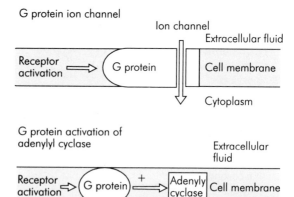

Figure PG.27 G protein signal transduction

Intracellular transduction

Lipophlic first messengers, such as steroids, can cross the phospholipid bilayer and activate intracellular receptors in the following ways (Figure PG.28):

- Ligand crosses cell membrane to form complex with cytosol receptor. This complex moves into nucleus and binds to promoter region of gene
- Ligand moves across cell and nuclear membranes to form complex with nuclear receptor. This complex binds to promoter region of gene

SECOND CHEMICAL MESSENGERS

This term refers to substances released intracellularly, following G protein activation of effector proteins (enzymes such as adenylyl cyclase and guanylyl cyclase). The second messengers released diffuse through the cytosol and exert wide ranging effects, usually by activation of a protein kinase (Figure PG.29). The kinase in turn activates or inhibits a range of cellular functions by enzyme phosphorylation. This sequence of events can be thought of as a cascade

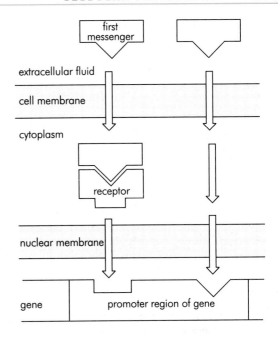

Figure PG.28 Intracellular signal transduction

SECOND MESSENGERS AND THEIR FUNCTIONS

Second messenger	Precursor or origin	Mediator	Examples of cell functions influenced
Cyclic AMP	ATP	Adenyl cyclase	Protein synthesis Calcium ion transport DNA synthesis RNA synthesis Lipid breakdown Glycogen breakdown Glycogen synthesis Ion channels Active transport
Cyclic GMP	GTP	Guanylyl cyclase	Physiology of vision
Inositol triphosphate (IP_3)	Phosphotidyl inositol diphosphate (PIP_2)	Phospholipase C	Release of calcium from endoplasmic reticulum
Diacylglycerol (DAG)	Phosphatidyl inositol diphosphate (PIP_2)	Phospholipase C	Activation of protein kinase C used in membrane protein regulation
Calcium	Entry via calcium channels	G proteins	Activation of protein kinases via calmodulin or directly Skeletal, smooth and cardiac muscle contraction
	Release from endoplasmic reticulum	G proteins	Synaptic function Protein synthesis

Figure PG.29 Second messengers and their functions

triggered by a single messenger. The cascade effectively amplifies and processes the effect of low concentrations of a ligand to produce widespread cellular changes, tailored to the needs of different tissues.

The second messengers cyclic AMP and cyclic GMP are metabolized by phosphodiesterase, which can be inhibited by methylxanthines (caffeine, theophylline). These compounds thus augment the second messenger effects.

Intracellular calcium

The extracellular-to-cytosol concentration gradient of calcium is $> 10^4$. Thus, calcium enters the cytosol readily via calcium channels that are controlled by ligand or voltage gating. Alternatively, calcium can be released internally from the endoplasmic reticulum that acts as a store. Active decrease of intracellular calcium levels is mediated by a $Ca^{2+}H^+ATPase$, a Na^+Ca^{2+} anti-port system and re-uptake into the endoplasmic reticulum.

Calcium exerts wide ranging effects intracellularly by binding to a group of proteins including calmodulin, troponin and calbindin.

Calmodulin is one of the most prominent of these proteins with wide-ranging activation of protein kinases involved in many aspects of cellular function (Figure PG.30).

AGEING

Ageing is a physiological process that involves general changes in the body systems that are distinct from the pathological changes associated with disease. These changes are illustrated by the following physiological parameters of a 70-year-old male expressed as a percentage of the equivalent young adult values (Figure PG.31).

The changes usually reflect a decline in function. This functional deterioration occurs in all of the physiological systems and includes the following (Figure PG.32).

AGEING AND DYSHOMEOSTASIS

The deterioration normally associated with the ageing process leads to a reduction in the effectiveness of homeostatic control mechanisms or dyshomeostasis. This contributes to an increased prevalence of certain conditions with age. These include:

- Dehydration
- Hypokalaemia
- Hyponatraemia
- Ankle oedema
- Diabetes mellitus
- Hypothyroidism
- Hypothermia

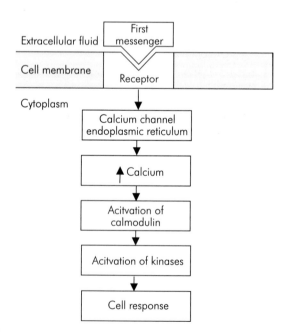

Figure PG.30 Calcium as second messenger

CHANGES IN PHYSIOLOGICAL PARAMETERS DUE TO AGEING	
Parameter for a 70 year-old male	**% of young adult value**
Muscle mass	74
Total body water	87
Cardiac output at rest	64
Cardiac reserve	50
PaO$_2$	90
Oxygen consumption at rest	74
Maximal oxygen consumption	65
Renal blood flow	60
Max urine concentration	64
Cerebral blood flow	80

Figure PG 31

EFFECTS OF AGEING ON PHYSIOLOGICAL SYSTEMS

System	Change due to ageing
Cardiovascular	↓cardiac output and reserve ↓heart rate ↓stroke volume ↓LV compliance
Respiratory	↓PaO_2 ↓lung elasticity ↓chest wall compliance ↓vital capacity ↑residual volume
Gastro-intestinal secretion	↓sense of smell and taste ↓co-ordination of swallowing and peristaltic reflexes ↓gastric and pancreatic ↓large bowel motility
Endocrine	↑norepinephrine levels ↓renin and aldosterone levels ↓carbohydrate tolerance ↑ADH levels ↓oestrogen in female ↓testostrone levels in male
Renal	↓kidney mass ↓ability to concentrate urine ↓renal response to ADH ↑prostate mass
CNS	↓brain mass ↓acetylcholine activity ↓cerbral blood flow ↓short-term memory and learning ability ↑reaction time
Musculoskeletal	↓bone and muscle mass ↓muscle effectiveness
Immunity	↓cellular and humoral immunity

Figure PG.32

THEORIES OF AGEING

Three theories on the origins of ageing have been put forward, wear and tear, adaptive evolution and non adaptive evolution.

'Wear and tear'

This states that the ageing process is a natural deterioration as a result of the continuous functioning of a highly complex organism

Adaptive evolution

adaptive evolution suggests that ageing is a genetically programmed termination of life in the interests of evolutionary selection

Non adaptive evolution

Non adaptive evolution suggests that the ageing process has evolved as an optimum balance between the limited energy sources available to the organism and the demands of normal function and repair.

Several cellular mechanisms are associated with ageing. It is unclear at present whether any of these predominate in determining the rate and extent of the process. The more important processes are:

- Accumulation of cells with random DNA mutations
- Increased cross-linking of collagens and proteins by glycosylation
- Accumulation of cytoplasmic lipofucsin granules
- Accumulation of oxidant radicals
- Genetic clock determining the number of cell reduplications
- Pleiotropic genes with 'good' effects early in life and 'bad' effects later in life

In general, it remains fair to say that the ageing process is incompletely understood at present.

SECTION 2: 2
BODY FLUIDS

J. Skoyles

FLUID COMPARTMENT VOLUMES
Total body water (TBW)
Intracellular fluid (ICF)
Extracellular fluid (ECF)
Plasma
Measurement of compartment volumes

SOLUTIONS AND SEMIPERMEABLE MEMBRANES
Concentration of a solution
Membranes separating fluid compartments
Movement of water across a membrane
Distribution of a solute across a membrane

COMPOSITION OF BODY FLUIDS
Intracellular fluid
Interstitial fluid
Plasma
Transcellular fluids

DISORDERS OF WATER AND ELECTROLYTE BALANCE
Sodium and water
Potassium
Calcium
Magnesium

SPECIAL FLUIDS
Lymph and the lymphatic system
Cerebrospinal fluid (CSF)
Intra-ocular fluid
Pleural fluid

FLUID COMPARTMENT VOLUMES

TOTAL BODY WATER (TBW)

Water comprises the major part of body weight, forming about 60% of the body weight of a young adult male. This percentage varies with build, sex and age in the following manner:

- TBW in the adult can range from 45 to 75% of body weight. This large variation is the result of individual differences in adipose tissue which contains relatively little water
- TBW in the female adult is less than in the male of the same age. In the young adult female TBW only forms about 50% of body weight. This difference between the sexes disappears below puberty and decreases in old age due to a reduction in adipose tissue
- TBW as a proportion of body weight may be as high as 80% in the neonate

TBW is divided into several fluid compartments (Figure FL.1) the main division being between intracellular fluid (ICF) and extracellular fluid (ECF).

The variations of TBW (% body weight) and ECF (% body weight), with age are shown in Figure FL.2.

INTRACELLULAR FLUID (ICF)

The ICF compartment contains about 60% of TBW. The volume of the ICF compartment, including red blood cell contents (2 litres), amounts to about 27

VARIATION OF TBW (% BODY WEIGHT) AND ECF (% BODY WEIGHT), WITH AGE

Age	TBW	ECF
Neonate	80	45
6 months	70	35
1 year	60	28
5 years	65	25
Young adult	60	22
Elderly	50	20

Figure FL.2

litres. The water content and composition of ICF varies according to the function of the tissue. As noted above, adipose tissue will have much lower water content than lean body tissue which contains about 70 ml/100 g water.

EXTRACELLULAR FLUID (ECF)

About one-third of total body water is ECF. Although ECF as a percentage of body weight, varies with age (Figure FL.2), when expressed as an index of body surface area it remains relatively constant throughout life. The ECF volume to body surface area index is about 7.5 litre/m^2.

ECF is composed of several components (Figure FL.3).

COMPONENTS OF ECF IN A 70 KG ADULT

Fluid	% Body weight	Volume (litres)
Interstitial fluid	15	10.5
Plasma	5	3.5
Transcellular fluid	1	0.7
Total ECF	21	14.7

Figure FL.3

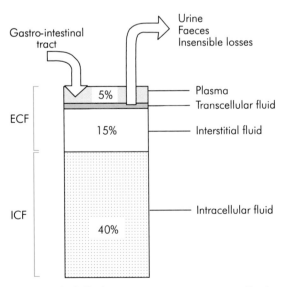

Figure FL.1 Body fluid compartments as percentage of body weight

PLASMA

Plasma volume equates to the intravascular component of ECF and amounts to about 5% of body weight. The total blood volume is composed of plasma and the red blood cell volume. Plasma volume (V_{PL}) can be measured using a dilution technique. The fractional red blood cell volume is readily available as the haematocrit (%). Given these values, the total blood volume (V_{BL}) can be calculated:

$$V_{PL} \ = \ 3.5 \text{ litres}$$

$$\text{Haematocrit (Hct)} \ = \ 45\%$$

$$\text{Total blood volume } (V_{BL}) \ = \ \frac{V_{PL} \times 100}{(100 - \text{Hct})}$$

$$= \ 6.4 \text{ litres}$$

TRANSCELLULAR FLUID

The transcellular fluid compartment is composed of fluids that have been secreted but are separated from the plasma by an epithelial layer. These include:

- Cerebrospinal fluid
- Intra-ocular fluid
- Gastro-intestinal fluid
- Bile
- Pleural, peritoneal and pericardial fluid
- Sweat

The composition of transcellular fluid differs from both plasma and interstitial fluid since it is controlled by the secretory cells.

MEASUREMENT OF FLUID COMPARTMENT VOLUMES

Compartment volumes are estimated by dilutional techniques. In these methods, an indicator dye that is freely distributed (but contained) within the compartment being estimated, is injected into the compartment. The mass of indicator used and the concentration in the fluid are measured. Then the size of the compartment can be determined using the formula:

$$\text{Volume of compartment} \ = \ \frac{\text{mass of indicator}}{\text{concentration in compartment}}$$

In reality, this method calculates the volume of distribution of the injected indicator. The mass of indicator must be corrected for excretion and metabolism during the time allowed for distribution.

Indicator methods used to estimate the volume of various compartments are summarised in Figure FL.4.

MEASUREMENT OF FLUID COMPARTMENT VOLUMES

Compartment	Indicator	Comments
Total body water (TBW)	Antipyrine D_2O	Tendency to underestimate uniform distribution
Extracellular fluid (ECF)	Radio isotopes of Na^+, Br^-, Cl^-	These enter cells and so overestimate
	Saccharides (mannitol, inulin)	Incomplete distribution and so underestimate
Plasma volume (V_{PL})	Radio isotope ^{131}I albumin	Total blood volume (V_{BL}) may be derived from V_{PL} and haematocrit (Hct)
Red cell volume (VRBC)	Red cells tagged with radio isotope ^{51}Cr	Measures fraction of red blood cells tagged to determine V_{RBC} measures concentration of tagged cells to determine V_{BL}
Intracellular fluid (ICF)		Derived from: ICF = TBW − ECF
Interstitial fluid volume (V_{INT})		Derived from: V_{INT} = ECF − V_{PL}

Figure FL.4

SOLUTIONS AND SEMIPERMEABLE MEMBRANES

CONCENTRATION OF A SOLUTION

The concentration of a solution is usually expressed in terms of the amount of solute present in a given amount of solvent. In the body, concentrations can be varied in fluid compartments by the movement of solute or solvent (water) into a compartment. The concentrations of various substances can be critical for normal function (e.g. extracellular potassium). Several units are used to express concentration and the following definitions should be noted.

Amount of solute

A given amount of any substance can simply be measured by its mass (g, kg). In chemical reactions, it is more useful to use the unit 'moles' since this relates to the number of molecules present:

1 mole (mol)   = gram molecular weight

1 millimole (mmol)   = (gram molecular weight) 10^{-3}

1 micromole (μmol)   = (gram molecular weight) 10^{-6}

1 mole contains 6.0247×10^{23} molecules (Avogadro's number)

Chemical and electrochemical activity of a solution

The effects exerted by a solution are related to concentration. This is most commonly expressed as mass per unit volume (mg/ml, g/l, kg/m^3). However, the chemical and electrochemical activity of a solution is more closely related to the number of molecules present in a given amount of solution. Concentration of a solution is thus better expressed in terms of its 'molarity' or its 'molality':

- Molarity – moles of solute per litre of solution (solute plus water) (mol/l)
- Molality – moles of solute per kg of solvent (water) (mol/kg H$_2$O)

Interpretation of laboratory values depends on how electrolyte concentrations are indexed (with reference to either litres of plasma water or total plasma volume). The latter includes the volume of proteins, about 7% of total plasma volume, as 93% of plasma volume is water. It follows that laboratory values expressed as mmol/l plasma water will be greater than results expressed as mmol/l plasma volume. This discrepancy will be increased when plasma volume is occupied by other particles such as in hyperlipidaemia.

Equivalent weight

Chemical reactions between elements occur with fixed proportions of different elements by weight. A gram equivalent weight can be defined for each element. This is the weight of an element that reacts with 8.000 g O$_2$. An electrical equivalent weight can also be defined for an ion, which is equal to the atomic weight divided by its valency. Thus, the electrical equivalent weight of Na$^+$ (atomic weight = 23) is 23/1 = 23, while the electrical equivalent weight of Ca^{2+} (atomic weight = 40) is 40/2 = 20. The concentration of a solution may thus be measured in terms of its 'normality', where a normal solution (1 N solution) contains 1 g equivalent solute per litre solution.

MEMBRANES SEPARATING FLUID COMPARTMENTS

Membranes separate the fluid compartments of the body. They differ widely in structure and function. The membrane separating the ICF and ECF compartments is the plasma membrane surrounding cells, a complex structure based on a bi-phospholipid structure, with highly active functions determining membrane permeability to different particle species, and hence maintaining significant differences between the compositions of ICF and ECF. The membrane separating interstitial fluid from intravascular fluid is the capillary wall in which the permeability to water and solutes is mainly dependent on passive mechanisms. The movement of both solutes and water across these membranes determines the composition of fluid in the different compartments.

MOVEMENT OF WATER ACROSS A MEMBRANE

The membranes separating the fluid compartments generally allow the free passage of water, but not solutes across them. Such membranes are known as semipermeable membranes. If a semipermeable membrane separates two aqueous solutions of different concentrations, water molecules will diffuse across the membrane to equalise the concentrations. 'Osmosis' describes this diffusion process. The solutions on each side of the membrane do not have to be of identical solutes, since the osmotic activity of the solutes is dependent on the number and not the type of free particles in solution.

Osmotic pressure

The osmotic activity of solute particles in an aqueous solution can be visualised as exerting an 'osmotic pressure', which would potentially draw water into the solution. This can be demonstrated as a hydrostatic pressure difference between two compartments separated by a semipermeable membrane, one containing solution and the other containing water alone. Osmotic pressure can thus be defined as the pressure required to prevent osmosis when the solution is separated from pure solvent by a semipermeable membrane (Figure FL.5).

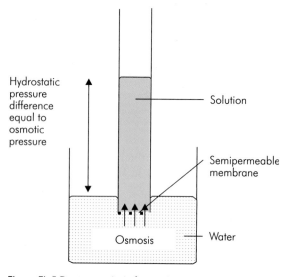

Figure FL.5 Demonstration of osmotic pressure

Calculation of osmotic pressure from molality of a solution

The osmotic pressure of a solution can be calculated from the solution molality. In a dilute solution, with a solute which does not dissociate or associate, osmotic pressure (π) is dependent on temperature and molal concentration. This can be expressed as:

$\pi \propto$ absolute temperature (T)

at a given concentration.

Also, $\pi \propto$ concentration (C)

at a given temperature.

van't Hoff equation for osmotic pressure

In 1877, van't Hoff noted the similarity of behaviour between dilute solutions and gases. Combining the two relations above gives the van't Hoff equation for the osmotic pressure exerted by a dilute solution as:

osmotic pressure (π) = RTC (Pascals),

where:

R = universal gas constant (= 8.32 J/K)

T = absolute temperature (K)

C = osmolality (mosm/kg H_2O)

This can be applied to find the osmotic pressure of plasma at body temperature (T = 307 K, C = 290 mosm/kg H_2O), thus:

Osmotic pressure of plasma = 8.32 × 307 × 290 Pa

= 740729.6 Pa

= 740.7 kPa

The osmole

The concentration of solute particles in solution can be expressed in osmoles, to reflect the osmotic activity of the solution, where:

1 osmole = amount of solute that exerts an osmotic pressure of 1 atm when placed in 22.4 litres of solution at 0°C.

For a substance that does not associate or dissociate in solution (e.g. glucose),

1 osmole = 1 mole.

For a substance which dissociates into two osmotically active particles (e.g. NaCl → Na⁺ + Cl⁻),

1 osmole = 1 mole/2.

For a substance that dissociates into three osmotically active particles (e.g. $CaCl_2 \rightarrow Ca^{2+} + 2 Cl^-$), then

1 osmole = 1 mole/3.

Osmolality and osmolarity of a solution

Osmolarity is concentration of a solution expressed in osmoles of solute per litre of solution (solute plus water). The units of osmolarity are thus osmoles per litre (osm/l) or milliosmoles per litre (mosm/l)

Osmolality is concentration of a solution expressed as osmoles of solute per kg solvent (water alone). The units of osmolality are thus osmoles per kg water (osm/kg H_2O) or milliosmoles per kg water (mosm/kg H_2O). Osmolality is, thus, independent of temperature and the volume occupied by the solute. Note particularly:

- As osmolality is independent of temperature, and independent of the volume taken up by the solutes within the solution, it is the preferred term in most physiological applications
- Equivalent osmolal (or osmolar) concentrations will exert the same osmotic pressures, even though the molality (or molarity) of the solutions may differ

The molality of a solution can be converted to its osmolality by multiplying molality by the number of discrete solute particles formed when a molecule of solute is in solution (e.g. for $CaCl_2$ solutions multiply by 3).

Osmolality of body fluids

The osmolality of a body fluid is usually higher than its osmolarity because of protein and lipid content, which occupy a small but finite volume. In practice this difference is insignificant except in cases of gross hyperproteinaemia or hyperlipidaemia.

Plasma osmolality ranges from 280 to 295 mosm/kg H_2O, and is maintained constant at about 290 mosm/kg H_2O throughout the body. The similar osmolality of all major body fluids is due to the free permeability to water of the endothelium and plasma membranes, which separate the various fluid compartments. The distribution and number of osmotically active particles contained by each primarily determine the size of these compartments.

Regulation of body fluid osmolality

The regulation of body fluid osmolality is inextricably linked to the control of total body water (TBW). It involves the secretion of anti-diuretic hormone (ADH, vasopressin) in response to an increase in osmolality or a decrease in TBW. Although osmoreceptors appear sensitive enough to respond to small changes in osmolality, their response can be overridden by the haemodynamic response to changes in effective circulating volume. An outline of these responses is shown in Figure FL.6.

Measurement of osmolality

The osmolality of a solution can be estimated in practice by measuring depression of freezing point of the solution, when compared with the pure solvent. This depression of freezing point depends on the number and not the type of particle in solution. A solution of 1 osm/kg H_2O freezes at $-1.86°C$. Normal plasma freezes at $-0.54°C$. This, therefore, corresponds to a plasma osmolality as determined by the relationship:

$$\text{Plasma osmolality} = \frac{0.54}{186} \times 10^3 \text{ mosm/kgH}_2O$$

$$= 290 \text{ mosm/kgH}_2O$$

Estimation of osmolality from solute concentration

Plasma osmolality can also be estimated from the

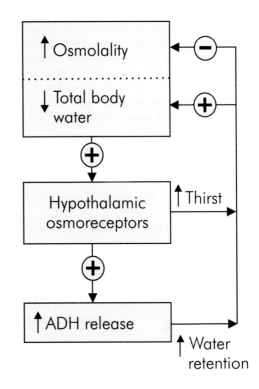

Figure FL.6 Regulation of body fluid osmolality

molality of the major solutes: sodium, chloride, urea and glucose:

$$\text{Plasma osmolality} = 2 \times [Na^+] + [\text{glucose}] + [\text{urea}]$$

$$= 2 \times 140 + 5.0 + 5.0$$

$$= 290 \text{ mosm/kg H}_2O.$$

Similarly the osmolality of IV solutions can also be estimated from their concentration. Thus, for normal saline:

$$0.9\% \text{ NaCl} = 9 \text{ g/l} = 9 \text{ g/kg H}_2O$$

$$= 9/(23 + 35.5) \times 10^3 \text{ mmol/kg H}_2O$$

$$= (154 Na^+ + 154 Cl^-) \text{ mosm/kg H}_2O$$

$$= 308 \text{ mosm/kg H}_2O.$$

Tonicity of a solution

Solutions with different osmolalities separated by a semipermeable membrane can result in significant physiological effects due to the passage of water from the lower osmolality side to the higher osmolality side. An example is provided by the swelling and haemolysis of red blood cells placed in water, which occurs due to the movement of water into the red blood cells.

'Tonicity' describes the relative osmolality between two fluid compartments. Thus, if one compartment contains solution of lower osmolality, it is hypotonic compared with the higher osmolality compartment. Similarly, the higher osmolality compartment is hypertonic relative to the lower osmolality side. This terminology is most commonly applied to the ECF surrounding cells e.g. plasma around red blood cells.

- Isotonicity describes a solution within which cells can be suspended without a change in cell volume
- Cells placed in a hypertonic solution will shrink in volume
- Cells placed in a hypotonic solution will swell in volume
- A 0.9% solution of NaCl is approximately isotonic (308 mosmol/kg H_2O)

Plasma colloid osmotic pressure

The plasma proteins, albumin and globulins do not normally pass out of the capillaries into the interstitium since they are reflected by the capillary endothelium. The retained plasma proteins raise the plasma osmotic pressure above that of the interstitial fluid by an amount referred to as the 'colloid osmotic pressure' (or oncotic pressure). Quantitatively, the most important protein contributing to the colloid osmotic pressure is albumin which is responsible for up to 75% of the total 25 mmHg colloid osmotic pressure.

DISTRIBUTION OF A SOLUTE ACROSS A MEMBRANE

Solute particles are distributed between fluid compartments according to the permeability of the separating membrane to each type of particle. Both passive and active mechanisms determine the movement of solutes across a membrane. Active processes such as carrier proteins or ion channels selectively transport or allow the diffusion of substances across a membrane. Passive movement of particles can occur through 'pores' or 'fenestrations', or even through the membrane depending on lipid solubility.

The distribution of different solute particles across cell plasma membranes is determined by their complex functions and structure. The mechanisms involved are both active and passive.

Movement of solute across a capillary wall generally occurs in the 'filtrate' as it passes from the capillary lumen into the interstitium. Large protein molecules remain in the capillary plasma unable to be filtered out because of their size. This capillary filtration process

and the balance of forces (Starling forces) driving it, is described on p 357–359.

The structure of capillaries and the composition of fluid passing across the capillary walls, differs between tissues. These differences reflect the variation in function between vessels such as glomerular capillaries in the kidneys, and capillaries found, for example, in skeletal muscle.

The main transport mechanisms involved across capillary endothelium are:

- Filtration, which describes the action of hydrostatic pressure forcing fluid out of the capillaries. It is opposed by the plasma colloid osmotic pressure
- Diffusion, which is the passive movement of substances under the influence of concentration gradients, and occurs through fenestrations and intercellular junctions. The main diffusion barrier is the basement membrane
- Transcytosis, which is the active transfer of substance by endocytosis from the capillary lumen, followed by exocytosis out of the endothelial cells. It only represents a small fraction of the total transport across capillary endothelium

Gibbs–Donnan effect

Passive movement of solute particles usually occurs under the influence of a chemical concentration or electrical gradient. Consider the case of two compartments (A and B) each containing NaCl but separated by a semipermeable membrane. The diffusion of Na^+ and Cl^- occurs between the compartments to equalise chemical concentration gradients and to maintain electrical neutrality on either side of the membrane (Figure FL.7a).

If protein is trapped in one of the compartments it can affect the distribution of the diffusible ions by the Gibbs–Donnan effect. This occurs due to the negative charge on protein molecules, which acts by holding Na^+ back on one side of the membrane to preserve electroneutrality in the compartment (Figure FL.7b). The chemical gradient of Na^+ across the membrane will then redistribute Na^+ (followed by Cl^- to preserve electroneutrality) between the compartments until an equilibrium is reached (Figure FL.7c), when:

$$[\text{cation}]_A \times [\text{anion}]_A = [\text{cation}]_B \times [\text{anion}]_B$$
$$[Na^+]_A \times [Cl^-]_A = [Na^+]_B \times [Cl^-]_B$$
$$9 \times 4 = 6 \times 6.$$

This mechanism is referred to as the Gibbs–Donnan effect and, in vivo, affects the distributions of Na^+ and Cl^- between the intravascular and interstitial compartments in the body.

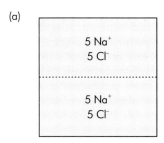

(a)

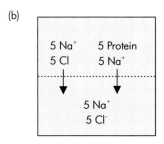

(b)

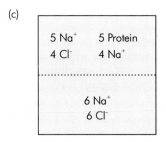

(c)

Figure FL.7 Gibbs–Donnan equilibrium

In this situation the Gibbs–Donnan effect gives rise to:

- Unequal distributions of diffusible ions, Na^+ and Cl^-, between intravascular and interstitial compartments
- Higher Na^+ concentration in the protein containing plasma compartment and higher Cl^- concentration in the interstitial compartment
- A small electrical potential difference across the membrane

The Gibbs–Donnan effect is significant in the distribution of diffusible ions across a largely passive semipermeable membrane such as capillary endothelium separating intravascular and interstitial compartments.

The Gibbs–Donnan equilibrium described above results when the diffusion of the ions down their chemical concentration gradients is balanced by the electrostatic attraction of the protein molecules trapped in one compartment of the model. This balance between chemical and electrostatic forces produces an electrical potential difference across the membrane. The magnitude of this potential difference can be calculated using the Nernst equation and is dependent on the ratio of the diffusible ion concentrations on either side of the membrane at equilibrium. Thus, applying the Nernst equation to a capillary wall:

$$\text{capillary wall potential} = \frac{RT}{FZ_{Na}} \times \log_e \frac{[Na^+]_{INT}}{[Na^+]_C}$$

$$= 62 \times (145/153)$$

$$= -3.24 \, mV.$$

Thus, there is a potential difference across the capillary wall of about 3mV, the endothelial surface being negative with respect to the interstitium.

COMPOSITION OF BODY FLUIDS

The compositions of the major body fluids – plasma, interstitial and intracellular – are shown in Figure FL.8.

INTRACELLULAR FLUID

ICF composition varies according to cell function. There are general differences between ICF and interstitial fluid. These include low intracellular Na^+, Cl^- and HCO_3^- concentrations compared with the extracellular values. The predominant cation is K^+ and

COMPOSITIONS OF PLASMA, INTERSTITIAL AND ICF (MMOL/L)

Substance	Plasma	Interstitial fluid	Intracellular fluid
Cations			
Na^+	153	145	10
K^+	4.3	4.1	159
Ca^{2+}	2.7	2.4	< 1
Mg^{2+}	1.1	1	40
Total	161.1	152.5	209
Anions			
Cl^-	112	117	3
HCO_3^-	25.8	27.1	7
Proteins	15.1	< 0.1	45
Others	8.2	8.4	154
Total	161.1	152.5	209

Figure FL.8

the organic phosphates and proteins are the principle intracellular anions.

The composition of ICF is maintained largely by the cell plasma membrane in a stable but dynamic state of flux. Membrane transport occurs by passive mechanisms such as diffusion and osmosis, which do not require energy expenditure, as well as active transport.

INTERSTITIAL FLUID

The composition of interstitial fluid is dependent on the filtration of plasma through the capillary wall. This is largely a passive process driven by the balance of hydrostatic and colloid osmotic pressures. The diffusible ions are, therefore, of approximately equal concentrations in plasma and interstitial fluid. The retention of protein however in the capillaries, results in a small discrepancy due to the Gibbs–Donnan effect.

PLASMA

The distinguishing component in plasma is the retained plasma protein. There is a total protein content in plasma of about 7 g/100 ml. The various plasma proteins are outlined in Figure FL.9.

Albumin

Albumin accounts for 60% of plasma protein. One of its main functions is to act as a transport protein binding free fatty acids and bilirubin. It is also the principal component responsible for plasma colloid osmotic pressure. Of plasma albumin, 5% circulates through the interstitial fluid compartment each hour, while 60% of the total mass of albumin is actually extravascular. The intravascular half-life of albumin is 19 days.

Immunoglobulins

Immunoglobulins form about 20% of plasma proteins and are split into five groups, each with differing functions and structures. IgG, IgD and IgE are monomers with molecular weights between 150 000 and 190 000 Daltons. IgA is secreted as a dimer with a molecular weight of 400 000; IgM is a pentamer with a molecular weight of 900 000. IgM immunoglobulin is completely confined to the intravascular space.

TRANSCELLULAR FLUIDS

Some of the transcellular fluids differ considerably from plasma in composition. Excessive losses of different transcellular fluids can give rise to significant water and electrolyte disturbances, when disease is present. Some examples of transcellular fluid composition are given below in Figure FL.10.

PLASMA PROTEINS

Plasma protein group	Name
Proteolytic systems	Kinins
Carrier proteins	Albumin
	Haptoglobulin
	Transferrin
	Ceruloplasmin
	Pre-albumin
	Transcortin
	Transcobalamin
Protease inhibitors	α_1 anti trypsin
	α_2 macroglobulin
	Anti thrombin III
Acute phase proteins	Interleukin I
	Tumour necrosis factor
	C-reactive protein
Immunoglobulins	IgG, IgA, IgM, IgD, IgE

Figure FL.9

COMPOSITION OF SOME TRANSCELLULAR FLUIDS

Substance (mmol/l)	Saliva	Gastric juice	Bile	Sweat
Na^+	33	60	149	45
K^+	20	9	5	5
Cl^-	34	84	101	58
HCO_3^-	0	0	45	0
pH	6.6	3	8	5.2

Figure FL.10

DISORDERS OF WATER AND ELECTROLYTE BALANCE

SODIUM AND WATER

The regulation of total body sodium is inextricably linked to the loss or retention of water, and, thus, disturbances in total body sodium content will be compensated for by changes in total body water. Similarly compensation for a disturbance of TBW will include re-adjustment of body sodium levels.

Disturbances of total body water

Some examples of body water disturbances are outlined in Figure FL.11.

Abnormalities of plasma sodium

Although total body sodium and total body water are different physiological entities, they are interdependent, so that a disturbance in one quantity will activate compensatory mechanisms which affect both. In practice, they are not readily measured and the clinical management of sodium/water disturbances often relies on the measurement of plasma sodium levels and osmolalities.

HYPERNATRAEMIA

Hypernatraemia occurs when plasma sodium > 145 mmol/l. It often presents with an altered sensorium, this being dependent on the speed of plasma sodium change and plasma osmolality. Coma ensues at plasma osmolalities > 350 mosm/kgH$_2$O. Hypernatraemia may occur with decreased or increased ECF volume (ECFV) and increased or decreased total body sodium depending on the cause of the original disturbance

FEATURES OF HYPERNATRAEMIA

Cause	ECFV	Total body free water	Total body sodium
Diuresis, vomiting, pyrexia	Low	↓↓	↓
Over transfusion with hypertonic sodium solutions	High	↑	↑↑

Figure FL.12

(Figure FL.12). Thus, the clinical signs and symptoms accompanying hypernatraemia may reflect hypervolaemia or hypovolaemia. Where hypovolaemia is present, sodium deficit can be replaced relatively rapidly compared with the replacement of free water. Free water deficits should be replaced gradually to avoid an increased risk of cerebral oedema.

HYPONATRAEMIA

Hyponatraemia occurs when plasma sodium is < 135 mmol/l. There are different clinical syndromes associated with hyponataemia that depend on the underlying cause (Figure FL.13).

DISTURBANCES OF TOTAL BODY WATER

Condition	Definition	Cause
Dehydration	A decrease in total body water (TBW) with or without a loss of sodium	↓intake e.g. nil by mouth, dysphagia
		↑insensible loss e.g. pyrexia, hyperhidrosis, hyperventilation
Water deficiency	A decrease in TBW without a comparable decrease in body sodium	↑urinary loss e.g. diabetes insipidus, diabetes mellitus
		↑Gastro-intestinal losses e.g. vomiting, diarrhoea
Water intoxication	An increase in TBW without a comparable increase in body sodium	Renal failure, inappropriate ADH secretion, hepatic failure, IV infusion of dextrose

Figure FL.11

FEATURES OF HYPONATRAEMIA

Cause	ECFV	Total body free water	Total body sodium	Urinary sodium
Cardiac failure, renal failure, hepatic failure, TURP syndrome	High	↑↑↑	↑	< 20 mmol/l
Inappropriate ADH secretion	Normal ECFV, Plasma osmolality < 290 mosm/kgH$_2$O	↑	→	< 20 mmol/l, Urine osmolality > 100 mosm/kg H$_2$O
Adrenal failure	Low	↓	↓↓↓	> 20 mmol/l

Figure FL.13

- Hyponatraemia will be associated with water intoxication, which is described above, and is due to excessive water intake or excessive water retention due to inappropriate ADH secretion
- Hypervolaemia will accompany hyponatraemia when the primary disturbance is an increase in TBW, and regulatory mechanisms attempt to maintain plasma osmolality by sodium retention
- Hypovolaemia and hyponatraemia occur when the primary disturbance is an excessive loss of water and sodium with inappropriate (hypotonic fluids) and inadequate resuscitation

Clinical signs and symptoms of hyponatraemia are those of hypovolaemia or hypervolaemia depending on the underlying disturbance. Central signs range from mild lethargy to seizures and respiratory arrest. Rapid correction can lead to central pontine myelinolysis.

POTASSIUM

Potassium is the main intracellular cation and plays an important role intracellularly in protein synthesis, acid–base balance and maintaining osmolality. Although extracellular concentrations are comparatively low, extracellular levels are also important because of they affect membrane potentials and plasma acid base balance. Some details of potassium excess (hyperkalaemia) and potassium deficit (hypokalaemia) are outlined in Figure FL.14.

CALCIUM

Calcium is quantitively the most common mineral in the body, with a total body content of about 1200 g. Of calcium, > 99% is in bone, the remainder being in body fluids partially ionised and partially protein bound. Ionised calcium is important as a co-factor, particularly in the coagulation cascade. Calcium is central in maintaining excitability of the myocardium, skeletal muscle, smooth muscle and nerves. It also has a significant role in the regulation of membrane permeability. See Figure FL.14 for some details of calcium imbalance.

MAGNESIUM

The total body content of magnesium is about 25 g, of which one-half is contained in bone and teeth. The normal plasma levels are about 1.1 mmol/l. The most important function of magnesium systemically is its role as a co-factor, since it is essential for the activity of all kinases. These enzymes catalyse phosphorylation reactions by ATP. Since this is the main mechanism for the transfer of chemical energy in intermediate metabolism, magnesium plays a key role in functions such as muscle contraction as well as pathways such as glycolysis. Regulation of magnesium levels in the body is not clear but may involve parathormone and aldosterone. Figure FL.14 details the effects of magnesium imbalance.

SPECIAL FLUIDS

LYMPH AND THE LYMPHATIC SYSTEM

The lymphatics are a system of blind-ending tubules with endothelium similar to blood capillaries. There is neither basement membrane nor intercellular gaps and pinocytosis makes the vessels permeable to proteins.

DISORDERS OF POTASSIUM, CALCIUM AND MAGNESIUM BALANCE

Disorder	Cause	Symptoms and signs
Hypokalaemia	Acute – administration of insulin and glucose, familial periodic paralysis, vomiting, diarrhoea	Tachycardia, extra systoles cardiac dilatation
	Chronic – dietary insufficiency, malabsorption, diuretics, hyperaldosteronism, Cushing's syndrome	Weakness, hypotonia and paralysis of muscle, metabolic alkalosis
Hyperkalaemia	Renal failure, Addison's disease, iatrogenic (spironolactone, administration of potassium supplements)	Cardiac arrhythmias, heart block, cardiac arrest in diastole
		Weakness, numbness paraesthesiae, listlessness confusion
Hypocalcaemia	Hypoparathyroidism, post thyroidectomy, vitamin D deficiency, renal failure, hyperventilation	Tetany, convulsions, cataracts, ectopic calcification in CNS
Hypercalcaemia	Hyperparathyroidism malignancy, sarcoidosis multiple myeloma, vitamin D toxicity, milk-alkali syndrome	Nephrolithiasis, personality changes, muscle weakness and atrophy, abdominal discomfort, corneal calcification
Hypomagnesaemia	Diarrhoea, malabsorption hyperaldosteronism	'Calcium-resistant' tetany muscular weakness depression, irritability convulsions
Hypermagnesaemia	Renal failure, iatrogenic administration	Prolonged AV and intra-ventricular conduction rates

Figure FL.14

Lymph nodes are encapsulated collections of specialised tissue situated along the course of the lymphatic vessels. They are populated by phagocytic cells lining medullary and cortical sinuses. These engulf bacteria so that under normal conditions the lymph exiting the nodes is sterile.

Ultimately two main vessels, the right lymphatic and thoracic duct, drain into the subclavian veins. The 24 H production of lymph is 2–4 litres. The low resistance of the lymphatic branching system the presence of valves and positive intrathoracic pressures promote forward flow. There is also a high resistance to return back into the interstitial space.

The lymphatic capillaries supplement the venous capillaries in the drainage of tissue fluid. Lymph pumps augment fluid removal. These take the form of adjacent arteriolar pulsations compressing and dilating the lymph vessels as is found in skeletal muscle. Excessive accumulation of tissue fluid is oedema. Other functions of the lymphatics include the return and absorption of nutrients. Plasma lipids are transported as lipoproteins and neutral fat as chylos and concentrations vary with dietary intake.

Lymph has the following features:

- Protein content is lower than plasma and depends on the drained organ

- Contains all coagulation factors especially hepatic lymph
- Antibodies are found in high concentrations
- Electrolyte composition similar to plasma
- Lymphocytes are common, red cells and platelets are rare

CEREBROSPINAL FLUID (CSF)

About 150 ml cerebrospinal fluid surrounds the structures of the CNS and fills the cerebral ventricles. This fluid is continually produced at 600 ml/24 H, it circulates and is re-absorbed back into the cerebrovenous system. The majority of CSF (70%) is produced by the choroid plexuses within the cerebral ventricles; the remaining 30% is produced in the endothelium of cerebral capillaries. The choroid plexuses are networks of cerebral blood vessels exposed to the cerbrospinal fluid in the third and lateral ventricles. They produce the CSF by modified ultrafiltration from the plexus capillaries into the ventricles. The filtration barrier consists of capillary endothelium, basement membrane and choroid epithelium, which also actively modifies the composition of the CSF produced.

Circulation of CSF

The CSF flows through the lateral ventricles to the brainstem where it passes via the third and fourth ventricles, aided by ciliated ependymal cells, which line the ventricles. From the fourth ventricle the CSF exits to the subarachnoid space via the lateral foramina of Luschka and the median foramen of Magendie. It then circulates around the brainstem, brain and spinal cord in the subarachnoid space, finally to be re-absorbed by arachnoid villi in the venous sinuses of the skull. The rate of re-absorbtion is proportional to CSF outflow pressure. This is normally 112 mmH$_2$O. Re-absorption ceases if this is < 70 mmH$_2$O.

Composition of CSF

As noted, the filtration process producing the CSF in the choroid plexuses is ultrafiltration, which is modified (by active secretion) by the ependymal cells. The concentrations of the major constituents in CSF are given in Figure FL.15.

Functions of CSF

The main functions of CSF are:

- Providing buoyancy and protection
- Ionic homeostasis
- Respiratory control

CONCENTRATIONS OF MAJOR SUBSTANCES IN CSF AND PLASMA

Substance		CSF	Plasma
Protein	(g/l)	0.3	70
HCO$_3^-$	(mmol/l)	23	25
Glucose	(mmol/l)	4.8	8
Na$^+$	(mmol/l)	147	150
K$^+$	(mmol/l)	2.9	4.6
Cl$^-$	(mmol/l)	112	100
pH		7.32	7.4
Osmolality	(mosm/kgH$_2$O)	290	290
PCO$_2$	(kPa)	6.6	5.3

Figure FL.15

IONIC HOMEOSTASIS

The ionic composition of interstitial fluid in the CNS is tightly controlled. Both the CSF and the cerebral capillaries contribute to the formation of interstitial fluid. CSF is in free communication with the interstitial fluid in the brain and has the same composition but there can be a significant time lag in the equilibration of changes between CSF and interstitial fluid. The formation of interstitial fluid and the CSF, occurs across a 'blood-brain barrier' located in the cerebral capillaries and the choroid plexuses respectively. This barrier separates the cerebral circulation from the cerebral tissue and serves several functions, which are to:

- Provide tight control over ion concentrations in the CNS
- Protect the brain from transient changes in plasma glucose
- Protect the brain from endogenous and exogenous toxins
- Prevent the release of central neurotransmitters into the systemic circulation

CNS chemoreceptor respiratory control

The central chemoreceptors involved in respiratory control are situated on the ventral surface of the medulla and the floor of the fourth ventricle. The chemoreceptors are bathed in interstitial fluid, which as noted is in communication with the CSF, as well as being formed by cerebral capillaries. The blood brain barrier is freely permeable to CO_2 but relatively impermeable to H^+ and HCO_3^-. Thus, CO_2 diffuses across into the CSF and interstitial fluid in proportion to arterial PCO_2. The low protein concentration in CSF and interstitial fluid, limits its buffering capacity and pH changes are greater than those in plasma for a given change in PCO_2.

The initial response to increasing plasma pCO_2, is formation of H^+ and HCO_3^- in the epithelial cells, catalysed by carbonic anhydrase. Compensation then takes place through the secretion of HCO_3^- buffering CSF and interstitial pH. The concentration of HCO_3^- in CSF and cerebral interstitial fluid is always lower than in plasma, because of the lack of protein buffering in these fluids. The chemoreceptor response to H^+ is to stimulate hyperventilation.

INTRA-OCULAR FLUID

Aqueous and vitreous humour are formed from plasma. Aqueous is a plasma diasylate with a continuous hourly turnover and provides the metabolic and respiratory substrate for the anterior chamber. Specialised cells in the ciliary body actively secrete aqueous humour. The principal route of drainage is via the canal of Schlemm. Production and drainage maintains intra-ocular pressure at 15–18 mmHg. Vitreous humour in the posterior chamber contains the gelatin like protein vitrein.

PLEURAL FLUID

Capillaries on the surface of highly vascular visceral and parietal pleurae form a thin lubricating layer of fluid. The forces of ultrafiltration and re-absorption apply as in the formation of any transcellular fluid discussed above. The hydrostatic pressure in pulmonary capillaries is low compared with a high plasma colloid pressure. The Starling shifts are in favour of re-absorption leaving a thin intrapleural layer of fluid.

SECTION 2: 3
HAEMATOLOGY AND IMMUNOLOGY

J. R. Neilson
J. K. Wood

RED BLOOD CELLS
Haemoglobin
Sickle cell disease
Thalassaemias

TRANSFUSION MEDICINE
ABO system
Rh system
Other red cell antigens
Group and screen
Transfusion reactions

HAEMOSTASIS
Extrinsic pathway
Intrinsic pathway
Final common pathway
Natural inhibitors of coagulation
Fibrinolysis
Platelets
von Willebrand's factor

THE IMMUNE SYSTEM
Mononuclear phagocyte system
Antigen presentation
Antibody-mediated response
Cell-mediated immunity

THE INFLAMMATORY RESPONSE
Mediators of inflammation

THE COMPLEMENT CASCADE
Classical pathway
Alternative pathway
Formation of membrane attack complex

HYPERSENSITIVITY
Type I
Type II
Type III
Type IV

RED BLOOD CELLS

Red blood cells (erythrocytes) provide the system for oxygen delivery from the lungs to the tissues and evolution has produced one of the most specialised cells for this purpose. The erythrocyte lacks organelles and a nucleus and instead is no more than a membrane enclosing a solution of protein and electrolytes. Over 95% of the protein is the oxygen transport protein haemoglobin, the remainder being enzymes required to maintain haemoglobin in a functional, reduced state and enzymes for glycolysis. The bi-concave shape of erythrocytes increases the surface area-to-volume ratio, making gas exchange more efficient and also makes the cell more deformable (compared with a sphere), therefore, more able to navigate the microvasculature. Under normal circumstances the average survival of erythrocytes is 120 days.

Haemopoiesis starts in the yolk sac in the 2-week-old embryo. At 6 weeks the liver, and to a lesser extent the spleen, start to produce haemopoietic cells and by 12–16 weeks the liver is the main haemopoietic tissue. The bone marrow starts to produce blood cells at 20 weeks. At birth haemopoietic (red) marrow occupies all bones. Fat gradually replaces the red marrow until in adults red marrow is confined to the axial skeleton only.

Manufacture of erythrocytes (erythropoiesis) occurs predominantly in the bone marrow from the seventh month of gestation. A homeostatic mechanism ensures that, under physiological conditions, the rate of production equals the rate of destruction but at the same time there is a capability to respond to demands such as hypoxia, haemorrhage or haemolysis by increasing production. Erythropoietin (EPO) is a glycoprotein produced mainly in the kidney but also in the liver, and is one of the most important erythropoietic stimuli. Specialised cells in the renal and hepatic parenchyma have been shown by in situ hybridisation studies to manufacture EPO. In the kidney, the cells are located outside the tubular basement membrane mainly in the inner cortex and outer medulla. Serum levels increase in response to hypoxia, anaemia and increased metabolism (due to effects of corticosteriods, androgens, thyroxine and growth hormone). The bone marrow is among the most highly proliferative tissues in the body and, therefore, requires an uninterrupted supply of nutrients, those particularly needed for erythropoiesis include iron (for haem), vitamin B_{12}, folate and pyridoxine (for DNA synthesis), riboflavin, vitamin E and copper.

HAEMOGLOBIN

Eighteen times more energy is available if glucose is metabolised aerobically than anaerobically. Hence, the transition to aerobic life was a major step in evolutionary terms. The acquisition of oxygen carrying molecules became necessary to overcome the relative insolubility of oxygen in water. The oxygen carriers in vertebrates are haemoglobin and myoglobin. Haemoglobin increases the oxygen carrying capacity of 1 litre blood > 50-fold, it also is involved in the transport of CO_2 and hydrogen ion (H^+). Myoglobin is present in skeletal muscle and serves as an oxygen store, releasing oxygen when needed.

Structure and function of haemoglobin

The haemoglobin A molecule has four polypeptide chains (2 α and 2 β chains), each of which has a covalently bound haem group consisting of a porphyrin ring with a central iron atom in the ferrous (Fe^{2+}) state. A single oxygen molecule can bind to the central iron atom of each haem group. The cross links between the polypeptide chains consist of non covalent electrostatic interactions (salt links). There are two distinct types of salt link in the haemoglobin molecule (Figure HA.1).

- The $\alpha_1\beta_1$ ($\alpha_2\beta_2$) interaction is responsible for stabilisation of the molecule
- The $\alpha_1\beta_2$ ($\alpha_2\beta_1$) interaction is located close to the haem group and undergoes conformational change with oxygenation, this causing the β chains to rotate apart by about 0.7 nm

The breathing molecule

The haemoglobin molecule is said to 'breath' during oxygen uptake and release. Deoxyhaemoglobin is in the taut (T) configuration while the binding of oxygen produces a more relaxed (R) configuration by breaking salt links in the $\alpha_1\beta_2$ and $\alpha_2\beta_1$ interactions. The first oxygen molecule binds relatively weakly to haemoglobin, since more salt links must be broken

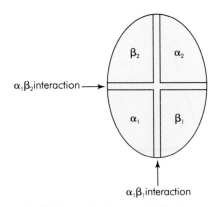

Figure HA.1 Relationship between globin chains in haemoglobin

(and, therefore, more energy is required) compared with the subsequent two oxygen molecules and less energy still is required for the binding of the fourth oxygen molecule. This sequential increase in oxygen affinity explains the sigmoid shape of the oxygen dissociation curve of haemoglobin (Figure HA.2). Myoglobin being a single chain molecule has a hyperbolic oxygen dissociation curve.

EFFECT OF CO_2, H^+ AND 2,3-DPG

CO_2 binds to the terminal amino groups of haemoglobin as bicarbonate, which is formed in the red cell by the action of carbonic anhydrase:

$$CO_2 + H_2O \rightleftharpoons HCO_3^- + H^+$$

This lowers the oxygen affinity of haemoglobin, shifting the oxygen dissociation curve to the right. Much of the hydrogen ion generated by this reaction is taken up by deoxyhaemoglobin which has a higher affinity for H^+ than oxyhaemoglobin:

$$HbO_2 + H^+ \rightleftharpoons HbH^+ + O_2$$

Hence, under acid conditions the equilibrium between deoxy- and oxyhaemoglobin shifts in favour of deoxyhaemoglobin – this is called the Bohr effect. Acidic conditions, therefore, reduce the oxygen affinity of haemoglobin and shift the oxygen dissociation curve to the right. In the highly oxygenated environment of the alveolar capillaries of the lungs the above reactions are reversed.

2,3-Diphosphoglycerate (2,3-DPG) is produced in a side reaction of the Embden–Meyerhof pathway, the Rapaport–Leubering shunt. Binding to haemoglobin in the ratio of one molecule of 2,3-DPG per tetramer, it reduces the oxygen affinity of haemoglobin 26-fold (oxygen dissociation curve moves to the right). In the absence of 2,3-DPG, haemoglobin would unload little oxygen in the capillaries.

Part of the 'storage lesion' of blood for transfusion is a fall in 2,3-DPG levels to about 30% of normal after 3 weeks storage in whole blood in CPD-A medium (citrate-phosphate-dextrose-adenine). This is improved with storage in plasma reduced blood in SAGM (saline-adenine-glucose-mannitol). The clinical significance of the low 2,3-DPG is only likely to be of importance in recipients with severe anaemia or cardiac ischaemia. 2,3-DPG levels are restored to at least 50% of normal in 24 H and 95% normal at 72 H after transfusion.

An increase in body temperature is capable of shifting the oxygen dissociation curve to the right and is an appropriate response to exercise. The converse is also true but in hypothermic individuals their oxygen requirement also falls.

Genetic control of haemoglobin synthesis and the haemoglobinopathies

The genes for the α-globins are located on the short arm of chromosome 16. The order of the genes on the chromosome is determined when they appear during development (Figure HA.3). There are also pseudogenes that during evolution have acquired mutations and are not expressed (ψ ζ, ψ $α_1$ and ψ $α_2$). After 8 weeks of embryonic development there are two functional α chain genes per chromosome ($α_1$ and $α_2$) which are normally expressed equally. Hence, there are four functioning α genes in each erythroid precursor.

The β-globin gene cluster is located on the short arm of chromosome 11, there is a single pseudogene in this cluster (ψ β). While there are two genes controlling expression of γ-chains (γ G and γ A), which are present in foetal haemoglobin, there is only a single functional β-chain gene per chromosome. The chain structure of human haemoglobins is given in Figure HA.4.

Alteration of the coding regions (exons) of the globin genes is likely to alter the amino acid sequence of the corresponding globin chain, the end result is a haemoglobinopathy (e.g. sickle cell disease). On the other hand, if there is lack of expression of a globin chain as a result of deletion or mutation at critical control regions (e.g. RNA splice sites) then a thalassaemia results. Although sickle cell and thalassaemia are the two most common anomalies of haemoglobin, there are other abnormal forms:

- Haemoglobin C – homozygotes have a mild haemolytic anaemia and splenomegaly. Heterozygotes are asymptomatic

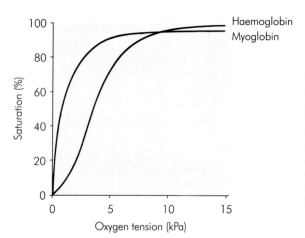

Figure HA.2 Oxygen-haemoglobin dissociation curve

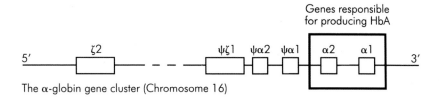

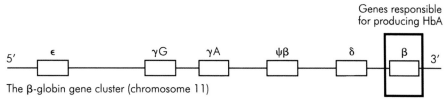

Figure HA.3 Genes responsible for haemoglobin synthesis

CHAIN STRUCTURES OF HUMAN HAEMOGLOBIN

- Embryonic (up to 8 weeks)
  - $\zeta_2\epsilon_2$ – Hb Gower I
  - $\zeta_2\gamma_2$ – Hb Portland
  - $\zeta_2\epsilon$ – Hb Gower II

- Fetal (from 8 weeks)
  - $\alpha_2\gamma_2$ – HbF   85%
  - $\alpha_2\beta_2$ – HbA   5–10%

- Adult (from 5 months of infancy)
  - $\alpha_2\beta_2$ – HbA   97%
  - $\alpha_2\delta_2$ – HbA$_2$ 2.5%
  - $\alpha_2\gamma_2$ – HbF   0.5%

Figure HA.4

- Haemoglobin D – similar to C
- Haemoglobin E – homozygotes have mild anaemia with thalassaemic indices (low MCV, low MCH). Heterozygotes have thalassaemic indices
- Haemoglobins with altered oxygen affinity (rare) – if increased, polycythaemia results (e.g. Hb Chesapeake) and if decreased mild (asymptomatic) anaemia is noted (e.g. Hb Kansas)
- Unstable haemoglobins (rare) – autosomal-dominant traits that present as congenital Heinz body haemolytic anaemia or after oxidant stress, e.g. after treatment with sulphonamides, e.g. Hb Zurich
- M Haemoglobins (rare) – favour the oxidised iron state (Fe^{3+}) and, therefore, have congenital methaemoglobinaemia. Present as familial cyanosis.

SICKLE CELL DISEASE

Pathophysiology

Sickle cell disease is a result of a single DNA base change (adenine to thymidine) which results in the substitution of valine for glutamic acid at position 6 of the β-globin chain. Sickle haemoglobin (HbS) polymerises into microfibrils (crystals) in the deoxygenated state. It is thought that the formation of parallel HbS microfibrils causes red cell membrane damage which results in the classical sickle cell deformity. The effect of this is to shorten the survival of sickle red cells (to 5–15 days in homozygous sickle cell disease) causing haemolytic anaemia. In addition, the deformed red cells are more rigid and less capable of passing through the microcirculation. The result is obstruction clinically manifest as 'crises', e.g. bone pain, pulmonary syndrome and stroke.

The rate of polymerisation of HbS is related to the 50th power of its concentration. Polymerisation is also affected by the presence of other haemoglobins, in that they inhibit this process but to varying degrees. Haemoglobin C and D are not sickling haemoglobins, but inhibit the sickling of HbS much less than HbA and HbF (Figure HA.5). Hence, persons with double heterozygosity for HbS and HbC or HbD have a sickling disorder, whereas heterozygotes for HbS do not.

Geography

β^S exists widely throughout Africa and in parts of Asia, the Arabian peninsula and Southern Europe. The high prevalence of this debilitating disease is a result of balanced polymorphism driven by the relative resistance of heterozygotes to malaria. The majority of sickle cell disease seen in the UK is found in African-Caribbean populations in large cities, where up to 10%

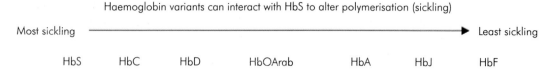

Figure HA.5 Effect of haemoglobin variants on sickling

of individuals carry the β^S gene. In parts of Africa this is as high as 45%.

Clinical features-sickle trait (AS)

Persons with sickle trait have normal growth, development, exercise tolerance and life expectancy. Black American football players, for example, have the same prevalence of sickle trait as the general population. There are rare reports of high altitude splenic infarction, though it must be stressed that most persons with sickle trait tolerate high altitude with impunity.

Clinical features-sickle cell disease

The clinical features of sickle cell disease can be summarised as follows:

- Anaemia – universal, most patients have a haemoglobin level between 5 and 10 g/dl. It is generally well tolerated and does not require therapy
- Vaso-occlusive (painful) crises – the most common manifestation that brings the person into contact with medical services. There is sudden onset if severe pain, usually in bones and joints which reflects bone marrow ischaemia due to sickling in the bone marrow sinusoids. It may be precipitated by infection or exposure to cold, though often no precipitant is identified. Abdominal crises may present as an acute abdomen and can be difficult to distinguish from biliary colic clinically. The absence of bowel sounds, however, should alert the physician to a disorder requiring surgical intervention
- Acute chest syndrome – features include pleuritic chest pain, fever, tachypnoea, pulmonary infiltrates and leucocytosis. It is difficult to distinguish infection, infarction due to sickling and pulmonary embolism. Hypoxia is common and ventilatory support is sometimes needed
- Stroke – perhaps the most important complication with the majority occurring in children. Infarction is the usual pathology. High recurrence rate, which is abrogated by transfusion regimens, but restored on their discontinuation

- In children – aplastic crises (parvovirus), splenic sequestration (major cause of death in children < 2 years old), dactylitis, delayed growth and development
- Long-term complications in adults – include cholelithiasis, sickle retinopathy, leg ulcers (more common in tropics), renal impairment, chronic bone damage from recurrent crises

Diagnosis

Figure HA.6 shows the conditions that can manifest as sickle cell disease. The presence of sickle haemoglobin (HbS, HbC Harlem, HbS Travis but **not** HbC or HbD) is proved in the sickle solubility test. To obtain an exact diagnosis haemoglobin electrophoresis should be performed.

SICKLING DISORDERS

- HbSS – homozygous sickle cell disease
- $S\beta^0$ thalassaemia – compound heterozygote – S and β thalassaemia
- $S\beta^+$ thalassaemia]
- SD – compound heterozygote – S and D
- SC – compound heterozygote – S and C
- SO Arab – compound heterozygote – S and O Arab
- HbS-HbLepore – compound heterozygote

Figure HA.6

Management

Ideally all patients should be managed in centres with experience in managing haemoglobinopathies. Management of specific problems is as follows:

- Vaso-occlusive crises – adequate and prompt pain relief is essential. Opioids are often required, though pethidine should be avoided if possible in view of its short half-life, poorer analgesic profile and risk of convulsions with repeated dosing or continuous infusion. Concerns regarding addiction should not result in patients receiving inadequate analgesia. Adequate hydration is essential and this usually means IV fluids. Broad-spectrum antibiotics should be given if infection is suspected. Hypoxia is the only proven indication for oxygen therapy

- Surgery – to reduce the risk of acute chest syndrome, patients with sickle cell disease should be transfused to reduce the HbS level to about 30% and to raise the Hb > 10 g/dl before major surgery. Transfusion for minor procedures (e.g. myringotomy) is not indicated
- Pregnancy – transfusion therapy during pregnancy reduces the incidence of painful crises but has not been shown to alter pregnancy outcome
- Prophylaxis – penicillin V 250–500 mg b.d. (important in hyposplenic status), vaccination against pneumococcus, *Haemophilus influenzae* and meningococcus is recommended

Genetic counselling and prenatal diagnosis is offered to all women known to be at risk of producing a child with sickle cell disease. Universal screening programmes attempt to detect at risk pregnancies at booking and at delivery. Early diagnosis reduces mortality.

THALASSAEMIAS

The thalassaemias are genetic disorders of globin chain synthesis (α or β). The genetic lesion results in failure of expression of the globin chain gene involved. In the α thalassaemias gene deletion is the usual mechanism and in the β thalassaemias gene mutation resulting in abnormal processing is most often responsible. Heterozygotes are said to have thalassaemia trait and are asymptomatic but may have characteristic blood count abnormalities.

The α thalassaemias

In α thalassaemias there is reduced or absent α chain synthesis. It is critical in the understanding of these disorders to recall that there are two α-chain genes on each chromosome and, therefore, four genes in any diploid cell. Either one gene is deleted on the same chromosome (α^+) or both are (α^0). The homozygous condition in which no α chains are produced (—/— or $\alpha^0\alpha^0$) is not compatible with life, the foetus being stillborn at 28–40 weeks or surviving a few hours after birth. It is termed the Hb Barts–Hydrops syndrome.

α THALASSAEMIA TRAIT

This may be suspected in persons having thalassaemic indices (MCH < 27 pg, low MCV, raised RBC) with normal HbA$_2$ level and who are iron replete. Globin chain synthesis studies can show a reduced α:β chain ratio but this is rarely performed, molecular analysis being preferred.

Carriers of α^0 deletions (– –/α α) are confined to South East Asian and Mediterranean races. They generally have a thalassaemic blood picture. α^+ carriers (α-/α α) are usually silent but persons homozygous for this abnormality (α-/α-) show a similar picture to α^0 carriers.

HAEMOGLOBIN H DISEASE

This corresponds to the genotype $\alpha^0\alpha^+$ (α-/– –) and results in anaemia and splenomegaly associated with normal development. Transfusion is usually not required. The diagnosis is readily apparent by finding Hb Barts (γ_4) at birth by electrophoresis or staining a blood film for HbH (β_4) after 6 months. It most often occurs in South East Asia.

β thalassaemias

In β thalassaemia there is reduced or absent β chain synthesis. Each diploid cell has two β chain genes. Mutation is the usual abnormality at the DNA level which results in transcriptional dysfunction, RNA processing error or non functional mRNA. This can result in either reduced β chain production from that gene (β^+) or absent production (β^0). Each racial group affected has its own repertoire of mutations. Affected populations originate from the Mediterranean, Indian subcontinent or South East Asia.

HOMOZYGOUS B THALASSAEMIA – THALASSAEMIA MAJOR (COOLEY'S ANAEMIA)

There is absent or greatly reduced β chain synthesis. This becomes apparent with the natural fall in foetal haemoglobin ($\alpha_2\gamma_2$) levels due to the switch from γ to β chain production. The infant presents with anaemia during the first 6 months of life. If transfusion therapy is not instituted then the infant may demonstrate the typical thalassaemic facies (frontal bossing, maxillary hyperplasia). With transfusion therapy there is normal development for the first decade, but iron overload then becomes clinically apparent in the absence of chelation therapy (desferrioxamine) and death occurs in the second or third decade. Chelation is usually started in infancy and with good compliance patients can expect to live well into their 30's and perhaps longer. In a select group of children bone marrow transplantation is an option, but not without risk of transplant-related death.

β THALASSAEMIA TRAIT

This is asymptomatic with a thalassaemic blood picture. The HbA$_2$ ($\alpha_2\delta_2$) level is elevated due to a relative reduction in β chain synthesis with normal δ chain synthesis. Iron deficiency can reduce HbA$_2$ levels into the normal range and, therefore, HbA$_2$ should be measured for diagnostic purposes when the individual is iron replete.

TRANSFUSION MEDICINE

Transfusion medicine involves the procurement, processing, testing and administration of blood and its components. It is also concerned with the prevention, investigation and treatment of transfusion-related complications.

To many disciplines this translates into the provision of safe red cells for transfusion as soon as possible. While emphasis is rightly placed on virological safety, the important objective of serological compatibility is the responsibility of the laboratory and clinicians, and deaths still occur as a result of ABO incompatability, most often as a result of clerical error. The reader is referred to the *Handbook of Transfusion Medicine* (McClelland 1996), which is essential reading for all clinicians involved in prescribing blood components.

The blood group systems were recognised following a reaction between the recipient's serum and donor red cells. Historically, this occurred in vitro and/or in vivo as a transfusion reaction or haemolytic disease of the newborn (HDN), such reactions being simple antibody–antigen reactions. If the particular antibody is able to fix complement (IgM, IgG), then lysis occurs. If this occurs in vivo, an immediate (intravascular) haemolytic transfusion reaction occurs.

ABO SYSTEM

The ABO system is the most important because of the presence of naturally occurring IgM antibodies to groups A and B in subjects lacking these antigens. These antibodies are active at 37°C and readily cause immediate haemolytic transfusion reactions in ABO incompatability. They are not present at birth and are thought to arise after exposure to foreign antigens in infancy. Figure HA.7 gives the frequencies of the ABO groups in the UK. Among blood group A and AB individuals approximately one-quarter have a lower density of A antigen on the surface of the red cells and such subjects are referred to as A$_2$ and A$_2$B (the rest are A$_1$/A$_1$B). Some A$_2$ and A$_2$B people have low levels of anti-A$_1$ in their serum, though this is rarely of clinical significance as it is not active at 37°C.

The majority (80%) of individuals can secrete ABO substances in their saliva and other bodily secretions. Persons who are group O and are secretors secrete a precursor substance (H) in the saliva, group A secrete A and H, and so on.

RHESUS SYSTEM

This is the second most important system, not because of naturally occurring antibodies as in the ABO system, but because Rhesus D (Rh D) antibodies are readily formed when blood from a Rh D-positive donor is infused into a Rh D-negative recipient or when a Rh D-negative mother bears a Rh D-positive infant. These

RELATIVE FREQUENCIES OF ABO GROUPS IN DIFFERENT POPULATIONS

Blood group	Naturally occurring antibodies (IgM)	UK (%)	Bengalese (%)	Vietnamese (%)
O	Anti-A, anti-B	47	22	45
A	Anti-B	42	24	21
B	Anti-A	8	38	29
AB	None	3	16	5

Figure HA.7

NOMENCLATURE AND FREQUENCY OF RH HAPLOTYPES

CDE nomenclature	Frequency
CDe	0.4076
cde	0.3886
cDE	0.1411
cDe	0.0257
CDe	0.0129
cdE	0.0119
Cde	0.0098
CDE	Rarer
CdE	Rarer

Figure HA.8

antibodies are IgG and can, therefore, cross the placenta to cause haemolytic disease of the newborn (HDN).

Alongside the D antigen there are four other Rh antigens of importance – C, c, E, e – although a total of 48 Rh antigens have been described. The antigens C and c are allelic, as are E and e. There is no d antigen; the letter is used to indicate a lack of D antigen. Each diploid cell has two sets of three Rh genes that are closely linked. Hence, some Rh haplotypes are commoner than others and there is some racial variation. Figure HA.8 shows the frequency of various haplotypes.

D is the most important of the Rh antigens as it is > 20 times more immunogenic than c, the next most important antigen. Because of the Rh D testing of all donor and recipients and immunoprophylaxis with anti-D, during pregnancy and at delivery, the relative frequency of anti-D compared with other Rh antibodies has declined significantly in recent years. Red cell units are still labelled Rh D-positive or -negative but a proportion will also have a Rh genotype label. The reason for this is to indicate a lack of certain antigens (c and e in the examples given); these units are, therefore, suitable for patients whose serum contains the corresponding antibodies.

OTHER RED CELL ANTIGENS

There are 21 blood group systems that have been given numbers by a working party of the International Society of Blood Transfusion. The number of antigens in each system varies from 1 to 48.

The importance of a particular blood group antigen relates to the frequency of development of antibodies and the clinical relevance of these antibodies. Space does not permit even brief descriptions of all the blood group systems of clinical relevance. Guidelines in the UK require that red cell antibody screening procedures can detect antibodies to C, c, D, E, e, K, k (Kell), Fy^a, Fy^b (Duffy), Jk^a, Jk^b (Kidd), S, s, M, N (MNS system), P$_1$, Le^a, Le^b (Lewis). This is done by ensuring that the screening cells used in the transfusion laboratory express between them all of the above antigens. Figure HA.9 shows the relative clinical importance of various red cell allo-antibodies.

RELATIVE FREQUENCY OF ALLOANTIBODIES OCCURRING POST TRANSFUSION AND RESPONSIBLE FOR IMMEDIATE AND DELAYED HAEMOLYTIC TRANSFUSION REACTIONS

Alloantibody	Post transfusion (%)	Associated with immediate haemolytic transfusion reaction (%)	Associated with DHTR (%)
Rhesus (excluding anti-D)*	52	42	34
Kell	29	30	15
Duffy	10	18	16
Kidd	4	9	33
Other	5	1	2

* mainly anti-E and anti-c.
ABO, Lewis, P, M and N excluded as they are only rarely of clinical significance

Figure HA.9 (modified from Mollinson et al. 1993)

GROUP AND SCREEN

It is of critical importance that blood samples for compatibility testing are correctly identified. The ABO and Rh D groups are established by using monoclonal typing reagents (anti-A, anti-B, anti-A + B and anti-D). In ABO grouping, the reverse group is also performed by mixing the patient's serum with A_1 and B red cells. Then an antibody screen is performed. The patient's serum is tested against red cells that between them carry the antigens listed above. If there is a positive reaction in the antibody screen, then the antibody is then identified by testing the patient's serum against a panel of red cells. This is done either in the hospital blood bank or the regional transfusion centre. Once an allo-antibody is identified, appropriate red cell units, lacking the red cell antigen, are selected.

Red cell selection and cross matching

If a red cell allo-antibody is detected then blood should be selected that is known to be negative for that antigen and is ABO- and Rh-compatible. A cross match follows where the patient's serum is tested against red cells from the units to be transfused. If the cross match is negative, then a compatibility label, giving patient details, is attached to the unit and the blood and a compatibility report issued.

Emergency situations

If the situation is life-threatening then group O blood is issued. If the patient is a pre menopausal female, O Rh D-negative must be issued. There is generally a shortage of O Rh D-negative blood due high demand for universal usage in emergency situations. Usually, there is sufficient time to perform ABO and Rh D groups on the patient sample by rapid techniques and to do an immediate spin cross match before issue. This may take 10–15 min. An antibody screen is then performed by the laboratory retrospectively. A label stating that standard pre transfusion testing has not been performed is attached to the blood bag. In massive transfusion where one blood volume has been given within 24 H, ABO- and Rh D-compatible blood can be issued without further serological testing, provided no allo-antibodies were present by earlier testing.

TRANSFUSION REACTIONS

Immediate and life-threatening reactions

IMMEDIATE HAEMOLYTIC TRANSFUSION REACTIONS

Most often due to ABO incompatability due to clerical error. Less commonly, due to antibodies against Rh D, Duffy, Kidd and Kell antigens. The antibodies (IgM, IgG1 and IgG3) fix complement and this causes intravascular haemolysis. Features include pain at infusion site, chest and back pain, hypotension, DIC, and haemoglobinuria. The mortality rate is 10%.

BACTERIAL CONTAMINATION

This is rare but is usually fatal if red cells are contaminated. One of the most frequent organisms responsible is *Yersinia enterocolitica*. There is rapid development of septic shock and collapse. The contaminated blood may be clotted or have a purple discoloration. Platelets can sometimes be contaminated with bacteria, most often gram-positive organisms such as *Staphylococcus epidermidis*. This relates to storage of platelets at 22°C.

Life-threatening reactions associated with dyspnoea

ANAPHYLAXIS

Anaphylaxis is rare and but may be fatal. It is most often related to IgA deficiency in the recipient associated with complement fixing anti-IgA.

TRANSFUSION-ASSOCIATED ACUTE LUNG INJURY (TRALI)

This is rare. It is due to anti-leukocyte antibodies in donor plasma, and most often seen associated with FFP. Hypoxia develops during or in the hours following transfusion. There are associated bilateral lung infiltrates radiographically. This syndrome is easily confused with ARDS and in the critical care setting TRALI may be overlooked as a cause of this clinical picture. Respiratory support is often required and IV methyprednisolone should be given. In contrast with ARDS, recovery is usual within 48 H. Recurrence is not a problem as the antibodies existed in the donor plasma.

CONGESTIVE CARDIAC FAILURE (usually LVF)

This is a common adverse effect of transfusion in the elderly and can be late in onset. Patients with ischaemic heart disease are most at risk. It can be avoided by prophylactic diuretics and transfusion of ≤ 2 units/day by slow infusion – 1 unit in 3 H.

Non life-threatening transfusion reactions

FEBRILE NON HAEMOLYTIC TRANSFUSION REACTIONS (FNHTR)

This is the most common type of transfusion reaction. It is due to recipient anti-leukocyte antibodies. These may be acquired following pregnancy or after transfusion of cellular blood components. The patient may experience a rigor, but the temperature may rise without one. There are no signs or symptoms to suggest a haemolytic reaction, however severe FNHTRs may be associated with moderate hypotension, nausea, vomiting, cyanosis and collapse. If FNHTRs have already been experienced, further reactions can be prevented by paracetamol before transfusion. Leucodepletion of blood components may be indicated if reactions persist despite this measure. Primary prevention of FNHTR by leucodepletion is appropriate in some situations, e.g. Aplastic anaemia, renal transplant candidates, patients living transfusion lives.

URTICARIAL REACTIONS

Urticarial reactions to donor plasma proteins may be treated with anti-histamines. If there are repeated reactions unresponsive to anti-histamines, washed red cells should be given.

Delayed haemolytic transfusion reactions

These occur in patients who have been transfused previously or have had a previous pregnancy, and who have developed a red cell antibody, the titre of which has fallen to undetectable levels. Re-exposure to the corresponding antigen in a later transfusion results in an amenestic immune response and haemolysis of the transfused cells. IgG antibodies are generally responsible and haemolysis is generally extravascular, though occasionally can be intravascular.

Clinical features include fever and a fall in haemoglobin level associated with jaundice between 4 and 14 days following transfusion. If the haemolysis is intravascular, then there may be haemoglobinuria. The clinical severity is related to the volume of incompatible blood transfused. Diagnosis requires a positive direct anti-globulin test (demonstrates antibody coating of red cells) and the demonstration of an allo-antibody either in the serum or in an red cell eluate, which is antibody eluted from the red blood cells.

Use of blood components

Guidelines are available for the use of platelets and fresh frozen plasma (FFP). Figures HA 10–12 give indications for the use of platelets, FFP and cryoprecipitate respectively.

HAEMOSTASIS

The arrest of bleeding following an injury is a rapid and complex process that involves changes in the involved

INDICATIONS FOR THE USE OF PLATELET CONCENTRATES

- Bone marrow failure – if this is reversible (e.g. after chemotherapy), prophylaxis to maintain platelets $> 10 \times 10^9/l$ is appropriate. In chronic bone marrow failure platelets are generally given if the patient is haemorrhagic
- Platelet function disorders – very occasionally required prior to surgery
- Massive blood transfusion – clinically significant dilutional thrombocytopenia occurs after the transfusion of about 1.5 blood volumes. The platelet count should be maintained $> 50 \times 10^9/l$
- Cardiopulmonary bypass surgery – platelet functional abnormalities and thrombocytopenia are common in this situation. Platelet transfusion should be reserved for patient with non surgical bleeding. Prophylaxis is not indicated
- Disseminated intravascular coagulation (DIC) – in acute DIC with haemorrhage and thrombocytopenia. Fibrin degradation products (FDPs) impair platelet function. In the absence of bleeding and in chronic DIC platelet transfusion is not indicated
- Prior to surgery and invasive procedures – platelet count should be raised to $50 \times 10^9/l$. For operations on critical sites (e.g. brain and eye) the platelet count should be raised to $100 \times 10^9/l$

Note that a 'standard dose' of platelets in an adult may be considered as 4 units/m^2.

Figure HA.10

vessel (smooth muscle constricts and the endothelium becomes procoagulant), platelets (become activated and aggregate) and the plasma (fibrin formation). Simultaneous inhibitory mechanisms ensure these processes are confined to the site of injury and do not propagate to, or occur in, normal vasculature. Subsequently, the removal of the clot (fibrinolysis) occurs as part of tissue remodelling.

Abnormal coagulation tests are among the commonest reasons for seeking haematological advice, both inside and outside normal working hours. In many cases, the underlying coagulation abnormality and its treatment can be deduced from a basic knowledge of the coagulation mechanism. The classical theory of blood coagulation that describes intrinsic and extrinsic systems is particularly useful for understanding in vitro coagulation tests. More modern theories have managed

INDICATIONS FOR THE USE OF FFP

- Replacement of single coagulation factor deficiencies where a specific concentrate is not available
- Immediate reversal of warfarin effect – but in life-threatening bleeding due to warfarin prothrombinase complex concentrates (PCC = intermediate purity factor IX) and factor VII concentrates are indicated together with vitamin K (5 mg IV)
- DIC if there is haemorrhage and coagulation abnormality – if there is no haemorrhage or the condition is chronic FFP is not indicated
- Thrombotic thrombocytopenic purpura – a rare disorder which is treated with plamapheresis using cryoprecipitate-poor FFP
- Massive transfusion if there are abnormal coagulation tests (PT and/or APTT ratio ≥ 1.5) and fibrinogen > 1.5g/l (if < 1.5 g/l cryoprecipitate indicated). Coagulation tests need to be repeated frequently to assess the need for further components
- Liver disease – if there is bleeding or prior to surgery/procedures if the PT ratio is prolonged ≥ 1.5
- Cardiopulmonary bypass if there is non surgical bleeding and a coagulation abnormality with normal platelet count and function

Note that a 'standard' dose of FFP in an adult may be consider as four units.

Figure HA.11

INDICATIONS FOR THE USE OF CRYOPRECIPITATE

- Emergency treatment of haemophilia and von Willebrand's disease when specific concentrates are not available and on the advice of a haematologist
- Dysfibrinogenaemia associated with bleeding
- Massive transfusion if the fibrinogen level is < 1.5 g/l
- DIC if there is bleeding and the fibrinogen level is <1.5 g/l
- Bleeding associated with renal failure
- Bleeding following thrombolytic therapy. Inhibitors of fibrinolysis (e.g. tranexamic acid) may also be required if the situation is life-threatening, but may result in the formation of large clots at the site of bleeding

Note that a 'standard' dose of cryoprecipitate in an adult may be considered as 10–15 units.

Figure HA.12

to explain some of the apparent paradoxes of the classical theory such as why haemophiliacs bleed and patients with factor XII deficiency do not.

The coagulation cascade is shown in Figure HA.13. Such cascade reactions allow for considerable amplification as well as many opportunities for control of the process.

EXTRINSIC PATHWAY

The extrinsic pathway is so called because to activate coagulation via this pathway a substance (i.e. tissue factor) which is normally present outside the vascular system is required. Tissue factor is a ubiquitous lipoprotein found in particularly high concentration in placenta, brain and lung. It is also in monocytes and endothelial cells but is only expressed when these cells

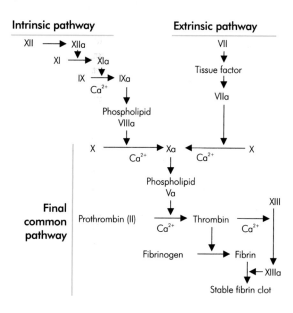

Figure HA.13. Classical coagulation cascade

are activated, e.g. by endotoxin. Tissue factor is not an enzyme, but a co-factor serving to increase the catalytic activity of factors VII and VIIa in the cleavage of factors X–Xa.

Prothrombin time (PT)

This tests the integrity of the extrinsic pathway. A source of tissue factor (thromboplastin) is added to citrated plasma, calcium chloride is then added to overcome the anti-coagulant effect of citrate and the time taken for a clot to form measured. Thromboplastin is usually derived from rabbit brain or lung but recently recombinant human thromboplastins have become available. In some laboratories the PT is expressed as an INR (international normalised ratio), this is a device to standardise the PT between laboratories for the purpose of monitoring anti-coagulation with coumarins. The INR is the ratio of the PT: mean normal PT to the **power** of the ISI (international sensitivity index) of the thromboplastin used in the system. Since sensitive thromboplastins (ISI close to 1.0) are usually used in the UK the INR often approximates to the PT ratio. The commonest causes of a prolonged PT are given in Figure HA.14.

INTRINSIC PATHWAY

The intrinsic pathway was thought to activate blood coagulation by involving only substances present in the plasma. Initiation of coagulation via this pathway requires 'contact activation'. This occurs when pre kallikrein (PK) and factors XII and XI are activated in the presence of high molecular weight kininogen (HMWK) on exposure to certain surfaces; in vivo to negatively charged surfaces such as collagen, in vitro to glass or kaolin (Figure HA.15). The sequential activation of factors XI and IX then occurs culminating

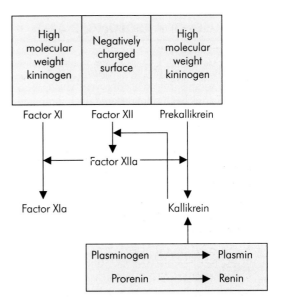

Figure HA.15 Initiation of the intrinsic coagulation pathway

in the activation of factor X by factor IX with factor VIII as a co-factor.

Activated partial thromboplastin time (APTT)

This was designed to assess the potential of the intrinsic pathway. It is also known as the PTTK (partial thromboplastin time with kaolin) and the KCCT (kaolin clotting time). The plasma is pre incubated with kaolin and phospholipid to activate the contact factors, calcium chloride is then added and the time recorded for a clot to form. The sensitivities of different phospholipid reagents to deficiencies of the clinically important factors (VIII and IX) in the intrinsic pathway vary. APTT is used to monitor heparin therapy; unfortunately, it has not yet been possible to standardise these reagents for the monitoring of heparins in the same way that thromboplastins have been for oral anti-coagulant control, making local derivation of therapeutic ranges for heparin necessary. The most frequent causes of a prolonged APTT are shown in Figure HA.16.

FINAL COMMON PATHWAY

The final common pathway sees the conversion of prothrombin to thrombin by factor Xa with factor Va as a co-factor. Thrombin has a central role in coagulation. Critically it cleaves fibrinogen to form fibrin monomers that then spontaneously aggregate to form fibrin strands that are subsequently cross-linked by

---

CAUSES OF A PROLONGED PROTHROMBIN TIME

Oral anticoagulant drug administration.

Liver disease, hepatocellular, (decreased production of factors II and VII obstructive (decreased absorbtion of vitamin K)

Vitamin K deficiency

Disseminated intravascular coagulation

Hypofibrinogenaemia

Massive transfusion

Inherited deficiency of factor VII, X or V.

Heparin

Figure HA.14

CAUSES OF A PROLONGED APTT

Heparin therapy

Sample contamination by heparin, e.g. by taking sample from a line through which heparin has been administered (including 'Hepflush')

Liver disease

Disseminated intravascular coagulation

Hypofibrinogenaemia

Massive transfusion

Coagulation inhibitor, e.g. lupus anti-coagulant, acquired factor VIII inhibitor

Inherited deficiency of factors xI, VIII, IX, x, PK or HMWK

Figure HA.16

CAUSES OF A PROLONGED TT

• Hypofibrinogenaemia

– Disseminated intravascular coagulation

– Fibrinolytic therapy

– Massive transfusion

– Inherited deficiency (rare)

• Dysfibrinogenaemia (abnormal fibrinogen molecule)

– Inherited (rare)

– Acquired (liver disease most common cause)

• Raised FDP levels – DIC or liver disease

• Heparin

Figure HA.17

factor XIIa resulting in a stable clot. Factor XII is activated by thrombin, as are the co-factors factor V and VIII, thrombin induces platelet aggregation and, by combining with thrombomodulin, activates protein C, an anti-coagulant protein, which results in the inactivation of factors V and VIII.

Deficiency of factors X, V, II and fibrinogen cause prolongation of both the PT and the APTT. Hence, the function of the final common pathway can be monitored by using both tests. In reality, since isolated deficiency of factors X or V are rare, the commonest reason for prolongation of both tests in a patient not receiving oral anti-coagulants is hypofibrinogenaemia.

Thrombin time (TT)

The TT tests the key reaction in the coagulation cascade; the conversion of fibrinogen to fibrin. Conceptually it is the most simple of all the coagulation tests as it consists of simply adding a solution of thrombin to platelet poor plasma and measuring the time taken for a clot to form, the addition of calcium is not necessary. TT is very sensitive to low levels of heparin, this probably being the most common reason for a prolonged TT, other reasons are shown in Figure HA.17. In many laboratories, the TT is not performed as part of a routine coagulation screen, instead the fibrinogen is measured. This can be done in an assay based loosely on the TT (Clauss method), but increasingly with the introduction of automation into the coagulation laboratory, fibrinogen is estimated during the performance of the PT by optometrical analysis of clot formation.

A revised view of in vivo coagulation (Figure HA.18) takes into account the paradoxes offered by the above scheme, for example; while patients severely deficient in factors VIII and IX (haemophiliacs) bleed spontaneously those with factor XII, PK or HMWK deficiency do not have a bleeding diathesis but do have considerably prolonged APTTs. So it is clear that the classical cascade theory is important to understand what is occurring in the screening coagulation tests, but comprehension of in vivo coagulation requires alternative explanations.

It is important to realise that coagulation reactions occur on surfaces, e.g. platelets, activated endothelium,

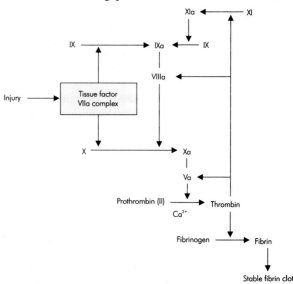

Figure HA.18 A revised coagulation hypothesis

subendothelial collagen. When coagulation is initiated thrombin is formed in the absence of activated factors V and VIII, trace amounts of thrombin then activate factors V and VIII. These are large molecules that act as co-factors in their respective reactions and localise reactions to surfaces, the overall result is an increase by many thousand-fold in the efficiency of the coagulation mechanism.

It is tissue factor that initiates coagulation in vivo by forming a complex with factor VIIa and then activating factor X (it is not clear how factor VII is activated); however, this complex also activates factor IX which is a significant departure from the classical hypothesis. The importance of this is only realised upon activation of factors V and VIII: the predominant action of factor VIIa/TF becomes activation of factor IX and massive amplification of the coagulation mechanism then occurs via two highly efficient reactions resulting in thrombin formation. Factor VIIa/TF complex is quickly inhibited by tissue factor pathway inhibitor, so factor Xa generation must occur via factor VIIIa/IXa. This is augmented by factor XIa, which is activated by thrombin, this being a late step in the pathway. The critical roles of factors XIa and VIIIa in this scheme reflect the severity of the bleeding when these factors are deficient. Contact activation has no place in in vivo coagulation.

NATURAL INHIBITORS OF COAGULATION

The cascade structure of the coagulation system ensures very rapid activation of coagulation, for example, it has been estimated that 10 ml plasma can generate sufficient thrombin to clot all the body's fibrinogen in 30 s; clearly this may be deleterious, so equally powerful inhibitors of coagulation in the plasma ensure that the haemostatic response is confined to the vicinity of the platelet plug and vascular injury. Tissue factor pathway inhibitor has already been mentioned, but there are two other broad groups of coagulation inhibitors: serine protease inhibitors the most important of which is anti-thrombin (previously called anti-thrombin III) and the coagulation co-factor (VIIIa and Va) inhibitors which are proteins C and S.

Anti-thrombin

Anti-thrombin complexes with the serine protease coagulation factors (thrombin, Xa, XIIa, XIa, and IXa but not VIIa) and inactivates them. The resulting inhibitor-protease complex is rapidly removed by the liver. The affinity for thrombin is highest followed by factor Xa. Heparin binds to anti-thrombin and induces a 2300-fold increase in thrombin inactivation.

Endothelial glycosaminoglycans act in a similar fashion. Reduction in plasma anti-thrombin levels results in a tendency to venous thrombosis.

Other serine protease inhibitors include heparin co-factor II, α_1-anti-trypsin, C_1 esterase inhibitor, α_2 anti-plasmin and α_2 macroglobulin. Deficiency of these inhibitors has not been clearly associated with thrombosis.

Protein C system

The protein C system is responsible for the inactivation of the activated co-factors Va and VIIIa. Protein C and S are vitamin K-dependent factors. The system is represented in Figure HA.19.

Thrombin behaves as an anti-coagulant when it binds to thrombomodulin, which is present on the endothelial surface. The resulting complex activates protein C, which in the presence of protein S inactivates factors Va and VIIIa by cleavage. Thus thrombosis is prevented from propagating along normal vessel close to a point of injury.

Reduced plasma levels of protein C and S are associated with thrombosis and can be inherited in an autosomal dominant fashion. Deficiency of thrombomodulin has not been described and probably results in non viability. The most common inherited cause of a thrombotic tendency is a mutation of factor V (Factor V-Leiden) which alters the activated protein C (APC) cleavage site, this results in reduced APC induced cleavage and demonstrated in vitro by the APC resistance (APCR) test. Once again this is an autosomal dominant trait.

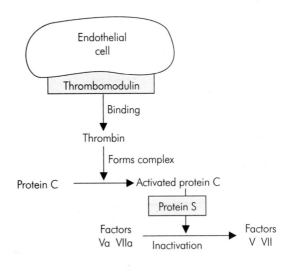

Figure HA.19 Protein C system

FIBRINOLYSIS

A scheme for the fibrinolyic system is shown in Figure HA.20. Intrinsic activation of fibrinolysis, via kallikrein, is possible but the physiological relevance is uncertain. Tissue-type plasminogen activators (t-PA) are of greatest importance; t-PA is synthesised by endothelial cells. Its release is stimulated by venous occlusion, thrombin, epinephrine, vasopressin and strenuous exercise. Its biological activity increases dramatically when bound to fibrin.

In vivo activity of the fibrinolytic system is routinely assessed in clinical situations by measuring fibrin degradation products (FDPs) which usually include the products of fibrinogen degradation and, therefore, does not rely on the presence of fibrin. D-dimers, on the other hand, are only produced by digestion of cross-linked fibrin and are, therefore, a more specific indicator of fibrinolysis which has been exploited recently in the assessment of suspected pulmonary embolism.

PLATELETS

Platelets are responsible for forming the primary haemostatic plug following injury. They are produced in the bone marrow by the cytoplasmic budding of megakaryocytes. They are bi-convex discs with a diameter of 2–4 μm and volume of 5–8 fl. The normal life span of a platelet is between 8 and 14 days. They contain granules of which the most numerous are α granules (the contents of which are listed in Figure HA.21). Dense bodies are less numerous but of

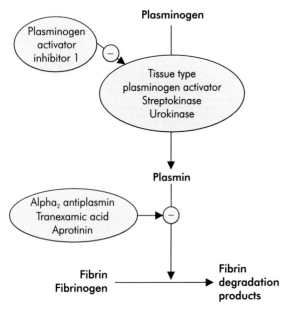

Figure HA.20 Fibrinolytic system

CONTENTS OF PLATELET ALPHA GRANULES

- Coagulation factors – V, X, protein S.
- Adhesive proteins – von Willebrand's factor, fibrinogen, fibronectin, vitronectin
- Growth factors
  - platelet-derived growth factor (PDGF)
  - platelet factor 4 (PF4)
  - β thromboglobulin

Figure HA.21

---

importance as their deficiency (storage pool disease) can result in significant haemorrhage. Dense bodies contain platelet nucleotides (ADP, ATP, 5-HT).

Platelets function by adhesion to sites of injury, they change shape and release their granules and then aggregate together forming the platelet plug. They also provide the surfaces that enhance the coagulation reaction and growth factors contained in the α granules stimulate tissue repair. Global platelet function can be tested by measuring the bleeding time, which is best performed by experienced laboratory staff using the template method (normal < 9 min). It should be remembered that thrombocytopenia results in prolongation of the bleeding time. Qualitative platelet defects can be assessed by platelet aggregometry to various stimuli.

Platelet adhesion

Blood vessel injury results in exposure of subendothelial collagen and microfibrils. Larger von Willebrand's factor (vWF) molecules bind to the microfibrils and platelets adhere to the vWF via platelet glycoprotein (GP)1b. Following this, the glycoprotein IIb–IIIa complex becomes exposed which increases adhesion (and is also involved in aggregation).

Platelet shape change

This occurs within seconds of adhesion; the platelet becomes more spherical and spikey which enhances interaction between platelets. The platelet granules migrate towards the surface.

Platelet release reaction

This follows immediately and involves the release of the contents of platelet granules, it is sustained for several minutes. Thus coagulation factors, adhesive proteins, growth factors and nucleotides are delivered to the site of injury.

Platelet aggregation

At the site of injury ADP is released from damaged cells (and following platelet release reaction), this binds to platelets and exposes the GP IIb–IIIa complex. Fibrinogen binds to this receptor, and as it is a dimeric molecule is capable of forming bridges between platelets. The other main physiological inducer of platelet aggregation is thromboxane A$_2$, this is a product of arachidonic acid metabolism in the platelet.

Prostaglandin metabolism in platelets

This is a critical part of platelet activation, because blocking it (with aspirin) prevents the release reaction. Arachidonic acid is released from membrane phospholipid by phospholipase A$_2$. Prostaglandin metabolism in the platelet and endothelial cell is shown in Figure HA.22.

von WILLEBRAND'S FACTOR

von Willebrand's factor consists of large molecules (multimers) made up of a variable number of subunits. It is produced in endothelial cells and megakaryocytes, then stored in Weibel–Palade bodies of endothelial cells and α granules of platelets. The main function of vWF is in platelet adhesion; however, it also acts as a carrier of factor VIII. vWF deficiency results in the most common inherited bleeding tendency – von Willebrand's disease, which is estimated to occur in up to 1% of the population. It is most commonly a mild quantitative (type 1) deficiency but type 2 (qualitative) and type 3 (severe quantitative) also occur. Deficiency of vWF produces two haemostatic defects – a prolonged bleeding time due to failure of platelet adhesion and a coagulation defect due to reduced levels of factor VIII.

THE IMMUNE SYSTEM

MONONUCLEAR PHAGOCYTE SYSTEM

Previously referred to as the reticuloendothelial system when endothelial cells, fibroblasts and granulocytes were included, the mononuclear phagocyte system is composed of cells derived from the bone marrow.

It has been demonstrated that the cells of the mononuclear phagocyte system can be generated from bone marrow stem cells or from peripheral blood monocytes. The two main types of cells are:

- Professional phagocytes
- Antigen presenting cells (APCs)

Figure HA.23 lists the cells of the mononuclear phagocyte system.

Phagocytic function

Human monocyte/macrophages have specific

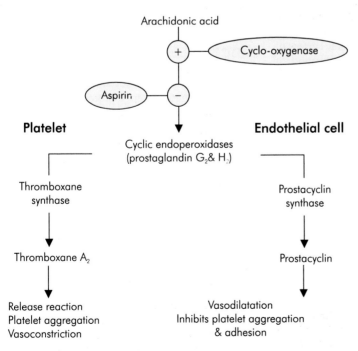

Figure HA.22 Prostaglandin metabolism in the platelet and endothelial cell

CELLS OF THE MONONUCLEAR PHAGOCYTE SYSTEM

Professional phagocytes	Antigen presenting cells
Circulating monocytes	Langerhans cells (skin)
Kupffer cells (liver)	Interdigitating cells (lymph node)
Mesangial macrophage (kidney)	Follicular dendritic cells (lymph node, thymus)
Alveolar macrophage (lung)	Macrophages
Serosal macrophage (pleura, peritoneum)	
Splenic sinus macrophage	
Lymph node sinus macrophage	

Figure HA.23

receptors on their surface that allow them to bind to micro-organisms. These include the mannosyl-fucosyl receptors (MFRs) which bind to microbial saccharides and a lipopolysaccharide binding protein (LBP) which binds gram-negative bacteria. Once bound, the microbes are ingested to form a phagosome. Lysosomes then merge with the phagosome, the micro-organism is killed and digested. The lysosome contents include proteolytic enzymes, peroxidase, elastase and collagenase. The exact enzymes present vary according to the type of macrophage, e.g. peritoneal macrophages are peroxidase-negative. The presence of complement receptors on macrophages and neutrophils improve phagocytic efficiency if micro-organisms are opsonised (coated) with complement. Fc_γ receptors are present on the surface of monocyte/macrophages and bind the Fc portion of IgG, which also serves as an opsonin. There are three types of receptor: $Fc_\gamma RI$, $Fc_\gamma RII$ and $Fc_\gamma RIII$ that have high, intermediate and low affinity for the Fc portion of IgG and probably have different functions, e.g. triggering extracellular killing, opsonisation and phagocytosis. Phagocytosis also occurs by receptor-independent mechanisms.

Intravenous immunoglobulin (IVIg) is thought to block reticuloendothelial Fc receptors and is used in auto-immune thrombocytopenia and auto-immune haemolytic anaemia.

ANTIGEN PRESENTATION

Macrophages are capable of presenting antigen to T-lymphocytes but there are also other specialised cells for this purpose. Foreign protein is digested into small peptides that are processed and expressed on the cell surface in conjunction with HLA class II molecules, which are found only on APCs and B-lymphocytes. The specialist antigen presenting cells have many fine, long projections (dendrites) which maximise the surface area over which interaction with T-cells can occur. They are found in the T-cell rich areas of lymphoid tissue. Other cell types, when stimulated, can function as antigen-presenting cells and these include endothelial and epithelial cells. Here antigen is presented in association with major histocompatibility (MHC) molecules, which are present on the surface of all nucleated cells.

Interaction between antigen presenting cells and T-lymphocytes

Linear peptide fragments bind to the peptide groove of MHC molecules in the rough endoplasmic reticulum of antigen presenting cells and then these molecules are expressed on the cell surface. Only a minority of peptide fragments from a protein antigen (from any source) are capable of being processed in this way.

The antigen is 'recognised' by specific T-helper cells (T_H). The T cell receptor (TCR) binds to the antigen-MHC molecule complex. Further molecular interactions occur once the cells are brought into close proximity by this interaction (Figure HA.24). The result is an exchange of cytokines including interleukin 1 (IL-1), produced by macrophages, which stimulates T_H proliferation and expression of interleukin 2 (IL-2) receptors on T_H-cells. Activation of T-cells also results in the production of interferon γ that stimulates the expression of MHC molecules on macrophages, producing positive feedback.

These processes are the first events following challenge by a new antigen and the development of an effective immune response depends on the production, by proliferation, of adequate numbers of T_H-cells. An

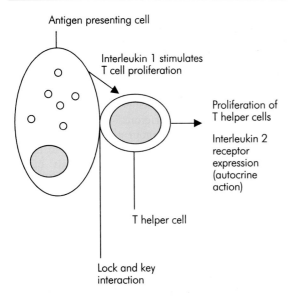

Figure HA.24 Interaction between antigen presenting cell and helper T cell

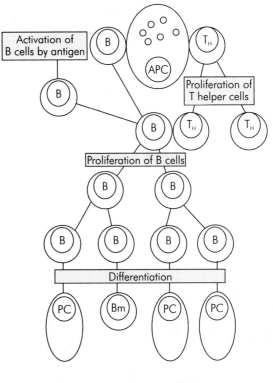

APC	Antigen presenting cell
B	B cell
T_H	T helper cell
PC	Plasma cell
Bm	B memory cell

Figure HA.25 B cell activation and interaction with T cells

immune response follows and this can be antibody-mediated (a B lymphocyte function) or cell-mediated (a T cell and macrophage function).

ANTIBODY-MEDIATED RESPONSE

Antigen binds to the surface immunoglobulin of specific B lymphocytes. It is processed and expressed in association with MHC molecules. The B cell is now capable of interacting with specific T_H-cells, which will have been activated by interaction with APCs. This B-T interaction results in delivery of stimulatory cytokines by the T_H-cells, the result is the proliferation and then differentiation of B cells to produce plasma cells and then antibody (Figure HA.25). B cells can also be activated by interacting with antigen presented by APCs, with subsequent proliferation and differentiation signals coming from T_H-cells. A proportion of B-cells, rather than differentiating to form plasma cells, enters a resting phase to become memory B-cells (B_M). Similarly a subpopulation of the stimulated T_H population will become T_H-memory cells.

Antibody structure, subtypes and diversity

Immunoglobulins are composed of four peptide chains – two heavy chains (IgH) and two light chains (Figure HA.26). There are five structural heavy chain variants to produce IgG, IgM, IgA, IgD and IgE. IgM is pentameric and IgA dimeric. There are two structural light chain variants – κ and λ. Most of the molecule consists of framework on which the highly variable

antigen binding site is located. Diversity of antigen binding sites is achieved by immunoglobulin gene rearrangement at the DNA level where a variable gene (V, one of several hundred), joining gene (J, one of six) and diversity gene (D, one of 30) are combined to produce a unique gene in each developing B cell, which then produces the unique antigen binding site. More refinement is achieved with point mutation of the VDJ recombination and this may occur during B cell activation and proliferation. Subsequently the best antigen–antibody matches selectively proliferate, enhancing the overall response. The relatively frequent occurrence of re-combinational inaccuracy of the VDJ adds a further mechanism of diversity generation.

Primary and secondary antibody responses

Following an initial antigen challenge there is a lag phase where no antibody is detectable. Then there is a logarithmic increase in antibody levels to a plateau and there follows a decline to low or undetectable levels. Such a primary response consists predominantly of

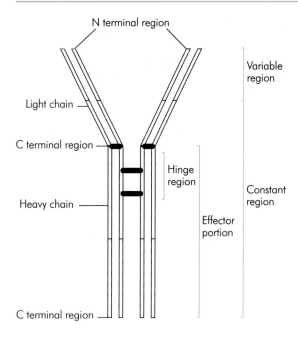

Figure HA.26 Antibody structure

IgM with IgG present but appearing slightly later. If the individual is challenged again, then there is a shorter lag phase before antibody is detected, the rise in antibody titre is up to 10 times greater than the primary response, the plateau is more prolonged and decline slow. The secondary response consists almost entirely of IgG and the affinity of the antibodies is greater, a process called antibody maturation.

A typical example of primary and secondary antibody responses occur with a delayed haemolytic transfusion reaction. Initial exposure to the foreign red cell antigen results in no clinical effects, but low level antibody is produced and subsequently declines. Antibody screening after the decline may miss a low level antibody, but should the individual be exposed to the antigen again, a brisk secondary response occurs which results in the destruction of the antibody coated transfused red cells by the mononuclear phagocyte system. Clinically this is apparent after 4–14 days when the patient presents with anaemia, fever and jaundice.

CELL-MEDIATED IMMUNITY

T-cell independent mechanisms

The two T-cell independent mechanisms are phagocytosis and cytokine release.

- Phagocytosis – macrophages and granulocytes are capable of migrating to sites of infection stimulated

by chemotactic components released by micro-organisms. They can then bind, engulf and kill pathogens utilizing oxidant free radicals and peroxides
- Cytokine release – cytokines are peptide or glycopeptide mediators released from stimulated cells. Examples include the interleukins (lymphokines), interferons, colony stimulating factors (CSFs) and tumour necrosis factor (TNF). Macrophages release TNF in response to micro-organisms and are an important part of the inflammatory response (below). TNF also enhances granulocyte and macrophage microbicidal capacity

T-cell-dependent mechanisms

CYTOTOXIC T CELLS (T_C)

A subpopulation of peripheral blood lymphocytes form cytotoxic T-cells. These recognise antigen when presented in association with the relevant MHC molecules. It is thought that T_C-cells are important in recognizing and destroying virus infected cells.

The antigen associated with a MHC molecule is recognised by the T-cell receptor (TCR) in the same way that T_H-cells recognise antigen presented by APCs. The TCR is analogous to the immunoglobulin molecule expressed on the surface of B cells in that diversity is generated by similar mechanism.

OTHER CYTOTOXIC CELLS

- Natural killer cells (NK cells) do not have rearranged TCR genes. It is thought that they recognise tumour-associated antigens. They also have F_C receptors on their surface and can destroy antibody coated cells
- Lymphokine activated killer cells (LAK cells) are formed by the culture of peripheral lymphocytes in IL-2. Enhanced tumour killing results. It is thought that LAK cells are activated NK cells
- Antibody-dependent cell-mediated cytotoxicity (ADCC) requires effector cells to have a F_C receptor. Antibody-coated cells are thus recognised and destroyed. Cell capable of such killing are T_C-cells, NK cells, mononuclear phagocytes and granulocytes

The role of T_H-cells in cell-mediated immunity is very important as T_H-cells provide cytokines necessary for activation and proliferation.

THE INFLAMMATORY RESPONSE

The clinical signs of inflammation are heat, redness,

swelling, pain, and reduced function. Inflammation is a response to injury or invasion by pathogens. Three fundamental events are involved:

- Hyperaemia – there is an increase in blood supply to the affected area. This is a result of arteriolar relaxation
- Exudation – there is an increase in capillary permeability resulting from retraction of endothelial cells. Larger molecules are allowed to pass across the endothelium and thus plasma enzyme systems reach the site of inflammation
- Emigration of leucocytes – initially phagocytes and then lymphocytes migrate between endothelial cells into the surrounding tissues along chemotactic gradients

Pathologically inflammation is diagnosed when there are increased numbers of granulocytes, macrophages and lymphocytes in a tissue section.

MEDIATORS OF INFLAMMATION

The Kinin system

The products of this system mediate the immediate vasoactive response (Figure HA.27).

Histamine and leukotrienes (B_4 and D_4)

These are released by basophils and their tissue equivalent, mast cells, after stimulation by microbes

and result in increase vascular permeability. Leukotrienes together with neutrophil chemotactic factor (also produced by mast cells) stimulate the migration of granulocytes to sites of invasion or injury. Leukotrienes are products of arachidonic acid metabolism via the lipoxygenase pathway.

Neutrophil adhesion and migration across the endothelium

Under normal, steady-state conditions, while leucocytes flow in close proximity to the endothelium they do not adhere to it (Figure HA.28a). At sites of inflammation, endothelial cells become activated by mediators such as TNF_α, one of the effects of this is adhesion molecule synthesis and expression on the surface of endothelial cells. One of the first to be expressed is E-selectin (4–12 H), later intercellular adhesion molecule-1 (ICAM-1) is produced (Figure HA.28b).

Neutrophils, upon stimulation by inflammatory mediators, express pre formed adhesion molecules such as LFA-1 and CR3. The result is neutrophil adhesion (Figure HA.28c). The neutrophil then, attracted by chemotactic agents, migrates between endothelial cells (Figure HA.28d) and migrate along the subendothelial matrix of collagen, laminin, etc. using different adhesion molecules, to sites of injury (Figure HA.28e). Lymphocytes and macrophages migrate in a similar way, but later than neutrophils.

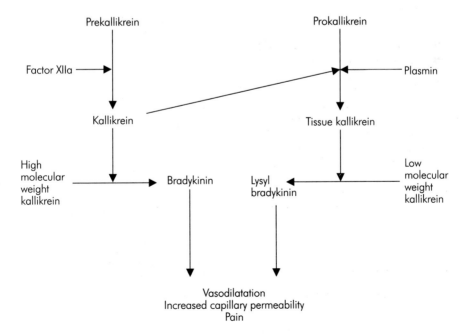

Figure HA.27 Kinin system

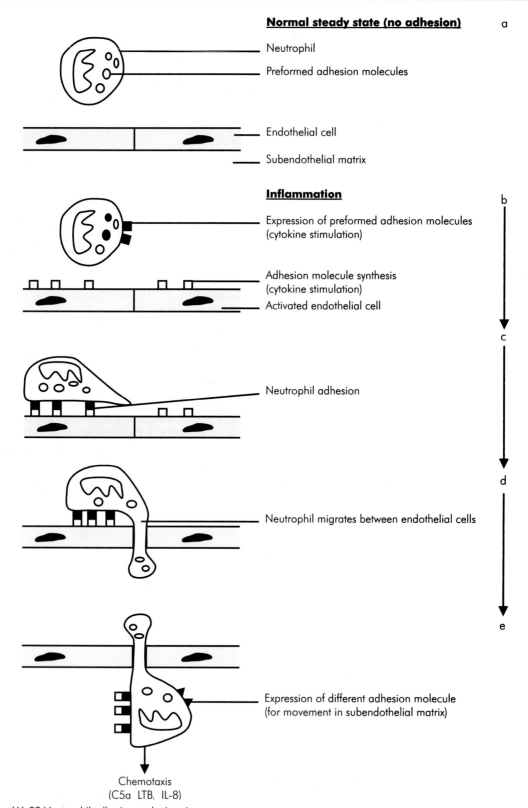

Normal steady state (no adhesion) a

— Neutrophil

— Preformed adhesion molecules

— Endothelial cell

— Subendothelial matrix

Inflammation b

— Expression of preformed adhesion molecules (cytokine stimulation)

— Adhesion molecule synthesis (cytokine stimulation)
— Activated endothelial cell

c

— Neutrophil adhesion

d

— Neutrophil migrates between endothelial cells

e

— Expression of different adhesion molecule (for movement in subendothelial matrix)

Chemotaxis
(C5a LTB, IL-8)

Figure HA.28 Neutrophil adhesion and migration

Once present at the site of injury, neutrophils release mediators including platelet activating factor (PAF), which stimulates mediator release from platelets, increases vascular permeability and smooth muscle contraction. PAF also activates other neutrophils. Macrophages and monocytes also migrate along the same chemotactic gradients and engulf microbes, they also present antigens to T and B lymphocytes as described above. Mononuclear cells and lymphocytes release cytokines.

Tumour necrosis factor

TNF is a mediator of inflammation released by macrophages and lymphocytes in the presence of bacterial pathogens. It activates endothelial cells and enhances phagocytic function. Activated endothelium becomes procoagulant, adhesive, more permeable and produces increased nitric oxide resulting in smooth muscle relaxation and vasodilation. TNF and nitric oxide are important mediators of septic shock.

Complement

Complement components C3a and C5a are inflammatory mediators and their production is described below. Both stimulate mast cell de-granulation and smooth muscle contraction. C5a also increases capillary permeability, activate neutrophils and stimulates phagocyte chemotaxis.

Other plasma enzyme systems are also involved in inflammation, namely the coagulation cascade and the fibrinolytic system. FDPs are capable of increasing vascular permeability and stimulating neutrophil and macrophage chemotaxis.

THE COMPLEMENT CASCADE

'Complement', coined by Ehrlich, refers to the activity in serum which when combined with antibody results in the lysis of bacteria. It has since been realised that complement performs three major functions:

- Opsonisation (coating) of bacteria and immune complexes
- Activation and attraction (chemotaxis) of phagocytes
- Lysis of target cells

There are many proteins involved in the complement system and a detailed account of all of these is not appropriate here. An outline of complement activation is given in the classical and alternative pathways below. The central event of the complement pathway is the cleavage of C3 to form C3b and C3a (Figure HA.29). C3b attaches to micro-organisms or immune complexes and acts as a site of membrane attack complex formation. It also acts as an opsonin. The small peptide cleaved from C3; C3a, stimulates mast cell de-granulation and smooth muscle contraction.

CLASSICAL PATHWAY (FIGURE HA.30)

This forms part of the specific immune response. C1q can bind to the F_C regions of aggregates of IgG1 or IgG3 molecules bound to antigen (immune complexes). C1q also attaches to single antigen bound IgM molecules, which are by nature pentameric. C1r and C1s are also components of the C1 complex. Binding of C1q leads to conformation change in the C1

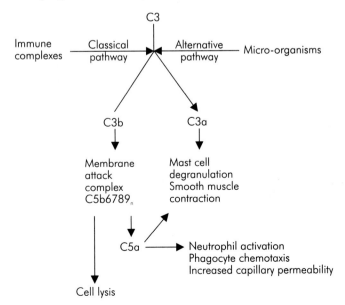

Figure HA.29 Central role of C3 in the complement pathway

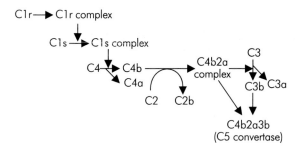

Figure HA.30 Classical complement pathway

complex resulting in auto-activation of C1r, which in turn activates C1s. The next step is activation of C4 with the production of C4b, which avidly binds surface carbohydrates or proteins, thus complement activation is localised to a surface. Like the coagulation cascade, the large number of steps ensures amplification and offer opportunity for regulation. The C4b2a complex catalyses the central step; the cleavage of C3.

Inhibitors of the classical pathway help ensure localisation of complement activation. C1 inhibitor in the serum inactivates C1r and C1s. Complement control proteins (such as decay accelerating factor) are present on the surface of cells and interfere with the C4b–C2 interaction, preventing complement activation and damage to nearby normal cells.

ALTERNATIVE PATHWAY (FIGURE HA.31)

This is a non specific immune function and relies on continual low level complement activation. This is

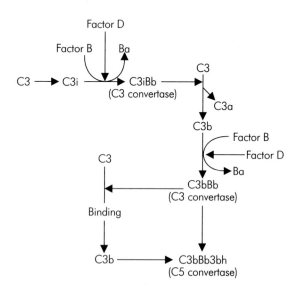

Figure HA.31 Alternative complement pathway

achieved by hydrolysis of C3 to form C3i, which in the presence of magnesium is able to associate with Factor B. The C3iB complex is then itself cleaved by Factor D to form C3iBb and Ba. C3iBb is able to act as a C3 convertase (i.e. catalyses C3 → C3b + C3a). The above reactions occur in the fluid phase but C3b attaches itself to any adjacent surface. Autologous cells can inactivate C3b. The surface of micro-organisms, however, stabilise C3b and facilitate C3 binding to Factor B and, as above, Factor D cleaves the resulting complex to form C3bBb and Ba. C3bBb is a C3 convertase and also combines to C3b to act as a C5 convertase, which initiates membrane attack complex formation. Here again is a system in which a large number of reaction steps occurring on a surface produces considerable amplification. Bacteria with surface bound C3b, C3i or C4b (which implies immunoglobulin binding also) are said to be opsonised and are readily phagocytosed by neutrophils or macrophages. This is initiated by binding to complement receptors on the phagocyte's surface. Otherwise lysis may occur as outlined below.

FORMATION OF THE MEMBRANE ATTACK COMPLEX

This is the final common pathway of complement activation. The first step is cleavage of C5 to C5a (a mediator of inflammation) and C5b. C5b can then aggregate with C6 and C7 to produce C5b67 which, being hydrophobic, attaches to plasma membranes. C8 then binds to a site on C5b and penetrates the membrane. The resulting C5b678 complex polymerises a number of C9 molecules to form the membrane attack complex ($C5b6789_n$) which is essentially a pore in the cell membrane; lysis is thus produced.

Once the C5b67 complex is formed it can attach to any nearby membrane and produce lysis – this is sometimes called 'the innocent bystander' effect. This is prevented in the fluid phase by proteins such as vitronectin inactivating this complex. On cell membranes a protein (MIRL = membrane inhibitor of reactive lysis) performs a similar function against membrane attack complex.

HYPERSENSITIVITY

Hypersensitivity occurs when an otherwise beneficial immune response is inappropriate or exaggerated resulting in tissue damage. It occurs on re-exposure to the antigen concerned and the damage may be due to one or more of four mechanisms – referred to as type I, II, III and IV hypersensitivity.

MEDIATORS RELEASED BY TISSUE MAST CELLS AND THEIR ACTIONS

Mediator	Action
Histamine	Vasodilatation
	Increases vascular permeability, smooth muscle contraction
Platelet activating factor (PAF)	Platelet degranulation & aggregation leading to microthrombi formation neutrophil chemotaxis
Tryptase	Protease acting to cleave C3 to C3a and C3b
Kininogenase	Activates kinin system
Cytokines e.g. IL-5, TNF_α IL-8	Granulocyte chemotaxis including eosinophils & basophils
Leukotriene B_4	Basophil chemotaxis
Leukotriene C_4 & D_4	Smooth muscle contraction
	Mucosal oedema increased mucus secretion

Figure HA.32

TYPE I

Type I hypersensitivity, also referred to as immediate hypersensitivity is an IgE-mediated response. IgE is synthesised by specific B cells with APC and T_H cells critically involved as described above. IgE is released and binds to tissue mast cells via their F_C receptors. If the antigen is subsequently encountered, it binds to the mast cell bound IgE and this stimulates mast cell de-granulation and release of pre formed mediators (Figure HA.32). The clinical effects depend on the site the where antigen is encountered. In the skin eczema or urticaria will result, if the antigen is inhaled asthma occurs and in the nasal passages allergic rhinitis (hay fever) develops.

In severe cases the reaction can be generalised producing anaphylactic shock. The mechanism is the same but there is widespread mediator release. This occurs most commonly on exposure to certain drugs or foods (e.g. penicillin, peanuts) in response to insect stings (e.g. bee and wasp) and on exposure to blood components (e.g. plasma in an IgA deficient individual). This response should be distinguished from the anaphylactoid reaction that can be induced by certain drugs (e.g. codeine and morphine) which act on mast cells directly and not via IgE.

TYPE II

This occurs when IgG and/or IgM molecules interact with complement to produce target cell damage. An example of this is Goodpasture's syndrome where an anti-basement membrane immunoglobulin is produced. This together with complement is deposited on the glomerular and pulmonary basement membranes and neutrophils attach via their F_C and complement receptors. As they are unable to phagocytose, they discharge their lysosomal contents which results in damage to the basement membrane. The clinical effects are renal failure and pulmonary haemorrhage. Auto-immune haemolytic anaemia and myasthenia gravis are further examples of type II hypersensitivity reactions.

TYPE III

This is a result of the production of large quantities of immune complex that cannot be adequately cleared by the mononuclear phagocyte system. There is often widespread deposition of these immune complexes that activate complement via the classical pathway. There are numerous diseases that are immune complex-related (Figure HA.33) and their clinical features reflect the sites of deposition.

TYPE IV

Type IV hypersensitivity reactions are produced by cell-mediated mechanisms and generally take > 12 H

EXAMPLES OF IMMUNE COMPLEX-RELATED DISEASES

Infections
- Bacterial endocarditis
- Hepatitis B
- Dengue fever

Autoimmune diseases
- Rheumatoid arthritis
- SLE
- Polyarteritis nodosa and microscopic polyarteritis
- Polymyositis
- Cutaneous vasculitis
- Fibrosing alveolitis
- Cryoglobulinaemia

Figure HA.33

to develop. Previously called delayed hypersensitivity, three types are described:

- Contact hypersensitivity, which is a cutaneous reaction, maximal at 48–72 H. Most commonly this is in response to a hapten, which is a molecule too small to induce an immune response. Instead, it combines with normal proteins to produce a neo-antigen. Examples include metals such as nickel and chromate. Antigen is presented to Langerhans' cells that interact with sensitised T_H-cells which then release cytokines, activating keratinocytes that release further cytokines to produce the eczematous lesions
- Tuberculin-type hypersensitivity which is maximal at 48–72 H is the reaction that occurs after intradermal injection of tuberculin. The antigen

presenting cells are thought to be predominantly macrophages. The cells responsible for the reaction are T_H and T_C-cells, macrophages and monocytes. Granuloma formation may follow due to persistence of antigen
- Granulomatous hypersensitivity is most important clinically because it is responsible for diseases such as tuberculosis, leprosy, schistosomiasis, leishmaniasis and sarcoidosis. Again, T_H-cells are critical in the production of these reactions that result from a continuous antigen stimulus or where macrophages are unable to destroy the antigen. The result is granuloma formation in the presence of antigen. Granulomas consist of macrophages, epithelioid cells, giant cells and lymphocytes

References and further reading

BCSH. Guidelines for platelet transfusions. *Transfusion Medicine* 1992; 2: 311–318.

BCSH. Guidelines for the use of fresh frozen plasma. *Transfusion Medicine* 1992; 2: 57–63.

Hathaway WE, Goodnight SC. *Disorders of Hemostasis and Thrombosis. A Clinical Guide*. McGraw-Hill, 1993.

Hoffbrand AV, Lewis SM (eds). *Postgraduate Haematology*, 3rd edn. Heinemann Medical, London, 1990.

Lee GR, Bithell TC, Foerster J, Athens JW, Lukens JH (eds). *Wintrobe's Clinical Hematology*, 9th edn. Lea & Febiger, Philadelphia, 1993.

McClelland B (ed.). *Handbook of Transfusion Medicine*, 2nd edn. HMSO, London, 1996.

Mollinson PL, Engelfriet CP, Contreras M. Blood *Transfusion in Clinical Medicine*, 9th edn. Blackwell, Oxford, 1993.

Roitt I, Brostoff J, Male D. *Immunology*, 3rd edn. Mosby, 1993.

SECTION 2: 4
MUSCLE PHYSIOLOGY

I. T. Campbell
D. Liu

Microscopic structure
Muscle contraction
Muscle metabolism
Neuromuscular transmission
Central control of muscle tone and movement

SMOOTH MUSCLE

Structure
Types
Smooth muscle contraction
Properties
Extrinsic control

**COMPARISON BETWEEN SKELETAL,
CARDIAC AND SMOOTH MUSCLE**

SKELETAL MUSCLE

Skeletal muscle fibres are attached to bone by tendons of strong connective tissue. The proximal attachment is known as the 'origin' and the distal attachment is the 'insertion', the two being connected by the muscle 'belly'. The precise shape and distribution of a muscle, or muscle group, about a joint depends on its particular function. In summary the functions of skeletal muscle are to provide:

- A mechanical response to environmental stimuli
- A short term store of glycogen and glucose
- A long term metabolic reserve of protein for gluconeogenesis

MICROSCOPIC STRUCTURE

Muscle cell

Muscle cells or fibres are quite large, typically about 100 μm in diameter and may run the full length of the muscle. They are multinucleated, are surrounded by a membrane, the endomysium, and are bound into fascicles. These fascicles are surrounded by the perimysium and combine to make up the whole muscle. This, in turn, is covered by connective tissue sheet, the epimysium (Figure MP.1).

Myofibril

The muscle cells or fibres are made up of myofibrils enclosed by the cell membrane (sarcolemma). The myofibrils consist of two types of myofilaments. There

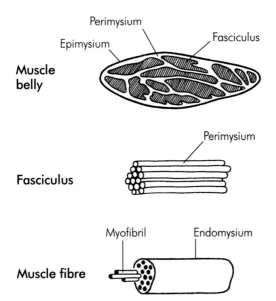

Figure MP.1 Skeletal muscle structure

are thick filaments composed of myosin and thin filaments that are made up of actin.

Sarcomere

The myofibril is made up of basic contractile units called sarcomeres. The microscopic appearance of the sarcomere identifies various regions, which are known by letters (Figure MP.2).

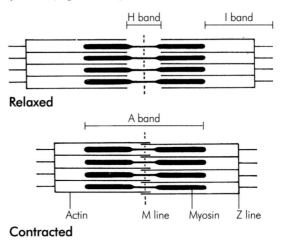

Figure MP.2 Structure of sarcomere

The sarcomere is composed principally of myosin filaments and actin filaments. The myosin filaments occupy the central part of the sarcomere and comprise the A band. The A band is transected by the M line, which keeps the myosin filaments in side by side alignment. The myosin filaments interdigitate with the thin actin filaments whose ends are joined to the Z line or disc which maintains their spatial arrangement. The area of myosin filaments in the middle of the sarcomere not overlapped by actin filaments is known as the H zone. A cross section of the sarcomere in areas where the two types of filaments overlap shows that the two types of filament are arranged in a hexagonal pattern (Figure MP.3). The myoplasm between the filaments contains glycogen, myoglobin, the enzymes involved in glycolysis and mitochondria.

Myofilaments

THIN MYOFILAMENT

The thin actin filament is a helical structure composed of two chains of actin molecules wound around each other. It is about 5.5 nm in diameter and the two chains are structured so that they make a half turn of the helix every 35–37 nm. A long, thin fibrous protein, tropomyosin, lies between the two strands of actin. Associated with the tropomyosin at each half turn of

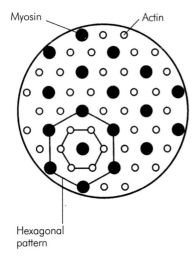

Figure MP.3 Cross-section of a myofibril

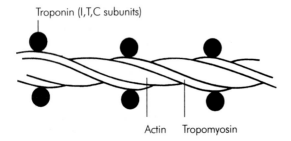

Figure MP.4 Thin myofilament

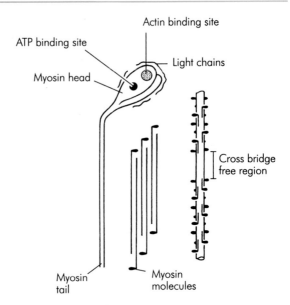

Figure MP.5 Thick myofilament

myosin filament. The assembled filaments are all held in place by the Z discs, the M line and associated accessory proteins, nebulin and titin.

SARCOTUBULAR SYSTEM

The sarcoplasmic reticulum is a network of intracellular membranes and tubules which extends throughout the muscle cell, wrapping itself around the myofibrils. It encloses a space containing calcium ions (Ca^{2+}), which play a key role in the contractile mechanism of muscle. The sarcoplasmic reticulum has enlarged terminal sacs or 'cisternae' which lie close to the T tubules at the A–I junction (Figure MP.6). The bulk of the contained Ca^{2+} accumulates within these sacs. The T tubules are essentially a continuation of the extracellular space and conduct the wave of depolarisation along the sarcolemma into the depths of the cell. The combination of a T tubule and two adjoining terminal cisternae on either side is termed a triad (Figure MP.7).

MUSCLE CONTRACTION

Muscle contracts by movement of the actin and myosin filaments past each other. The A band (composed of myosin filaments) remains the same size, but the Z lines move inwards and the width of the H zone and the I bands diminish. The distance between the two groups of actin filaments diminishes and at maximum contraction they overlap.

Myosin–actin interaction

Contraction of a sarcomere is caused by interaction

the actin/tropomyosin strand is a protein complex called troponin consisting of 3 subunits: troponin I, troponin T and troponin C (Figure MP.4).

THICK MYOFILAMENT

The thick myosin filament is made up of myosin molecules that consist of two parts, a rod shaped 'tail' section and a head portion consisting of two globular heads with ATP and actin binding sites. Associated with each of the heads are two protein molecules called myosin 'light' chains because of their low molecular weight. They have a regulatory function in muscle contraction.

The myosin filaments are packed together with the tail regions making up the structure of the thick filament (Figure MP.5). The heads project from the side of the myosin filament in a helical fashion with one turn of the helix every six molecules so that the heads project at 60° to each other and at a distance from each others 14.3 nm. Each myosin filament is constructed of two groups of myosin molecules with their tails abutting. There is, thus, an area bare of myosin heads, or cross bridge-free region that constitutes the mid point of the H zone. The heads are thus at opposite ends of the halves of the

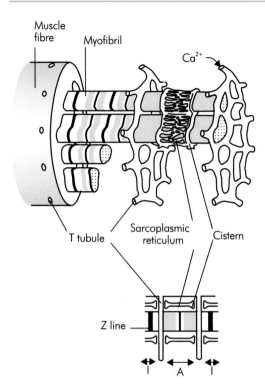

Figure MP.6 Separated components of the sarcotubular system

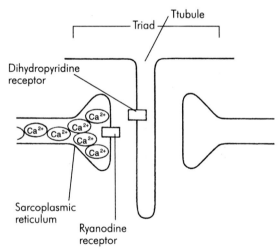

Figure MP.7 Sarcotubular triad

between the myosin and actin filaments. This is a cyclical sequence of events repeated triggered by stimulated release of calcium ions. The reaction producing the movement between the filaments occurs between the myosin heads and the actin filaments and can be referred to as the 'powerstroke' (Figure MP.8).

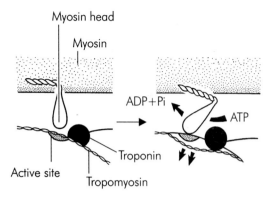

Figure MP.8 The powerstroke

Myosin–actin powerstroke

In the powerstroke the myosin heads attaches to the actin at 90° and subsequently bend to 45° producing relative movement between the filaments. The myosin then detaches from the actin and the process starts again. Each power stroke shortens the muscle by about 1%; the thick filaments each have about 500 myosin heads and during a rapid contraction these move at 5/s. This whole process uses energy in the form of ATP and requires the presence of the calcium contained by the sarcoplasmic reticulum. When a myofibril is stimulated Ca^{2+} is released into the myoplasm from the sarcoplasmic reticulum, principally from the terminal cisternae. This binds to the C unit of the troponin regulating complex, which is attached to the tropomyosin. This causes a conformational change in the other subunits of troponin (I and T) which in turn results in movement of the tropomyosin strand within the groove of the actin molecule, revealing active sites on the actin filament to which myosin can attach. When this happens, the power stroke of the myosin head is initiated and the two filaments move past each other.

Myosin–actin contraction cycle

The myosin–actin cycle involves the consumption of energy provided by ATP. In resting muscle a molecule of ATP, split into ADP and inorganic phosphate (Pi) is bound to each myosin head. The cycle of events making up the myosin–actin interaction cycle can be considered in the following stages, the numbers of which refer to Figure MP.9.

- Stage 1 – at the completion of the power stroke myosin is still attached to actin. ATP then binds to myosin causing its release from actin and also release of Ca^{2+}
- Stage 2 – ATP is hydrolysed, energising myosin but ADP and Pi remain bound to myosin

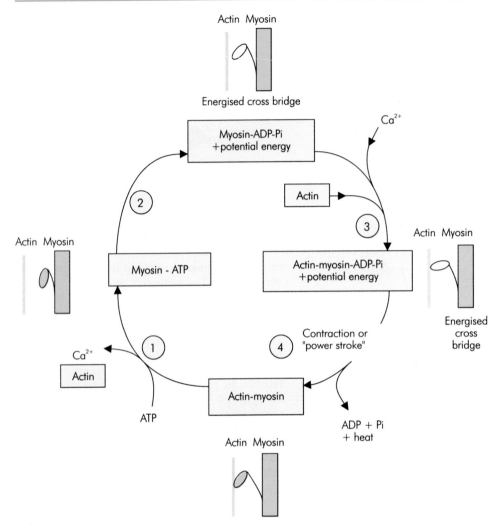

Figure MP.9 Actin–myosin cycle

- Stage 3 – in presence of Ca^{2+} and actin, re-attachment of the energised myosin head occurs
- Stage 4 – power stroke occurs as ADP and Pi are released.

Muscle contraction is initiated by the release of calcium ions from the sarcoplasmic reticulum into the myoplasm resulting from depolarisation of the sarcolemma (initiated by the motor nerve) at the motor end plate. The process is termed 'excitation contraction coupling' and for a nerve stimulus to ensure an adequate release of calcium throughout the whole length and depth of a fibre the process has to be efficient.

Membrane depolarisation is initiated at a motor end plate and a wave of depolarisation spreads along the sarcolemma in the same way as it does in a peripheral nerve. It is carried into the depths of the fibre by a system of invaginations of sarcolemma found in association with the junction of the A and I bands of the myofibril.

Excitation–contraction coupling

Resting Ca^{2+} concentration in the myoplasm is between 10^{-7} and 10^{-8} mol/l. The resting state is maintained by the storage of Ca^{2+} in the sarcoplasmic reticulum where it binds to a specific Ca^{2+}-binding protein called calsequestrin. Calcium ions are released when the sarcolemma is depolarised and the wave of depolarisation spreads into the depths of the cell via the T tubules. A calcium release channel in the sarcoplamic reticulum opens and Ca^{2+} passes from the sarcoplasmic reticulum into the myoplasm; myoplasmic Ca^{2+} concentrations increase to 10^{-5} mol/l. The calcium binding sites on troponin C are occupied and muscle contraction takes place by the mechanisms discussed above.

The Ca^{2+} release channel is also known as the ryanodine receptor (after a plant alkaloid). It has a transmembraneous part and a section that projects into the myoplasm where it bridges the gap between the sarcoplasmic reticulum and the sarcolemma. It also lies close to the dihydropyridine receptor (a slow Ca^{2+} channel) of the T tubular system and the two proteins may be coupled.

Relaxation occurs when myoplasmic Ca^{2+} falls due to re-uptake by the sarcoplasmic reticulum and this is an energy consuming process. Troponin C loses its Ca^{2+} and the myosin head detaches from the actin filament. Factors that diminish the re-uptake of Ca^{2+} such as profound fatigue and ischaemia decrease the ability of the muscle to relax and it tends towards the rigidity seen in rigor mortis.

Single muscle fibre contraction

A muscle contraction is the result of the combined responses of many individual muscle fibres of different types. It is also the temporal summation of the response of these fibres to multiple action potentials transmitted by the motor nerve. Consider the mechanical response of a single muscle fibre and its response to repeated action potentials. When a muscle contracts, the tension developed varies with time and its length may change depending on the load it is attached to. Three different types of muscle contraction can be described:

- Isometric – a contraction with no change in length
- Isotonic – a contraction with constant load but shortening length
- Lengthening contraction – a contraction in which the external load is greater than the tension developed by the muscle, causing the muscle to increase in length in spite of its contraction

Single fibre twitch

A muscle fibre responds to a single stimulus with a single brief contraction mediated by the release of Ca^{2+}. This is called a twitch. Isometric and isotonic twitches are illustrated in Figure MP.10a and b. The following characteristics can be seen:

- There is a latent period between stimulus and onset of developed tension. This varies between fibre types
- Contraction time is that time between onset of tension development and maximum tension, which differs between fibre types
- The shortening profile of isotonic contractions depends on the applied load

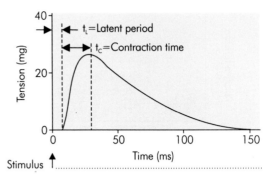

(a) **Isometric twitch of single muscle fibre**

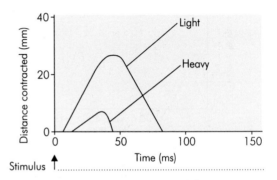

(b) **Isotonic twitch of single muscle fibre with light load and heavy load**

Figure MP.10 Single fibre-twitch response

Relaxation follows with the immediate re-uptake of Ca^{2+} by the sarcoplasmic reticulum. This re-uptake starts before maximal contraction has taken place, so the muscle fibre does not develop the strongest force of which it is capable. Muscle tissue has the properties of absolute and relative refractoriness seen in most excitable tissue, but the time periods of de- and repolarisations are shorter than the time usually taken for contraction and relaxation.

Repeated action potentials produce different results according to the interval between stimuli. If a second stimulus may come along before complete re-uptake of the Ca^{2+}, it elicits a contraction stronger than the first (Figure MP.11a).

A series of stimuli repeated rapidly produces a gradual augmentation of contraction until the tension developed reaches a maximum which is then sustained. This is called a tetanic contraction and it is significantly stronger than that produced by a single twitch (Figure MP.11b).

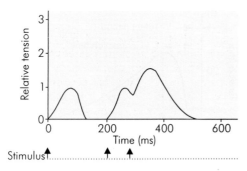

(a) Repeated isometric twitches of single muscle fibre

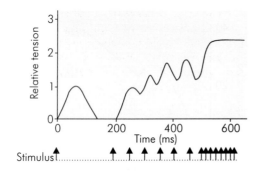

(b) High frequency twitches of single muscle fibre giving tetany

Figure MP.11 Single fibre-repeated twitch response

MUSCLE METABOLISM

Energy for muscle contraction

Adenosine triphosphate (ATP) is the immediate energy source for muscle contraction. There are three main pathways forming ATP for contraction:

- Phosphorylation of ADP by creatine phosphate (CP) – very rapid and occurs at the onset of contraction. It is limited by the content of CP in the cell, only lasts a few seconds and lasts until OP and GP can take over
- Oxidative phosphorylation (OP) in mitochondria – requires oxygen and supplies most of ATP requirements during moderate exercise levels
- Glycolytic phosphorylation (GP) in the cytoplasm – does not require oxygen and normally only produces small numbers of ATP molecules per mole of glucose, but can produce greater quantities if the enzymes and substrate are available. Glycolytic phosphorylation produces lactic acid and incurs an 'oxygen debt' which may be repaid by a prolonged elevation of oxygen usage after muscle activity has ceased

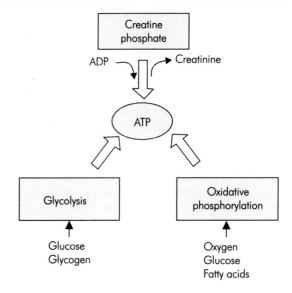

Figure MP.12 Metabolism and substrates in muscle contraction

The energy sources and substrates used during muscle contraction are summarised in Figure MP.12.

Metabolic substrates during contraction

The principal fuel for muscle metabolism is glycogen. The following points summarise substrate utilisation:

- Glycogen mobilisation is stimulated by Ca^{2+} and epinephrine
- Muscle glycogen only lasts about 10 min during moderate exercise
- For the next 30 min blood glucose and fatty acids provide substrate equally
- After this fatty acids become the predominant fuel

Muscle fibre types

Muscle fibres are classified according to their mechanical performance and their metabolic performance. Mechanical performance is reflected by maximal shortening velocity, which is dependent on the myosin–ATPase activity in the fibre. Metabolic performance is determined by whether ATP formation is mainly oxidative or glycolytic. A high oxidative capacity in a fibre will give it the ability to resist fatigue, since this will avoid the accumulation of an oxygen debt during prolonged contraction. On this basis three main types of fibre may be identified:

- Type I – slow oxidative fibres which are red in colour
- Type II – fast glycolytic fibres which are white in colour
- Type III – fast oxidative fibres

Type I fibres are metabolically and mechanically relatively slow compared with type II fibres, but they have greater oxidative capacity and are capable of sustained work rates over prolonged periods without incurring a significant oxygen debt. Type II fibres, on the other hand, are fast metabolically and mechanically, capable of intense work rates but only for short periods as they readily accumulate a significant oxygen debt. Functionally, type I fibres predominate in muscles associated with continuous slow sustained contractions, such as the paraspinal muscle columns responsible for maintaining posture. Type II fibres are found mainly in muscles performing short, rapid movements such as the oculomotor muscles and the small muscles of the hand. A comparison of the properties of these muscle fibres is given in Figure MP.13.

In practice, few muscles are made up exclusively of red or white fibres. Classically, sprinters have relatively more white fibres and marathon runners relatively more red. With periods of inactivity there is a relative increase in the number of white fibres.

NEUROMUSCULAR TRANSMISSION

Electrical impulses are transmitted from the motor neurone to the muscle by the release of acetylcholine (Ach). This transducer process is similar to that of synaptic transmission. Ach is the only neuro-transmitter involved in skeletal neuromuscular transmission. It diffuses across the junctional gap and interacts with specific receptors on the post junctional membrane of the motor end plates.

Neuromuscular junction (NMJ)

When the motor neurone reaches its termination, it becomes unmyelinated and branches into a number of terminal buttons or endfeet. At the same time the muscle membrane, opposite the endfeet, become thickened and invaginated to form junctional folds. Between the endfeet and the motor end plate is the junctional gap, structurally similar to the synaptic cleft. The whole structure is known as the NMJ (Figure MP.14).

Acetylcholine receptors

Ach receptors in the post junctional membrane of the

COMPARISON OF TYPE I, II AND III MUSCLE FIBRES			
Property	**Type I**	**Type II**	**Type III**
Colour	Red	White	Red
Diameter	Small	Large	Intermediate
Formation of ATP	Oxidative phosphorylation	Glycolysis	Oxidative phosphorylation
Mitochondria	Many	Few	Many
Glycogen content	Low	High	Intermediate
Glycolytic enzymes	Low	High	Intermediate
Myosin-ATPase activity	Low	High	High
Contraction speed	Slow	Fast	Fast
Myoglobin content	High	Low	High
Fatigue rate	Slow	High	Intermediate
Mitochondria	Many	Few	Many

Figure MP.13

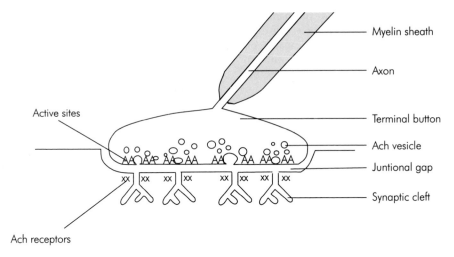

Myelin sheath

Axon

Terminal button

Ach vesicle

Juntional gap

Synaptic cleft

Active sites

Ach receptors

Figure MP.14 Structure of the NMJ

motor endplate are of the nicotinic type. A normal neuromuscular endplate on average contains about 50 million Ach receptors. They are situated at the crests of the junctional folds. The nicotinic Ach receptor is a protein with a molecular weight of about 250 000 Daltons and is made up of five polypeptide subunits: two identical α subunits, one β, one γ (replaced by ε in adult mammals) and one δ subunit. Each subunit is encoded by a different gene and has similar overall structure. The five subunits are arranged in a cylindrical fashion surrounding a central funnel-shaped pore, which is the ion channel (Figure MP.15). The receptor spans the membrane and possesses both hydrophilic and hydrophobic regions.

When Ach molecules bind to the receptors, they do so by binding onto specific binding sites on the α subunits. As a result, they induce a change in the configuration to the receptor so that the central pore opens, allowing Na^+ and other ions to pass down their concentration and electrical gradients. This sudden influx of Na^+ ions into the cell results in depolarisation.

Acetylcholine synthesis and storage (pre-junctional)

Synthesis of acetylcholine involves the reaction of acetyl-coenzyme A (acetyl-CoA) and choline, catalysed by the enzyme choline acetyltransferase. Acetyl-CoA is synthesised in the mitochondria of the axon terminals from pyruvate. About 50% of the choline is derived from the breakdown of Ach; the remaining is extracted from the extracellular fluid by a Na^+-dependent active transport process in the cell membrane which is the rate-limiting step in Ach synthesis. Choline

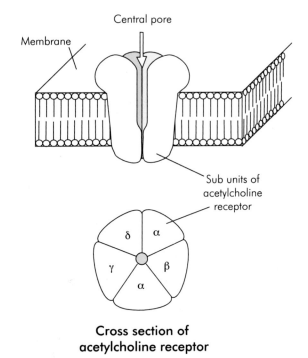

Central pore

Membrane

Sub units of acetylcholine receptor

δ α

γ β

α

Cross section of acetylcholine receptor

Figure MP.15 Acetylcholine receptor structure

acetyltransferase is originally synthesised on the ribosomes in the cell bodies of motor neurones and transported distally by axoplasmic flow to the nerve terminals, where high concentration can be detected. Enzyme activity is inhibited by acetylcholine but enhanced by nerve stimulation (Figure MP.16).

Ach molecules are stored in the vesicles situated in the nerve endings. Each vesicle contains about 4000

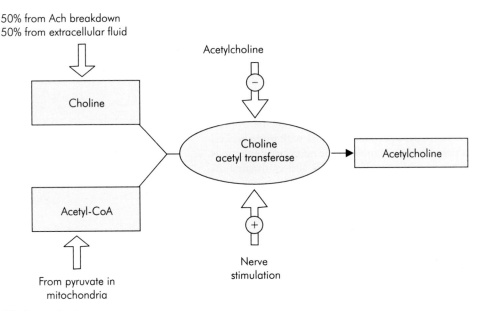

Figure MP.16 Acetylcholine synthesis

molecules of Ach. There appears to be different stores of vesicles that differ in their availability for release, depending on the level of demand (nerve stimulation). Thus there are the readily releasable store (80%) and the stationary store (20%).

Mechanism of neuromuscular transmission (junctional)

The vesicles situated in the active zone (that part of the terminal endfoot immediately opposite the junctional folds) spontaneously and randomly fuse with the pre-synaptic membrane and release Ach molecules into the NMJ. This process is known as exocytosis. Acetylcholine then diffuses across the NMJ and interacts with Ach receptors located on the post synaptic folds of the muscle membrane. This small spontaneous discharge is only sufficient to produce small transient electrical changes in the post synaptic membrane known as 'miniature end plate potential' or MEP. However, when the motor neurone is adequately stimulated, action potentials increase the permeability of nerve endings to Ca^{2+} ions. This increase in intracellular Ca^{2+} ion concentration triggers a marked increase in exocytosis of vesicles. This leads to an explosive release of Ach across the junctional gap increasing the Na^+ and K^+ conductance of the membrane. The sudden influx of Na^+ produces a de-polarising potential, known as 'end plate potential'.

Acetylcholine inactivation (post junctional)

For repolarisation to occur, it is necessary to remove Ach rapidly from the junctional gap. Ach is hydrolysed to choline and acetate. This reaction is catalysed by the enzyme acetylcholinesterase, also known as true acetylcholinesterase. This is found specifically at nerve endings, unlike pseudocholinesterase which is present in the plasma and does not involve in Ach breakdown at the NMJ.

Action potential generation and transmission in muscle

Each nerve impulse releases about 60 Ach vesicles. This amount is sufficient to activate about 10 times the number of Ach receptors required to produce a propagatable end plate potential. Thus, there is usually a 10-fold safety margin to protect normal neuromuscular transmission.

The electrical events and changes in ion permeability in skeletal muscle induced by the arrival of an action potential are similar to that in nerve tissue. However, the resting membrane potential of skeletal muscle is about –90 mV. The action potential lasts 2–4 ms and is conducted along the muscle fibre at about 5 m/s.

The potential change at the end plate depolarises the adjacent muscle membrane to its firing level, by transiently increasing Na^+ and K^+ conductance. Action potentials are generated on either side of the end plate and are conducted away from the end plate to the rest of the muscle. The muscle action potential then leads to depolarisation along the T-tubules and finally result in muscle contraction.

CENTRAL CONTROL OF MUSCLE TONE AND MOVEMENT

Skeletal muscle fibres contract in response to activity in α motor neurones of the anterior horn of the spinal cord. One motor axon innervates a number of fibres, the precise number depending on the task performed by that particular muscle. Muscle controlling fine movement such as the small muscles of the eye has fewer fibres per neurone than those with more general functions. In the eye muscles the neurone:fibre ratio is 1:15 whereas the anterior tibialis and gastrocnemius have ratios of 1:2000.

There is a strict order of recruitment of fibres in a given muscle contraction and for that particular contraction it is always the same. Oxidative fibres are innervated by the smaller neurones and it is these that are recruited first, the larger neurones and the glycolytic fibres coming in as the size or strength of the muscle contraction increases.

Muscle spindles and the γ efferent system

Good control of muscle tone and stretch is essential for the maintenance of posture and for accuracy of movements. This control is mediated by stretch receptors in the skeletal muscles, called 'muscle spindles'. These fusiform structures are scattered throughout the fibres of a skeletal muscle. They are small specialised structures composed of 4–20 intrafusal (within spindle) fibres and are supplied by both sensory (Ia and IIa afferents) and motor (γ efferent) nerves.

In the control of muscle tone and movement the spindles provide a feedback signal which tends to maintain a skeletal muscle at a desired length, or controls the rate at which a muscle lengthens or shortens. Thus the spindles provide a static signal (via IIa afferents) helping to maintain posture, and a dynamic component (via Ia afferents) controlling the rate of contraction and, hence, smoothness of movements. When the position of a muscle is disturbed by stretching, the spindles are also stretched which increases their feedback signal to the spinal cord. This increases α motor output and skeletal muscle tone opposing the original disturbance (Figure MP.17).

The γ efferent motor nerves to the spindles pre-tension the intrafusal fibres, which effectively sets their sensitivity. γ efferent tone is under the influence of higher centres in the central nervous system such as the cortex, basal ganglia and cerebellum. If γ efferent tone is high the spindles are taut and slight disturbances in skeletal muscle length elicit reflex contraction of the skeletal muscle. The skeletal musculature then appears

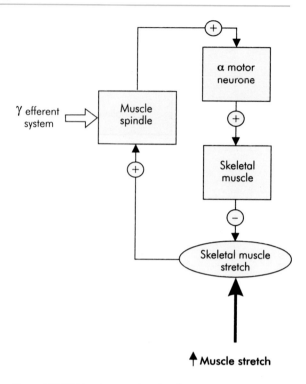

Figure MP.17 Muscle control and γ efferent system

to be clinically hypertonic. This can occur with upper motor neurone lesions such as those following cerebrovascular accidents. When γ efferent tone is low, muscular hypotonia results, as may occur with some cerebellar lesions.

Golgi tendon organ reflex

Another reflex that modulates contraction and relaxation of skeletal muscles is mediated by the Golgi tendon organs. These are situated in the muscle tendon just adjacent to the muscle fibres. The Golgi tendon organs also respond to muscle stretch but supply a feed back signal (via Ib afferents) to inhibitory neurones in the spinal cord. These neurones synapse with the α motor neurones, inhibiting them and reducing skeletal muscle tone during contraction. The Golgi tendon feedback signal also stimulates antagonist muscles of opposing groups to the inhibited muscle (Figure MP.18). The result is to smooth rapid or jerky muscle contraction. If a muscle is subjected to an excessive stretching force the Golgi tendon organ reflex can cause virtual relaxation of the muscle, thus helping to protect it against mechanical rupture. The Golgi tendon organ reflex is thus an example of a positive feedback loop.

The combination of Golgi tendon organ and muscle

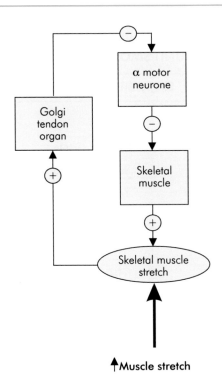

↑Muscle stretch

Figure MP.18 Golgi tendon organ reflex

spindle activity provides a dynamic balance of two opposing signals, which controls the α motor neurone output. This control has a static component helping to maintain posture and a dynamic component providing smooth and accurate movements.

SMOOTH MUSCLE

As the name implies, smooth muscles do not possess cross striations that are characteristics of the skeletal and cardiac muscles. Smooth muscles are innervated by the autonomic nervous system and thus are not under voluntary control. They play a vital role in the functioning of most hollow viscera and, in particular, the regulation of vascular resistance.

STRUCTURE

Each smooth muscle fibre is a spindle-shaped cell consisting of a single nucleus capable of cell division. Cell diameter varies between 2 and 10 μm. Smooth muscle fibre contains myosin, actin and tropomyosin, but unlike skeletal muscle there is no regular arrangement between these fibrils. There is also an absence of troponin and only a poorly developed sarcoplasmic reticulum. Compared with skeletal muscle, smooth muscle contains only one-third as much myosin but twice as much actin; however, the maximal tension achievable per unit of cross sectional area by smooth muscles is similar to that of skeletal muscle. Smooth muscles contain only a few mitochondria and cellular metabolism depends largely on glycolysis.

TYPES

Based on the electrical characteristics, smooth muscles can generally be divided into two prototypes: single or multi-unit. However, these only represent the two extremes of a spectrum exhibited by smooth muscles.

Single-unit smooth muscles

The membranes can propagate action potentials from cell to cell through low resistance bridges (or gap junctions) and may exhibit spontaneous action potentials. All muscle fibres may undergo electrical and mechanical activity in a synchronous manner. In other words, the whole muscle responds to stimulation as a single unit. In addition, the contractility of this type of muscle is also influenced by neurohumoral factors. The nerve terminals are often restricted to regions of the muscle that contain the pacemaker cells. By regulating the activity of the pacemaker cells, the activity of the entire muscle can thus be controlled. Single unit smooth muscles are characteristically found in the gastro-intestinal tract, uterus, ureters and small-diameter blood vessels.

Multi-unit smooth muscles

Multi-unit smooth muscles rarely contain gap junctions, compared with single unit smooth muscles, but are densely innervated by autonomic nerve fibres. Each muscle fibre responds independently of its adjacent fibre and therefore behaves as independent multiple units. Contractility of the whole muscle depends on the number of muscle fibres activated and on the frequency of nerve stimulation. Spontaneous action potentials do not usually occur in multi-unit smooth muscles. Stretching does not induce contraction in this type of muscle. Examples of this type of muscle can be located in the large airways, most blood vessels, the iris and ciliary body.

SMOOTH MUSCLE CONTRACTION

Action potential will either release Ca^{2+} from the sarcoplasmic reticulum or open up voltage gated Ca^{2+} channels in the cell membrane. As in the case of striated muscle, the latter may trigger off further Ca^{2+} release from the sarcoplasmic reticulum. It is this change in the intracellular Ca^{2+} concentration that plays a pivotal role in the contractile activity of smooth muscle. Unlike skeletal muscle where calcium binds to troponin, calcium binds to calmodulin in the cytoplasm in smooth muscle. The calmodulin–Ca^{2+} complex then activates myosin light chain kinase, which uses ATP to phosphorylate the myosin cross bridges. The latter then binds to actin filaments to produce contraction.

In single unit smooth muscle, the membrane potential is often unstable and recurrent de-polarisation leads to continuous, irregular contractions. Because of this instability, there is no constant 'resting' potential. The smooth muscle cell depolarises until it reaches the threshold potential and produces an action potential. During depolarisation, voltage-gated Ca^{2+} channels open, generating calcium action potentials rather than sodium action potentials as in the case of skeletal muscle.

PROPERTIES

Certain smooth muscle cells have the propensity to de-polarise spontaneously. In the absence of extrinsic neurohumoral stimulation these cells are known as pacemaker cells. The change in membrane potential is known as pacemaker potential. This property is not unique to smooth muscles, occurring also in cardiac pacemaker cells and a few neurones in the central nervous system.

A series of such action potentials may occur leading to a tonic state of contractile activity. This tonic state is also known as 'smooth muscle tone'.

Stretching of the muscle causes depolarisation and reinforces the existing tone. Stretching opens mechano-sensitive ion channels, which may lead to membrane de-polarisation and induces contraction. It is this property that is involved in autoregulation of blood flow. However, if the muscle is held at the greater length after stretching, the tension gradually decreases. It can be demonstrated that the tension generated by a particular length of smooth muscle progressively decreases when the muscle is kept stretched. This property is referred to as the plasticity of smooth muscle.

The similarities and differences between single unit and multi-unit smooth muscle are summarised in Figure MP.19.

EXTRINSIC CONTROL

Unlike striated muscle whereby contraction is an all or

DIFFERENCES BETWEEN SINGLE AND MULTI-UNIT SMOOTH MUSCLE

Property	Single-unit SM	Multi-unit SM
Gap junctions	Yes	Few
Pacemaker potentials	Yes	No
Tone	Yes	No
Neuro-control	Yes	Yes
Hormonal control	Yes	Yes
Stretch induced contraction	Yes	No

Figure MP.19

none response, in the case of smooth muscle, the contractile state is graded according to the concentration of intracellular calcium, which in turn is controlled by graded changes in the membrane potential, not just to action potentials. These graded changes are influenced by extrinsic factors as follows:

- Autonomic nervous system – post ganglionic fibres from sympathetic and parasympathetic nerves innervate smooth muscle. A single smooth muscle fibre may be influenced by neurotransmitter from more than one neurone. Both excitatory or inhibitory response can be elicited depending not only on the type of neurotransmitter but also on the type of receptors present on the membrane
- Hormones – the plasma membrane of smooth muscle cells contains receptors for a variety of hormones. Binding of a hormone to the membrane receptors may result in the opening or closure of ion channels. In addition, it may release second messengers that may result in the release of calcium from the sarcoplasmic reticulum. This in turn may increase or decrease contractile activity
- Local humoral factors – local factors such as paracrine agents, oxygen concentration, pH, osmolarity and ionic composition of the ECF surrounding the smooth muscle may also exert marked influence on the intracellular calcium concentration

COMPARISON BETWEEN SKELETAL, CARDIAC AND SMOOTH MUSCLE

Although the basic contractile mechanisms of the

various types of muscle are based on interaction between myosin and actin filaments, their ultimate physiological functions differ significantly. This variation is reflected in gross as well as microscopic differences between skeletal, cardiac and smooth muscle. Figure MP.20 highlights some differences in structure and function between the different types of muscle:

COMPARISON BETWEEN SKELETAL, CARDIAC AND SMOOTH MUSCLE

	Skeletal muscle	Cardiac muscle	Smooth muscle
Structure			
Motor endplate	Present	None	None
Mitochondria	Few	Many	Few
Sarcomere	Yes	Yes	None
Sarcoplasmic reticulum	Extensively developed	Well developed	Poorly developed
Syncytium	None	Yes	Yes
Function			
Pacemaker	No	Yes (fast)	Yes (slow)
Response	All or none	All or none	Graded
Tetanic contraction	Yes	No	Yes

Figure MP.20

SECTION 2: 5
CARDIAC PHYSIOLOGY

J. L. C. Swanevelder

THE HEART
Cardiac muscle
Excitation–contraction coupling

CARDIAC ACTION POTENTIALS
Fast response action potentials
Slow response action potentials
Conduction system
Conduction system defects

THE ELECTROCARDIOGRAM
ECG waves and the cardiac cycle
ECG leads
Calculation of the heart rate
Calculation of the cardiac axis
Physiological arrhythmias
Effects of electrolyte changes on the ECG

THE CARDIAC CYCLE
Ventricles
Systolic function
Diastolic function
Cardiac valves
Heart sounds and murmurs
Central venous pressure

THE CARDIAC PUMP
Ventricular pressure–volume loop
End diastolic pressure–volume relationship
End systolic pressure–volume relationship
Cardiac output

CONTROL OF CARDIAC PUMP FUNCTION
Stroke volume
Heart rate

CARDIOVASCULAR COUPLING
Ventriculo-arterial coupling
Ventriculovenous coupling

CARDIAC FAILURE

THE HEART

The cardiovascular system acts as a transport system for the tissues and has the following functions:

- Supply of oxygen and removal of CO_2
- Delivery of nutrients and removal of metabolic waste products
- Delivery of hormones and vaso-active substances to target cells

The heart is the driving force behind this system and can be considered a transducer that converts chemical energy into mechanical energy. It consists of a right-sided low-pressure pump and a left-sided high-pressure pump. Each of these pumps is composed of an atrium and a ventricle. The atria prime the ventricles, which in turn eject the cardiac output (CO) into either the pulmonary or the systemic circulation.

CARDIAC MUSCLE

Cardiac muscle is striated, the striations being due to the structure of the contractile intracellular myofibrils. The myofibrils are composed of sarcomere units which are identical to those of skeletal muscle, composed of thick and thin filaments arranged to give the characteristic Z line, A band and I band striations. The thick filaments are composed of myosin molecules, whose tails are linked to form the filament leaving the actin binding 'heads' of the molecules free. Each thick filament is surrounded by six thin filaments composed of a double spiral of actin molecules in combination with tropomyosin and troponin. These thin filaments form a hexagonal tube around the thick myosin filament. Contraction of the sarcomere is then produced by a coupling and de-coupling reaction between the myosin heads and actin filaments, which results in a 'walking' action of the myosin heads along the thin filaments and causes the thick filaments to slide along the axis of the actin tubes. The actin–myosin coupling and de-coupling reaction lies at the heart of the contractile process and is fuelled by ATP and Ca^{2+}.

Each cardiac muscle cell is surrounded by a cell membrane, the sarcolemma. This forms invaginations penetrating deeply into the cell, which are called transverse or T tubules. These tubules are located at the Z-lines and spread the action potential (AP) into the interior of the muscle cell. A system of closed cisterns and tubules, the sarcoplasmic reticulum (SR), surrounds each myofibril, the cisterns being closely related to the T tubules. The SR acts as a reversible intracellular store for calcium ions.

Differences between cardiac muscle and skeletal muscle

Cardiac muscle differs from skeletal muscle in that the individual cells or fibres are tightly coupled, mechanically and electrically, to form a functional syncytium. This is achieved by branching and interdigitation of the cells and specialised end-to-end membrane junctions called intercalated disks. Intercalated disks are located at positions corresponding to Z lines (Figure HE.1). Functionally the result is an all-or-nothing contractile response of the myocardium when stimulated. Cardiac muscle is not a true syncytium as each cardiac muscle cell has a single nucleus and is surrounded by the sarcolemma. A further difference lies in the electrically conductive characteristics of the cardiac muscle fibres that offer a low resistance to the propagation of AP along the axis of muscle cells due to the intercalated disks. The intercalated disks allow rapid transmission of AP between cells via gap junctions that are composed of connections or open channels connecting the cytosol of adjacent cells. Cardiac muscle cells contain much greater numbers of packed mitochondria and are more richly supplied with capillaries than skeletal muscle, since the myocardium cannot afford to incur an oxygen debt by using anaerobic metabolism.

EXCITATION–CONTRACTION COUPLING

This term describes the events initially triggered by an AP and which culminate in contraction of a myofibril. Propagation of an AP along the sarcolemma and into the muscle cell through the T tubule system causes calcium ions (Ca^{2+}) to enter the cell through voltage-dependent channels, receptor-dependent channels and also by passive diffusion across the sarcolemma. This initial rise in Ca^{2+} triggers further release of Ca^{2+} from the sarcoplasmic reticulum. As a result, intracellular Ca^{2+} levels increase from resting values of 10^{-7} mmol/l to concentrations of 10^{-4} mmol/l (Figure HE.2). The released calcium acts on the thin filaments, binding to troponin and causing tropomyosin to move and reveal the actin binding sites for the myosin heads. This enables the myosin heads to attach themselves to the actin filaments and contraction commences. Contraction proceeds by a 'walk-along' or 'ratchet' process, in which ATP is hydrolysed to ADP by ATPase in the myosin head. The energy released produces the 'powerstroke' that slides the myosin on the actin.

The strength of cardiac muscle contraction is highly dependent on the calcium concentration in the extracellular fluid. At the end of the AP plateau the

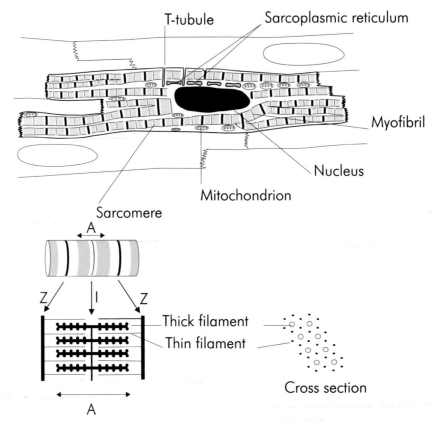

Figure HE.1 Cardiac muscle structure

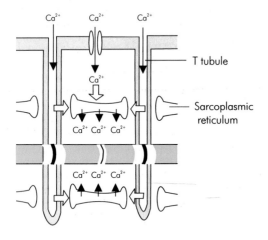

Figure HE.2 T tubule and sarcoplasmic reticulum structure

calcium flow into the cell decreases, and the intracellular Ca^{2+} is actively pumped back into the sarcoplasmic reticulum and T tubules by a $Ca^+Mg^+ATPase$ pump. The chemical interaction between actin and myosin ceases and the muscle relaxes until the next AP.

CARDIAC ACTION POTENTIALS

An action potentials (AP) is a spontaneous depolarisation of the membrane of an excitable cell, usually in response to a stimulus. Two different types of AP are found in the heart: fast and slow responses. In the myocardium two cell types produce fast response AP: contractile myocardial cells and conduction system cells. Slow response AP are normally produced by the pacemaker cells in the sinoatrial (SA) node and the atrioventricular (AV) node. These pacemaker cells spontaneously depolarise to produce slow response AP, exhibiting a property called automaticity.

FAST RESPONSE ACTION POTENTIALS

The fast response AP of the cardiac muscle cell can be divided into five distinct phases (Figure HE.3):

- Phase 0 – initial rapid depolarisation/upstroke
- Phase 1 – early rapid repolarisation
- Phase 2 – prolonged plateau phase
- Phase 3 – final rapid repolarisation
- Phase 4 – resting membrane potential (RMP)

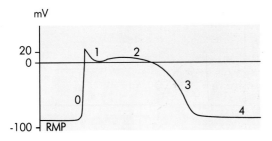

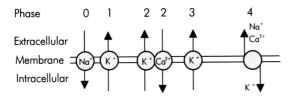

Figure HE.3 Fast response action potential

Resting membrane potential

The RMP is the electrical potential across the cell membrane during diastole and is about –90 mV, the intracellular membrane surface being negative with respect to the extracellular surface. RMP is maintained by the permeability properties of the cell membrane that retains negative ions in the cell but allows positive ions to diffuse out. The cell membrane is impermeable to negatively charged ions such as proteins, sulphates and phosphates, which, therefore, remain intra-cellularly. In contrast, membrane permeability to potassium is higher, allowing it to diffuse out of the cell under its concentration gradient of about 30:1. Potassium diffuses out of the cell until an equilibrium is reached at which the electrostatic attraction of the retained anions balances the chemical force moving the potassium down its concentration gradient out of the cell. This equilibrium is expressed mathematically by the Nernst equation in the following way:

$$\text{Electrostatic force} = \text{Chemical force}$$

or

$$\text{Equilibrium potential} = \frac{RT}{FZ_K} \times \log_e \frac{[K^+_I]}{[K^+_o]}$$

where

$[K^+_I]$ = potassium concentration inside cell membrane
$[K^+_o]$ = potassium concentration outside cell membrane
R = gas constant
T = absolute temperature

F = Faraday's constant
Z_K = valency of potassium

Thus the membrane potential due to

$$K^+ = 62 \times \log_e \frac{[K^+_I]}{[K^+_o]}$$

Thus, as RMP is due mainly to the distribution and diffusion of potassium ions (below), it can be said that:

$$RMP = 62 \times \log_e \frac{[5]}{[150]}$$
$$= -94 \text{ mV.}$$

The intracellular–extracellular concentration gradient of potassium must be maintained if RMP is to stay constant. This is achieved by the active transport of potassium from the extracellular fluid to the intracellular space by a Na$^+$K$^+$ATPase pump.

Other ions also contribute to RMP by producing transmembrane potentials due to the balance between chemical and electrostatic forces acting on them. For instance, sodium will diffuse across the cell membrane in the opposite direction to potassium (i.e. extra- to intracellular) because of the normal resting sodium concentration gradient. Accordingly, this movement of sodium into the cell will reduce the membrane potential set up by potassium. However, because membrane permeability to sodium under resting conditions is relatively low, this effect is small, merely reducing the membrane potential by about 4 mV. Similarly, the cell membrane is relatively impermeable to other ions in the resting state, and, therefore, the RMP is primarily determined by the intra-extracellular distribution of potassium ions.

To summarise, RMP is maintained by three mechanisms:

- Retention of many intracellular anions (proteins, phosphates and sulphates) to which the cell membrane is not permeable
- The resting cell membrane is almost 100 times more permeable to potassium than sodium, allowing potassium to flow down its concentration gradient out of the cell while keeping sodium extracellular
- Maintenance of an intracellular–extracellular concentration gradient for potassium ions by a Na$^+$K$^+$ATPase pump. This transports potassium actively into the cell and sodium out of the cell (three Na$^+$ ions for every two K$^+$ ions) and is dependent on energy supplied by the hydrolysis of ATP

The fast response AP is described by the following phases:

Phase 0 – rapid depolarisation

An AP is produced when an electrical stimulus increases RMP (causes it to become less negative) to a threshold potential (TP). At this value, fast sodium channels open for a very short period and potassium channels close. Sodium rapidly enters the cell under the influence of its concentration gradient and the electrostatic attraction of the intracellular anions, to make the inside positive in comparison with the outside by +20 mV. At the end of this stage, the sodium channels close. This phase coincides with the 'all-or-nothing' depolarisation of the myocardium and the QRS complex of the ECG

Phase 1 – early rapid repolarisation

This phase describes a brief fall in membrane potential towards zero following the rapid rise in phase 0. This occurs due to the start of potassium flow out of the cell under the positive intracellular electrical gradient and chemical gradients. At the same time slow, L type, Ca^{2+} channels open, providing a prolonged influx of calcium ions which maintains the positive intracellular charge There is also movement intracellularly of chloride following sodium into the cell along the electrical gradient. This leads to an initial rapid repolarisation of the cell membrane to just above 0 mV.

Phase 2 – plateau phase

During this phase, the continued influx of calcium via the slow L type Ca^{2+} channels is balanced by the continued efflux of potassium commenced in phase 1. This maintains the zero or slightly positive membrane potential and corresponds in time with the ST segment of the ECG.

Phase 3 – final rapid repolarisation

Potassium permeability rapidly increases at this stage and potassium flows out to restore the transmembrane potential to –90 mV. Although repolarisation of the membrane is complete by the end of phase 3, the normal ionic gradients have not yet been re-established across the membrane.

Phase 4 – restoration of ionic concentrations and resting state

During this phase ATPase-dependent ion pumps exchange intracellular sodium and calcium ions for extracellular potassium, thus, restoring the resting ionic gradients. When an equilibrium state is reached

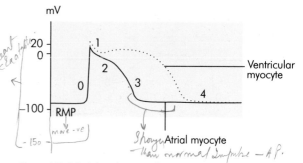

Figure HE.4 Atrial and ventricular myocyte action potentials

electrostatic forces equal the chemical forces acting on the different ions and RMP is re-established. This phase corresponds to diastole.

Atrial cell action potentials

Atrial myocyte AP are also of the rapid response type but vary from the ventricular AP in having a shorter duration plateau (phase 2). This effect is due to a much greater early repolarisation current (phase 1) in the atrial AP than in the ventricular case (Figure HE.4).

Excitability of cardiac cells

Excitability describes the ability of cardiac tissue to depolarise to a given electrical stimulus. It is dependent on the difference between RMP and TP, and, thus, changes in RMP will alter myocardial excitability. When RMP decreases (becomes more negative) this difference becomes greater and the heart becomes less excitable. Similarly, excitability is increased as the difference between RMP and TP decreases. Various factors affect excitability including:

- Catecholamines
- β-blockers
- Local anaesthetic agents
- Plasma electrolyte concentrations

Refractoriness

During rapid depolarisation (phase 0) and the early part of repolarisation (phases 1, 2 and initial part of 3), the cell cannot be depolarised to produce another AP regardless of stimulus strength. The sodium and calcium channels are inactivated and repolarisation must occur before they can open again. This is called the absolute refractory period. During the latter part of phase 3 and early phase 4 a stronger than normal impulse can lead to an AP. This is called the relative refractory period. For the duration of this period the heart is particularly vulnerable because an impulse at this time might produce repetitive, asynchronous depolarisation (e.g. ventricular fibrillation or tachycardia). The absolute and relative refractory periods together form the effective refractory period.

Pacemaker cells

The heart continues to beat after all nerves to it are sectioned. This happens because of the specialised pacemaker tissue (P-cell) that makes up the conduction system of the heart. These cells are found in the SA and AV nodes and also in the His–Purkinje system. Pacemaker cells exhibit automaticity (ability to depolarise spontaneously) and rhythmicity (ability to maintain a regular discharge rate). Normally atrial and ventricular myocardial cells do not have pacemaker ability and they only discharge spontaneously when injured. There are, however, latent pacemakers in other parts of the conduction system that can take over when conduction from the SA and AV nodes is blocked.

SLOW RESPONSE ACTION POTENTIALS

The AP produced when a pacemaker cell depolarises spontaneously is called a slow response AP (Figure HE.5). The most negative potential reached just before depolarisation is called the 'maximum diastolic potential' (MDP), which is only –60 mV compared with the RMP of –90 mV for a myocardial muscle cell. The reason for this is that the pacemaker cell membranes are more permeable to sodium ions in their resting state. Phases can be identified in the slow response AP which corresponding superficially to some phases of the rapid response, as detailed below although the underlying events differ.

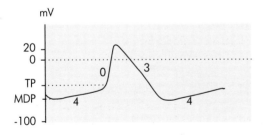

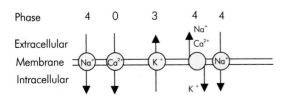

Figure HE.5 Slow response action potential

Phase 4 – restoration of ionic gradients and resting state

Pacemaker cells do not maintain a stable RMP, but instead depolarise spontaneously because of increased membrane permeability to cations during this phase. Sodium and calcium slowly 'leak' into the cell. Although potassium diffuses out simultaneously during this phase the inward 'leak' of sodium predominates to cause the membrane potential to gradually increase until a TP is reached at about –40 mV. This property is called spontaneous diastolic de-polarisation or pacemaker automaticity, and is directly related to the positive slope of phase 4.

Phase 0 – rapid depolarisation

Rapid depolarisation occurs at TP and is mainly due to calcium influx through transient or (T type) Ca^{2+} channels, which are slower than the rapid sodium channels responsible for phase 0 in the myocardial cell AP. The slope of phase 0 is, therefore, less steep than in the rapid AP case. The phase 0 slope in these cells is also reduced because of onset at a less negative transmembrane potential.

Phase 3 – repolarisation

In the slow response AP, repolarisation is effectively a single-phase equivalent to phase 3 in the rapid response. Effectively phase 1 is absent and phase 2 is very brief resulting in the absence of a plateau effect.

Differences between pacemaker and myocardial cell action potential

Pacemaker AP have the following features which differ from those of the myocardial cells:

- Less negative phase 4 membrane potential
- Less negative TP
- Spontaneous depolarisation in phase 4
- Less steep slope in phase 0 (dependence on T type Ca^{2+} channels)
- Absence of phase 2 (plateau)

Ion channels and action potentials

AP owe their basic characteristics to voltage controlled changes in membrane permeability to different ions. The main ions concerned are potassium, sodium and calcium, whose membrane permeabilities are dependent on various types of ion diffusion channel. These ion channels have been described in vitro by controlling and varying membrane potentials in different ion solutions, using a technique called 'patch clamping'. Different channels can then be identified by the changes in current produced as the channels open

VOLTAGE-CONTROLLED ION CHANNELS IN ACTION POTENTIALS

Action potential	Phase	Ion	Channel/gating mechanism
Rapid response (ventricular)	0	Na$^+$	Fast channels with 'm' activation and 'h' inactivation gates
	1,2,3	K$^+$	Transient outward current (i_{to}) channel
	2,3,4	K$^+$	Inward rectifier K$^+$ current (i_{K1}) channel
	2,3,4	K$^+$	Delayed rectifier K$^+$ current (i_K) channel
	2	Ca^{2+}	Slow (long lasting, L-type) Ca^{2+} channel blocked by calcium antagonists
Slow response (pacemaker)	0	Ca^{2+}	Transient (T-type) Ca^{2+} channel
	4	Na$^+$	Specific channels 'leaking' sodium current (i_f) into pacemaker cells

Figure HE.6

and close according to their control potentials. Some of these channels are outlined in Figure HE.6.

Automaticity of pacemaker cells

Automaticity is the ability of pacemaker cells to maintain a spontaneous rhythm and depends mainly on the leakage of sodium into the cell in phase 4 of the AP. This occurs via specific sodium channels that are activated when the membrane potential has become hyperpolarised i.e. reached about –50 mV during repolarisation. These channels then allow an inward hyperpolarisation current (i_f), which commences the spontaneous depolarisation of phase 4. The sodium current (i_f) is aided to a small extent by overlap of the decaying rapid depolarisation calcium current and opposed by extracellular diffusion of potassium. Automaticity is dependent on the slope of phase 4 of the AP which is influenced by the autonomic system and various drugs.

PACEMAKER DISCHARGE RATE

Pacemaker discharge rate is controlled primarily by the autonomic system. Control is mediated by changes in AP characteristics. The following characteristics are associated with variation of the discharge rate (Figure HE.7):

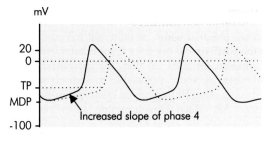

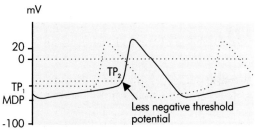

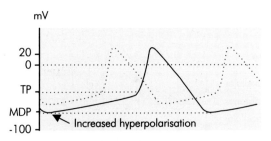

Figure HE.7 Changes in pacemaker action potential causing variation of discharge rate

- Slope of phase 4 in AP – an increase in the slope of phase 4 reduces the time to reach TP during spontaneous depolarisation and, thus, increases pacemaker rate. Similarly, a decrease in the phase 4 slope results in a slower pacemaker rate. Phase 4 slope can be varied by the autonomic nervous system
- Threshold potential – if this becomes less negative the pacemaker rate will decrease, drugs such as quinidine and procainamide have this effect
- Hyperpolarisation potential – if hyperpolarisation is increased, i.e. the membrane potential becomes more negative, spontaneous discharge will take longer to reach TP during phase 4 and the pacemaker rate will decrease. This occurs with increases in acetylcholine levels

CONDUCTION SYSTEM

The conduction system of the heart is composed of specialised cardiac tissues that form the following structures (Figure HE.8):

- SA node
- Atrial conduction pathways
- Atrioventricular node
- Bundle of His
- Bundle branches
- Purkinje fibres

The SA node is the normal cardiac pacemaker with a resting rate of between 60 and 100 per min. It is a group of modified myocardial cells located close to the junction of the superior vena cava with the right atrium. Blood supply is usually from a branch of the right coronary artery. Depolarisation spreads from the SA node through the atria and converges on the AV node.

The two atria are electrically separated from the two ventricles except for three internodal communication pathways, the anterior (Bachmann), middle (Wenckebach) and posterior (Thorel) bundles which

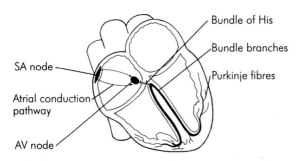

Figure HE.8 Anatomy of the conduction system

connect the SA node to the AV node. Th AV node is located in the right posterior part of the right atrium close to the tricuspid valve and the coronary sinus opening. Anomalous accessory pathways (like the bundle of Kent) can sometimes connect the atria directly to the ventricle or other areas of the conducting system and cause a pre-excitation syndrome with arrhythmias. Blood supply to the AV node is also from a branch off the right coronary artery. The AV node is connected to the bundle of His that distributes the impulse to the ventricles via the left and right bundle branches in the interventricular septum. There is a slight delay (about 0.13 s) of the impulse before it enters the AV node, inside the AV node and in the bundle of His. This delay permits completion of both atrial electrical activation and conduction before ventricular activation is started. The left bundle branch divides into the anterior and posterior fascicles. These bundles and fasicles run subendocardially down the septum and into the Purkinje system which spreads the impulse to all parts of the ventricular muscle. Conduction velocity through the bundle branches and the Purkinje system is the most rapid of the conduction system. The AP also begins endocardially and spreads out to the outside of the heart. However, repolarisation occurs from the outside to the inside. Ventricular activation is earliest at the apex and latest at the base of the heart, giving it an apical to basal contraction pattern.

CONDUCTION SYSTEM DEFECTS

Defects can arise in any part of the conduction system. Some examples of arrhythmias occurring due to lesions in different parts of the conduction system are shown in Figure HE.9.

THE ELECTROCARDIOGRAM

In an electrophysiological sense the heart consists of two chambers. The two atria function as a single electrophysiological unit and are separated from the bi-ventricular unit by the fibrous AV ring. Electrical communication between these two units is only possible through the specialised conduction system. The main electrical events of the cardiac cycle are the mass de- and repolarisation of the atria and ventricles. These can be thought of as waves of depolarisation (or repolarisation) that propagate through the cardiac tissues. As they propagate they generate potentials that can be sensed by electrodes on the skin surface. The electrocardiogram (ECG) is a recording of the signals picked up by a standard pattern of skin electrodes over the chest. When an electrode detects depolarisation

ARRHYTHMIAS DUE TO CONDUCTION SYSTEM DEFECTS

Site	Arrhythmia	Features
Sino-atrial node	Sick sinus syndrome	Sinus arrest, sinus bradycardia, tachycardias
Atrial conduction pathways	Wolff–Parkinson–White syndrome	Supraventricular tachycardia
Atrioventricular node	AV junctional rhythm	Bradycardia with abnormal P waves
Bundle of His	Complete (3° block) AV block	Bradycardia with dissociated P waves
Bundle branches	Bundle branch block	abnormal broad QRS complexes (> 0.12 s)

Figure HE.9

moving towards it, a positive deflection on the ECG is produced. Alternatively, if depolarisation is moving away from the electrode, it produces a negative deflection.

ECG WAVES AND THE CARDIAC CYCLE

The normal ECG consists of P, QRS, T and U deflections (Figure HE.10). Electrical activity precedes corresponding mechanical events during the cardiac cycle as follows:

- The P wave is associated with atrial depolarisation and contraction. The atria repolarise at the same time as ventricular depolarisation; therefore, the atrial repolarisation wave is usually obscured by the prominent QRS complex
- The P–R interval is between the beginning of the P wave and the start of the QRS complex. This represents the time from onset of atrial contraction to the beginning of ventricular contraction. The normal P–R interval is about 0.16 s but varies with heart rate
- The QRS complex reflects ventricular depolarisation and precedes ventricular contraction. A normal QRS complex has smooth peaks with no notches or slurs and has a duration < 0.12 s. The amplitude is dependent on multiple factors

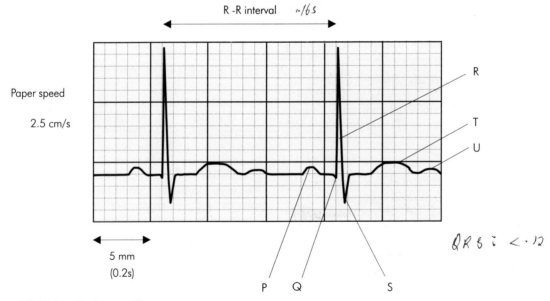

Figure HE.10 Sample electrocardiogram trace

including myocardial mass, the cardiac axis, the distance of the sensing electrode from the ventricles and the anatomical orientation of the heart

- The Q–T interval lies between the beginning of Q wave and the end of the T wave. This is about 0.35 s at a normal resting heart rate. The Q–T interval shortens with tachycardia and lengthens with bradycardia and can be normalised to a heart rate of 60 bpm, by using Bazett's formula for the corrected interval, Q–Tc,

$$Q\text{–}Tc = \frac{Q\text{–}T}{\sqrt{R\text{–}R}}$$

where:

R–R = interval measured between two R waves.

- The ST segment and T wave are associated with ventricular repolarisation. The ventricles remain contracted until a few milliseconds after repolarisation ends
- The U wave remains controversial in its origin. It may represent the slow repolarisation of the papillary muscles

Electrical axis of the heart

Electrical activity in the heart can be represented by a vector, since it possesses both amplitude and direction. A single or resultant vector can be drawn showing the magnitude and direction of the electrical activity in the heart at any instant. This will change continuously throughout the cardiac cycle. Thus, a vector can be drawn to represent maximum electrical activity for any wave of the ECG. During the QRS complex, a maximum vector is normally produced pointing downwards and to the left. This vector reflects peak electrical activity during mass depolarisation of the ventricles, and its direction is referred to as the electrical axis of the heart or the cardiac axis. Various factors may vary the direction of this axis including the anatomical position of the heart and different pathological conditions (e.g. left ventricular hypertrophy).

ECG LEADS

An electrical signal is a potential difference detected between two points. In the ECG, signals are recorded between two active surface electrodes or an active electrode and a common or indifferent point. Each signal recorded is called a lead and may have an amplitude of several millivolts. There are 12 conventional ECG leads that may be divided into two groups:

- Frontal plane leads

- Unipolar limb leads aVR, aVL and aVF

Standard limb leads I–III

These leads are recorded with a combination of two active electrodes at a time and are, therefore, bipolar leads. Each signal is recorded in the direction of the sides of an equilateral triangle with an apex on each shoulder and the pubic region, and the heart at its centre. This is called Einthoven's triangle (Figure HE.11).

- Lead I – the negative electrode is placed on the right arm and the positive electrode on the left arm
- Lead II – the negative electrode is placed on the right arm and the positive electrode on the left foot
- Lead III – the negative electrode is placed on the left arm and the positive electrode on the left foot

The ECG traces from these three leads are very similar to each other. They all record positive P waves, positive T waves and positive QRS complexes.

Unipolar limb leads aVR, aVL, aVF

Unipolar leads record the difference between an active limb electrode and an indifferent (zero potential) electrode at the centre of Einthoven's triangle (Figure HE.11). These signals are of lower amplitude than other leads and require increased amplification (hence referred to as augmented leads):

- aVR – the augmented unipolar right arm lead faces the heart from the right side and is usually orientated to the cavity of the heart. Therefore, all the deflections P, QRS and T are normally negative in this lead

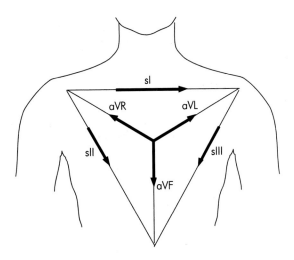

Figure HE.11 Einthoven triangle

- aVL – the augmented unipolar left arm lead faces the heart from the left side and is orientated to the anterolateral surface of the left ventricle
- aVF – the augmented unipolar left leg lead, orientated to the inferior surface of the heart

Precordial chest leads

These are horizontal plane, unipolar leads, placed as follows:

- V_1 – fourth intercostal space immediately right of the sternum
- V_2 – fourth intercostal space immediately left of the sternum
- V_3 – exactly halfway between the positions of V_2 and V_4
- V_4 – fifth intercostal space in the mid-clavicular line
- V_5 – same horizontal level as V_4 but on the anterior axillary line
- V_6 – same horizontal level as V_4 and V_5 on the mid-axillary line

Anatomical orientation of ECG electrodes

Although there is considerable variation in the position of the normal heart the atria are usually positioned posteriorly in the chest while the ventricles form the base and anterior surface. The right ventricle is anterolateral to the left ventricle. The ventricles consist of three muscle masses. These are the free walls of the left and right ventricles and the interventricular septum. Electrical activity in the left ventricle and the interventricular septum are predominant. ECG electrodes will pick up signals from the closest structures and those producing the greatest electrical signals. Therefore, ECG signals recorded from the anterior aspect of the heart are mainly due to activity in the interventricular septum with only a small contribution from the right ventricular wall. Since ECG lead signals reflect activity in different parts of the heart because of their position, they are said to 'look' at different aspects of the heart:

- sII, sIII and aVF look at the inferior surface of the heart
- sI and aVL are orientated towards the superior left lateral wall
- aVR and V_1 face the cavity of the heart and the deflections are mainly negative in these leads
- Leads V_{1-6} are orientated towards the anterior wall. V_1 and V_2 are anterior leads, V_3 and V_4 are septal leads, V_5 and V_6 are lateral leads
- V_1 and V_2 examines the right ventricle, while V_{4-6} are orientated towards the septum and left ventricle

There is no lead orientated directly to the posterior wall of the heart.

CALCULATION OF THE HEART RATE

The heart rate (bpm) can be determined from the ECG by measuring the time interval (s) between two successive beats (R–R interval), and dividing this into 60 s. Thus,

if R–R interval = 0.6 s
heart rate = 60/0.6
= 100 bpm.

The time scale of the ECG depends on the recording paper speed. Normal paper speed is 2.5 cm/s, meaning that each large square (5 mm) of the ECG trace represents 0.2 s (Figure HE.10). In the above example, the R–R interval is three large squares (15 mm), which is equal to 0.6 s. If the R–R interval were to become five large squares (1 s) this would give a heart rate of 60 bpm.

CALCULATION OF THE CARDIAC AXIS

The direction of the electrical axis of the heart is usually calculated in the frontal plane only and can be done using two of the frontal ECG leads (these are the standard limb and unipolar limb leads). It is determined as an angle referred to the axes shown in Figure HE.12, the normal range lying between 0 and $+90°$.

The cardiac vector, like any vector, can be resolved to give an effect or 'component' in any given direction. The amplitudes of the QRS complexes in the frontal leads represent components of the cardiac vector in the direction of the leads. The cardiac axis can, therefore,

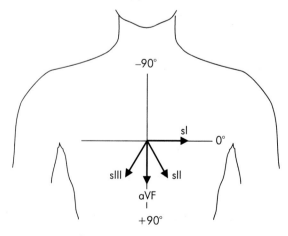

Figure HE.12 Reference axes and leads sI–III

be found by the vector summation of any two of these components to find their resultant (here sI and aVF are taken for convenience since they lie at 0 and 90° respectively). The direction of the cardiac axis is then given by the angle (theta), of the resultant. A simple algorithm is presented to determine the cardiac axis from sI and aVF.

Calculation algorithm for cardiac axis

An example illustrating the calculation of the cardiac axis from ECG leads sI and aVF is shown in Figure HE.13. To obtain the axis:

- Determine the amplitudes of the QRS complexes in sI and aVF by subtracting the height of the S wave from the height of the R wave in each lead
- Construct a rectangle with the sides in proportion to the amplitudes of sI and aVF. The diagonal then represents the resultant of sI and aVF (i.e. the cardiac vector)
- Determine the direction of the cardiac axis is from

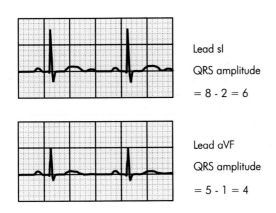

Lead sI

QRS amplitude

= 8 - 2 = 6

Lead aVF

QRS amplitude

= 5 - 1 = 4

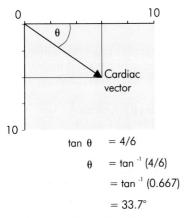

$$\tan \theta = 4/6$$
$$\theta = \tan^{-1} (4/6)$$
$$= \tan^{-1} (0.667)$$
$$= 33.7°$$

the angle θ by taking the tangent of θ as the ratio of

Figure HE.13 Calculation of cardiac axis

[amplitude of aVF]/[amplitude of sI]

Cardiac axis estimation by inspection of standard limb leads

In practice, a rapid estimation of the cardiac axis can be made simply by inspection of the frontal ECG leads. Convenient leads to use are the standard limb leads sI, sII, sIII and aVF, which lie at 0, 60, 120 and 90° respectively.

Initially, some basic facts about the relationship between a vector and its components should be noted. The QRS amplitudes in these leads are components of the cardiac vector. The amplitude of a component depends on the angle between the component and the vector it is derived from. As this angle increases the amplitude of the component decreases. Note that:

- For angles < 90° the component is positive
- When the angle between vector and component is zero, i.e. the component is acting in the direction of the vector, the component is maximum and equal to the vector
- At 60° the amplitude of the component is half of the vector
- At 90° the amplitude of the component becomes zero
- For angles > 90° the component becomes negative

Applying these simple principles will confirm the following estimations. If:

- sII = 0, the cardiac axis is at –30° (left axis deviation)
- aVF = 0, the cardiac axis is at 0°
- sI = sII, then the cardiac axis is at +30° bisecting the angle between them
- sI and sIII are each half of sII, the cardiac axis is at +60°
- sI = 0, the cardiac axis is at +90°
- sIII > sII the cardiac axis is at >90° (right axis deviation)

MONITORING IN THE OPERATING THEATRE

During routine non cardiac surgery standard II and V_5 are usually used as continuous monitoring leads. The P wave is best detected in standard II that facilitates detection of junctional or ventricular arrhythmias. Chest lead V_5 is most sensitive to S–T segment changes and can warn of possible ischaemia. During cardiac surgery all six limb leads are connected for intermittent S–T segment examination and this can increase sensitivity for the detection of ischaemia.

PHYSIOLOGICAL ARRHYTHMIAS

A cardiac rhythm is defined by three characteristics:

- The anatomical origin – a description of where the rhythm originates anatomically, e.g. SA node, atria, AV node or ventricles
- The discharge sequence – a description of the pattern of electrical discharge, e.g. sinus rhythm, tachycardia, bradycardia, fibrillation
- The conduction sequence – a description of abnormalities in conduction of the discharge impulses to the myocardium, e.g. 2:1 SA block, complete AV block

Abnormal cardiac rhythms or arrhythmias can arise as a primary or secondary disorders. Acute arrhythmias occurring during the peri-operative period can seriously compromise perfusion. An arrhythmia must be correctly diagnosed and the precipitating causes should be removed before treatment is considered. Acute arrhythmias are more likely to be reversible. Chronic arrhythmias are usually disease related and relatively stable.

Some departures from a perfectly regular cardiac rhythm occur as a result, of normal physiological responses, as opposed to having an underlying pathological cause. These are outlined below.

Sinus rhythm

This is the normal rhythm for the heart. All other rhythms are arrhythmias by definition. In the normal adult heart sinus rhythm originates in the SA node, has a regular pattern of discharge at a resting rate of between 60 and 80 bpm. The conduction sequence occurs on a 1:1 basis from SA node to atria to AV node and to the ventricles. The resting rate for neonates varies between 110 and 180 bpm and gradually decreases with increasing age until it reaches the adult rate at about ten years of age.

Sinus arrhythmia

In healthy young patients with a regular breathing rate, the heart rate increases with inspiration and decreases with expiration. This is a normal finding called sinus arrhythmia. It is caused by an irregular fluctuating discharge of the SA node. During inspiration the stretch receptors in the lungs send impulses via the vagus nerves to inhibit the cardio-inhibitory centre in the medulla oblongata. This stimulates the sinus node increasing the heart rate. Sinus arrhythmia is characterised by normal P–QRS–T complexes with alternating periods of gradually lengthening and shortening P–P intervals.

Sinus bradycardia

This rhythm occurs when the SA node discharges at a rate lower than 60 per min, with normal P–QRS–T complexes. This is a normal phenomenon in fit, young athletes and may also occur during sleep. Sinus bradycardia can be associated with pathological conditions that include myxoedema, uraemia, glaucoma and increased intracranial pressure. Various drugs such as β-blockers, digitalis or volatile anaesthetic agents may also cause sinus bradycardia. Occasionally during sinus bradycardia, a ventricular ectopic pacemaker site can take over. This may cause premature ventricular contractions that will usually disappear when the sinus rate speeds up again. When the heart rate goes < 40 bpm it is likely to cause hypotension or decreased perfusion, and should be treated immediately with an anti-muscarinic drug, β agonist or pacemaker as required.

Sinus tachycardia

Sympathetic stimuli such as emotion, exercise, pain and fever increase the SA discharge rate to > 100 per min although the P–QRS–T complexes remain normal. It commonly occurs during the peri-operative period. Hypovolaemia can often causes a sinus tachycardia through the baroreceptor reflex. Certain pathological conditions such as anxiety, thyrotoxicosis, toxaemia and cardiac failure may also cause it. The administration of drugs like epinephrine, atropine, isoprenaline and many others may lead to sinus tachycardia. When the heart rate > 140 bpm there is not enough time for left ventricular filling and the patient becomes haemodynamically compromised. This should be initially treated by removal of the cause and thereafter pharmacologically.

EFFECTS OF ELECTROLYTE CHANGES ON THE ECG

The AP of the heart is dependent upon the sodium and potassium ion distribution across the cell membrane. Electrolyte abnormalities can often produce ECG changes. Some common electrolyte disturbances are described below with their effects on the ECG.

Hypokalaemia

Hypokalaemia makes the RMP of the cardiac muscle fibres more negative. The heart becomes less excitable, but automaticity increases. Moderate hypokalaemia (3–3.5 mmol/l) causes a prolonged PR interval, flattening of the T wave and a prominent U wave. In severe hypokalaemia (2.5 mmol/l) ST depression can be seen and late T wave inversion occurs in the precordial leads. The QT interval is often prolonged. None of these changes are exclusively associated with hypokalaemia.

Hyperkalaemia

Hyperkalaemia (> 5.5–6 mmol/l) is a potentially life-threatening condition, especially when the onset is acute. As the extracellular potassium concentration increases, the RMP of the cardiac cell membrane progressively becomes less negative moving towards TP. Initially this makes the cardiac muscle more excitable. However, a deterioration of the AP also occurs, with a reduction in rapid depolarisation and a loss of the plateau phase. This results in poor contraction of the cardiac muscle. At plasma levels of 6–8 mmol/l, ventricular tachycardia and fibrillation readily occur. As the RMP approaches the TP (plasma levels > 8–10 mmol/l) the muscle fibres become unexcitable and the heart finally stops in ventricular diastole.

The ECG starts to change when serum potassium level reaches 6.0 mmol/l. Initially a shortened QT interval and narrow, peaked T wave appears. Further potassium increases produce widening of the QRS complex and PR interval prolongation until the P wave disappears.

Hypocalcaemia   QT↑↑ , Vent Ectopics, V. Tach
                    ST↑↑

Hypocalcaemia produces a flat prolonged ST segment and QT interval. Advanced stages of hypocalcaemia may lead to increased ventricular ectopic activity and ventricular tachycardia.

Hypercalcaemia ← ↓ Conduction V'
                     shortens Reg period
                     VT, VF.

Hypercalcaemia makes the TP of cardiac muscle fibres less negative, decreases conduction velocity and shortens the refractory period. This increases the likelihood of coupled beats, ventricular tachycardia and ventricular fibrillation.

In acute hyperkalaemia immediate treatment with an IV bolus of calcium opposes the effects of the high potassium levels. At very high calcium levels (animal experiments) the heart will relax less during diastole and will eventually stop in systole (calcium rigor). ECG changes produced by hypercalcaemia are prolongation of the PR interval, widening of the QRS complex and shortening of the QT interval. The T wave is also broadened.

>PR, >QRS, ↓QT.

Hypomagnesemia → ↑↑ HR

Hypomagnesemia promotes cell membrane depolarisation and tachyarrhythmias since magnesium is necessary for the normal functioning of the cardiac cell membrane pump. ECG changes produced by hypomagnesaemia include low voltage P waves and QRS complexes, prominent U waves and peaked T waves.

Hypermagnesemia

Hypermagnesemia is associated with delayed AV conduction and, therefore, presents with a prolonged PR interval, wide QRS complex and T wave elevation at plasma levels > 5.0 mmol/l. Levels > 10 mmol/l may lead to a complete heart block and cardiac arrest.

THE CARDIAC CYCLE

Each cardiac cycle consists of a period of relaxation (diastole) followed by ventricular contraction (systole). During diastole the ventricles are relaxed to allow filling. In systole the right and left ventricles contract ejecting blood into the pulmonary and systemic circulations respectively.

VENTRICLES

The left ventricle pumps blood into the systemic circulation via the aorta. The systemic vascular resistance (SVR) is 5–7 times greater than the pulmonary vascular resistance (PVR). This makes it a high-pressure system (compared with the pulmonary vascular system) which requires a greater mechanical power output from the left ventricle (LV). The free wall of the LV and the interventricular septum form the bulk of the muscle mass in the heart. A normal LV can develop intraventricular pressures up to 300 mmHg. Coronary perfusion to the LV occurs mainly in diastole when the myocardium is relaxed.

The right ventricle receives blood from the vena cavae and coronary circulation, and pumps it via the pulmonary vasculature into the LV. Since PVR is a fraction of SVR, pulmonary arterial pressures are relatively low and the wall thickness of the right ventricle (RV) is much less than that of the LV. The RV, thus, resembles a passive conduit rather than a pump. Coronary perfusion to the RV occurs continuously during systole and diastole because of the low intraventricular and intramural pressures.

In spite of the anatomical differences, the mechanical behaviour of the RV and LV are very similar.

The cardiac cycle can be examined in detail by considering the ECG trace, intracardiac pressure and volume curves and heart valve function (Figure HE.14).

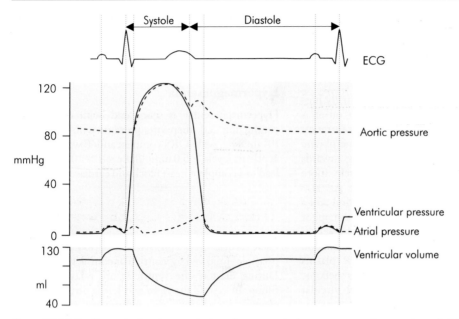

Figure HE.14 Cardiac cycle showing ventricular volume, ventricular pressure, aortic pressure and atrial pressure

SYSTOLIC FUNCTION

Systole can be broken down into the following stages:

- Isovolumetric ventricular contraction
- Ventricular ejection

Systole commences with a period of isovolumetric contraction initiated by the QRS complex of the ECG. During this brief period the volume of the ventricle does not change since both the AV and semilunar valves are closed. Isovolumetric contraction ends when the semilunar valve opens and ejection begins. The events during systole are described below and should be considered along with the ventricular pressure, aortic pressure and ventricular volume curves.

Left ventricular pressure

The QRS complex of the ECG initiates ventricular contraction. As the pressures in the left ventricle increases during isovolumetric contraction, it comes to exceed the pressure in the aorta. At this point the aortic valve opens and ejection begins. The aortic valve opens at about 80 mmHg. Ejection continues as long as ventricular pressure exceeds aortic pressure. The total volume ejected into the aorta is the stroke volume (SV). The ventricular pressure increases initially during ejection, but then starts to decrease as the ventricle relaxes. The gradient between ventricle and aorta starts to reverse at this point, since LV pressure has started to fall but aortic pressure is maintained by the momentum of the last of the ejected blood. When the

ventricular to aortic pressure gradient has reversed, the aortic valve closes and isovolumetric relaxation begins. The dicrotic notch on the aortic pressure curve (below) marks this point. The LV pressure normally reaches a systolic maximum of 120 mmHg. At the end of systole the LV pressure is described as the end systolic pressure and the LV volume is at its smallest (end systolic volume) about 40–50 ml.

Right ventricular pressure

This follows a similar course to LV pressure described above. The tricuspid and pulmonary valves dictate events, with ejection occurring into the pulmonary artery. Right ventricular pressure reaches a maximum of about 20–24 mmHg during systole.

Ventricular volume

Diastole commences in the left side of the heart with closure of the aortic valve and relaxation of the left ventricle. Since the mitral and aortic valves are both closed at this time the relaxation is described as isovolumetric. The ventricle contains 40–50 ml blood at this stage (end systolic volume). Isovolumetric relaxation ends with opening of the mitral valve, when a period of rapid filling of the ventricle begins, which lasts for the first third of diastole. After the initial period of rapid filling follows a period of passive filling called diastasis and flow continues passively into the ventricle providing up to 75% (60 ml) of the filling volume. During the last third of diastole the P wave of the ECG initiates atrial contraction which contributes the remaining 25% of filling to give an end diastolic volume of about 120 ml. The end diastolic volume of the ventricle is not always 120 ml, but can vary due to changes in venous return to the heart, contractility and the heart rate. A similar sequence of events occurs on the right side of the heart controlled by the pulmonary and tricuspid valves (Figure HE.14).

Aortic pressure curve

Ejection of blood into the aorta begins when the aortic valve opens. During ejection the aortic pressure follows the ventricular pressure curve apart from a small pressure gradient. This gradient is about 1–2 mmHg when the aortic valve normal. As ejection proceeds aortic pressure increases to a maximum (systolic pressure) and starts to fall as the LV relaxes. When the ventricular pressure has fallen below the aortic pressure, the aortic valve closes and ejection ceases. Following closure of the aortic valve, elastic rebound of the aorta walls gives rise to a small hump in the aortic pressure curve forming the dicrotic notch. This notch marks the beginning of diastole. During diastole the aortic pressure gradually falls to a minimum (diastolic pressure), due to the run off of blood into the systemic circulation.

Atrial pressure

Normally blood fills the right atrium (RA) via the superior and inferior venae cavae, continuously throughout the cardiac cycle. This flow is returned from the peripheral circulation and is called the venous return to the heart. On the left side of the heart, the left atrium (LA) receives blood from the pulmonary vascular bed via the pulmonary veins.

Passive filling of the atria produces RA pressures between 0 and 2 mmHg and LA pressures of 2–5 mmHg. During diastole atrial pressures follow ventricular pressures since the AV valves are open and both chambers are joined. Three waves or peaks are produced in the atrial pressure curve during the cycle. At the end of diastole the atria prime the ventricles by contracting and developing pressures between 0 and 5 mmHg. Atrial contraction is shown on the atrial pressure curve as a smooth peak immediately preceding systole, the 'a' wave. As systole begins the AV valves close and a brief period of isovolumetric contraction occurs, producing a second low-pressure peak, the 'c' wave. This is due to the AV valve bulging back into the atrium.

As blood is ejected during systole the atrium continues to fill with the AV valve closed and atrial pressure increases until early diastole when the AV valve opens.

At this point rapid filling of the ventricles commences and a sudden fall in atrial pressure follows. This gives rise to the 'v' wave (Figure HE.14).

DIASTOLIC FUNCTION

Diastole can be broken down into the following stages:

- Isovolumetric ventricular relaxation
- Rapid ventricular filling
- Slow ventricular filling (diastasis)
- Atrial contraction

Although diastole appears to be a passive part of the cardiac cycle it has some important functions.

- Myocardial relaxation – a metabolically active phase. One essential process is the re-uptake of calcium by the sarcoplasmic reticulum. Incomplete re-uptake leads to diastolic dysfunction due to decreased end diastolic compliance. The negative slope of the ventricular pressure–time curve during isovolumetric relaxation (termed [dp/dt max]) indicates myocardial relaxation. Increased sympathetic tone or circulating catecholamine levels give rise to an increased [dp/dt max]. This is known as positive lusitropy
- Ventricular filling – provides the volume for the cardiac pump. Most of the ventricular filling occurs during early diastole. There is only a small increase in ventricular volume during diastasis. As the heart rate increases diastasis is shortened first. When the heart rate > about 140 bpm, rapid filling in early diastole becomes compromised and the volume of blood ejected during systole (stroke volume, SV) is significantly decreased
- Atrial contraction – contributes up to 25% of total ventricular filling in the normal heart. This atrial contribution can become of greater importance in the presence of myocardial ischaemia or ventricular hypertrophy
- Coronary artery perfusion – greater part of left coronary blood flow occurs during diastole

CARDIAC VALVES

The cardiac valves open and close passively in response to the changes in pressure gradient across them. These valves control the sequence of flow between atria and ventricles and from ventricles to the pulmonary and systemic circulations. Valve timing in relation to the ventricular pressure curve is shown in Figure HE.15.

The AV valves are the mitral and tricuspid valves. These prevent backflow from the ventricles into the atria during systole. The papillary muscles are attached

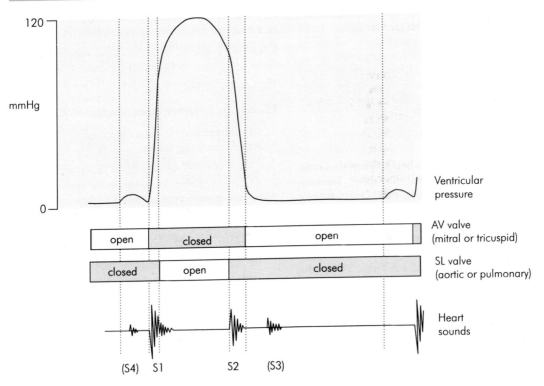

Figure HE.15 Heart sounds and timing

to the AV valves by chordae tendinae. They contract together with the ventricular muscle during systole, but do not help to close the valves. They prevent excessive bulging of the valves into the atria and pull the base of the heart toward the ventricular apex to shorten the longitudinal axis of the ventricle, thus, increasing systolic efficiency.

The semilunar (SL) valves are the aortic and pulmonary valves. These prevent backflow from the aorta and pulmonary arteries into the ventricles during diastole. The SL valves function quite differently from the AV valves because they are exposed to higher pressures in the arteries. They are smaller (normal aortic valve area is 2.6–3.5 cm^2 while normal mitral valve area is 4–6 cm^2), therefore, the blood velocity through them is greater. Disease in the cardiac valves may cause them to leak when they are meant to be closed, thus, allowing backflow or regurgitation. This situation leads to inefficiency in producing cardiac output (CO), since the work done by the heart has to increase to compensate for the backflow and yet maintain adequate CO. Mitral and aortic regurgitation are the most common regurgitant lesions.

Alternatively, the orifice of a valve may become narrowed or stenotic. This obstructs the flow of blood through it and requires increased pressure gradients to be generated across the valve to achieve adequate blood flows. In mitral stenosis the valve area can be reduced by > 50%. This causes the left atrium to contract more forcefully to maintain ventricular filling. In severe cases a valve area of 1 cm^2 can require the left atrium to produce peak pressures of 25 mmHg to produce normal CO. Aortic stenosis obstructs left ventricular output and increases the workload of the left ventricle. The stenosis can multiply the normal pressure gradient across the aortic valve during systole by ten times or more. When the aortic valve area decreases by 70% (< 0.8 cm^2), the stenosis becomes critical and systolic pressure gradients across the valve of > 50 mmHg may be required, to produce normal CO.

Differences in timing between left and right sides of the heart

Although the sequence of events on each side of the heart is similar, events occur asynchronously. This disparity in timing reflects differences in anatomy and working pressures between left and right sides of the heart. RA systole precedes LA systole; however, RV contraction starts after LV contraction. In spite of contracting later, the RV starts to eject blood before the LV because pulmonary artery pressure is lower than aortic pressure. Differences of timing also occur in the closure of the heart valves. These differences in valve timing lead to 'splitting' of the heart sounds.

HEART SOUNDS AND MURMURS

In the normal individual two heart sounds can be heard during each cardiac cycle. They are produced by closure of the valves that causes the ventricular walls and valve leaflets to vibrate, and also produces turbulence of the interrupted blood flow. The first sound (S1) occurs when the AV valves close at the start of ventricular systole and is best heard over the apex of the heart. The mitral valve normally closes earlier than the tricuspid by 10–30 ms. Thus, S1 is split with the mitral component occurring before the tricuspid component. The second sound (S2) corresponds to closure of the SL valves and is heard at the beginning of diastole. During inspiration the aortic valve closes before the pulmonary valve due to increased venous return which delays RV ejection. During expiration aortic and pulmonary valve closure is simultaneous, and S2 appears to be a single sound. S2 is louder when the diastolic pressure is elevated in the aorta or pulmonary artery.

Abnormal heart sounds can be heard under pathological conditions. Heart failure can cause a third heart sound (S3) to be heard in mid-diastole. This is due to rapid filling of a dilated non compliant ventricle following the opening of the AV valves. In conditions where stronger atrial contraction develops to help ventricular filling, a fourth heart sound (S4) may occur immediately before S1 (systole). This is thought to be due to ventricular wall vibration in response to forceful atrial filling.

When the cardiac valves undergo pathological changes abnormal sounds called murmurs can sometimes be heard. Under normal conditions blood flow is not turbulent but remains laminar up to a critical velocity. When blood flows across a narrowed valve, flow velocities are higher and turbulent, giving rise to a murmur. In the case of a 'leaking' or incompetent valve, turbulent regurgitant flow is produced which also creates a murmur. The most common murmurs occur due to faults in the mitral and aortic valves. The valve involved and the type of lesion (stenotic or regurgitant) can be identified by the timing of the murmur and the site on the chest wall where it is loudest. In normal individuals without cardiac disease (especially children) soft physiological systolic murmurs can often be heard.

CENTRAL VENOUS PRESSURE (CVP)

CVP is usually monitored in the large veins feeding the superior vena cava, i.e. the internal jugular or subclavian veins. The CVP waveform reflects right atrial pressure and, therefore, consists of 'a', 'c' and 'v' waves that correspond to atrial contraction, isovolumetric contraction and opening of the tricuspid valve, as described above. There are also two labelled downward deflections, the 'x' and 'y' descents, which occur after the 'c' and 'v' waves respectively (Figure

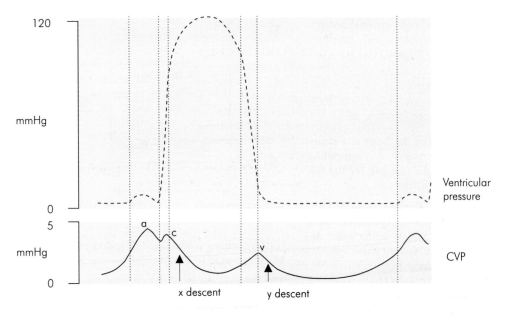

Figure HE.16 Central venous pressure waveform

SOME FACTORS AFFECTING THE CENTRAL VENOUS PRESSURE WAVEFORM

Factor	Change in CVP
Depleted intravascular volume	↓ mean CVP
Excessive intravascular volume ('overloading' with intravascular fluid)	↑ mean CVP
Cardiac failure	↑ mean CVP
Pericardial tamponade	↑ mean CVP
Bradycardia	More distinct 'a', 'c' and 'v' waves
Tachycardia	Fusion of 'a' and 'c' waves
AV junctional rhythm	Regular 'cannon' 'a' waves
3° AV block	Irregular 'cannon' 'a' waves
Tricuspid regurgitation	Loss of 'c' wave and 'x' descent Prominent 'v' waves

Figure HE.17

HE.16). The 'x' descent reflects the fall in right ventricular pressure when the pulmonary valve opens. The 'y' descent corresponds to the initial drop in atrial pressure caused by rapid ventricular filling when the AV valves open. Various pathological conditions affect mean CVP or alter the CVP waveform. For example, if the timing of atrial and ventricular contraction become dissociated (as in 3° block) the right atrium contracts against a closed tricuspid valve and produces prominent or cannon 'a' waves (Figure HE.17).

THE CARDIAC PUMP

VENTRICULAR PRESSURE–VOLUME LOOP

The mechanical performance of the heart as a pump can be summarised using a ventricular pressure–volume (PV) loop. An example for the left ventricle is shown in Figure HE.18.

The cycle starts at the end diastolic point (EDP). Isovolumetric contraction follows, represented by a vertical ascending segment which ends with the opening of the aortic valve. The ejection phase segment passes across the top of the loop from right to left. Ejection ends at the end systolic point (ESP) when the aortic valve closes. Isovolumetric relaxation follows next as a vertical descending segment ending when the mitral valve opens. The final lower segment

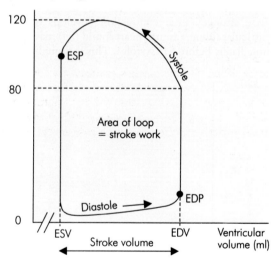

Figure HE.18 Pressure–volume loop for the ventricle

corresponds to ventricular filling and ends when the MV closes at EDP.

The PV loop can be used to derive several parameters reflecting ventricular function including SV, stroke work (SW), end diastolic volume (EDV) and end systolic volume (ESV).

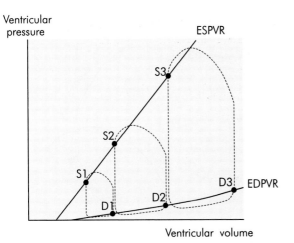

Figure HE.19 End diastolic and end systolic pressure–volume relationship curves

END DIASTOLIC PRESSURE–VOLUME RELATIONSHIP

On the ventricular pressure PV loop, the EDP records volume and pressure at the end of diastole. If different PV loops are plotted for a given ventricle, different EDP are obtained (D1, D2, and D3; Figure HE.19).

These points form a PV relationship for the ventricle at end diastole when plotted. This is called the end diastolic PV relationship (EDPVR). EDPVR is a useful indicator of diastolic function, and in particular ventricular filling performance, since its gradient is equal to the elastance or (compliance⁻¹), of the ventricle during filling. The steeper this gradient, the lower the compliance of the ventricle during filling. Over the normal range of ventricular filling volumes the EDPVR gradient is approximately linear and the ventricle is relatively compliant. As EDV increases and

the ventricle becomes more distended at the end of diastole, the EDPVR gradient becomes steeper showing a marked decrease in ventricular compliance to filling. Pathological conditions such as ischaemic heart disease and ventricular hypertrophy can shift the EDPVR up and to the left, demonstrating ventricular diastolic dysfunction (Figure HE.20).

END SYSTOLIC PRESSURE–VOLUME RELATIONSHIP

The ESP from several ventricular PV loops (S1, S2, S3) may be plotted to give an end systolic PV curve (Figure HE.21). This curve is the ESPVR. The gradient of the ESPVR curve represents the elastance of the contracted ventricle at the end of systole. This is partially dependent on how forcefully the ventricle contracts, and, hence, is related to ventricular contractility. The ESPVR curve is approximately linear under normal conditions. Increased non linearity is introduced under ischaemic or hypercontractile conditions and appears as a change in gradient and shift in the curve up or down.

Frank–Starling curve

The function of the heart as a pump is based on cardiac muscle. The contractile properties of cardiac muscle not only provide the engine to drive the cardiac pump but also give the heart an intrinsic ability to adapt its performance to a continually varying venous return. The mechanism underlying this adaptive ability is the Frank–Starling relationship.

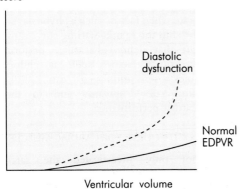

Figure HE.20 Effects of diastolic dysfunction on the end diastolic pressure–volume relationship curve

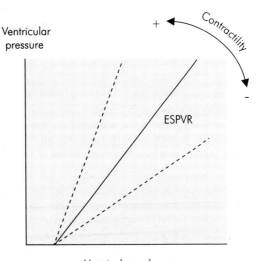

Figure HE.21 Effects of contractility on the end diastolic pressure–volume relationship curve

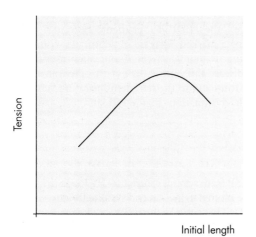

Figure HE.22 Frank curve for isolated muscle fibre

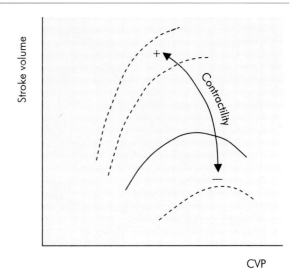

Figure HE.23 Ventricular function curve

THE FRANK CURVE

Frank demonstrated in isolated muscle fibre preparations that the tension developed on contraction, was dependent on the initial length of the fibre. As initial length increased from resting value, the tension developed during contraction, increased and reached a maximum. Above this, the tension declined as the sarcomeres became over extended (Figure HE.22).

THE STARLING CURVE

The above property of isolated cardiac muscle fibres can be applied to the muscle fibres in the walls of an intact ventricle, where the length of muscle fibres is related to the volume of the ventricle. In this case the tension per unit cross section (ventricular wall stress, T), developed in the wall during contraction, is dependent on the end diastolic volume. Laplace's law relates the wall stress to internal pressure in an elastic sphere; thus, the Frank relationship for an isolated muscle fibre translates into a relationship between intraventricular pressure and EDV during isovolumetric contraction. Effectively, the greater the ventricular filling volume, the stronger the contraction of the ventricle. A mechanism that gives the intact heart its built in ability to adjust to varying levels of venous return.

Starling confirmed in ejecting mammalian hearts that with a constant aortic pressure, an increase in EDV produces a more forceful contraction and an increase in SV.

THE FRANK–STARLING RELATIONSHIP

In the intact heart, a ventricular function curve (Frank–Starling curve) can be plotted to demonstrate the ability of the ventricle to vary its mechanical output according to its filling volumes. An index of mechanical output (such as SV) can be plotted against a measure of filling pressure (such as CVP) (Figure HE.23).

THE FRANK–STARLING CURVE AND CARDIAC FAILURE

The normal ventricle never fills to an EDV that would place it on the descending limb of the Frank–Starling curve. This is because of a decreased compliance of the ventricle that occurs at high filling pressures. Sarcomere length at optimum filling pressures (about 12 mmHg) is 2.2 μm; however, even if filling pressures are increased four-fold (> 50 mmHg) sarcomere length will not increase beyond about 2.6μm.

If the heart becomes pathologically dilated as in cardiac failure, ventricular function may then shift to the descending portion of the Frank–Starling curve and cardiac de-compensation ensues. Cardiac function can also deteriorate when factors such as hypoxia, acidosis or β-blockers shift the Frank–Starling curve down and to the right that depresses cardiac performance. Alternatively, other factors such as endogenous catecholamines or inotropes can shift the Frank–Starling curve upwards and to the left enhancing cardiac performance.

FORCE–VELOCITY CURVE FOR CARDIAC MUSCLE

Starling not only investigated the sarcomere tension–length relationship, but also looked at the interaction between muscle force and velocity. The force–velocity curve demonstrates that the force generated and the velocity of muscle shortening is

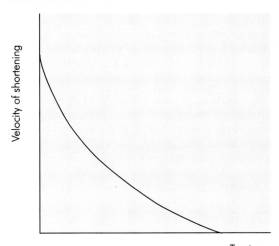

Figure HE.24 Force–velocity curve for isolated muscle fibre

inversely related. Changes in pre-load and contractility will influence this relationship by shifting the force–velocity curve (Figure HE.24).

Stroke volume and ejection fraction

SV is the volume of blood ejected by the ventricle with a single contraction and can be defined as the difference between the end-diastolic volume and the end-systolic volume in the following equation:

$$SV = EDV - ESV.$$

The normal SV is between 70 and 80 ml and may be normalised to take account of body size by dividing by body surface area (BSA). This gives a stroke index (SI) which is for a 70 kg normal person (BSA = 1.7 m²) is 30–65 ml/beat/m². SV can also be given as a percentage of the EDV. It is then called ejection fraction (EF), a formula for is:

$$\text{Ejection Fraction} = \frac{EDV - ESV}{EDV} = \frac{SV}{EDV} \times 100\%.$$

The normal EF is about 60–65% and is a useful index of ventricular contractility.

Measurement of stroke volume

VENTRICULOGRAPHY

This has been the Gold Standard for measuring ventricular volumes, to which less invasive measurement methods have been compared. However, it is a cumbersome procedure done in the catheter suite and is not appropriate for repeated estimations. Other techniques to measure LV volume and size include computed tomography, magnetic

resonance imaging and radionuclide scans, but none is practical in the peri-operative setting.

ECHOCARDIOGRAPHY

The end-systolic and end-diastolic areas can be measured by two-dimensional echocardiography to give an estimate of the SV. SV is then multiplied by the heart rate to obtain the CO. This technique is limited by the approximation made to transform the two-dimensional images of the ventricular into volumes.

TRANSOESOPHAGEAL ECHOCARDIOGRAPHY

A recent development has been the introduction of transoesophageal echocardiography (TOE). Several studies have found a good correlation between left ventricular areas measured by TOE and LV areas or volumes obtained by other techniques. The two-dimensional transgastric short axis view of LV at the level of the papillary muscles reflects LV filling reasonably well. Modern echocardiography includes the automated border detection method that displays the LV area throughout the cardiac cycle, together with the fractional area change (FAC) calculation, where:

$$FAC = \frac{\text{End diastolic area} - \text{End systolic area}}{\text{End diastolic area}}$$

The normal value for FAC varies between 50% and 70%.

THORACIC IMPEDANCE

A small alternating current of low amplitude and high frequency is introduced between two sets of electrodes around the neck and lower thorax. The resultant electrical impedance between the neck and thoracic electrodes is measured and represents the transthoracic impedance. Both ventilation and pulsatile blood flow produce changes in thoracic impedance. SV can be estimated by considering the pulsatile cardiac component of the impedance signal only. Cardiac output can then be calculated by measuring the heart rate and taking the product HR × SV. Although this technique is non invasive and can provide a continuous reading of CO, a significant degree of inaccuracy is present.

CARDIAC OUTPUT

Cardiac output gives a measure of the performance of the heart as a pump. It is defined as the volume of blood pumped by the LV (or RV) per min and is equal to the product of the SV and heart rate:

$$CO = SV \times HR$$

With a normal HR = 70–80 bpm and SV = 70–80 ml, the average CO of a 70 kg person varies between 5 and 6 l/min under resting conditions. To compare patients of different body sizes, CO can be divided by the patient's body surface area to give a normalised parameter called the cardiac index (CI):

$$CI = \frac{CO}{BSA}$$

BSA can be estimated from the height (cm) and weight (kg) of an individual and is quoted in m^2. The average 70 kg adult has a BSA = 1.7 m^2 and a CI = 3–3.5 l/min/m^2.

When the oxygen demand of the body increases during exercise, the CO of a young, healthy individual can increase up to five-fold. CO should always be evaluated with reference to the oxygen demand at the time.

Cardiac output measurement

In animal models CO can be measured directly by cannulating the aorta, pulmonary artery or any of the great veins and then using an electromagnetic or ultrasonic flowmeter. However, this is not appropriate in a clinical situation and CO is usually measured by indirect methods.

INDICATOR DILUTION TECHNIQUES

Thermodilution is at present the most commonly used method to measure CO at the bedside. A pulmonary artery catheter (PAC) is inserted, cold saline injected into the RA, and the change in blood temperature is measured by the PAC thermistor in the PA. The PAC is connected to an analogue computer, which calculates CO by using the modified Steward–Hamilton equation:

$$CO = \frac{V(T_B - T_I) \times K_1 \times K_2}{\int_0^\infty T_B(t)\, dt}$$

where:

V	=	volume of injectate
T_B	=	initial blood temperature (°C)
T_I	=	initial injectate temperature (°C)
K_1	=	density constant
K_2	=	computation constant

and

$$\int_0^\infty T_B(t)\, dt \;=\; \text{integral of blood temperature change}$$

CO is inversely proportional to the area under the temperature–time curve. This technique is popular because multiple CO estimations can be made at frequent intervals without blood sampling. The accuracy of the technique is influenced by several factors, which include intracardiac shunts, tricuspid regurgitation and positive pressure ventilation.

A modification of this principle is used in the 'continuous' CO monitor. A pulse of electrical current heats up a proximal part of the PAC creating a bolus of warmed blood. The temperature rise is sensed when the warmed blood passes a thermistor in the PA. A computer then calculates the 'area under the curve' and, hence, CO.

DYE DILUTION

This was the most popular technique prior to thermodilution. Indocyanine green is injected into a central vein, while blood is continuously sampled from an arterial cannula. The change in indicator concentration over time is measured, a computer calculates the area under the dye concentration curve, and CO is computed. Unfortunately recirculation and build up of the indicator results in a high background concentration, which limits the total number of measurements that can be taken. The dye is non toxic and rapidly removed from circulation by the liver.

FICK METHOD

The Fick principle states that the amount of a substance taken up by an organ (or the whole body) per unit time, is equal to the arterial concentration of the substance minus the venous concentration (a–v difference), times the blood flow. This can be applied to the oxygen content of blood to determine CO.

First, the steady state oxygen content of venous (CvO_2), and arterial blood (CaO_2), are measured. Then oxygen uptake in the lungs is measured over 1 min ($\dot{V}O_2$). Finally, the Fick principle is applied to calculate the blood flowing in 1 min:

$$\text{Cardiac output} = \frac{\dot{V}O_2}{(CaO_2 - CvO_2)}$$

Errors in sampling, and the inability to maintain steady state conditions limit this technique.

DOPPLER TECHNIQUES

Ultrasonic Doppler transducers have been incorporated into pulmonary artery catheters, endotracheal tubes, suprasternal probes and oesophageal probes. These probes can then be used to measure mean blood flow velocity through the aorta or any valve orifice. Using an estimation for the cross

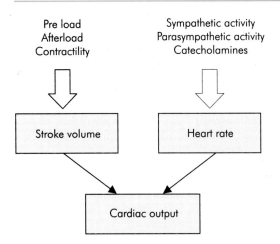

Figure HE.25 Control of cardiac output

sectional area of flow, the flow velocity–time integral, heart rate and a constant, CO can be calculated.

CONTROL OF CARDIAC PUMP FUNCTION

The product of SV and heart rate gives CO. The factors determining CO can, thus, be divided into those affecting HR and those that determine SV. Overall control of CO is a combination of the mechanisms controlling SV and HR. This is illustrated in Figure HE.25 and the individual control of SV and HR is considered in detail below.

Several factors determine SV. The three major determinants of SV are:

- Pre load
- Afterload
- Contractility

Overall control of SV is summarised in Figure HE.26. The above factors are based on physiological concepts arising from the performance of isolated muscle preparations. They have become useful in clinical practice when applied to the intact heart, but are difficult or impractical to measure directly. Hence more easily monitored parameters are used as practical indices. A summary definition for each of the above factors is given which consists of:

- Physiological definition – a theoretical definition for the parameter.
- Physiological index – a measurement from which the physiological definition can be derived
- Practical concept – a description of the parameter suitable for clinical use
- Practical index – a measurement used clinically for the parameter

Pre load

In clinical circumstances, 'pre load' remains loosely defined and has become synonymous with a range of parameters including CVP, venous return and pulmonary capillary wedge pressure.

A strict definition for pre load can be obtained from the Frank relationship between muscle fibre length and

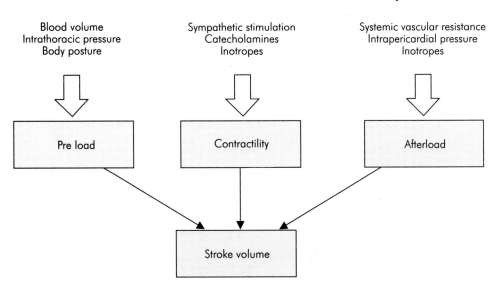

Figure HE.26 Control of stroke volume

SUMMARY DEFINITION OF PRE LOAD

- Physiological definition – Pre-systolic length of cardiac muscle fibres
- Physiological index – End diastolic volume
- Practical concept – Filling pressure of ventricles
- Practical index – CVP or PCWP

Various factors affecting EDV include:

Total blood volume

Body position

Intrathoracic and intrapericardial pressures

Venous tone and compliance

Pumping action of skeletal muscles

Synchronous atrial contribution to ventricular filling

Ventricular end diastolic compliance

Figure HE.27

developed tension. Here pre load is the initial length of the muscle fibre before contraction. In the intact ventricle the pre load would, therefore, be equivalent to the end diastolic volume, since the pre-systolic length of the myocardial fibres will be directly related to EDV. See Figure HE.27.

MEASUREMENT OF PRE LOAD

There are no convenient or practical methods of measuring EDV directly. Because of this EDP is often used when assessing the filling conditions of the intact ventricle. EDP is related to EDV by the ventricular end diastolic PV curve and is sometimes referred to as the 'filling pressure' of the ventricle. EDPVR is approximately linear at normal filling pressures, but the gradient (ventricular elastance = compliance^{-1}) gradually increases as filling pressure increases. EDP is, therefore, only a reasonable index of pre load under normal conditions.

In practice, EDP can be estimated on the left side of the heart, by measuring left atrial pressure (LAP), pulmonary capillary wedge pressure (PCWP) or pulmonary artery diastolic pressure (PADP). On the right side, preload is reflected by right atrial pressure (RAP) or central venous pressure. These measurements can be made using a pulmonary artery catheter, but the most common measurements used are CVP and PCWP as indices of right and left preload respectively. Interpretation of these estimates is subject to the following limitations:

- Ventricular compliance may not be normal as it can be reduced by factors such as myocardial ischaemia, ventricular hypertrophy or pericardial tamponade. In a non compliant ventricle, higher than normal filling pressures may be required to provide adequate preload
- The AV valve may be abnormal. The presence of mitral stenosis may require higher than normal filling pressures to achieve adequate preload in the left ventricle
- Positive intrathoracic pressures can be transmitted through to a pulmonary artery catheter and increase the mean PCWP reading. In the case of a ventilated patient, positive end expiratory pressure (PEEP) and the inspiratory pressure cycles can affect the PCWP signal
- Placement of the PAC in the dependent part of the lung can add a hydrostatic pressure component to a PCWP signal
- Increased pulmonary vascular resistance as in pulmonary hypertension can lead to higher than normal pulmonary artery diastolic pressures (PADP). This reduces the accuracy of the PADP as an estimate of left-sided pre load

Afterload

In an isolated muscle fibre preparation, afterload is defined as the tension developed during contraction. Thus, afterload is related to the mechanical resistance to shortening of the muscle fibre. In the intact heart, after-load becomes the tension per unit cross section (T), developed in the ventricular wall during systole.

SUMMARY DEFINITION OF AFTERLOAD

- Physiological definition – Ventricular wall stress developed during systole
- Physiological index – Systolic ventricular wall stress
- Practical concept – Intraventricular pressure developed during systole
- Practical index – SVR and MAP, PVR and MPAP

Factors which affect afterload include:

Systemic or pulmonary vascular resistance

Factors stimulating or depressing cardiac contraction

Intrathoracic pressure or intrapericardial pressure

Preload

Ventricular wall thickness

Figure HE.28

This can be related to the intraventricular pressure during systole, by applying Laplace's law for pressure in an elastic sphere as follows:

Intraventricular pressure $= \dfrac{2hT}{r}$

where:

h = ventricular wall thickness
r = radius of the ventricular cavity.

Afterload is, thus, a measure of how forcefully the ventricle contracts during systole to eject blood (Figure HE.28).

The normal ventricle has an intrinsic ability to increase its performance in response to increases in afterload, to maintain SV. If the afterload increases suddenly, it causes an initial fall in SV. The ventricle then increases its EDV in response to the change, which in turn restores the SV. This is called the Anrep effect.

MEASUREMENT OF AFTERLOAD

SVR, SV index and elastance may be used to give an estimate of afterload.

- Arterial pressure or ventricular pressures during systole normally follow each other and are indirect indices of ventricular wall tension. Arterial systolic pressure is often the available measurement, but its accuracy is limited if there is a significant gradient between aorta and ventricle, e.g. as in aortic stenosis
- Systemic vascular resistance is the most commonly used index of afterload in clinical practice and can be calculated from mean arterial pressure (MAP), central venous pressure and CO, as follows:

$$\text{SVR} = \frac{\text{MAP} - \text{CVP}}{\text{CO}} \times 80 \text{ dynes.s/cm}^5$$

The normal values for SVR ranges from 900 to 1400 dynes.s/cm^5. SVR is not a good estimate of after-load, since it is only one component determining after-load, and does not provide any index of intraventricular pressures generated during systole (i.e. how hard the ventricle is contracting). Clearly, if the ventricle only generates low intraventricular pressures by contracting softly, the afterload is low irrespective of SVR.

In a similar manner the pulmonary vascular resistance (PVR) may be calculated as an index of RV afterload, using mean pulmonary arterial pressure (MPAP), pulmonary capillary wedge pressure and CO:

$$\text{PVR} = \frac{\text{MPAP} - \text{PCWP}}{\text{CO}} \times 80 \text{ dynes.s/cm}^5$$

The normal PVR ranges from 90 to 150 dynes.s/cm^5.

CO, PAP and PCWP have to be obtained with a PAC to calculate SVR and PVR.

- Systemic vascular impedance is the mechanical property of the vascular system opposing the ejection and flow of blood into it. This is composed of two components. One is the resistive or steady flow component, which is the SVR (see above). This component is mainly due to the frictional opposition to flow in the vessels. The other component is the reactive or frequency dependent component which is due to the compliance of the vessel walls and inertia of the ejected blood. This component is dependent on the pulsatile nature of the flow and rapidity of ejection. A major part of this reactive component is formed by the arterial elastance (Ea).
- Arterial elastance is the inverse of arterial compliance and is a measure of the elastic forces in

SUMMARY DEFINITION OF CONTRACTILITY

- Physiological definition – Systolic myocardial work done with given pre- and afterload
- Physiological index – Ventricular stroke work index or maximum slope (dp/dt) of ventricular isovolumetric contraction curve
- Practical concept – Ejection fraction for given CVP and MAP
- Practical index – Ejection fraction

Figure HE.29.

the arterial system that tends to oppose the ejection of blood into it. Determination of Ea involves plotting a PV curve for the arterial system using different SV and recording end systolic pressures. The slope of the curve then gives the effective elastance (compliance^{-1}) of the arterial system.

Contractility

Contractility is a poorly defined term describing the intrinsic ability of a cardiac muscle fibre to do mechanical work when it contracts with a pre-defined load and initial degree of stretch. In the intact ventricle contractility reflects the amount of work that can be done for a given pre- and afterload (Figure HE.29).

Contractility can be increased by various factors including:

- Increased serum calcium levels
- Sympathetic stimulation

- Parasympathetic inhibition
- Positive inotropic drugs

Contractility can be decreased by various factors including:

- Decreased serum calcium levels
- Parasympathetic stimulation
- Sympathetic blockade
- Myocardial ischaemia or infarction
- Hypoxia and acidosis
- Mismatched ventriculo-arterial coupling

MEASUREMENT OF CONTRACTILITY

Contractility is an index of work performance at a given pre- and afterload. Ideally these parameters should be controlled during measurement, which is often impractical. Accordingly, pre- and afterload should be recorded during assessment of contractility. The interpretation of contractility measurements is then made at the given pre- and afterload.

The calculation of ventricular work done during systole requires an integral of the ventricular PV loop area. This is not a practical measurement, but an index loosely reflecting systolic work is stroke work, obtained from the following product:

SW = (SV) × (mean arterial pressure – filling pressure).

Figure HE.30 illustrates how this product approximates to the PV loop area for the left ventricle.

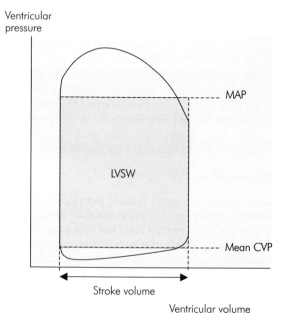

Figure HE.30 Left ventricular stroke work estimate for ventricular pressure–volume loop area

SV work index (SVWI) is a more useful indicator of contractility and is derived in the following way. SV work index is calculated by normalising stroke work for body surface area by using stroke index in its calculation. Thus, for the left ventricular stroke work index (LVSWI):

$$\text{LVSWI} = \frac{(\text{MAP} - \text{PCWP}) \times \text{SI}}{100} \times 1.36\,\text{g.m/m}^2$$

Normal values for LVSWI are 45–60 g.m/m².

While for the right ventricle (right ventricular stroke work index, RVSWI):

$$\text{RVSWI} = \frac{(\text{MPAP} - \text{CVP}) \times \text{SI}}{100} \times 1.36\,\text{g.m/m}^2$$

Normal values for right ventricle SVWI are 5–10 g.m/m².

Other measures of contractility include ejection fraction and ventricular function curves.

Ejection fraction is measured by radionuclide ventriculography or transthoracic echocardiography. It is often derived from the fractional area change measurement. EF and FAC are both sensitive to pre- and afterload. These latter parameters should also be evaluated with EF or FAC. There is a clear association between EF and prognosis in cardiac patients.

Ventricular function curves can be plotted between an index of ventricular filling (e.g. CVP or PCWP) and an index of ventricular performance (e.g. CO or SV). Factors increasing contractility will shift the curve upwards and to the left while those decreasing contractility will shift it downwards and to the right.

HEART RATE

The heart rate is normally determined by the spontaneous depolarisation rate of the SA node pacemaker cells. The normal heart rate of 60–80 bpm is much slower than the intrinsic rate of the denervated heart (110 bpm). This is because of the dominant parasympathetic tone in the intact cardiovascular system (Figure HE.31).

Autonomic control of pacemaker discharge rate

In vivo, control of the pacemaker rate is mediated peripherally via the autonomic nervous system. Central control of pacemaker rate lies in parasympathetic and sympathetic nuclei of the medulla. These are responsible for cardiovascular reflexes, and are influenced by higher centres including

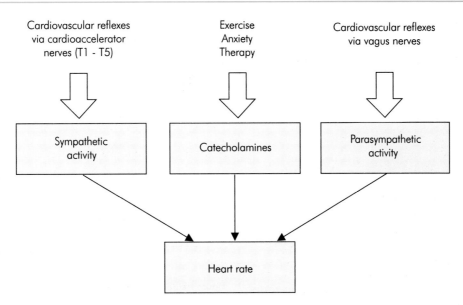

Figure HE.31 Control of heart rate

the posterior hypothalamus and cortical areas. Relevant autonomic pathways may be categorised as follows:

- Parasympathetic – parasympathetic fibres to the heart originate in the dorsal motor nucleus of the vagus and the nucleus ambiguus in the medulla oblongata. These parasympathetic fibres travel to the heart via the right and left vagus nerves. During embryological development the right vagus nerve becomes connected to the SA node, while the left vagus supplies the AV node. Vagal stimulation (parasympathetic activity) decreases the slope of phase 4 and also increases hyperpolarisation, thus, slowing the heart rate
- Sympathetic – sympathetic innervation to the heart originates in the sympathetic chain (T1–T5 fibres) passing via the stellate ganglion to all parts of the heart, with a strong representation to the ventricular muscle. The right side distributes to the SA node, while the left side primarily supplies the AV node. Sympathetic activity increases the slope of phase 4 and, hence, heart rate. This effect occurs in exercise, anxiety and febrile illness
- Mixed – direct interconnections exist between the parasympathetic and sympathetic cardiac supplies which enable both systems to inhibit each other directly

Cardiovascular reflexes

Some recognised cardiovascular reflexes controlling heart rate include:

- Lung volume stretch receptor reflex – moderate

increases in lung volume increase HR via the vagus nerves
- Chemoreceptor reflexes – the primary effect of carotid chemoreceptor stimulation is to activate vagal centres in the medulla giving a decrease in HR. However, this is modified by a secondary effect exerted by concomitant excitation of respiratory centres in the medulla which oppose the primary effect
- Atrial stretch receptor reflex (Bainbridge reflex) – stimulation of atrial stretch receptors by increases in venous return or blood volume gives rise to acceleration of the HR
- Baroreceptor reflexes – stimulation of baroreceptors in the aortic arch or carotid sinus, by an increase in blood pressure lead to a decrease in HR. Similarly, a drop in blood pressure causes an increase in HR

EFFECTS OF HEART RATE ON CARDIAC OUTPUT

Heart rate affects CO in the following ways:

- An increase in heart rate will lead to a progressive increase in CO up to about 140 bpm. When heart rate increases, SV decreases due to shorter diastolic filling time, but this only becomes significant at higher rates > 140 bpm
- When HR > 150 bpm the decrease in diastolic filling time reduces the CO significantly because it encroaches on rapid filling time. Diastolic time is affected by a tachycardia to a much greater extent than systolic time
- The Bowditch phenomenon ('Treppe' or staircase

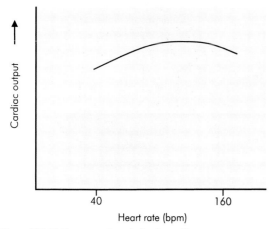

Figure HE.32 Treppe or Bowditch effect of heart rate on cardiac output

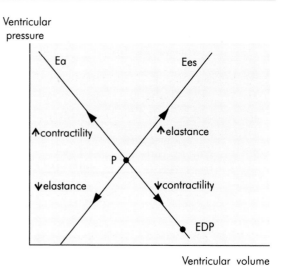

Figure HE.33 Ventriculo-arterial coupling diagram

effect) is increased inotropy in response to increased chronotropy. This occurs above 40 bpm and is due to the greater availability of intracellular calcium for excitation–contraction coupling which follows the reduced diastolic time available for calcium re-uptake (Figure HE.32)

- During a tachycardia in a normal heart, EDPVR will move to the left and downwards, i.e. smaller filling volumes at lower EDP. In an ischaemic heart, however, a tachycardia will move EDPVR to the left, but upwards, i.e. smaller filling volumes at higher EDP
- Tachycardia will increase the ventricular systolic elastance (Ees) due to the increased contractility
- A pronounced bradycardia < 40 bpm will cause a fall in CO, because the compensatory increase in SV is not enough to make up for the decrease in ejection rate

CARDIOVASCULAR COUPLING

In clinical practice assessment of cardiac function often relies on the available measurements of filling pressures (CVP and PCWP), arterial pressures (pulmonary and aortic) and CO. These measurements are dependent on two sets of characteristics that reflect:

- Contractile performance of the heart
- Elastance (PV relationship) of the vascular system

Assessing the relative effects of cardiac contractility and vascular system elastance on pressure measurements is important clinically, since it can influence therapeutic decisions.

Interpretation of pressure and CO measurements is aided by a consideration of the interaction or coupling between the heart and the vascular system. This can be performed at the arterial side (ventriculo-arterial coupling) for arterial pressures, or on the venous side of the heart (ventriculovenous coupling) for CVP.

VENTRICULO-ARTERIAL COUPLING

Coupling between the ventricle and arterial system is illustrated by plotting the ventricular elastance and arterial elastance on the same diagram. The ESP (P) then lies at junction of the curves that are approximately at right angles to each other. Changes in arterial pressure are reflected by a shift in the position of P. If pre load (EDP) is maintained constant, then the direction of displacement of P identifies the degree to which ventricular contractility or arterial elastance is responsible (Figure HE.33).

The left ventricle and arterial system can be seen as two elastic chambers with opposing elastances, Ees and Ea respectively. The distribution of blood is determined by the individual elastances of the two chambers. Theoretical analysis suggests that the LV will deliver maximal work when Ees = Ea but will work with maximal mechanical efficiency when Ees = 2 × Ea. The implication is that there is an optimum ventriculo-arterial coupling ratio for these elastances. If these elastances are mismatched the ventricle may fail, e.g. should the ventricle eject for a prolonged period against a very low afterload.

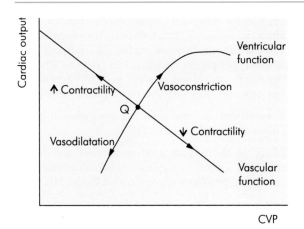

Figure HE.34 Ventriculovenous coupling diagram

VENTRICULOVENOUS COUPLING

Description of cardiovascular coupling at the venous side of the heart requires the use of a vascular function curve. This curve describes the changes occurring in CVP as venous return is removed at different rates by the heart. It is obtained by varying the CO and recording the resulting CVP, at constant intravascular volume. The vascular function curve is a pressure–flow relationship at the venous side of the vascular system, dependent on the balance between vascular tone and intravascular volume. Changes in the gradient reflect alterations in vascular tone. Thus, vasodilatation causes a decreased gradient, while an increased gradient is associate with vasoconstriction. Changes in the intercept reflect altered intravascular volume.

A ventriculovenous coupling diagram can be drawn by plotting a vascular function curve and a ventricular function curve on the same axes. The ventricular function curve is described earlier and in Figure HE.23. These curves intersect at an operating point (Q). When Q becomes displaced by cardiovascular changes, the direction of displacement indicates the relative contributions of vascular tone and ventricular contractility effects to the changes (Figure HE.34).

Ventricular interdependence

Right and left ventricles are situated inside the same

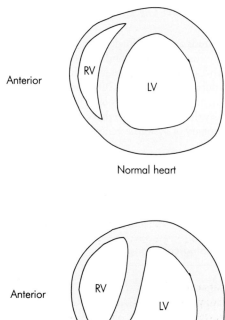

Figure HE.35 Ventricular interdependence

non compliant pericardium. This means that they are both exposed to the same intrathoracic and intraalveolar pressures. Changes in volume and pressure of one ventricle will directly affect the other. Normally LV pressure is greater than RV pressure and the interventricular septum bows into the RV. However, the thin free wall of the RV makes it more sensitive to increases in afterload than the LV, and any increase in afterload (e.g. pulmonary hypertension) will lead to dilatation of the RV. Under these circumstances the trans-septal pressure gradient can reverse and the septum can shift to the left compromising LV filling during diastole. Interaction between the two ventricles occurs during systole and diastole, and is called ventricular interdependence (Figure HE.35).

CARDIAC FAILURE

Cardiac failure is a state of inadequate circulation due to cardiac dysfunction. The condition manifests itself through two aspects. First, there is a failure to provide adequate arterial pressure and CO ('forward failure') into the systemic circulation. Second, there is a failure to pump away the venous return that causes congestion in the pulmonary or systemic venous beds ('backward failure').

The course of cardiac failure may be acute or chronic. The commonest cause of acute cardiac failure is myocardial infarction, while chronic failure often arises in ischaemic heart disease, hypertension and valvular disease. In acute cardiac failure hypotension without peripheral oedema may occur. While in chronic failure, blood pressure is usually maintained, but signs and symptoms due to congestion develop.

Some of the common signs and symptoms of cardiac failure are shown in Figure HE.36.

Many of the physiological parameters and indices reflecting aspects of cardiac performance change in cardiac failure. These are outlined in Figure HE.37.

SIGNS AND SYMPTOMS OF CARDIAC FAILURE

Physiological change	Sign or symptom
Congestion in the pulmonary vascular system	Pulmonary oedema
	Dyspnoea on exertion
	Orthopnoea
	Paroxysmal nocturnal dyspnoea
Congestion in the systemic vascular system	Dependent oedema (e.g. ankle)
	Hepatomegaly
	Raised jugulovenous pressure
Inadequate systemic circulation	Fatigue
	Sodium retention
	Increased intravascular volume

Figure HE.36

CHANGES IN PHYSIOLOGICAL INDICES IN CARDIAC FAILURE

Change in heart	Change in physiological index
↓ Ventricular contractility	↓ decreased CO
	Shift of ventricular function curve down
Ventricular dilatation	↑ CVP
	↑ systolic ventricular wall stress
	↑ EDV
Ventricular diastolic dysfunction	Shift of EDPVR curve up and left
Altered cardiovascular coupling	Displacement of operating point on ventriculo-arterial and ventriculovenous coupling diagrams

Figure HE.37

SECTION 2: 6
PHYSIOLOGY OF THE CIRCULATION

E. S. Lin

BLOOD VESSELS
Structure and function

PRESSURE AND FLOW IN THE VASCULAR SYSTEM
Flow and flow velocity
Vascular resistance
Flow in a single vessel
Blood viscosity

ARTERIAL SYSTEM
Arterial factors
Determinants of systolic and diastolic pressures

VENOUS SYSTEM
Venous circulation
Thoracic pump

MICROCIRCULATION AND LYMPHATIC SYSTEM
Structure of a capillary network
Capillary exchange
Starling forces and filtration
The lymphatic system

CONTROL OF THE CIRCULATION
Resistance and capacitance vessels
Vascular smooth muscle
Local mechanisms controlling blood flow
Systemic humoral control of blood flow
Systemic neurological control of blood flow

BLOOD VOLUME
Control of blood volume

CIRCULATORY CONTROL UNDER SPECIAL CIRCUMSTANCES
Haemorrhage
Valsalva manoeuvre
Exercise

SPECIAL CIRCULATIONS
Coronary circulation
Cerebral circulation
Foetal circulation

BLOOD VESSELS

The circulation can be divided into the systemic and the pulmonary circulation. The systemic circulation receives oxygenated blood from the left side of the heart via the aorta and returns desaturated blood to the right side of the heart in the vena cavae. The desaturated blood is delivered to the pulmonary circulation from the right ventricle via the pulmonary artery to be oxygenated and to exchange carbon dioxide. Oxygenated blood is then returned to the left atrium via the pulmonary veins (Figure CR.1).

STRUCTURE AND FUNCTION

Blood vessel walls are basically structured in three layers. The adventitia is the outer layer and is made up of connective tissue with nerve fibres. The middle layer or media is of varying thickness and contains mainly smooth muscle. The innermost layer is the intima and consists of the endothelium, basement membrane and supporting connective tissue (Figure CR.2). The composition of blood vessel walls is mainly a mixture of elastic tissue, fibrous tissue and smooth muscle. This mixture again varies according to the type of vessel. The aorta walls are predominantly elastic and fibrous

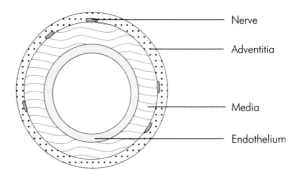

Figure CR.2 Blood vessel structure

tissue with little smooth muscle, whereas the vena cava walls consist largely of smooth muscle and fibrous components. The composition of vessel walls reflects their function.

Figure CR.3 lists functional aspects relating vessel characteristics to function.

Blood vessel diameter and wall thickness

A major factor determining thickness is mean arterial pressure. Some typical values for vessel diameter, wall thickness and mean arterial pressure are given below in Figure CR.4.

Blood vessel function

The arteries transport blood under high pressure to the tissues where they divide into smaller arterioles, which in turn release the blood into capillaries. There the exchange of fluid, nutrients, electrolytes and other substances between the interstitial fluid and the blood take place. The venules collect blood from the capillaries, join together into veins which transport the blood back to the heart.

Blood vessels also function to smooth the pulsatile pressure waveform in the aorta, to control pressure at the capillary beds and to store blood volume. The control of regional perfusion is dependent on reflexes and autoregulation that rely on arteriolar control. The functions of the different types of vessel in the circulatory system are summarised in Figure CR.5.

PRESSURE AND FLOW IN THE VASCULAR SYSTEM

FLOW AND FLOW VELOCITY

Function of the organ systems depends on the volume of blood flowing per unit time through them, or the

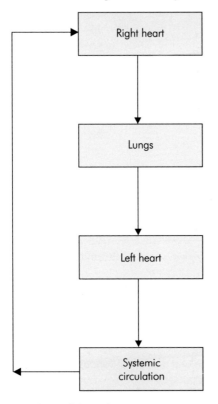

Figure CR.1 Adult circulation system

FUNCTIONAL ASPECTS OF BLOOD VESSEL WALL CHARACTERISTICS

Characteristic	Functional aspect
Wall thickness	Thick walls provide tensile strength to withstand pressure in arteries Thin walls in capillaries allow exchange with interstitial fluid
Elastic component in walls	Smoothing of pulsations, storage of energy to maintain flow in diastole
Smooth muscle component in walls	Control of vessel diameter by autonomic reflex and humoral activity
Fibrous component in walls	Mechanical strength

Figure CR.3

BLOOD VESSEL DIAMETERS AND MEAN PRESSURES

Vessel	Diameter	Wall thickness	Mean pressure (mmHg)
Aorta	25 mm	2 mm	100
Artery	4 mm	1 mm	95
Arteriole	20 μm	6 μm	50
Terminal arteriole	10 μm	2 μm	45
Capillary	8 μm	0.5 μm	30
Venules	20 μm	1 μm	20
Veins	5 mm	0.5 mm	8
Vena cava	30 mm	1.5 mm	3

Figure CR.4

BLOOD VESSELS AND THEIR FUNCTIONS

Vessel	Function
Aorta	Storage of energy to maintain delivery in diastole, and damping of pressure pulses
Arteries	Delivery, distribution and damping of pressure waveform
Arterioles	Resistance to control pressure and distribution to capillaries
Capillaries	Microcirculation and exchange
Venules and small veins	Collection
Large veins and vena cava	Collection, storage capacitance and delivery of venous return (or portal circulations)

Figure CR.5

volume flow rate. This is often shortened to the term 'flow'. Flow can be measured in ml/s (or l/min). The total flow through the systemic circulation or the lungs is equal to the cardiac output.

Flow should be differentiated from flow velocity. Flow velocity defines how fast fluid is moving at any given point and has units of cm/s. In a blood vessel the flow velocity of blood varies between the centre of the vessel and the vessel wall. If the flow pattern of the blood is described as laminar (i.e. without turbulence) the blood moves smoothly in the direction of the axis of the vessel. The velocity of the blood varies in a predictable pattern with maximum velocity in the centre of the vessel and minimum velocity next to the wall, as if the blood is moving in concentric layers (Figure CR.6).

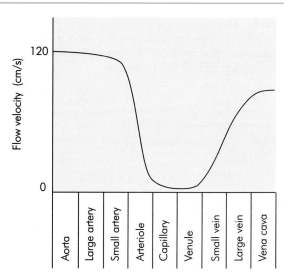

Figure CR.7 Flow velocity in different vessels

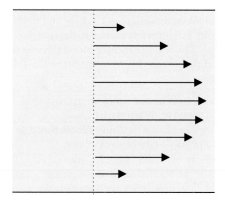

Figure CR.6 Physics of laminar flow

Consider a vessel with cross sectional area A. The mean flow velocity (v) can be taken across the cross section. The flow (Q) is then related to the mean flow velocity (v) by:

$$Q = vA$$

This relationship can be applied to the vascular system as a whole since the number and diameter of any type of blood vessel determines the total cross sectional area presented to flow at that stage in the vascular system. The greater the total cross sectional area of any given generation of vessels, the slower the velocity of blood flow through those vessels. The cross sectional area of the aorta is about 4.5 cm^2 with peak flow velocities of > 120 cm/s. In contrast, the flow velocity in the several billion capillaries of the vascular system is usually between 0 and 1 cm/s due to a total capillary cross sectional area of > 4500 cm^2 (Figure CR.7). These flow velocities reflect the functions of delivery and distribution in the aorta and arteries, as opposed to perfusion and exchange in the capillaries.

In an individual vessel if the cross sectional area is reduced by a constriction such as a valve or an atheromatous plaque, the flow velocity increases through the constriction. Such increases in flow velocity can affect the characteristics of the blood flow making it turbulent and leading to an increased tendency towards thrombus formation. The motion of blood across the stationary surface of the vessel wall produces a viscous drag or shear stress along the surface of the vessel wall. This shear stress is increased with increased flow velocity producing a force that tends to pull endothelium and plaques away from the wall, leading to dissection or emboli. Increased flow velocity also produces bruits or murmurs (Figure CR.8).

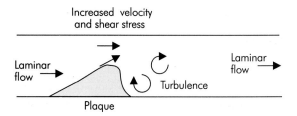

Figure CR.8 Turbulent flow and drag in vessels

Flow through the systemic circulation

The energy imparted to blood within the circulation by the heart and the elastic recoil of the great vessels causes it flow through the systemic and pulmonary circulations. There are additional contributions of energy to flow from skeletal muscle contraction and negative intrathoracic pressure during inspiration. These mechanisms create a pressure difference across the vascular system that produces the total flow (cardiac output) through the vascular system. A simple electrical analogy lies in Ohm's law where a potential difference (V) produces an electrical current (I) through a resistance (R). In this case:

$$V = I \times R.$$

Thus the pressure difference between mean arterial pressure (MAP) and central venous pressure (CVP) is related to cardiac output (CO) and systemic vascular (SVR) by:

$$(MAP) - (CVP) = (CO) \times (SVR)$$

This is often approximated to:

$$(MAP) = (CO) \times (SVR)$$

VASCULAR RESISTANCE

'Vascular resistance' is a clinical term used to represent the effect of all the forces opposing blood flow through a vascular bed. It may be applied to the systemic vascular circulation, the pulmonary circulation or a given visceral circulation. The forces opposing blood flow through a vascular system are composed of two main components. First, those which dissipate energy due to frictional effects. This resistance arises as a result of drag between fluid layers and friction between fluid and vessel walls. The viscosity of the blood is a major determinant of this component of resistance.

The second component of opposing forces arises from the conversion of pump work into stored energy. This occurs when potential energy is stored by the elasticity of distended vessel walls or by gravity as blood is pumped to a greater height within the body. In addition, inertial effects store kinetic energy when blood is accelerated. This component is referred to as the 'reactive' component and is dependent on the pulsatile component of the pressure waveform. If the pressure difference applied across a vascular bed were constant the reactive component would be minimal.

In vivo the systemic vascular resistance (SVR) and the pulmonary vascular resistance (PVR) can be estimated using pulmonary artery catheterisation.

FLOW IN A SINGLE VESSEL

Blood flow through larger vessels (> 0.5 mm diameter) can be approximated to the case of an idealised or Newtonian fluid (such as water) flowing though a tube. Under laminar flow conditions with a steady pressure gradient, the flow (Q) between any two points, P_1 and P_2, is dependent on the pressure difference, ΔP, between the points, and inversely dependent on the resistance to flow (R) (Figure CR.9).

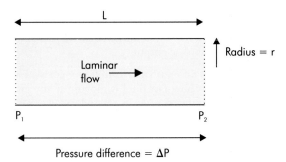

Figure CR.9 Poiseuille's law

$$Q = \frac{\Delta P}{R}$$

According to the Hagen–Poiseuille law, which describes laminar flow in tubes, the flow resistance, R, is dependent on the length of the tube and the viscosity of the fluid, but inversely related to the fourth power of the radius. The real situation of blood flowing through a vessel differs from this ideal model in the following respects:

- Blood vessels are not uniform in cross section
- Blood vessel walls are elastic
- Pressure gradients pushing blood through vessels have a pulsatile component
- Blood as a fluid behaves differently from a Newtonian fluid due to the cellular components and its flow properties are not solely determined by viscosity

BLOOD VISCOSITY

The rheological properties of blood describe its flow resistive properties. In a Newtonian fluid these resistive properties are dependent on a constant, the coefficient of viscosity. Blood, however, is a suspension of cells, and although the viscosity can be determined to give an apparent value, this value varies significantly with blood composition and flow conditions. The factors causing this variation in apparent viscosity include:

- Haematocrit – an increase in haematocrit to 0.7 (normal haematocrit = 0.45) can double the apparent viscosity (Figure CR.10)
- Diameter of the vessel – apparent blood viscosity can be measured in vitro using a capillary tube viscometer, and decreases as tube diameter decreases < about 0.3 mm
- Red blood cell streaming – in smaller diameter vessels red blood cells stream centrally along the axis of the vessel. This effectively reduces the

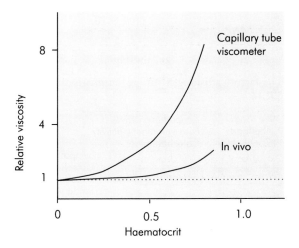

Figure CR.10 Haematocrit related to viscosity

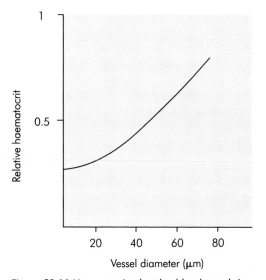

Figure CR.11 Haematocrit related to blood vessel size

haematocrit in these vessels. The haematocrit in capillaries may be 25% of the value in larger vessels (Figure CR.11)

- In vivo – apparent blood viscosity is lower in vivo than in vitro. At normal haematocrit the in vivo blood viscosity may only be half of the equivalent in vitro value
- Flow velocity – apparent viscosity decreases at higher flow velocities and increases at low flow velocities. This is due to increased red cell aggregation and leucocyte adherence to vessel walls at low flow velocities

ARTERIAL SYSTEM

The main function of the arterial system is to distribute and deliver blood to the capillary beds throughout the peripheral vascular system. A secondary arterial function is to convert the high-pressure pulsatile blood flow of the aorta, into the low-pressure steady flow of the capillary beds. This modification of the flow and pressure profiles is achieved by the elasticity of the arterial system and is sometimes referred to as hydraulic filtering, or the 'Windkessel' effect (Windkessel – volume of air trapped in a pump reservoir to smooth out pressure variations).

ARTERIAL FACTORS

Flow velocity

In systole, the heart ejects a stroke volume of 70–90 ml blood into the aorta. The heart generates an average flow velocity of 70 cm/s, with a peak velocity of 120 cm/s that makes flow in the aorta turbulent. There is transient backflow at the end of systole until the aortic valve closes. The aorta and arteries distend in systole due to the elasticity of their walls, then subsequent elastic recoil during diastole maintains forward flow distally into the peripheral vascular system.

Pressure wave

In the aorta and arteries the pressure is pulsatile. The maximum pressure is the systolic arterial pressure (about 120 mmHg) and the minimum is the diastolic arterial pressure (about 70 mmHg). The difference between diastolic and systolic is the pulse pressure, normally about 50 mmHg.

The aortic pressure wave changes in magnitude and shape occur as it travels through the arterial system. The shape of the pressure wave narrows and high frequency features such as the incisura (end systolic notch) become dampened as it moves distally. Initially systolic pressures increase as the pressure waves travel from aorta distally through the large arteries. At the femoral arteries systolic pressures have risen by 20 mmHg, and by the time pressure waves have reached the foot systolic pressures are 40 mmHg higher than in the aorta. Pressure pulsations begin to become attenuated in the smaller arteries and are finally reduced to a steady pressure with a mean level of 30–35 mmHg by the arterioles, ready for the capillary beds (Figure CR.12). The changes in the shape of the pressure waves are mainly due to the visco-elastic properties of the arterial walls. While the increases in systolic pressure are thought to be due to factors affecting the propagation of the pressure waves through the vessels, such as reflection, resonance and changes in the velocity of propagation.

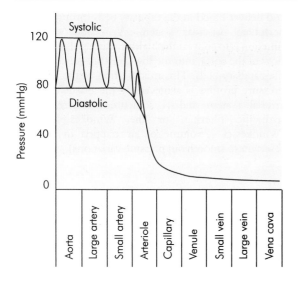

Figure CR.12 Pressure related to vessel size

Mean arterial pressure

Mean arterial pressure (MAP) is the value obtained when the pressure is averaged over time and can be obtained from the product of cardiac output and systemic vascular resistance. Since the pressure varies cyclically, MAP can be determined by integrating a pressure signal over the duration of one cycle (this gives the shaded area shown in Figure CR.13). The mean pressure is then given by the value of this integral divided by time. An estimate of mean arterial pressure may be made by taking the diastolic plus one-third of the pulse pressure. Thus, for a systolic pressure of 120 mmHg and a diastolic of 70 mmHg, the mean pressure (MAP) is given by:

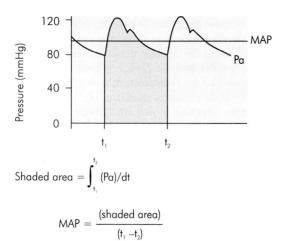

$$\text{Shaded area} = \int_{t_1}^{t_2} (Pa)/dt$$

$$MAP = \frac{(\text{shaded area})}{(t_1 - t_2)}$$

Figure CR.13 Calculation of mean arterial pressure

$$MAP \approx 70 + \frac{(120 - 70)}{3}$$

$$= 86.7 \text{ mmHg.}$$

The factors affecting MAP are summarised in Figure CR.14.

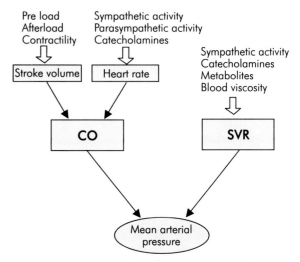

Figure CR.14 Factors affecting mean arterial pressure

Compliance

The elasticity of the arterial walls provides an essential mechanism for maintaining forward blood flow during diastole. When the aorta and arteries are distended during systole the elasticity of the walls store kinetic energy from the ejected blood. This stored energy is then returned in diastole by the recoil of the vessel walls. A useful measure of arterial elasticity is the arterial compliance (Ca). Compliance (as in the respiratory system) is the change in arterial blood volume produced by a unit change in arterial blood pressure. Thus, easily distended arteries have a high compliance, and stiff arteries have a low compliance. The reciprocal relationship between Ca and arterial elastance (Ea) should be noted as Ea is used in describing left ventricular performance.

DETERMINATION OF ARTERIAL COMPLIANCE

In vitro – the pressure–volume curves of post mortem aorta preparations have been plotted for different age groups. This is approximately linear in the young normal subject, the gradient of the curve being equal to Ca. With age the arterial walls increase in stiffness and the gradient decreases to a fraction of its value in young subjects. In addition, the compliance curve becomes curvilinear in the working arterial pressure range (Figure CR.15)

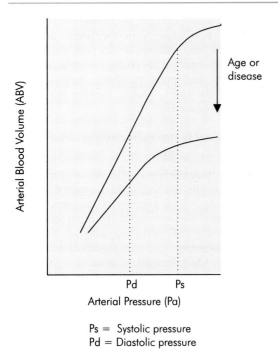

Ps = Systolic pressure
Pd = Diastolic pressure

Figure CR.15 Arterial compliance curves

In vivo – the end systolic points from different ventricular pressure–volume loops can be plotted for a given subject. This gives an arterial elastance curve in which the gradient is equal to Ea.

DETERMINANTS OF SYSTOLIC AND DIASTOLIC PRESSURES

The factors determining systolic and diastolic pressures are summarised in Figure CR.16:

- Arterial blood volume (ABV)
- Stroke volume
- Systemic vascular resistance (SVR)
- Arterial compliance (Ca)

The arterial system can be visualised as an elastic vessel containing a varying volume of blood. This volume (ABV) varies with the injection of each stroke volume injected by the left ventricle (LV), and the 'run off' of blood into the peripheral vessels. The arterial pressure at any instant (Pa), is then dependent on the relationship between ABV, Ca and SVR. Pa should be differentiated from mean arterial pressure (MAP), which is averaged over time (Figure CR.13).

The determination of systolic and diastolic pressures can be examined by extending the electrical circuit analogy used previously to relate MAP to cardiac output and systemic vascular resistance (SVR). Arterial compliance (Ca) is added as a 'shunt' capacitance across

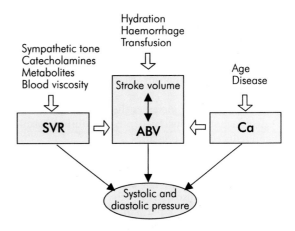

Figure CR.16 Factors affecting systolic and diastolic pressure

SVR to give a parallel resistance–capacitance (RC) circuit (Figure CR.17). This is fed by a continual series of current pulses (stroke volumes). Each pulse of current divides between the SVR and Ca. Ca charges to a maximum voltage (systolic pressure) during a current pulse and discharges to a minimum (diastolic pressure) in between pulses. For a given pulse amplitude these maximum and minimum values will be determined by the parallel RC time constant. The effects of SVR and

(a) Systole

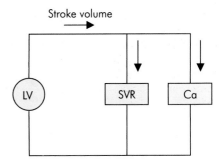

(b) Diastole

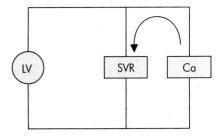

Figure CR.17 Circuit demonstrating shunt arterial compliance

Ca on systolic and diastolic arterial pressures are illustrated by the following notes:

- Ca reduces the peak current through SVR by 'shunting' current away from SVR. Thus, increasing Ca (compliant arteries) leads to reduced systolic pressures
- Increased Ca also increases the RC time constant, giving a more gradual fall of pressure during diastole and reduced pulse pressures
- Decreased Ca (stiff arteries) gives reduced shunted current, giving increased peak current through SVR and higher systolic pressures
- Decreasing Ca also decreases the RC time constant, allowing a more rapid fall in pressure during diastole and increased pulse pressures
- When arterial compliance is decreased as with age or disease, the arterial pressure–volume curve becomes non linear. The effect of this on systolic and diastolic pressures can be seen by comparing the arterial pressure waves produced (P_0 and P_1) by the same stroke volume, using the normal and decreased arterial compliance curves shown in Figure CR.18. Projecting the stroke volume variation on the normal compliance curve produces the pressure signal, P_0. Repeating this with the decreased compliance curve gives arterial pressure signal P_1. It can be seen that systolic pressure is increased disproportionately compared with diastolic pressure

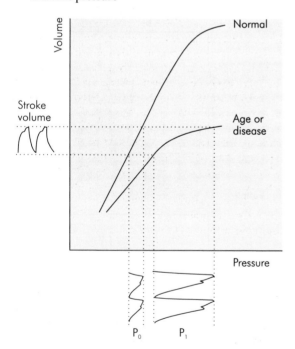

Figure CR.18 Effect of compliance on systolic and diastolic pressures

- Increased SVR as occurs in chronic hypertension, produces non linearity in the pressure–volume curve like the effects of age on the arterial compliance curve. This produces similar increases in systolic and pulse pressures. Increased SVR increases the time constant slowing the rate of diastolic pressure fall

Technological factors affecting arterial blood pressure

The value obtained for arterial blood pressure is dependent on the method of measurement and the anatomical site where pressure is sampled. Arterial blood pressure measurements are often made non invasively using an occluding cuff as with the sphygmomanometer or oscillotonometer. Alternatively, intra-arterial cannulation may be performed and the arterial pressure measured using a piezoresistive transducer.

VENOUS SYSTEM

VENOUS CIRCULATION

Venous blood flow is primarily driven by pressure transmitted from the capillary beds. Venous pressure falls from 15 to 20 mmHg at the venous end of capillaries to 10–15 mmHg in small veins, and 5–6 mmHg in large extrathoracic veins. Flow in the venules and small veins is continuous. In the great veins, pressure changes due to respiration and the heart beat cause fluctuations in the venous pressure wave. There are three identifiable peaks in the central venous pulse, the 'a', 'c' and 'v' waves which are related to events in the cardiac cycle. The central venous pulse waveform is described on page 317.

Other secondary mechanisms also assist venous blood flow back to the heart. These are gravity, the thoracic pump and the muscle pump. Unidirectional venous flow is maintained by the presence of valves in the peripheral veins.

Gravity and the venous system

The pressure in the venous system is largely determined by gravity since the system can be visualised as a simple manometer (Figure CR.19). In the erect position, a hydrostatic gradient is produced from head to toe. The hydrostatic pressure difference between any two points in the venous system can be calculated by taking the product of the difference in height between the points (h), the density of blood (ρ = 1.050 g/cm³), and the acceleration due to gravity (g = 980 cm/s). These figures give a pressure difference

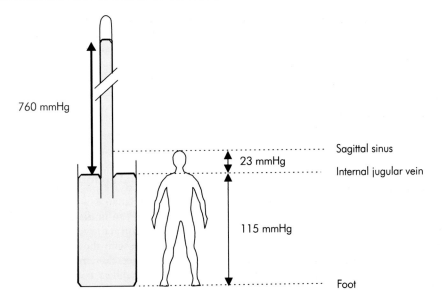

Figure CR.19 Gravity and venous pressure

equivalent to 0.77 mmHg for every centimetre difference in height.

The venous pressure in the internal jugular vein is normally atmospheric at neck level if the vein is collapsed. Venous pressure above the neck may be less than atmospheric and can be estimated, e.g. 30 cm above the neck (sagittal sinus) venous pressure is less than atmospheric by $30 \times 0.77 = 23$ mmHg.

Similarly in the foot, 150 cm below neck level, venous pressure is greater than atmospheric by $150 \times 0.77 = 115$ mmHg.

Such hydrostatic pressure differences are reduced significantly by the primary and secondary mechanisms outlined above and the presence of valves or venous obstruction. Thus, in the foot venous pressures may only be 80 mmHg when standing and decrease further to < 30 mmHg when walking.

Jugular venous pressure (JVP)

The superior vena cava (SVC) and internal jugular vein effectively form a manometer connected to the right atrium, and are usually collapsed being approximately at atmospheric pressure in the neck. In the erect position, the level of blood in the internal jugular vein represents the filling pressure in the right atrium and is not normally visible above the clavicle. The jugular venous pulse may become visible as a pulsatile distension of the internal jugular vein in a reclined or supine position, or when the CVP is increased. The jugular venous pulsations correspond to those of the central venous pulsations as described above. This

correlation between jugular venous pulse and central venous pulse is limited if there are any anatomical obstructions to drainage of blood from the superior vena cava.

Cerebral venous pressure and air embolism

In the brain, venous pressure can become sub atmospheric, since the skull is a rigid container and the cerebral veins are held open by surrounding tissue. These veins are therefore susceptible to air embolism during surgery or if punctured by needles or cannulae open to air. The air embolus forms bubbles that are compressible compared with blood. If a large enough volume (> 10 ml) of air becomes trapped in the heart ventricles cardiac output can be reduced significantly with serious effects. Small amounts of air may pass through the heart to become trapped in pulmonary capillaries and be eliminated by diffusion without ill effects. On the other hand a few millilitres of air if shunted into the left ventricle and systemic circulation could have disastrous or even fatal effects. Gas embolism may also occur under positive pressure during laparoscopic surgery.

THORACIC PUMP

Normal respiration produces cyclical changes in intrathoracic pressure which increase the venous return to the heart. During inspiration intrapleural pressure falls from its resting value of –2 to –6 mmHg. This increase in negative intrathoracic pressure is transmitted to the central veins reducing CVP, and augmenting the pressure gradient between abdomen and thorax, allowing blood to pool in the pulmonary circulation. Central venous blood flow into the thorax may double during inspiration from its resting expiratory level of about 5 ml/s. Diaphragmatic displacement caudally during inspiration also contributes to increased venous return by increasing intra-abdominal pressure and consequently the abdominothoracic venous pressure gradient. Pooling of blood in the pulmonary circulation during inspiration produces a small decrease in arterial pressure and increase in heart rate. Forced inspiration against a closed glottis (Muller manoeuvre), accentuates these changes.

During expiration, which is normally passive, the diaphragm relaxes, intrapleural pressure returns to resting value, pulmonary blood volume is reduced and blood flow in the large veins decreases. Forced expiration against a closed glottis (Valsalva manoeuvre) can produce positive intrathoracic pressures with marked changes in heart rate and blood pressure, see page 353.

MICROCIRCULATION AND LYMPHATIC SYSTEM

STRUCTURE OF A CAPILLARY NETWORK

Capillaries and venules form an interface with a surface area > 6000 m² for the exchange of water and solutes between the circulation and tissues. Arterioles feed capillary networks via smaller metarterioles and the capillaries drain into venules. Metarterioles possess smooth muscle contractile elements in their walls and give rise to capillaries through smooth muscle pre-capillary sphincters (Figure CR.20). While arterioles are supplied by the autonomic system, the innervation

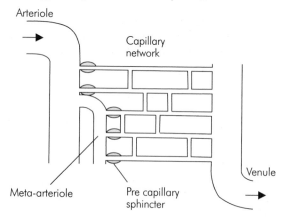

Figure CR.20 Capillary network

of metarterioles and pre-capillary sphincters is uncertain, and these vessels may only be responsive to local or humoral agents. Capillary blood flow varies according to the activity of the tissue. At rest the majority of capillary beds is collapsed and arteriovenous anastomoses allowing direct communication between arterioles and venules, shunt blood away from the tissues. These anastomotic channels are widespread in skin and play a prominent role in thermoregulation.

Capillaries and endothelium

Capillaries contain 6% of the circulating blood volume and measure 5 μm in diameter at their arteriolar end widening to 9 μm at the venous end. These dimensions are comparable with the 7 μm diameter of red blood cells, which decrease in diameter when traversing capillaries. A capillary consists of a tube formed by a single sheet of endothelial cells resting on a basement membrane. Associated with capillaries and venules are interstitial cells called pericytes, akin to renal mesangial cells. These cells release chemicals that mediate capillary permeability and also secrete the basement membrane (Figure CR.21).

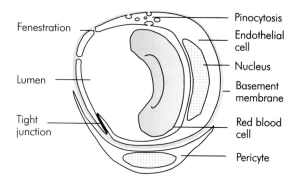

Figure CR.21 Capillaries and pericytes

CAPILLARY EXCHANGE

Capillaries have differing structures and permeabilities according to the tissues they serve. Most capillaries comprise a continuous layer of endothelial cells. Intercellular junctions and small pores representing about 0.02% of the capillary surface area permit the diffusion of small molecules < 8 nm in size. Larger molecules may cross through cell cytoplasm in vesicles and fat soluble molecules; water, oxygen and CO_2 pass directly across the cell membrane. Fenestrations, gaps of 20–100 nm diameter, appear in the endothelial cells of endocrine glands, renal glomeruli and intestinal villi to facilitate secretion, filtration and absorption. In the sinusoids of the liver and in the spleen, the endothelium is discontinuous with gaps of > 1000 nm. As a result albumin escapes from hepatic sinusoids much more readily than in other tissues.

In summary, transfer of water and solutes across the endothelium occurs by several mechanisms:

- Diffusion – the main mechanism mediating the exchange of gases, and for the movement of small molecules such as glucose, urea, electrolytes and between circulation and tissues. It occurs at endothelial defects such as pores and fenestrations. Diffusion of gases and lipid soluble molecules also occurs directly across cell membranes
- Filtration – the movement of water and small size solutes across the endothelium under the influence of hydrostatic and osmotic gradients. Transport of substances this way is only a fraction of that occurring by diffusion; however, a significant flow of water circulates between the circulation and interstitial fluid by filtration. About 2% of capillary plasma flow is filtered (20–40 ml/min)
- Pinocytosis – transports larger (> 30 nm) lipid insoluble molecules across the endothelium. Pinocytotic vesicles form at the cell membrane (endocytosis), migrate across the cell, and expel their contents at the opposite cell membrane (exocytosis). The numbers of pinocytotic vesicles seen varies between tissues and is greater at the arteriolar end than the venous end of capillaries
- Direct passage of lipid soluble compounds and gases occurs by diffusion across cell membranes, through the cells and into the interstitial fluid

Diffusion across capillary walls

Diffusion is the movement of substances down a concentration gradient. Across the capillary endothelium the diffusion of lipid insoluble molecules and ions occurs at defects such as intercellular junctions, pores, fenestrations and larger gaps. Gases and lipid soluble molecules diffuse directly across cell membranes as well as at these endothelial defects. The rate of diffusion of a substance is dependent on concentration gradient ($C_O - C_I$), capillary permeability (k), capillary surface area (A), and capillary wall thickness (D). This is given by Fick's law:

$$\text{Rate of diffusion} = \frac{kA\,(C_O - C_I)}{D}$$

where

C_O = concentration in the capillary

C_I = concentration in the interstitial fluid.

The capillary permeability is a constant combining the various factors that affect the diffusion of different substances such as:

- Molecular size
- Charge
- Lipid solubility
- Diffusion across membranes as well as pores and fenestrations
- Interactions between solutes

Substances that diffuse readily such as gases, reach equilibrium close to the proximal end of capillaries and their exchange rate is said to be 'flow limited' since it is dependent on the capillary flow rate. Alternatively, the movement of substances which diffuse slowly and do not reach equilibrium with the interstitial fluid over the length of the capillary, is 'diffusion limited'. Capillary permeability not only varies between tissues but is also greater at the venous end and in the venules, than at the proximal end of the capillaries.

STARLING FORCES AND FILTRATION

The balance of hydrostatic and colloid osmotic (oncotic) pressures between capillary plasma and interstitial fluid, causes fluid to be filtered out of a capillary at the arteriolar end and re-absorbed at the venous end. These forces acting to move fluid in and out of a capillary are sometimes referred to as Starling forces.

In a capillary hydrostatic pressure (P_C) falls from 33 mmHg at the arterial end to 15 mmHg at the venous end. Interstitial hydrostatic pressure (P_{IF}) can vary from 9 to –9 mmHg, depending on the tissue. In solid tissues it is usually near zero or slightly positive (1 mmHg). Loose areolar connective tissue, such as in the epidural space, tends to have a negative hydrostatic pressure.

Colloid osmotic pressure in the capillaries (π_C) is 25 mmHg, while in the interstitial fluid colloid osmotic pressure (π_{IF}) is usually zero. The Starling forces are summarised in Figure CR.22.

The pressure acting to force fluid out of the capillary is made up of the hydrostatic pressure in the capillary and the colloid osmotic pressure in the interstitial fluid:

$$\text{Outward pressure} \quad = \quad P_C + \pi_{IF}$$

Similarly the pressure acting to force fluid back into the capillary is made up of the interstitial hydrostatic pressure and the colloid osmotic pressure in the capillary:

$$\text{Inward pressure} \quad = \quad P_{IF} + \pi_C$$

The resultant pressure gradient is the difference between outward and inward pressures (Figure CR.22):

$$\text{Pressure gradient} \quad = \quad (P_C + \pi_{IF}) - (P_{IF} + \pi_C)$$

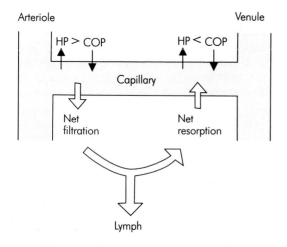

HP = Hydrostatic pressure

COP = Colloid osmotic pressure

Figure CR.22 Starling forces

The rate of filtration is proportional to this pressure gradient and is given by:

$$\text{Rate of filtration} = [(P_C + \pi_{IF}) - (P_{IF} + \pi_C)] \times K$$

where:

K = filtration coefficient of isotonic fluids (i.e. volume rate filtered per unit of pressure) and is about 0.01 ml/min/mmHg/100 g tissue at 37°C.

Assuming an interstitial hydrostatic pressure (P_{IF}) of 1 mmHg, and an interstitial colloid osmotic pressure (π_{IF}) of zero, it can be seen that at the arterial capillary end:

$$\text{Pressure gradient} = 33 - (1 + 25)$$
$$= + 7 \text{ mmHg.}$$

Therefore, pressure gradient acts outwards, filtering fluid out of the capillary. While at the venous capillary end:

$$\text{Pressure gradient} = 15 - (1 + 25)$$
$$= -11 \text{ mmHg.}$$

Here the pressure gradient is negative acting inwards, re-absorbing fluid back into the capillary.

The total volume of fluid filtered through the capillaries is dependent on capillary blood flow, but estimates have been made of between 1 and 3 litres per h. The filtered fluid exceeds the amount of fluid re-absorbed by about 10 %, the difference being absorbed by the lymphatic system.

Capillary filtration equilibrium

In a capillary there is normally a dynamic equilibrium between the fluid filtered out, the fluid re-absorbed

FACTORS DISTURBING CAPILLARY FILTRATION EQUILIBRIUM	
Change	**Effects**
Vasodilatation pressure	↑ proximal capillary hydrostatic pressure ↑ filtration
↑ Intravascular volume	↑ proximal capillary hydrostatic pressure ↑ filtration
Vasoconstriction	↓ proximal capillary hydrostatic pressure ↓ filtration
↓ Intravascular volume	↓ proximal capillary hydrostatic pressure ↓ filtration
Hypo-albuminaemia	↓ capillary colloid osmotic pressure ↑ filtration ↓ reabsorption
↑ Venous pressure	↑ distal capillary hydrostatic pressure ↓ reabsorption

Figure CR.23

and the fluid absorbed by lymphatics. Disturbance of this equilibrium either dehydrates tissue or makes it oedematous. The equilibrium can be disturbed by various changes. Some examples are shown in Figure CR.23.

THE LYMPHATIC SYSTEM

The functions of the lymphatic system include:

- Drainage of interstitial fluid – the total lymph drainage for an adult is about 2–4 litres per 24 H
- Return of 'leaked' protein in the interstitial fluid to the systemic circulation. Lymph from most tissues contains a protein concentration of 20 g/l
- Absorption of particles, proteins and other large molecular weight molecules accumulated in inflamed tissues
- Absorption of protein and fat derived from metabolism and gastro-intestinal absorption. The protein concentration is two-to-three times higher in lymph draining from liver and intestine

Lymphatic vessels

Lymph flows from lymphatic capillaries with a single layer of lymphatic endothelial cells, into lymphatic vessels that contain smooth muscle in their walls. This smooth muscle contracts in response to distension by the presence of lymph. Valves within lymph vessels maintain unidirectional flow towards the thoracic ducts, which drain into venous blood at the junction of internal jugular and subclavian veins. External compression from adjacent pulsatile arteries and skeletal muscle contractions augment lymph flow through larger lymphatic vessels.

Tissue oedema

The accumulation of abnormal amounts of interstitial fluid results in tissue swelling and is referred to as oedema. The common mechanisms underlying oedema formation include:

- Increased capillary filtration (raised venous pressure as in congestive heart failure, incompetent venous valves, venous obstruction)
- Decreased capillary colloid osmotic pressure (hypo-albuminaemia from any cause)
- Increased capillary permeability (inflammation, hypersensitivity, systemic inflammatory response syndrome)
- Decreased lymphatic drainage (lymphatic obstruction by lymphadenopathy, Milroy's disease, filiariasis)

CONTROL OF THE CIRCULATION

Control of the circulation ensures that adequate blood flow reaches the tissues to supply their metabolic demands. This is achieved by simultaneous regulation of the cardiac pump and the peripheral vascular system. Pump control varies the cardiac output. Control of the peripheral vascular system regulates the relative intravascular volume providing venous return for the pump, varies vascular resistance to maintain perfusion pressures, and distributes appropriate flows to the various vascular beds.

Multiple control mechanisms have evolved to regulate the circulation. These may be local (intrinsic) or systemic (extrinsic). Most areas of the peripheral vascular system are under both local and systemic control, but may be dominated by one set of mechanisms more than the other. Circulation in the heart and brain are mainly regulated intrinsically to maintain perfusion independently of systemic disturbances. On the other hand perfusion of the skin and gut are largely controlled extrinsically, increasing the flexibility to maintain vital organ perfusion under adverse conditions.

RESISTANCE VESSELS AND CAPACITANCE VESSELS

Control of the vascular system is mediated via:

- Resistance vessels – these vessels are the arterioles. Increasing or decreasing the tone of the smooth muscle in arterioles (vasoconstriction or vasodilatation), varies the perfusion pressure across a vascular bed. Changes in these vessels also affect flow rates through the capillaries and alter vascular resistance
- Capacitance vessels – these comprise the venous system. Increasing or decreasing the tone of smooth muscle in the venous system (venoconstriction or venodilatation) varies the relative intravascular volume since the venous system contains > 60% of the blood volume. Changes in these vessels have little effect on vascular resistance

Arterioles

Resistance vessels or arterioles, possess a high proportion of smooth muscle in their walls. The smooth muscle fibres are arranged circumferentially in the media, and the effects of varying the muscle tone can range from complete obliteration of the vessel lumen to maximal dilatation.

VASCULAR SMOOTH MUSCLE

Vascular smooth muscle differs from both skeletal muscle and cardiac muscle both structurally and functionally. Vascular smooth muscle characteristics include:

- Contractions are mediated by actin–myosin interaction dependent on calcium influx, release from the sarcoplasmic reticulum and re-uptake. However, actin and myosin filaments are not arranged to give striations
- Contractions are relatively slow, develop high forces and are maintained for longer durations when compared with striated muscle fibres
- There are no action potentials generated. Contraction occurs in response to systemic and locally released agents such as catecholamines, acetylcholine, and prostaglandins
- The majority of vascular smooth muscle is innervated by sympathetic fibres that maintain a basal level of vascular tone. Sympathetic stimulation increases vascular resistance
- The parasympathetic system supplies a small fraction of visceral vessels which can produce a decrease in vascular resistance when stimulated

LOCAL MECHANISMS CONTROLLING BLOOD FLOW

Autoregulation

The blood flow to certain organs (e.g. brain or kidney) is adjusted locally to respond to their activity levels and meet their metabolic demands. This process is known as autoregulation and is achieved by various mechanisms. These mechanisms include mechanical responses of smooth muscle, the accumulation of metabolites or products of injury, and the release of factors by the endothelium.

Metabolic regulation

This is the most important control mechanism since it determines the balance of oxygen supply and demand for individual tissues and organs. Exposure of tissue to hypoxia or injury results in the release of factors or accumulation of metabolites, which increase capillary permeability and blood flow. These override central and hormonal control of capillary blood flow. Some examples are:

- Tissue hypoxia or the accumulation of carbon dioxide and hydrogen ions by diffusion around an arteriole causes vasodilatation. Lactic acid, and to a lesser extent pyruvic acid, produced in anaerobic metabolism, vasodilate by reducing tissue pH

- Adenosine, ATP, ADP and AMP are also strong vasodilators. Adenosine dilates hepatic arteries in response to a fall in flow in the hepatic portal vein
- The accumulation of potassium and phosphate in exercising muscle augments blood flow to the muscle. This is sometimes referred to as 'active hyperaemia'
- 'Reactive hyperaemia' occurs when the blood supply to a tissue is occluded, and then the occlusion is released. There follows an immediate vasodilatation and increase in flow to the tissue
- Local mechanical damage to tissues usually produces localised constriction of vessels associated with serotonin release from platelets at the site of injury
- An alternative local response to local injury is the 'triple response'. There is an initial red reaction due to arteriolar dilatation caused by the mechanical stimulus. An axon reflex causes a rapid, more widespread brighter red reaction due to further vasodilatation. Later local oedema raises a wheal caused by capillary damage

Mechanical responses of smooth muscle

MYOGENIC MECHANISM

Vascular smooth muscle contracts or relaxes in response to changes in transmural pressure. When perfusion pressure in a vessel varies, although blood flow may change initially, the vessel subsequently constricts or dilates in response to the altered transmural pressure maintaining constant blood flow. Isolated muscle preparations suggest this local response can maintain constant blood flow over perfusion pressures from 20 to 120 mmHg.

ENDOTHELIAL MECHANISM

When flow through a vessel is varied without changes in transmural pressure, increases in flow velocity are associated with dilation of the vessel. This response may be due to an endothelial derived factor (e.g. nitric oxide) as it is abolished by removal of the endothelium.

Endothelial factors

Endothelial cells release various local factors that affect blood flow:

- Prostacyclin and thromboxane A_2 – these are arachidonites dependent on the cyclo-oxygenase pathway. Prostacyclin is a vasodilator and inhibits platelet aggregation, while thromboxane A_2 is a vasoconstrictor that promotes platelet aggregation. Regular administration of aspirin causes a predominance of prostacyclin effects, providing prophylaxis against myocardial infarction and stroke

- Endothelium-derived relaxing factor (EDRF) – original term for nitric oxide (NO), which has been identified as a potent vasodilator. NO is synthesised from arginine by NO synthase and is inactivated by haemoglobin. NO is released from endothelium by multiple factors such as acetylcholine, bradykinin and various polypeptides. Its role is uncertain but it may act locally to maintain perfusion in different parts of the circulation

- Endothelins – these polypeptides are potent vasoconstrictors that are produced by endothelium though out the tissues of the body, including the central nervous system, the kidneys and the gut. The endothelins have multiple physiological effects although their exact role remains uncertain. These effects include contraction of vascular smooth muscle, positive inotropy and chronotropy, reduction of glomerular filtration rate, bronchoconstriction and stimulation of cell growth. Three endothelins have been identified ET-1, ET-2, and ET-3, together with two G protein coupled receptors

SYSTEMIC HUMORAL CONTROL OF BLOOD FLOW

Humoral factors affecting the vascular system include both vasodilators and vasoconstrictors. Some examples are shown in Figure CR.24.

Catecholamines

Under physiological conditions the most powerful humoral agents affecting the systemic vessels are the catecholamines. Epinephrine is released from the adrenal medulla and exerts its primary effect on cardiac muscle. It also dilates resistance vessels in skeletal muscle via β-adrenergic fibres at low concentrations. At higher concentrations α-adrenergic effects predominate causing vasoconstriction. Norepinephrine is a powerful vasoconstrictor and is controlled mainly via its release from sympathetic nerve endings as opposed to its release from the adrenal medulla.

Vasopressin

This nine amino acid peptide is also called antidiuretic hormone (ADH) because of its primary action in the kidney of causing the retention of free water from the glomerular filtrate in the collecting ducts. In supranormal doses vasopressin increases blood pressure by systemic vasoconstriction. It also stimulates ACTH secretion from the anterior pituitary and promotes glycogenolysis in the liver.

SOME ENDOGENOUS SYSTEMIC VASOCONSTRICTORS AND VASODILATORS

Action	Agent	Origin
Vasoconstrictors	Norepinephrine	Adrenal medulla, post ganglionic nerve endings
	Epinephrine	Adrenal medulla
	Vasopressin	Posterior pituitary
	Angiotensin II	Conversion of angiotesin I in the lung
Vasodilators	Histamine	Mast cells
	Kinins	Pancreas, salivary glands, sweat glands
	Atrial natriuretic peptide (ANP)	Atria
	Vasoactive intestinal peptide (VIP)	Autonomic nerve endings Gastro-intestinal tract nerves

Figure CR.24

Angiotensin

The juxtaglomerular apparatus of the kidney synthesizes and stores renin. Low renal perfusion stimulates the juxtaglomerular apparatus to release renin which splits the α_2-globulin angiotensinogen to produce angiotensin I. Angiotensin converting enzyme (ACE) then cleaves angiotensin I to angiotensin II in the lung. Angiotensin II has central and peripheral vasoconstrictor effects as well as participating in the control of thirst and stimulating the release of aldosterone from the adrenal cortex. Aldosterone increases tubular re-absorption of sodium and, by osmotic effects, water and stimulates the excretion of potassium and hydrogen ions. Aldosterone also enhances excitability of vascular smooth muscle, augmenting the action of angiotensin II.

Atrial natriuretic peptide (ANP)

This is a 17 amino acid polypeptide containing a ring formed by a disulphide bond between two cysteine residues. It causes natriuresis, lowers blood pressure and inhibits vasopressin secretion; thus, opposing the action of angiotensin II. The rate of release from atrial muscle cells is proportional to the stretch of the atria obtained by changes in central venous pressure.

Kinins

Kinins are peptides originating from the exocrine glands. Bradykinin (9 amino acids) and lysylbradykinin (10 amino acids) are recognised vasodilators. The kinins are formed by kallikreins from protein precursors, and are metabolised by kininases. One kininase is angiotensin converting enzyme (ACE) which gives this enzyme a pivotal role in the control of blood pressure.

Histamine

This amine is derived from the decarboxylation of histidine, and is produced in the CNS, gastric mucosa and mast cells. Regulation of histamine release is via inhibitory H_1, H_2 and H_3 receptors. Histamine is a potent vasodilator. Hypersensitivity reactions can result in a massive release of histamine with a disastrous drop in blood pressure due to generalised vasodilatation.

Polypeptides

Other polypeptides have roles in blood pressure control. At cholinergic neurones, vasoactive intestinal peptide causes vasodilatation. Neuropeptide Y causes constriction at sympathetic post ganglionic neurones. In association with sensory neurones, substance P causes vasodilatation and increases capillary permeability.

SYSTEMIC NEUROLOGICAL CONTROL OF BLOOD FLOW

All blood vessels except capillaries and venules possess smooth muscle in their walls and are supplied by sympathetic motor fibres. The fibres supplying blood vessels form a plexus in the adventitia, and then extend to the outer layers of smooth muscle cells in the media. These sympathetic fibres possess a normal resting firing rate or tone, which may be increased or decreased. The vascular smooth muscle is innervated by noradrenergic sympathetic fibres, in which increased activity produces vasoconstriction. However, blood vessels in skeletal muscle are also supplied by cholinergic sympathetic fibres, which cause vasodilatation when stimulated. Constriction of arterioles (vasoconstriction) increases systemic vascular resistance, whereas constriction of veins (venoconstriction), especially splanchnic veins, increases the relative intravascular volume, and, hence, venous return to the heart. Systemic vascular resistance does not change significantly with venoconstriction when compared with vasoconstriction.

Autonomic reflexes mediate neurological control of the peripheral vascular system. In these reflexes peripheral receptors feed impulses into the vasomotor centres in the CNS via afferent pathways. There the sensory information is used to modulate sympathetic tone that is relayed back to the peripheral vessels via efferent pathways. Some reflexes are mediated at spinal level while others involve higher centres.

Vasomotor centres in the CNS

The vasomotor centres are areas of the reticular formation in the medulla oblongata and bulbar parts of the pons. The pressor region is located rostrally in the ventrolateral medulla, and provides a tonic output that maintains a background level of vascular smooth muscle tone. When the pressor centre is stimulated it causes increased vasoconstriction, increased heart rate and increased myocardial contractility. The depressor region is caudal and ventromedial to the pressor area. When stimulated the depressor region decreases blood pressure by inhibiting the pressor area and also inhibiting sympathetic outflow directly at spinal level. Sympathetic tone is, thus, set by the balance between these two centres, which not only respond to afferents from peripheral reflexes, but are also influenced by central chemoreceptors and higher centres in the brain.

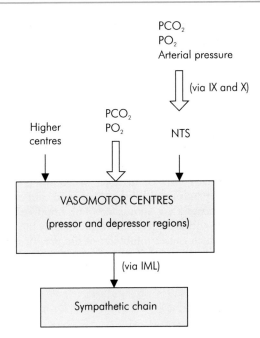

NTS = nucleus tractus solitarius
IML = intermediolateral grey column

Figure CR.25 Factors affecting the vasomotor centre

The various influences on the vasomotor centres are summarised in Figure CR.25.

Efferent pathways

The vasomotor centres project directly to pre-ganglionic neurones in the intermediolateral (IML) grey columns of the spinal cord. There is continuous tonic activity in sympathetic noradrenergic but not cholinergic neurones. Pre-ganglionic fibres pass from the IML columns to the paravertebral sympathetic chain, from which post ganglionic fibres carry the sympathetic outflow to the heart, vessels and adrenal medullae.

Afferent pathways

Baroreceptors in the carotid sinuses and chemoreceptors in the carotid bodies feed afferent impulses into the CNS via branches (nerve of Hering) of the glossopharyngeal nerves. Cardiac baroreceptors, aortic arch baroreceptors and aortic body chemoreceptors, relay afferent impulses centrally in fibres (cardiac depressor nerves) of the right and left vagus nerves. The nucleus tractus solitarius (NTS) is the sensory nucleus for the glossopharyngeal and vagus nerves, and is located in the dorsomedial medulla. Inhibitory connections pass from the NTS to the pressor centre.

Influence of higher centres on vasomotor tone

The vasomotor centres also respond to higher centres in the brain. These include:

- Hypothalamus – stimulation of the anterior hypothalamus decreases blood pressure and heart rate, while stimulation of the posterolateral hypothalamus increases blood pressure and heart rate. The hypothalamus also controls cutaneous vasodilatation and vasoconstriction in response to environmental or body temperature changes
- Cerebral cortex – stimulation of the motor and pre-motor areas is associated with increased blood pressure and heart rate
- Limbic system – emotional stimuli can produce depressor responses such as fainting and blushing

Baroreceptors

Baroreceptors are irregularly branched and coiled nerve endings located in the walls of the carotid sinus, the aorta and the heart. The carotid sinus is an enlargement of the internal carotid artery just above its origin. They respond to the degree of stretch in the vessel or heart wall and, hence, to the pressure (or more strictly the transmural pressure) in the vessel or heart. When intraluminal pressure increases, wall stretch increases and the frequency of impulses discharged by baroreceptors increases. If stretch decreases baroreceptor output frequency decreases. The baroreceptor impulses exert an inhibitory influence on the pressor centre and, thus, baroreceptor control represents a negative feedback control system to maintain cardiovascular stability. The baroreceptor response curve is sigmoidal but is linear over a pressure range of 80–180 mmHg (Figure CR.26).

Baroreceptors not only respond to pressure magnitude but also rate of change of pressure. The impulse discharge rate is, thus, greater during early systole than diastole. At low pressures there are few discharges during the upstroke of arterial pressure. At higher

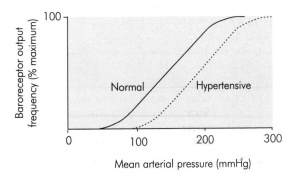

Figure CR.26 Baroreceptor response curve

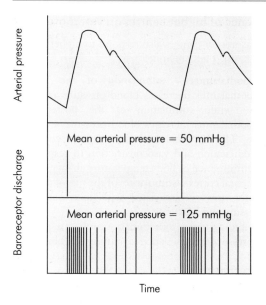

Figure CR.27 Baroreceptor activity during the cardiac cycle

mean arterial pressures, discharges are present throughout more of the cycle. The frequency remains higher early in the cycle. At very high mean arterial pressures, discharges occur continuously, achieving maximum inhibition of the vasomotor centre (Figure CR.27). This means that baroreceptors not only respond to changes in pressure but also to changes in pulse pressure and heart rate.

Baroreceptors can reset their working range and sensitivity, or are 'adaptive', in response to sustained pressure changes. During chronic hypertension, the baroreceptors adapt to higher pressures and the response curve is shifted to the right. These changes are reversible.

Carotid and aortic baroreceptor reflex

Baroreceptors in the carotid sinus and the arch of the aorta monitor arterial pressure, arterial pulse pressure and heart rate. They play a key role in maintaining cardiovasular homeostasis against acute disturbances as occur in trauma or exercise. Carotid sinus baroreceptors are more sensitive to blood pressure changes than aortic baroreceptors. The carotid baroreceptors also respond to external mechanical stimulation, which increases their firing rate eliciting an inhibitory vasomotor response. In susceptible individuals this may reduce blood pressure sufficiently to induce syncope. Therapeutically, carotid sinus massage can sometimes be effective in slowing a supraventricular tachycardia.

Cardiopulmonary baroreceptor reflex

Stretch receptors exist in the atria, ventricles and pulmonary vessels. These receptors protect against rapid changes in intravascular volume by varying their tonic discharge, which exerts an inhibitory influence over the medullary pressor centre. They also play a part in controlling heart rate.

There are two types of stretch receptor in the atria. Type A discharge predominantly during atrial systole, while type B discharge during atrial filling, particularly over the later part of diastole. When intravascular volume expands atrial filling is increased, and both A and B receptors are stimulated. The impulses from these receptors are relayed to the medulla by the vagus nerves, which causes inhibition of the pressor centre and stimulation of the sinus node. This results in vasodilatation, a fall in blood pressure, increased renal blood flow, increased urine output, and a rise in heart rate.

Bainbridge reflex

This reflex was described by the English physiologist Bainbridge in 1915, who noted an increase in heart rate in response to rapid intravascular infusion of fluid into anaesthetised animals. The receptors are the atrial A and B receptors described above. The afferent limb of the reflex is the vagus nerves, while the efferent limb consists of sympathetic nerves to the sinus node. Heart rate is, thus, influenced by the two opposing actions of the arterial baroreceptor reflex and the Bainbridge reflex. Whether the heart rate increases or decreases with a sudden increase in intravascular volume is thought to be dependent on the initial heart rate, if it is high it tends to decrease (arterial baroreceptor reflex), while if the initial heart rate is low it tends to increase (Bainbridge reflex).

Pulmonary stretch receptors

Stretch receptors in the lung, although mainly concerned with respiratory control also inhibit the vasomotor centres when stimulated. Thus, inflation of the lungs results in systemic vasodilatation and a decrease in blood pressure.

Chemoreceptor reflexes

These reflexes are mediated centrally by receptors in the medulla, and peripherally by the carotid and aortic bodies. The chemoreceptors can respond to parameters that reflect hypoxia, hypercapnia, acidaemia or ischaemia. Chemoreceptor reflexes are mainly directed towards respiratory control but do exert some effects over cardiovascular parameters. Afferent pathways are mainly via the glossopharyngeal or vagus nerves, although coronary and pulmonary chemoreceptors may also possess sympathetic afferents.

- Peripheral chemoreceptor reflexes – chemoreceptors are in the carotid and aortic bodies. The carotid bodies are small masses of chromaffin tissue situated on the medial aspects of the carotid sinuses, while the aortic bodies are similar organs located over the anterior and posterior aspects of the aortic arch. The chemoreceptors respond primarily to a reduction in arterial oxygen tension (PaO_2), but are also sensitive to a rise in arterial carbon dioxide tension ($PaCO_2$) or a fall in pH. Both respiratory and circulatory centres in the brain stem receive the afferent impulses. The main effects of peripheral chemoreceptor reflexes are on the respiratory centre but a minor effect is exerted on the pressor centre with hypoxia and hypercapnia producing increases in blood pressure and a transient bradycardia
- Central chemoreceptor reflexes – the vasomotor centres as well as other medullary receptors respond to changes in $PaCO_2$ and pH. These central reflexes predominate over the peripheral receptors, stimulating the respiratory centres and causing an increase in pressor tone and decrease in heart rate, following a rise in $PaCO_2$ or a fall in pH. Central chemoreceptors are relatively insensitive to hypoxia, hypoxic reflexes being mediated primarily through the carotid and aortic bodies. Concomitant peripheral vasodilatation often leaves arterial blood pressure unchanged
- Cushing reflex – a vasomotor centre reflex caused by a direct response of pressor cells to ischaemia. This results in reflex vasoconstriction and decreased heart rate. This increases blood pressure at the expense of cardiac output, but sustains cerebral perfusion pressure
- The Bezold–Jarisch reflex – a response of coronary artery chemoreceptors to ischaemia causing hypotension and bradycardia but increasing coronary blood flow
- Pulmonary chemoreceptor reflex – chemoreceptors also exist in the lung which cause apnoea, hypotension and bradycardia when stimulated by ischaemic metabolites

Pain reflexes

Cutaneous painful stimuli evoke the somatosympathetic reflex. Afferent impulses stimulate the rostral ventrolateral medulla to cause a rise in blood pressure. Prolonged or severe pain may cause vasodilatation and syncope.

Visceral pain often produces a depressor response due to stimulation of vagal or pelvic parasympathetic afferents. In contrast, large bowel has a significant degree of sympathetic innervation and can produce a pressor response when stimulated.

BLOOD VOLUME

The volume of blood in the body is about 70 ml/kg in adults and 80 ml/kg in infants. Various types of blood vessel contain different proportions of the total blood volume. Distribution of blood volume in the vascular system is summarised in Figure CR.28.

Central venous pressure and blood volume

The venous system contains about two-thirds of the blood volume and can be visualised as a 'venous reservoir' supplying blood flow to the heart. Central venous pressure (CVP) is therefore a balance between blood volume, venomotor tone and the demands of the cardiac pump. At a given blood volume, as cardiac output increases, the rate at which blood is removed from the venous reservoir increases and central venous pressure falls. Similarly when cardiac output decreases a rise in CVP is produced. This relationship reflects the passive pressure–volume characteristics of the venous system, and can be described by the vascular function curve (Figure CR.29) which plots CVP against cardiac output with a fixed blood volume. Alterations in blood volume, e.g. haemorrhage or transfusion will shift the vascular function curve up or down.

This relationship should be differentiated from the

DISTRIBUTION OF BLOOD IN THE CIRCULATORY SYSTEM

Location	Volume (%)
Heart	5
Systemic circulation	
Aorta and arteries	11
Capillaries	6
Veins and venules	66
Pulmonary circulation	
Arteries	3
Capillaries	4
Veins and venules	5

Figure CR.28

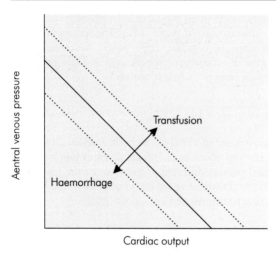

Figure CR.29 Vascular function curve

situation in which blood volume is actively increased to increase cardiac output. This is an application of the Frank–Starling relationship and is described by a ventricular function curve that plots cardiac output against CVP. A combination of the vascular function curve and the ventricular function curve describes ventriculovenous coupling (see page 329), which has a potential clinical application in balancing the use of IV infusion and inotropes when optimising cardiac output.

CONTROL OF BLOOD VOLUME

The haemodynamic effects of blood volume depend on the volume in the venous reservoir. This is controlled acutely by reflex venoconstriction and redistribution from other areas of the circulatory system. Blood can be diverted from 'reservoirs' such as cutaneous vascular beds, splanchnic vessels and the liver. Longer term control of blood volume is set by the balance between intravascular fluid and interstitial fluid compartments, fluid intake and renal loss. These mechanisms are illustrated by considering the events occurring in response to haemorrhage.

CIRCULATORY CONTROL UNDER SPECIAL CIRCUMSTANCES

HAEMORRHAGE

An acute loss of about 5% or more, of the blood volume is accompanied by immediate physiological changes, which can cause a patient to become pale and sweaty with a rapid thready pulse. A rapid respiratory rate and

mild cyanosis may also be present. The underlying physiological changes include:

- Decreased systolic and diastolic blood pressures
- Reduced pulse pressure
- Increased heart rate and contractility
- Increased vasoconstriction and venoconstriction
- Diversion of blood centrally from cutaneous, muscular and splanchnic circulations
- Adrenal medulla stimulation with increased circulating catecholamine levels
- Tachypnoea

These initial haemodynamic changes may reverse over about 20 min, depending on the extent of the blood loss. If blood loss is excessive, compensatory mechanisms can only produce transient improvement and haemorrhagic shock ensues, with continued haemodynamic deterioration. Compensation for acute blood loss is mediated via a series of mechanisms:

- The baroreceptor reflex gives rise to selective vasoconstriction of arterioles which increases systemic vascular resistance and preserves cerebral and coronary blood flow
- Chemoreceptor reflexes augment the baroreceptor reflex particularly at lower arterial pressures (< 60 mmHg) where the baroreceptor response is limited by its threshold effect
- Cerebral ischaemic response. At mean arterial pressures below 40 mmHg cerebral ischaemia is associated with direct stimulation of the adrenal medulla augmenting the effects produced by baroreceptor and chemoreceptor reflexes
- Re-absorption of interstitial fluid – vasoconstriction reduces capillary hydrostatic pressures which increases net re-absorption of interstitial fluid. About 0.25 ml/kg/min tissue fluid can be gained through increased re-absorption. Ultimately fluid is also shifted from the intracellular compartment to the interstitial space, this balance probably being influenced by raised cortisol levels stimulated during haemorrhage
- Release of catecholamines. Activation of the sympathetic system via the baroreceptor and chemoreceptor reflexes produces stimulation of the adrenal medulla and increased levels of circulating catecholamines
- Renal conservation of water and salt. Decreased renal perfusion produces secretion of renin from the juxtaglomerular apparatus. The renin converts plasma angiotensinogen, to angiotensin I, which in turn becomes angiotensin II, a potent vasoconstrictor. Stimulation of the adrenal cortex also increases aldosterone levels leading to renal retention of sodium. Reduced intravascular volume

decreases firing of atrial stretch receptors and produces increased secretion of antidiuretic hormone (ADH) from the posterior pituitary. This results in the retention of water in the renal collecting ducts. ADH is also a potent vasoconstrictor at higher concentrations. The overall effects are retention of water and sodium which help to restore extracellular fluid volume

Over 6 weeks increased erythropoietin secretion from the kidney stimulates bone marrow to produce more red blood cells and replace haemoglobin lost during haemorrhage.

VALSALVA MANOEUVRE

The Valsalva manoeuvre is forced expiration against a closed glottis, and provides a good demonstration of autonomic reflex control of heart rate and blood pressure. The manoeuvre produces a square wave rise in intrathoracic pressure of about 40 mmHg (Figure CR.30). The cardiovascular response can be considered in the following stages:

- Initially there is an immediate increase in arterial blood pressure as the step in intrathoracic pressure is transmitted to the pressure in the aorta. The increased intrathoracic pressure also compresses pulmonary veins, forcing their contents into the left atrium, and producing a transient rise in cardiac output

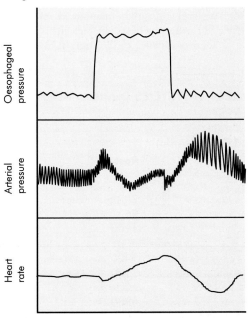

Figure CR.30 Valsalva manoeuvre

- The sustained increase in intrathoracic pressure is also accompanied by higher intra-abdominal pressure due to contraction of the abdominal wall muscles. Raised pressure in the abdomen and thorax compresses the venae cavae reducing the venous return to the right and left sides of the heart. This causes a decrease in arterial and pulse pressures
- The fall in arterial and pulse pressures results in diminished stimulation of baroreceptors, causing a tachycardia and increased systemic vascular resistance. This restores mean arterial and pulse pressures to about resting values recorded before the manoeuvre
- Opening the glottis releases the positive intrathoracic pressure, producing a sudden fall in aortic pressure. The resulting drop in arterial pressure is maintained briefly as blood fills the pulmonary vessels and central veins, rather than providing venous return to the heart. Baroreceptor reflexes again respond to this sudden drop in arterial pressure, and act to restore venous return and cardiac output
- Finally, as venous return to both sides of the heart increases again, cardiac output is restored, but ejects into a peripheral vascular system already constricted by baroreceptor reflexes. Blood pressure, thus, overshoots its original resting value, until increased stimulation of baroreceptors causes reflex bradycardia and vasodilatation to restore blood pressure to normal once again

The events described above occur even after sympathectomy, because reflex activity can still be mediated if the vagus nerves remain intact. However, in the case of autonomic neuropathy, a persisting fall in blood pressure is caused by the high intrathoracic pressure, and there is no reflex tachycardia. Then, on release of the intrathoracic pressure, no overshoot of arterial blood pressure occurs.

A. M. Valsalva (1666–1723) was an Italian anatomist who described the above manoeuvre for clearing the Eustachian tube.

EXERCISE

Exercise activates reflex mechanisms that enhance cardiovascular performance. These include:

- Cerebrocortical activation of the sympathetic system due to anticipation of physical activity. This is sometimes referred to as 'central command'
- Cardiovascular reflexes due to stimulation of muscle mechanoreceptors during contraction. The afferent limb is via small unmyelinated fibres which relay centrally by unidentified connections, to

activate sympathetic fibres to the heart and peripheral vessels
- Local reflexes stimulated by rapid accumulation of metabolites during muscle contraction
- Baroreceptor reflexes

Peripheral chemoreceptors do not play a significant part during exercise as arterial pH, $PaCO_2$ and PaO_2 remain about normal. In addition to the cardiovascular reflexes outlined above, pulmonary reflexes increase the depth and rate of breathing.

Moderate exercise levels

Prior to commencing exercise, anticipation of activity increases sympathetic discharge and inhibits the parasympathetic system. Mild to moderate degrees of exercise lead to graded changes which:

- Increase cardiovascular performance
- Redistribute blood flow to active areas
- Maintain cerebral blood flow
- Increase oxygen consumption
- Increase the efficiency of oxygen extraction

Regional blood flow during exercise

Blood flow is diverted to active muscle from skin, splanchnic regions, kidneys and inactive muscles. Cutaneous blood flow although decreased initially gradually increases during exercise with rising body temperature. As exercise severity increases further and oxygen consumption increases to maximum levels, cutaneous vasoconstriction occurs and blood flow to the skin starts to decrease. Myocardial blood flow increases concomitantly according to metabolic

demands. Cerebral blood flow remains unchanged during exercise. These changes in the distribution of blood flow are summarised in Figure CR.31.

Skeletal muscle during exercise

Blood flow to the active muscles increases progressively in keeping with the work rate of the tissues. Locally accumulating substances and conditions, such as potassium and adenosine together with a reduction in pH, produce arteriolar dilatation and blood flows up to 20 times resting values. Capillary recruitment increases dramatically. Net movement of fluid into the interstitial compartment occurs and lymph flow increases aided by muscle contractions. Oxygen extraction can rise by as much as sixty times, outstripping increases in blood flow and leading to greater arteriovenous oxygen differences. This higher degree of extraction is mediated by the right shift in the haemoglobin oxygen dissociation curve, which is associated with the accumulation of lactic acid, decreased pH, increased $PaCO_2$ and increased temperature.

Cardiac output in exercise

The enhanced cardiac output during exercise is achieved mainly through the heart rate, which follows increased sympathetic and decreased parasympathetic drive of the sino-atrial node. At mild to moderate work rates the heart rate increases proportionately to an appropriate level and is then maintained. As work rate is increased further the heart rate plateaus at about 180 bpm. In trained athletes, cardiac output may increase

DISTRIBUTION OF BLOOD FLOW TO DIFFERENT ORGAN SYSTEMS DURING MODERATE EXERCISE AND REST

Organ system	Blood flow (ml/min)	
	Exercise	Rest
Brain	750	750
Heart	750	250
Skeletal muscle	12 500	1200
Skin	1900	500
Abdominal viscera	600	1400
Kidneys	600	1100
Other	400	600
Total	17 500	5800

Figure CR.31

by seven times resting values but stroke volume may only increase to twice the resting value.

Venous return and blood volume in exercise

The increase in cardiac output during exercise is accompanied by a commensurate increase in venous return. As a result central venous pressure does not change significantly. Thus, the Frank–Starling mechanism does not normally play a major part in increasing stroke volume during moderate exercise; however, when exercise becomes maximal, central venous pressure tends to rise and the Frank–Starling mechanism starts to contribute significantly. The mechanisms augmenting venous return include:

- Increased venomotor tone
- Increased muscle pump activity
- Redirection of blood from cutaneous, renal and splanchnic circulations
- Enhanced thoracic pump action due to increased respiratory rate and tidal volume

Intravascular volume is usually slightly reduced during exercise due to increased insensible losses from the respiratory tract and skin. In addition, there is increased net capillary filtration into the interstitial muscle space. As a result there is often a slight rise in haematocrit during exercise.

Arterial pressure

Both systolic and diastolic blood pressures increase during exercise, although systolic pressure increases relatively more than diastolic. This results in an increased pulse pressure, which is attributed to an increased stroke volume and higher ejection velocity from the left ventricle.

This increased arterial pressure occurs in the face of a decreased systemic vascular resistance (mainly due to vasodilatation in active muscle), and reflects the greatly increased cardiac output (up to seven times resting value).

The sympathetic system is important in maintaining blood pressure during exercise and if compromised by drugs (β blockers) or disease (autonomic neuropathy) effort induced hypotension or syncope can result. Similarly a restricted cardiac output (aortic stenosis) can produce the same effect.

Severe exercise and exhaustion

When exercise is taken to the point of exhaustion, the compensatory reflexes fail and de-compensatory changes occur. These include:

- Heart rate rises to plateau of about 180 bpm
- Stroke volume plateaus and may even decrease
- Blood pressure begins to fall
- Dehydration occurs
- Vasoconstriction due to excessive sympathetic activity
- Body temperature continues to rise due to decreased heat loss
- Lactic acid and CO_2 accumulate giving rise to decreased tissue pH
- Muscle cramps and pain
- Subjective feelings of weariness and lack of drive to continue activity

SPECIAL CIRCULATIONS

Cardiac output is distributed between the various organ systems as shown in Figure CR.32.

Circulation to the lungs, kidneys and liver are described on pages 413, 363 and 489 respectively.

BLOOD FLOW TO DIFFERENT ORGAN SYSTEMS AT REST		
Organ system	Blood flow (ml/min)	% Cardiac output
Brain	750	13
Heart	250	4
Skeletal muscle	1200	20
Skin	500	9
Abdominal viscera	1400	24
Kidneys	1100	20
Other	600	10
Total	5800	100

Figure CR.32

This section discusses the circulations of the heart, the brain and the foetus.

CORONARY CIRCULATION

In the root of the aorta, the right coronary artery arises behind the right cusp of the aortic valve, and supplies the right atrium and ventricle. The left coronary artery arises behind the posterior cusp of the aortic valve, and divides close to its origin into circumflex and anterior descending branches, before supplying the left atrium and ventricle. Some overlap of the territory supplied by each main artery usually occurs. Epicardial arteries originate from these main coronary arteries, and branch to form end arteries that penetrate the myocardium. The blood flow through each main artery is equal in 30% of people, but the right coronary artery is dominant in 50%. Two-thirds of coronary blood flow drains into the right atrium via the coronary sinus and anterior coronary veins. The remainder drains directly into the chambers of the heart through small thebesian veins, arteriosinusoidal vessels and arterioluminal vessels. Venous drainage into left sided chambers constitutes true shunt and makes a small contribution to arterial desaturation.

Coronary blood flow

Total coronary blood flow at rest is about 250 ml/min. The myocardium normally extracts about 70% of the oxygen content of coronary blood at rest; thus, increasing coronary perfusion is the only way to increase oxygen delivery. At rest the oxygen requirement of the myocardium is 10 ml/min/100 g at rest giving a total basal oxygen requirement of 30 ml/min for an adult. Cardiac muscle is versatile in its use of substrate, normally using 60% fatty acid and 40% carbohydrate as fuel. It may adapt to use different proportions and include ketone bodies as substrate.

Coronary blood flow and its distribution can be studied using:

- Coronary angiography – radiopaque dye is used to outline coronary vessels and radioactive xenon to quantify regional perfusion
- Thallium scan – radioactive thallium uptake is used as a marker of regional distribution of perfusion in the myocardium
- Technetium scan – selective uptake of radioactive technetium marks infarcted areas

Factors determining coronary blood flow

Since the coronary arteries originate in the root of the aorta, aortic pressure provides the main driving force for coronary blood flow. Normally, this pressure is controlled by baroreceptor reflexes and, thus, regulation of coronary blood flow is achieved through coronary vasodilatation or vasoconstriction. Coronary vascular resistance is mainly controlled by local factors. Some of the factors affecting coronary blood flow are detailed below:

- Extravascular compression (extracoronary resistance) – this describes the external compression produced by myocardial contraction during the cardiac cycle. Coronary blood flow is reduced to zero in early systole and may even be transiently reversed (Figure CR.33). This 'squeezing' effect is greatest at endocardial levels and least towards the epicardium. However, in the normal heart endocardial and epicardial blood flows are about equal in the cardiac cycle. The bulk of coronary blood flow, thus, occurs during diastole. However, since diastole decreases as heart rate increases, coronary blood flow can become compromised by tachyarrhythmias. Counterpulsation or 'balloon pumping' assists coronary blood flow by inflating an aortic balloon cyclically during diastole
- Metabolic demands – the correlation between metabolic activity in the heart and coronary blood flow is fixed. Metabolites or an unidentified vasoactive agent, act to increase or decrease the oxygen supply if demand is varied. Alternatively, if the oxygen supply is limited cardiac activity adapts. Likely substances responsible for this effect include potassium ions and adenosine
- Autonomic system – activation of the sympathetic system tends to produce an increase in coronary blood flow. This occurs as a net result of increased

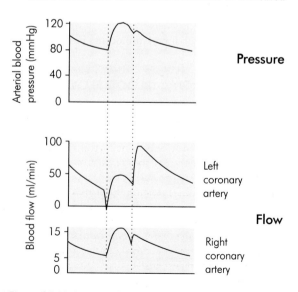

Figure CR.33 Coronary blood flow and the cardiac cycle

metabolic demand in the face of the negative effects of increased contractility and heart rate on coronary blood flow. Under β blockade coronary vessels constrict in response to sympathetic stimulation. Stimulation of the vagus nerves produces slight coronary vasodilatation

- Coronary perfusion pressure (CPP) – this is the pressure across the coronary arteries and equals the difference between aortic pressure and intraventricular pressure. Autoregulation operates over a range of CPP between 60 and 180 mmHg. If CPP changes suddenly, coronary vessels respond by dilating or constricting to dampen dramatic surges or falls in coronary blood flow

Figure CR.34 Summarises the factors affecting coronary vascular resistance

SUMMARY OF FACTORS AFFECTING CORONARY VASCULAR RESISTANCE

Factor	Effect on coronary vascular resistance
Sympathetic activity	
alpha-receptors	↑
beta-receptors	↓
Vagal activity	↓
Systolic compression	↑
Coronary perfusion pressure	↑ or ↓
Adenosine	↓
Other metabolic factors	
CO_2, O_2, H^+, K^+	↓ or ↑

Figure CR.34

Cardiac ischaemia

When the oxygen demands of the myocardium outstrip the oxygen supply, myocardial dysfunction and tissue damage follow. The oxygen requirements are related to the cardiac work rate, which in turn is dependent on systolic arterial pressure and cardiac output. Oxygen requirements are increased disproportionately by increases in systolic pressure, compared with cardiac output. Thus, if cardiac work is increased by increasing systolic pressure, oxygen requirements are much greater than if the increase in cardiac work were achieved by increasing cardiac output. 'Pressure' work is therefore more expensive than 'volume' work in terms of oxygen consumption. This is a major factor underlying the mortality associated with aortic stenosis. Clinically myocardial ischaemia results in the chest pain of angina pectoris and ultimately the tissue necrosis occurring in myocardial infarction.

Myocardial blood flow may be increased in ischaemic heart disease by:

- Coronary vasodilators (glyceryl trinitrate)
- Coronary thrombus dissolution (streptokinase)
- Coronary angioplasty (dilatation by catheter balloon)
- Coronary bypass graft
- Coronary laser endarterectomy

CEREBRAL CIRCULATION

The left and right carotid arteries join the basilar artery to form the circle of Willis from which the left and right anterior, middle and posterior cerebral arteries arise. The basilar artery is formed by the anastomosis of the two vertebral arteries. Each carotid artery supplies its own side of the brain, and there is no significant perfusion of the opposite side by a carotid. Cerebral venous drainage is via the internal jugular veins that are fed by the dural sinuses or directly by cerebral veins.

Brain cells are intolerant of hypoxia and require uninterrupted perfusion. Several seconds of total ischaemia can produce unconsciousness and several minutes may result in irreversible damage. Cerebral vessels are innervated by sympathetic fibres that enter the skull around the carotid arteries. These fibres originate in the superior cervical ganglia. There are also cholinergic fibres from the sphenopalantine ganglia and facial nerve. Cerebral vessels are supplied by sensory fibres originating in the trigeminal ganglia. The stimulation of sensory fibres on vessels by metabolites is thought to cause migraine.

Cerebral blood flow

Mean cerebral blood flow is about 55 ml/100 g/min and is maintained within a relatively narrow range compared with other organs. It varies between the anatomical structures of the brain with grey matter in general receiving more than twice (70 ml/100 g/min) the blood flow of white matter (30 ml/100 g/min).

The brain consumes about 3.5 ml/100 g/min oxygen leaving the jugular venous blood 65% saturated. Structures such as the colliculi and basal ganglia receive much greater blood flows than the brain stem and cerebellum. Cortical blood flow is dependent on activity and perfusion of specific areas reaches high levels (> 130 ml/100 g/min) when activated.

Cerebral blood flow can be estimated by:

- Kety method – an application of the Fick principle that determines the total cerebral blood flow in ml/100 g/min. Nitrous oxide is used as the transported substance because it has partition coefficient = 1, which ensures that the brain concentration becomes equal to the jugular venous concentration, after an equilibration time of 10 min. A subject breathes 15% nitrous oxide for 10 min. The total nitrous oxide transferred to 100 g brain tissue per min (Q) can be determined from the final nitrous oxide content of 100g of jugular venous blood divided by 10. The average arteriovenous difference (D) in nitrous oxide content per ml is determined from arterial and venous samples during equilibration. The blood flow can then be calculated from the ratio Q/D
- Scintillography – using radioactive tracers (xenon) to trace regional blood flow
- SPECT scanning – scintillography enhanced by CT or MRI scanning
- PET scanning – use of 2-deoxyglucose labelled with a positron emitter
- Doppler – crude but readily available for clinical use in ICU or operating theatre

Regulation of cerebral blood flow

Control of cerebral circulation is primarily through autoregulation due to local metabolic factors. Neural control is thought to play a minor role. Total cerebral blood flow is maintained constant over a range of mean arterial pressure and in the face of varying levels of $PaCO_2$ and PaO_2. This is achieved by control of total cerebrovascular resistance and cerebral perfusion pressure (Figure CR.35).

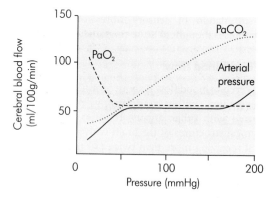

Figure CR.35 Autoregulation of cerebral blood flow

Regional cerebral blood flow on the other hand, is highly variable and varies according to activity and local metabolic factors. The factors affecting total cerebral blood flow include:

- Cerebral perfusion pressure – pressure across the cerebral vessels, given by the difference between the mean arterial pressure – (venous pressure + intracranial pressure). Raised intracranial pressure may reduce cerebral perfusion pressure
- $PaCO_2$ – arterial CO_2 tensions have a marked influence over cerebral blood flow. Low $PaCO_2$ vasoconstricts and raised $PaCO_2$ vasodilates cerebral vessels. Hyperventilation reduces blood volume within the brain and is used to reduce raised intracranial pressure after head injury
- PaO_2 – low PaO_2 vasodilates and high PaO_2 vasoconstricts but the effect of oxygen tension on cerebral vessels occurs to a far lesser degree than with $PaCO_2$
- pH – cerebral vessels are also sensitive to pH independently of $PaCO_2$. A decreased pH causes vasodilatation
- Metabolites – adenosine and potassium have both been implicated in adjusting local cerebral perfusion. Any event causing decreased PaO_2 or increased oxygen demand, produces raised local levels of adenosine in the brain, which are sustained throughout the event. A similar transient rise in potassium ion concentration is also produced. These substances are thought to be instrumental in linking regional blood flow to activity in the brain

RAISED INTRACRANIAL PRESSURE (ICP)

The skull is a rigid bony enclosure that contains 1400 g brain tissue (80%), 75 ml blood (10%) and 75 ml cerebrospinal fluid (10%). These contents are effectively incompressible; therefore, any increase in one component produces a reciprocal decrease in the others (Monro–Kellie doctrine) and an increase in ICP. Cerebral oedema will, thus, be accompanied by a reduction in cerebral blood volume and compression of the ventricles. Brain injury secondary to raised ICP occurs when cerebral blood flow is compromised, or when the increase in ICP is asymmetrical and brain shift occurs. Normal ICP is 0–10 mmHg, while > 15 mmHg is considered significantly raised. As ICP continues to rise, cerebral blood flow is increasingly reduced and brain tissue becomes ischaemic. Vital centres respond by increasing systemic arterial blood pressure, slowing the heart rate and respiratory rate. The blood pressure response attempts to restore cerebral blood flow by restoring the cerebral perfusion pressure. Ultimately herniation of the cerebellar tonsils through the foramen magnum causes compression of the brainstem and death.

Blood-brain barrier

The blood-brain barrier exists between the circulation

and the interstitial fluid in the brain. It consists of the ultrafiltration barrier in the choroid plexuses and the barrier around cerebral capillaries. The latter consists of capillary endothelium, basement membrane and a fenestrated layer of astrocyte endfeet. Tight junctions, impermeable to solutes, join capillary endothelial cells and form a basic component of the blood-brain barrier. Water, carbon dioxide and oxygen diffuse freely across the blood-brain barrier, but the transport of glucose, the principal brain substrate, and ionised molecules is controlled. Proteins and some drugs cannot cross the endothelium unless it is inflamed. The blood-brain barrier has the following functions:

- To provide tight control over ionic (H$^+$, Na$^+$, K$^+$, Ca^{2+}, Mg^{2+}) concentrations in the interstitial fluid because brain cells are extremely sensitive to ion changes
- To protect the brain from transient changes in plasma glucose, the main substrate for the brain
- To protect the brain from endogenous and exogenous toxins in the plasma
- To prevent release of central neurotransmitters into the systemic circulation

FOETAL CIRCULATION

The foetus and placenta form a unit in which the placenta enables the foetus to exchange carbon dioxide and metabolic waste products for oxygen and nutrients from the maternal circulation. In the foetus the left and right sides of the heart work in parallel, unlike the adult circulation where the ventricles work in series. The foetal ventricles acting in parallel, pump blood through the systemic vessels and the placenta, which are also arranged in parallel. The output of the foetal heart is split about 60:40, with the majority passing through the placenta, for oxygenation and nutrient – waste exchange (Figure CR.36). The oxygenated blood returns from the placenta, about half of it entering the liver with the portal circulation, while the rest joins the inferior vena cava (IVC) directly. IVC blood is therefore relatively well oxygenated and passes back to the heart where it divides between right and left sides, the majority passing to the left atrium. The right atrium receives superior vena caval blood from the head and upper limbs which mixes with its portion of the oxygenated IVC blood. The right side of the heart provides two-thirds of the foetal cardiac output that goes to supply the lower half of the foetus. The blood filling the left ventricle is nearly all from the IVC, which is therefore better oxygenated than the blood in the right ventricle. The left ventricle output goes to supply the head and upper limbs. The above pattern of foetal circulation is due to the following vascular

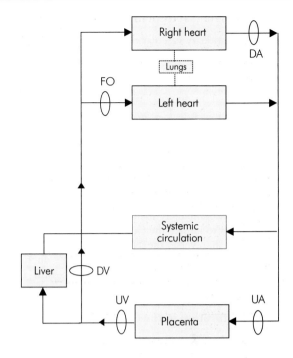

= Foetal vessels which close at or after birth

DA = Ductus arteriosus
FO = Foramen ovale
UA = Umbilical arteries
UV = Umbilical vein
DV = Ductus venosus

Figure CR.36 Foetal circulation

features in the foetus, which ultimately convert to the adult configuration immediately or soon after birth:

- Umbilical arteries – two arteries that arise from the internal iliac arteries and carry 60% of the cardiac output to the placenta
- Umbilical vein – carries oxygenated blood from the placenta back to the foetal liver and IVC
- Ductus venosus – splits off 50% of the oxygenated blood from the umbilical vein to bypass the liver and enter the IVC directly
- Foramen ovale – communication between right and left atria allows about two-thirds of the oxygenated IVC blood to pass directly to the left atrium
- Pulmonary vasculature – foetal lungs are collapsed and have a high pulmonary vascular resistance only allowing about 10% of the right ventricular output to pass through the lungs
- Ductus arteriosus – connects pulmonary artery to the aorta, allowing the right ventricular output to bypass the lungs and flow down the aorta to the lower foetal body and placenta

Changes in foetal circulation at birth

At birth, pulmonary vascular resistance falls markedly as the lungs expand and become aerated. This reduces pulmonary arterial pressures and increases blood flow to the left atrium. Umbilical vessels constrict strongly when exposed to trauma, tension, catecholamines, angiotensin and PaO_2. These stimuli occur at birth and placental circulation ceases resulting in a rise in systemic vascular resistance and arterial pressure. These changes make left atrial pressure higher than right atrial pressure and tend to close the foramen ovale. The ductus arteriosus closes soon after birth usually within 48 H. The mechanism for this closure has not been completely identified, although a high PaO_2 appears to initiate the closure and exposure to a low PaO_2 can reverse the closure in the neonate. Prostaglandins maintain the patency of the ductus arteriosus and indomethacin may be successful in closing a patent ductus arteriosus in a neonate.

Oxygen saturation in the foetus

The foetal blood is oxygenated from venous pools in the placenta. Thus, oxygen saturations at various points in the foetal circulation are lower than their equivalents in the adult. Some oxygen saturation levels are shown in Figure CR.37.

OXYGEN SATURATION IN THE FOETUS

Site	Foetal O_2 saturation
Umbilical vein	80%
IVC/SVC deoxygenated	25%
IVC oxygenated (mixed with placental blood)	67%
Pulmonary artery	52%
Left ventricle	65%
Aorta	62%

Figure CR.37

SECTION 2: 7
RENAL PHYSIOLOGY

C. J. Lote

MORPHOLOGY AND CELLULAR ORGANISATION OF THE KIDNEY

GLOMERULAR FILTRATION

RENAL CLEARANCE AND ITS APPLICATIONS

REGULATION OF RENAL BLOOD FLOW AND GLOMERULAR FILTRATION RATE

TUBULAR TRANSPORT

THE PROXIMAL TUBULE

THE LOOP OF HENLE

THE DISTAL TUBULE AND COLLECTING TUBULE

RENAL EFFECTS OF ANTI-DIURETIC HORMONE

REGULATION OF BODY FLUID VOLUME AND SODIUM RE-ABSORPTION

RENAL REGULATION OF BODY FLUID pH

RENAL REGULATION OF pH IN ACID BASE BALANCE DISTURBANCES

MICTURITION

MORPHOLOGY AND CELLULAR ORGANISATION OF THE KIDNEY

Each human kidney has 1–1.5 million functional units called nephrons. The nephron is a blind ended tube, the blind end forming a capsule (Bowman's capsule) around a knot of blood capillaries (the glomerulus). The other parts of the nephron are the proximal tubule, loop of Henle, distal tubule and collecting duct, although in transport terms the nephron has been divided into additional segments (Figure RE.1).

The glomeruli, proximal tubules and distal tubules are in the outer part of the kidney, the cortex, whereas the loops of Henle and the collecting ducts extend down into the deeper part, the medulla.

Cortical nephrons possess glomeruli located in the outer two-thirds of the cortex and have very short loops of Henle, which only extend a short distance into the medulla or may not reach the medulla at all. In contrast, nephrons whose glomeruli are in the inner third of the cortex (juxtamedullary nephrons) have long loops of Henle that pass deeply into the medulla. In man, about 15% of nephrons are long looped but there are also intermediate types of nephron.

RENAL BLOOD SUPPLY AND VASCULATURE

The kidneys receive 20–25% of the cardiac output but account for only 0.5% of the body weight. Of the blood to the kidney, > 90% enters via the renal artery and supplies the renal cortex, which is perfused at about 500 ml/min/100 g tissue (100 times greater than resting muscle blood flow). The remainder of the renal blood supply goes to the capsule and the renal adipose tissue. Some of the cortical blood passes to the medulla; the outer medulla having a blood flow of 100 ml/min/100 g tissue, while the inner medulla receives 20 ml/min/100 g tissue.

Almost all of the blood that enters the kidneys does so at the renal hilum, via the renal artery. The renal artery

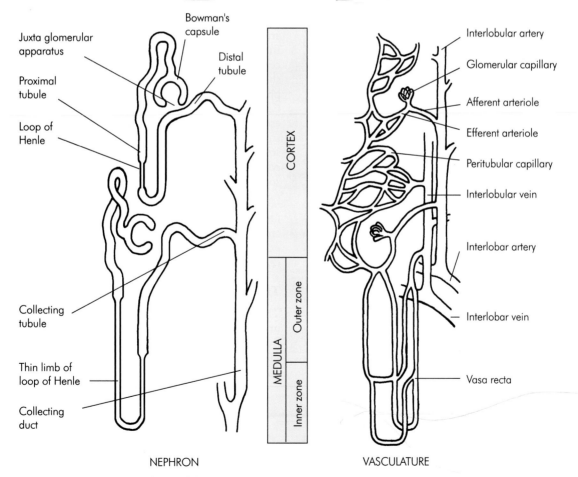

Figure RE.1 Anatomy and vasculature of the kidney

branches to form several interlobar arteries, which themselves branch to give rise to arcuate (or arciform) arteries, which pass along the boundary between cortex and medulla. From these arcuate arteries, branches travel out at right angles, through the cortex towards the capsule. These are interlobular arteries, and the afferent arterioles that supply the glomerular capillaries branch off from the interlobular arteries.

The glomerular capillaries are the site of filtration of the blood, the filtrate entering the Bowman's capsule of the nephron. Glomerular capillaries drain into a second arteriole, the efferent arteriole.

Efferent arterioles are portal vessels, since they carry blood from a capillary network directly to a second capillary network. The efferent arterioles from nephrons in the outer two-thirds of the cortex branch to form a dense network of peritubular capillaries, which surround all the cortical tubular elements. The efferent arterioles in the inner one-third of the cortex give rise not only to some peritubular capillaries, but also to capillaries that have a hairpin course into and out of the medulla, where they are adjacent to the loops of Henle and collecting tubules. These medullary capillaries are vasa recta (Figure RE.1). Vasa recta and peritubular capillaries eventually drain into the renal vein which leaves the kidney at the hilum.

renal cortex → O_2 supply
renal medulla → a-v diff: 1-2%
O_2 supply

FUNCTIONS OF THE RENAL BLOOD SUPPLY

In most organs and tissues of the body, the main purpose of the blood supply is to provide oxygen and to remove CO_2 and other products of metabolism. In the kidney the blood supply not only provides for the metabolic demands of renal tissues but also has to maintain GFR and provide oxygen for the active re-absorption of sodium. The kidneys have a very high oxygen consumption, but because of the high blood flow, the arteriovenous oxygen difference across the kidney is small.

The renal cortex receives far more oxygen than it requires, so that the arteriovenous O_2 difference is only 1–2%. However, the medullary blood supply is only just adequate for the oxygen requirements of medullary cells, because the vasa recta arrangement causes oxygen to short circuit the loops of Henle.

In the cortex, the main function of the blood supply is to provide flow for glomerular filtration and oxygen for sodium re-absorption. Of cortical O_2 consumption, > 50% is used for sodium re-absorption. If renal blood flow is reduced GFR decreases together with sodium re-absorption and oxygen demand. Thus, a reduction in cortical blood flow does not necessarily produce an

increase in oxygen uptake and arteriovenous O_2 difference, until the cortical flow is down to about 150 ml/min/100 g tissue.

RENAL LYMPH DRAINAGE

Renal lymph vessels begin as blind ended tubes in the renal cortex (close to the corticomedullary junction) and run parallel to the arcuate veins to leave the kidney at the renal hilum. Other lymph vessels travel towards the cortex and may pass through the capsule. The importance of the renal lymphatic drainage is frequently overlooked, but in fact the volume of lymph draining into the renal hilum per min is about 0.5 ml, i.e. the kidney produces almost as much lymph per min as urine. Its function is probably to return protein (re-absorbed from the tubular fluid) to the blood.

GLOMERULAR FILTRATION

mesangial cells: (1) prevent macromol
(2) holds B.M in place
(3) act like s.m

THE GLOMERULUS

A glomerulus is a knot of capillaries fed by an afferent arteriole and drained by an efferent arteriole. Its function is to produce ultrafiltrate of the plasma. In the central part of the glomerular tuft are irregularly shaped cells, termed mesangial cells. These are phagocytic and may prevent the accumulation, in the basement membrane, of macromolecules that have escaped from the capillaries. The cells may also have a structural role in holding the delicate glomerular structure in position and, in addition, are capable of contraction (i.e. behave like smooth muscle cells) and so may modify the surface area of the glomerular capillaries available for filtration.

Outside the glomerular area, close to the macula densa, are cells identical to mesangial cells, termed extraglomerular mesangial cells, or 'Goormaghtigh cells' (Figure RE.2).

The glomerular filter

The glomerular ultrafiltrate forms the basis of the urine ultimately produced by the kidney. In moving from the capillary into the Bowman's capsule, the filtrate must traverse three layers, which are:

- The endothelial cell lining of the glomerular capillaries – in this layer adjacent endothelial cells are in contact with each other, and the cells have many circular fenestrations (pores), with a diameter of about 60 nm. The capillary endothelium acts as a screen to prevent blood cells and platelets from coming into contact with the main filter, which is the basement membrane

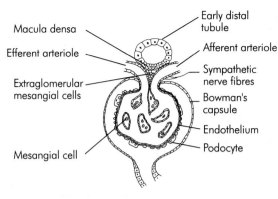

Macula densa

Efferent arteriole

Extraglomerular
mesangial cells

Mesangial cell

Early distal
tubule

Afferent arteriole

Sympathetic
nerve fibres

Bowman's
capsule

Endothelium

Podocyte

Figure RE.2 Structure of the glomerulus

- The glomerular basement membrane – immediately beneath the glomerular endothelium. It forms a continuous layer and is the main filtration barrier allowing the passage of molecules according to their size, shape and charge. It consists of collagen and other glycoproteins, including large amounts of heparan sulphate proteoglycan, with a large number of negative charges
- The visceral epithelial cells of the Bowman's capsule – the third layer of the filter. These cells are podocytes and have a complex morphology. The cell body has projections (trabeculae) that encircle the basement membrane around the capillary. From the trabeculae, many smaller processes (pedicels) project. Substances passing through the slits (slit pores) between adjacent pedicels must pass close to the surface coating of the pedicels, and this could influence the filtration behaviour of large charged molecules, since the pedicels are coated with negatively charged sialoglycoproteins. This layer is thought to maintain the basement membrane by the phagocytosis of macromolecules. It may also play a role in permselectivity which supplements that of the basement membrane

GLOMERULAR FILTRATION AND THE ULTRAFILTRATE

The glomerular filtration rate (GFR) is about 180 l/day (125 ml/min). Since the filtrate is derived from plasma, and the average person has only 3 litres plasma, it follows that this same plasma is filtered (and re-absorbed in the tubules) many times in the course of a day.

Molecular size is the main determinant of whether a substance is filtered or retained in the capillaries. The molecular weight cut-off for the filter is about 70 000 Daltons. Plasma albumin, with a molecular weight of 69 000 Daltons, passes through the filter in minute quantities (retarded also by its charge, as mentioned above). Smaller molecules pass through the filter more easily, but the filter is freely permeable only to those molecules with a molecular weight < about 7000 Daltons (Figure RE.3).

Molecular shape and charge also influence filtration but mainly of large molecules. For example, the rate of filtration of albumin, which has a negative charge, is only about 1/20 that of uncharged dextran molecules of the same molecular weight. This due to the negative charges of the heparan sulphate proteoglycan in the glomerular basement membrane, and the sialoglycoproteins on the foot processes, which repel anionic macromolecules.

The ultrafiltrate passing into Bowman's capsule from the glomerular capillaries is almost protein-free and contains small molecules and ions in virtually the same concentrations as in the afferent arteriole. Similarly, the efferent arteriolar concentrations of such substances are not significantly altered by the filtration process.

GLOMERULAR FILTRATION FORCES

The forces determining filtration are similar to those forces determining the formation of tissue fluid through capillaries elsewhere in the body and depend on the balance between hydrostatic pressure (P_C) and colloid osmotic (π_C) pressure. The balance between P_C and π_C in a normal capillary is shown in Figure RE.3a, which illustrates the drop in P_C (solid line) along a capillary from the arteriolar end to the venous end, and also π_C (broken line), which remains constant along the length of the capillary. At the arteriolar end, $P_C > \pi_C$ causing fluid to leave the capillary forming interstitial fluid. At the venous end of the capillary, $\pi_C > P_C$ leading to net tissue fluid re-absorption. There is an approximate balance between the formation and re-absorption of tissue fluid, any excess being drained by lymphatics.

In a glomerulus, the arrangement of the capillaries as portal vessels alters the magnitude of the filtration forces. The presence of a second resistance vessel (the efferent arteriole) following the glomerular capillary bed produces a higher hydrostatic pressure (45 mmHg), than in other capillary beds (32 mmHg). In addition, the fall in pressure along the glomerular capillary length is less marked (P_G in Figure RE.3b). The filtration rate depends on the difference between forces the pushing fluid out of the capillaries (favouring filtration) and forces tending to draw fluid back into the capillaries (opposing filtration). This relationship can be expressed as:

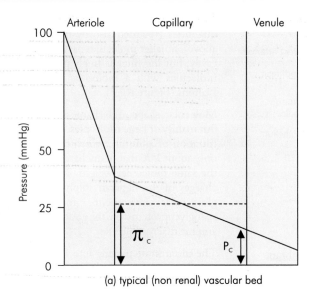

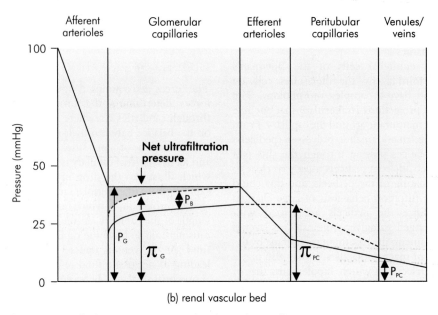

Figure RE.3 Hydrostatic and colloid osmotic pressures in the glomerular capillary

GFR ∝ Forces favouring filtration – Forces opposing filtration.

Alternatively put:

$$(P_G + \pi_B) - (P_B + \pi_G)$$

where:

P_G = hydrostatic pressure in the glomerular capillaries

P_B = colloid osmotic pressure in Bowman's capsule

π_B = hydrostatic pressure in Bowman's capsule

π_G = colloid osmotic pressure in the glomerular capillaries.

Since only very small amounts of protein enter the Bowman's capsule, π_B is effectively zero, and, therefore, it can be said that:

$$GFR \propto P_G - (P_B + \pi_G)$$

Initially at the afferent end of the glomerular capillaries the colloid osmotic pressure, π_G, is initially about 25 mmHg. As the filtration process occurs along the length of the glomerular capillaries, plasma proteins become progressively more concentrated and π_G increases towards the efferent end. Eventually, when π_G reaches about 35 mmHg, the net ultrafiltration pressure is reduced to zero, and there is filtration equilibrium (Figure RE.3b).

The permeability of glomerular capillaries is about 100 times greater than the permeability of capillaries elsewhere in the body. There is only a small quantity of protein filtered at the glomerulus, but its loss in the urine would represent a considerable wastage over the course of a day. Essentially, all of the filtered protein (about 30 g/day) is re-absorbed in the proximal tubule and enters the renal lymph vessels.

Filtration coefficient

To evaluate GFR, K_F, the filtration coefficient, must be introduced:

$$GFR = K_F (P_G - P_B - \pi_G)$$

where:

K_F = (glomerular capillary permeability) × (capillary filtration area).

In man, filtration pressure equilibrium is not quite achieved. A consequence of this disequilibrium, is that small changes in K_F have a considerable effect on GFR.

FILTRATION FRACTION

Renal blood flow is large in relation to the size of the kidneys (about 1.1 l/min), but only a relatively small fraction of this is filtered. Since red blood cells are not filterable, renal plasma flow is the total amount of fluid entering the kidney which is potentially filterable. Renal plasma flow is about 600 ml/min of which 120 ml/min forms the normal GFR. Thus, the filtration fraction is 120/600 or about 20%, i.e. of every 600 ml plasma arriving at the glomeruli, about 480 ml continues into the efferent arterioles.

GLOMERULAR FILTRATION PRESSURE

The net filtration pressure must be sufficient to move plasma out of the glomerular capillary and into the Bowman's capsule. The resulting pressure in the Bowman's capsule must be high enough to overcome the viscosity of the tubular fluid and its friction against the tubule walls, and to maintain the tubules in a patent form against the renal interstitial pressure tending to compress the tubules. Occlusion of the renal blood supply, so that filtration ceases, causes the collapse of the tubular lumina.

Tubulo-glomerular feedback

The filtration rate of individual nephrons; (the single nephron GFR, SNGFR) is greater in juxtamedullary nephrons than in cortical nephrons (50 compared with 30 nl/min). The SNGFR is determined or influenced by the composition of the tubular fluid in the distal nephron while the concentration itself is influenced by the filtration rate. The mechanism of this tubulo–glomerular feedback can be divided into:

- A luminal component, whereby some characteristic of the tubular fluid is recognised by the tubular epithelium
- A mechanism whereby the signal is transmitted to the glomerulus
- An effector mechanism to adjust the rate of glomerular filtration

Such a mechanism can be regarded as preventing the overloading of the re-absorptive capacity of individual nephrons, i.e. if the tubular NaCl load is too high, filtration by that nephron is decreased.

RENAL CLEARANCE AND ITS APPLICATIONS

Clearance is a key concept whose definition requires emphasis.

DEFINITION OF CLEARANCE

The clearance of any substance excreted by the kidney is the volume of plasma that is cleared of the substance in unit time. Thus, the units of clearance are those of volume per unit time (usually ml/min).

Considering the clearance of a substance x, clearance is given by the formula:

$$C_x = \frac{U_x V}{P_x}$$

where:

C_x = clearance of x

U_x = urine concentration of x

P_x = plasma concentration of x

V = urine flow (ml/min).

In fact, clearance only represents a theoretical volume of plasma, since no aliquot of plasma is completely cleared of any substance during its passage through the kidney. The clearance formula has considerable usefulness for assessing renal function. Clearances of two specific substances, inulin and para-aminohippuric acid (PAH), can be used to measure GFR and the renal plasma flow respectively.

MEASUREMENT OF CLEARANCE

To determine clearance of a substance in practice, the following measurements must be made:

- Plasma concentration of the substance – must either be constant or changing in a predictable way so that an accurate average concentration can be calculated. It, therefore, follows that clearance measurements are only suitable for average or steady-state determinations of GFR and RBF and cannot be used if rapid or transient changes are occurring
- Urine concentration of the substance – urine flow must be adequate for the assay in the clearance period (which is a minimum of 10–20 min).

INULIN CLEARANCE: THE MEASUREMENT OF GFR

Inulin is a polysaccharide with a molecular weight of about 5500 Daltons. It is not a normal constituent of the body, but can be injected (or, usually, infused) intravenously to measure inulin clearance. Inulin is small enough to pass through the glomerular filter without difficulty, but is not re-absorbed, secreted, synthesised or metabolised by the kidney. Thus, all the filtered inulin is excreted and all the inulin that is excreted has entered the urine only by filtration at the glomerulus.

If urinary inulin concentration is U_{in} (mg/ml), and urine flow is V (ml/min), then the amount of inulin excreted per min is:

$$= \quad (U_{in}V)$$

This is also the total amount of inulin that enters the nephrons contained in the filtered plasma per min. The volume of plasma containing this amount of inulin is therefore:

$$\frac{U_{in}V \text{ (mg)}}{P_{in} \text{ (mg/ml)}}$$

where:

P_{in} = plasma concentration of inulin.

This volume of plasma is equivalent to the volume cleared of inulin per min i.e. the inulin clearance. Thus, the inulin clearance (C_{in}) is equal to GFR. The inulin clearance measurement (and, hence, GFR measurement) is independent of the plasma inulin concentration. For an adult, the normal inulin clearance (GFR) is 125 ml/min. From day to day, GFR is remarkably constant in man. Variations in excretion of water and solutes are much more dependent on changes in tubular re-absorption and secretion than on GFR changes.

If a solute has a clearance value higher than the inulin clearance, then the solute must get into the renal tubules not only by glomerular filtration, but also by tubular secretion (PAH is such a substance, see below). However, if a solute has a clearance value less than that of inulin, there are two possibilities:

- The solute may not be freely filtered at the glomerulus
- The solute is freely filtered but is then re-absorbed from the tubule

CREATININE CLEARANCE

Because measurements of inulin clearance involve exogenous inulin administration it is rarely used clinically. An alternative way to measure GFR is by using creatinine clearance. Creatinine is a product of muscle metabolism, and as long as the subject remains at rest, the plasma creatinine level stays reasonably constant. Like inulin, it is freely filtered and not re-absorbed, synthesised or metabolised by the kidney, but creatinine is secreted to some extent by the tubules. This tends to make the value for creatinine clearance higher than that for inulin clearance, since the term (U.V) in the formula for clearance is artifactually high. However, as the plasma creatinine assay is not absolutely specific and overestimates the true plasma creatinine concentration, the two errors tend to cancel each other out, and creatinine clearance becomes a reasonable estimate of GFR.

PAH CLEARANCE: MEASUREMENT OF RENAL PLASMA FLOW

PAH is one of the groups of organic acids secreted by the proximal tubule. PAH is not only secreted, but also is filtered at the glomerulus. Thus, the total amount of PAH excreted is equal to the sum of the amount filtered plus the amount secreted. PAH is almost completely removed from the plasma by the kidneys, even though only a fraction of the plasma is filtered. The clearance of PAH, therefore, provides a measurement of the total renal plasma flow (RPF). (It should be noted that this relationship only holds as long as the tubular maximum, T_m, for the transport of PAH is not exceeded. T_m is reached at a plasma concentration of about 10 mg/100ml plasma.)

At plasma concentrations < 10 mg/100 ml:

PAH delivered to kidneys in plasma = PAH excreted in urine.

The amount of PAH excreted in the urine is given by:

(urinary concentration of PAH) × (urine flow),

which can be expressed as

$$U_{PAH} \times V$$

where:

U_{PAH} = urinary concentration of PAH

V = urine flow (ml/min).

Also, the PAH delivered to the kidneys is given by:

(renal plasma flow) × (plasma concentration of PAH)

which can be expressed as

$$RPF \times P_{PAH}$$

where:

P_{PAH} = plasma concentration of PAH

RPF = renal plasma flow.

Therefore, it follows that

$$RPF \times P_{PAH} = U_{PAH} \times V$$

So

$$RPF = \frac{U_{PAH} \times V}{P_{PAH}}$$

As can be seen, this is also the clearance formula for PAH. A typical value for RPF is 600 ml/min.

CALCULATION OF RENAL BLOOD FLOW

Given the haematocrit, renal blood flow (RBF) can be obtained. A typical haematocrit is 45%, which means that 45% of the total blood volume is cells and, therefore, 55% is plasma. So renal blood flow can be calculated by:

$$RBF = \frac{RPF \times 100}{55}$$

which gives about 1091 ml/min.

The clearance of PAH, although generally used as a measure of renal plasma flow, does not measure the plasma flow exactly, because PAH is not completely cleared from the blood during one passage through the kidney. The PAH extraction is only about 90% complete, due to that not all of the blood which enters the kidney goes to the glomeruli and tubules. Some goes to the capsule, the perirenal fat and the medulla (the blood in the vasa recta has had some PAH removed by filtration, but is not available for

secretion). PAH clearance approximates to cortical plasma flow and is usually called the effective renal plasma flow.

REGULATION OF RENAL BLOOD FLOW AND GLOMERULAR FILTRATION RATE

AUTOREGULATION

Over a wide range of mean arterial pressures (90–200 mmHg) renal blood flow is independent of the perfusion pressure. This is true even if the kidney is denervated. This property is, therefore, termed 'autoregulation' (Figure RE.4). GFR also autoregulates The relationship between blood pressure and renal blood flow demonstrated in Figure RE.4 implies that as the perfusion pressure increases, the resistance to flow also increases. Both afferent and efferent arterioles are capable of vasoconstriction. There is still controversy about the mechanisms underlying autoregulation of the kidneys. The most widely accepted explanation is the myogenic theory. According to this, the increase in wall tension of the afferent arterioles, produced by increased perfusion pressure, causes automatic contraction of the smooth muscle fibres in the vessel walls. This increases flow resistance and acts to maintain constant blood flow.

Renal response to increased sympathetic activity

Despite autoregulation, renal haemodynamics vary considerably. Autoregulation means that changes in blood pressure per se in the autoregulatory range have little effect on blood flow, but it does not mean that blood flow is always constant. In many circumstances (e.g. physical or mental stress, haemorrhage), there are increases in the sympathetic nervous activity to the

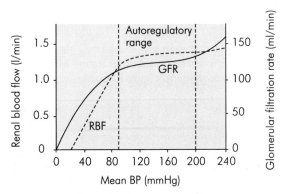

Figure RE.4 Autoregulation of renal blood flow

kidney (and to other parts of the body), causing vasoconstriction and, hence, a reduction in renal blood flow, even though the perfusion pressure is still in the autoregulatory range. This suggests that the kidneys play a part in maintaining systemic blood pressure, rather than reacting passively to it.

Other mechanisms include:

- Renal prostaglandin production – renal vasoconstriction in response to renal sympathetic nerve activity is attenuated to some extent by the intrarenal production of vasodilator prostaglandins
- Angiotensin II – when the renal blood flow is reduced, there is generally an increased filtration fraction, brought about by efferent arteriolar vasoconstriction (mediated by angiotensin II), so that GFR tends to be maintained
- Tubulo–glomerular feedback mechanism – this mechanism may also contribute significantly to renal autoregulation
- Vaso-active agents – the regulation of GFR also involves other vaso-active agents, which are present within blood vessel walls throughout the body, but may be of particular importance in the kidney, including endothelin (vasoconstrictor) and the vasodilator nitric oxide

TUBULAR TRANSPORT

The final urine that leaves the nephrons to enter the bladder and be excreted is very different from the initial glomerular filtrate, because the composition of the filtrate is modified by selective re-absorption and secretion processes. Transport of solutes and water across the renal tubular epithelium can occur between the cells (paracellular movement) or through the cells (transcellular movement). Transcellular movement occurs across two cell membranes, the apical and basal membranes of the cell. **Secretion** is movement from the blood, through or between the tubular cells, into the tubular fluid. **Re-absorption** is movement of a substance from the tubular fluid, into or between the tubular cells, and then into the blood. Neither term conveys any information about the nature of the forces causing the movement (Figure RE.5).

PRIMARY AND SECONDARY ACTIVE TRANSPORT

Conventionally, the transport of solutes has been regarded as 'active' if metabolic energy is required, and 'passive' if metabolic energy is not required. This distinction is too simplistic, since many transport processes that do not directly require metabolic energy

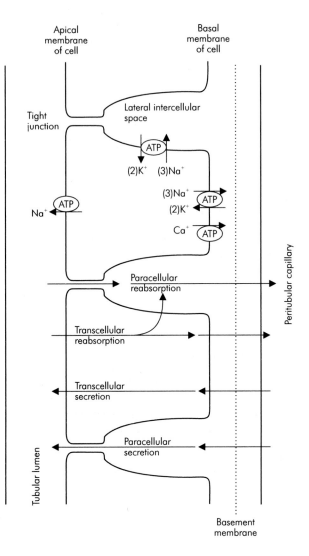

Figure RE.5 Solute transport mechanisms in tubular cells

would nevertheless not occur if metabolic energy were not available.

Primary active transport

This involves the direct coupling of ATP hydrolysis to a transport process in the cell membrane. The most important primary active process in the nephron is the $Na^+K^+ATPase$, located on the basal (and basolateral) side of the cells lining the nephron. The $Na^+K^+ATPase$ accounts for the majority of the oxygen consumption in the kidney and enables the nephrons to re-absorb > 99% of the filtered sodium.

Other primary active transport mechanisms in the nephron include a $Ca^{2+}ATPase$, an H^+ (proton)-ATPase, and an $H^+K^+ATPase$ (see p230).

Secondary active transport

This process uses ionic gradients that have been established across the nephron cell membranes by ATPases, to drive the transport process resulting in secretion or re-absorption of a solute. Although the transport of such solutes is not directly linked to ATP breakdown, nevertheless if primary active transport was not active, then secondary active transport could not occur. The sodium gradient provides the most important driving force for secondary active transport. When the solute that is being transported with Na^+ moves in the same direction as the Na^+ gradient, the process is termed **co-transport**; where the solute is transported against the Na^+ gradient the process is termed **countertransport** (see p231).

ION CHANNELS

In addition to ATPases and transporter molecules, epithelial cell membranes also contain proteins that constitute ion 'channels'. There are sodium ion channels in the apical membranes of cells throughout the nephron. These channels are closed by the drug amiloride and opened by a number of hormones. There are also both Cl^- and K^+ channels in the apical membranes. Ion channels allow much faster rates of transport than either ATPases or transporter molecules.

PARACELLULAR MOVEMENT

This is movement of substances through the spaces between the cells of the nephron. Driving forces for paracellular movement are concentration, osmotic or electrical gradients. Such movements are discussed below in relation to specific substances (Figure RE.5).

WATER ABSORPTION

There is no active water re-absorption. Water re-absorption along the nephron follows solute absorption and can be both trans- and paracellular. It has become clear in recent years that much of the water movement through epithelia is transcellular, and occurs via specific water channel proteins, termed aquaporins (AQP); several (five at present) different aquaporins have been identified.

- AQP1 (also called CHIP-28, or 28 kilodalton channel-forming integral protein) is abundant in the apical and basal membranes of renal proximal tubule cells, and the cells of the thin descending limb of Henle, as well as in many extrarenal tissues
- AQP2 is the vasopressin (ADH)-sensitive channel
- AQP3 is in the basolateral membranes of the collecting duct principal cells, where it provides an exit route for water
- AQP4 is abundant in the brain, and may be important in the hypothalamic osmoreceptor cells
- AQP5 has not yet been elucidated.

THE PROXIMAL TUBULE

MORPHOLOGY OF PROXIMAL TUBULE CELLS

Adjacent proximal tubule cells are in contact with each other at the luminal side (the tight junction), but there are gaps between the cells – lateral intercellular spaces – at the peritubular side (Figure RE.5). The luminal surface has a brush border of microvilli, which greatly increases the surface area available for absorption. There are some differences in the transport properties of the early proximal tubule (pars convoluta), compared with later parts (pars convoluta and pars recta), particularly in relation to Cl^- transport.

SODIUM RE-ABSORPTION IN THE PROXIMAL TUBULE

The proximal tubule is highly permeable to sodium in both directions; net re-absorption of sodium from the tubule into the peritubular capillaries, occurs as a result of the difference between an efflux of sodium from the tubule lumen, and a return of sodium back into it. Only about 20% of the sodium efflux from the tubular lumen is ultimately re-absorbed into the peritubular capillaries. Thus, the majority of the sodium efflux passes back into the tubular lumen as a backflux. This two-way movement of sodium occurs between the tubular lumen and the tubule cells and is linked with the transport of other substances. Some of the backflux is paracellular.

Sodium entry into tubule cells

The proximal tubule cells have a negative intracellular potential of –70 mV relative to both luminal fluid and peritubular fluid, and the cells have a low intracellular sodium concentration (< 30 mmol). So sodium movement from the luminal fluid into the cell is in the direction of a large electrical gradient as well as a chemical concentration gradient. Thus, sodium entry into the cell occurs passively. However, this entry of sodium is mediated by carrier proteins that also transport other solutes simultaneously. As noted above, these solutes may be transported with the sodium ions (symport) or in exchange for the sodium (antiport). Many solutes are transported by Na^+-linked symport and anti-port. Most of the sodium (80%) entering the tubule cells does so in exchange for H^+ secretion. In turn, H^+ secretion into the tubular lumen, leads to the re-absorption of both Cl^- and HCO_3^- (Figure RE.6a).

Sodium extrusion from tubular cells

The $Na^+K^+ATPase$ pump extrudes sodium from the cells against electrical and chemical gradients. The entry into the cells of potassium ions has little effect on

the intracellular K^+ concentration, since K^+ can readily cross cell membranes and so rapidly diffuses out of the cells. The ratio of transport is not 1:1, 3 Na^+ leave for 2 K^+ ions entering. The active extrusion of sodium from the tubule cells occurs almost entirely across the basolateral and basal surfaces of the cells, and much of this transport is directed into the lateral intercellular spaces.

CHLORIDE RE-ABSORPTION IN THE PROXIMAL TUBULE

The intracellular electrical potential opposes Cl^- entry into the cells from the tubular lumen. In the early proximal tubule Na^+ absorption is accompanied by HCO_3^- absorption (in the form of CO_2), so that although the tubular osmolality remains similar to that of plasma, the Cl^- concentration is increased. There are

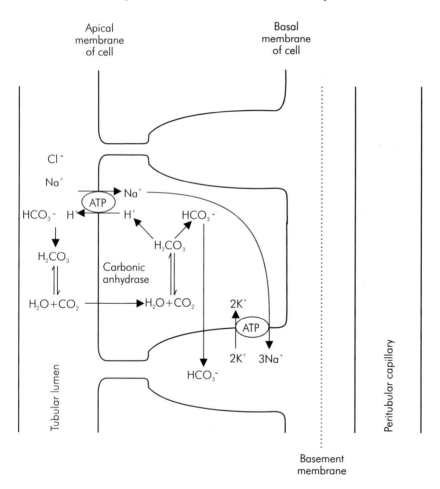

Figure RE.6a Sodium handling in the early proximal tubule

two main mechanisms by which Cl⁻ is absorbed from the tubular lumen into the tubule cells (Figure RE.6b). These are:

- By antiport in exchange for the secretion of organic anions. The main organic anions involved are bicarbonate (HCO_3^-), formate ($HCOO^-$) and oxalate. In Figure RE.6b, formate is used as an example. This shows Cl⁻ re-absorption into tubule cells in exchange for $HCOO^-$, which is secreted back into the tubule. In the lumen the $HCOO^-$ combines with H⁺ to form HCOOH, which readily diffuses back into the cells. There it dissociates into H⁺ and $HCOO^-$. The intracellular H⁺ is then antiported back into the tubule in exchange for Na⁺, while the $HCOO^-$ drives the antiport of Cl⁻. Thus, the net result of the Cl⁻ and Na⁺ anti-port systems is the re-absorption of equal amounts of Cl⁻ and Na⁺ from the lumen into the tubular cells

- In the final two-thirds of the proximal tubule, Cl⁻ handling differs between superficial nephrons and juxtamedullary ones. In superficial nephrons Cl⁻ permeability in the late proximal tubule, is greater than that for other anions (notably HCO_3^-). Hence Cl⁻ is re-absorbed from the lumen down its concentration gradient because of the high luminal Cl⁻ concentration established by HCO_3^- absorption. This occurs mainly by the paracellular route (Figure RE.6c). Na⁺ then follows passively down its electrical gradient. Up to 20% of NaCl re-absorption in the late proximal tubule occurs by this mechanism. In contrast, Cl⁻ and HCO_3^- permeabilities do not differ in the juxtamedullary nephron tubule.

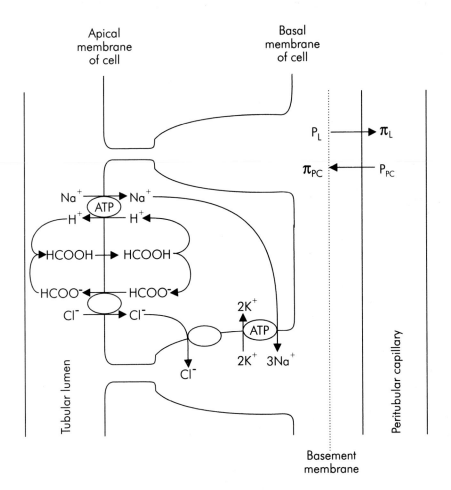

Figure RE.6b Sodium handling throughout the proximal tubule

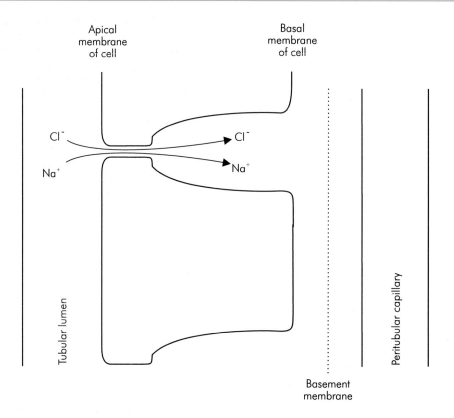

Figure RE.6c Sodium handling in the late proximal tubule

RE-ABSORPTION OF OTHER SOLUTES IN THE PROXIMAL TUBULE

Sodium re-absorption leads to electrical, concentration and osmotic gradients for the re-absorption of such solutes as chloride, potassium and urea, and also for water re-absorption. It is also important for the re-absorption of glucose, amino acids, phosphate and calcium and for the secretion of H^+.

Glucose

Normally, almost all of the filtered glucose is re-absorbed and a negligible amount is excreted. Since the normal plasma glucose concentration is between 3.3 and 5.5 mmol/l (60–100 mg/100 ml) and GFR is 125 ml/min, 0.4–0.7 mmol (or 75–125 mg) glucose is re-absorbed every min. Although most glucose re-absorption occurs in the proximal tubule, more distal parts of the nephron are also capable of re-absorbing glucose. Figure RE.7 shows the relationship between filtration, re-absorption and excretion of glucose, and the plasma glucose concentration. The amount of glucose filtered is directly proportional to the plasma glucose concentration. No glucose is excreted in the urine, unless the plasma glucose concentration exceeds about 11 mmol/l (200 mg/100 ml). At this plasma glucose concentration, those nephrons with the lowest capacity for glucose re-absorption (relative to their filtration rate) reach their glucose re-absorptive rate limit, and glucose begins to be excreted. Further increases in plasma glucose concentration saturate the glucose transport process of an increasing proportion of nephrons until, when the plasma glucose concentration is about 22 mmol/l. No nephrons can absorb their entire filtered glucose load. The fact that the curves for re-absorption and excretion are 'rounded' indicates the existence of nephron heterogeneity, i.e. that all the nephrons are not identical.

The type of transport process typified by glucose re-absorption is known as T_m-limited transport. 'T_m' means tubular maximum and refers to the maximum tubular transport rate for a particular solute. From Figure RE.7, it can be seen that the maximum rate of

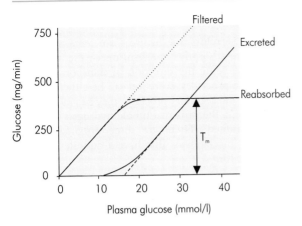

Figure RE.7 Glucose transport in the proximal tubule

glucose re-absorption is about 380 mg/min. This is the T_m for glucose. The most common abnormality of glucose excretion is that caused by a change in the plasma glucose concentration, so that the filtered load is altered: diabetes mellitus is caused by the relative or total absence of the pancreatic hormone, insulin, which regulates the blood glucose concentration. The filtered load of glucose can, therefore, be far in excess of the re-absorptive capacity of the nephrons, so that glucose is excreted in the urine. This excretion of osmotically active solute causes an osmotic diuresis resulting in water loss from the body and, hence, dehydration and thirst.

Relationship of glucose re-absorption to sodium re-absorption

Proximal tubular glucose absorption is linked to sodium re-absorption. The entry of glucose into the tubular cells is via symport. Symporter carrier proteins that possess both sodium and glucose binding sites, transfer sodium ions and glucose molecules simultaneously into the tubular cells. The movement of sodium occurs down its electrochemical gradient (co-transport), thus providing the energy to transfer glucose against its gradient (countertransport). Maintenance of the sodium gradient is, therefore, essential for glucose absorption. This in turn depends on the extrusion of sodium from the proximal tubule cells by the sodium pump.

Note that in the pars convoluta, the stoichiometry of the glucose sodium co-transport is one glucose molecule per sodium ion, but in the pars recta it is one glucose per two sodium ions.

AMINO ACIDS

The plasma concentration of amino acids is between 2.5 and 3.5 mmol/l. Amino acids in the plasma are in a dynamic equilibrium, since they enter the blood from the gut, as products of protein digestion, and are continually being used to restructure the body tissues. Amino acids are readily filtered at the glomeruli, but negligible quantities are excreted, because there are effective T_m-limited transport processes for amino acids in the proximal tubule. There are several proximal transport processes for amino acid re-absorption coupled with Na^+. These are for:

* Basic amino acids
* Glutamic and aspartic acids
* Neutral amino acids
* Glycine
* Cysteine and cystine
* β and γ amino acids

The functional characteristics of these transport processes are very similar to that for glucose. Amino acid entry into the proximal tubule cells from the lumen is a co-transport process with sodium, the driving force being the sodium gradient.

PHOSPHATE

Phosphate is an essential constituent of the body. Bones and teeth are salts of calcium and phosphate, and the skeleton accounts for about 80% of the body phosphate content. The other 20% is present mainly in intracellular fluid. The extracellular (plasma) phosphate concentration is 1 mmol/l and plasma phosphate is freely filtered at the glomerulus. In the nephron, tubular re-absorption and possibly secretion of phosphate occurs. Normally, the urinary phosphate excretion is < 20% of the amount filtered, but above a phosphate concentration of about 1.2 mmol/l increases in filtered phosphate are excreted in the urine, suggesting that there is a T_m for phosphate. Phosphate re-absorption occurs by electroneutral co-transport (i.e. two sodium ions per phosphate ion) across the apical membrane of tubular cells. Two distinct sodium-phosphate transporters are present in the membrane. The rate of phosphate uptake is hormonally regulated, being under the control of PTH (parathyroid hormone) and vitamin D.

UREA

The normal plasma urea concentration is 2.5–7.5 mmol/l. Only 40–50% of filtered urea is re-absorbed; 50–60% is excreted. Urea is the end produce of protein metabolism and clinically is measured as blood urea nitrogen. Because urea is a small molecule, it is re-absorbed in the proximal tubule as a consequence of sodium re-absorption. Thus, as sodium chloride and water are abstracted from the proximal tubule, the urea concentration in the tubular fluid tends to increase and so urea is re-absorbed passively by diffusing down its concentration gradient, out of the tubule. The urea handling of the more distal parts of the nephron plays an important part in the process of concentrating the urine, and is considered later.

BICARBONATE

Normal plasma HCO_3^- concentration is about 25 mmol/l. Bicarbonate has a key role in acid base balance, and the kidney contributes to acid base balance largely by regulating the plasma bicarbonate concentration.

About 90% of the filtered HCO_3^- is re-absorbed in the proximal tubule; the remainder is re-absorbed in the distal tubule and collecting ducts. In the proximal tubule, HCO_3^- re-absorption occurs as a result of H^+ secretion from tubular cells into the lumen. The bicarbonate re-absorption mechanism behaves as if there were a T_m for bicarbonate. However, this apparent T_m can be altered by the rate of H^+ secretion, which is itself loosely dependent on the rate of Na^+ re-absorption.

WATER

Water re-absorption occurs in the proximal tubule in the following manner:

- Some 60–70% of the filtered water is re-absorbed in the proximal tubules. About 20% of the re-absorbed water load occurs as a result of the chemical gradient provided by a small degree of hypotonicity (2–5 mosmol/l lower than plasma) in the tubular lumen, and the increased concentration of Na^+ caused by extrusion into the lateral intercellular spaces
- A further 40% of the water re-absorbed proximally is attributable to the different permeabilities of anions (primarily Cl^- and HCO_3^-) in superficial nephrons. As described above, tubular Cl^- concentration is increased by the end of the first part of the proximal tubule, due to HCO_3^- re-absorption. In addition, the distal parts of the proximal tubule are more permeable to Cl^- than to other solutes. This causes both Cl^- and water to be re-absorbed in this region
- The remaining 40% of the total proximal water re-absorption can be attributed to the existence of a hypertonic intermediate compartment – the lateral intercellular spaces

SECRETION IN THE PROXIMAL TUBULE

Tubular secretory mechanisms are very much like tubular re-absorptive mechanisms – the important difference being the direction of transport. Like re-absorptive processes, secretion can be either active or passive – and secretory processes may be gradient time limited (e.g. the proximal tubule hydrogen secretion) or T_m limited. There are three proximal tubular secretory mechanisms that have a definite T_m limit. These are for:

- Some organic acids – these include penicillin, chlorothiazide, hippurate, PAH and possibly uric acid
- Some strong organic bases, which include histamine, choline, thiamine, guanidine and probably creatinine
- EDTA (ethylene diamine tetra-acetic acid)

Although most of these substances do not occur endogenously, endogenous organic acids are also transported. There is some anatomical separation of the different secretory processes. Organic acid secretion (and uric acid secretion) takes place in the pars recta, but organic base secretion occurs in the pars convoluta.

When a substance is filtered and actively secreted, the total amount excreted in the urine is greater than the amount filtered due to transport from the peritubular capillaries into the tubular lumen. An example is shown in Figure RE.8 illustrating the results of PAH secretion in proximal tubule. This shows the relationship between the plasma concentration of PAH and the rates of filtration, tubular secretion and urinary excretion. For plasma concentrations up to 8 mg/100 ml, PAH is cleared completely from the peritubular capillaries. For concentrations greater than this the T_m for PAH is exceeded, and excretion rates only increase in step with filtration rates.

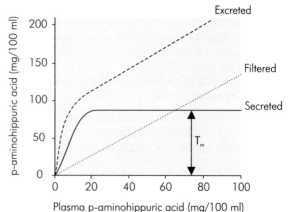

Figure RE.8 PAH secretion in the proximal tubule

The peritubular capillaries

The end result of the transport processes described above is the passage of essentially isotonic fluid from the tubule lumen, into the lateral intercellular spaces (LIS). This occurs mainly through tubular cell re-absorption and secretion, but some paracellular movement also occurs into the LIS, but mainly in the late proximal tubule. From here, the NaCl–NaHCO$_3$ solution can move in two possible directions; either into the peritubular capillaries, or back into the tubular lumen.

A proportion of the Na$^+$ always leaks back and, hence, the sodium re-absorption process can be called a 'pump-leak' system (it is also known as a gradient time-limited transport process). The rate of proximal tubular sodium re-absorption can be varied by changes in the rate of backflux into the tubule, as well as by changes in the rate of active sodium extrusion from the cells. The rate of backflux is affected by the rate of uptake from the lateral intercellular spaces into the capillaries. Re-absorption from the tubule is finally completed by the uptake of water and solutes into the peritubular capillaries. The faster the capillary uptake the lower the rate of backflux.

UPTAKE FORCES IN THE PERITUBULAR CAPILLARIES

The forces governing the movement of fluid across the walls of the peritubular capillaries are Starling forces, i.e. colloid osmotic pressure (COP) and hydrostatic pressure gradients.

The forces favouring capillary uptake are:

(capillary COP) + (LIS hydrostatic pressure)

or

$$\pi_{PC} + P_L$$

The forces opposing capillary uptake are:

(capillary hydrostatic pressure) + (COP in LIS)

or

$$P_{PC} + \pi_L$$

Therefore, rate of capillary uptake is related to:

(forces favouring uptake) – (forces opposing uptake)

$$\propto (\pi_{PC} + P_L) - (\pi_L + P_{PC})$$

where:

π_L and π_{PC} = COPs in the LIS and peritubular capillary respectively
P_L and P_{PC} = hydrostatic pressures in LIS and peritubular capillary respectively.

Effect of GFR on peritubular fluid uptake

The peritubular capillaries are branches of the efferent arterioles, which in turn arise from the glomerular capillaries. Consequently, the Starling forces in the peritubular capillaries can be modified by the glomerular filtration process. The peritubular capillary COP (π_{PC}) depends on the capillary plasma protein concentration. As plasma proteins are concentrated in the glomerular capillaries by the filtration process, COP in the peritubular capillaries increases with filtration fraction. The peritubular capillary COP is normally high compared with that in the glomerular capillaries, resulting in fluid re-absorption by the peritubular capillaries.

This dependence of π_{PC} on the filtration fraction is a mechanism that automatically adjusts proximal tubular re-absorption to compensate for changes in glomerular filtration. When GFR increases, the forces available to re-absorb the increased volume of filtrate also increase and vice versa. This glomerulo tubular mechanism normally ensures re-absorption of a fixed proportion of the gomerular filtrate by the proximal tubule, i.e. there is constant proximal tubular fractional re-absorption.

However, proximal tubular fractional re-absorption can be altered by other factors, e.g. by alterations in the effective circulating volume. Such alterations are considered later.

The peritubular capillary hydrostatic pressure (P_{PC}) is determined mainly by venous pressure. However, changes in tone of the afferent and efferent glomerular arterioles may also affect P_{PC} by varying the amount of arterial pressure transmitted to the peritubular capillaries.

THE LOOP OF HENLE

The loop of Henle (LOH) is continuous with the proximal tubule and originates in the renal cortex. It consists of a descending limb that passes into the medulla and loops round to become the ascending limb which passes back into the cortex. This limb then continues as the distal tubule (Figure RE.9).

The fluid entering the LOH is initially isotonic compared with plasma, but after traversing the loop the fluid entering the distal tubule is hypotonic. Thus, the tubular fluid is diluted during its passage through LOH. However, LOH plays a crucial role in the concentration of urine by functioning as a countercurrent multiplier. The salient process is emphasised below:

The loops of Henle do not concentrate the tubular

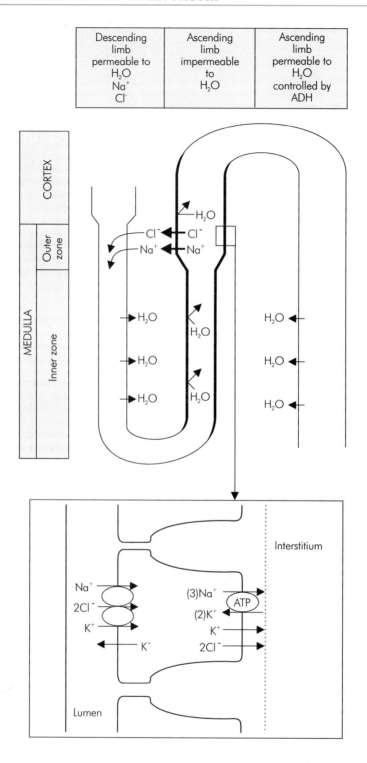

Figure RE.9 Sodium and water movement in the loop of Henle

fluid within them, but manufacture a hypertonic interstitial fluid in the renal medulla. Urine is then concentrated by osmosis from collecting ducts as they pass through the medulla.

THE COUNTERCURRENT MECHANISM

A proposed mechanism for countercurrent multiplication was described by Wirz, Hargitay and Kuhn in 1951. The hypertonic interstitium is produced by a small osmotic pressure difference between the ascending and descending limbs of the loops (i.e. a small transverse gradient). This small difference is then multiplied into a large longitudinal gradient by the countercurrent arrangement (i.e. flow in opposite directions) in the two adjacent limbs of the loop.

The ascending limb is not uniform in structure but possesses both a thin and a thick segment. This limb produces an increase in the osmolality of the surrounding interstitium by the extrusion of sodium and accompanying ions. Only the thick segment actively extrudes ions. Both thin and thick segments of the ascending limb are impermeable to water so that water is unable osmotically to follow the extruded ions. Consequently, the osmolality of the medullary interstitium is increased and the osmolality of the fluid in the ascending limb is decreased.

The extrusion process is performed by the tubular cells that take up ions from the tubular lumen through their apical membrane and extrude ions through their basal membrane. The entry of solutes into the cells across the apical membrane involves co-transport of sodium, chloride and potassium, with the stoichiometry of one Na^+, two Cl^- and one K^+, so the process is electrically neutral. The primary active transport on the basal cell membrane is performed by $Na^+K^+ATPase$. This basal membrane transport is also electrically neutral. The thin ascending limb has little $Na^+K^+ATPase$ activity, thus the thick segment is primarily responsible for the extrusion of sodium. Much of the K^+ leaks back into the tubular lumen, so that it is predominantly NaCl which accumulates in the medullary interstitium. This transport can be inhibited by loop diuretics, such as furosemide and bumetanide.

The descending limb is permeable to water and, to a lesser extent, is also permeable to NaCl. The fluid within the descending limb will, therefore, come to osmotic equilibrium with the interstitium. In effect, then, one can consider the transport of NaCl out of the ascending limb as being directed into the descending limb.

The sodium extrusion mechanism or 'sodium pump'

action in the ascending limb can maintain an osmolality gradient of 200 mosmol/kgH$_2$O between the ascending tubular lumen and the interstitium. In effect, since the descending limb is permeable and assumes the same osmolality as the interstitium, the 'sodium pump' can be thought of as maintaining a 200 mosmol/kgH$_2$O gradient between the tubular fluid in the adjacent sections of the ascending and descending limbs. The countercurrent arrangement of the limbs will then result in a gradually increasing interstitial (and descending limb) osmolality, as the LOH descends into the renal medulla. In man the osmolality at the papillary tips may reach 1400 mosmol/kgH$_2$O (Figure RE.10).

The fluid in the ascending tubule leaving the medulla and entering the cortex is hypotonic to plasma, with an osmolality of about 100 mosmol/kgH$_2$O. Thus, the ascending limb of the loop of Henle (and its continuation in the cortex as the distal tubule) can be called the 'diluting segment' of the nephron. However, some nephrons possess short loops of Henle, and these are unlikely to lower the osmolality of the ascending limb fluid to 100 mosmol/kgH$_2$O.

Long and short loops of Henle

Only 15% of the nephrons (the juxtamedullary nephrons) have long loops of Henle that pass deeply into the medulla. The remaining 85% of nephrons (cortical nephrons) have short loops of Henle that barely reach the medulla, and these nephrons do not make a significant contribution to the manufacture of medullary hypertonicity. However, the collecting tubules of all the nephrons (both cortical and juxtamedullary) pass through the medulla. Thus, only the long-looped nephrons, which form 15% of the total, produce the medullary gradient that concentrates the urine produced by all the nephrons. There are also differences in sodium re-absorption between the long and short looped nephrons.

THE DISTAL TUBULE AND COLLECTING TUBULE

THE DISTAL TUBULE

The 'distal tubule' although anatomically defined is not a distinct section of the nephron in terms of physiological function. Functionally, the distal tubule is a segment of the nephron in which the tubule cells undergo transition from 'ascending limb of Henle type' cells to 'collecting tubule type' cells. The walls of the former cell type have only a very low and essentially constant permeability to water, whereas the 'collecting

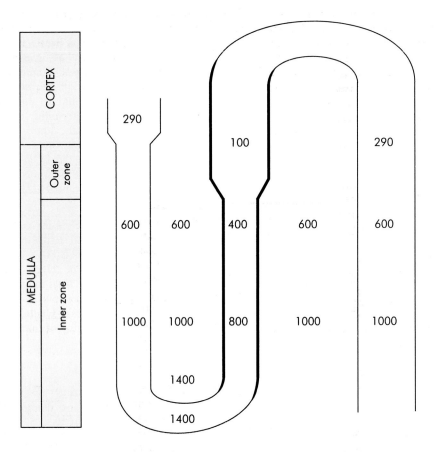

Figure RE.10 Osmolalities in the loop of Henle

tubule type' cells have a variable water permeability, which is regulated by the hormone ADH (anti-diuretic hormone, vasopressin).

The potential difference across the distal tubular wall, varies with distance along the tubule. In the early part, the lumen is positive with respect to the interstitium (as in the ascending limb of Henle), but in the later parts the luminal potential becomes negative and may reach –45 mV. This negative potential is caused by active sodium re-absorption.

THE COLLECTING TUBULES

The collecting tubules have cortical and medullary sections, each section having somewhat different properties. Both are relatively impermeable to water, urea and NaCl, but the water permeability is increased by ADH. Thus, ADH leads to urine concentration by permitting the osmotic abstraction of water into the interstitium. Theoretically the urine in the collecting tubule can achieve the same osmolality as the

medullary interstitium but in reality it is usually rather less than this.

ADH also increases the urea permeability of the **medullary** collecting tubules, but has no effect on the urea permeability of the **cortical** collecting tubules. This impermeability of the cortical part of the collecting tubule to urea, is one of the factors that make urea so important in the urine concentration mechanism.

Importance of urea in countercurrent multiplication

Previously, the countercurrent multiplication process has only been considered in terms of NaCl transport into the interstitium. However, a considerable fraction of the medullary interstitial osmolality, particularly in the papillary region is attributable to urea (up to 50%). This high interstitial urea concentration is obtained by diffusion of urea from the medullary collecting tubules, which have an ADH dependent permeability to urea.

The normal plasma concentration of urea is 2.5–7.5 mmol/l. Urea is freely filterable at the glomerulus, and about 50% of the filtered load is re-absorbed in the proximal tubule. As the tubular fluid passes down the descending limb into the medulla, it passes into the high interstitial urea concentration established by diffusion from the collecting tubules, as described above. The tubular urea concentration thus increases by diffusion from the interstitium in both the descending and ascending limbs, which are permeable to urea.

In the distal and cortical collecting tubules, the urea concentration rises further, as a result of water re-absorption, since these segments are almost impermeable to urea. Initially, when the medullary collecting tubule is reached, the high urea concentration in the tubule causes the diffusion of urea out of the tubule into the interstitium (under the influence of ADH), which maintains the high medullary urea concentration. Urea thus recycles between medullary collecting tubule and medullary interstitium via the tubular fluid. This produces a high interstitial urea concentration that helps to increase the final urea concentration in the urine. The maximum attainable urinary osmolality is greater when urea excretion is high because a proportion of this extra urea enters the medullary interstitium.

The role of the vasa recta

In most tissues, the selective permeability of capillaries ensures that the composition of interstitial fluid remains uniform. If medullary capillaries served this purpose, the osmotic gradient built up by the loop of Henle would be dissipated. However, this does not occur, because the hairpin arrangement of the vasa recta enables them to function as countercurrent exchangers (distinguished from countercurrent **multipliers** by the fact that no energy is necessary). This enables the vasa recta to exchange nutrients for waste products in the renal medulla, without washing away the solutes responsible for medullary hypertonicity.

The vasa recta, like capillaries elsewhere, are permeable to water and solutes. As the descending vasa recta passes into the medulla, water is osmotically abstracted from the capillary blood, into the interstitium, in exchange for solutes (NaCl and urea). More and more water is extracted, as the blood passes further into the medulla, until, at the tip of the loop, the plasma has almost the same osmolality as the surrounding interstitium. This makes the blood very viscous with a high plasma protein concentration. In the ascending vasa recta, the plasma regains water and loses solute.

Since the plasma concentrations of diffusible solutes and plasma osmolality in the vasa recta virtually assume interstitial values, the differences between descending and ascending limbs become very small. Although this minimises transport of water and solutes away from the interstitium, it also makes the exchange of oxygen and CO_2 very inefficient. The renal medulla is, therefore, susceptible to the effects of reduced perfusion.

RENAL EFFECTS OF ANTI-DIURETIC HORMONE

The main determinant of whether the urine will be copious and dilute, or low in volume and concentrated, is the level of circulating anti-diuretic hormone (ADH). Re-absorption of water in the nephron occurs at several sites. GFR = 180 l/day. About 70% of this is re-absorbed in the proximal tubule. A further 15% of the glomerular filtrate is re-absorbed by the loop of Henle. This leaves about 23 litres to enter the distal tubules and collecting tubules. It is these 23 litres that are mainly either excreted or re-absorbed, depending on the level of circulating ADH.

In the presence of ADH, the collecting tubule wall is permeable to water, so the hypertonic medullary interstitium leads to the osmotic abstraction of water from the tubule. ADH also makes the collecting tubules permeable to urea, which leaves the tubule in this region and contributes to the osmolality of the renal medulla. Normal levels of circulating ADH produce urine volumes of about 1.5 l/day, with an osmolality of 300–500 mosmol/kgH$_2$O. ADH levels may be increased to conserve body water and urine volumes in these circumstances can be as little as 400 ml/day.

In the absence of circulating ADH, water re-absorption in the proximal tubule and LOH remains unchanged, since ADH does not affect water absorption at these sites. However, the collecting tubules become impermeable to water, and the large volumes entering the medullary collecting tubules, pass through and are excreted. In addition, the collecting tubules also become impermeable to urea, preventing the attainment of maximal medullary interstitial osmolality. This in turn also reduces water re-absorption from the descending limb of the loop of Henle. Thus, when no ADH is present (diabetes insipidus), urine volume is about 23 l/day, with an osmolality as low as 60 mosmol/kgH$_2$O. Note that adrenal steroids (cortisol) must be present for ADH to have its maximum effect on water permeability.

OSMORECEPTORS AND THE CONTROL OF PLASMA OSMOLALITY

Osmoreceptors in the vicinity of the supra-optic and paraventricular areas of the anterior hypothalamus, supplied with blood by the internal carotid artery, regulate the release of the hormone ADH. These receptors, and others in the lateral pre-optic area of the hypothalamus, also affect thirst. Normal plasma osmolality is associated with a plasma ADH concentration of about 4 pg/ml. Lowering the plasma osmolality reduces ADH concentration and raising the plasma osmolality increases the plasma ADH concentration. This coupling of the ADH-sensitive concentrating mechanism to the precise control of ADH release through the osmoreceptors provides a very good regulatory mechanism for plasma osmolality.

SYNTHESIS AND STORAGE OF ANTI-DIURETIC HORMONE

ADH is synthesised in the hypothalamus (supra-optic nucleus) as part of a large precursor molecule. After synthesis this is transported to the neurohypophysis (posterior pituitary) within nerve fibres that constitute the hypothalamohypophyseal tract, and is cleaved progressively as it moves down the axons. In the nerve terminals, ADH and neurophysin are stored as insoluble complexes in secretory granules.

CELLULAR ACTIONS OF ADH CONTROLLING WATER PERMEABILITY

The renal ADH receptors (V_2 receptors) are on the basal membranes of the tubular cells. The V_2 receptor is a G-protein coupled receptor characterised by seven membrane-spanning regions. Binding of ADH to the receptor activates adenylate cyclase, which increases cyclic AMP formation from ATP. The cyclic AMP activates protein kinase that phosphorylates controlling proteins in water channels close to the apical membrane that increases water re-absorption from the tubular fluid. The ADH-sensitive water channel is known as aquaporin-2.

REMOVAL OF ADH FROM THE BLOOD

For precise regulation of plasma osmolality, not only is rapid control of ADH release required in response to changes in hydration, but also it is necessary that ADH is rapidly removed from the plasma. This removal occurs in the liver and in the kidneys. The kidneys remove about half of the total ADH, metabolising the

majority and excreting < 10% in the urine (plasma half-life of ADH is 15 min). A number of pharmacological agents may alter ADH release and thereby disturb osmoregulation.

ADRENAL STEROIDS AND THE RENAL RESPONSE TO ADH

Adrenal steroids (glucocorticoids) decrease the permeability of the collecting ducts to water. In the absence of adrenal steroids, collecting duct water permeability is above basal level, even if no ADH is present. Adrenal insufficiency also impairs the renal response to water loading, i.e. very dilute urine cannot be produced. In adrenal insufficiency the effect of ADH on water permeability appears to be reduced.

REGULATION OF BODY FLUID VOLUME AND SODIUM RE-ABSORPTION

Regulation of total body fluid volume is dependent on regulation of the extracellular fluid (ECF) volume. Control of ECF volume is mediated by osmoreceptors that affect ADH release.

ADH release responds to changes in ECF osmolality and the effective circulating volume (ECV) of blood. The ECV is the component of the ECF that actually perfuses tissues (this may not necessarily be identical to the intravascular volume, since there may be circumstances in which not all of the blood is involved in tissue perfusion). Reflexes controlling the release of ADH may be activated by changes in blood pressure, atrial filling, haemorrhage or stress. Thus, a response in ADH release takes place within minutes, and acts rapidly to correct a disturbance (Figure RE.11).

Osmoreceptors respond to changes in ECF osmolality. Since sodium salts are the main osmotically active solutes in the ECF, control of body fluid volume is dependent on the control of body sodium content. Man can conserve sodium very effectively, and urinary losses can be < 1 mmol/l. However, maximal sodium re-absorption can increase the excretion of K^+ and H^+, and so may disturb acid base balance. Changes in Na^+ excretion are normally brought about by changes in tubular re-absorption. When disturbances of body fluid osmolality occur, disturbances in body sodium content (and consequently in body fluid volume) may take hours or even days to correct.

Primary control of sodium re-absorption is mediated by the release of systemic hormones renin, angiotensin

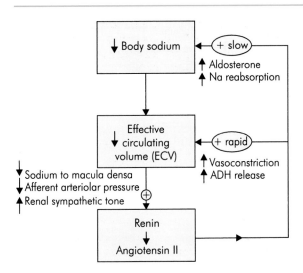

Figure RE.11 Regulation of body sodium and extracellular volume

and aldosterone. The effects of these hormones are modified by other mechanisms and also depend on changes in ECV. Overall regulation of sodium re-absorption is complex being influenced by the following factors:

- Systemic hormones
- Starling forces in the peritubular capillaries
- Neurological reflexes
- Renal prostaglandins
- Atrial natriuretic peptide
- Dopamine

JUXTAGLOMERULAR APPARATUS AND THE MACULA DENSA

In a nephron the ascending limb of the loop of Henle re-enters the cortex to become the distal tubule, passing very close to its own Bowman's capsule. At this point it comes into contact with the afferent and efferent arterioles from its own glomerulus. This region of contact is the juxtaglomerular apparatus, and consists of renin containing granular cells in the walls of the afferent arterioles, and specialised cells, the macula densa, in the wall of the early distal tubule.

RENIN

Renin is an enzyme synthesised and stored in the granular cells of the juxtaglomerular apparatus. It is released into the plasma when the body sodium content decreases. As noted above, body sodium content determines ECV and it is this relationship that determines renin release. There are three main ways in

which decreases in ECV elicit increases in renin release.

Increased sympathetic activity

When there is a reduction of the ECV, decreases in the systemic blood pressure, venous return and cardiac output result. These changes increase sympathetic activity so increasing arteriolar tone and promoting renin release, via stretch receptor and baroreceptor reflexes. The renin-containing granular cells of the renal afferent arterioles are innervated by sympathetic nerve fibres. Increased sympathetic activity in these causes renin release. This release of renin is mediated by β-adrenergic receptors and is important in maintaining renin release under basal conditions. It is also activated when assuming the upright posture, as well as during sodium depletion.

Decreased wall tension in the afferent arterioles

Decreased renal perfusion pressure in response to reduced ECV, leads to increased renin release from the granular cells. The immediate stimulus appears to be arteriolar wall tension and its rate of change (dependent on pulse pressure) at the granular cells. This is known as the afferent arteriolar baroreceptor reflex mechanism. Sympathetic vasoconstriction of the kidney will also increase renin release by this mechanism, since the afferent arteriole is constricted by renal sympathetic nerve activity and this constriction is 'upstream' from the granular cells. This occurs in addition to the release of renin by the β-receptor mechanism.

The macula densa mechanism

A decrease in the delivery of NaCl to the macula densa leads to renin release, but the details of this mechanism are not clear.

Following stimulation of the juxtaglomerular apparatus, renin is released into the blood, where it acts on an α_2-globulin (angiotensinogen) and splits off a decapeptide (angiotensin I). An enzyme on the surface of endothelial cells (converting enzyme) rapidly removes a further two amino acids from angiotensin I, to form the octapeptide, angiotensin II (Figure RE.12).

ANGIOTENSIN II

A primary action of angiotensin II is its action on the zona glomerulosa of the adrenal cortex to promote the release of aldosterone. Very little aldosterone is stored but stimulation of its release promotes further aldosterone biosynthesis.

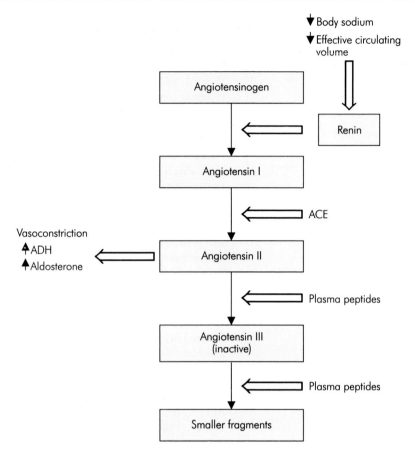

Figure RE.12 Renin–angiotensin system

Angiotensin II is an extremely potent vasoconstrictor. Normally this action plays a minor part in the maintenance of systemic blood pressure, but intrarenally this can alter the distribution of glomerular filtration

A third important role of angiotensin II is its direct effect on proximal tubular sodium re-absorption. Physiological concentrations of angiotensin II increase proximal tubular Na^+ re-absorption. This is mediated by inhibition of adenylate cyclase that increases Na^+-H^+ antiport.

Angiotensin II also inhibits renin release by negative feedback on the juxtaglomerular granular cells, and has various other actions (Figure RE.13).

ALDOSTERONE

Aldosterone is an adrenal cortical hormone necessary for normal sodium absorption and excretion. Its role in sodium regulation is exerted more via a permissive action than a controlling action. Changes in plasma aldosterone levels are usually accompanied by parallel changes in ADH and form part of the overall mechanism for regulating body fluid volume. The main actions of aldosterone are to promote Na^+ re-absorption from the distal nephron and to promote Hydrogen and potassium ion excretion. Actions of aldosterone are summarised in Figure RE.13.

STARLING FORCES AND PROXIMAL TUBULAR SODIUM RE-ABSORPTION

When body sodium content changes, the consequent changes in ECV that result, automatically adjust proximal tubular Na^+ re-absorption to correct the disturbance.

Re-absorption of sodium chloride and water from the proximal tubule passes to the peritubular capillaries via the lateral intercellular spaces (LIS). The overall rate of re-absorption is determined by the rate of uptake from the LIS into the capillaries. Starling forces govern this uptake and these are dependent on the hydrostatic

ACTIONS OF ANGIOTENSIN II AND ALDOSTERONE

Substance	Actions
Angiotensin II	Stimulates release of aldosterone
	Potent systemic and renal vasoconstrictor
	↑ Na^+ in proximal tubule
	↑ Na^+ in distal tubule
	Stimulates release of ADH
	Water retention
	Stimulates thirst
	Inhibits release of renin
Aldosterone	↑ renal Na^+ reabsorption
	↑ renal H^+/K^+ excretion
	↑ Na^+ and K^+ channels in tubule cells
	↑ ATPase synthesis and activity in tubule cells
	↑ gastro-intestinal Na^+ reabsorption
	↑ Na^+ re-absorption from sweat glands

Figure RE.13

pressure and colloid osmotic pressure (COP), in the peritubular capillaries and LIS. The acting Starling forces are summarised by the equation:

capillary uptake ∝ forces favouring uptake – forces opposing uptake

$$\propto (\pi_{PC} + P_L) - (\pi_L + P_{PC})$$

where:

π_{PC} = peritubular capillary COP
π_L = COP in LIS
P_{PC} = hydrostatic pressure in the peritubular capillaries
P_L = hydrostatic pressure in the LIS.

Both P_{PC} and π_{PC} vary with changes in body fluid volume. An increase in body fluid volume results in increased peritubular capillary hydrostatic (P_{PC}) due to an increased venous pressure. At the same time, the plasma proteins are diluted by increased body fluid volume, reducing the capillary COP (π_{PC}). These changes decrease proximal tubular re-absorption of NaCl and water, thus acting to correct the original disturbance.

LONG AND SHORT LOOPS OF HENLE IN SODIUM RE-ABSORPTION

Changes in the proximal re-absorption of sodium

affect its delivery to more distal parts of the nephron. Thus, if proximal sodium re-absorption is increased, the distal delivery of sodium to the loop of Henle is decreased. Similarly if proximal re-absorption is decreased more sodium is delivered to the LOH.

Consider a disturbance leading to an increase in body sodium and water. From the above discussion this will produce a decrease in proximal sodium re-absorption and an increase in sodium delivered to the ascending LOH. However, in the long LOH, re-absorption from the ascending limb is directly dependent on Na^+ delivery, and, hence, more Na^+ will be extruded into the interstitium. This would appear to be counterproductive towards correcting the original disturbance of increased body sodium and water. However, nephrons with shorts loops of Henle cannot extrude enough Na^+ from their ascending limbs to re-absorb the entire increased Na^+ load resulting from reduced proximal re-absorption. Thus, the final urinary composition of the short looped nephrons depends on proximal re-absorption to a much greater extent than that of the long looped nephrons. Effectively the short-looped nephrons can be thought of as 'sodium losing', while the long looped nephrons are 'sodium retaining' nephrons.

The response to changes in ECV, may, therefore, involve redistribution of the renal blood flow between the two populations of nephrons, to obtain the urine composition that would compensate for the original disturbance in ECV.

NEUROLOGICAL REFLEXES IN THE KIDNEY AND SODIUM RE-ABSORPTION

The nerve supply to the kidney is mainly sympathetic and is controlled by arterial baroreceptors. The sympathetic nerves of the kidney primarily supply the afferent arterioles. Decreased ECV will tend to reduce blood pressure, causing a reflex increase in renal sympathetic activity. Mild stimulation of the renal nerves reduces the blood flow to the superficial short-looped nephrons, and increases blood flow to the juxtamedullary long-looped nephrons, thus tending to conserve sodium. This baroreceptor mechanism also increases proximal tubular Na^+ re-absorption that also conserves sodium. Angiotensin II may mediate this effect, because renal nerve stimulation is known to release renin. This also causes sodium retention by promoting aldosterone release, but, in addition, catecholamines released from the renal sympathetic nerve endings (and from the adrenal medulla) stimulate sodium re-absorption in the proximal tubule by a direct action on sodium transport.

PROSTAGLANDINS

In the kidney, there are at least three distinct sites of prostaglandin synthesis:

- The cortex, including arterioles and glomeruli
- Medullary interstitial cells
- Collecting duct epithelial cells

The main prostaglandins synthesised by the kidney are PGE_2, PGI_2, $PGF_{2\alpha}$, PGD_2 and thromboxane A_2 (TXA_2).

Renal prostaglandins are synthesised from arachidonic acid, which is stored esterified in membrane phospholipids. The release of free arachidonic acid occurs enzymatically, and can be inhibited by steroids. Free arachidonic acid is converted by a cyclo-oxygenase enzyme into unstable endoperoxides, which then give rise to the renal prostanoids. The major arachidonate products are PGI_2 (prostacyclin) in the cortex, and PGE_2 in the medulla.

As with other prostaglandins, the renal prostaglandins act locally and have important intrarenal effects. PGE_2 and PGI_2 are produced in increased amounts when renal perfusion is threatened by vasoconstrictors such as norepinephrine, vasopressin and angiotensin II, or when hypotension occurs. These renal prostaglandins are vasodilators that minimise renal vasoconstriction. The use

of non steroidal anti-inflammatory drugs, such as aspirin or indomethacin, can reduce renal prostaglandin synthesis by inhibiting cyclo-oxygenase. This may have no effect on renal blood flow or GFR in normal individuals, but in patients with compromised renal perfusion (e.g. hypotension or receiving vasoconstrictors) these drugs can lead to large falls in GFR.

The anti-vasoconstrictor role of the renal prostaglandins is a cortical effect, PGI_2 is likely to be the most important prostanoid in this role. Hence decreased ECV leads to increased cortical prostaglandin synthesis.

The medullary prostaglandins (mainly PGE_2) have actions on the renal tubules, predominantly the collecting tubules. Their main actions are natriuretic and diuretic. They also impair the anti-diuretic action of ADH. These actions may also limit the extent to which Na^+ re-absorption (ATP-dependent) can be stimulated by aldosterone in the renal medulla, and, hence, protect the medullary tubule cells from excessive anoxia during hypovolaemia.

TXA_2 unlike the other renal prostanoids, is a vasoconstrictor. Little TXA_2 is normally produced, but its synthesis increases following prolonged ureteral obstruction.

ATRIAL NATRIURETIC PEPTIDE

Cardiac atrial cells contain granules in which the precursor of α-human atrial natriuretic peptide (ANP) is stored. The atrial genes code for a 'pre-prohormone' with 152 amino acids. The removal of a hydrophobic sequence from the N-terminal end of this leaves the 126 amino acid prohormone. The primary released form of the hormone is α-human ANP (28 amino acids), but smaller fragments have been isolated and similar peptides are released from the brain (brain natriuretic peptide BNP) and from the kidney itself (renal natriuretic peptide or urodilatin).

ANP can be detected in normal plasma and increased atrial stretch leads to an increased circulating level of ANP. Many of the effects of ANP are mediated via specific cell surface receptors, which when ANP binds to them, elicit an increase in the intracellular level of cyclic guanosine monophosphate (cyclic GMP). The major actions of ANP are:

- Activation of receptors on the inner medullary collecting duct cells, leading to closure of epithelial sodium channels, and inhibition of $Na^+K^+ATPase$, thereby decreasing Na^+ re-absorption at this nephron site
- Inhibition of aldosterone secretion by the zona glomerulosa of the adrenal cortex

- Reduction of renin release, which also causes a reduction in aldosterone secretion
- Vasodilatation, particularly of the afferent arterioles, leading to increased GFR
- Inhibition of ADH release by the posterior pituitary

All of these actions contribute to the natriuretic effect of ANP.

DOPAMINE

The kidneys synthesise dopamine, mostly in the cells of the proximal tubule and this dopamine synthesis reduces tubular sodium transport, by inhibiting the $Na^+K^+ATPase$ and by decreasing Na^+H^+ antiport activity. Dopamine is also a vasodilator, but the natriuretic effect is mainly due to its tubular action, since dopamine increases sodium excretion even when renal blood flow and GFR are unaffected.

KININS

Kinins are vasodilator peptides produced from precursor proteins ('kininogens') by the action of the enzyme kallikrein. The effects of renally produced kinins are very similar to those of the prostaglandins; they vasodilate the kidney, antagonise ADH-induced increases of urine osmolality and are natriuretic. Their significance in the overall control of sodium excretion is not clear. The haemodynamic effects of kinins are thought to be due to the increased production of nitric oxide.

NATRIURETIC HORMONE

There is thought to be an as yet unidentified 'natriuretic hormone', probably of hypothalamic origin, and released during volume expansion or in circumstances where the number of functioning nephrons is reduced, so that the remaining ones must increase the fraction of filtered sodium which they excrete.

ADH IN OSMOTIC AND VOLUME REGULATION

There are circumstances in which the maintenance of effective circulating volume is more important to survival than the maintenance of body fluid osmolality. When the effective circulating volume is threatened, volume regulation takes precedence over osmotic regulation.

Changes in effective circulating volume are detected by stretch receptors in atria and rapidly lead to appropriate alterations in urine flow, which is mediated by changes in ADH release (e.g. stretching the left atrial receptors produces a diuresis). These receptors exist in both the venous and arterial sides of the circulatory system. This enables changes in ADH secretion to occur in response to both volume and blood pressure changes.

Changes in ECV alter the range of plasma osmolalities over which ADH is released (Figure RE.14). It can be seen that the normal response curve of ADH to plasma osmolality is a straight line. Changes in ECV alter the gradient of this line, which is equivalent to altering the sensitivity of the ADH response. Thus, when ECV is decreased ADH levels are higher at a given plasma osmolality, giving rise to retained volume even at the expense of lower than normal osmolality. Under these circumstances of hypovolaemia the ADH response is more sensitive. When hypervolaemia is present, the ADH response becomes blunted and lower than expected ADH levels are found for any given plasma osmolality.

In summary it can be seen that the regulation of sodium excretion is complex.

RENAL REGULATION OF BODY FLUID pH

NORMAL BODY FLUID PH

The normal blood pH is kept within the range 7.35–7.45, although a range of 7.00–7.80 can be tolerated. Enzyme reactions in the body have a pH optimum, but the pH dependence of such reactions is much less sharply defined than the pH dependence of the whole organism. The pH notation tends to obscure the range of H^+ concentration tolerated, which is broad compared with some other biochemical parameters. To convert the normal pH range to H^+ concentration values:

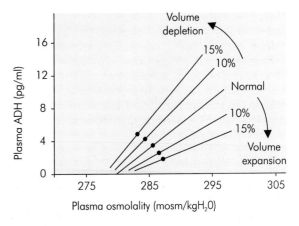

Figure RE.14 ADH response to changes in extracellular volume

Let concentration of $H^+ = [H^+]$

By definition $pH = -\log[H^+]$

As normal $pH = 7.4$

Therefore $-\log[H^+] = 7.4$

$$[H^+] = \log^{-1}(-7.4)$$
$$= \log^{-1}(-8) \times \log^{-1}(0.6)$$
$$= 10^{-8} \times 3.98$$
$$= 39.8 \times 10^{-9} \text{ mol/l}$$
$$= 39.8 \text{ nmol/l}.$$

A pH between 7.35 and 7.45 corresponds to an $[H^+]$ range of 45–35 nmol/l. This means a change of $> 20\%$ may be tolerated under normal conditions.

PHYSIOLOGICAL BUFFERS

A buffer solution minimises the change of pH, when acid or base is added to it. Buffer solutions consist of a weak acid and the conjugate base of that acid. Thus, in solution:

(acid) $\rightleftharpoons$ (hydrogen ion) $+$ (conjugate base)
HA $\rightleftharpoons$ H$^+$ $+$ A$^-$

When hydrogen ions are added to the buffer solution, the above reaction is driven to the left and the hydrogen ions (H$^+$) are 'neutralised' by combination with the conjugate base (A$^-$).

Definition of pK for a buffer

The equilibrium constant (K) for the above dissociation reaction is given by the equation:

$$K = \frac{[H^+][A^-]}{[HA]}$$

and $pK = -\log K$

From the above, and using the definition of pH, it can be seen that pK is the pH at which $[A^-] = [HA]$, i.e. when the weak acid, HA, is half dissociated.

HENDERSON–HASSELBACH EQUATION

In any buffer system consisting of a dissociating weak acid HA, the pH of the buffer solution is dependent on the ratio of conjugate base concentration $[A^-]$ to undissociated acid concentration $[HA]$.

Re-arranging the equation for K from above:

$$[H+] = \frac{K[A^-]}{[HA]}$$

So $$\frac{1}{[H^+]} = \frac{1}{K}\frac{[HA]}{[A^-]}$$

or $$-\log[H+] = -\log K + \log\frac{[A^-]}{[HA]}$$

therefore, $$pH = pK + \log\frac{[A^-]}{[HA]}$$

which can be expressed as

$$pH = pK + \log\frac{[\text{conjugate base}]}{[\text{acid}]}$$

which is known as the Henderson–Hasselbach equation.

BICARBONATE BUFFER SYSTEM

In the body fluids, there are several buffer systems. These are summarised in Figure RE.15.

MAIN PHYSIOLOGICAL BUFFER SYSTEMS	
Body compartment	**Buffer**
Blood	Bicarbonate/CO_2 Haemoglobin (HHb/Hb$^-$ and HHbO$_2$/HbO$_2$) Plasma proteins (H$^+$–protein/protein$^-$) Phosphate (H$_2$PO$_4^-$/HPO$_4^{2-}$)
Extracellular fluid	Bicarbonate/CO_2 Plasma proteins (H$^+$–protein/protein$^-$) Phosphate (H$_2$PO$_4^-$/HPO$_4^{2-}$)
Intracellular fluid	Plasma proteins (H$^+$–protein/protein$^-$) Phosphate (H$_2$PO$_4^-$/HPO$_4^{2-}$) Organic phosphates Bicarbonate/CO_2

Figure RE.15

Throughout the body fluids, the bicarbonate buffer system is the most important. The reaction sequence for this system is:

$$CO_2 + H_2O \rightleftharpoons H_2CO_3 \rightleftharpoons H^+ + HCO_3^-$$

The importance of the bicarbonate buffer system is due to the ready excretion of CO_2 by the lungs, which eliminates the carbonic acid formed when H^+ is neutralised. This is coupled with the continuous maintenance of buffer base levels through re-absorption of bicarbonate in the kidneys.

These actions continually drive the above equations to the left, neutralising H^+ as it is produced by intermediate metabolism.

Thus, for the bicarbonate buffer system (pK = 6.3), the Henderson–Hasselbach equation can be written as follows:

$$pH = 6.3 + \log \frac{[HCO_3^-]}{[H_2CO_3]}$$

$[H_2CO_3]$ is proportional to the pCO_2 (partial pressure of CO_2 in mmHg) and is about 2.0 mmol/l. Assuming a normal value of $[HCO_3^-]$ = 25 mmol/l, substitution in the above equation gives:

$$pH = 6.3 + \log\left(\frac{25}{2}\right)$$
$$= 7.39$$

This illustrates how the bicarbonate buffer system determines normal pH for the body fluids, by fixing its [conjugate base]:[acid] ratio. This pH will then determine the [conjugate base]:[acid] ratio for all the other buffer systems in the body.

The bicarbonate system, chemically, is a poor buffer, but physiologically it is extremely effective because of the physiological control over $[HCO_3^-]$ and PCO_2. Since bicarbonate is regulated by the kidneys and PCO_2 by the lungs, it is apparent that pH depends on the activity of both organs.

RENAL REGULATION OF PLASMA BICARBONATE CONCENTRATION

Intermediate metabolism generates a continuous load of H^+. This is buffered by the blood buffer systems, which prevent excessive levels of free H^+, but become depleted as their base reserves combine with the H^+. Thus, the buffer bases need to be constantly regenerated. The most important buffer is bicarbonate, since H^+ is readily neutralised by plasma HCO_3^- to give carbonic acid, which is easily excreted as CO_2 in the lungs. The bicarbonate reserve is regenerated continually by the re-absorption process in the kidney. The role of the kidney can thus be seen as the conservation of the remaining HCO_3^- and the generation of additional HCO_3^-.

Renal T_m for bicarbonate

Bicarbonate ion is freely filtered at the glomeruli; hence, the concentration of bicarbonate entering the nephron is 25 mmol/l.

The kidney behaves as if there is a T_m for bicarbonate re-absorption, with the T_m set close to the amount filtered at the normal plasma concentrations. In fact, the T_m for HCO_3^- is not constant but varies with the rate of H^+ secretion, and also directly with fractional sodium re-absorption. The T_m provides a means of dealing with increases in plasma $[HCO_3^-]$, since an increase will lead to T_m being exceeded and HCO_3^- being excreted until the plasma level reaches normal again.

H^+ AND BICARBONATE RE-ABSORPTION

In the proximal tubule 90% of the filtered bicarbonate is re-absorbed from the tubular fluid. This bicarbonate re-absorption is in fact brought about not by the transport of HCO_3^- ions, but by the luminal conversion of HCO_3^- into CO_2. H^+ is secreted from the proximal tubule cell into the lumen, where it associates with HCO_3^- to form H_2CO_3. This carbonic acid dissociates into CO_2 and H_2O. The reaction is catalysed by an enzyme, carbonic anhydrase, which is present in the brush borders of the cells, and so catalyses the luminal reaction without being lost in the urine. The CO_2 so formed can readily diffuse into the tubule cells, where intracellular carbonic anhydrase catalyses the re-hydration of CO_2 to H_2CO_3, which dissociates to H^+ and HCO_3^-. The H^+ thus regenerated in the tubular cells is then available for excretion back into the tubule lumen to enable further re-absorption of HCO_3^-. It can, therefore, be claimed that the purpose of H^+ excretion in the kidney, is to permit HCO_3^- re-absorption. Under normal circumstances, < 0.1% of filtered HCO_3^- is excreted in the final urine.

NaCl AND BICARBONATE RE-ABSORPTION

Although the entry of Na^+ into the proximal tubule cells is down the electrochemical gradient, Na^+ entry is coupled to H^+ excretion (via an antiport or countertransport process) and the transport is electroneutral. In addition, the luminal membrane has a primary H^+ secretory mechanism, using proton ATPase, although this is of little importance in the proximal tubule. However, there is evidence that most apical membrane Na^+ re-absorption is associated with H^+ excretion, which generates CO_2 in the tubular lumen. The CO_2 enters the cells and again forms HCO_3^- much of which then exchanges with luminal Cl^-, i.e. there is HCO_3^- secretion and Cl^- re-absorption, such that the overall effect is predominantly the re-absorption of NaCl.

Bicarbonate re-absorption in the distal tubule

The acid base regulating process that occurs in the 'distal tubule' and collecting duct is the same as that in the proximal tubule, being basically HCO_3^- re-absorption and H^+ excretion. The distal nephron processes are, quantitatively, much less important than those in the proximal tubule, since they account for only 10% of the total bicarbonate re-absorption. However, to achieve this, the distal tubule and collecting duct have to secrete H^+ against a much bigger gradient than that in the proximal tubule and this requires specific mechanisms.

The distal nephron cell types that are primarily involved in acid base regulation, are the intercalated cells that secrete H^+ across the apical membrane by an $H^+ATPase$. In addition, there is an $H^+K^+ATPase$, which pumps H^+ out in exchange for K^+. The linked Na^+H^+ transport of H^+ is of lesser importance in the distal nephron, but does occur in the proximal cells and is one of the means whereby aldosterone enhances H^+ secretion.

In both the proximal tubule and the distal nephron H^+ secretion is required not only for the re-absorption of filtered HCO_3^-, but also to remove H^+ produced in generating additional HCO_3^- to maintain plasma levels. In order for H^+ secretion to occur, there must be some way in which the secreted H^+ can be buffered in the tubular lumen, to provide a continuing gradient for secretion, or at least to prevent the gradient against which secretion is occurring from being too large. It is mainly filtered HCO_3^- which provides this H^+ buffering. However, there are other forms of buffering for the secreted H^+.

Alkaline/acid phosphate as a urinary buffer system

In the plasma there are two phosphate salts, disodium hydrogen phosphate (alkaline phosphate, Na_2HPO_4) and sodium dihydrogen phosphate (acid phosphate, NaH_2PO_4). The ratio of alkaline phosphate to acid phosphate in plasma is about 4:1. These phosphate salts form an additional buffer system in the plasma.

Both the acidic and basic forms of phosphate are also filtered at the glomerulus. These then form another system for buffering H^+ in the urine. When H^+ secretion occurs into the tubule, the ratio $[HPO_4^{2-}]:[H_2PO_4^-]$ in the luminal fluid is reduced, i.e. alkaline phosphate is converted into acid phosphate as buffering of the secreted H^+ occurs. Some phosphate buffering takes place in the proximal tubule (since there is a small fall in pH of the tubular fluid proximally), but it takes place mainly in the distal tubule. The $H_2PO_4^-$ constitutes the titratable acidity of the urine.

An important consequence of phosphate buffering in the urine, is that secretion levels of H^+ can be maintained. This in turn maintains the levels of HCO_3^- generated intracellularly, since for every H^+ one HCO_3^- is produced, and this HCO_3^- is then available for export to the plasma.

Ammonia is a form of excess nitrogen that is produced as a by-product of protein metabolism in the body. It does not circulate in its free form but forms a buffer system with the ammoniun ion:

$$NH_3 + H^+ \rightleftharpoons NH_4^+$$

The main circulating sources of NH_4^+ are glutamine and glutamic acid. The ultimate fate of NH_4^+ is to be excreted by the kidney either as ammonia or as urea.

NH_4^+ is produced by de-amination of glutamine to glutamic acid and to α-ketoglutarate in most parts of the nephron, but mainly in the proximal tubule cells. The NH_4^+ is then excreted into the tubular lumen. Transport of NH_4 across cell membranes requires the ammonium ion to split into NH_3, which is freely diffusible, and H^+.

The α-ketoglutarate left behind in the tubule cells reacts with H^+ to form glucose or CO_2, leaving bicarbonate to enter the plasma. Thus, the de-amination of glutamine, produces NH_4^+ and generates bicarbonate for the plasma. If the NH_4^+ were not excreted but remained in the body, then the liver could utilise NH_4^+ and HCO_3^- to produce urea for excretion, but with no gain of HCO_3^-. Thus, renal secretion of NH_4+ also regenerates HCO_3^- for the plasma.

About 50% of the NH_4^+ secreted into the lumen by the proximal tubule cells, is re-absorbed by the thick ascending limb of the loop of Henle, and accumulates in the medullary interstitium. This re-absorption occurs by $Na^+/NH_4^+/2\ Cl^-$ co-transport across the apical membrane. The NH_4^+ re-absorption lowers the luminal NH_4^+ concentration, and, hence, also lowers the luminal NH_3 concentration, which is freely diffusible, as the luminal fluid passes into the distal tubule. This also has the effect of maintaining a higher NH_4^+ concentration in the medullary interstitium, from where the NH_4^+ then passes into the cells of the collecting tubules to be excreted.

NH_4^+ excretion is increased in acidosis because:

- The enzymes in the proximal tubule which de-aminate glutamine are stimulated by acidosis
- NH_3 conversion to NH_4^+ in the collecting tubule is greater if H^+ excretion is greater
- Increased conversion of NH_3 to NH_4^+ in the collecting duct decreases the concentration of NH_3 in the duct. This increases the diffusion gradient for NH_3, and its rate of removal from the renal medulla

H^+ SECRETION IN THE NEPHRON

The secretion of H^+ in the nephron requires it to combine with ions in the tubular fluid in the following manner:

- Combination of H^+ with HCO_3^- leads to CO_2 absorption by the tubular cells and formation of HCO_3^- intracellularly. This can be viewed as re-absorption of the HCO_3^- from the tubular lumen
- Combination of H^+ with HPO_4^{2-} or NH_3, leads to formation of HCO_3^- in the tubular cells rather than re-absorption from the tubular lumen. This can be viewed as generation of HCO_3^-

The H^+ secreted causes the pH of the tubular fluid to fall progressively along the nephron. This fall is small in the proximal tubule (from 7.4 to about 6.9), but the pH may be as low as 4.5 in the collecting duct. Although the urine is usually acidic and can be titrated to determine the 'titratable acidity' this only constitutes a fraction of the total H^+ secreted. This is because:

Total H^+ secreted = (H^+ neutralised in HCO_3^- re-absorption)
+ (H^+ combined in $H_2PO_4^-$ excretion)
+ (H^+ combined in NH_4^+ excretion).

But only the $H_2PO_4^-$ excretion is 'titratable acidity'.

Points of emphasis for H^+ secretion in the nephron are:

- H^+ secreted must be combined with anions in the tubular fluid
- The main anions are HCO_3^-, HPO_4^{2-} and NH_3
- Combination with HCO_3^- leads to re-absorption of HCO_3^-
- Combination with HPO_4^{2-} or NH_3 leads to generation of HCO_3^-

RENAL REGULATION OF PH IN ACID BASE BALANCE DISTURBANCES

Acid base disturbances can be divided into disturbances of respiratory origin (respiratory acidosis and alkalosis) and non respiratory origin (metabolic acidosis and alkalosis). 'Metabolic' refers to acid base disturbances that affect the bicarbonate buffer system by a means other than an alteration of PCO_2. Metabolic acidosis is by far the most common metabolic disturbance, and is often associated with pathological conditions involving the excess production of acid. Examples of these are diabetic ketoacidosis or septicaemia. Alternatively failure to excrete acid as in renal failure can also lead to a metabolic acidosis.

In each of the four disturbances, there is initially a change in body fluid pH (i.e. a change in H^+ concentration). However, the buffer and compensatory systems are so effective that this change in pH may be barely measurable.

When changes in extracellular fluid pH occur, there are parallel, although not necessarily identical, changes in intracellular pH. Therefore, a change in arterial pH is reflected in the pH of all the cells of the body, including the renal tubule cells. The rate of H^+ secretion from the tubule cells varies inversely with pH (i.e. varies directly with H^+ concentration). This is vital for the compensation for, and correction of, acid base disturbances.

COMPENSATION AND CORRECTION IN ACID BASE DISTURBANCES

Normal acid base status comprises not only a pH of 7.4, but also a plasma $[HCO_3^-]$ of about 25 mmol/l and a PCO_2 of about 40 mmHg. An acid base disturbance disrupts at least two of these three variables.

Two definitions are important:

- **Compensation** which is the restoration of pH towards normal even though $[HCO_3^-]$ and/or PCO_2 are still disturbed
- **Correction** which is the restoration of normal pH, $[HCO_3^-]$ and PCO_2

The purpose of homeostatic acid-balance regulating mechanisms is the maintenance of normal pH. The process used for the immediate regulation of pH is adjustment of PCO_2 and $[HCO_3^-]$. The normal levels of these parameters are sacrificed initially to correct for pH disturbances. Ultimately long-term correction requires regeneration of buffer base reserves and secretion of H^+ by the kidneys.

In the following sections, a simplified version of the Henderson–Hasselbalch equation is used to show changes in pH, PCO_2 and HCO_3^-. The simplified form of the Henderson–Hasselbach equation used is as follows:

$$pH \quad \propto \quad \frac{[HCO_3^-]}{PCO_2}$$

Three types of arrow are used to indicate changes: $\Uparrow$ or $\Downarrow$ are the initial acid base defect; $\uparrow$ or $\downarrow$ are the consequence of the defect; $\uparrow$ or $\downarrow$ are compensatory changes.

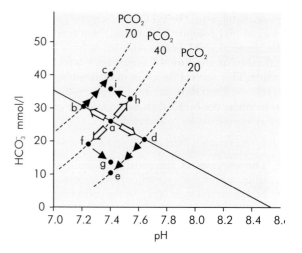

Figure RE.16. Acid base disturbances and compensation

RESPIRATORY ACIDOSIS

This is a disturbance of acid base balance that occurs when the respiratory system is unable to remove sufficient CO_2 from the body, giving rise to higher than normal PCO_2 levels (hypercapnia). This condition might be caused by failure to breathe adequately (hypoventilation) and results in an arterial partial pressure of CO_2 ($PaCO_2$) that > 6.0 kPa (45 mmHg). The following reaction becomes displaced to the right by the increased PCO_2:

$$CO_2 + H_2O \rightleftharpoons H_2CO_3 \rightleftharpoons H^+ + HCO_3^-$$

The consequence of this defect is an increased $[H^+]$ (i.e. acidosis – reduced pH), and an increased $[HCO_3^-]$. These changes are illustrated in Figure RE.16, which plots the three variables of $[HCO_3^-]$, pH and PCO_2. Normal acid base status is represented by 'a'. Respiratory acidosis producing the above disturbances in pH and $[HCO_3^-]$ shifts the acid base status to 'b'. Inserting these changes into the simplified Henderson–Hasselbach equation results in:

$$\downarrow pH \quad \propto \quad \frac{\uparrow [HCO_3^-]}{\Uparrow PCO_2}$$

A change in $[H^+]$ in the body fluids changes the rate of H^+ secretion from renal tubular cells. In respiratory acidosis, $[H^+]$ is increased; therefore, the rate of H^+ secretion also increases. This increased secretion is sufficient to re-absorb all of the filtered HCO_3^- even though the plasma $[HCO_3^-]$ is raised by the defect and, therefore, the amount of HCO_3^- filtered is increased. In addition, it is also sufficient to generate HCO_3^-, which increases plasma $[HCO_3^-]$ further.

This increased renal H^+ secretion leading to increased plasma $[HCO_3^-]$ is renal compensation for the respiratory acidosis. This compensation is demonstrated in Figure RE.16 by a shift of the

respiratory acidosis point 'b' to the compensated point 'c'. These compensatory changes can be added to the simplified Henderson–Hasselbalch equation:

$$\downarrow pH \uparrow \quad \propto \quad \frac{\uparrow [HCO_3^-] \downarrow}{\Uparrow pCO_2}$$

Although compensation restores the pH towards normal, PCO_2 remains raised due to the initial defect, and plasma $[HCO_3^-]$ is raised, both as a consequence of the defect, and by compensation. To restore normal $[HCO_3^-]$ and PCO_2 would require an alteration in respiration i.e. correction of the original defect.

RESPIRATORY ALKALOSIS

This is caused by the excessive removal of CO_2 from the body by the respiratory system. This may occur with excessively rapid breathing (hyperventilation). Under these circumstances the $PaCO_2$ falls below 4.6 kPa (35 mmHg). The reaction:

$$CO_2 + H_2O \rightleftharpoons H_2CO_3 \rightleftharpoons H^+ + HCO_3^-$$

is displaced to the left by the lowering of PCO_2 and leads to a decrease in $[H^+]$ (i.e. alkalosis), and a decrease in $[HCO_3^-]$. The changes are illustrated by a shift from the normal status point 'a' to 'd' in Figure RE.16.

In the simplified form the Henderson–Hasselbach equation can be seen:

$$\uparrow pH \quad \propto \quad \frac{\downarrow [HCO_3^-]}{\Downarrow PCO_2}$$

The decreased PCO_2 results in a decreased $[H^+]$ in the renal tubule cells and a reduced rate of H^+ secretion.

Thus, although plasma $[HCO_3^-]$ is reduced, which decreases the amount of HCO_3^- filtered by the kidney, the rate of H^+ secretion is insufficient to re-absorb all the filtered bicarbonate, or to generate more bicarbonate. Therefore, HCO_3^- is excreted in the urine, and the plasma $[HCO_3^-]$ falls further.

The reduced H^+ secretion in the renal tubules, leading to HCO_3^- excretion represents renal compensation for respiratory alkalosis. This compensation is demonstrated by the movement from point 'd' to 'e' in Figure RE.16, and can be added to the equation above resulting in:

$$\uparrow pH \sim \downarrow \quad \propto \quad \frac{\downarrow[HCO_3^-]\downarrow}{\Downarrow PCO_2}$$

The renal compensation restores pH towards normal, but lowers the plasma $[HCO_3^-]$ further, even though plasma $[HCO_3^-]$ has already been reduced by the original disturbance. In addition, PCO_2 remains lower than normal. The restoration of normal plasma $[HCO_3^-]$ and PCO_2 levels requires the removal of the respiratory defect, i.e. requires a reduction of ventilation.

The body's mechanisms for control of respiration maintain PCO_2 levels within normal limits (4.5 < $PaCO_2$ < 5.5 kPa). Increases in $PaCO_2$ results in increased $[H^+]$ in body fluid, which stimulates respiration via central and peripheral chemoreceptors. Decreases in $PaCO_2$ decrease ventilation. However, if the PO_2 in the inspired air is below normal, so that PaO_2 falls significantly, then oxygen lack, acting via chemoreceptors in the carotid body, increases ventilation. When this occurs, the $PaCO_2$ falls. This is respiratory alkalosis. Thus, hypoxia, leading to increased ventilation, can lead to hypocapnia and respiratory alkalosis. This occurs in normal people when they ascend to a high altitude (> 10 000 feet). Other causes of respiratory alkalosis include hyperventilation.

METABOLIC ACIDOSIS

Metabolic acidosis is an acidosis that is not caused by a change in the arterial PCO_2. So, in the reaction sequence:

$$CO_2 + H_2O \rightleftharpoons H_2CO_3 \rightleftharpoons H^+ + HCO_3$$
$$\searrow$$
$$H^+$$

The metabolic acidosis can be regarded as the addition of H^+ to the right of the reaction, so driving it to the left and depleting the plasma HCO_3^- as it does so. The direct loss of HCO_3^- can also cause metabolic acidosis,

as can be seen from the Henderson–Hasselbalch equation below. Initially since respiration is unimpaired, the original disturbance can be assumed to occur at a constant (normal) PCO_2.

Metabolic acidosis is illustrated in Figure RE.16 by a shift from normal at point 'a' to 'f'. The simplified Henderson–Hasselbach equation becomes:

$$\Downarrow pH \quad \propto \quad \frac{\downarrow[HCO_3^-]}{PCO_2}$$

The change in pH, acting on the peripheral chemoreceptors, stimulates respiration so that $PaCO_2$ falls. This is respiratory compensation for metabolic acidosis. However, the lowering of PCO_2 moves the reaction

$$CO_2 + H_2O \rightleftharpoons H_2CO_3 \rightleftharpoons H^+ + HCO_3^-$$

to the left thus lowering $[H^+]$ and so raising the pH towards normal, but also further lowering the plasma $[HCO_3^-]$. These compensatory changes can be seen by the movement from 'f' to 'g' in Figure RE.16, and are added to the simplified Henderson–Hasselbach equation as follows:

$$\Downarrow pH \uparrow \quad \propto \quad \frac{\downarrow[HCO_3^-]\downarrow}{PCO_2\downarrow}$$

Thus, the original disturbance initiates the corrective process to restore pH to normal. This occurs because the increased $[H^+]$ in the blood is reflected in an increased $[H^+]$ in the renal tubular cells. This increases the rate of H^+ secretion, and permits the re-absorption of all the filtered HCO_3^-, particularly as the filtered HCO_3^- load is below normal. In addition, the increased rate of H^+ secretion allows generation of more HCO_3^-, restoring the depleted plasma HCO_3^- reserve and returning pH to normal. The stimulated respiratory drive due to the original disturbed pH can then also be normalised.

It should be noted that in metabolic acidosis there is often nothing wrong with the kidneys. They simply cannot excrete an H^+ load instantaneously. The respiratory compensation, although restoring pH towards normal, also hampers the renal correction of the defect. This is because any decrease in pH also reduces H^+ secretion and, hence, reduces renal HCO_3^- re-absorption and regeneration. The exception to this is renal failure, where the kidneys' failure to excrete H^+ is the cause of metabolic acidosis.

METABOLIC ALKALOSIS

This is alkalosis that is not caused by a change in the arterial PCO_2. In the reaction sequence:

$$CO_2 + H_2O \rightleftharpoons H_2CO_3 \rightleftharpoons H^+ + HCO_3^-$$
$$\searrow \longrightarrow H_2O$$
$$OH^-$$

metabolic alkalosis can be regarded as the addition of base (OH⁻ in the equation, although it can be any H^+ acceptor) to the system. This removes H^+ from the right of the reaction and causes the reaction to move to the right, increasing plasma $[HCO_3^-]$. Initially this can be assumed to occur at a constant (normal) pCO_2, and is shown by a shift from point 'a' to 'h' in Figure RE.16. The simplified Henderson–Hasselbach equation then becomes:

$$\Uparrow pH \; \propto \; \frac{\uparrow[HCO_3^-]}{PCO_2}$$

The decreased $[H^+]$ acting on chemoreceptors, reduces ventilation and so increases the PCO_2. This is respiratory compensation for metabolic alkalosis. The compensatory changes are illustrated by movement from 'h' to 'I' in Figure RE.16, and can be added to the above equation as:

$$\Uparrow pH \downarrow \; \propto \; \frac{\uparrow[HCO_3^-] \uparrow}{PCO_2 \uparrow}$$

The compensation thus reduces the pH, but increases the plasma $[HCO_3^-]$ further, although the effect of respiratory compensation in metabolic alkalosis is normally of very minor importance. Correction of the original disturbance is initiated by the effects of the disturbance itself on renal H^+ secretion. The decreased $[H^+]$ in the body reduces the rate of H^+ secretion, and the increased plasma $[HCO_3^-]$ increases the filtered HCO_3^- load. Thus, H^+ secretion is inadequate to re-absorb all the filtered HCO_3^- or to generate more HCO_3^-. The plasma $[HCO_3^-]$, therefore, falls, causing the reaction below

$$CO_2 + H_2O \rightleftharpoons H_2CO_3 \rightleftharpoons H^+ + HCO_3^-$$

to move to the right and restoring $[H^+]$ to normal. As in the case of metabolic acidosis, the respiratory compensation hampers the renal correction of the defect. This fact again emphasises that it is the regulation of pH that is all-important, rather than the regulation of $[HCO_3^-]$ or PCO_2 *per se*.

MICTURITION

The smooth muscle of the bladder is arranged in spiral, circular and longitudinal bundles. This arrangement forms the detrusor muscle, which is responsible for emptying of the bladder. Two sphincters oppose emptying of the bladder. The first is an incomplete ring of smooth muscle around the urethra–internal urethral sphincter. The second is a ring of skeletal muscle around the membranous urethra–external urethral sphincter.

The process of micturition is a spinal reflex that is affected by higher centres. When micturition is initiated, relaxation of the perineal muscles and external urethral sphincter occurs, followed by contraction of the detrusor muscle which leads to voiding.

The precise mechanism of voluntary micturition remains unclear. Learned ability to exert higher control over the reflex emptying of the bladder when it becomes full is the most likely mechanism.

When the bladder reaches a certain threshold volume (normally about 400 ml) stretch receptors in the bladder wall initiate a voiding reflex. The pelvic nerves constitute the afferent limb of this reflex and the parasympathetic fibres the efferent limb. The threshold for voiding is controlled by the brainstem. A facilitatory area exists in the pons and an inhibitory area in the mid-brain. Other cortical areas are also thought to be of importance.

SECTION 2: 8
RESPIRATORY PHYSIOLOGY

B. L. Appadu
C. D. Hanning

FUNCTIONAL ANATOMY

LUNG VOLUMES

VENTILATION

RESPIRATORY MECHANICS

GAS EXCHANGE

PULMONARY CIRCULATION

CONTROL OF VENTILATION

NON RESPIRATORY LUNG FUNCTIONS

LUNG FUNCTION AT HIGH ALTITUDE

FUNCTIONAL ANATOMY

The primary function of the respiratory system is the exchange of oxygen and carbon dioxide between the body and the environment. In addition, the lungs also have a metabolic role, act as a filter for small emboli in the circulation, play a part in acid base balance and contribute to the immune defences of the body. These functions are all reflected in the anatomy of the components of the respiratory system.

UPPER AIRWAY AND LARYNX

In respiration, the function of the nose, mouth and pharynx is to conduct fresh gas to the larynx, which marks the entrance to the conducting airways. These structures also warm, humidify and filter the gases.

During quiet nasal breathing this section of the airway can provide two-thirds of the total resistance to airflow of the respiratory system. Since the pharynx is a muscular tube without rigid structures to maintain its patency, it can increase the flow resistance considerably, even to the point of total obstruction, depending on the tone of its muscular wall, the associated muscles and the transmural pressure.

The larynx has three main functions:

- Regulation of expiratory airflow (expiratory braking). This is important for vocalisation, coughing and control of end expiratory lung volume
- Protection of the lower airway. Vocal cord closure prevents aspiration of foreign material or objects and expiratory braking enables the cough reflex to expel foreign material and secretions
- Vocalisation

CONDUCTING AIRWAYS

The respiratory system is traditionally divided into gas-conducting and gas-exchanging components. The conducting system begins with its smallest cross-sectional area at the level of the larynx. The conducting system begins as the trachea and undergoes irregular dichotomous branching for about 16 generations forming bronchi and bronchioles (there are seven additional generations which are respiratory airways). The 23 generations are called Weibel's classification, after E. R. Weibel, a contemporary anatomist from Bern in Switzerland.

Adult trachea

This is about 18 mm in diameter and 11 cm in length. The trachea is lined with columnar ciliated epithelium containing many mucus-secreting goblet cells. It also contains a number of receptors that are sensitive to mechanical or chemical stimuli. These mediate respiratory and cough reflexes.

Major bronchi (generations 2–4)

The major bronchi are named after the lobe or segment supplied. Circumferential cartilage rings support them. The right bronchus is wider than the left and leaves the trachea at about 25° from the tracheal axis, while the angle of the left bronchus is about 45°. Inadvertent endobronchial intubation or aspiration of foreign material is, therefore, more likely to occur in the right lung than the left. The right upper lobe bronchus branches posteriorly at about 90° to the right main bronchus. Thus, foreign bodies or fluid that are aspirated by a supine subject usually enter the right upper lobe.

Small bronchi (generations 5–11)

These are smaller versions of the major bronchi and their mucosa tends to be more cuboidal than columnar towards the periphery. As the number of bronchi increases, the total cross-sectional area increases markedly with a reduction in the velocity of gas flow and a decrease in airway resistance.

Bronchioles (generations 12–16)

Bronchioles typically have diameters < 1 mm. They are devoid of cartilage and have a high proportion of smooth muscle in their walls in relation to intraluminal diameter. There are three-to-four bronchiolar generations, the final generation being the terminal bronchioles. Goblet cells are not found in bronchioles and there is a continued gradual transition from ciliated epithelial cells to cuboidal epithelium.

RESPIRATORY AREAS OF THE LUNG

Gas exchange begins in the smaller bronchioles and extends throughout the succeeding generations of airways to the most peripheral spaces, which are the alveoli.

Respiratory bronchioles (generations 17–19)

These are characterised by intermittent alveolar outpockets. Their cuboidal epithelium is thinning and a muscle layer is still present forming 'sphincters' around openings to alveoli.

Alveolar ducts and sacs (generations 20–23)

These are formed from the alveoli that line and form

their walls. The sacs differ from the ducts in being blind ended. The alveolus is the basic unit of gas exchange, being a thin walled pocket, about 0.3 mm in diameter. There are 300 million alveoli with a total surface area of 50–100 m². Three types of cells cover the alveolar surface:

- Type I alveolar cells occupy 80% of the surface for gas exchange. They provide a very thin layer of cytoplasm, spread over a relatively wide area (50 times that of a Type II cell). Type I cells are derived from Type II cells and are highly differentiated and metabolically limited, which makes them susceptible to injury
- Type II alveolar cells have extensive metabolic and enzymatic capacity and manufacture surfactant. Both Type I and II alveolar cells have tight intracellular junctions, providing a relatively impermeable barrier to fluids
- Type III alveolar cells are alveolar macrophages and form an important part of lung defences. They contain proteolytic enzymes which may be released during lung injury, thus contributing to pulmonary damage

Alveoli have holes in their walls called pores of Kohn (8–10 μm in diameter) which permit collateral ventilation between neighbouring alveoli. Similarly larger diameter (30 μm) ducts allow collateral ventilation between respiratory bronchioles.

ALVEOLAR-CAPILLARY MEMBRANE

The alveolar-capillary membrane exists between the alveolar space and the capillary lumen, and consists of alveolar epithelium, interstitial tissue and endothelium. This membrane must perform two conflicting functions:

- Gas exchange across the blood-gas barrier
- Fluid exchange between alveolar interstitial tissue and the capillary lumen

In order for these to take place, the capillaries are located asymmetrically in the alveolar walls, which gives them a 'thick side' and a 'thin side'. The 'thick side' is used for fluid exchange with the interstitium, while the 'thin side' forms the blood gas barrier (Figure RR.1).

Blood gas barrier

This is the barrier between alveolar gas and pulmonary capillary blood, across which gas exchange takes place. It consists of three components:

- Alveolar epithelium, which is a thin layer of Type I alveolar cell cytoplasm

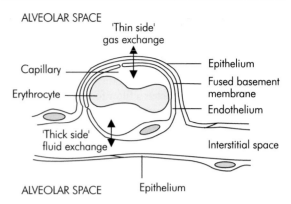

Figure RR.1 Alveolar-capillary membrane

- Interstitial tissue, consisting of fused alveolar and endothelial basement membranes
- Pulmonary capillary endothelium

Blood vessels and lymphatics

The lung is divided into lobes each supplied by its own artery, vein and bronchus. The arterioles form densely packed sheets of capillaries in the walls of the alveoli, thus matching the large ventilated surface area with an equivalent perfused area. Bronchi receive their own blood supply via bronchial arteries originating directly from the aorta.

Lymphatic drainage is important in the lung because of the magnitude of the perfused area and the effect accumulating interstitial fluid would have on gas exchange. Pulmonary lymphatics travel with blood vessels to the hila ultimately draining into the thoracic duct.

LUNG VOLUMES

The lung can be divided into various volumes. These are identified either by measurements made during lung function testing, or according to the function of the lung in gas exchange.

LUNG VOLUMES DERIVED FROM SPIROMETRY

During quiet breathing a small volume of gas is moved in and out of the lungs repeatedly. If a maximal inspiration is taken, followed by a maximal expiration, the volume changes occurring can be recorded using a spirometer. Figure RR.2 shows a typical spirometer trace of these changes.

Lung volumes vary with age, sex and body size (more related to height rather than weight). The lung volumes are:

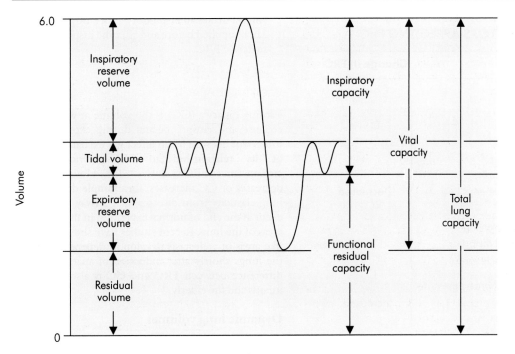

Figure RR.2 Spirometer trace of lung volumes

- Total lung capacity (TLC) – volume of gas present in the lungs at the end of maximal inspiration
- Tidal volume (VT) – amount of gas inspired and expired during normal quiet breathing
- Inspiratory reserve volume (IRV) – extra volume of gas that can be inspired over and beyond the normal VT
- Expiratory reserve volume (ERV) – amount of gas that can be forcefully expired at the end of normal tidal expiration
- Residual volume (RV) – amount of gas remaining in the lungs at the end of a maximum forced expiration
- Vital capacity (VC) – maximal volume of gas which can be expelled after a maximal inspiration
- Functional residual capacity (FRC) – lung volume following expiration during quiet breathing

Some typical values for the above volumes are given in Figure RR.3.

VITAL CAPACITY

Apart from body size, the major factors that determine VC are the strength of the respiratory muscles, and chest and lung compliance. It is an important clinical measure of respiratory sufficiency particularly in patients with restrictive diseases. VC < 10 ml/kg is indicative of impending respiratory failure.

VALUES FOR LUNG VOLUMES (ml)

Lung volume	Male	Female
TLC	6000	4200
VT	500	500
IRV	3300	1900
ERV	1000	700
RV	1200	1100

Figure RR.3

FUNCTIONAL RESIDUAL CAPACITY

From the spirometry trace in Figure RR.2 it can be seen that FRC is the lung volume at the end of normal quiet expiration, and is also equal to the sum of ERV + RV. The thoracic cage normally has a resting volume > FRC, while the normal lung has a volume < FRC. Thus, FRC represents the equilibrium point between the tendency of the lungs to collapse and of the thoracic cage to expand. It is not a fixed volume and varies with normal respiration as well as depending on gravity and other factors. FRC is decreased by 20–25% in the supine position and is further decreased by the head down posture and induction of anaesthesia. Some of the factors affecting FRC are shown in Figure RR.4.

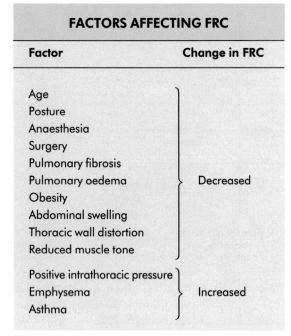

FACTORS AFFECTING FRC

Factor	Change in FRC
Age	
Posture	
Anaesthesia	
Surgery	
Pulmonary fibrosis	
Pulmonary oedema	Decreased
Obesity	
Abdominal swelling	
Thoracic wall distortion	
Reduced muscle tone	
Positive intrathoracic pressure	
Emphysema	Increased
Asthma	

Figure RR.4

Measurement of FRC

Spirometry does not give a value for TLC, FRC or RV. These can be derived if FRC is measured. Two common methods of determining FRC are:

- Helium dilution, which is used to obtain FRC using a spirometer, and an analyser to measure helium concentration. The subject is connected to the spirometer containing a known volume of fresh gas mixture (V_1) with a known initial concentration of helium (C_1). Normal breathing is allowed to take place through the spirometer until the helium becomes diluted and mixed in the larger combined volume (V_1 + FRC) of the spirometer and the respiratory system of the subject. Oxygen is fed into the spirometer to keep the spirometer reading constant, thus compensating for the difference between oxygen consumption and CO_2 production. Helium is used because it is virtually insoluble and not metabolised. FRC can be derived by measuring final helium concentration (C_2) and using the expression for the amount helium present before and after as follows:

$$\text{Amount of helium} = V_1 \times C_1 \text{ (before)}$$
$$= (V_1 + FRC) \, C_2 \text{ (after)}.$$

- Body plethysmograph – obtains FRC by placing the subject in a closed chamber and measuring the pressure and volume changes occurring when the subject makes an inspiratory effort. Boyle's Gas Law can be applied before and after the inspiratory effort to derive FRC.

CLOSING CAPACITY

Closing capacity (CC) is the volume at which airway collapse and closure occurs during expiration. It is important because it can affect gas exchange by virtue of its relationship to FRC. Under normal circumstances FRC is always > CC. However, if FRC decreases or CC increases, for example due to loss of lung elasticity from disease, then airway closure may occur at the end of normal expiration in the dependent areas of the lung. Recent studies have shown that plate like areas of atelectasis develop in dependent areas of the lungs shortly after induction of anaesthesia. The difference between FRC and CC is also reduced in infants and the elderly.

Dynamic lung volumes

Lung function can also be measured by its dynamic performance during active inflation or deflation. A common test is the recording of expired volumes during forced expiration of a maximal breath. The forced vital capacity (FVC) is the total volume of gas that can be forcibly expired after maximal inspiration. During forced expiration, dynamic compression of the intrathoracic airways occurs, limiting both the rate of expiration and the total amount of gas that can be expelled. The limiting effect may be seen from the expiratory curve of a VC breath, which is linear rather than exponentially declining and is described by the mid-expiratory flow rate which applies to the gas volume expired between 25 and 75% of the total ($MEFR_{25-75}$). In clinical practice the volume expired in the first second (FEV_1) is often measured as part of an FVC measurement. The ratio (FEV_1/FVC) can then be derived, which is a useful index of obstructive airways disease. Normally this ratio would be > 95% but it declines with age and 85% may be acceptable in an elderly subject (Figure RR.5).

VENTILATION

Ventilation describes the process of fresh gas reaching the areas of the lung where gas exchange takes place. Gas exchange is dependent on the volume of gas moved in and out of the lungs per min. This is referred to as total ventilation (minute ventilation). It is usually measured as the volume of gas expired per min and can determined for respiratory rate = n breaths/min and tidal volume = V_T:

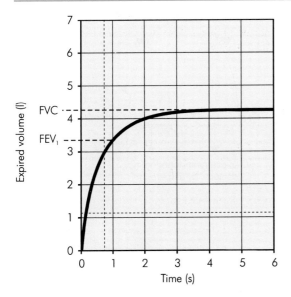

Figure RR.5 Vitalograph trace

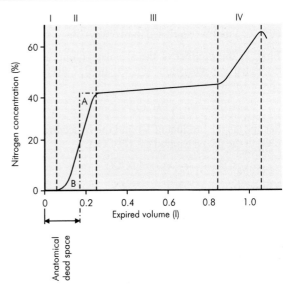

Figure RR.6 Fowler's method of dead space measurement

Total ventilation = (respiratory rate) × (tidal volume)
= n × V_T.

Not all the gas moving in and out of the lungs takes part in gas exchange. Since there are two main parts of the lung: **dead space**, which does not take part in gas exchange, and **alveolar space**, in which gas exchange does take place.

DEAD SPACE

Dead space can be subdivided into anatomical dead space, which corresponds to the conducting airways, and alveolar dead space. Alveolar dead space consists of those parts of the lung which are ventilated but not perfused. The sum of the anatomical and alveolar dead space is the physiological dead space.

Anatomical dead space

This is about 2 ml/kg (150 ml in an adult). Early measurements of the volume were obtained by taking casts of the conducting airways but it may be measured non invasively by Fowler's method.

In Fowler's method the patient takes a single VC breath of 100% oxygen and exhales through a rapid nitrogen analyser. Expired N_2 concentration is then plotted against expired volume (Figure RR.6). The initial gas from the dead space (Phase I) is free of nitrogen being pure oxygen, thereafter the nitrogen concentration increases with the introduction of alveolar gas (Phase II) until an 'alveolar' plateau is achieved (Phase III).

The dead space is found by dividing Phase II by a vertical line such that area A = area B and measuring the volume from zero.

Anatomical dead space will vary with changes in bronchial muscle tone and also with changes in position of the head and neck or the placing of an endotracheal tube. A functional decrease in anatomical dead space occurs at low V_T when gas flow in the airways is laminar.

ALVEOLAR VOLUME

Only fresh gas reaching the alveoli takes part in gas exchange. In each breath, only a portion of each V_T, will reach the alveoli due to anatomical dead space (V_D). This portion is the alveolar volume (V_A),

e.g. for V_T = 500 ml and V_D = 150 ml
$V_A = V_T - V_D$
= 350 ml

ALVEOLAR VENTILATION

Alveolar ventilation is the volume of gas per min reaching the alveolar spaces. It can be calculated from the respiratory rate (n) and alveolar volume (V_A),

e.g. for V_A = 350 ml and n = 15 breaths/min
alveolar ventilation = n × V_A
= 15 × 350
= 5250 ml/min

Physiological dead space

Under normal circumstances, physiological dead space differs very little from the anatomical and may be estimated with Bohr's equation.

The total volume of CO_2 expired in one breath ($VTCO_2$) may be expressed in two ways.

First, as the product of the alveolar volume and the fractional concentration of CO_2 in the alveolar gas ($FACO_2$):

$$VTCO_2 = VA \times FACO_2$$

Second, as the product of VT and the concentration of CO_2 in the mixed expired gas ($F\bar{E}CO_2$):

$$VTCO_2 = VT \times F\bar{E}CO_2$$

Thus

$$VA \times FACO_2 = VT \times F\bar{E}CO_2$$

Substituting, as

$$VA = VT - VD$$

gives

$$(VT - VD) \times FACO_2 = VT \times F\bar{E}CO_2$$

Rearrange to give:

$$\frac{VD}{VT} = \frac{FACO_2 - F\bar{E}CO_2}{FACO_2}$$

As the barometric pressure is the same for expired gas and alveolar gas, the partial pressures in the alveoli ($PACO_2$) and mixed expired gas ($P\bar{E}CO_2$) may be substituted instead, yielding:

$$\frac{VD}{VT} = \frac{PACO_2 - P\bar{E}CO_2}{PACO_2}$$

In practice, $P\bar{E}CO_2$ can be measured from a collection of mixed expired gas in a large bag, and $PACO_2$ may be taken as being equal to the $PaCO_2$.

Physiological dead space is dependent on both anatomical and alveolar dead space. Anatomical dead space varies as noted above. Alveolar dead space will be increased whenever areas of the lung become better ventilated than perfused.

RESPIRATORY MECHANICS

The movement of gas in and out of the lungs is a mechanical process, which is dependent on the following factors:

- The respiratory muscles and their actions
- The compliance of the chest wall and the lungs
- The gas flow in the airways

THE RESPIRATORY MUSCLES AND THEIR ACTIONS

Respiration can be divided into inspiration and

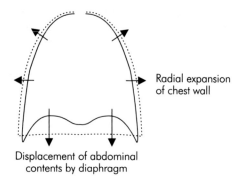

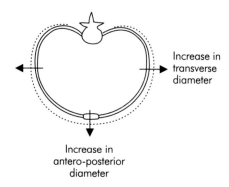

Figure RR.7. Movement of the chest wall during inspiration

expiration. Inspiration is normally active while expiration is passive.

Inspiration

During inspiration the lungs can be expanded with two degrees of freedom (Figure RR.7):

- Displacement of the abdominal contents by contraction of the diaphragm
- Radial expansion of the thoracic cage by the accessory respiratory muscles

DIAPHRAGM

This is the principal muscle of breathing, accounting for about 75% of the air that enters the lungs during spontaneous inspiration. Contraction of the diaphragm moves abdominal contents downward and forward during each inspiration. Two-thirds of the diaphragmatic fibres are slow twitch, making it relatively resistant to fatigue.

ACCESSORY RESPIRATORY MUSCLES

These comprise the external intercostal and strap muscles (sternocleidomastoid, anterior serrati, scalenes). During quiet breathing their contribution to inspiration is small. They act mainly to stabilise the upper rib cage and preventing indrawing. As respiration deepens, the contribution of these muscles increases by elevating the rib cage and expanding it in the lateral and antero-posterior directions.

Expiration

In contrast with inspiration, the diaphragm relaxes during exhalation and the elastic recoil of the lungs, chest wall and abdominal structures compresses the lungs. Forced expiration for a cough or when airway resistance is increased requires the abdominal muscles and the internal intercostals. Paralysis of abdominal muscles produced by regional anaesthesia does not usually influence alveolar ventilation.

COMPLIANCE OF THE CHEST WALL AND LUNGS

Mechanically the respiratory system consists of two main components, the lungs and thoracic cage (including the diaphragmatic surface), which expand and contract together. Thus, the lungs and chest wall move together as a unit. The lung expands in response to a pressure gradient produced across its surface, called the transpulmonary pressure. The transpulmonary pressure is equal to the difference between the airway pressure in the lungs and the pressure on the lung surface i.e. in between the lung and chest wall. This pressure is the intrapleural pressure.

Intrapleural pressure

The resting position of the lungs and chest wall occurs at FRC. If isolated, the lungs being elastic, would collapse to a volume < FRC. However, the isolated thoracic cage would normally have a volume > FRC. Since the chest wall is coupled to the lung surface by the thin layer of intrapleural fluid between parietal and visceral pleura, opposing lung and chest wall recoil forces are in equilibrium at FRC. This produces a pressure of about -0.3 kPa in the pleural space. Normal inspiration reduces intrapleural pressure further to -1.0 kPa, but with forced inspiration it can reach negative pressures of -4.0 kPa or more. Intrapleural pressure may be measured by an intrapleural catheter or from a balloon catheter placed in the mid-oesophagus.

Transpulmonary pressure

Normally during spontaneous respiration, airway pressures in the lung can be approximated to atmospheric pressure. The pressure on the lung surface is the intrapleural pressure, which may reach -1.0 kPa during inspiration. This is equivalent to a distending transpulmonary pressure of +1.0 kPa.

Lung compliance

The lungs expand in response to the transpulmonary pressures produced by the respiratory muscles. The amount of expansion for a given transpulmonary pressure represents the ease with which the lungs expand. This property is measured by the lung compliance, which is defined by:

$$\text{Lung compliance} = \frac{\text{Change in volume}}{\text{Change in transpulmonary pressure}}$$

A value for compliance can be obtained from the pressure–volume curve for a normal isolated lung undergoing inflation as shown in Figure RR.8. It can be seen that the curve is approximately linear over the 'working range' of the lung centred around FRC. At FRC, lung compliance is about 200 ml/cmH$_2$O. However, compliance is reduced at high lung volumes because the elastic fibres are fully stretched close to their elastic limit. While at low lung volumes compliance is reduced because airway and alveolar collapse occurs requiring greater pressures to open up the airways and alveoli. Lung compliance may also be reduced by other factors, see later.

Chest wall compliance

If a pressure–volume curve is plotted for the isolated thoracic cage (Figure RR.8) the chest wall compliance can be obtained from the gradient, and is also about 200 ml/cmH$_2$O at FRC. The chest wall compliance can be reduced by disease as in ankylosing spondylitis in which the chest wall can become virtually rigid giving an extremely low compliance value.

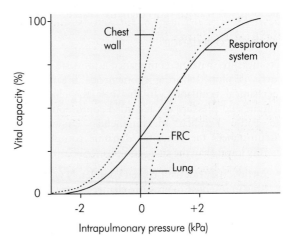

Figure RR.8. Lung and chest wall compliance

TOTAL RESPIRATORY SYSTEM COMPLIANCE

In the respiratory system the lungs and chest wall move together during inspiration and expiration. The respiratory system compliance is, therefore, the combination of chest wall and lung compliances, e.g. if lung compliance (C_L) = 200 ml/cmH$_2$O, and chest wall compliance (C_W) = 200 ml/cmH$_2$O, then respiratory system compliance (C_R) is given by:

$$\frac{1}{C_R} = \frac{1}{C_L} + \frac{1}{C_W}$$

$$\frac{1}{C_R} = \frac{1}{200} + \frac{1}{200} = \frac{1}{100}$$

$$\text{So } C_R = 100 \text{ ml/cmH}_2\text{O}$$

The effect of combining lung and chest wall compliances to give the overall respiratory system pressure–volume curve is shown in Figure RR.8. Here it can be seen how the respiratory system compliance at FRC (gradient of the curve) is less than the individual gradients for lung or chest wall.

Measurement of respiratory system compliance

Compliance can be obtained from the gradient of a pressure–volume curve plotted for the respiratory system. However, this leads to two different values depending on the measurement technique.

STATIC COMPLIANCE

To obtain static compliance a pressure–volume curve is plotted by applying known distending pressures to the respiratory system, and measuring the corresponding changes in volume produced. Appropriate time must be allowed between measurements, for equilibration of the lung, when all gas movement has ceased.

DYNAMIC COMPLIANCE

To measure dynamic compliance a pressure–volume curve is plotted during spontaneous breathing or mechanical ventilation. In this case the changes in volume and pressure are recorded continuously with no pause between measurements. Under these circumstances the value for dynamic compliance is usually lower than the static compliance because:

- Airflow may not have ceased completely within the lung in response to pressure changes, particularly in diseased lungs. Further volume increases can follow gas movement from less distensible areas of the lung to more distensible areas ('pendelluft')
- Relaxation of tissues occurs with applied pressures

that are sustained. This is due to the so called 'visco-elastic' nature of tissues. This property of tissues, which mimics the action of hydraulic dampers in mechanical systems, means that when stretching forces are applied to real tissues they do not respond instantaneously, but stretch gradually in a viscous manner

- The intrapulmonary pressure will be less than the applied airway pressure due to airway resistance and inertia of the respiratory system. This causes an underestimation of the compliance

The resultant effect of making dynamic measurements is that airway pressures in the dynamic case will be greater than those in the static case at any given lung volume. This means that the value for dynamic compliance will always be less than the static compliance.

Factors decreasing respiratory system compliance

Respiratory system compliance is usually maximum or optimal at FRC, and is decreased by both physiological factors and disease. Disease may affect both lung compliance (C_L) and chest wall compliance (C_W). Some examples of these factors are shown in Figure RR.9.

FACTORS DECREASING RESPIRATORY SYSTEM COMPLIANCE (C_R)	
Factor	**Change in C_R**
FRC	
Normal	Maximum
High	Decreased
Low	Decreased
Posture	
Standing	Maximum
Supine posture	Decreased
Age	
Infant	Decreased
Elderly	Decreased
Pregnancy	Decreased
Disease	
ARDS	Decreased ($\downarrow C_L$)
Pulmonary oedema	Decreased ($\downarrow C_L$)
Ankylosing spondylitis	Decreased ($\downarrow C_L$ and $\downarrow C_W$)

Figure RR.9

Pressure–volume loop for the respiratory system

If a pressure–volume curve for the respiratory system is plotted through a cycle of inspiration and expiration a 'loop' is obtained, as the inspiratory and expiratory limbs of the curve do not exactly coincide (Figure RR.10). This 'loop' effect is known as hysteresis, the area of the loop representing the energy expended or 'wasted' as heat in moving through the inspiratory-expiratory cycle. This wasted energy is a result of viscous losses during the stretching and recoil of the tissues, and also the frictional losses due to airway resistance. A factor that reduces this wasted energy and hence improving the efficiency of the breathing cycle is the lining of surfactant in the alveoli.

SURFACTANT

Surfactant is a phospholipid based substance secreted by the alveolar type II cells, which lines the alveoli and acts by markedly reducing surface tension. This action has the following effects:

- Reduction of surface tension, which helps to even out the distribution of compliance and hence ventilation, since if without surfactant, alveoli with low resting volumes are significantly more difficult to expand, than those with larger resting volumes. This effect is important in neonates, in whom deficiency of surfactant is associated with infant respiratory distress syndrome
- Stabilisation of small alveoli. In a bubble wall, surface tension acts to shrink or collapse the bubble. A similar effect is seen in an alveolus. The smaller the alveolus the greater the tendency to collapse. Because of this, small alveoli tend to collapse by forcing their gas into larger communicating alveoli. The reduction of surface tension by surfactant decreases this effect
- Reduction of the energy expended as heat during each inspiratory-expiratory cycle, i.e. the hysteresis area of the pressure–volume loop is decreased
- Surfactant also keeps the alveoli dry by reducing the 'suction' effect created by surface tension as it tries to collapse alveoli. Surface tension creates negative interstitial pressures as it tries to shrink alveoli, thus drawing fluid from capillaries into the air spaces

DISTRIBUTION OF VENTILATION

When inspiration occurs, the fresh gas entering the lung is not distributed evenly but the majority of the fresh gas passes to the most dependent regions of the lung.

The mechanism underlying this uneven distribution of ventilation lies in the variation of intrapleural pressure from top to base of the lung. Gravitational effects cause the lung in the thoracic cage to behave as a fluid volume, producing a hydrostatic pressure gradient due to the blood perfusing the lung. Thus, in the upright position intrapleural pressure at the base of the lung is greater than at the apex. In the upright adult there is a difference in intrapleural pressure of about 0.7 kPa between the apex and the base of the lung. This variation of intrapleural pressure means that the alveoli also vary in degree of distension, and hence position on the pressure–volume curve of the lung (Figure RR.11). The more dependent alveoli are less distended, and situated on the linear part of the pressure–volume curve, compared with the apical alveoli which are over distended and situated on the top part of the

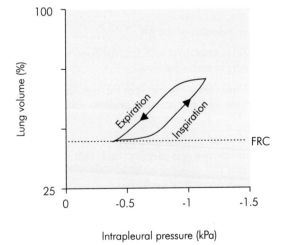

Figure RR.10 Inspiration–expiration loop showing hysteresis

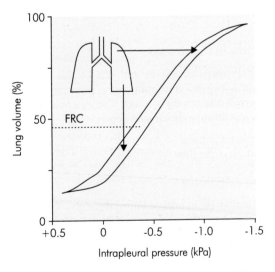

Figure RR.11 Compliance during spontaneous ventilation

pressure–volume curve. Thus, at the base of the lung the alveolar compliance (gradient of curve) is greater than at the apex. Consequently during inspiration, greater expansion of alveoli in the lower areas of the lung occurs, and ventilation is preferentially directed to the base. This preferential distribution of ventilation matches the relatively high pulmonary blood flow to the dependent parts of the lung, since perfusion is gravitationally determined. In addition, there is lower airway resistance to the dependent areas of the lung that enhances gas flow to these regions.

This distribution of ventilation during spontaneous breathing contrasts with the situation during artificial ventilation, when a reduced FRC tends to reverse the distribution of alveolar compliances, and gives preferential ventilation of non dependent areas (Figure RR.12).

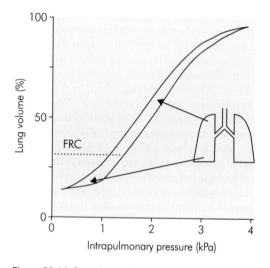

Figure RR.12 Compliance during mechanical ventilation

Gas flow in the airways

The movement of gas in and out of the lungs is produced by the transpulmonary pressure and is conducted through the airways. The ease with which gas moves through the airways depends on:

- Airway resistance
- Pattern of gas flow

AIRWAY RESISTANCE

The gas flow (F, in ml/s or l/min) through an airway is determined by the pressure difference between the ends of the airway (ΔP), and the resistance of the airway to gas flow (R). This is loosely analogous to the flow of electrical current through a conductor with electrical resistance. The case of laminar gas flow in an airway

can be approximated to fluid (i.e. gas or liquid) flow in a tube, in which:

$$F = \frac{\Delta P}{R}$$

This is modified in the Hagen-Poiseuille Law, which substitutes factors for the resistance R. These factors include radius, viscosity and length. R is inversely proportional to (radius)^4, but dependent on the viscosity of the gas and the length of the tube.

PATTERN OF GAS FLOW

Gas can flow through an airway can occur in a smooth fashion behaving as if in circumferential layers sliding across each other in the direction of flow. This is laminar flow, which occurs with a 'cone' shaped gas velocity profile across the airway cross-section, the velocity being faster in the centre than at the periphery.

Alternatively gas flow can be disorderly with random eddies and whirls occurring across the overall direction of flow. This is turbulent flow, which moves with a relatively flat velocity profile in the direction of flow. Both laminar and turbulent flow exist within the respiratory tract, usually in mixed patterns.

TURBULENT FLOW

In a given airway with a known gas and flow velocity, the likelihood of turbulent flow can be predicted from an index known as Reynold's number (Re), which is calculated from:

$$Re = \frac{2\,r\,v\,\rho}{\eta}$$

where:
  r = airway radius
  v = average velocity of gas flow
  ρ = gas density
  η = viscosity of the gas

Re < 1000 is associated with laminar flow, while Re > 2000 results in turbulent flow.

The pressure–flow relationship for turbulent flow is different because the pressure gradient producing the flow is:

- Proportional to (flow velocity)^2
- Dependent on gas density and independent of viscosity
- Inversely dependent on (radius)^5

The resultant effect of turbulence is to increase the effective resistance of an airway compared with laminar flow. Turbulent flow occurs at the laryngeal opening, the trachea and the large bronchi (generations 1–5) during most of the respiratory cycle. It is usually audible and almost invariably present when high resistance to gas flow is encountered.

LOCATION OF AIRWAY RESISTANCE

The principal sites of resistance to gas flow in the respiratory system, are the nose and the major bronchi rather than the small airways. Since the cross-sectional area of the airway increases exponentially as branching occurs, the velocity of the airflow decreases markedly with progression through the airway generations, and laminar flow becomes predominant below the fifth generation of airway.

FACTORS AFFECTING AIRWAY RESISTANCE

The factors affecting airway resistance are:

- Lung volume – the main factor affecting airway resistance. Increasing lung volume decreases airway resistance, thus patients with high airway resistance often increase their FRC by position or pursed-lip breathing
- Bronchial smooth muscle tone – airway smooth muscle is primarily under parasympathetic (vagal) control. Reflex constriction occurs with stimulation of the larynx, trachea or bronchi. Sympathetic influence is mediated mainly by β receptors in the airway smooth muscle
- Histamine release – H_1 receptors cause bronchoconstriction, while H_2 receptors cause bronchodilation. However, the predominant effect of histamine is bronchoconstriction
- Properties of inspired gas – flow resistance dependent on the density and viscosity of the inspired gas. Use of a helium-oxygen mixture improves ventilation in some cases of severe bronchospasm
- Lower airway obstruction, which may be due to mucosal oedema, mucous plugging, epithelial de-squamation, and foreign bodies
- Upper airway obstruction secondary to decreased conscious level, drugs, position of head, neck, or jaw, tonsils or adenoids
- Anaesthesia – airway resistance doubles during anaesthesia due mainly to a reduction in FRC but also to increased upper airway resistance in some patients. Inappropriate selection of breathing systems may also contribute to increased total airway resistance. It is often forgotten that the upper airway contributes significantly to total airway resistance

Measurement of airway resistance

Airway resistance can be measured during spontaneous breathing by simultaneous recording of air flow, and the pressure gradient between mouth and alveoli. In practice the alveolar pressure is difficult to obtain since it must be derived using a body plethysmograph. Intrapleural pressure can be used instead, but will include the pressure gradient required to overcome lung tissue resistance and inertial properties. Thus, this technique measures the resistance to air flow, the viscous resistance due to the lung tissue and the inertia of the lung. Under normal circumstances, these factors are negligible, but tissue viscous resistance may become more significant in pulmonary oedema and fibrosis. Inertia of the lung may be of importance during high frequency ventilation.

In clinical practice airway resistance can be assessed using, forced expiratory flow rates such as FEV_1, peak expiratory flow rate (PEFR), and mid expiratory flow rate. These indices are more easily measured, but they rely upon expiratory muscle activity in addition to airway resistance, and are affected by patient technique.

WORK OF BREATHING

Work is normally expended in inspiration, expiration being passive. The work of inspiration can be subdivided into:

- Work required to overcome the elastic forces of the lung (compliance), which is stored as elastic energy
- Work required to overcome airway resistance during the movement of air into the lung
- Work required to overcome the viscosity of the lung and chest wall tissues (tissue resistive work)

During quiet breathing, most of the work performed is elastic. This inflates the lungs but provides a store of elastic energy to be returned during expiration, and is, therefore, useful work done.

The effect of overcoming tissue resistance and airway resistance is dissipated as heat and can be viewed as wasted energy. Figure RR.13 shows an idealised loop inspiration occurring along the path AGB and expiration along BEA. The following points illustrate the relationship between the wasted work done and the useful work done.

- In an ideal elastic lung with no tissue or airway losses, the work stored in inspiration would be completely returned in expiration. Inspiration and expiration would then occur along the straight line AFB, with equal amounts of inspiratory work done and expiratory work, represented by the area AFBCD
- In the real lung with tissue and airway losses, inspiration occurs along curve AGB. The inspiratory work done (AGBCD) is thus greater

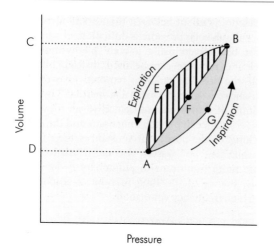

Figure RR.13 Work of breathing loop

In lung diseases all three types of work are increased. Compliance work and tissue resistive work are greatly increased during restrictive diseases such as fibrosis of the lungs whereas airway resistance work is increased in pulmonary obstructive diseases.

Expiration does not normally entail active work, but may be necessary in forced breathing or when airway resistance or tissue resistance are increased. In some circumstances, expiratory work may be greater than inspiratory work, for example in asthma.

GAS EXCHANGE

The oxygen tension in air (at sea level) is about 20 kPa, falling to 0.5 kPa in the mitochondria where it is utilised. The transport of oxygen down this concentration gradient is described as the oxygen cascade (Figure RR.14). It involves different transport mechanisms, convection, diffusion through gas and liquid media and transport bound to Hb. The same process occurs in the reverse direction for CO_2.

The fractional concentration of oxygen in dry ambient air ($F_{AMB}O_2$) is 0.21 and at sea level with a barometric pressure (P_B) of 101.3 kPa the partial pressure of oxygen ($P_{AMB}O_2$) is given by:

$$P_{AMB}O_2 = 0.21 \times 101.3$$
$$= 21.3 \text{ kPa}$$

than the ideal case (by the shaded area AGBF). This wasted work is only a fraction of the inspiratory work
- In the real lung, expiration occurs along BEA. The expiratory work returned (BEADC) is thus less than the ideal case by (hatched area BEAF)
- The total 'wasted' energy due to tissue and airway losses is thus the sum of the shaded and hatched areas, or the area of the loop

Factors influencing oxygen cascade

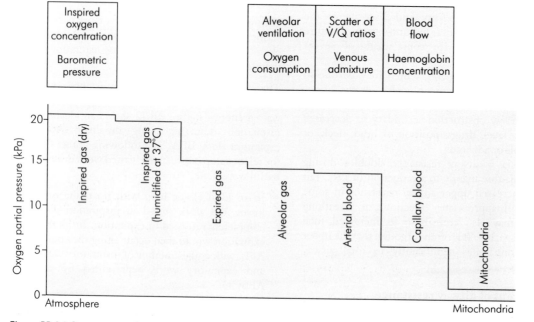

Figure RR.14 Oxygen cascade

The addition of saturated water vapour (PSVP) by the upper airway mucosa, reduces the tension of inspired gas (PIO$_2$) by a small amount:

$$PIO_2 = (PB - PSVP) \times FAMBO_2$$
$$= (101.3 - 6.3) \times (0.21) = 20 \text{ kPa}$$

ALVEOLAR OXYGEN TENSION

The alveolar oxygen tension (PAO$_2$) is less than the inspired oxygen tension (PIO$_2$) because some oxygen is absorbed in exchange for CO$_2$ excreted. Thus, the PAO$_2$ is determined by:

- The rate at which oxygen is introduced in to the alveoli (dependent on alveolar ventilation and inspired oxygen concentration)
- The rate of removal by absorption into pulmonary capillary blood (oxygen consumption, $\dot{V}O_2$)
- The rate of delivery of CO$_2$ ($\dot{V}CO_2$) by pulmonary capillary blood

The decrease in oxygen tension caused by oxygen absorption, is estimated by using the tension of CO$_2$ excreted (about PACO$_2$), which must be corrected by the respiratory quotient (because less CO$_2$ is excreted than O$_2$ absorbed).

The alveolar gas equation thus becomes:

$$PAO_2 = PIO_2 - \frac{PACO_2}{RQ}$$

where RQ is the respiratory quotient, and

$$RQ = \frac{\dot{V}CO_2}{\dot{V}O_2}$$

which in a normal subject on a mixed diet is about 0.8. For PIO$_2$ = 20 kPa and PACO$_2$ = 5 kPa,

$$PAO_2 = 20 - (5 \div 0.8)$$
$$= 13.8 \text{ kPa}.$$

To summarise:

PAO$_2$ is intermediate between the inspired oxygen tension (PIO$_2$) and the arterial oxygen tension (PaO$_2$), due to oxygen being absorbed in exchange for CO$_2$. Its value is given by the alveolar gas equation, which is based on:

PAO$_2$ = (inspired oxygen tension) – (tension decrease due to oxygen absorbed).

The importance of PAO$_2$ in practice is that it determines the partial pressure gradient driving oxygen across the alveolar-capillary membrane. It is not easily measured directly, but an awareness of its value in clinical practice is useful in patient management. The following points should be noted:

- PAO$_2$ is most easily increased by increasing inspired oxygen fraction (FIO$_2$)
- PAO$_2$ will fall with hypoventilation, but it only falls rapidly below alveolar ventilation levels of about 4 l/min assuming normal oxygen consumption (about 250 ml/min). Figure RR.15a illustrates how varying alveolar ventilation rate affects PAO$_2$
- Hypermetabolic states (sepsis, malignant hyperthermia) will significantly increase the susceptibility to hypoxaemia by increasing oxygen consumption ($\dot{V}O_2$), and by increasing the rate of CO$_2$ delivery into the alveoli. Thus, both FIO$_2$ and alveolar ventilation may need to be increased in such patients
- PAO$_2$ can be decreased iatrogenically by sodium bicarbonate infusion since this increases body CO$_2$ levels, and hence CO$_2$ delivery to the alveoli
- PAO$_2$ can be used to calculate the alveolar-arterial PO$_2$ difference which is a useful index of gas exchange efficiency in the lungs

ALVEOLAR CO$_2$ TENSION

PACO$_2$ is determined by the balance between:

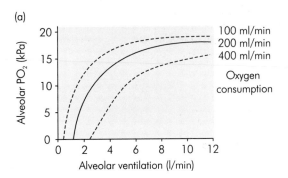

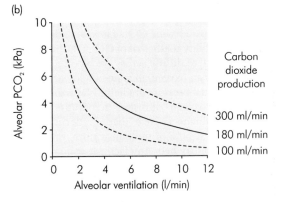

Figure RR.15. Variation of alveolar gas tensions with alveolar ventilation

- Rate of delivery of CO_2 ($\dot{V}CO_2$) into the alveoli by pulmonary capillary blood
- Rate of removal by alveolar ventilation

Alveolar CO_2 tension ($PACO_2$) can be varied by controlling alveolar ventilation. This effect is most noticeable at rates of alveolar ventilation < about 6 l/min, given normal rates of CO_2 production (about 200 ml/min). Hyperventilation above this level produces a more gradual reduction in $PACO_2$. Figure RR.15b illustrates the variation of $PACO_2$ (which correlates well with $PaCO_2$ in the normal subject) with alveolar ventilation.

GAS DIFFUSION FROM ALVEOLI TO BLOOD

Gases diffuse between alveoli and pulmonary capillary blood across the blood gas barrier, which is effectively a membrane with a total surface area about 70 m². Over this membrane about 60–140 ml blood is spread as a thin sheet. The rate of gas transfer across this membrane will depend on:

- Properties of the gas (solubility and molecular weight)
- Properties of the membrane (surface area, A, and thickness, D)
- Partial pressure gradient (ΔP) across the membrane

Then according to Fick's Law:

$$\text{Rate of gas transfer} \propto \frac{k \times A \times \Delta P}{D}$$

Where:

$$\text{Diffusion constant, k} \propto \frac{\text{solubility}}{\sqrt{\text{molecular weight}}}$$

The lower molecular weight of oxygen, and its greater alveolar to capillary partial pressure gradient favour its diffusion compared with CO_2. However, the higher blood/gas solubility coefficient of CO_2 (24 times that of O_2) causes CO_2 to diffuse across the blood gas barrier more readily than oxygen, in spite of a lower capillary to alveolar partial pressure gradient. Nevertheless, the efficiency of oxygen diffusion across the alveolar capillary membrane is such that a red cell is fully oxygenated in < 50% of the transit time through the pulmonary capillary bed. Any factor that increases the thickness of the membrane such as pulmonary oedema interferes with the diffusion of oxygen more than that of CO_2.

OXYGEN TRANSPORT IN THE BLOOD

Most of the oxygen (97%) in the blood is transported in combination with Hb. Once the Hb is saturated, oxygen content can only be marginally increased by dissolved oxygen. Dissolved oxygen is a linear function of PaO_2 and is 0.023 ml/kPa/100 ml plasma. Thus, for a PaO_2 = 13 kPa, only 0.3 ml oxygen (3%) is carried in a dissolved state. Even breathing pure oxygen, where it is possible to increase PaO_2 to about 80 kPa, the dissolved arterial oxygen content would be only about 2.0 ml/100 ml blood.

Haemoglobin

Oxygen is transported and delivered to the tissues by haemoglobin (Hb). Hb is a conjugated protein with a molecular weight of 66 700 Daltons, and is composed of four haem subunits. Each subunit has a central ferrous (Fe^{2+}) atom and is conjugated to a polypeptide chain. The four polypeptide chains collectively form the globin moiety. Different forms of Hb exist, identified by their polypeptide chains. Normal adult Hb consists of HbA_1 (98%) containing 2α and 2β polypeptide chains, and HbA_2 (2%) containing 2α and 2δ chains.

Foetal erythrocytes contain HbF with 2α and 2γ chains. HbF is also modified by having a lower affinity for binding 2,3-diphosphoglycerate (2,3-DPG) than adult forms of Hb. 2,3-DPG is a highly anionic intermediate of glycolysis. It binds to the de-oxygenated form of Hb significantly reducing the affinity of Hb for oxygen. This facilitates the 'unloading' of oxygen in tissues with low oxygen tensions. HbF thus has an increased affinity for oxygen, which adapts its transport and delivery characteristics to the lower oxygen tensions in the placento-foetal circulation. After birth the production of β chains starts and HbA replaces HbF during the first year of life.

Oxygenation of haemoglobin

Each molecule of Hb can bind four molecules of oxygen. This is not a chemical reaction as in oxidation, but is a readily reversible bond. The following are characteristics of Hb oxygen binding:

- It is determined primarily by local oxygen tension (PaO_2)
- It is affected by local tissue conditions (e.g. pH, temperature) and local concentrations of substances (e.g. 2,3-DPG, CO_2)
- It produces an allosteric change in the structure of Hb to a 'Relaxed' form, while deoxygenated Hb has a 'Tense' form. This switching between R and T forms underlies the oxygenation and delivery mechanisms
- It is 'cooperative' meaning that binding O_2 at each site promotes binding at the remaining sites due to allosteric changes. This increases the amount of O_2

delivered under physiological conditions, compared with a carrier having independent binding sites
- De-oxygenation of Hb increases the affinity of several proton-binding sites on its molecule. This enhances its ability to transport CO_2 from the tissues to the lungs (Haldane effect) and underlies the role of Hb as a major buffer in acid base regulation

Oxyhaemoglobin dissociation curve

The percentage of Hb saturation with oxygen (SO_2) at different partial pressures of oxygen in blood is described by the oxyhaemoglobin dissociation curve (ODC). This is a sigmoid curve whose shape is determined by the cooperativity of the oxygen binding process (Figure RR.16). The position of the curve is best described by the P_{50}, which is the PO_2 at which Hb is 50% saturated (normally 3.56 kPa). Various factors can 'shift' the ODC to the left or right, altering the characteristics of oxygen uptake and delivery.

'LEFT SHIFT' OF THE ODC

This represents an increase in the affinity of Hb for oxygen in the pulmonary capillaries but requires lower tissue capillary PO_2 to achieve adequate oxygen delivery. P_{50} is reduced by factors causing a left shift, which include:

- Alkalosis
- Decreased PCO_2
- Decreased concentration of 2,3-DPG
- Decreased temperature
- Presence of HbF rather than adult forms of Hb

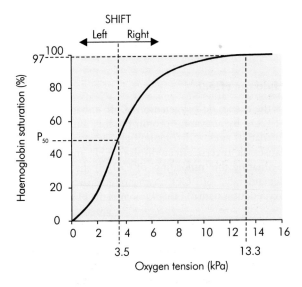

SHIFT

Figure RR.16 Oxyhaemoglobin dissociation curve

'RIGHT SHIFT' OF THE ODC

This represents an increase in the affinity of Hb for oxygen. In this situation P_{50} is increased requiring higher pulmonary capillary saturations to saturate the Hb, but enhancing delivery at the tissues. Factors causing a right shift of the ODC include:

- Acidosis
- Increased PCO_2
- Increased concentration of 2,3-DPG
- Increased temperature

Bohr effect

The shift in position of the ODC caused by CO_2 entering or leaving blood is known as the Bohr effect. It enhances the 'unloading' of oxygen in the tissues, where PCO_2 levels are high compared with the pulmonary capillaries. In the tissues CO_2 enters the red cells, combining with water and dissociating into H^+ and HCO_3^-. The increased $[H^+]$ shifts the ODC to the right facilitating the release of oxygen from Hb. The HCO_3^- diffuses out of the cells and is matched by an inward movement of chloride. The reverse change occurs in the lungs enhancing the uptake of oxygen.

Oxygen content of blood

The theoretical maximum oxygen carrying capacity is 1.39 ml O_2/g Hb but direct measurement gives a capacity of 1.34 ml O_2/gHb.

The oxygen content of blood is the volume of oxygen carried in each 100 ml blood. It is calculated by:

$$(O_2 \text{ carried by Hb}) + (O_2 \text{ in solution})$$
$$= (SO_2 \times 1.34 \times Hb \times 0.01) + (0.023 \times PO_2)$$

where:

SO_2 = percentage saturation of Hb with oxygen
Hb = Hb concentration in grams per 100 ml blood
PO_2 = partial pressure of oxygen.

For a normal male adult the oxygen content of arterial blood can be calculated.

Given arterial oxygen saturation (SaO_2) = 100%, Hb = 15 g/100 ml, and arterial partial pressure of oxygen (PaO_2) = 13.3 kPa, then oxygen content of arterial blood (CaO_2):

$$CaO_2 = 20.1 + 0.3 = 20.4 \text{ ml}/100 \text{ ml}$$

Similarly the oxygen content of mixed venous blood can be calculated. Given normal values of mixed venous oxygen saturation ($S\bar{v}O_2$) = 75%, and venous partial pressure of oxygen ($P\bar{v}O_2$) = 6 kPa, so:

$$C\bar{v}O_2 = 15.1 + 0.1 = 15.2 \text{ ml}/100 \text{ ml}$$

Oxygen delivery ($\dot{D}O_2$) and oxygen uptake ($\dot{V}O_2$)

Oxygen delivery is the amount of oxygen delivered to the peripheral tissues, and is obtained by multiplying the arterial oxygen content (CaO_2) by the cardiac output ($\dot{Q}$). For $CaO_2 = 20.1$ ml/100 ml and $\dot{Q} = 5.0$ l/min,

$$\text{oxygen delivery } (\dot{D}O_2) = 1005 \text{ ml/min.}$$

Oxygen uptake is the amount of oxygen taken up by the tissues that can be calculated from the difference between oxygen delivery and the oxygen returned to the lungs in the mixed venous blood. The oxygen return is given by the product of mixed venous oxygen content ($C\bar{v}O_2$) and cardiac output. For $C\bar{v}O_2 = 15.2$ ml/100 ml and $\dot{Q} = 5.0$ l/min:

$$\text{oxygen return} = 760 \text{ ml/min.}$$

Thus

$$\begin{aligned}\text{oxygen uptake } (\dot{V}O_2) &= (\text{oxygen delivery}) - \\ &\quad (\text{oxygen return}) \\ &= 1005 - 760 = 245 \\ &\quad \text{ml/min.}\end{aligned}$$

To summarise:

The primary goal of the cardiorespiratory system is to deliver adequate oxygen to the tissues to meet their metabolic requirements, a balance between $\dot{V}O_2$ and $\dot{D}O_2$.

The balance between oxygen uptake by the body tissues, and oxygen delivery to them, is assessed by:

- The oxygen content of mixed venous blood $C\bar{v}O_2$, which is normally about 15 ml/100 ml
- The oxygen extraction ratio, which is the ratio of $\dot{V}O_2$ to $\dot{D}O_2$ expressed as a percentage. Normally the extraction ratio is about 25% but can double to 50% if tissue demand increases

Both of the above indices are dependent on mixed venous saturation ($S\bar{v}O_2$), and cardiac output.

Increased tissue demand due to exercise or disease, is normally compensated for by increased oxygen delivery. This has to be mediated by increasing cardiac output, since the ability to increase SaO_2 and Hb is limited. However, under extreme conditions (severe exercise, sepsis, malignant hyperthermia) tissue demand can increase 12-fold (requiring a $\dot{V}O_2$ of up to 3000 ml O_2/min). Cardiac output can usually be increased by a maximum of up to seven times, and thus under extreme conditions, tissue demand can outstrip the body's capacity to increase delivery. In such a case $S\bar{v}O_2$ falls, extraction ratios increase and tissue hypoxia ensues. This susceptibility towards tissue hypoxia will be greatly increased in conditions where cardiac output is limited or compromised.

CARBON DIOXIDE TRANSPORT

CO_2 diffuses passively down its concentration gradient from the mitochondria to the capillaries. Although partial pressure gradients are low between tissues and blood, transfer is rapid due to the high solubility of CO_2. Partial pressures of CO_2 (PCO_2) in the tissues equilibrate with capillary blood to produce a veno-arterial PCO_2 difference of about 0.7 kPa. This corresponds to a CO_2 content difference of about 4 ml/100 ml blood, depending upon RQ.

The 4 ml CO_2 that is added to each 100 ml arterial blood as it passes through the tissues consists of (Figure RR.17):

- 2.8 ml (70%) that enters erythrocytes to form carbonic acid (H_2CO_3). This reaction is catalysed by carbonic anhydrase, which, if inhibited, produces a marked increase in the alveolar/capillary PCO_2 gradient. The H_2CO_3 formed dissociates to give H^+ and HCO_3^-. As noted above, de-oxygenation of Hb activates H^+ acceptor sites increasing its buffering capacity. This encourages the dissociation of H_2CO_3 and as a result enhances the 'loading' of CO_2 in the tissues. The HCO_3^- formed diffuses out of the erythrocytes in exchange for chloride (Cl^-), which enters the red cells to maintain electroneutrality (the 'chloride shift'). The increase in osmotically active ions HCO_3^- and Cl^- in venous red blood cell leads to an increase in their size. This is probably the reason for the venous haematocrit being about 3% greater than that of arterial blood
- 0.9 ml (22%) carried as carbamino compounds, which are formed by reactions of CO_2 with terminal and side chain amino groups of proteins. Haemoglobin provides most of the amino groups, reduced Hb having at least 3 times more active sites than oxyhaemoglobin
- 0.3 ml (8%) carried in solution

Haldane effect

In the tissues de-oxygenation of Hb enhances carriage of CO_2, by activating proton binding and carbamino formation sites. Correspondingly, oxygenation of Hb causes the reverse effect, displacing H^+ and CO_2, thus facilitating the 'unloading' of CO_2 in the lungs. This dependency of CO_2 carrying capacity on the oxygenation state of Hb is known as the Haldane effect.

Body stores of oxygen and CO_2

The oxygen stores of the body are relatively small in comparison to the consumption (around 250 ml/min for an adult). Total body oxygen is about 1.5 litres, which is held as:

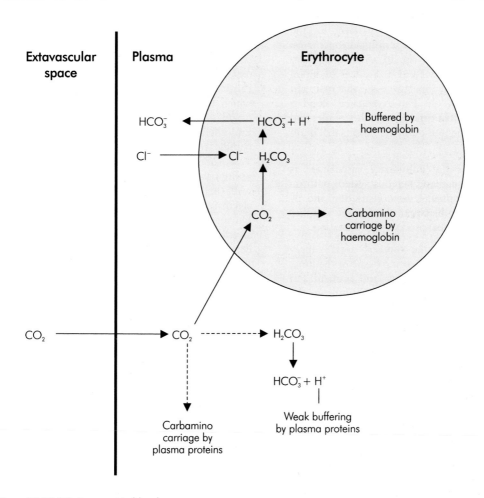

Figure RR.17 CO_2 transport in blood

- 50% in combination with Hb
- 30% in the lungs
- 20% in combination with myoglobin

Not all stored oxygen is available for use since severe hypoxaemia occurs before even half of the oxygen stored in combination with Hb and myoglobin is released. These available stores will last only for 3–4 min of apnoea, assuming air breathing and normal oxygen consumption. Breathing 100% O_2 increases the oxygen stores to about 4.25 litres, mainly by increasing the O_2 contained in the lungs.

In contrast, total body stores of CO_2 are about 120 litres. During apnoea, $PaCO_2$ increases by about 1 kPa in the first min. This initial rise in $PaCO_2$ then decreases to a rate of 0.4 kPa/min, as alveolar PCO_2 levels build up and CO_2 elimination by diffusion through the airways increases.

PULMONARY CIRCULATION

The pulmonary circulation is a low pressure, low resistance system in series with the right ventricle. The cardiac output from the right ventricle passes through the lungs into the left atrium. The cardiac output from the right ventricle is almost the same as that from the left ventricle.

Blood passes through pulmonary capillaries in about 0.5–1.0 s, depending on the cardiac output, during which time it is oxygenated and excess CO_2 is removed. The distribution of blood flow and ventilation throughout the lungs are generally very well matched, but this may vary markedly during anaesthesia or disease.

The pulmonary artery is a thin walled structure which arises from the right ventricle and divides immediately into left and right branches and then divides successively following a similar pattern to the conducting airways down to the terminal bronchioles. These small branches give rise to a dense capillary network which may be viewed as a sheet of blood broken up by 'pillars' of connective tissue that maintain the stability of the alveoli. The oxygenated blood is collected by venules that run between the lobules and then unite to form the four pulmonary veins that drain into the left atrium.

The innervation of the pulmonary vasculature is supplied by the sympathetic nervous system with α-adrenergic fibres producing vasoconstriction and β-adrenergic fibres vasodilatation. The vagus supplies parasympathetic fibres that produce vasodilatation.

Bronchial arteries from the thoracic aorta supply oxygenated blood to the supporting tissue of the lung, including connective tissue, septa, and bronchi and drains into the pulmonary veins contributing to the anatomical shunt. An average of 1–2% of the total cardiac output passes through the bronchial arteries, thus making the left ventricular output slightly greater than the right.

Pressures in the pulmonary circulation are about 20% of those in the systemic circulation. Normal pulmonary arterial pressure has a systolic value 25 mmHg, a diastolic value of 8 mmHg, and a mean of 15 mmHg. The mean pulmonary capillary pressure is 10 mmHg with a pulmonary venous pressure of 4 mmHg at heart level. Pulmonary arterial and right ventricular pressures are not greatly influenced by increases in cardiac output in normal subjects demonstrating the distensibility of the pulmonary vasculature.

PULMONARY VASCULAR RESISTANCE

Pulmonary vascular resistance (PVR) is influenced by the following factors:

- Autonomic innervation – vasomotor tone is minimal in the normal resting state and pulmonary vessels are maximally dilated. The autonomic system exerts a relatively weak influence on PVR, increases in sympathetic tone giving rise to vasoconstriction
- Nitric oxide (NO), which is an important mediator of pulmonary vascular tone causing vasodilatation (it is also active in systemic vessels). Nitric oxide has been identified as endothelium-derived relaxing factor, which also mediates other processes by the relaxation of smooth muscle. It is derived from L-

arginine and increases intracellular concentrations of cGMP. Its actions as a potent vasodilator have led to its use in severe acute lung disease where inhaled concentrations of 5–80 ppm can improve oxygenation
- Prostacyclin (prostaglandin I_2), is an arachidonate, which is a potent vasodilator also of endothelial origin
- Endothelins, these are potent vasoconstrictor peptides released by the pulmonary endothelial cells
- Vascular transmural pressure – important in the pulmonary circulation because the thinner vessel walls make them more prone to collapse when alveolar pressure exceeds intravascular pressure. During positive pressure ventilation, high positive alveolar pressures can cause increased PVR and decrease perfusion in some areas of the lung
- Lung volume, which also determines the calibre of the vessels embedded in the lung parenchyma. PVR is least at FRC. As the lung increases in volume, the vessels become narrowed and elongated and, as it decreases in volume, the vessels become tortuous
- Lung disease – both acute and chronic lung disease can result in significant increases in PVR. Long-term increases in PVR due to chronic disease can lead to right sided heart failure
- Hypoxic vasoconstriction – a powerful physiological reflex which diverts perfusion away from hypoxic areas of the lung

HYPOXIC PULMONARY VASOCONSTRICTION

Hypoxic pulmonary vasoconstriction (HPV) is an important mechanism, designed to improve the match between perfusion and ventilation by diverting blood from poorly ventilated areas to better ventilated areas. HPV maintains this balance of ventilation to perfusion on a breath-to-breath basis. The predominant site of HPV lies in the small pulmonary arteries (30–50 μm) with the remaining resistance arising from the capillary bed and venous system.

HPV may also affect the pulmonary vessels in general rather than on a regional basis. Low PaO_2 levels are responsible for generalised HPV in the foetus, reducing blood flow through the pulmonary vascular bed to about 10–15% of the foetal cardiac output. This generalised response also causes a significant increase in PVR at high altitude.

The exact mechanism of HPV is unknown. It is potentiated by acidosis and modified by various drugs (Figure RR.18).

DRUGS MODIFYING THE HPV REFLEX

Drugs	Effect on HPV
Volatile anaesthetic agents Nitrates Nitroprusside Calcium channel blockers Bronchodilators	Attenuate HPV
Cyclo-oxygenase inhibitors Propanolol Almitrine	Potentiate HPV

Figure RR.18

CAUSES OF PULMONARY HYPERTENSION

Mechanism	Clinical condition
Intracardiac shunt	Atrial septal defect Ventricular septal defect
↑ Left ventricular end- diastolic pressure	Mitral stenosis Constrictive pericarditis
Obliteration	Pulmonary fibrosis
Obstruction	Pulmonary embolism
Vasoconstriction	Sleep apnoea syndrome High altitude
Idiopathic	Primary pulmonary Hypertension

Figure RR.19

Pulmonary hypertension

Increased pulmonary arterial pressures can be caused by various pathological mechanisms. These are listed in Figure RR.19 together with examples of associated clinical conditions.

Distribution of perfusion

As outlined above, the pulmonary vascular resistance (PVR) is influenced by various factors. Although PVR determines the overall blood flow through the lungs, this blood flow is not evenly distributed throughout each lung, but is preferentially directed to the bases by gravity.

This effect is mediated by the pressure difference across the walls (transmural pressure) of the pulmonary blood vessels (arteries, capillaries and post capillary veins). When the extravascular pressure is greater than the hydrostatic pressure in the vessel, the vessel collapses obstructing flow. If the transmural pressure is reversed (intravascular greater than extravascular pressure) the vessel remains patent.

In the lung, gravity gives rise to an intravascular hydrostatic pressure gradient that increases from the top of the lung to the base. Thus, the arterial (Pa) and venous (Pv), pressures in the base are greater than those in the apex by about 23 mmHg. In contrast, extravascular pressure is effectively equal to alveolar pressure (PA), which is approximately atmospheric pressure and is the same throughout the lung.

Functional zones of the lung

The relative magnitudes of the above pressures, PA, Pa and Pv, define different functional zones in the lung (Figure RR.20):

ZONE 1

In zone 1 alveolar pressure (PA) is greater than the arteriolar pressure (Pa) and venular pressure. Both

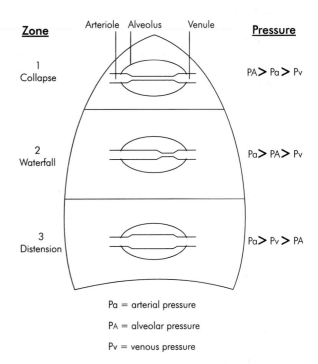

Pa = arterial pressure

PA = alveolar pressure

Pv = venous pressure

Figure RR.20 Functional zones of the lung

arterioles and venules will collapse obstructing blood flow completely. In this case:

$$PA > Pa > Pv$$

Arterial pressures (Pa) are minimal in the lung apex, and are just adequate to provide perfusion to these areas. In practice, Pa in the apical areas, although low, is not normally less than alveolar pressure (PA) and zone 1 does not exist. Usually this can only occur under conditions of reduced pulmonary arterial pressure (e.g. hypovolaemia, decreased cardiac output), or increased alveolar pressure (e.g. positive pressure ventilation of the lungs, positive end-expiratory pressure). In such a case, perfusion to this part of the lung is zero and alveolar dead space increases significantly.

ZONE 2

In zone 2 alveolar pressure is greater than the venous pressure but less than the arterial pressure. The veins collapse but the arteries remain patent, and blood flow will be partially obstructed. In this case:

$$Pa > PA > Pv$$

Below the apical regions of the lung, alveolar pressure is less than arterial pressure, but greater than the venous pressure. In these areas the post capillary veins are collapsed, offering high resistance to flow. The collapsed vessels can open up during systole or if pulmonary arterial pressure increases. This model of a collapsible tube with variable flow resistance due to downstream occlusion by external pressure, is sometimes referred to as the Starling resistor or 'waterfall' effect.

ZONE 3

Alveolar pressure is less than venous pressure in zone 3, and both arteries and veins will remain patent and blood flow will be unobstructed. In this case:

$$Pa > Pv > PA$$

In the more dependent regions of the lung arteries, capillaries and veins are patent and pulmonary blood flow is continuous. This zone extends from about 7 to 10 cm above the heart to the lowermost portions of the lung. There is some increase in perfusion moving down the zone, as pulmonary arterial pressure increases due to the gravitational pressure gradient. This increase in blood flow is achieved by:

- Recruitment of closed pulmonary vessels
- The perfusion of open but not perfused vessels
- Dilation of vessels already perfused

These mechanisms enable zone 3 blood flow to increase in response to increases in pulmonary arterial pressure. Their overall result is a decrease in pulmonary vascular resistance.

Delineation of the functional zones is variable and affected by different conditions, which alter the relationship between Pa, Pv and PA. In the supine position, nearly all portions of the lung become zone 3, with pulmonary blood flow being more evenly distributed. During exercise pulmonary artery pressures increase and recruit previously under perfused capillaries, thus converting most of the lung to a zone 3 pattern of pulmonary blood flow.

A zone 4 is sometimes described for regions in the most dependent parts of the lung where intravascular pressures are highest but blood flow is reduced.

Ventilation:perfusion ratio

Efficient gas exchange in the lung requires the gas flow in and out of each functional unit to be matched by the blood flow through it i.e. ventilation ($\dot{V}$) must match perfusion ($\dot{Q}$). At rest the overall ratio of total alveolar ventilation (about 5250 ml/min) to total pulmonary blood flow (about 5000 ml/min) is about 1. Thus, it is normally assumed that the optimum ventilation:perfusion ($\dot{V}/\dot{Q}$) ratio for any unit of lung tissue is also 1.

When a unit of lung tissue is inadequately ventilated ($\dot{V}/\dot{Q} < 1$), some of the pulmonary capillary blood perfusing it, effectively bypasses the lungs, since there is too much perfusion for the blood gases to equilibrate adequately with alveolar gas. This increases the 'shunt' effect in the lungs (see below).

When a lung unit is under perfused ($\dot{V}/\dot{Q} > 1$), the expired gas from the unit contains a lower than normal concentration of CO_2, since excess fresh gas is supplied which does not exchange gases with pulmonary capillary blood. This increases the 'alveolar dead space' effect in the lungs.

To summarise:

Ventilation:perfusion ($\dot{V}/\dot{Q}$) ratio for any area of lung tissue is an index that reflects the efficiency of gas exchange in that region. It has an optimum value of 1.

In an area of lung tissue:

- If $\dot{V}/\dot{Q} < 1$, it increases the 'physiological shunt'
- If $\dot{V}/\dot{Q} > 1$, it increases the 'alveolar dead space'

Distribution of $\dot{V}/\dot{Q}$ ratios in the lung

In the normal lung, although ventilation and perfusion are both distributed to favour the dependent areas, the $\dot{V}/\dot{Q}$ ratios are not uniform and vary from the lung apices to the bases. At the top of the lung $\dot{V}/\dot{Q}$ ratios have been estimated to be about 3.3, and this value decreases passing down the lung to the bottom where the $\dot{V}/\dot{Q}$ ratios are about 0.6. $\dot{V}/\dot{Q}$ ratios vary in three dimensions, so that a distribution of values will be found across a horisontal section of the lung as well as from apex to base.

In diseased lungs $\dot{V}/\dot{Q}$ ratios vary over a wider range as there is greater non homogeneity of the lung tissue. The effects on gas exchange of increased $\dot{V}/\dot{Q}$ mismatch is reflected by a deterioration in the following indices from their normal values, so there is:

- An increase in shunt fraction
- An increase in the alveolar-arterial PO_2 difference ($P_AO_2 - PaO_2$)
- An increase in alveolar dead space
- A decrease in PaO_2 or increase in $PaCO_2$

Alveolar-arterial PO_2 difference

In the normal lung there is a small alveolar-arterial partial pressure gradient for oxygen ($P_AO_2 - PaO_2$) of 0.5 – 1.0 kPa. This difference is the sum of the PO_2 gradient across the alveolar-capillary membrane and the effect of admixture of shunted blood. Any increase in the thickness of the diffusion barrier (e.g. pulmonary oedema or fibrosis) or the shunt effect due to $\dot{V}/\dot{Q}$ mismatch in the lungs will, therefore, produce an increase in this value.

PHYSIOLOGICAL SHUNT (VENOUS ADMIXTURE, SHUNT FRACTION)

Arterial blood may be less well oxygenated than blood leaving the alveoli for several reasons, for example:

- Venous blood may bypass the lungs entirely (e.g. intracardiac shunts, thebesian veins, bronchial circulation)
- Blood may pass through parts of the lung which are not ventilated adequately, in which case $\dot{V}/\dot{Q} < 1$ (e.g. pneumonia)

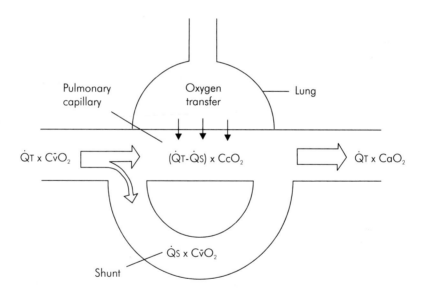

CaO_2 = arterial oxygen content

$C\bar{v}O_2$ = mixed venous content

CcO_2 = pulmonary capillary oxygen content

$\dot{Q}T$ = cardiac output

$\dot{Q}s$ = shunt flow

$(\dot{Q}T-\dot{Q}s)$ = pulmonary capillary blood flow

Figure RR.21 Diagram of shunt in the lung

alkalosis. The second more gradual increase occurs due to, renal elimination of bicarbonate, bicarbonate shift out of the cerebrospinal fluid compartment and de-sensitisation of the chemoreceptors.

ACCLIMATISATION

Acclimatisation describes the adaptive physiological changes that occur when a person moves from sea level to high altitude. There are physiological differences between peoples who live their whole lives at high altitude and those who live at sea level, which are referred to as 'adaptation'. The main changes occurring in acclimatisation are:

- Hyperventilation, an immediate and sustained response
- Polycythaemia – Hb levels reach 20 g/100 ml or more increasing the oxygen content of blood to > 22 ml O_2/100 ml
- Right shift of the oxyhaemoglobin dissociation curve which is due to increased levels of 2,3-DPG
- Increased capillary density – in peripheral tissues, particularly muscle
- Increased mitochondrial density – and increased concentration of respiratory chain enzymes
- Increased pulmonary arterial pressures, due to hypoxic vasoconstriction
- Increased ventilatory capacity that is aided by the decreased density of air. Maximum ventilation rates of 200 l/min or more may occur

- More even distribution of perfusion

VENTILATION–PERFUSION MATCHING AT ALTITUDE

The distribution of perfusion is more even throughout the lung due to higher pulmonary arterial pressures and lower alveolar pressures. This has the effect of reducing the transmural pressure of the capillaries and post capillary venules in perfusion zones 1 and 2. As described above perfusion in these zones is dependent on the Starling resistor effect of these vessels, which is reduced by the changes at high altitude.

HIGH ALTITUDE DISEASE

Additional physiological changes to those described in acclimatisation may develop. These include:

- Right ventricular hypertrophy
- Muscle atrophy and catabolism
- Anti-diuresis and oedema formation
- Increased thyroid activity
- Sleep disturbance and periodic breathing
- Impaired central nervous system performance

These changes may develop into acute and chronic mountain sickness, pulmonary oedema and cerebral oedema.

SECTION 2: 9

PHYSIOLOGY OF THE NERVOUS SYSTEM

A. K. Gupta
A. M. Sardesai

STRUCTURE AND FUNCTION OF NEURONES

IONIC BASIS OF MEMBRANE POTENTIAL

SYNAPTIC TRANSMISSION

FUNCTION ORGANISATION OF THE CNS

REFLEX ARC

MOTOR FUNCTION

CONTROL OF POSTURE

CEREBROSPINAL FLUID

INTRACRANIAL PRESSURE

SPECIAL SENSES

AUTONOMIC NERVOUS SYSTEM

THE LIMBIC SYSTEM

NOCICEPTION AND PAIN

STRUCTURE AND FUNCTION OF NEURONES

The main excitable cell in the nervous system is the neurone. Non-excitable cells or glial cells support neurones and perform various other functions (see Figure NE.1). Neurones specialise in processing and transmitting information. The human nervous system contains between 1011 and 1012 neurones. Functionally, neurones are classified as sensory, motor and interneurone. A typical neurone is structurally made up of three parts: a cell body, an axon and terminal buttons (Figure NE.2). The cell body consists of intracellular organelles by which the cell maintains its functional and structural integrity. The axon originates from the cell body and divides into terminal branches; each branch terminates in enlarged endings called terminal buttons. The axon is a long projection surrounded by supporting cells (oligodendrocytes or Schwann cells). When there is a layer of lipid–protein complex deposited within the Schwann cell membrane, the neurone is said to be myelinated, otherwise it is unmyelinated. Myelination allows saltatory conduction with an accompanying increase in speed of propagation of a nerve impulse. Mammalian neurones have varying fibre diameters and speeds of conduction which are summarised in Figure NE.3.

FUNCTIONS OF DIFFERENT CELLS IN THE NERVOUS SYSTEM

Cell	Function
Neurones	Generation, transmission and processing of potentials
Astrocytes	Support neurones and contribute to blood brain barrier
Oligodendrocytes	Insulate neurones in CNS
Ependymal	Line ventricles and spinal canal
Schwann	Insulate axons in PNS

Figure NE.1

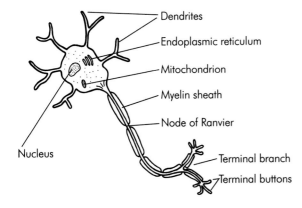

Figure NE.2 A typical neurone

TYPES OF NEURONE AND THEIR CHARACTERISTICS

Fibre Type	Function	Fibre Diameter (μ)	Conduction Speed (m/s)
Aα	Proprioception somatic motor	12–20	70–120
Aβ	Touch, pressure	5–12	30–70
Aγ	Muscle spindle motor	3–6	15–30
Aδ	Pain, temperature, touch	2–5	12–30
B	Pre-ganglionic ANS	3	3–15
C dorsal root	Pain, temperature mechanoreceptors, reflex responses	0.4–1.2	0.5–2
C sympathetic	Post-ganglionic	0.3–1.3	0.7–2.2

Figure NE.3 Classification of mammalian neurones

THE IONIC BASIS OF MEMBRANE POTENTIAL

MEMBRANE POTENTIAL AT REST

Like other excitable tissues in the body, the electrical potential of a neurone in the resting state is more negative on the inside of the cell compared with the outside. This polarity is maintained by the active transport of Na$^+$ ions out of the cell, together with the active transport of K$^+$ ions into the cell. However, there is a tendency for both ions to diffuse passively down their concentration gradient through leaky ion channels. During its resting state, the membrane is more permeable to K$^+$ than to Na$^+$ ion, thus more K$^+$ ions leak out of the neurone than Na$^+$ ions enter the cell. At the same time, the resting membrane is not permeable to anions. The result is that the interior of the neurone is more electronegative (-70 mV) than the outside – this is the resting membrane potential.

CHARACTERISTICS OF THE ACTION POTENTIAL

Neurones respond to a stimulus by transiently producing changes in ion permeability or conductance in the cell membrane. Ion conductance is defined as the reciprocal of electrical resistance of the membrane to a given ion and, therefore, reflects permeability. When the stimulus is below the threshold potential, the changes produced remain localised. However, when the stimulus reaches the threshold, the membrane becomes depolarised. When this depolarisation is propagated along the axon, it gives rise to an action potential. The latter can be divided into a number of Phases (Figure NE.4).

At the beginning of an action potential, the rate of de-polarisation increases so that the inside of the cell becomes increasingly positive until it rises to a peak, then falls when repolarisation begins. This sharp rise and decline is called the spike potential. The sharp rise is due to an increase in Na^+ conductance, so that Na^+ ions diffuse down their electrical and concentration gradients. However, there are three factors which limit the depolarisation process: first, the Na^+ channels open only very transiently; second, as the inside of the cell becomes increasingly more electropositive, the initial gradients which facilitate Na^+ influx disappear; and finally K^+ conductance also increases. The rate of repolarisation slows down when the process is about 70% complete; this phase is known as after-depolarisation.

During the final recovery phase, there is a slight but prolonged overshoot after the resting potential is reached. This is due to the slow return of K^+ conductance to normal (Figure NE.5). This phase is called the after-hyperpolarisation,

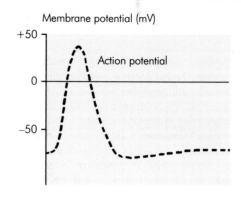

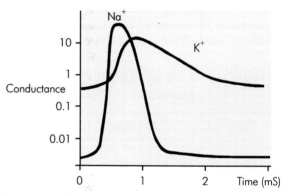

Figure NE.5 Changes in Na^+ and K^+ conductance during the course of an action potential

A neurone is said to be in the absolute refractory period when it is totally unresponsive to any stimulus regardless of its strength. This corresponds to the period between the threshold being reached and when repolarisation is one third completed. The relative refractory period starts at this point until the beginning of after-depolarisation. During this period, a stronger than normal stimulus may lead to excitation.

SYNAPTIC TRANSMISSION

Nerve impulses are transmitted from one neurone to another through junctions known as synapses. Synapses are formed between the terminal buttons of a neurone and the cell body or axon of another neurone. The number of terminal buttons forming synapses with a neurone varies from one to several thousand. Synapses almost invariably allow unidirectional impulse conduction, i.e. from pre-synaptic to the postsynaptic neurone. This ensures nerve impulses are transmitted in an orderly fashion. Most synaptic

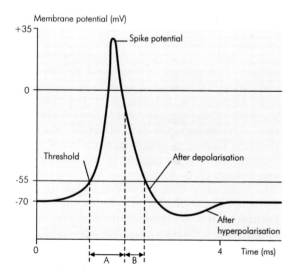

A= absolute refractory period
B= relative refractory period

Figure NE.4 Different phases of an action potential

transmissions are chemical in nature, others are either electrical or mixed. In electrical synapses, the membranes between the pre-synaptic and postsynaptic neurones meet to form gap junctions, which contain channels that facilitate diffusion of ions.

STRUCTURE OF A SYNAPSE

Chemical synapses consist of a small gap known as synaptic cleft. The synaptic cleft measures about 20 nm wide and contains extra cellular fluid across which the neurotransmitters diffuse. There are three essential structures that can be found in the cytoplasm of the terminal button: synaptic vesicles, mitochondria and endoplasmic reticulum (see Figure NE.6). The synaptic vesicles, containing the neurotransmitters, are usually found in large concentrations in the release zone adjacent to the synaptic cleft. The endoplasmic reticulum is responsible for the production of new, and recycling the used vesicles. Mitochondria provide the energy required for chemical transmission and the formation of synaptic vesicles by the endoplasmic reticulum.

SYNAPTIC MECHANISM

When an action potential is transmitted down an axon, the depolarisation opens the voltage-gated calcium channels, allowing an influx of Ca^{2+} ions into the terminal button. In the release zone the Ca^{2+} ions bind with groups of protein molecules in synaptic vesicle membranes. These protein molecules spread apart,

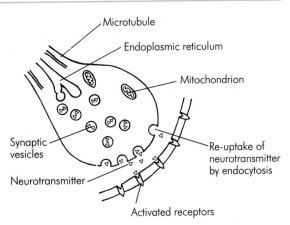

Figure NE.6 Structure of a chemical synapse

allowing fusion between vesicle and terminal button membranes. This releases neurotransmitter into the synaptic cleft. The amount of neurotransmitter released is directly proportional to the Ca^{2+} influx. The postsynaptic receptors are activated by the binding of neurotransmitters which lead to the opening of ion channels, resulting in postsynaptic potentials. Postsynaptic potentials are transient in action because of two mechanisms: first and predominantly, by transmitter re-uptake and, second, by enzymatic de-activation. The terminal buttons at the end of the transmission rapidly and actively takes up neurotransmitters. Figure NE.7 summarises the different types of neurotransmitter found in the CNS.

DIFFERENT TYPES OF NEUROTRANSMITTER, LOCATION AND FUNCTION

Neurotransmitter	Location	Function
Acetylcholine	Cerebral cortex, thalamus, limbic system	Likely to be involved in memory, perception, cognition, attention and arousal functions
Norepinephrine	Locus ceruleus Cerebellum Hypothalamus	Descending pain pathway Inhibits Purkinje cells Regulates secretion of anterior pituitary hormones
Epinephrine	Medulla	Functions uncertain
Dopamine	Substantia nigra Hypothalamus	Control of motor functions Regulates prolactin secretion
Serotonin	Neocortex and limbic system	Alters mood and behaviour
	Hypothalamus Nucleus raphe magnus and spinal cord	Increases prolactin secretion Pain modulation

Figure NE.7

The events following the generation of postsynaptic potentials depend mainly on two conditions: first, the amount of neurotransmitter released and, second, the type of ion channel that is being opened. Not all postsynaptic potential changes are propagated as action potentials in the postsynaptic neurone. When an insufficient amount of neurotransmitter becomes bound to the post synaptic receptor, the change in membrane potential may not reach the firing threshold of the neurone, thus only giving rise to local potential changes. When sodium channels are open, there is a sudden influx of Na^+ ions down its concentration and electrical gradients producing an excitatory postsynaptic potential (EPSP). However, when K^+ or Cl^- channels are open, K^+ and Cl^- ions move down their concentration gradients making the inside of the neurone more electronegative with respect to the outside of the neurone, i.e. hyperpolarised, resulting in an inhibitory post synaptic potential (IPSP) (Figure NE.8). When the postsynaptic potential reaches threshold an action potential occurs.

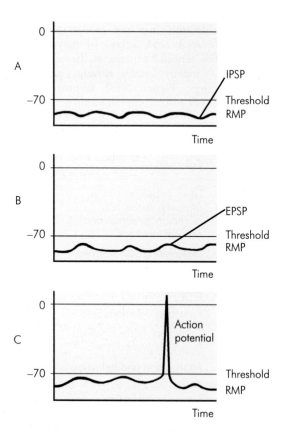

Figure NE.8 Synaptic transmission

SENSORY RECEPTORS

Sensory receptors are specialised structures that receive and transmit information from the external and internal environment to the CNS. A sensory receptor may be part of a neurone such as nerve endings or a separate structure that is capable of generating and transmitting action potentials to a neurone. They are essentially transducers that respond to different forms of energy, such as mechanical or thermal energy, and convert them into electrical signals. Special sense organs such as the eye are a collection of sensory receptors supported by highly organised structural and connective tissue.

Sensory receptors may be classified according to whether they perceive visceral or somatic sensory changes. Visceral receptors are primarily concerned with perceiving changes in the internal environment; such information does not usually reach consciousness. These include chemoreceptors which are sensitive to changes in glucose level, oxygen tension, osmolality and acidity in the plasma. Stretch receptors in the lungs and pressure receptors in the carotid sinus are other examples of visceral receptors.

Somatic receptors are sensory receptors that respond to external stimuli such as temperature, light touch and pressure. Pain is initiated by noxious or potentially damaging stimuli; pain receptors are, therefore, also known as nociceptors. Information from the somatic receptors usually reaches consciousness and is represented at the cerebral level, giving rise to a variety of sensations. Sensory pathways are multi-synaptic and thus involve a first-order neurone (for example a dorsal root ganglion) which then synapses with a central chain of second order and third order neurones as outlined in Figure NE.9.

FUNCTIONAL ORGANISATION OF THE NERVOUS SYSTEM

The nervous system is divided into two main parts; the central nervous system, consisting of the brain (cerebral cortex, the basal ganglia, cerebellum, brain stem) and the spinal cord, and the peripheral nervous system, which includes the cranial and spinal nerves and their ganglia. The autonomic nervous system also forms an important part of the nervous system and can be subdivided into the sympathetic and parasympathetic nervous system.

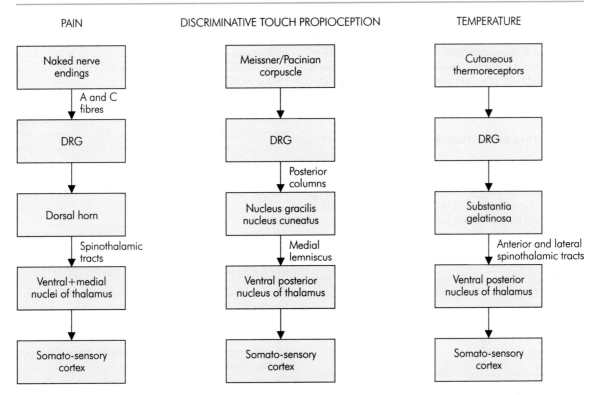

Figure NE.9 Somatic sensory perceptions and their afferent pathways to the CNS

CORTEX

The cerebral cortex is topographically the highest level of the central nervous system and always functions in association with the lower centres. The surface of the cerebral cortex is thrown into convolutions called gyri, which are separated by the sulci.

The cortex is divided into various lobes namely frontal, temporal, occipital and parietal which have different functions.

The frontal lobe lies in front of the central sulcus and is divided into the precentral area and prefrontal cortex. The precentral area is further divided into anterior and posterior regions. The posterior region is referred to as the primary motor area or Brodmann's area 4 and the anterior region is known as the premotor area. The supplemental motor area is also situated in the frontal lobe. The rest of the frontal lobe or the prefrontal cortex is divided into superior, middle and inferior frontal gyri. Broca's speech area is situated in the inferior frontal gyrus of the dominant hemisphere. The prefrontal cortex is concerned with personality, initiative and judgement. The frontal cortex controls motor function of the opposite side of the body, insight and control of emotions. Broca's area in the categorical

(dominant) hemisphere is also involved in output of speech.

The temporal lobe contains primary and secondary auditory areas. The ability to locate the source of sound is impaired with the destruction of the primary auditory area. Bilateral destruction leads to complete deafness. The secondary auditory area is necessary for the interpretation of sounds. Wernicke's area, which is the sensory speech area, is located in the categorical (dominant) hemisphere and is associated with comprehension of speech.

The parietal lobe houses the primary sensory area in the postcentral gyrus. The majority of sensations reach the cortex from the contralateral side of the body, although some signals from the oral region go to the same side, and those from the pharynx, larynx, and perineum go to both sides. A secondary sensory area is situated in the wall of the Sylvian fissure. Loss of the primary sensory cortex leads to inability to judge shape or form (astereognosis), degree of pressure or weight of an object. Problems occur with position sense and in localising different sensations occurring in different parts of the body. The secondary sensory area is involved in receiving information and relating it to past experience so that the information can be interpreted.

The occipital lobe contains the primary visual area (area 17) close to the occipital pole. The macula lutea of the retina is represented on the cortex in the posterior part of area 17 and accounts for a third of the visual cortex with the remaining cortex accounting for the rest of the retina. Lesions of the occipital pole produce central scotomas.

Higher functions of cerebral cortex

CONSCIOUSNESS

There are different levels of consciousness ranging from alertness to coma. The level of consciousness is determined by activities of both the cerebral cortex and the reticular-activating system (RAS). The latter is a diffuse network of neurones situated in the brainstem reticular formation. It receives sensory information from ascending sensory tracts as well as auditory, visual, olfactory and trigeminal tracts. The reticular formation projects to the cerebral cortex directly and indirectly via the thalamic nuclei. RAS activity is closely related to the electrical activity of the cerebral cortex.

Electrical activity of the cerebral cortex can be recorded by scalp electrodes as an Electro-encephalogram (EEG). Various EEG rhythms can be identified:

α **rhythm** is seen in an adult human at rest with eyes closed. It is more common in parieto-occipital areas and has a frequency of 8–12 Hz with amplitude of 50–100 μV.

β **rhythm** is a lower amplitude wave with a frequency of 18–30 Hz and is seen over the frontal region and is seen in a normal alert adult.

γ **rhythm** has a large amplitude with a frequency of 4–7 Hz, normally seen in the very old and very young.

δ **rhythm** shows are large slow waves with a frequency of less than 4 Hz.

Two basic sleep patterns are seen; Rapid eye movement sleep (REM) and non-rapid eye movement sleep (NREM).

NREM has four stages. From stage 1 to 4 there is progressive slowing of the EEG with associated increase in EEG amplitude. Stage 1 sleep occurs at the beginning of sleep while stage 4 sleep represents deep sleep. In stage 2 bursts of α - like rhythm known as sleep spindles are seen. In REM sleep the NREM pattern of EEG is replaced by fast low voltage electrical activity similar to that seen in alert individuals. However sleep is not disturbed and in fact the threshold for arousal is increased. This kind of sleep is associated with rapid eye movements hence the name.

Large phasic potentials are seen, there is decrease in muscle tone during REM sleep, and it is also associated with dreaming.

LANGUAGE

Wernicke's area in the categorical hemisphere receives auditory and visual information and is concerned with comprehension of this information. It communicates via the arcuate fasciculus with Broca's area. Broca's area is concerned with output of speech. It processes the information from Wernicke's area to produce appropriate movements of the vocal apparatus.

MEMORY

Memory is the process of retention and storage of acquired information and can be further divided into explicit and implicit memory.

Explicit memory involves hippocampus and medial temporal lobes of the brain. It requires conscious retrieval or awareness and can be further divided into Episodic memory (memory of events) and Semantic memory which is memory of words, rules, language and the world around us.

Implicit memory does not require conscious awareness and is not processed in the hippocampus. It is associated with skills required for day to day activities and habits. When learning certain tasks like driving or cycling, explicit memory is used but once these tasks are well learned then implicit memory is used to perform these tasks.

Both forms of memory can also be divided into short-term memory which lasts from a few seconds to hours. Information is processed in the hippocampus and then stored as a long-term memory which lasts for years. Short-term memory is easily affected by drugs and trauma.

It is thought that short-term memory is a transient store of limited capacity which permits instantaneous encoding and retrieval, but when the material is no longer the focus of conscious attention, only some of this material may pass on to long-term memory. The latter represents a long-term storage of indefinite capacity that requires effortful encoding and retrieval. The more elaborate and effortful the encoding process, the better the memory of the material.

At the cellular level, it is thought that information is stored in the short-term memory as reverberating electrical activity in the brain, whereas long-term memory is stored in a more robust form. It is thought that memory formation may lead to an alteration in the transmission of electrical signals through parts of the brain. However, it is not clear whether this is the result of facilitation of existing synapses or due to the formation of new synapses. In both situations, however, protein synthesis is thought to be ultimately involved in the formation of long-term memory and this is brought about through either structural or enzymatic changes in the neurones. The hippocampus is primarily involved in memory storage, since pathological lesions in this area result in both anterograde and retrograde amnesia.

THE BASAL GANGLIA

The basal ganglia consist of interconnected deep nuclei including the caudate, globus pallidum, substantia nigra and putamen. The basal ganglia are involved in control of posture and movement.

THE CEREBELLUM

The cerebellum consists of two cerebellar hemispheres and a central structure. In contrast to the cerebral hemispheres the cerebellar hemispheres control the structures on the same side of the body. The central cerebral structures control gait and balance while a person is seated.

THE BRAIN STEM

Included in the brain stem are the midbrain, pons and medulla. The brain stem contains the reticular formation, which maintains consciousness and the nuclei of all the cranial nerves except I and II. It also has ascending and descending tracts from cerebral structures and spinal cord. The corticospinal tract (one of the main descending tracts) and the dorsal columns, which are the ascending tracts, cross over in the medulla. Thus a lesion in the brain stem can produce cranial nerve lesions on the same side but limb signs on the other side.

The brain stem contains control centres for respiration, cardiovascular homeostasis, gastro-intestinal function, balance, equilibrium and eye movements. Irreversible brain stem lesions are therefore frequently incompatible with life without artificial support.

THE SPINAL CORD

The spinal cord extends from the lower part of medulla and ends at birth at the lower border of the third lumbar vertebra and in the adult between first and second lumbar vertebral bodies. The spinal cord is an elongated cylinder with cervical and a lumbar enlargement corresponding to the origins of brachial and lumbosacral plexuses. The spinal cord tapers into the conus medullaris.

The spinal cord has three covering membranes also known as meninges- the dura mater, arachnoid and pia mater. The dura mater, which covers the brain, has two layers – the inner or the meningeal layer of the cerebral dura and the outer endosteal layer, which at the foramen magnum merges with the periosteum of the skull. The outer layer of the cerebral dura is represented in the vertebral canal by its periosteum while the inner layer continues down to cover the spinal cord. The dural sac usually ends at the level of the second sacral vertebra in adults. Dura covering the spinal cord is attached to the edges of the vertebral canal except posteriorly where it is completely free. Arachnoid mater closely lines the dural sheath while the pia mater closely covers the brain and the spinal cord. Due to the arrangement of the meninges, the following compartments are formed:

- Subarachnoid space
  This contains the cerebrospinal fluid and is traversed by three incomplete trabeculae – a single posterior subarachnoid septum and the ligamentum denticulatum on either side.
- Subdural space
  This is a potential space only between the arachnoid and the dura mater and contains a thin film of serous fluid.
- Extradural space
  A space between the dura and the spinal canal which extends from the foramen magnum downwards as the dura covering the spinal cord fuses with the edges of the foramen magnum .It ends at the sacral hiatus and contains fat, lymphatics, arteries, and veins which are valveless and form the venous plexus of Bateson communicating between the pelvic veins and cerebral veins.

Anterior and posterior spinal roots emerge at the lateral surface of the spinal cord and are covered by the pia and arachnoid mater. They then pierce the dura mater and are subsequently covered by the dura which fuses with the epineurium of the spinal nerve. Spinal nerves then travel through the epidural space and come out through the intervertebral foramen into the paravertebral space. Paravertebral spaces on either side of the vertebral column are in communication with each other through the epidural space

Structure of the spinal cord

The spinal cord has an anterior median fissure and a posterior median sulcus which extends as a posterior median septum into the spinal cord. Posterior roots emerge along the postero-lateral sulci which are on either side of the posterior median sulcus. Anterior roots emerge as a series of nerve tufts at the front of the cord.

The spinal cord has a central canal, which is the continuation of the IVth ventricle and contains the CSF. An 'H' shaped zone of grey matter, which contains nerve cells, surrounds the central canal. It has an outer zone of white matter, which contains myelinated nerve cells and forms ascending and descending tracts (see Section 1 Chapter 10).

DESCENDING TRACTS

Descending pathways, which start in the cerebral cortex, are usually made of three neurones (See Figure NE.10). The first order neurone lies in the cells of the cerebral cortex. The axons of these cells synapse on the second order neurone situated in the anterior grey column of the spinal cord. The second order neurone is known as the internuncial neurone, the axon of which is shorter than the axon of the first order neurone. It synapses with the third order neurone,

known as the lower motor neurone. The lower motor neurone also lies in the anterior grey column of the spinal cord. The axon of this lower motor neurone innervates the skeletal muscle through the anterior root and the spinal nerve. Figure NE.11 gives examples of descending tracts.

ASCENDING TRACTS

In common with descending tracts ascending tracts have three neurones (Figure NE.12). The first order neurone lies in the posterior root ganglia. The peripheral process of this neurone receives the sensory information from the sensory receptor. The central process of this neurone enters the spinal cord via the posterior root and synapses with the second order neurone. The axon of the second order neurone crosses the midline and synapses with the third order neurone in the thalamus. The third order neurone projects to the sensory cortex. Figure NE.13 details important ascending tracts.

Spinal cord transection

COMPLETE TRANSECTION

In man, cord transection is followed by a variable period of spinal shock. In this period all spinal reflexes are profoundly depressed or absent. All muscles innervated by spinal nerves below the level of the cord lesion become paralysed. The initial phase of spinal shock is followed by recovery of reflex function but the voluntary control is lost forever. The time of reflex recovery can be variable in man and can be delayed for up to 6 weeks, although the most frequent interval is about 2 weeks from initial injury. The first reflexes to return are flexor responses to touch and ano-genital reflex responses. Reflex responses are hyperactive in the early recovery phase. Tendon reflexes are the slowest to recover. Hyperactivity of tendon reflexes can be accompanied by clonus. In paraplegic patients over time, a mass reflex response develops. This can occur even after a minor noxious stimulus is applied to the skin. This results in evacuation of bladder and bowel, along with signs of autonomic hyperactivity such as sweating, pallor and swings in blood pressure. In complete transection there is total loss of sensation in the dermatomes supplied by the cord below the level of injury.

HEMISECTION OF THE SPINAL CORD (BROWN SEQUARD SYNDROME)

This affects the pyramidal tracts and posterior columns of the ipsilateral side while the spinothalamic tracts which have crossed over from the opposite side are also

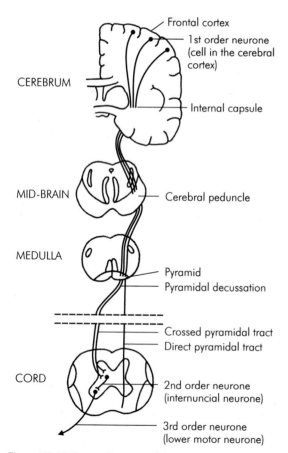

Figure NE.10 Descending tract of the spinal cord

CEREBRUM

Frontal cortex
1st order neurone (cell in the cerebral cortex)
Internal capsule

MID-BRAIN

Cerebral peduncle

MEDULLA

Pyramid
Pyramidal decussation

Crossed pyramidal tract
Direct pyramidal tract

CORD

2nd order neurone (internuncial neurone)

3rd order neurone (lower motor neurone)

DETAIL OF DESCENDING TRACTS OF THE SPINAL CORD

TRACT	DETAIL
Corticospinal Tract (Pyramidal tract)	First order neurones originate in the pyramidal cells of the motor cortex. Axons descend, enter the medulla and group to form the pyramid. At the junction of medulla and cord 80% decussate toform the lateral cortocospinal tract, the remainder cotinue as the anterior cortico spinal tract. The axons synapse in the anterior grey column with internuncial neurones which in turn synpase with lower motor neurones that innervate skeletal muscle
Reticulospinal Tracts	Originate in the reticular formation, pons and medulla. Fibres synapse in the anterior grey column and influence alpha and gamma motor neurones. The reticulospinal tract also carries descending autonomic fibres.
Tectospinal Tract	Arises int he superior colliculus of midbrain. Axons decussate and end in the anterior grey column in the cervical cord. Mediates reflex postural movement secondary to visual stimuli.
Rubrospinal Tract	Originates in the red nucleus of midbrain and decussates. Affects alpha and gamma motor neurones int he anterior grey columns of the cord to facilitate flexor groups of muscles and inhibit extensors.
Vestibulospinal Tract	Associated with posture and balance having a facilitation of extensor muscle groups and inhibition of flexors
Olivospinal Tract	Originates in the olivary nucleus in the pons
Descending Autonomic Fibres	Minor significance only

Figure NE.11

affected. Thus there is paralysis of muscles on the same side along with loss of touch, pressure, joint and vibration sense. The pain and temperature fibres coming from the opposite side are also affected.

Blood supply of the spinal cord

Blood supply of the spinal cord arises from a single anterior spinal artery and two small posterior spinal arteries.

The anterior spinal artery is formed by the union of a branch from each vertebral artery and runs along the midline of the cord, supplying the anterior 2/3rd of spinal cord. Thrombosis of this artery can cause anterior spinal artery syndrome in which there is paralysis due to ischaemia of the pyramidal tract although there is sparing of the posterior columns so that sensation conveyed by these columns remains intact.

The two smaller posterior spinal arteries lie on each side of the cord posteriorly. They are derived from posterior inferior cerebellar arteries and supply the posterior third of the spinal cord. Blood vessels known as vaso corona communicate between the anterior and posterior spinal arteries. Various radicular arteries (which arise from deep cervical, intercostal and lumbar arteries) supply the anterior and posterior spinal arteries along the spinal canal. The arteria radicularis magna (major anterior radicular artery) is the principal arterial blood supply of the lower two thirds of the spinal cord (usually found between T 11 and L 3). In case of occlusion of the anterior spinal artery the blood supply of the lower two third of the spinal cord may be compromised.

Anterior and posterior spinal arteries do not anastomose with each other than within the spinal cord itself.

THE REFLEX ARC

Stimulation of the reflex arc by a specific sensory stimulus produces a repetitive, specific response. The reflex arc begins with a sense organ (e.g. muscle spindle), which transmits information via the afferent neurone to the spinal cord entering via the dorsal root or cranial nerve. The ganglia of these neurones act as a central co-ordinating station. The efferent nerve leaves the central station via the ventral roots or a motor cranial nerve and innervates an effector organ such as a voluntary muscle. The activity in this reflex arc is influenced by the central nervous system.

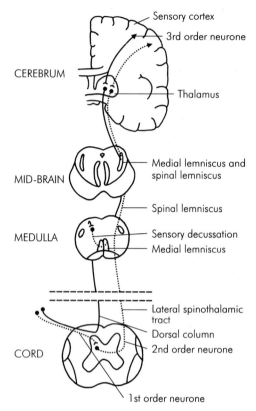

Figure NE.12 Ascending tract of the spinal cord

The reflex arc can be monosynaptic i.e. a single synapse between the afferent and efferent neurone (Figure NE.14) or polysynaptic where two or more synapses occur between afferent and efferent neurone (Figure NE.15). The stretch reflex is an example of a monosynaptic reflex. The sense organ for this reflex is the muscle spindle. Skeletal muscle consists of two types of muscle fibres, namely the extrafusal and intrafusal fibres. Contraction of the extrafusal fibres is controlled by α motor neurones located in the anterior horn of the spinal cord. These contractions result in contraction of a muscle. The number of muscle fibres controlled by a single motor neurone varies according to the precision of the movement involved. The finer the movement the less the number of extrafusal fibres; the ratio is < 1:10 for muscles controlling finger movement whereas for lower limb muscle it is about one to several hundred.

STRUCTURE OF MUSCLE SPINDLES

The intrafusal fibres form specialised sensory organs called muscle spindles, which are arranged in parallel with the extrafusal fibres. These spindles respond to the change in length of surrounding extrafusal fibres and form part of the control system for maintaining posture and limb position. Each spindle consists of up to a dozen intrafusal fibres whose ends are attached to

DETAIL OF ASCENDING TRACTS OF THE SPINAL CORD	
TRACT	DETAIL
Spinothalamic Tract	Originate from free nerve endings in the skin carrying pain and temperature sensation. First order neurones are A delta and C fibres which enter the cord and synapse with second order neurones in the posterior grey columns. Second order neurones cross to the opposite side within one segment and ascend as the lateral spinothalamic tract. Fibres synapse with third order neurones in the ventral posterolateral nucleus of the thalamus. Termination is the sensory area of the postcentral gyrus.
Gracile and Cuneate Tracts	Fibres from receptors for touch, vibration and joint proprioceptors enter the cord via the posterior root ganglia and travel in the posterior white columns of the ipsilateral side. Descending branches affect intersegmental reflexes. Ascending fibres synapse with cells in the posterior grey horn, internuncial neurones and anterior horn cells before travelling up as the Gracile and Cuneate tracts. Fibures synapse with second order neurones in the Gracile and Cuneate nuclei of the medulla, which then decussate to travel as the medial lemniscus. The third order neurones lie in the ventral posterolateral nucleus of the thalamus and terminate in the post central gyrus of the sensory cortex.
Anterior and Posterior Spinocerebellar Tracts	Relay information from muscle and joins to the cerebellum
Spinotectal Tract	Transmits pain, temperature and touch sensation to the superior colliculus of the midbrain. Facilitates spino-visual reflexes.
Spinoreticular Tract	Relays various information to the reticular formation. Affects consciousness.
Spino-Olivary Tract	Minor afferent path to cerebellum

Figure NE.13

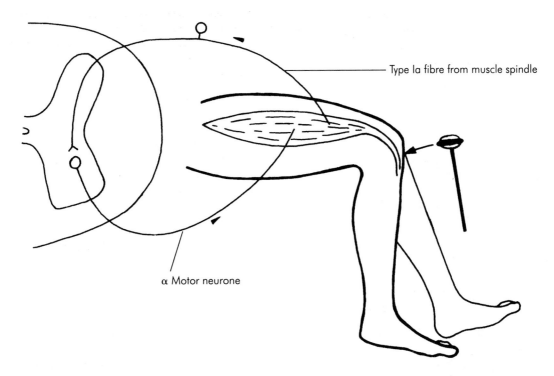

Type la fibre from muscle spindle

α Motor neurone

Figure NE.14 Monosynaptic stretch reflex

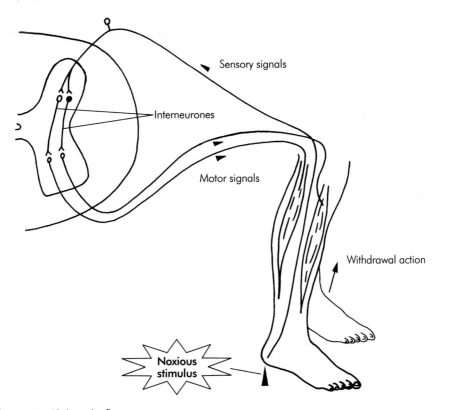

Sensory signals

Interneurones

Motor signals

Withdrawal action

Noxious
stimulus

Figure NE.15 Polysynaptic withdrawal reflex

the extrafusal fibres. Each intrafusal fibre consists of two portions: the central non contractile region and a contractile muscle fibre portion at either end. The efferent control of these contractile portions is supplied by the γ motor neurones. The central portion of the intrafusal fibres can take two forms, either a nuclear bag or a nuclear chain. The former consists of an expanded central portion containing a collection of nuclei whereas the latter consist of nuclei arranged in a chain. Two types of sensory nerve fibres innervate the central portion of the intrafusal fibres: Type Ia (or annulospiral) and type II fibres. Type Ia fibres innervate both the nuclear bag fibres and nuclear chain fibres, but the type II fibres only innervate the nuclear chain fibres. See Figure NE.16.

FUNCTION OF MUSCLE SPINDLES

The central portion of the muscle spindle detects the change in length of the muscle. When the whole muscle contracts, the muscle spindle relaxes and firing in its afferent axon stops. However, the opposite occurs when the muscle relaxes or is stretched passively. In other words, the muscle spindle acts as muscle length detector. This should not be confused with the Golgi tendon apparatus, which are stretch receptors within tendons and respond to the tension, not length, within muscle. One of the most basic functions of the muscle spindle, therefore, is to maintain muscle length (see stretch reflex below). Furthermore, the sensitivity of the muscle spindle is adjustable. When the muscle spindles are relaxed, they are relatively insensitive to

stretch. However, when the motor neurones are active, they become shorter and become much more sensitive to changes in muscle length. Therefore by establishing a rate of firing in the motor system, the higher centres control the length of the muscle spindles and indirectly the length of the entire muscle.

During normal movements, both the α and γ motor neurones are activated at the same time. If little resistance is encountered, both the extrafusal and intrafusal muscle fibres will contract at approximately the same rate, and as a result the central portion of the muscle spindle retains its original length before the contraction and little change in activity will be detected in the afferent axons of the spindle. If, however, the limb meets with resistance, the intrafusal muscle fibres will shorten more than the extrafusal muscle fibres, the centre of the muscle spindle becomes stretched and the rate of firing in the afferent axons increases. This will stimulate the motor neurone and thereby increase contraction of the motor unit.

The inverse stretch reflex implies that the harder a muscle is stretched, the stronger is the reflex contraction. If the muscle tension increases excessively, the Golgi tendon organs, which are attached in series with the muscle, inhibit the activity of the motor neurone, providing an inhibitory feedback mechanism to prevent muscle damage. The relaxation in response to strong stretch is called the inverse stretch reflex. Thus, the muscle spindles and the Golgi tendon organs work hand in hand to make sure that length and tension in a muscle is appropriate to perform a particular task.

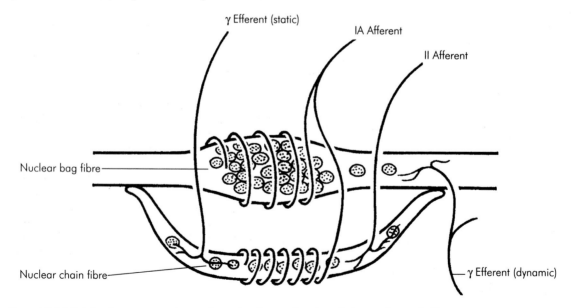

Figure NE.16 Details of nerve connections to the nuclear bag and nuclear chain muscle spindle fibres

The resistance of a muscle to stretch is known as tone. When a motor nerve is cut, the muscle it supplies becomes flaccid. The muscle is hypotonic if the rate of efferent discharge is low and hypertonic when it is high. Another phenomenon seen in the hypertonic state is clonus. This occurs when a sustained and sudden force is applied to a muscle, resulting in regular rhythmic contractions of the stretched muscle.

The Withdrawal Reflex is a polysynaptic reflex. Contraction of flexor muscles and relaxation of the extensors in response to a painful stimulus, results in withdrawal of the stimulated part. When a noxious stimulus is applied to a limb, the signal is first transmitted via sensory fibres to the interneurone(s) in the spinal cord and then onto the motor neurones. This is an example of a polysynaptic withdrawal reflex (Figure NE.15). The neuronal circuitry involves not only activation of muscle(s), which carry out the withdrawal, but also the inhibition of the antagonist muscles. Other muscle groups may also be stimulated or inhibited so that the withdrawal of the limb and movement of the rest of the body are coordinated to move safely away from the noxious stimulus.

MOTOR FUCTION

The structures involved in the control of movement are the cerebral cortex, cerebellum and the basal ganglia.

CEREBRAL CORTEX

The motor cortex is situated in the frontal lobe. It is divided into three parts:

Primary motor cortex is situated in the precentral gyrus. Different areas of the body are represented in the primary cortex. Parts of the body performing the finer functions have largest representation. The facial area is represented bilaterally.

The premotor area lies anterior to the primary motor cortex immediately superior to Sylvian fissure. It is concerned with postural adjustment at the beginning of a voluntary movement.

The supplemental motor area is concerned with planning of complex movements.

Motor signals are transmitted directly from the cortex to the spinal cord through the corticospinal tract and indirectly through multiple accessory pathways that involve the basal ganglia, the cerebellum, and the various nuclei of the brain stem.

CEREBELLUM

The cerebellum is situated in the posterior fossa and has two lateral lobes that are joined in the centre by the vermis. It is functionally divided into three parts:

The vestibulocerebellum has connections with the vestibule of the middle ear and maintains the body's equilibrium during motion.

Spinocerebellum is mainly concerned with proprioception. It receives information from the whole body as well as the motor cortex. Voluntary movements are co-ordinated here depending on the sensory information received. The central portion of the cerebellum is concerned with axial and proximal limb muscles whilst the lobes control the distal musculature.

The Neocerebellum is involved in planned execution of voluntary movements. Fast co-ordinated activity is affected in cerebellar disease. Dysdiadochokinesia (the inability to perform rapid alternating movements) is a feature of cerebellar dysfunction. Other signs of cerebellar dysfunction include ataxia, scanning speech and intention tremor.

BASAL GANGLIA

The term basal ganglia refers to the following structures: Caudate nucleus, Putamen, Globus pallidus, subthalamic nucleus and substantia nigra.

The Caudate nucleus and Putamen are together called the 'striatum'. The basal ganglia form a loop with the cortex (Figure NE.17). The cortex projects to the striatum via the corticostriate projections, the striatum in turn sends efferents to the globus pallidus which in turn sends efferents to the thalamus. The thalamus then communicates with the primary motor cortex via accessory motor areas.

Command for voluntary action originates in the cortical association area. It is further planned in the cortex, basal ganglia and lateral portion of the cerebellar cortex. The efferents to muscle travel in the corticospinal tract (Pyramidal system) and bring about the voluntary action. The cerebellum and basal ganglia both influence voluntary action. The cerebellum by enhancing the stretch reflex, fine tuning of rapid movements preventing oscillations, and the basal ganglia help by carrying out various subconscious movements which are required to carry out a voluntary activity.

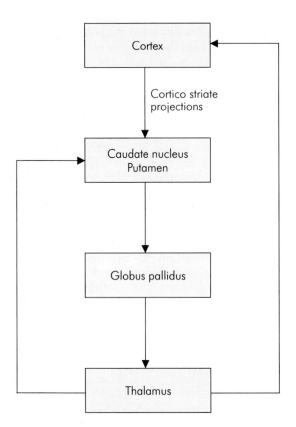

Figure NE.17 connections of the basal ganglia

CONTROL OF POSTURE

Posture regulating mechanisms involve structures in the spinal cord, the brain stem, and the cerebral cortex.

A voluntary action requires smooth co-ordinated activity in different muscle groups so that posture is maintained. The postural reflexes involved are co-ordinated at the level of spinal cord and are influenced by higher centres. When the influence of these higher centres is removed at different levels it is possible to understand the postural reflexes involved.

SPINAL CORD COMPONENTS

The stretch Reflex has already been described in detail earlier. Additionally proprioceptors in flexors and extensor group of muscles respectively, keep an animal standing upright resisting gravity. Placing a foot on the ground stiffens the leg so that the body can be supported. This is the positive supporting reaction. The disappearance of this is known as negative supporting reaction.

BRAIN STEM COMPONENTS

These components can be studied by transection of the brain stem at the superior border of the pons. This is known as decerebration which causes increased rigidity. In the brain stem there are areas that facilitate and inhibit stretch reflexes. After decerebration the influence of the inhibitory area is reduced whilst that of the facilitatory area is increased resulting in increased efferent discharge. This facilitates the stretch reflex and causes rigidity. Spasticity produced by decerebration is most marked in the extensor group of muscles as these are the antigravity muscles helping the animal to maintain its posture. In humans decerebrate rigidity causes extension in all four limbs.

The scale of rigidity of the limbs in a decerebrate animal is position related. In the prone position the rigidity is minimal whilst if the animal is on its back the rigidity is maximal. This is known as the 'tonic labyrinthine reflex'. The receptors for this reflex are in the otolithic organs.

When the head of the decerebrate animal is turned to one side, the limbs on that side become more rigidly extended and the limbs on the opposite side become less rigid. Flexion of the neck causes flexion of the forelimbs and hindlimbs. The reverse happens with the extension of the head. This is known as the 'tonic neck reflex' and is initiated by the stretch receptors in the neck.

MIDBRAIN COMPONENTS

Midbrain components can be studied by interrupting the neural pathways at the superior border of the midbrain. In the midbrain animal, the phasic postural reflexes are intact so that the animal can stand, walk and correct its position. Rigidity is seen only when the animal is at rest as it is due to static postural reflexes.

The Righting reflexes, such as the labyrinthine righting reflex, body on head righting reflex, neck righting reflex, and body on body righting reflex are essential for maintaining normal position of the animal. These reflexes are co-ordinated by the nuclei in the midbrain.

CORTICAL COMPONENTS

Removal of the cerebral cortex is called decortication. In the decorticate animal there is loss of the cortical area that inhibits gamma efferent discharge The increased (gamma) efferent discharge causes facilitation of the stretch reflex leading to rigidity. This is only seen at rest due to the presence of phasic postural reflexes. Postural reactions like hopping and placing reaction are seriously affected by decortication.

CEREBROSPINAL FLUID (CSF)

CSF is present in the cerebral ventricles and the subarachnoid space. The total volume of CSF is about 150 ml. Approximately 550 ml of CSF is produced per day in an adult. Most (50–70%) of the CSF is produced in the choroid plexuses of the lateral, third and forth ventricles, which are highly vascular invaginations of pia mater, covered by single layered ependymal epithelium. It is formed by secretion and filtration of plasma. Formation of CSF is not affected by intracranial pressure but removal of CSF increases with increasing pressure. CSF from the lateral ventricles drains into the IIIrd ventricle via the foramina of Monro. From IIIrd ventricle it travels to IVth ventricle via aqueduct of Sylvius.It enters cerebral subarachnoid space through the median foramen of Magendie and lateral foramina of Lushka. CSF is absorbed into the venous sinuses by the arachnoid villi. Arachnoid villi are projections of arachnoid into the venous sinuses which are covered by a single layered endothelium of the venous sinuses. Composition of the CSF and its circulation is detailed more fully in Section 2, Chapter 2-Body Fluids.

Larger molecular weight substances do not pass from blood into the CSF or the interstitial spaces of brain due to presence of 'tight junctions' between the endothelium of cerebral capillaries. This 'Blood-Brain Barrier' is highly permeable to water, carbon dioxide, oxygen and most lipid soluble substances such as volatile anaesthetic agents. The barrier is impermeable to plasma proteins and large molecular weight substances.

INTRACRANIAL PRESSURE (ICP)

Intracranial pressure (ICP) is the pressure inside the cranial vault relative to atmospheric pressure. Normal intracranial pressure ranges between 5 – 15 mmHg, although this varies with arterial pulsation, breathing, coughing and straining. The intracranial contents can be divided into four compartments: Solid material (≈ 10%), tissue water (≈ 75%), CSF (150 ml ≈ 10%), blood (50–75 ml ≈ 5%).

These compartments are all contained within the rigid cranial vault, and a change in volume of one compartment is accompanied by a reciprocal change in another compartment (The Monro-Kelly Doctrine).

CONTROL OF ICP

Raised ICP causes brain damage by reducing cerebral perfusion pressure (CPP) or by focal compression of brain tissue due to distortion and herniation of intracranial contents. Control of ICP depends on compensatory mechanisms involving the four compartments described above.

Volume buffering is illustrated in Figure NE.18. With an increase in intracranial volume, compensatory mechanisms maintain ICP within the normal range (between point 1 and point 2 on the figure). At point 2, further increases in volume cause a slight rise in ICP. As volume increases, there is a steady decline in compliance which increases the ICP even more (point 3) until a small rise in volume is associated with a marked rise in ICP causing a fall in the perfusion pressure and ultimately cerebral ischaemia (between points 3 and 4).

The CSF plays a major part in compensating for an increase in intracranial volume. As a space-occupying lesion expands, it will cause progressive reduction of the CSF space (reduced size of the ventricles and basal cisterns). CSF outflow into the spinal canal increases, and its absorption into the venous system is also increased. Rapid rises in intracranial volume (e.g. acute intracranial haematoma) exhaust spatial compensation quickly resulting in a rapid rise of ICP.

Another important compensatory mechanism is provided by changes in cerebral blood volume (CBV). Most of the intracranial blood volume is contained in venous sinuses and the pial veins and only a small change in CBV could have a profound effect on ICP. A rise in ICP decreases cerebral perfusion pressure (CPP). CPP is related to ICP by the formula:

$$CPP = Mean\ Arterial\ Pressure - (ICP + JVP).$$

Thus a reduction in CPP triggers pressure autoregulation which causes vasodilatation to maintain

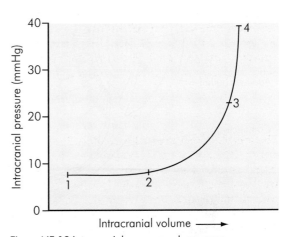

Figure NE.18 Intracranial pressure-volume curve

a constant CBF. This results in a rise in CBV and consequently a rise in ICP in a non-compliant or swollen brain. Conversely, a rise in mean arterial pressure will within autoregulatory limits cause cerebral vasoconstriction, resulting in a reduction in CBV and ICP.

Arterial blood gas values also have a major contribution to CBF and CBV. Both CBF and CBV increase with raised $PaCO_2$, but the CBV response curve is flatter than the CBF curve. A reduction in $PaCO_2$ from 5.3–2.7 kPa results in a 65% reduction in CBF but only a 28% reduction in CBV. This small change in intracranial volume will have a significant reduction in ICP in the presence of intracranial hypertension because the system operates on the steep part of the pressure volume curve. A reduction in arterial oxygen tension causes cerebral vasodilation resulting in a rise in CBV.

Increased metabolic demand increases CBF, CBV and ICP due to flow metabolism coupling. Reduction in cerebral metabolism (using intravenous anaesthetic agents for example) will reduce CBV and is a useful therapeutic intervention in patients with raised ICP.

A rise in cerebral venous blood volume will also increase CBV and ICP. Venous distension is a common cause of increased cerebral venous volume and can occur from jugular venous obstruction, increased intrathoracic pressure, raised central venous pressure, head down tilt etc. For detail see Section 2 Chapter 6, Figure CR.35.

SPECIAL SENSES

VISION

STRUCTURE OF THE EYE

Before reaching the photoreceptors on the retina, light must pass through the optical apparatus that is made up of the cornea, aqueous humour, lens and vitreous humour (Figure NE.19). The globe is protected by the sclera, which becomes transparent in the anterior part of the eye known as the cornea. Aqueous humour is produced by the ciliary processes and catalysed by the action of carbonic anhydrase; it passes from the posterior chamber through the pupil into the anterior chamber of the eye. It is then drained into a vein via the canal of Schlemm (located at the angle of the anterior chamber).

Pupillary size is determined by the activities of the smooth muscle fibres in the iris: the circular fibres constrict (miosis) while the radial fibres dilate (mydriasis) the pupil. The interior surface of the globe

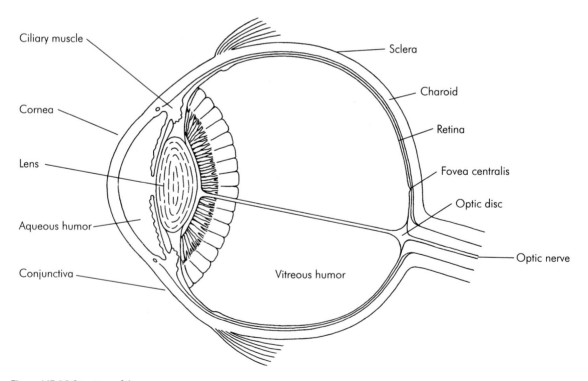

Figure NE.19 Structure of the eye

is lined by the retina, except where the optic nerve leaves the eye and where the ciliary muscle begins. The ciliary muscle changes the tension of the suspensory ligaments that alters the convexity of the lens and thereby achieves accommodation.

The retina

The retina is made up of photoreceptors – rods and cones. These are located along the outer surface of the retina adjacent to the pigment epithelium. The blood supply of the photoreceptors is derived from the choroid and not from blood vessels on the inner retinal surface. There are about 120 million rods and only 7 million cones in each eye. Rods are uniformly distributed throughout the retina and are responsible for night and monochromatic vision. They contain the pigment rhodopsin. Cones, however, are concentrated in the fovea and are responsible for bright and colour vision. Cones contain opsins that are sensitive to red, green and blue.

The visual pathway

Electrical potential is generated when light reaches the photoreceptors on the retina. This potential is then transmitted to the ganglion cells either via the bipolar and/or the horizontal and amacrine cells. Axons from the ganglion cells converge at the blind spot of the optic disc to form the optic nerve. The axons coming from the nasal half of the retina decussate at the optic chiasm while those situated on the temporal half remain on the ipsilateral side (Figure NE.19) These then synapse in the lateral geniculate nuclei. From here, synaptic connections are made via the optic radiation to the primary visual cortex giving rise to a topographical projection of the visual field around the calcarine fissure. Some fibres of the optic tracts relay to the superior colliculi, which are involved in the control of eye movements or posture. Lesions in the visual pathway will give visual field defects according to their position. Thus as shown in Figure NE.20, the following lesions will give rise to their corresponding defects:

- Lesion 1 – right eye blindness,
- Lesion 2 – bi-temporal hemianopia
- Lesion 3 – right homonymous hemianopia

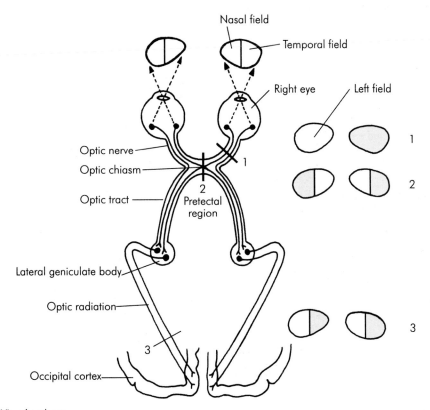

Figure NE.20 Visual pathway

HEARING

STRUCTURE OF THE EAR

The ear is divided into the external, middle and internal compartments. The external compartment consists of the pinna that directs sound waves via the external auditory meatus to the tympanic membrane. Vibrations of the tympanic membrane transmit sound energy to the middle ear that consists of the ossicles: malleus, incus and stapes. The latter stimulates the inner ear through the oval window. The middle ear is air-filled and is connected to the pharynx via the Eustachian tube, which allows equilibration of pressure to occur between the middle ear and the environment. The inner ear consists of the cochlea, which is a bony coiled tube, and is divided lengthwise into three canals by two membranes: the scala vestibuli and scala media (or cochlear duct) is separated by Reissner's membrane whereas the scala media and scala tympani is separated by the basilar membrane (Figure NE.21). The scala tympani communicates with the middle ear via the round window. The inner ear is fluid-filled: the scala media is filled with endolymph, while the scala vestibuli and tympani, being joined at the helicotrema, are filled with perilymph. The sound receptors are found in the organ of Corti (Figure NE.22), which is located on the basilar membrane within the cochlear duct. The organ of Corti is made up of an epithelium of hair cells and supporting cells. Each hair cell is anchored on the basilar membrane and has a bundle of hairs projecting from its tip into the scala media. Directly opposite to these hair cells is the tectorial membrane. The hair cells synapse with dendrites of the ganglion cells which in turn synapse with fibres from the cochlear nerve. The latter traverses the subarachnoid space and enters the brainstem at the pontomedullary junction.

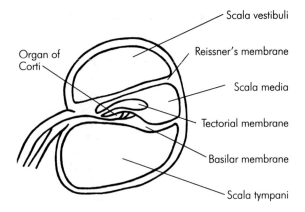

Figure NE.22 Organ of Corti

Mechanism of hearing

Sound waves produce vibrations of the tympanic membrane that lead to movements of the ossicles. Movements of the footplate of the stapes in the oval window are converted to pressure waves in the scala vestibuli. These pressure waves are then transmitted in the endolymphatic canal to reach the basilar membrane. Such oscillations cause displacements of the tectorial membrane with respect to the basilar membrane. The hair cells situated on the latter are thus stimulated and become depolarised. The resulting receptor potential is then transmitted via the underlying ganglion cells to the cochlear nerve. All the cochlear nerve fibres terminate at the cochlear nucleus in the brainstem. From here, second-order fibres project mainly to the contralateral (and to a lesser extent to the ipsilateral) inferior colliculus via the lateral lemniscus. From the inferior colliculus, connections are projected, via the medial geniculate body, to the primary auditory cortex in the temporal lobe.

TASTE AND OLFACTION

TASTE

Taste buds are made up of specialised epithelial cells (taste cells) and supporting cells, which are located on the surface of the tongue, soft palate and oropharynx.

Most taste buds are found on protuberances called papillae at the back of the tongue. Taste cells have a half-life of about 2 weeks and are constantly being replenished by division of the underlying basal cells. There are four basic tastes: sweet, sour, salty and bitter. All complex tastes are thought to be composed of different combinations of the basic tastes. Nearly all tastes are the combined result of taste and smell. The

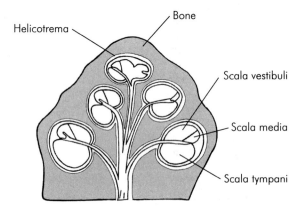

Figure NE.21 Cochlea in cross-section

transduction process of taste is poorly understood: it is thought that chemicals in food interact with chemoreceptors on the surface membrane of taste cells induce a change in membrane permeability to Na^+ ions. This leads to depolarisation of taste cells which then leads to the production of generator potentials in the afferent nerve fibres. Taste buds are innervated by the chorda tympani (anterior two-thirds of the tongue), glossopharyngeal (posterior third of the tongue), vagus (epiglottis), and greater petrosal (soft palate), nerves. These then relay in the tractus solitarius in the medulla before projecting to the thalamus and cortex.

OLFACTION

Olfactory cells are specialised bipolar neurones found in the olfactory epithelium in the roof of the nasal cavity. The olfactory epithelium also contains basal and supporting cells. Olfactory cells are the only neurones in the body known to be replaced continually by division of the underlying basal cells. Situated at the apical region of these cells are long cilia embedded in a layer of mucus, produced by the supporting cells. Odoriferous compounds reach the olfactory epithelium by diffusion, which is facilitated by sniffing to increase the airflow. These compounds must first dissolve in the mucus; the chemical interaction between odoriferous chemicals and the chemoreceptors on the cilia trigger off changes in ion conductance in the olfactory cell, resulting in the generation of action potentials in the olfactory neurones. The axons of the olfactory nerve pass through the cribriform plate and enter the olfactory bulb. Here there is complex signal processing in that there is marked convergence of afferent inputs and also the presence of interneurones. From here second-order neurones project to the olfactory cortex and also to other regions such as the thalamus and the limbic system.

AUTONOMIC NERVOUS SYSTEM

The autonomic nervous system (ANS) is that part of the nervous system which controls the visceral activities of the body. This control is involuntary and enables the body to adjust to varying physiological demands. For example, one cannot consciously increase cardiac output, but when physical threat is detected, the ANS will initiate changes in various systems of the body which enable the individual to deal with the physical demand. The ANS is controlled mainly by centres in the brain stem and hypothalamus. Sensory inputs are relayed to these areas and reflex responses are effected in the visceral organs. Acting in concert with the hypothalamus and the endocrine

system, the ANS is largely responsible for the control of the internal environment of the body.

There are two subdivisions: the sympathetic and the parasympathetic nervous system. In general, the two systems are antagonistic to each other. It is not always predictable whether sympathetic or parasympathetic stimulation will produce inhibition or excitation in a particular organ, but most organs are predominantly controlled by one or the other system. This background activity is known as the sympathetic or parasympathetic tone. For example, arteriolar smooth muscle has a predominant sympathetic tone, whereas the basal tone in the gut is mainly parasympathetic.

SYMPATHETIC NERVOUS SYSTEM

Neurones of the sympathetic nervous system originate in the thoracic and lumbar segments (from T 1 to L 2) of the spinal cord, the so-called thoraco-lumbar outflow (Figure NE.23). These synapse in a paired chain of ganglia, the sympathetic ganglia, situated on either side of the vertebral column. The nerve fibres which run from the spinal cord to the sympathetic ganglia are known as preganglionic fibres, while those which leave the ganglia to reach their effector organs are known as postganglionic fibres. A few of the preganglionic fibres pass through the sympathetic chain without forming synapses until they arrive at a more peripheral location in the coeliac and mesenteric ganglia or the adrenal medulla. The adrenal medulla is unique in that it is innervated by sympathetic preganglionic fibres but has no postganglionic nerve fibres.

PARASYMPATHETIC NERVOUS SYSTEM

The parasympathetic nervous system leaves the central nervous system via cranial nerves (III, VII, IX and X) and sacral nerves (S 2,3,4). This is called the cranio-sacral outflow. Approximately three-quarters of all parasympathetic fibres are located in the two vagus (X) nerves. Like the sympathetic pathway, the parasympathetic system has both preganglionic and postganglionic neurones. However, the cell bodies of the parasympathetic ganglia are located within the effector organs themselves, and so the preganglionic fibres travel long distances from the spinal cord and the postganglionic fibres are therefore relatively short.

Neurotransmitters and receptors in the autonomic nervous system

The sympathetic and parasympathetic nerve fibres

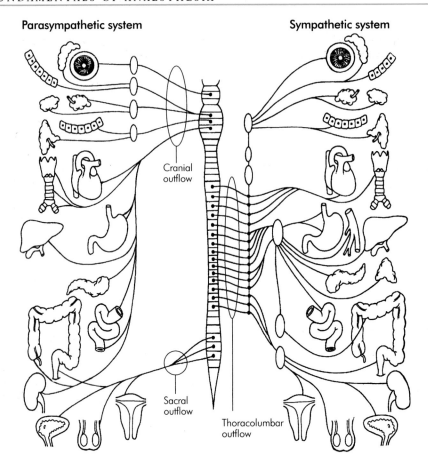

Parasympathetic system

Sympathetic system

Cranial
outflow

Sacral
outflow

Thoracolumbar
outflow

Figure NE.23 Distribution of the autonomic nervous system

release either acetylcholine or norepinephrine in the nerve endings. All preganglionic fibres are cholinergic in both the sympathetic and parasympathetic ganglia. Nearly all the postganglionic neurones of the parasympathetic system are also cholinergic but a few may release vasoactive intestinal polypeptide (VIP). Most of the postganglionic sympathetic fibres are noradrenergic, except in sweat glands, piloerector muscles and a few blood vessels where they are cholinergic.

Sympathetic stimulation to the adrenal medulla releases epinephrine and norepinephrine into the circulation. In general, about 80% of the secretion is epinephrine and 20% is norepinephrine but this proportion may change considerably depending on physiological conditions. There are two major types of adrenoreceptors: alpha and beta receptors. Norepinephrine acts predominantly on alpha receptors, whereas epinephrine acts on both alpha and beta adrenoreceptors. Alpha receptors can also be divided into two types: $alpha_1$ and $alpha_2$ and there are three subtypes of beta adrenoreceptors.

There are two types of cholinergic receptors: nicotinic and muscarinic. Nicotinic receptors are found in both the sympathetic and parasympathetic ganglia. On the other hand, muscarinic receptors are located in the postganglionic parasympathetic synapses. Although five distinct subclasses of muscarinic receptors have been identified by gene cloning, functionally there are three subtypes: M_1 receptors are found mainly in the CNS, M_2 receptors are located in the heart and M_3 are found in exocrine glands and vascular endothelium.

Consequences of autonomic stimulation

In life threatening situations, the sympathetic nervous system discharges almost as a complete unit, a phenomenon known as mass discharge. This may occur when the hypothalamus is activated by fear, noxious stimulus or severe pain. There is stimulation of different systems and organs simultaneously to prepare the individual for survival. The resulting sympathetic "stress" response is summarised in Figure NE.23.

'STRESS' RESPONSES DUE TO SYMPATHETIC MASS DISCHARGE

Tachycardia

Raised arterial pressure

Sweating

Pupillary dilation

Increase in blood glucose concentration

Increase in glycolysis and gluconeogenesis

Redistribution of blood flow from splanchnic to cerebral and coronary circulation

Increase in cellular metabolism throughout the body

Increase in mental alertness

Figure NE.24

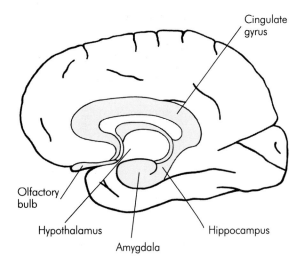

Figure NE.25 Paramedian sagittal section of the brain showing different components of the limbic system

The parasympathetic nervous system, on the contrary, is more organ-specific. For example, stimulation of the heart by the parasympathetic system is quite separate from that of gastric secretion. Nevertheless, there is some association between closely related functions; for example, although salivary secretion can occur separately from gastric secretion, they are often co-ordinated and occur together.

THE LIMBIC SYSTEM

The limbic system is made up of a number of cortical and subcortical structures situated around the basal regions of the cerebrum. It is principally involved in the control of instinctive and learned behaviour, emotions, sexual and motivational drives. The limbic system has extensive neuronal connections with the frontal and temporal cortex. The most important components of the limbic system consist of the hypothalamus, amygdala and hippocampus (Figure NE.25).

HIPPOCAMPUS AND AMYGDALA

Similar to other structures within the limbic system, stimulation of different areas of the hippocampus also lead to behavioural and emotional changes such as increased sex drive, rage and placidity. In addition, when the hippocampi have been surgically excised, the end result is anterograde amnesia and some degree of retrograde amnesia. It is therefore suggested that hippocampus may be involved in the short and long term memory processes. Due to the extensive neuronal connections between it and various areas of the brain, stimulation of the amygdala not only causes effects

similar to that of the hypothalamus, but widespread behavioural patterns. It is thought that the amygdala project into the limbic system the current behavioural status in relation to both the surroundings and thoughts of the individual. It is believed to help pattern the behavioural response of the individual so that it is appropriate for each occasion.

HYPOTHALAMUS

The hypothalamus is situated just rostral to the brain stem in the basal region of the brain. Inferior to it is the pituitary gland. It has extensive neuronal connections to the brain stem, pituitary gland and cerebrum. Together with other limbic structures and the endocrine system, the hypothalamus controls the vegetative and endocrine functions of the body as well as many aspects of emotional behaviour. The hypothalamus maintains homeostatic control of the internal environment and as such it plays a central role in the control of body temperature, control of pituitary secretion, osmolality of body fluids and the drive to eat and drink (Figure NE.26).

Control of body temperature

The hypothalamus receives and processes information from both the central thermoreceptors, situated in the preoptic area (anterior part) of the hypothalamus, and the peripheral thermoreceptors found on the skin. Physiological changes are initiated in response to temperature changes so that a nearly constant body temperature is maintained. For example, in response to cold the hypothalamus will initiate peripheral

FUNCTIONS OF THE HYPOTHALAMUS

Control of body temperature

Regulate water balance

Control food intake

Control over endocrine system via pituitary gland

Behavioural and emotional influence

Figure NE.26

vasoconstriction and shivering. At the same time, behavioural changes also occur so that a lowering of environmental temperature will lead to an increase in muscular activity to generate heat and extra layers of clothes may be added to conserve heat.

Control of pituitary secretion

Anterior pituitary secretion is controlled by releasing and inhibiting hormones carried in the portal hypophyseal vessels from the hypothalamus to the pituitary gland. These chemical agents are secreted by nerve endings in the median eminence of the hypothalamus. These nerve endings are in close proximity to the capillary loops from which the portal vessels are formed. There are seven hypothalamic releasing and inhibiting hormones summarised in Figure NE.27.

The posterior pituitary gland secretes the hormones oxytocin and vasopressin. They are synthesised in the neurones in the supraoptic and paraventricular nuclei of the hypothalamus and are transported down the axons to their endings in the posterior pituitary where they are released into the circulation. Oxytocin is released when the breast is suckled and is responsible for milk ejection. It also causes contraction of the uterine smooth muscle. The release of vasopressin depends on the osmolality of the plasma. Even small changes in osmolality may cause significant changes in vasopressin release. The main effect of vasopression is water retention by the kidneys. It increases the permeability of the collecting ducts of the kidney so that more water is reabsorbed.

Water balance

The hypothalamus maintains water balance by controlling both water intake and water loss. Electrical stimulation or injection of hypertonic saline into the anterior hypothalamus leads to the desire to drink. Drinking is regulated by changes in plasma osmolality and extracellular fluid (ECF) volume. Depletion in

HYPOTHALAMIC-RELEASING AND -INHIBITING HORMONES

Corticotropin-releasing hormone

Thyrotropin-releasing hormone

Growth hormone-releasing hormone

Luteinising hormone-releasing hormone

Follicle-stimulating hormone-releasing hormone

Prolactin-releasing hormone

Prolactin-inhibiting hormone

Figure NE.27

ECF volume leads to thirst. The thirst sensation is mediated partly by vasopressin release from the hypothalamus and also via the renin-angiotensin system. When an individual is dehydrated, plasma osmolality increases and volume of the ECF (therefore plasma volume) decreases. As a consequence, the hypothalamic osmoreceptors and stretch receptors in the large vessels are stimulated and vasopressin is released from the hypothalamus. However, the stimuli for vasopressin release as a result of changes in plasma osmolality and plasma volume may override one another. For instance, during haemorrhage the resulting hypovolaemia increases vasopressin release even when the plasma is hypotonic.

FOOD INTAKE

Two hypothalamic centres, namely the feeding centre and the satiety centre, control food intake. Animal studies suggest that the two centres are antagonistic. Electrical stimulation of the feeding centre results in feeding behaviour while stimulation of the satiety centre stops feeding behaviour. It is also suggested that the feeding centre is constantly active and its activity is only temporarily inhibited by the satiety centre after food intake. The level of blood glucose probably controls the activity of the satiety centre. After a meal, blood glucose rises and the satiety centre is activated and inhibits the feeding centre.

BEHAVIOURAL FUNCTIONS

Apart from the functions described above, animal studies suggest that stimulation of or lesions in the hypothalamus lead to significant changes in behaviour. For instance, stimulation in the ventromedial hypothalamus leads to placidity and satiety whereas stimulation in the lateral hypothalamus leads to increased rage, restlessness and fighting behaviours. Stimulation of the extreme anterior and posterior areas of hypothalamus increases sexual drive. Destructive lesions such as tumours usually lead to the opposite effects.

NOCICEPTION AND PAIN

- Pain is defined as an unpleasant emotional and sensory experience associated with actual or potential tissue damage. It is a subjective phenomenon.
- Chronic Pain is defined as pain, which persists even when the noxious stimulus is removed.
- Nociception is a process by which the painful stimulus is conveyed to the brain.

PAIN TRANSMISSION

Nociceptors are the sensory receptors for pain, and are naked nerve endings that exist in almost all tissues of the body. These receptors respond to different type of stimuli, mechanical, thermal or chemical. Chemical stimuli (algogens) can be exogenous (e.g. capsaicin) or endogenous. Endogenous algogens are released when cell membranes are damaged or with inflammation, examples of such substances include bradykinin, H^+, substance P, histamine and K^+ ions. Nociceptors are classified according to their sensitivity to various types of stimuli. Unimodal receptors respond to either mechanical distortion or to heat, and polymodal receptors to mechanical distortion, heat, cold or chemical stimuli. The thermal and mechanical stimuli need to be of sufficient intensity to have the potential to injure skin. For thermal receptors a temperature above 45–50°C is sufficient.

Various receptor subtypes have been isolated:
- Vanilloid receptors. These include VR1 and Vanilloid receptor-like protein (VRL-1). VR1 receptors transduce noxious heat and are expressed exclusively on C fibres. Capsaicin and H^+ ions reduce the threshold of VR1 receptors
- ASIC (acid-sensing ion-channel) receptors, which respond to the low pH of an acidic environment. Some subtypes are mechanosensitive as well
- Purinergic receptors which are stimulated by adenosine and its metabolites

Stimulation of these receptors opens ion channels involving Na^+ and Ca^{2+}. The drug gabapentin acts at Ca^{2+} channels.

Aβ fibres which are myelinated large diameter, fast conducting fibres carry touch sensation. Peripheral pain is transmitted to the CNS by two fibre systems; small myelinated Aδ fibres conduct fast pain, whereas unmyelinated C fibres conduct slow pain. According to gate control theory, pain transmission in the Aδ and C fibres is inhibited by activity in the Aβ fibres (See Figure NE.28). Thus rubbing a painful area relieves the pain.

In the dorsal root ganglia there are large and small diameter cells. Aβ and some of Aδ fibres terminate in the large diameter cells while the C fibres and remaining Aδ fibres terminate in the small diameter cells. The large diameter cells express tyrosine kinase receptors trkB and trkC which have high affinity for brain-derived neurotrophic factor (BDNF) and neurotrophin-3. The small diameter cells are divided into two groups. One group responds to nerve growth factor (NGF) while other group responds to glial cell line-derived neurotrophic factor (GDNF).

The dorsal horn of the spinal cord is divided into various laminae. The small diameter cells terminate in the superficial laminae I and II of the dorsal horn of the spinal cord while the large diameter cells terminate in laminas III and IV. The lamina V is the zone of convergence of both these inputs. The impulses generated by the nociceptor input are then transferred, via the spinothalamic tracts, to the ventral and medial parts of the thalamus and are then transmitted to the sensory cortex. Neurones in the medial thalamus

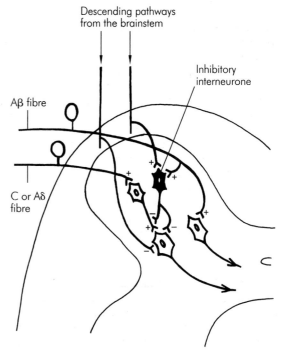

Figure NE.28 'Gating' mechanism

respond specifically to noxious peripheral stimuli. Pathological lesions in the medial thalamus may produce analgesia whereas similar lesions in the sensory cortex do not, although the affective component of pain sensation may be altered.

DESCENDING INHIBITORY PATHWAYS

Descending pathways can act to inhibit pain transmission via the gating mechanism. It has been demonstrated in rats that electrical stimulation in the peri-aqueductal grey (PAG) region of the midbrain produces surgical analgesia sufficient for abdominal operations. In man, electrical stimulation of the anterior hypothalamus and periventricular grey (PVG) areas can also produce effective analgesia. The PAG is believed to be the main descending inhibitory control on the 'gate' mechanism in the dorsal horn. It receives inputs from hypothalamus, thalamus and cortex and delivers several projections which are central to its role in descending inhibition. An important projection goes to the nucleus raphe magnus (NRM) which is situated in the medulla close to the midline. From here, fibres form synaptic connections with the interneurones in the dorsal horn. Another significant descending pathway originates at the locus ceruleus (LC) and also descends to exert an inhibitory influence on the dorsal horn neurones. Figure NE.29 shows a schematic diagram of the pain pathway.

Different neurotransmitters occur in each descending inhibitory pathway; for example, there is an abundance of opioid receptors and neuropeptides (β-endorphin and met-enkephalin) in the PAG region. Met-enkephalin and 5-HT can be found in the NRM mediated pathway. Norepinephrine, on the other hand, is the predominant neurotransmitter in the LC pathway. The clinical implication of this is that a number of different therapeutic agents may be employed to achieve pain control.

NOCICEPTIVE PAIN

Pain can be broadly classified as 'Inflammatory or nociceptive pain' due to tissue damage or inflammation and 'Neuropathic pain' due to primary lesion or dysfunction in the nervous system.

The nervous system is not a hard-wired system but adapts and changes according to its environment. This is called 'plasticity'. The changes in the nervous system are designed to protect the injured part. If these changes persist it can lead to chronic and persistent pain. Allodynia and hyperalgesia are some of the features seen in chronic pain. Allodynia refers to a painful response to a normally non-painful stimulus. In hyperalgesia there is increased response to a normally painful stimulus. Hyperalgesia can be further classified as primary and secondary. Primary hyperalgesia occurs within the zone of tissue injury and is due to changes at the site of injury and secondary hyperalgesia occurs within and around the zone of tissue injury and results from neuroplasticity.

The mechanism of primary hyperalgesia is as follows:

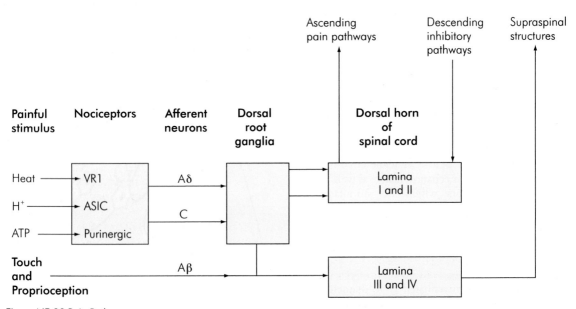

Figure NE.29 Pain Pathway

- Following tissue damage there is release of K^+, H^+ ions, bradykinin, histamine, 5-HT, ATP and nitric oxide. These inflammatory mediators modify the response of primary afferent neurons to subsequent stimuli. This occurs due to changes in either receptor molecules or the voltage gated ion channels.
- Prostaglandins and leukotrienes are also produced through the activation of the arachidonic acid pathways.
- There is recruitment of immune cells that release cytokines and growth factors. NGF is an important growth factor involved in this sensitisation process. It binds to trkA receptors expressed on primary afferent nociceptive neurones and the NGF-trkA complex is internalised and then transported to cell bodies of nociceptors where it regulates further production of neuropeptides like CGRP. NGF also causes mast cells to degranulate further releasing the inflammatory mediators.
- Bradykinin acts on B1 receptors that are expressed during inflammation and contribute to sensitisation of neuron.
- There is altered expression of neuronal Na^+ channels on the nociceptors so the threshold for their stimulation falls.

Secondary hyperalgesia is a different phenomenon, due to neuroplasticity of the neurons of the dorsal horn in response to persistent pain. In response to persistent afferent input the dorsal horn cells show the following changes:

- Increased excitability of dorsal horn cells
- Excitation thresholds of these cells for mechanical stimuli falls and they show increased response to subsequent stimuli
- Expansion of the receptive field size

Glutamate plays a central role in transmission of pain at the dorsal horn of the spinal cord. Under acutely painful conditions glutamate acts via the AMPA receptors. In chronic pain states glutamate also acts via the NMDA receptor. Substance P released by the central terminals of the afferent neurons acts on the neurokinin1 receptor and phosphorylates the NMDA receptor which increases its activity. The NMDA receptors are normally held in a state of physiological block by the presence of Magnesium ions. This block is removed by activation of AMPA receptors by glutamate. Thus there is increased activity of NMDA receptors. Calcium channels linked to NMDA receptors subsequently open, leading to increased intracellular calcium. In addition to substance P there is increased release of BDNF (brain derived neurotrophic factor) at the central terminals of afferent

neurones. All these changes contribute to the neuroplasticity observed at the dorsal horn.

NEUROPATHIC PAIN

Neuropathic pain is initiated by a primary lesion or dysfunction within the nervous system. It is often described as a burning or lancinating type of pain, occurring spontaneously associated with allodynia, hyperalgesia, and hyperpathia which is pain in response to stimulation inspite of sensory impairment in that part. Some of the examples of neuropathic pain are post-herpetic neuralgia, polyneuropathy, central post stroke pain etc. A number of peripheral and central mechanisms have been described for neuropathic pain:

- Following nerve injury there is an increased level of spontaneous and ectopic discharge from the injured nerve. This ectopic activity can be detected in the injured nerve and its surrounding uninjured neurones. This response is due to down regulation of certain types of Na^+ and Ca^{2+} channels.
- Sensory axons from the normal area sprout into the denervated area of the skin. Local release of NGF is responsible for this.
- Abnormal communication develops between the sympathetic nervous system and the sensory nervous system such that increased activity in the sympathetic nervous system leads to increased perception of pain in the sensory nervous system.
- Bradykinin binding sites at the level of dorsal root ganglion are increased.
- There is rewiring of neurones in the dorsal horn of the spinal cord. $A\beta$ fibres carrying touch and proprioception terminate in lamina III and IV of the spinal cord. Following nerve damage they sprout in lamina I and II of the dorsal horn where fibres carrying pain normally terminate. Due to this abnormal communication touch is perceived as very painful.
- There is increased activity of glutamate in the dorsal horn of the spinal cord as discussed earlier with secondary hyperalgesia. Increase in response to C fibre stimulation is seen. This phenomenon is known as 'Wind-up'.
- Opioid sensitivity is reduced, In contrast to nociceptive pain. There is down regulation of opioid receptors at the dorsal root ganglion and an increase in cholecystokinin receptors (CCK_B) at the dorsal horn of the spinal cord. Note that CCK is an opioid antagonist.

SECTION 2: 10
GASTRO-INTESTINAL PHYSIOLOGY

A. Ogilvy

GASTRO-INTESTINAL MOTILITY
Nervous control
Chemical control

MOTILITY CHARACTERISTICS OF THE SPECIALISED REGIONS OF THE GI TRACT
Oesophagus
Gastric motility
Small and large bowel motility

SECRETORY FUNCTIONS OF GASTRO-INTESTINAL TRACT
Salivary glands
Gastric secretion
Pancreatic secretion
Biliary secretion

DIGESTION AND ABSORPTION
Carbohydrate
Protein
Lipid

NAUSEA AND VOMITING
Mechanisms
Post operative nausea and vomiting (PONV)

The primary functions of the gastro-intestinal (GI) tract are the digestion of ingested food, the absorption of water, nutrients, electrolytes and vitamins, and the excretion of indigestible and waste products. The GI tract should not be thought of as a single organ, but a series of organs each with specialised functions. Each section of the GI tract has characteristic motor and secretory properties to accomplish a particular role in the overall function of the gut.

GASTRO-INTESTINAL MOTILITY

Apart from the proximal part of the oesophagus, the GI tract has a remarkably uniform structure consisting of three layers of smooth muscle. These are arranged as an outer longitudinal layer, a middle circular layer and an inner submucosal layer (muscularis mucosa) (Figure GI.1).

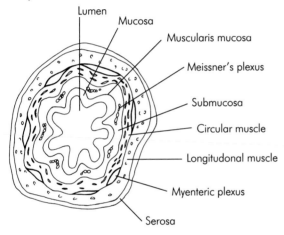

Figure GI.1 Muscle structure of the gastro-intestinal tract

The basic contractile unit of the circular and longitudinal muscle layers is the smooth muscle cell. Across each cell membrane a transmembrane potential of between –40 and –70 mV (negative intracellular charge) is maintained by an ATP-dependent Na$^+$/K$^+$ ATPase pump. In most areas of the GI tract, the transmembrane potential of smooth muscle cells rhythmically depolarises and repolarises, which is called basic electrical rhythm, slow wave activity or electrical control activity (ECA). Gap junctions between individual cells allow transmembrane ionic movements to be conducted from cell to cell. Slow wave activity is conducted along lengths of bowel in a synchronised pattern due to this electrical continuity between cells. Segments of intestine with similar electrical activity, therefore, behave as a functional syncitium.

Contraction of smooth muscle only occurs when the transmembrane potential activity reaches a threshold voltage during slow wave activity. Ion channels in the cell membrane open allowing a rapid influx of sodium and calcium ions with subsequent depolarisation and myocyte contraction. Electrophysiologically, this is recognised as a series of rapid and repeating action potentials known as spikeburst activity (Figure GI.2).

The frequency and amplitude of slow wave activity varies throughout the GI tract and is altered by factors including nervous system control, hormones and pharmacological agents. Inhibition of slow wave activity hyperpolarises the smooth muscle cell membrane and reduces the likelihood of spikeburst activity occurring. Conversely stimulatory factors increase the transmembrane potential towards zero and make contraction more likely.

The relative density of gap junctions between smooth muscle cells is not constant throughout the intestine. In regions of the gut rich in gap junctions (oesophagus, stomach, upper small bowel) slow wave activity is easily conducted in an orderly co-ordinated fashion.

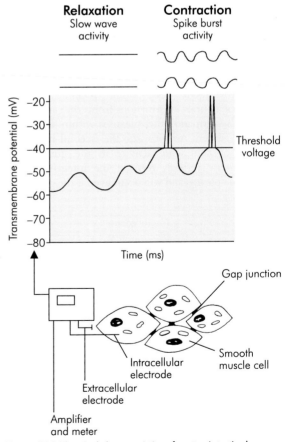

Figure GI.2 Electrical characteristics of gastro-intestinal smooth muscle

However, other areas (e.g. colon) have relatively fewer gap junctions leading to poor intercellular conduction with apparently disorganised and poorly transmitted slow wave activity.

Gut motility is controlled by the nervous and endocrine systems which are illustrated in Figure GI.3. At any one time, different parts of the gut exhibit different patterns of motility that are due the integration of several different signals from the nervous and endocrine systems.

NERVOUS CONTROL

Neurological control of intestinal motility is modulated by intrinsic and extrinsic nervous systems.

The intrinsic (enteric) nervous system is a complicated latticework of neurons within the bowel wall. It contains nearly as many neurones as the CNS and is organised into a number of plexuses and ganglia, which contain the cell bodies. The most important intrinsic plexus regarding control of bowel motility is the myenteric (Auerbach's) plexus that lies between the longitudinal and circular muscle layers. Neurones within the myenteric plexus are classified as cholinergic (stimulatory), adrenergic (inhibitory) and non adrenergic-non cholinergic (NANC) inhibitory neurons. Neurotransmitters in the last group include substance P, vasoactive intestinal polypeptide (VIP) and nitric oxide (NO). The myenteric plexus integrates neural information from the autonomic nervous system and other plexuses within the enteric nervous system to provide the second-by-second control of contractile activity in the gut. Several enteroenteric reflexes rely on the integrity of the myenteric plexus, and will occur even if the gut has no extrinsic nerve supply. The classic example is the peristaltic reflex where stretching of a segment of bowel by a bolus of food leads to proximal contraction (cholinergic) and distal relaxation (NANC) causing propulsion of the bolus in a distal direction. It is unlikely that this reflex is important in the normal propulsion of chyme through the bowel, but it neatly demonstrates the circuitry of the enteric nervous system (Figure GI.4).

Extrinsic nervous control of intestinal motility is through the somatic (voluntary) and autonomic (involuntary) nervous systems, which includes sympathetic and parasympathetic fibres.

Voluntary control of GI motility only occurs in the pharynx during the initial stages of swallowing and at the anus during defaecation.

Parasympathetic innervation of the oesophagus, stomach, small intestine and first half of the colon is by the vagus nerve. The pelvic parasympathetic fibres from the second, third and fourth sacral segments supply the rest of the colon, rectum and anus. These are pre-ganglionic fibres that synapse within the enteric nerve plexuses and have both inhibitory and stimulatory actions within the gut. Sympathetic innervation of the gut arises from the spinal cord between T 5 and L 3. Pre-ganglionic fibres pass through the paravertebral ganglia without synapsing to form the splanchnic nerves which then synapse at the superior, middle and inferior pre-vertebral mesenteric plexuses. Post ganglionic fibres run with the mesenteric vessels supplying all areas of the gut where they terminate in the enteric nervous system.

CHEMICAL CONTROL

Chemical mediators affecting GI motility may be

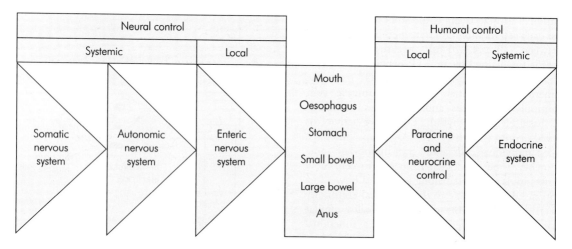

Figure GI.3 Control of gastro-intestinal motility

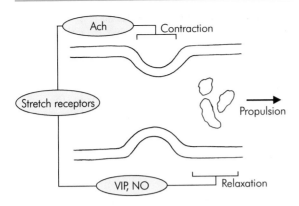

Figure GI.4 Mechanism of peristalsis

released locally from nerve endings (neurocrine), from endocrine or inflammatory cells within the gut wall (paracrine), or from endocrine glands remote from their site of action (endocrine). Figure GI.5 summarises the effects of some of the common mediators on GI motility.

It is somewhat artificial to consider the control mechanisms individually because in the intact intestine several control systems, both neuronal and chemical, operate simultaneously. In addition, they often have complementary effects on the secretary functions of the intestine which are closely coupled to its contractile state at any one time.

MOTILITY CHARACTERISTICS OF SPECIALISED REGIONS OF THE GI TRACT

OESOPHAGUS

The adult oesophagus is about 30 cm long. Its main functions are to transmit boluses of food and liquid from the mouth to the stomach and to prevent reflux of gastric contents out of the stomach.

The anatomy of the oesophagus is similar to the rest of the GI tract except that the upper 6 cm consists of striated skeletal muscle. The rest of the oesophagus is smooth muscle but has no slow wave activity and, therefore, has no spontaneous contractile activity.

The oesophagus has two sphincters, upper and a lower. The upper oesophageal sphincter (UOS) at the level of the fifth and sixth cervical vertebrae, consists of the cricopharyngeal and pharyngeal constrictor muscles. It is supplied by branches of the vagus nerve and is usually in a state of tonic contraction to prevent entrainment of air during respiration.

The lower oesophageal sphincter (LOS) is functionally a zone of increased intraluminal pressure (15–25 mmHg) in the lower 2–4 cm of the oesophagus. Macroscopically this area of smooth muscle is indistinguishable from the rest of the oesophagus. Electrophysiologically, the smooth muscle of the LOS displays continuous spike burst activity and, therefore, the sphincter is usually closed to prevent reflux of gastric contents into the oesophagus. During swallowing the LOS relaxes before a peristaltic wave, but quickly constricts again after a food bolus has entered the stomach. **Barrier pressure** is the pressure difference between that exerted by the LOS and the intragastric pressure. Any decrease in LOS or increase in intragastric pressure will reduce barrier pressure and make reflux more likely. Factors effecting LOS pressure and hence barrier pressure are listed in Figure GI.6. The flutter-valve action of the oesophagus below the diaphragm also helps to prevent reflux whenever the intragastric pressure is increased.

FACTORS AFFECTING GI MOTILITY				
Factor	Gastric Motility	Gastric Emptying	Intestinal Motility	Gallbladder Emptying
Gastrin	Increased	Decreased	Increased	—
Cholecystokinin (CCK)	Increased	Decreased	Increased	Increased
Secretin (augments CCK)	Increased	Decreased	Decreased	Increased
Gastric Inhibitory Peptide*	Increased	Decreased	—	—
Motilin	Increased	Increased	Increased	—
Somatostatin	Decreased	Decreased	Decreased	Decreased

* also called glucose-dependent insulinotrophic polypeptide

Figure GI.5

FACTORS AFFECTING LOWER OESOPHAGEAL SPHINCTER TONE

Increased Tone	Decreased Tone
Cholinergic stimulation	Cholinergic inhibition
Dopaminergic inhibition	Dopaminergic stimulation
Histamine	Oestrogen
α adrenergic stimulation	α adrenergic inhibition
β adrenergic blockade	β adrenergic stimulation
Gastrin	Cholecystokinin
Motilin	Secretin
Prostaglandin F$_2$	Prostaglandin E$_1$

Figure GI.6

Swallowing

Swallowing is a motor reflex that transmits food from the mouth to the stomach. It is controlled by the deglutination centre in the reticular formation and is divided into voluntary, a pharyngeal and oesophageal stages.

In the voluntary stage, masticated food is voluntarily squeezed into the pharynx by upward and backward pressure of the tongue against the hard palate. This initiates a reflex arc that begins with the pharyngeal stage of swallowing.

The soft palate is elevated to close off the nasopharynx and the palatopharyngeal folds are pulled into the midline forming a narrow slit through which boluses of food must pass. The upper airway is protected by the vocal cords closing and by an upward and anterior movement of the hyoid and larynx, which allow the epiglottis to cover the larynx. The upper oesophageal sphincter relaxes and the superior constrictor muscle of the pharynx begins a wave of contraction that passes down through the middle and inferior constrictors and into the oesophagus. The pharyngeal stage lasts about 1–2 s during which time respiration is temporarily halted.

The peristaltic wave started in the pharyngeal stage, known as primary peristalsis, progresses along the oesophagus preceded by a wave of relaxation aiding the movement of food down the oesophagus. It normally takes 8–10 s to complete a single swallow. If primary peristalsis fails, a secondary wave of peristalsis (secondary peristalsis) is generated within the oesophagus by stimulation of stretch receptors.

NERVOUS CONTROL OF SWALLOWING

Swallowing is a reflex arc with an afferent and efferent limb. Once initiated it cannot be interrupted or terminated. Afferent impulses from the pharynx are transmitted via the trigeminal and vagus nerves to the tractus solitarius. Afferent nerves from the upper middle and lower oesophagus run in the superior laryngeal, recurrent laryngeal and vagus nerves to converge in the tractus solitarius. Efferent motor signals are transmitted by the vagus, trigeminal, facial and spinal accessory nerves.

GASTRIC MOTILITY

Functionally the stomach has a proximal portion, the gastric fundus and upper one-third of the corpus, and a distal portion which is the lower two-thirds of the corpus and the antrum.

The proximal stomach stores ingested food and controls intragastric pressure that is important for controlling the rate of gastric emptying for fluids. During a swallow, the fundus relaxes (receptive relaxation) to prevent large increases in intragastric pressure during a meal. The proximal stomach has no phasic contractile activity because there is no slow wave activity. Instead, muscle activity consists of prolonged tonic contractions lasting between 1 and 6 min, which allows stored food in the proximal stomach to be gradually released into the distal stomach for digestion.

The distal portion of the stomach mixes food with gastric juices and grinds it down to a fine paste called chyme. The smooth muscle cells in the distal stomach exhibit slow wave activity with a resting membrane potential of between –50 and –60 mV. Towards the antrum and pylorus the smooth muscle cells are more polarised with less frequent slow wave activity. Owing to the abundance of gap junctions between the cells, the corpus acts as the pacemaker region of the stomach whereby slow wave activity is propagated distally in an orderly fashion.

The contractile status of the stomach alters between the 'fed' and 'fasted' state. For several hours after a meal, rings of peristalsis are generated every 15–20 s in the pacemaker centre on the greater curve and sweep down to the pylorus, mixing ingested food with digestive enzymes. The pylorus contracts in concert with the peristaltic waves of the distal stomach to prevent undigested stomach contents entering the duodenum. Food particles are squeezed down the walls of the stomach towards the pylorus and then return in an eddy current to a more proximal region of the stomach. The pylorus does not close completely during a contraction and food particles that are < 1 mm in diameter can pass through into the duodenum during a contraction. Indigestible particles, such as vegetable fibre, are too large to pass through the pylorus and are removed during the fasted state when the contractile characteristics of the stomach change.

The fasted state begins when the majority of the stomach contents reach the caecum. During fasting, the stomach and small bowel exhibit a regular and co-ordinated progressive contraction known as the interdigestive migratory motor complex (MMC). Usually this migratory contraction occurs every 90–120 min and starts in the antrum of the stomach. It then progresses down the small bowel at 6–8 cm/min. This specialised contraction probably acts as a 'house-keeper', periodically sweeping undigested contents, sloughed mucosa, secretions and bacteria along the intestine in a distal direction.

Control of gastric motility and emptying

The rate at which chyme is released from the stomach into the duodenum is carefully controlled so that the small bowel is presented with partially digested material at the optimum rate to allow further digestive and absorption processes to occur. Several factors affect the tone of the proximal stomach. The activity of the distal stomach and the tone of the pylorus are particularly important in controlling the mixing of gastric contents, and the rate of gastric emptying. The overall integration of these inputs determines the rate of gastric emptying. Although the exact mechanisms that control gastric motility are incompletely understood, it is clear both neuronal and hormonal factors are important (Figure GI.7).

The regulation of the fasting MMC is incompletely understood but motilin, a 22 amino acid peptide released from the duodenal mucosa, is thought to be an important stimulus. Both stomach and duodenal smooth muscle have receptors for motilin that produce an increase in proximal stomach tone, initiation of the MMC and relaxation of the pylorus.

The 'fed' pattern of gastric motility is triggered by the sight or smell of food, the ingestion of food or gastric distension. The duration of the fed pattern of motility depends on the nutrient content of the stomach and is longer after fatty meals. Liquidised meals induce infrequent low amplitude antral contractions, whereas solid material produces frequent high amplitude contractions to aid breakdown into smaller more digestible particles.

The rate of gastric emptying is controlled by central and peripheral mechanisms. Pain, anxiety and stress reduce gastric emptying by activation of the sympathetic nervous system. Peripheral mechanisms include both neuronal and hormonal mechanisms activated in the stomach and small bowel. Distension of the stomach leads to the release of gastrin and stimulation of vagal and local enteric reflexes. The sum effect of these responses is an increase in the secretion of gastric acid and an increase in antral peristaltic activity, thereby increasing the production of chyme.

The composition of chyme entering the duodenum has an important regulatory role in the control of gastric emptying. Receptors within the duodenum are activated by stretch, increasing acidity or osmolarity, and large concentrations of fatty or amino acids (which indicate that stomach emptying is occurring too

EFFECTS OF HORMONES ON GASTRIC MOTILITY

Hormone	Proximal stomach	Distal stomach	Pylorus	Effect
Gastrin	↓ tone	↑ frequency of pacemaker and amplitude	Constricts	↑ peristalsis and chyme production
Cholecystokinin	↓ tone	↑ frequency of pacemaker and amplitude	Constricts	↑ peristalsis and chyme production
Motilin	↑ tone	MMC activity	Relaxes	↑ gastric emptying in fasted state
Gastric inhibitory peptide	No effect	↓ frequency of pacemaker	Constricts	Decreased emptying

Figure GI.7

rapidly). Receptor activation initiates reflex arcs that reduce gastric emptying and include, vago-vagal and local enteric inhibitory reflexes as well as the release of several inhibitory peptides which act on receptors in the stomach.

If small bowel contents rich in fat reach the ileum, an inhibitory reflex termed the ileal brake occurs whereby gastric emptying, pancreatic secretion and small bowel transit are all reduced to improve further digestion and absorption. This is another hormonally mediated reflex probably involving neurotensin and enteroglucagon.

SMALL AND LARGE BOWEL MOTILITY

The small bowel is about 5 m long in the adult. It has specialised contractile properties to promote the digestion of food, the absorption of nutrients and propulsion of non digested material along its lumen. Slow wave activity is present throughout the small bowel but the duodenum acts as the pacemaker. Transit times for intestinal contents are more rapid in the proximal small bowel due to the higher density of gap junctions compared with the distal small bowel. Contractile activity of the small bowel is categorised into several types of contraction (Figure GI.8).

On average, transit of intestinal contents through the large bowel on average takes 33 H. The colon is important for the absorption of water and electrolytes from the chyme, fermentation of complex carbohydrates by colonic bacteria and the storage of faeces until a convenient time arises for defaecation.

CONTRACTILE ACTIVITY OF SMALL AND LARGE BOWEL	
Small Bowel	
Interdigestive migratory motor complex	Similar waveform to gastric MMC acting as 'housekeeper' to the small bowel. Takes 2 hours to traverse small bowel
Migratory Clustered Contractions	Highly propulsive contractions over 10 to 30 cm of bowel. Prominent in terminal ileum to propel viscous contents into caecum
Retrograde Giant Contractions	Empty upper small bowel contents into stomach prior to vomiting
Giant Migrating Contractions	Infrequent large amplitude long duration contractions in the terminal ileum to return refluxed faecal contents into the ileum. Increased in some disease states
Large Bowel	
Individual phasic contractions (long and short duration).	Mix and knead faecal contents. Poorly co-ordinated with little propulsive action. Two to thirteen short duration and up to two long contractions per minute
Organised groups of contractions	Periodic co-ordinated peristaltic wave passing along length of colon. Not related to fed or fasted state
Ultrapropulsive contractions	Occur once or twice a day. Responsible for mass movement of faeces in colon and rectum
Defaecation	Distension of rectum by faeces produces reflex relaxation of internal anal sphincter (rectosphincteric reflex) followed by reflex contraction of descending and sigmoid colon

Figure GI.8

The contractile properties of the colon are designed to mix the semi-solid chyme to allow adequate contact with the colonic mucosa, slowly to propel it along the colon and at certain times to produce mass movements of faeces, e.g. during defaecation.

SECRETORY FUNCTIONS OF THE GASTRO-INTESTINAL TRACT

Figure GI.9 gives an overview of the composition of fluids secreted into the GI tract.

COMPOSITION OF GASTRO-INTESTINAL SECRETIONS

	Daily volume secreted	Electrolyte content (low-high secretion rates)	Enzyme content
Saliva	1000–1500 ml pH 6.0–7.0	Na^+ 40–140 mmol/l K^+ 40 mmol/l HCO_3^- 40–80 mmol/l	Amylase Lipase Mucus Lactoferrin IgA Lysozyme
Gastric secretion	1500–2500 ml pH 1–3.5	Na^+ 100–150 mmol/l K^+ 10–20 mmol/l H^+ 20–130 mmol/l Cl^- 20–160 mmol/l	Pepsin Lipase Mucus Intrinsic factor
Pancreatic secretion	1000–1500 ml pH 8.0–8.3	Na^+ 150 mmol/l K^+ 5 mmol/l HCO_3^- 40–115 mmol/l Cl^- 110–30 mmol/l	Trypsin Chymotrypsin Elastase Carboxypeptidase A and B lipase Amylase Ribonuclease Deoxyribonuclease Phospholipase A_2
Bile	700–1200 ml pH 7–8	Na^+ 130–140 mmol/l K^+ 5–12 mmol/l HCO_3^- 10–28 mmol/l Cl^- 25–100 mmol/l Ca^{2+} 5–23 mmol/l	Bile pigments Bile salts Cholesterol Inorganic salts Fatty acids Lecithin Fat
Small bowel secretion	1800 ml pH 7–8	Concentrations from proximal to distal small bowel Na^+ 140–125 mmol/l Cl^- 110–60 mmol/l K^+ 5–9 mmol/l HCO_3^- 100–74 mmol/l	Mucus Peptidases Lipase Sucrase Maltase Isomaltase Lactase
Large bowel secretion	200 ml pH 7–8	Na^+ 40 mmol/l K^+ 90 mmol/l Cl^- 15 mmol/l HCO_3^- 40 mmol/l	

Figure GI.9

SALIVARY GLANDS

The three paired salivary glands produce between 0.5 and 1.5 litres saliva a day, which consists of water, mucus, digestive enzymes, sodium chloride, potassium, chloride and bicarbonate. The parotid and submandibular glands secrete about 90% of the total volume of saliva.

The electrolyte composition of saliva varies with flow rates. Salivary potassium concentrations are 20 times those of the plasma at low flow rates but decrease at higher rates. Bicarbonate secretion increases at higher flow rates to produce alkaline saliva. Sodium and chloride concentrations are always less than plasma levels but increase at higher flow rates. The functions of saliva are:

- Lubrication to aid swallowing and speech
- Buffering and dilution of irritants
- Antibacterial/anti-viral properties due to secretion of lysozyme, lactoferrin and IgA
- Digestion of starch by salivary amylase (optimal pH 7.0, therefore, inactivated in the stomach)
- Digestion of fats by salivary lipase (not pH-dependent)

The rate of saliva secretion is entirely controlled by the autonomic nervous system although anti-diuretic hormone and aldosterone can modify its electrolytic content by decreasing sodium and increasing potassium secretion. Both parasympathetic and sympathetic stimulation produce in increase in salivary gland secretion although the sympathetic response is less pronounced. Parasympathetic fibres release acetylcholine, which binds to muscarinic receptors with subsequent activation of inositol triphosphate and calcium ion release. Norepinephrine released by sympathetic fibres acts via the cAMP pathway. The common response of the salivary gland is an increase in production and secretion of saliva and local vasodilation.

GASTRIC SECRETION

The stomach secretes about 1.2–2.5 litres gastric juice a day with a pH between 1 and 3.5. The stomach contains principally two type of secretory gland: oxyntic and pyloric. The oxyntic glands are tubular pits of mucosa located all over the gastric mucosa except the lesser curve and are lined by three different types of cell: chief cells that secrete pepsinogen, mucus cells that secrete mucus and oxyntic (parietal cells) that secrete acid. Pyloric glands are in the pyloric region of the stomach and contain G-cells that secrete the hormone gastrin and mucus cells.

Hydrochloric acid secretion (parietal cells)

Gastric acid aids protein digestion, activates pepsin, has anti-bacterial actions and stimulates biliary and pancreatic secretions in the duodenum. A simplified diagram of acid production by parietal cells is given in Figure GI.10.

Gastrin, acetyl choline and histamine stimulate gastric acid secretion by binding to specific receptors on the basolateral membrane of the parietal cell, with subsequent activation of intracellular second messenger systems. The final common pathway is an increase in protein phosphorylation and activation of ATP-dependent H^+/K^+ pump, which is summarised in Figure GI.11.

Pepsinogen secretion (chief cells)

Pepsinogens are secreted mainly by chief cells and are converted to the active enzyme pepsin by gastric acid. There are eight types of pepsinogen that are classified depending on the optimal pH for their activation. In normal health, 85% of pepsin secreted is pepsin 3. Pepsinogens are stored in secretory granules within the chief cells, which when stimulated fuse with the apical membrane to release the pepsinogens. In general, stimuli that activate acid secretion also stimulate pepsin secretion.

Mucus secretion

Mucus is secreted throughout the GI tract where it coats and lubricates food particles, protects epithelial surfaces from digestive enzymes and has a small buffering capacity against acid or alkalis. It is also important in the formation of solid faeces by its binding action on faecal particles.

In the stomach mucus is secreted by mucus cells covering the entire mucosa as well as from the pyloric glands in the antrum. Mucus consists of 70% water,

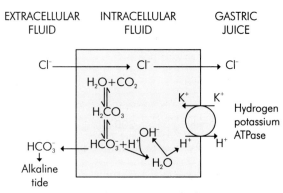

Figure GI.10 Acid production in parietal cells

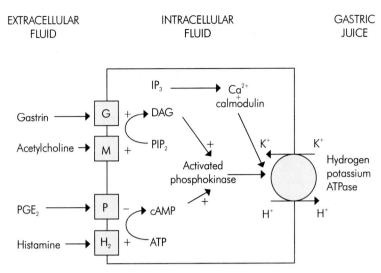

Figure GI.11 Modulators of gastric acid production

electrolytes, sloughed cells and complex glycoproteins called mucins which are important for the viscous and gel-forming properties of mucus. In the normal stomach, the epithelium is covered by a 0.2–0.6-mm layer of viscous mucus which is continually eroded away by the action of pepsins and replaced by newly secreted mucus. Cholinergic stimulation results in an increase in mucus secretion by mobilisation of intracellular calcium. Prostaglandin E_2 stimulates the production of mucus by a cAMP-mediated pathway.

Bicarbonate secretion

Gastric secretion of bicarbonate accounts for about 5–10% of total gastric secretions. Secretion is both an active and passive process and requires the presence of intraluminal chloride with which it is exchanged. Bicarbonate alone would be an ineffectual epithelial defence against intraluminal acid; however, in combination with mucus it provides improves the buffering capacity of mucus. In the stomach this mucus-bicarbonate layer is only effective at pH > 1.5 and is considered as a weak first line defence. In the duodenum it is a more important mechanism in preventing villous injury.

Intrinsic factor

Intrinsic factor is a mucoprotein essential for the absorption of vitamin B_{12}. It is secreted by parietal cells in the stomach and forms a complex with the vitamin which is actively absorbed in the distal ileum.

Control of gastric secretion

Following a meal there is a rapid increase in gastric secretion which normally peaks after 30 min to 1 H. Gastric secretion is divided into three stages: cephalic and gastric stages which are stimulatory and the intestinal stage which is inhibitory.

The cephalic stage commences even before food enters the stomach and causes increased gastric secretion in response to the sight, smell, taste or thought of food by vagal stimulation of oxyntic glands. Vagal stimulation of gastrin producing cells in the pylorus (G cells) leads to an increase in gastrin production which then stimulates further gastric acid production.

The gastric stage begins when food enters the stomach. Gastric distension and an increase in luminal peptides promote the release of gastrin. Secretion of acid ceases when the pH of stomach contents reaches 2.0 to allow the optimum conditions for pepsin activity whereas > pH 3.5 acid secretion recommences.

Gastric secretion usually declines about one hour after eating due to a decrease in the stimulatory factors and an increase in the inhibitory factors controlling gastric secretion which include:

• Distension of the duodenum, or the presence of acid, lipids or carbohydrate in the upper small bowel reducing gastric secretion and stomach emptying by entero-gastric reflex
• Cholecystokinin released from the duodenum in response to an increase in the fat, protein or carbohydrate content will antagonise the effects of gastrin, decrease gastric tone, stimulate gallbladder contraction and pancreatic secretion and augment the effects of the hormone secretin
• Other hormones may be released in response to

nutrients in the small bowel including gastric inhibitory peptide, secretin, neurotensin and enteroglucagon, all of which reduce gastric secretion

PANCREATIC SECRETION

The pancreas is a complex alveolar gland similar in structure to salivary glands with acini draining into small ductules which then drain into larger ducts and finally the main pancreatic duct. The pancreas has a huge functional reserve where up to 80% of pancreatic tissue can be removed with no effect on digestion. Normally the pancreas produces about 1500 ml a day of alkaline fluid (pH 8.0), which consists of digestive enzymes secreted by the acina and bicarbonate produced by the epithelial cells of the ducts.

Pancreatic enzymes are synthesised as inactive pro-enzymes and stored in secretory granules in the acina. The following enzymatic processes occur:

- Trypsinogen is converted to active trypsin in the duodenum by the presence of enteropeptidase (enterokinase) released from duodenal epithelium, and by the presence of previously activated trypsin. Trypsin is the predominant enzyme produced by the pancreas and splits ingested proteins into smaller peptide chains and activates most of the pro-enzymes secreted by the pancreas
- Chymotrypsinogen is converted to chymotrypsin by trypsin in the small bowel and has a similar action to trypsin
- Carboxypeptidase cleaves carboxyl groups from peptides to produce free amino acids
- Ribonuclease and deoxyribonuclease split ribonucleic and deoxyribonucleic acids
- Fat is digested by pancreatic lipase, which converts it into fatty acids and monoglycerides, cholesterol esterase which hydrolyses esters and phospholipase which cleaves phospholipids into fatty acids
- Pancreatic amylase hydrolyses starch, and other carbohydrates into tri- and disaccharides
- Bicarbonate and water are secreted entirely by the epithelial cells of the pancreatic ducts

Other electrolytes secreted by the pancreas include zinc, magnesium and calcium in small amounts although their functional significance is unknown.

Control of pancreatic secretion

Pancreatic secretion fluctuates throughout the day. Following a meal production of pancreatic fluid increases and during fasting secretion is dormant except during an interdigestive MMC, when secretion temporarily increases. The dietary content of ingested food determines the magnitude and duration of the pancreatic response to a meal. Intestinal fats and proteins are the main stimuli for pancreatic secretion and produce the biggest response (carbohydrates induce only a weak pancreatic response). Calcium and magnesium are also stimuli for pancreatic secretion and alcohol may have both inhibitory or stimulatory effects.

Two hormones are responsible for stimulating pancreatic secretion, secretin and cholecystokinin.

- Secretin is released from S cells in the upper small intestine in response to a reduction in duodenal pH < 4.5. Its main effect is stimulation of the ductile systems of the pancreas to produce large volumes of fluid rich in bicarbonate but low in chloride. Bicarbonate neutralises acid in the small bowel protects intestinal mucosa and provides the optimal pH for the activation of pancreatic enzymes.
- Cholecystokinin released from duodenal mucosa in response to duodenal amino acids, peptides and fats stimulates the release of pancreatic enzymes from acina cells. It also augments the actions of secretin on the ductal epithelium.

Several neuronal reflexes are also important in the control of pancreatic secretion. These include a cephalic phase of pancreatic secretion mediated by the vagus nerve. In addition, several enteropancreatic reflexes are probably involved in initiating pancreatic secretion in response to nutrients in the small bowel.

Little is known of the inhibitory control of pancreatic secretion. Glucagon secretion, which increases in the post prandial state, may have an influence, as might somatostatin and vaso active intestinal polypeptide (VIP). The presence of intraluminal pancreatic enzymes may have a negative feedback effect by reducing the release of cholecystokinin.

BILIARY SECRETION

The liver produces between 700 and 1200 ml bile a day of which between 30 and 60 ml can be stored and concentrated in the gallbladder. Bile is a complex mixture of water, bile salts, pigments and other organic and inorganic compounds.

Bile salts are synthesised in the liver by the conversion of cholesterol to the bile acids, cholic and deoxycholic acid. These are then conjugated with glycine and taurine to form bile salts that are secreted in the bile. Over 94% of bile salts secreted by the biliary system are actively re-absorbed in the distal ileum and re-excreted as bile in the liver. This enterohepatic circulation of bile salts is an important mechanism in maintaining an adequate concentration of bile salts in the upper small necessary for adequate digestion. Approximately 24 g bile salts are required a day for the complete digestion and absorption of fat. As the total body reserves of bile salts is only 6 g and the daily synthesis of bile salts is 0.5 g, the importance of the enterohepatic circulation can be appreciated (Figure GI.12).

Bile salts emulsify fatty globules in the small bowel by decreasing their surface tension, thereby breaking them down into smaller particles. They then bind with fats to form micelles that are readily absorbed in the small bowel. The fat-soluble vitamins A, D, E and K indirectly rely on this mechanism for absorption.

The colour of bile is due to the presence of bile pigments (mainly bilirubin) formed from the breakdown products of haemoglobin. Bile pigments have no role in the digestion of fat but are responsible for the normal colour of faeces and urine.

Control of biliary secretion

The secretion of bile into the duodenum varies throughout the day. During fasting, the smooth muscle of the gallbladder and biliary tree exhibits activity similar to the interdigestive MMC seen in the GI tract. Approximately every 2 H a contraction of the gallbladder expresses about 10 ml bile into the duodenum in the fasted individual.

Gallbladder contraction within a few minutes of starting eating and bile output reaches a maximum at

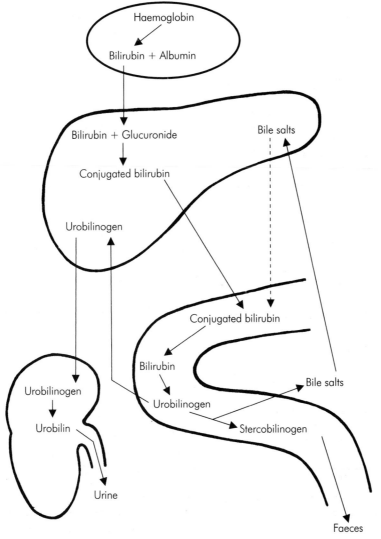

Figure GI.12 Physiology of bile

about 1 H after ingestion of food. Thereafter it reaches a plateau and remains constant until gastric emptying has been completed. The initial rise is due to gallbladder contraction that empties about two-thirds of the bile stored. Thereafter, during the plateau phase there is a constant secretion of bile by the liver that bypasses the gallbladder and enters the small bowel through a relaxed sphincter of Oddi. Owing to the enterohepatic circulation, it is estimated that the total pool of bile salts is re-circulated two-to-three times every meal.

The initial gallbladder contraction in response to a meal is vagally mediated. There are also enteric nervous system reflexes that stimulate gallbladder contraction in response to gastric distension. Biliary secretion is affected by the following factors:

- Cholecystokinin is the main hormone controlling biliary secretion. The presence of intraluminal fat in the duodenum stimulates the release of cholecystokinin which causes relaxation of the sphincter of Oddi and gallbladder contraction
- Biliary secretion is also stimulated by increasing concentrations of bile salts returning to the liver in the portal circulation which occurs in the post prandial phase due to the enterohepatic circulation
- Secretin released in response to acid in the duodenum increases the production of watery alkaline bile and probably augments the action of cholecystokinin

DIGESTION AND ABSORPTION

Digestion is the chemical breakdown of ingested food by GI enzymes into substances that can then be absorbed from the intestines into the systemic circulation. The organ principally responsible for these functions is the small intestine, although some digestion and absorption may occur in the mouth and stomach.

CARBOHYDRATE

The small bowel can only absorb the carbohydrates glucose, fructose and galactose. Therefore, all dietary carbohydrate must be broken down to one of these monosaccharides. Cellulose is a complex polysaccharide with β-glucose linkages, the human does not possess enzymes capable of breaking these linkages and, therefore, is indigestible and forms dietary fibre.

Starch is broken down to oligo- and disaccharides by salivary and pancreatic amylase. Small bowel brush border enzymes cleave larger sugars to

monosaccharides, which can then be absorbed. The functional reserve of the enzymes involved in carbohydrate digestion is such that the digestive tract can handle huge carbohydrate loads and still achieve complete hydrolysis by the proximal jejunum. Detail of carbohydrate absorption is shown in Figure GI.13.

PROTEIN

Ingested proteins are broken down by digestive enzymes to free amino acids and small di- and tripeptides in the stomach by pepsin, and in the small bowel by pancreatic peptidases. Pancreatic peptidases are either endopeptidases (trypsin, chymotrypsin, elastase) that hydrolyse interior peptide bonds or exopeptidases (carboxypeptidase) which hydrolyse external peptide bonds. The individual peptidases differ in their ability to cleave peptide bonds containing different classes of amino acid, e.g. neutral or basic, aromatic or aliphatic. The pancreatic peptidases are rapidly inactivated in the duodenum by trypsin. Free amino acids, monopeptides and dipeptides are absorbed by epithelial cells of the small intestine and the remaining larger peptides further hydrolysed by brush border peptidases to smaller peptides with subsequent absorption. Detail of protein absorption is shown in Figure GI.14.

LIPID

Of dietary fat, 90% is triglyceride with the remainder consisting of phospholipids, cholesterol and cholesterol esters, and fat-soluble vitamins (A, D, E, K). Lingual lipase and pancreatic lipase hydrolyse triglycerides to free fatty acids and monoglycerides.

In combination with bile salts, free fatty acids, glycerides and cholesterol form micelles that fuse with the unstirred layer of the intestinal epithelium to allow the absorption of fats. Phospholipids are metabolised by pancreatic phospholipase A_2 to free fatty acids and lysophospholipids which are taken up into micelles.

In the intestinal epithelial cell the free fatty acid and monoglycerides are re-constituted back into triglycerides, which are then incorporated into large lipoproteins called chylos. These consist of a hydrophobic core of triglycerides, cholesterol esters and fat-soluble vitamins surrounded by a hydrophilic shell of phospholipid, free cholesterol and protein (synthesised by the rough endoplasmic reticulum as apoprotein). The chylos enter the extracellular fluid by pinocytosis and enter the circulation via the lymphatic system.

The absorption of the fat-soluble vitamins A, D, E and

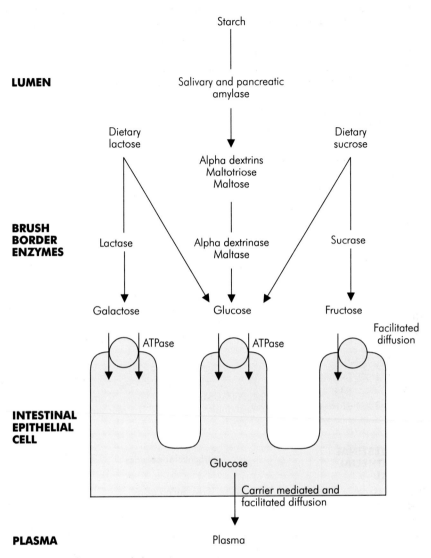

Figure GI.13 Carbohydrate digestion and absorption

K depends on micelle uptake. With regard to the absorption of water-soluble vitamins:

- Thiamine (B_1) is absorbed in the jejunum by sodium-dependent active transport
- Vitamin C is absorbed by both active and passive processes in the small bowel
- Folic acid is actively absorbed from the whole small intestine
- Vitamin B_{12} requires intrinsic factor for absorption. Initially, the vitamin combines with glycoprotein (R protein) in the stomach. The combination is then digested in the duodenum by peptidases to release the free vitamin, which then binds to intrinsic factor. In the terminal ileum the complex is finally absorbed probably by pinocytosis

Detail of lipid absorption is shown in Figure GI.15.

Sodium and chloride re-absorption

The intestine re-absorbs between 25 and 35 g sodium a day, which accounts for about 15% of the total body sodium. Most of this sodium is from intestinal secretions with dietary sodium contributing about 5–8 g. Chloride ions are absorbed through out the intestine especially the colon.

Water absorption

Dietary fluid and intestinal secretions account for 7.5–10 litres water handled by the intestine per day. Of this, only 200 ml is excreted in the faeces daily, the

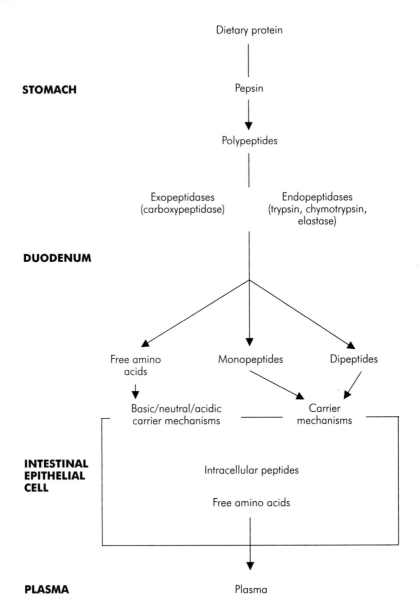

Figure GI.14 Protein digestion and absorption

majority being re-absorbed in the small intestine and about 400 ml in the colon.

Water absorption can be regulated to some extent by the autonomic nervous system by its effects of sodium and chloride absorption. Sympathetic stimulation or cholinergic inhibition leads to an increase in sodium and water absorption. In addition to its renal effects, the mineralocorticoid aldosterone also has effects on sodium and water absorption in the intestine, particularly the colon. Aldosterone increases the number of sodium channels on the epithelium and the number of Na^+/K^+ pumps on the basolateral membrane, therefore, increasing sodium and water absorption.

Iron absorption

Iron is primarily absorbed in the duodenum and jejunum either as haem (derived from meat) or as free iron. Absorption is related to the total body iron stores and normally the amount absorbed is a small fraction of the amount ingested. Haem is absorbed by pinocytosis and broken down to free iron within the enterocyte.

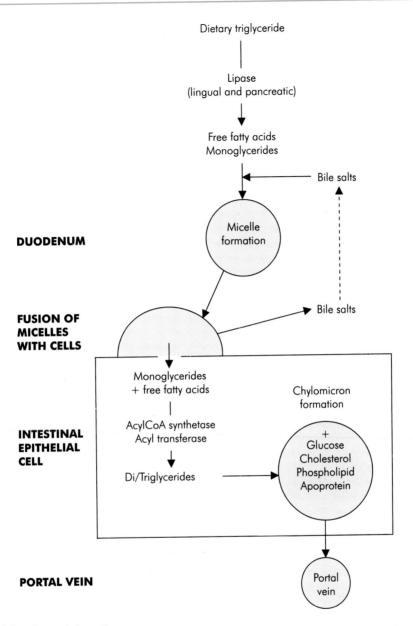

Figure GI.15 Lipid digestion and absorption

Free iron is absorbed using a specific receptor and once inside the cell it binds with a specific protein, apoferritin, to form ferritin, an intracellular storage complex for iron. Most iron in the form of ferritin is lost in the normal sloughing of epithelial cells. Ferritin-bound iron enters the circulation by cleaving from ferritin and then binding to a intracellular transport protein which then crosses the basal membrane to release iron into the circulation where it is bound to a β_1-globulin, transferrin. Iron absorption increases if total body iron is reduced by increasing the number of iron receptors in the intestine, and by increasing the amount of the intracellular carrier protein. Iron absorption is summarised in Figure GI.16.

Calcium absorption

Calcium absorption occurs mainly in the duodenum and is regulated by the hormone 1,25-dihydroxycholecalciferol, synthesised from vitamin D (cholecalciferol) in a series of steps occurring in the skin, liver and kidneys. The action of 1,25-

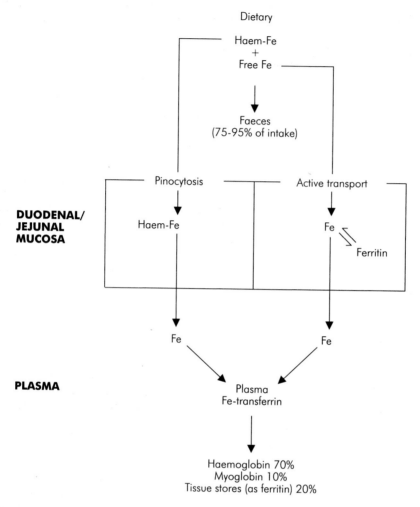

Figure GI.16 Iron absorption

dihydroxycholecalciferol on the intestinal epithelial cells is probably to stimulate the synthesis of a calcium-binding protein which is inserted in the apical membrane of the cells. Intestinal calcium then enters the cell down a concentration gradient through channels gated by the binding protein when it is taken up into intracellular stores to prevent a rise in free intracellular concentrations. Calcium is released from the cell into the circulation by the action of a calcium ATPase pump and by countertransport with sodium.

NAUSEA AND VOMITING

Nausea is an unpleasant but not painful sensation often relating to the pharynx and abdomen associated with the desire to vomit. It can be transient or prolonged and often occurs in 'waves'. Vomiting is forceful expulsion of the contents of the upper GI tract out of the mouth. It is an active process as opposed to re-gurgitation, which is a passive reflux of stomach contents into the oesophagus. In the animal kingdom, most poisons are ingested orally; therefore, vomiting serves as a protective mechanism in which ingested toxins are detected and expelled from the body. Diarrhoea serves the same purpose except that it clears the lower half of the GI tract. In man, and especially with post operative nausea and vomiting, the perceived toxin frequently has not been ingested via the oral route although the basic response is to purge the GI system.

MECHANISMS

Vomiting can be considered as a reflex with a sensory afferent and a motor efferent limb connected by a central integrative centre located in the brain stem. The afferent limb may be activated by a wide range of stimuli using a variety of pathways which include fibres form the GI tract, the chemoreceptor trigger zone (CTZ) in the brain stem, the vestibular system and other miscellaneous inputs.

GI tract afferents

Vagal fibres are the main afferent nerve fibres in the GI tract associated with the vomiting reflex. These fibres supply two types of receptor within the GI tract: mechano and chemo. Mechanoreceptors are activated by excessive stretching of the gut such as occurs after overeating or in bowel obstruction. Chemoreceptors detect changes in the intraluminal environment, which may indicate the ingestion of a potential toxin including excess alkalinity or acidity, certain irritants or bacterial endo- or exotoxins.

Chemoreceptor trigger zone (CTZ)

This is a specialised chemoreceptor region situated in the area postrema in the caudal part of the fourth ventricle. It lies both outside the blood-brain barrier and the cerebrospinal fluid brain barrier and is ideally situated for the detection toxins in the plasma and CSF which may have been absorbed from the gut or administered by other routes. Cells of the CTZ contain many types of receptor including muscarinic, histaminic, serotonergic ($5\text{-}HT_3$), dopaminergic (D_2), opioid (μ) and α_1 and α_2 adrenoceptors, which may be activated by different chemicals including drugs, or biochemical and endocrine changes such as hypoglycaemia or pregnancy.

Vestibular system

Stimulation of the labyrinthine system is a potent stimulus for vomiting (e.g. vertigo) although it is unclear what protective mechanism this has in man.

Central co-ordination of the vomiting reflex

The act of vomiting is a highly complex co-ordinated series of actions involving the GI, respiratory, cardiovascular, somatic and autonomic nervous systems. 'Vomiting centre', which describes the area of the brain stem responsible for the control of vomiting, is a gross over simplification. In reality, it is probably several discrete areas of the brain stem with complex interconnections that co-ordinate the reflex. These areas probably include the dorsal and ventral respiratory groups, the dorsal motor vagal nucleus, the nucleus tractus solitarius and the parvicellular reticular formation.

Motor components of vomiting

Vomiting can be divided into two distinct phases: pre-ejection and ejection.

PRE-EJECTION

The early stages of vomiting usually start with a sensation of nausea, followed by signs of sympathetic activity including peripheral vasoconstriction, hyperventilation, sweating, pupillary dilatation, tachycardia and reduction in gastric secretion. Salivation occurs in response to parasympathetic activity. Vagal impulses arising from the dorsal motor vagal nucleus cause a profound relaxation of the proximal stomach followed by a retrograde giant contraction beginning in the mid-small intestine which propels small bowel contents proximally back into the stomach in preparation for ejection.

EJECTION

Usually, vomiting is preceded by retching, which involve the synchronous contraction of the abdominal wall muscles and diaphragm producing a rapid rise in intragastric pressure. As the peri-oesophageal portion of the diaphragm contracts during this phase, the oesophagus is tightly compressed preventing the escape of gastric contents. The exact function of retching is unknown. Vomiting involves exactly the same actions except the peri-oesophageal area of the diaphragm relaxes allowing gastric contents to be expelled into the oesophagus and out of the mouth. Respiration temporarily ceases during this phase to protect the airway from aspiration.

POST OPERATIVE NAUSEA AND VOMITING (PONV)

The aetiology of post operative nausea and vomiting is extremely complicated and almost certainly multifactorial. Various factors are associated with an increased risk of PONV that can be broadly categorised into patient, anaesthetic and surgical factors. For details, see anti-emetic pharmacology, Section 3, Chapter 10.

SECTION 2: 11
METABOLISM AND TEMPERATURE REGULATION

S. Graham
E. S. Lin

NUTRITION
Carbohydrates
Proteins
Lipids
Vitamins and minerals

ENERGY BALANCE
Metabolic rate
Basal metabolic rate

METABOLISM
Organization
Adenosine triphosphate (ATP)
Activated carriers
Control of metabolism

CARBOHYDRATE METABOLISM
Glycolysis
Glycogenolysis
Gluconeogenesis
Citric acid cycle
Oxidative phosphorylation

PROTEIN METABOLISM
Amino acid pool
Transamination and de-amination
Nitrogen balance
Urea cycle
Creatine and creatinine
Purines and pyrimidines

LIPID METABOLISM
Fatty acids
Cholesterol
Eicosanoids
Ketones

STARVATION

THE LIVER
Structure
Metabolic functions

BODY TEMPERATURE AND THERMOREGULATION

NUTRITION

Food provides basic energy requirements, and provides the structural building blocks to maintain metabolic integrity. A normal diet consists of carbohydrates, proteins and fats. In addition, small quantities of vitamins and minerals are also required for good health. Nutritional status may be assessed by measurement of skin fold thickness with callipers (the area overlying the triceps muscle is often used) or by calculation of the body mass index (BMI). BMI is obtained by dividing weight (kg) by the square of the height (m²). Values between 20 and 24 are normal with > 30 indicating obesity and > 40 severe obesity. BMI is also called Quetelet's Test after Adolphe Quetelet (1796–1874), a Belgian mathematician who came up with the concept of the 'average' man.

The average calorific requirement for 24 H in a fit 70-kg man is about 3000 kcal, but this varies greatly with occupation.

CARBOHYDRATES

Dietary carbohydrates may be in the form of simple or complex carbohydrates. Complex carbohydrates, mainly plant starches, are acted upon by salivary amylase, with the production of oligosaccharides. The intestinal mucosa secretes maltase, lactase and sucrase to complete the conversion of these oligosaccharides to simple hexoses. The products of carbohydrate digestion are rapidly absorbed in the small intestine. Pentoses are absorbed by diffusion, although glucose utilises a sodium-driven active transport mechanism, with a limit of around 120 g/H. The average daily requirement of carbohydrate for an adult is between 5 and 10 g/kg.

PROTEINS

Dietary proteins may be classed as grade I protein (containing all the essential amino acids) usually derived from animal sources. Grade II protein is almost always of plant origin and lacks one or more of the essential amino acids. Pepsin in the stomach and trypsin and chymotrypsin in the small intestine break down protein into peptides. The peptides are then further degraded to free amino acids by peptidases in the small intestine where they are absorbed. The average daily requirements of protein are 0.5–1 g/kg.

LIPIDS

Dietary lipids are usually in the form of neutral fats (fatty acids condensed with glycerol to produce an uncharged triglyceride) but may also include phospholipids and cholesterol. Ingested fats are digested by pancreatic lipase to produce free fatty acids, mono- and diglycerides. These are absorbed by simple diffusion, and reconstituted within the mucosal cell. Some lipid crosses the mucosal barrier by uptake as small lipid micelles. Reformed triglycerides, carrier proteins, phospholipids and cholesterol are then combined as chylos. The average intake of fat in the diet is 1–2 g/kg although much lower intakes are well tolerated. A small percentage of the lipid intake must consist of essential fatty acids, which cannot be synthesised by the body. These include linoleic, linolenic and arachidonic acids.

VITAMINS AND MINERALS

Vitamins are organic molecules essential for life, but which can no longer be synthesised by higher organisms. Vitamins are only required in small amounts, but fulfil key functions. They are divided loosely into the water-soluble (C, B complex) and fat-soluble vitamins (A, D, E, and K).

Minerals are single elements also essential to life. They include calcium, phosphorus, magnesium, zinc, iron and iodine, all of which have minimal recommended daily intakes for an adult.

In addition, there are also minute quantities of other elements essential to life, such as copper, cobalt, manganese, nickel, molybdenum and chromium, which are known as trace elements.

Deficiencies of vitamins or minerals can produce a wide range of clinical syndromes. Some of these are outlined in Figure MT.1.

ENERGY BALANCE

Energy in the body is obtained by breaking down the larger molecules of digested food or alternatively using stored carbohydrate, fat or protein from body reserves. The degradation of these larger molecules is referred to as catabolism and is accompanied by the release of energy as the chemical bonds are broken. The energy released is either used to perform work or appears as heat. Approximately 60% of the energy released during catabolism appears as heat; only 40% produces useful work. The work done may be external work, such as that performed by skeletal muscles. Alternatively, internal work can be done, either mechanically, as in cardiac contraction, or biochemically in the synthesis of larger molecules and high-energy compounds such

VITAMIN AND MINERAL DEFICIENCIES

Substance	Function or Co-enzyme derivative	Deficiency
Water-soluble vitamins		
Vitamin C (ascorbic acid)	Anti-oxidant maintaining collagen integrity	Scurvy
Vitamin B1 (thiamine)	Thiamine pyrophosphate	Beri-beri, congestive Heart failure
Vitamin B2 (riboflavin)	Flavine adenine dinucleotide	Angular stomatitis
Vitamin B3 (niacin)	Nicotinamide adenine dinucleotide	Pellagra, dermatosis Mental disorders
Vitamin B6 (pyridoxine)	Pyridoxal phosphate	Peripheral neuropathy Convulsions
Panthothenic acid	Co-enzyme A	Fatigue, sleep Disturbance
Biotin	Carboxylases	Fatigue, depression Dermatitis
Folate	Tetrahydrofolate	Macrocytic anaemia Stomatitis, diarrhoea
Vitamin B12 (cyanocobalamin)	Cobamide co-enzymes	Macrocytic anaemia Optic neuritis
Fat-soluble vitamins		
Vitamin A	Retinal precursor	Night blindness Xerophthalmia
Vitamin D	Regulation of calcium metabolism	Rickets, Osteomalacia
Vitamin E	Anti-oxidant	Anaemia
Vitamin K	Coagulation cascade	Bleeding diathesis
Minerals and trace elements		
Iron	Component of haemoglobin myoglobin, cytochromes,	Microcytic, hypochromic anaemia
Zinc	Alcohol dehydrogenase Alkaline phosphatase Carbonic anhydrase Superoxide dismutase	Growth restriction hypogonadism
Copper	Cytochrome c oxidase Superoxide dismutase	Microcytic, hypochromic anaemia

Figure MT.1

as adenosine triphosphate (ATP). Similarly cellular processes such as the active transport of substances across membranes and mucosa also use energy internally.

This energy balance in the body can be summarised as:

Total energy expenditure = Heat produced by the body + External work done + Energy stored.

METABOLIC RATE

The continuous energy expenditure per unit time in a person, is supplied by metabolism, and is known as the metabolic rate. This is measured in kilocalories per H and is dependent on various factors, which include:

- Age and sex
- Height, body weight and body surface area
- Pregnancy, menstruation and lactation
- Body temperature or environmental temperature
- Muscular activity
- Emotional state
- Circulating levels of hormones, e.g. thyroxine and epinephrine
- Recent ingestion of food
- Conscious level
- Presence of sepsis or other disease

BASAL METABOLIC RATE

The basal metabolic rate (BMR) is the metabolic rate of a subject under standardised conditions at mental and physical rest, in a comfortable environmental temperature and fasted for 12 H. The BMR is not necessarily the minimum metabolic rate since this may occur with the subject asleep. Under these conditions the BMR can be visualised as the basic metabolic cost of living. For an average young adult the BMR is about 70–100 kcal/H.

Measurement of BMR

Under the specified steady-state conditions BMR can be measured directly using a whole body calorimeter. The subject is placed in the calorimeter chamber and the heat produced per H is determined by the temperature rise of a steady flow of water through the calorimeter. Since the total energy expenditure of the body ultimately appears as heat in the absence of any external work done, the heat produced per H equals the BMR of the subject.

The BMR can be estimated indirectly, by measuring the oxygen consumption per h of a subject at rest. The oxygen consumption is then multiplied by 4.8 kcal/H.

of heat produced per litre oxygen, to give the heat produced per H. This is an empirical figure representative of heat production regardless of substrate used. The oxygen usage can be measured using a modified spirometer containing oxygen and a carbon dioxide absorber.

METABOLISM

This term is used to describe the complex mass of biochemical reactions which breakdown the absorbed products of digestion to extract chemical energy, synthesise substances for structural maintenance and growth, and synthesise or detoxify waste products.

ORGANISATION

The organisation of metabolism can be visualised as being composed of three sets of interlinked pathways. These deal with the three main types of molecule fed into the system, and are often referred to separately, as carbohydrate metabolism, protein metabolism and fat metabolism. The three areas of metabolism are linked by the main energy-producing machinery, which comprises the citric acid cycle and the oxidative phosphorylation cascade. This is illustrated in Figure MT.2.

The extraction of energy is a primary function of metabolism and provides the driving force that determines the direction taken by the different biochemical pathways. The universal energy currency used to move and supply energy to various pathways is a high-energy compound, adenosine triphosphate (ATP). Figure MT.2 also shows how there are three levels of reactions involved in harvesting energy:

- Level 1 – breakdown of proteins, fats and carbohydrates into their simple molecules of fatty acids and glycerol, amino acids and glucose and other sugars. No energy is produced at this level
- Level 2 – degradation of these simpler molecules to a common smaller molecule acetyl-CoA. A small amount of ATP is produced at this stage
- Level 3 – passage of acetyl-CoA through the citric acid cycle, and an oxidative phosphorylation pathway, which generates > 90% of the finally harvested ATP

The generation and supply of energy for various reactions is the key to maintaining the complex metabolic pathways and keeping them in balance. Most metabolic reactions are potentially reversible, but are directed by the energy released or absorbed during the reaction. The energy exchanged during a reaction is

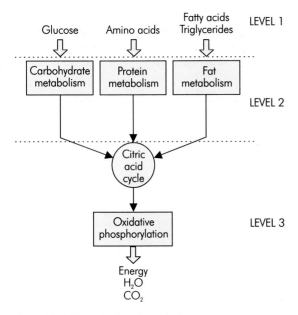

Figure MT.2 Organisation of metabolism

called the free energy of the reaction, (ΔG). All reactions include a free energy component as well as the reagents. Thus, the reaction of reagents A and B to give products C and D can be written thus:

$$A + B + \Delta G \rightleftharpoons C + D$$

If energy is released, ΔG is negative, and the reaction proceeds spontaneously. If energy is absorbed, ΔG is positive, and the reaction has to be driven by supplying energy.

In general terms, metabolism tends to proceed spontaneously in the direction of catabolism, oxidation and the production of protons. The processes and reactions reversing these trends i.e. anabolism, reductive reactions and the maintenance of acid base balance, require energy. Thus, the supply of chemical energy for these reactions is the key to maintaining the life process.

Chemical energy may be supplied in different forms, which are outlined below.

ADENOSINE TRIPHOSPHATE (ATP)

The majority of reactions and processes requiring chemical energy to drive them use it in the form of ATP. This compound is used in processes such as the myosin–actin interaction in muscle or the active transport of substances across cell membranes, and is sometimes referred to as the common energy currency of metabolism. ATP delivers its energy when it is

hydrolysed to adenosine diphosphate (ADP), since its useable energy is carried in a high-energy phosphoryl bond (Figure MT.3). The ADP is 'recharged' by various reactions including the citric acid cycle, oxidative phosphorylation and phosphorylation by creatine phosphate. There is a continuous turnover of ATP and at rest an adult can use 40 kg ATP in 24 H.

ACTIVATED CARRIERS

Although ATP has a universal role in supplying energy to drive reactions, other compounds also have the ability to drive reactions that require energy. The energy in these cases may be carried in the form of a high potential electron or an activated group. In the case of an electron carrier donation of an electron to one of the reagents constitutes a chemical reduction, which reverses the spontaneous tendency of the metabolic pathways towards oxidation. ATP can be regenerated with the use of a major electron carrier nicotinamide adenine dinucleotide (NADH). Figure MT.4 shows some of the known activated carriers operating in metabolic pathways.

CONTROL OF METABOLISM

Metabolic reactions are regulated via three basic mechanisms:

- The amounts of enzymes present – enzyme levels are regulated by varying the transcription rate of the genes that encode them. An example of this mechanism is the induction of β-galactosidase by lactose, which can increase enzyme levels by 50 times
- The availability of substrates. Substrate levels intracellularly can be controlled by hormones that affect the transport of substrates across cell

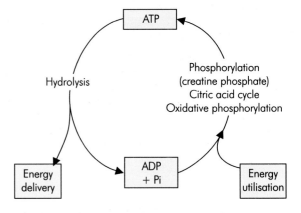

Figure MT.3 ATP cycle

SOME ACTIVATED CARRIERS

Carrier molecule	Group carried
Adenosine triphosphate (ATP)	Phosphoryl
Nicotinamide adenine dinucleotide (NAD)	Electrons
Nicotinamide adenine dinucleotide phosphate (NADPH)	Electrons
Flavine adenine dinucleotide (FADH$_2$)	Electrons
Co-enzyme A	Acyl
Thiamine pyrophosphate (TPP)	Aldehyde
Creatine phosphate	Phosphoryl

Figure MT.4

COMPARTMENTATION OF METABOLIC REACTIONS BETWEEN CYTOPLASM AND MITOCHONDRIA

Reaction site	Reaction pathway
Cytoplasm	Glycolysis
	Pyruvate oxidation
	Glycogenloysis
	Fatty acid synthesis
Mitochondria	Citric acid cycle
	Oxidative phosphorylation
	β oxidation

Figure MT.5

membranes. An example of this mechanism is the action of insulin in promoting glucose entry into cells.

- The activity of the enzymes – enzyme activity is subject to regulation via different biochemical mechanisms. A common mechanism is allosteric modulation in which the active site of an enzyme is structurally altered by the attachment of a modulator molecule to a separate modulator site (see page 236). In many synthetic pathways, the final product of the pathway inhibits the first stage reaction in this way, by reversible allosteric control
- Additional control of metabolism is provided by maintaining separate synthetic and degradative pathways. This may be achieved by physical separation of the pathways as in intracellular 'compartmentation'. In such a case, for example, fatty acid breakdown (β oxidation) occurs in mitochondria while fatty acid synthesis takes place in the cytoplasm (Figure MT.5)

Systemic control of metabolic responses is mainly mediated by hormones. Various hormones such as the catecholamines, insulin, cortisol and thyroxine produce their physiological responses through wide ranging changes in the metabolism of different tissues. Some examples are outlined below while a summary of endocrine effects on metabolism is given on pages 495–510.

Insulin

Insulin secretion is stimulated by glucose and amino acid uptake, and by parasympathetic innervation.

Within the liver it increases glycogen synthesis, prevents gluconeogenesis and stimulates the glycolytic production of fatty acid precursors, with resultant increase in fat storage. In the gut it increases the uptake of branched chain amino acids, and is a stimulant to formation of protein.

Amylin, co-secreted with insulin, may promote lactate transfer back to the liver, and support generation of fat stores.

Glucagon

Released by the pancreas in response to hypoglycaemia, glucagon acts on the liver to inhibit glycogen synthesis and promote gluconeogenesis and glycogen breakdown. In adipose tissue it results in the activation of lipases and fatty acid mobilisation.

Epinephrine and norepinephrine

Secreted as a response to stress or hypoglycaemia, these catecholamines promote glycogenolysis (greater in muscle than liver), while reducing muscle uptake of glucose. Fatty acids are mobilised from adipose tissue to provide fuel for the increase in muscle activity.

CARBOHYDRATE METABOLISM

Carbohydrate metabolism is mainly concerned with the generation of energy and the storage of carbohydrate as glycogen. The transportable form of carbohydrate throughout the body is the hexose sugar glucose (six carbon, termed C6), which can be thought of as a universal fuel for all cells. The circulating levels of this are derived from:

- Dietary intake of carbohydrate
- Breakdown of stored carbohydrate in the form of glycogen, i.e. glycogenolysis
- Synthesis from smaller precursor molecules derived from other pathways, i.e. gluconeogenesis

The energy produced by the metabolism of one mole of glucose can be measured by the number of moles ATP produced. Under aerobic conditions there is a net gain of 38 moles ATP per mole glucose. Each ATP molecule provides the energy from one activated phosphoryl group (7.6 kcal), which gives a total yield of 288 kcal chemical energy per mole glucose. If 1 mole glucose undergoes complete combustion in a calorimeter, it liberates about 686 kcal heat. The efficiency of carbohydrate metabolism is, therefore, 42%.

The main pathways in carbohydrate metabolism are:

- Glycolysis
- Gluconeogenesis
- Glycogenolysis and glycogenesis
- Hexose monophosphate (HMP) shunt

These pathways and their relationship to each other are illustrated in Figure MT.6 and their functions are outlined below.

GLYCOLYSIS

Glycolysis (also called the Embden–Meyerhof pathway) breaks down glucose (C6) to the triose, pyruvate (C3). Its main function is to produce pyruvate for oxidation to acetyl-CoA to feed the citric acid cycle. Glucose is activated to glucose 6-phosphate to enter the pathway. This activated form may also be utilised to generate glycogen or for conjugation, but most enters into glycolysis (Figure MT.7).

This pathway uses up 2 ATP, but generates 4 ATP and 2 NADH per molecule glucose. Thus, overall there is a net gain of 2 ATP and 2 NADH. Under aerobic conditions, the 2 NADH can be oxidised through oxidative phosphorylation to generate further ATP. Glycolysis can also proceed under anaerobic conditions, but the net energy gain is then only 2 ATP and lactate accumulates. Anaerobic glycolysis is important to the white muscle fibres of skeletal muscle. These are capable of intense activity disproportionate to their oxygen supply, which incurs an 'oxygen debt' in the form of the accumulated lactate. Lactate itself can be used as a substrate by some tissues. Pyruvate is oxidised to acetyl-CoA, which enters the citric acid cycle (also known as Krebs' cycle after the biochemist who elucidated it), or can be used in other pathways.

GLYCOGENOLYSIS

Glycogen is a branched polymer of glucose and is the storage form of carbohydrate in the body. Total body

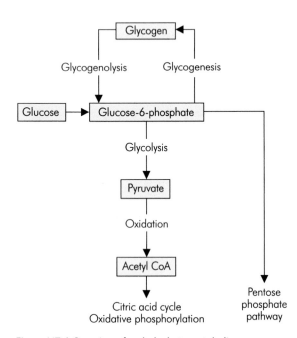

Figure MT.6 Overview of carbohydrate metabolism

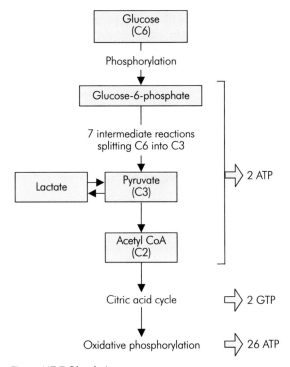

Figure MT.7 Glycolysis

reserves are about 325 g and these are distributed between skeletal muscle and liver in the ratio of 3:1. The pathways for the breakdown of glycogen, (glycogenolysis), and its synthesis, (glycogenesis, are different employing different enzymes and controls. They are illustrated in Figure MT.6. Glucose is activated by phosphorylation and combination with uridine triphosphate. It is then added to a pre-existing glycogen chain by glycogen synthetase. Branching of the glycogen chains requires a branching enzyme. Glycogenolysis requires a phosphorylase to activate and split off the terminal glucose unit from a glycogen chain. A debranching enzyme is also required to deal with branching points in the glycogen polymer. The enzymes in the glycogenesis and glycolytic pathways are distinct and respond individually to hormonal control. Storage of glucose as glycogen is highly efficient. The energy cost of storage and retrieval is a little over 3% of the total energy available from glucose.

GLUCONEOGENESIS

Gluconeogenesis is the generation of glucose from substrates such as pyruvate. And lactate. These in turn may be produced from amino acids by de-amination, and consequently muscle mass also serves as a large potential glucose source. This is predominantly a liver function, although it does occur to some extent in the renal cortex. The much smaller mass of the kidney, however, means that the overall renal contribution is small. The purpose of gluconeogenesis is to allow maintenance of plasma glucose for those tissues that preferentially use glucose as an energy source. An outline of the gluconeogenesis pathway is shown in Figure MT.8. Gluconeogenesis from pyruvate is not simply a reverse of glycolysis, since the energetics so greatly favour pyruvate formation from the breakdown of glucose. Instead, pyruvate is converted to oxaloacetate at the cost of a single ATP by pyruvate carboxylase, and then phosphorylated and decarboxylated using GTP as an energy source, to give phospho-enolpyruvate. The net cost of glucose synthesis from pyruvate is 6 ATP, whereas only 2 ATP are generated in glycolysis.

Pentose phosphate pathway (PPP) or hexose monophosphate shunt

This is an alternative pathway for the activated form of glucose, glucose 6-phosphate. It is important in tissues that require reductive power for anabolic processes such as cell membrane repair, the synthesis of amino acids, fatty acids and steroids, and the production of nucleic acids.

The PPP is a cyclic pathway that takes in activated glucose units and produces CO_2, ribose 5-phosphate and NADPH. The NADPH is important as an activated reducing agent in certain tissues such as the liver, adipose tissue, erythrocytes and the testes.

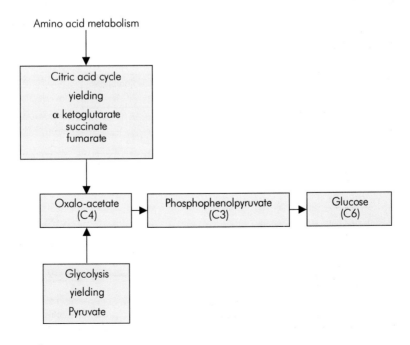

Figure MT.8 Gluconeogenesis

The cyclic process involves the transfer of a C2 fragment between pentoses (C5) and also provides a source of ribose 5-phosphate, an aldopentose required in the production of nucleic acids (Figure MT.9).

Oxidation of pyruvate to acetyl-CoA

This step in carbohydrate metabolism occurs inside the mitochondria and is important because it irreversibly funnels pyruvate (C3) into the citric acid cycle. The net reaction is:

Pyruvate + CoA + NAD$^+$ = acetyl-CoA + CO$_2$ + NADH

It is a complex reaction requiring pyruvate dehydrogenase (an enzyme complex composed of three different types of enzyme) and several co-factors (including TPP and NAD). This key reaction is subject to feedback control, in which the presence of high levels of energy in the form of NADH, ATP and acetyl-CoA 'switch off' the pyruvate dehydrogenase complex. There is, thus, a net energy gain in this step of NADH, which can be converted to ATP through oxidative phosphorylation.

CITRIC ACID CYCLE

The citric acid cycle and oxidative phosphorylation process both form the core of the energy producing machinery in metabolism. They take place in the mitochondria and are not exclusive to carbohydrate metabolism, but form a common end pathway for the products of carbohydrate, lipid and protein metabolism. Carbohydrate metabolism and the breakdown of lipids feed acetyl-CoA into the cycle, while protein metabolism can feed into the cycle via several intermediates, including oxaloacetate (C4), α-ketoglutarate (C5) and fumarate (C4).

The main entry to the citric acid cycle is via acetyl-CoA, which is essentially an activated C2 (acetyl) group

bound to a carrier (Co-enzyme A). This C2 fragment is loaded onto a C4 molecule (oxaloacetate) to form citrate (C6), which passes around a cycle of intermediate compounds. Two decarboxylation reactions take place to regenerate the oxaloacetate (C4). Energy production from each cycle is in the form of:
- Three NADH
- One high energy phosphoryl bond in guanosine triphosphate (GTP)
- One FADH$_2$

The NADH and FADH$_2$ are high potential electron carriers and enter the oxidative phosphorylation process to generate ATP (Figure MT.10).

OXIDATIVE PHOSPHORYLATION

Oxidative phosphorylation is a biochemical process in the mitochondria in which ATP is generated by the high potential electrons carried by NADH and FADH$_2$. 'High potential' refers to the tendency for electrons to be transferred from these activated carriers to a cascade of 'lower potential' carriers (NADH-Q reductase, cytochrome reductase and cytochrome oxidase) which are located in the inner mitochondrial membrane, and are sometimes referred to as 'the respiratory chain'.

These mitochondrial membrane carriers are basically proton pumps activated by the flow of electrons

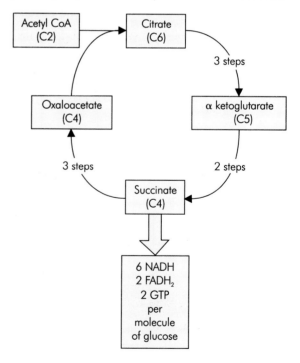

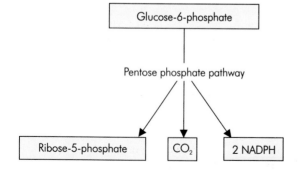

Figure MT.9 Pentose phosphate pathway

Figure MT.10 Citric acid cycle

through them. They pump H⁺ out of the inner mitochondrion to give an H^+ gradient across the inner membrane. This H^+ gradient then generates ATP by driving H^+ back across the inner membrane through channels of ATP synthase. The passage of H^+ through these channels catalyses the synthesis of ATP (Figure MT.11).

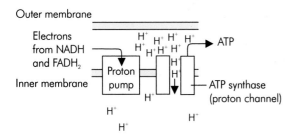

Figure MT.11 Oxidative phosphorylation

Defects in carbohydrate metabolism

Inborn errors in the metabolism of carbohydrates can be grouped as follows:

- Intestinal defects
- A deficiency of an enzyme in the intermediary metabolic pathways, without accompanying lactic acidosis
- A deficiency of an enzyme in the intermediary metabolic pathways, with accompanying lactic acidosis
- Glycogen storage disease

Some examples are shown Figure MT.12.

PROTEIN METABOLISM

The basic building block of a protein is the amino acid. Amino acids are characterised by the presence of carboxyl and amine groups on a carbon atom. Also attached is a group, R as shown below:

$$H_2N - \overset{\overset{\displaystyle H}{|}}{\underset{\underset{\displaystyle R}{|}}{C}} - COOH$$

R may be simple as in glycine, where R = H; or complex as in glutamic acid, where R = $(CH_2)_2COOH$.

Amino acids can be condensed into chains to form peptides and these chains can increase in size to form proteins. Protein chains can form a secondary structure by winding and twisting together. Such twisted chains can form more complex molecules by assuming a tertiary structure resulting in sheets or fibres. In a

EXAMPLES OF DEFECTS IN CARBOHYDRATE METABOLISM		
Disease	Biochemical defect	Clinical features
Intestinal defect		
Lactose intolerance (non familial type)	Gastro-intestinal lactase deficiency	Diarrhoea, flatulence abdominal discomfort
Enzyme deficiency with lactic acidosis		
von Gierke disease	Glucokinase deficiency	Large liver and kidneys stunted growth, 'doll's face' lactic acidosis
Enzyme deficiency without lactic acidosis		
Galactosaemia	Galactokinase deficiency	Cataracts, hepatomegaly mental retardation
Glycogen storage disease		
Pompe disease	Lysosomal debranching enzyme deficiency	Infantile cardiomegaly, hepatomegaly, hypotonia

Figure MT.12

quaternary structured protein, the amalgamation of several tertiary proteins or subunits form a final complex protein molecule. Examples of such quaternary structures are haemoglobin (formed by four globin subunits connected to a haem core) and apoferritin (20 sub units arranged to form a hollow sphere).

AMINO ACID POOL

Body proteins undergo a continual turnover by being broken down into amino acids and resynthesised from the same amino acids. This creates a metabolic 'amino acid pool', which provides precursors not only for protein synthesis but also many other compounds and pathways including:

- Purines and pyrimidines
- Hormones
- Neurotransmitters
- Creatine
- Gluconeogenesis
- Fatty acid synthesis
- Citric acid cycle

Interconversion of different amino acids, or between amino acids and intermediates of carbohydrate and lipid metabolism, enable specific pathways to link into the amino acid pool. These interconversions occur via transamination, amination or de-amination reactions, which are active in many tissues. The metabolic amino acid pool is replenished by the absorbed products of ingested protein.

Excess amino acids from the amino acid pool have their amino groups removed leaving carbon skeletons. These residues enter other pathways (such as the citric acid cycle) while the excess amino groups are ultimately excreted as urea and creatinine. Figure MT.13 gives a simple overview of protein metabolism.

TRANSAMINATION AND DEAMINATION

Transamination is the transfer of an NH_2 group to another molecule, usually a keto acid. This common reaction allows excess amino acids to be degraded to intermediates that can be metabolised to give energy. Alternatively these intermediates can be used in gluconeogenesis or the synthesis of fatty acids. An example is the transfer of NH_2 from alanine to a-ketoglutarate as follows:

alanine + α-ketoglutarate = pyruvate + glutamate.

Pyruvate can then be oxidised to acetyl-CoA and enter the citric acid cycle.

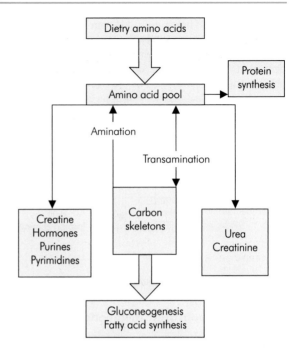

Figure MT.13 Overview of protein metabolism

Deamination is the removal of the amino group from an amino acid to leave a carbon skeleton that can be metabolised. An example of deamination occurs with serine, which can be deaminated to give pyruvate:

$$serine = pyruvate + NH_4^+$$

In this way many of the amino acids can be converted to relatively few intermediate molecules (Figure MT.14).

Defects in amino acid metabolism

Congenital syndromes are recognised that are due to the disruption of specific amino acids pathways. These are usually rare but illustrate the importance of individual amino acids. Some examples are shown in Figure MT.15.

NITROGEN BALANCE

Although amino acids are continually recycled from the amino acid pool, a daily loss occurs from the gastro-intestinal tract and in the urine. Normally, therefore, protein intake is required to compensate for these losses. The intake and losses of protein may be assessed by their nitrogen content and these should be balanced in the healthy adult. Normal nitrogen requirements for an adult are a daily intake of about 10 g (approximating to 46 g protein). Dietary intake should be decreased in

CONVERSION OF SOME AMINO ACIDS TO METABOLIC INTERMEDIATES

Amino acid	Intermediate
Isoleucine Leucine Tryptophan	Acetyl CoA (C2)
Alanine Cysteine Glycine Serine	Pyruvate (C3)
Aspartate Phenylalanine Tyrosine	Fumarate (C4)
Methionine Threonine Valine	Succinyl CoA (C4)
Arginine Glutamate Histidine Proline	Alpha-ketoglutarate (C5)

Figure MT.14

the presence of hepatic or renal dysfunction since the capacity of the body to produce and excrete urea is compromised. In the case of hypermetabolic and hypercatabolic illness the body requirements are increased.

Negative balance occurs if losses exceed intake as in illness or starvation. Positive balance, when intake is greater than losses, occurs in growth, convalescence or the use of drugs such as anabolic steroids. Urinary nitrogen losses are mainly contained in the excreted urea, although small amounts of nitrogen are also excreted as creatinine, uric acid and amino acids.

UREA CYCLE

Excess amino acids are deaminated to release NH_4^+. This reaction occurs mainly in two tissues:
- The kidneys where the NH_4^+ dissociates into NH_3 and H^+ for excretion into the urine
- The liver where the NH_4^+ is converted to carbamyl phosphate which then contributes to the formation of urea

The formation of urea is a cyclic process that takes place in the mitochondria. In a normal adult, about 30 g urea is produced daily. In hepatic failure, this conversion is less likely to occur, and an accumulation of ammonia occurs. The formation of urea is illustrated in Figure MT.16, which shows how urea, which has two nitrogen atoms, obtains one from carbamyl phosphate and the other by transamination from aspartate. The synthesis of one molecule of urea requires the energy from 3 ATP. This process is sometimes referred to as the ornithine cycle.

CREATINE AND CREATININE

Creatine is present in muscle, brain and blood. It is particularly important in its phosphorylated form as an immediate store of high-energy phosphoryl bonds for the generation of ATP from ADP. The chemical energy for the first few seconds of muscle contraction are supplied by ATP generated from this source.

EXAMPLES OF DEFECTS IN AMINO ACID METABOLISM

Condition	Biochemical defect	Clinical features
Phenylketonuria	↓ conversion of phenylalanine to tyrosine	1 in 10 000 births mental retardation
Homocystinuria	↓ levels of cysteine and cystine ↑ levels of homocystine and methionine	Tall, thin body, subluxation of lens mental retardation
Alkaptonuria	↑ levels of homogentisic acid	Ochronosis (pigmented connective tissues), arthritis

Figure MT.15

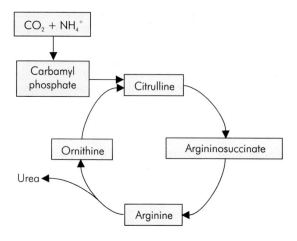

Figure MT.16 Urea cycle

Creatine is phosphorylated by creatine kinase. The serum levels of this enzyme are used as a marker of muscle damage following trauma or myocardial infarction. Creatine kinase activity may also be raised however simply as a result of violent exercise.

Creatinine is the anhydride of creatine and is formed as a metabolite for excretion in the urine. The 24 H urinary excretion of creatinine is relatively constant for any given individual, while renal tubular re-absorption is small. This means that the value for creatinine clearance can be used as an approximation to glomerular filtration rate.

PURINES AND PYRIMIDINES

These substances are ring-based structures that occur widely throughout the body. They form the base components in the ribonucleotides and deoxyribonucleotides, i.e. the 'alphabet' triplets that code RNA and DNA strands. Purines and pyrimidines occur throughout the tissues as carriers of high-energy phosphoryl bonds, e.g. adenosine triphosphate (ATP), guanosine triphosphate (GTP) and uridine triphosphate (UTP). These molecules are also ubiquitous as the functional parts of many co-factors.

Purines

Purines are double-ringed molecules with six- and five-membered nitrogenated rings, commonly occurring examples being adenine and guanine. When metabolised, purines ultimately give rise to uric acid, which is excreted in the urine. The average excretion rate for an adult being between 400 and 600 mg over 24 H. Uric acid and sodium urate are found in the plasma and urine. They have relatively limited solubility at

body pH and urine pH, and it requires only a moderate increase in uric acid levels to precipitate the deposition of urate crystals in the tissues or in the kidneys. The clinical syndrome of gout is associated with hyperuricaemia and deposition of urate in soft tissues and joints. The underlying defect is usually a combination of overproduction and increased breakdown of purines, but the cause may range from an enzyme deficiency to a hypercatabolic state.

Pyrimidines

Pyrimidines are based on a six-membered nitrogenated ring. Common pyrimidines in the body are cytosine, thymine and uracil. Breakdown of pyrimidines occurs in the liver and results in highly soluble products, β-alanine and β-aminoisobutyric acid.

LIPID METABOLISM

The lipids occurring in the body can be classified into the following groups:

- Fatty acids – chains of saturated or unsaturated carbon atoms with a terminal carboxyl group. These form the body's main energy store, and are also components of many structural molecules
- Triglycerides – storage form for fatty acid chains, in which three chains are attached to a glycerol (C3) mole by ester linkages. Triglycerides are not free in the plasma but are transported as lipoproteins in chylomicra
- Plasma lipoproteins – 95% of plasma lipids are transported in combination with protein to make them soluble. These lipoproteins have different roles and are targeted to specific tissues
- Phospholipids and glycolipids – form building blocks for membranes and tissues
- Cholesterol – precursor of steroid hormones and a component of membranes

FATTY ACIDS

Fatty acids have the following important functions:

- Fuel molecules
- Components of phospholipids and glycolipids
- Components of hormones and intracellular messengers

Free fatty acids (FFA) only form about 5% of the lipids in the plasma, but this group of lipids is the most active metabolically. They are stored as triglycerides and metabolised to yield energy by β oxidation in the mitochondria. The energy yield from fatty acid oxidation is about 9 kcal/g compared with 4 kcal/g for carbohydrates and protein. In addition, because triglycerides are hydrophobic they are effectively anhydrous compared to glycogen which binds twice its weight in water. This means weight for weight triglycerides contain more than six times the energy of carbohydrates. A 70 kg man possesses about 11 kg triglycerides representing a reserve of 100 000 kcal stored energy compared with 25 000 kcal stored as protein and only 600 kcal stored as carbohydrate. The synthesis of fatty acids takes place in the cytoplasm by using acetyl-CoA to elongate fatty acid chains in C2 steps. An overview of lipid metabolism is shown in Figure MT.17.

β oxidation of fatty acids

The breakdown of fatty acid chains to give energy is a cyclic process called β oxidation, which takes place in the mitochondrial matrix. Free fatty acids in the cytoplasm are first activated by esterification with acetyl-CoA. The activated fatty acid is then loaded on to a carrier protein called carnitine at the outer mitochondrial membrane. This complex is then transported across the inner mitochondrial membrane into the mitochondrial matrix where it is unloaded by recombination with acetyl-CoA. This is performed by an inner membrane protein called carnitine acyl-transferase. Carnitine is then returned to the outer membrane where it is available to pick up more

activated fatty acid. This cyclic process is sometimes known as the 'carnitine shuttle'. In the matrix C2 fragments are split off from the fatty acid in repeated steps, each C2 fragment producing acetyl-CoA to feed into the citric acid cycle. In this way a molecule of a C16 fatty acid (palmitoyl) can produce 106 molecules ATP.

Fatty acid synthesis

Fatty acid synthesis takes place in the cytoplasm, in contrast with β oxidation which is mitochondrial. This is also a cyclic process that builds up fatty acid chains by the addition of activated C2 fragments (acetyl-CoA). These C2 fragments are obtained from the mitochondria and are transferred out to the cytoplasm by a citrate carrier. The acetyl-CoA is removed from the citrate in the cytoplasm, leaving the citrate, which is then converted to pyruvate. The pyruvate passes back into the mitochondria where it is re-converted back to citrate.

Reducing power in the form of NADPH is required for FA synthesis. Some of this is generated by the citrate-pyruvate carrier cycle, while the pentose phosphate pathway provides the rest.

Fatty acid synthesis is regulated by a key enzyme, acetyl-CoA carboxylase, to ensure that synthesis and degradation occur appropriately for the body's needs.

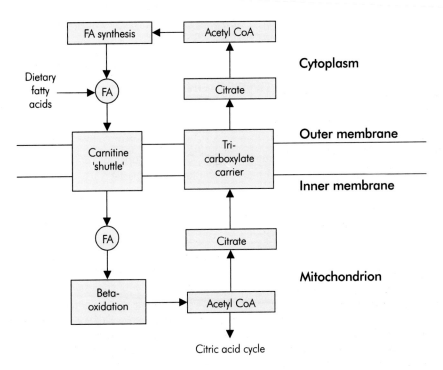

Figure MT.17 Overview of lipid metabolism

This control responds to biochemical feedback as well as hormones such as insulin and the catecholamines.

Plasma lipoproteins

Plasma triglycerides and cholesterol combine with proteins to form a range of lipoprotein particles, the largest being chylos (100–1000 nm diameter), while the smallest are the high-density lipoproteins (7.5–20 nm diameter). These macromolecular aggregates have different lipid contents and are metabolised by specific tissues. Their basic structure consists of a lipid core coated with protein and phospholipid to solubilise them. Specific apoproteins in the particle coatings act as cellular signals for target tissues. The lipoproteins are classified according to density and have different metabolic functions (Figure MT.18).

CHOLESTEROL

Cholesterol is a component of all cell membranes and produces membrane fluidity by its interaction with membrane phospholipids. It possesses a steroid-based structure and is also a precursor of the steroid hormones. Cholesterol is, therefore, essential for the growth and viability of the tissues. Tissues outside the liver obtain cholesterol from the plasma low-density lipoprotein (LDL) particles, using membrane LDL receptors to mediate uptake. Normal plasma levels of cholesterol are < 240 mg/100 ml, and are contributed to by both diet (normal daily intake is about 1 g) and endogenous synthesis. Abnormally high levels of cholesterol result in disease due to deposition of cholesterol in soft tissues and formation of cholesterol containing plaques in arteries (atherosclerosis).

EICOSANOIDS

The eicosanoids are C20 unsaturated fatty acids containing a five-carbon ring. They are derived from arachidonic acid that is synthesised from linoleic acid, one of the essential fatty acids. The eicosanoids include the following compounds:

- Prostaglandins
- Leukotrienes
- Thromboxanes
- Prostacyclin

These substances are local hormones with short-lived and highly localised effects, depending on the tissue in which they are released. Their effects are wide ranging and include stimulation of the inflammatory response, regulation of local blood flow, control of membrane transport, modulation of synaptic transmission and modulation of platelet adhesion. A key step in the synthesis of prostaglandins is cyclo-oxygenase, which can be inhibited by non steroidal anti-inflammatory drugs such as aspirin.

KETONES

When excessive levels of acetyl-CoA are present, the acetyl-CoA is diverted to form acetoacetate and

PLASMA LIPOPROTEINS		
Lipoprotein	**Major core lipid**	**Function**
Chylomicrons	Dietary triglyceride	Carries dietary triglycerides to tissues for fuel (e.g. muscle)
Chylomicron remnants	Dietary cholesterol	Taken up by liver for metabolism
Very low-density lipoprotein (VLDL)	Endogenous triglyceride	Exported form of excess triglyceride and cholesterol from liver
Low-density lipoprotein (LDL)	Endogenous cholesterol	Major carrier of cholesterol to peripheral tissues for metabolism
High-density lipoprotein (HDL)	Endogenous cholesterol	Cholesterol from dying cells and membrane repair, for recycling

Figure MT.18

γ hydroxybutyric acid. These compounds are known as ketone bodies and accumulation of ketone bodies results in the clinical syndrome of ketosis or ketoacidosis (Figure MT.19).

Acetyl CoA represents a crossroads between major metabolic pathways. It can be produced either by glycolysis or β oxidation. Normally glycolysis is responsible for supplying the acetyl-CoA for the citric acid cycle, but of the glycolytic pathway fails as in uncontrolled diabetes or starvation, acetyl-CoA is obtained from β oxidation. Under such circumstances excessive levels can result because of:

- Insulin deficiency, leading to increased free fatty acid levels
- Increased glucagon levels, which stimulate β oxidation
- Decreased levels of oxaloacetate, due to increased gluconeogenesis

(a) Normal metabolism

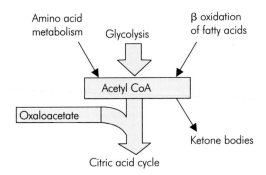

(b) Ketosis

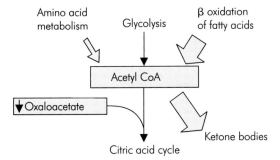

Figure MT.19 Ketosis

STARVATION

Starvation is a complete absence of dietary intake and can result in death after about 60 days. This should be differentiated from malnutrition in which some calorific intake may be present, but which follows a more protracted course accompanied by the effects of chronic lack of protein, fats and essential vitamins and minerals.

In starvation, glucose supplies to the brain are a priority since it is largely dependent on glucose as an energy substrate. Initially there is an increase in glycogenolysis. However, as glycogen reserves are depleted, blood glucose falls to subnormal levels. Mobilisation of fatty acids occurs to provide energy, and the liver ceases to use glucose as a substrate but uses fatty acids instead. Muscle also adapts to use fatty acids as an energy source.

With the depletion of glycogen, gluconeogenesis increases using amino acid residues derived from the breakdown of muscle protein. Gluconeogenesis takes place in the liver, which also uses glycerol from lipolysis and oxaloacetate. The use of these substrates leads to the accumulation of acetyl-CoA and hence the formation of ketone bodies. Thus, starvation is associated with ketosis. Most tissues including the brain can ultimately adapt to the use of ketone bodies as a fuel source. Therefore, protein catabolism is quite rapid in early starvation, but as the body shifts to the use of ketone bodies, the rate of protein breakdown decreases. After three days approximately a third of the brain's energy requirements are derived from ketone bodies and ultimately this proportion increases to a half. The total reserves of an average adult are sufficient to provide the calorie requirements for about 3 months.

THE LIVER

STRUCTURE

The liver weighs 1.5–2 kg and is divided into right and left lobes, the right lobe being much larger than (up to six times) the left lobe in size. The functional unit of the liver is the hepatic lobule. These are roughly hexagonal in cross section and possess a central vein from which cords of hepatocytes radiate outwards. In between the lobules are portal spaces through which run branches of the hepatic artery, portal vein and a bile duct. The radial spaces between the hepatocytes are called sinusoids and carry a mixture of arterial and portal blood supplied by the vessels in the portal spaces, towards the centre of the lobule where it drains into the central vein. The central veins join to form the hepatic vein which drains into the inferior vena cava.

As the blood flows though the sinusoids it is exposed

over a large surface area to the hepatocytes which are highly active metabolically. The walls of the sinusoids are also lined by macrophages known as Kupffer cells, which are an active part of the reticulo-endothelial system.

The cords of hepatocytes are closely apposed to bile cannaliculi which drain centrifugally towards the bile ducts in the portal spaces. These carry the bile secreted by the hepatocytes to the gallbladder and common bile duct (Figure MT.20). For detail of bile formation and content see pages 464–465.

METABOLIC FUNCTIONS

The metabolic functions of the liver may be divided into:

- Formation of bile
- Protein metabolism
- Carbohydrate metabolism
- Lipid metabolism
- Detoxification
- Excretion

Protein synthesis

The major proteins synthesised by the liver include:

ALBUMIN

Albumin is synthesised at about 200 mg/kg/day in a normal adult. This is about 4% of the total body albumin pool. Plasma albumin correlates well with liver synthetic activity, but with a half-life of about 20 days, it is a poor marker for acute liver injury. Albumin

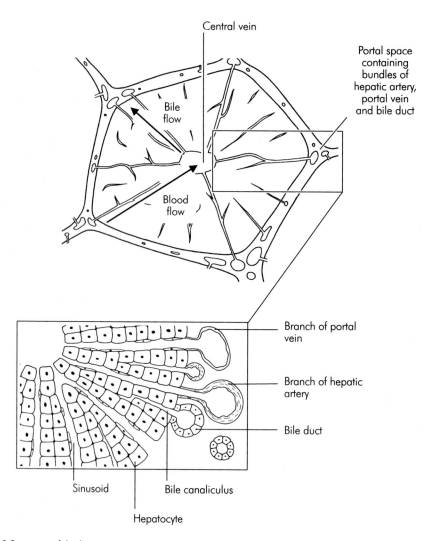

Figure MT.20 Structure of the liver

is important in the maintenance of plasma colloid oncotic pressure, and in the transport of drugs, bilirubin and some hormones.

GLOBULINS

These are a range of lipo- and glycoproteins with transport functions (e.g. ferritin, caeruloplasmin). The liver is the principal site for synthesis and recycling of haptoglobin, which serves to bind and conserve free haemoglobin.

CLOTTING FACTORS

Most clotting factors are synthesised exclusively by the liver. Half-lives vary widely, up to 28 days for prothrombin. Coagulopathies may occur either due to failure of hepatic synthesis directly or because of failure of bile excretion leading to a reduction in the absorption of Vitamin K, necessary for the synthesis of factors II, VII, IX and X. Factor VII has one of the shortest half lives, at about 4 H.

Protein catabolism

The liver is involved in protein catabolism either directly, in turnover of proteins in the hepatocyte, or indirectly, in handling the products of the absorption of dietary proteins or amino acids from peripheral protein turnover. Amino acids or dipeptides from portal or systemic circulations are absorbed by the liver. They may be used as substrates for new protein synthesis or be used for gluconeogenesis. The conversion of amino acids to carbon skeletons may involve transamination, deamination or modification to primary amines. The by-product from deamination is ammonia, which may be converted by the ornithine cycle to ammonia. In a normal adult, about 30 g urea is produced daily. In hepatic failure, this conversion is less likely to occur, and an accumulation of ammonia occurs.

Carbohydrate metabolism

The liver's main role in carbohydrate metabolism is in maintaining glucose homeostasis during periods of fasting. It accomplishes this by glycogenesis, storing glycogen and glycogenolysis. When glycogen reserves are depleted it is the site of gluconeogenesis.

Lipid metabolism

The liver synthesises fatty acids and lipoproteins for export. It also is a major site of endogenous cholesterol and prostaglandin synthesis.

Detoxification

The liver has a major function in the detoxification of steroid hormones. The mechanisms for detoxification are also used for the metabolism of exogenous substances, in particular therapeutic drugs.

DRUG METABOLISM

Drug metabolism in the liver is divided into two phases:

- Phase 1 – covers modification of the drug to increase its polar nature and make it hydrophilic. It also provides reactive end groups to act as conjugation sites
- Phase 2 – involves conjugation of the modified drug with hydrophilic groups to increase its solubility and aid renal excretion

Phase 1 metabolism is almost entirely oxidative. There is a little reductive metabolism in the gut, and in isolated hepatocytes, as most of the liver is relatively hypoxic, with periportal hepatocytes running at a normal PO_2 of about 3 kPa. This oxidative activity is carried out by a diverse enzyme superfamily known collectively as cytochrome P_{450}, which occur in many tissues. A large part of first-pass metabolism may be due to cytochrome activity in the gut mucosa. Similarly, nephrotoxicity after the metabolism of volatile anaesthetic agents may be due to intrarenal metabolism by cytochromes, rather than a consequence of elevated plasma fluoride levels.

Phase 2 metabolism is conjugative. Drugs that have been modified by phase 1 metabolism are usually left with reactive end groups (such as hydroxyl). These groups provide sites for conjugation with more hydrophilic compounds, such as glucuronic acid, acetate, sulphate or glutathione (Figure MT.21).

HEPATIC METABOLISM OF DRUGS

Phase	Reaction
Phase 1	Oxidation
	Hydrolysis
	Hydration
	Dealkylation
	Reduction
	n-oxidation
	Isomerisation
Phase 2	Glucuronidation
	Sulphation
	Acetylation
	Glutathione conjugation

Figure MT.21

The overall result of phase 1 and 2 metabolism is to produce a modified drug structure which is hydrophilic and rapidly eliminated by the kidneys.

BODY TEMPERATURE AND THERMOREGULATION

Body temperature is tightly regulated. Many enzyme and transport systems cannot tolerate excessive temperature changes. Normal body temperature is 37°C and thermoregulatory mechanisms maintain this temperature with a standard deviation of about 0.2°C. There are normal variations within this range, such as a circadian variation of up to 0.7°C. A variation during the menstrual cycle produces a rise in temperature at ovulation. Body temperature may be altered by various factors including exercise, feeding, thyroid disease, infection and drugs.

PHYSIOLOGICAL MECHANISMS

The hypothalamus processes temperature information from skin, central tissues, and neural tissues. Cold signals travel via A fibres, and warm signals via C fibres in the spinothalamic tracts. This temperature information is integrated and compared to temperature thresholds. Thermoregulation is currently thought based on a series of thresholds that activate thermoregulatory responses when crossed by the integrated temperature information. The further the crossed threshold is from the 'normal' temperature, the greater is the response pattern.

If the warm threshold is exceeded, heat loss responses are initiated, which include:

- Behavioural modification, e.g. removal of clothes
- Cutaneous vasodilation
- Sweating
- Panting

If the cold threshold is exceeded, thermogenic activities are initiated. These include:

- Behavioural (turning on heat sources, adding more clothes)
- Exercise
- Cutaneous vasoconstriction
- Shivering
- Non shivering thermogenesis

THERMOREGULATORY RESPONSES

There are several effective thermoregulatory responses in the normal human. These include:

- Behaviour – in a conscious adult, this is the major regulator of heat loss. The options to move away from heat sources, modify local temperature, or add or remove clothing make this a very powerful mechanism
- Cutaneous blood flow – skin blood flow is a combination of capillary flow and extracapillary shunts. Vasoconstriction minimally reduces capillary flow but has major effects on the shunts, which act as thermoregulator mechanisms. Vasodilation can increase capillary blood flow up to about 7 l/min
- Shivering – can increase metabolic activity by up to 600% in adults. The effectiveness of this heat source is reduced by the fact that muscle activity also increases blood flow to peripheral tissues, dissipating the heat generated. Non shivering thermogenesis. Specialised areas of brown fat are able to increase metabolic output by fat oxidation. This can increase heat production by up to 100% in infants, but is much less effective in adults
- Sweating – in stressed athletes sweating can account for the loss of about 2 litres per H, and increase heat loss by a factor of 10 times

DISTURBANCES OF THERMOREGULATION

Fever

This is one of the most common manifestations of disease. It is due to the production of endogenous pyrogens, which are most likely to include certain interleukins, interferons and tumour necrosis factor (TNF). These cytokines are thought to act by causing the local release of prostaglandins in the hypothalamus. The anti-pyretic effect of aspirin and other non steroidal anti-inflammatory agents is due to the inhibition of cyclo-oxygenase a key enzyme in prostaglandin synthesis.

Malignant hyperpyrexia

A genetic condition that causes widespread persistent muscle contraction when triggered by stress or specific anaesthetic agents. The result is massive heat production and a rapid uncontrolled body rise in body temperature with metabolic acidosis and myoglobinuria. The underlying lesion is a defect in the gene coding for the ryanodine receptors in the sarcoplasmic triads, which leads to excessive Ca^{2+} release.

Hypothermia

Hypothermia is said to be present when body core

temperatures are less than 36°C. It may be associated with:

- Exposure
- Near drowning
- The elderly
- Hypothyroidism
- Prolonged surgery

Normal metabolic and physiological processes are slowed down resulting in hypotension, bradycardia, bradypnoea and loss of consciousness. In severe cases, pulmonary oedema and ventricular fibrillation may occur. Re-warming can be active or passive and with adequate physiological support humans can be resuscitated from 20 to 25°C without permanent sequelae.

Hypothermic effects of anaesthesia and surgery

Anaesthesia has a number of effects on thermoregulation. Behavioural responses are totally abolished. An individual is unable to control their environment, clothing levels, or level of voluntary muscle activity. Cutaneous vasoconstriction is antagonised by vasodilator anaesthetics. In addition, thresholds are directly affected by anaesthesia, which tends to increase the displacement of the thresholds from normal temperature. The hyperthermic threshold are increased by about 1°C, while hypothermic thresholds are markedly reduced, by up to 3–4°C. This effect also appears to be dose-dependent. Thus, thermoregulatory responses to heat loss are impaired or abolished.

The physical mechanisms during anaesthesia and surgery causing heat loss are:

- Conduction – heat loss due to contact with an object at a lower temperature such as a cold operating table. The rate of heat loss is dependent on the temperature gradient between the body and the table, the surface area of contact, and the thermal conductance of the tissues
- Convection – heat loss due to the movement of air away from the exposed body surfaces and will be increased by imposed air flow currents such as in laminar flow operating theatres
- Radiation – heat loss by infra red radiation from exposed portions of the body to neighbouring objects not in contact. This may be reduced by the use of reflective coverings over the exposed surfaces such as a space blanket, or by increasing the ambient temperature
- Evaporation of sweat from skin or body fluids from mucosal or tissue surfaces – heat loss is due to the latent heat of evaporation lost when fluid changes phase from liquid to vapour. The rate of heat loss is dependent on the mass of fluid evaporated per unit time, since the latent heat of evaporation is a constant.

SECTION 2: 12
ENDOCRINOLOGY

T. A. Leach

ENDOCRINE FUNCTION
Cellular mechanisms of hormone action
Control mechanisms regulating hormone release

PITUITARY GLAND
Structure
Anterior pituitary hormones
Posterior pituitary hormones
Abnormalities of secretion

THYROID GLAND
Structure
Thyroid hormones
Abnormalities of secretion

ADRENAL GLAND
Structure of the adrenal cortex
Mineralocorticoids
Glucocorticoids
Adrenal androgens
Abnormalities of adrenocortical secretion
Structure of the adrenal medulla
Catecholamines
Control of catecholamine secretion
Abnormalities of catecholamine secretion

PARATHYROID GLAND AND CALCIUM HOMEOSTASIS
Regulation of calcium
Parathyroid hormone
Vitamin D
Calcitonin
Abnormalities of secretion

PANCREAS
Structure
Insulin
Glucagon
Somatostatin
Abnormalities of secretion

ENDOCRINE FUNCTION

Endocrinology encompasses the regulation, mechanism of action and effects of hormones. Hormones are secreted into the circulation by endocrine glands, and are then transported in the blood to numerous organs and tissues. Hormones produce physiological effects by various cellular mechanisms, which operate at the target tissues. These physiological changes play a major part in homeostasis.

CELLULAR MECHANISMS OF HORMONE ACTION

A hormone produces its physiological changes by a spectrum of actions on different tissues. These physiological changes may also follow a characteristic time course. Cellular mechanisms which enable a single substance to produce such a complex result include:

- Attachment to cell membrane receptors, which in turn activate intracellular second messengers such as cyclic AMP. These hormones include peptides and catecholamines.
- Diffusion across cell membrane to activate receptors intracellularly and modify genetic expression. Hormones such as steroids and thyroxine come into this category.
- Upregulation or down regulation of cell membrane receptors.
- Interaction with other hormones by displaying permissiveness. In such a case, one hormone in low concentration produces a permissive effect on the receptors of a second hormone thus enabling the second hormone to exert full activity. An example of this is the permissive effect of thyroid hormones on epinephrine receptors in fat tissue promoting the release of fatty acids.

CONTROL MECHANISMS REGULATING HORMONE RELEASE

Control of secretion in the endocrine system is important because of the primary role hormones play in homeostatic reflexes. Various mechanisms regulate the secretion of a hormone. The most important type of control is negative feedback control, which attempts to maintain a constant circulating level of the hormone or a substance controlled by the hormone. Thus high circulating levels of hormone act on the secreting cells to reduce subsequent release. Other regulating factors include:

- Plasma concentrations of inorganic ions (e.g. sodium)
- Plasma concentrations of organic substances (e.g. glucose)
- The action of neurotransmitters released by stimulated nerves (e.g. acetyl choline)
- Another hormone or paracrine agent (e.g. prostaglandins)
- Direct chemical or physical stimulation (e.g. release of gut hormones)

PITUITARY GLAND

The pituitary gland secretes a wide range of hormones and is both anatomically and functionally linked to the hypothalamus. As a result, the hypothalamus is able to regulate several aspects of endocrine function.

STRUCTURE OF THE PITUITARY GLAND

The pituitary gland is located immediately below the hypothalamus to which it is connected by both hypophyseal portal blood vessels and neuronal tissue contained within the pituitary stalk. The pituitary gland consists of two embryologically distinct parts, **anterior** and **posterior**.

Anterior Pituitary

The activity of the anterior pituitary is regulated by hormones secreted from the hypothalamus and transported in the hypophyseal portal blood (see Figure EP. 1). These hypothalamic factors are peptides, which

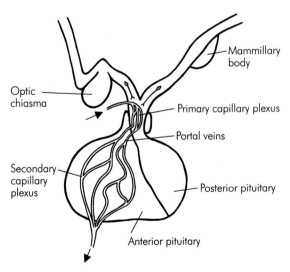

Figure EP.1 Portal system of the pituitary gland

can either stimulate or inhibit the secretion of a given pituitary hormone. Secretion of these regulating hormones is influenced by neurological inputs and feedback control as shown in Figure EP. 2. Thus, the hypothalamus acts as a link between the central nervous system and the endocrine glands.

ANTERIOR PITUITARY HORMONES

The anterior pituitary secretes six peptide hormones, ACTH, TSH, FSH, LH, Prolactin and growth hormone. Prolactin acts on the breast, the others are at least in part tropic hormones, i.e. they stimulate the secretion of hormonally active substances by other glands or tissues (see later).

Adrenocorticotropic Hormone (ACTH)
ACTH is formed from a large precursor protein, which is cleaved to form a family of hormones. ACTH is principally responsible for regulating secretions of the adrenal cortex, especially cortisol. Secretion of ACTH is under the control of corticotrophin-releasing hormone (CRH), which is released from the hypothalamus, as well as a negative feedback mechanism dependent on the circulating concentration of cortisol.

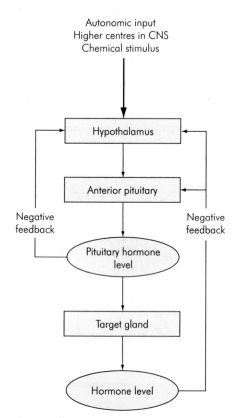

Figure EP.2 Feedback control of the pituitary gland

Exogenous administration of steroids can lead to suppression of the hypothalamic-pituitary axis. Sub-physiological levels of cortisol can lead to haemodynamic instability in situations of stress, for example in the perioperative period. Therefore, it has been common practice to administer supplementary exogenous corticosteroids if the pituitary axis is thought to be suppressed, for example after long-term oral steroid therapy.

Thyroid stimulating hormone (TSH)
TSH is secreted from the anterior pituitary in response to thyrotrophin-releasing hormone (TRH) released from the hypothalamus, as well as a negative feedback mechanism depending on the plasma concentration of thyroid hormone. It stimulates thyroid secretion and general follicular activity is increased.

Follicle-stimulating hormone (FSH) and luteinising hormone (LH)
FSH and LH are secreted in response to their appropriate releasing hormones. FSH stimulates ovarian follicle growth in the female, and spermatogenesis in the male. LH stimulates ovulation and luteinisation of ovarian follicles in female and testosterone secretion in the male.

Prolactin
Prolactin secretion is mainly controlled by prolactin-inhibiting hormone (PIH), which is probably dopamine. Stimuli which reduce PIH release, raise prolactin levels. Secretion increases during pregnancy, reaching a peak at parturition, resulting in development of the breasts ready for lactation. Plasma prolactin levels fall in the week following delivery. Suckling leads to an increase in prolactin secretion, but the magnitude of this rise decreases with time. Raised prolactin levels reduce ovarian function, leading to a degree of sub-fertility during breast-feeding.

Growth hormone (GH)
Secretion of GH is controlled by releasing and inhibiting factors regulated by the hypothalamus. GH is a major anabolic hormone, which stimulates growth of all tissues in the body, particularly bones, and is therefore especially important in children although GH continues to have important metabolic functions even after the epiphyses have fused. Protein synthesis is increased; fat stores are broken down and used for energy, whilst blood glucose levels tend to rise.

The growth hormone receptor is a cytokine, having 620 amino acids. There is a large extracellular portion, a transmembrane domain, and a large cytoplasmic portion. It has two binding sites and dimerisation is essential for receptor activation.

The effects of GH on target tissues are mediated by a group of polypeptide factors secreted by the liver and other tissues in response to GH. These growth factors are known as somatomedins. The two main circulating somatomedins are Insulin-like Growth Factor I (IGF-I) and IGF-II. Both of these factors are related to insulin in structure. IGF-I is mainly responsible for skeletal and cartilage growth, while IGF-II exerts its effects on foetal growth.

Figure EP.3 details the actions of growth hormone and the somatomedins

Posterior pituitary

The posterior pituitary secretes two peptides, vasopressin (antidiuretic hormone, ADH) and oxytocin, which are synthesised in the hypothalamus and then transported down axons within the pituitary stalk to be stored in vesicles ready for subsequent release into the bloodstream in response to appropriate stimuli (see Figure EP.4).

POSTERIOR PITUITARY HORMONES

Vasopressin (antidiuretic hormone, ADH)
ADH is produced in the supraoptic nucleus of the hypothalamus. It is then transferred in vesicles along axons to the posterior pituitary for subsequent release in response to appropriate stimuli. Release of ADH is triggered whenever the osmolarity of the extracellular fluid rises or if blood volume or blood pressure falls.

Painful stimulation and haemorrhage, such as that associated with surgery, are potent triggers for evoking the release of ADH. The resulting increase in ADH

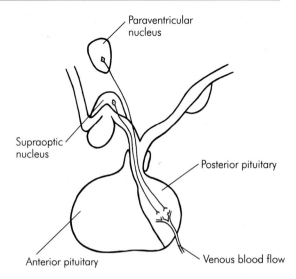

Figure EP.4 Posterior pituitary innervation

promotes water reabsorption from the distal renal tubules and collecting ducts in the renal medulla. This tends to reduce plasma osmolarity and expand the volume of extracellular fluid, due to water retention. The resultant urine produced is of low volume and concentrated. ADH is thought to act at a specific aquaporin type receptor in the distal tubule (see section 2 chapter 7). ADH activity is also affected by the metabolites of volatile anaesthetic agents. Fluoride ions produced from the metabolism of methoxyflurane, and to a lesser extent, enflurane, interfere with the normal receptor response to ADH resulting in the potential for high output renal failure. ADH also increases peripheral resistance through arteriolar constriction, which helps to maintain arterial pressure.

Oxytocin
Oxytocin is produced by cells in the paraventricular nucleus of the hypothalamus. Its primary role is to stimulate ejection of milk through contraction of the myoepithelial cells surrounding the milk ducts during lactation. Oxytocin also stimulates uterine contraction and reduces the likelihood of postpartum haemorrhage.

The principal actions of the pituitary hormones are summarised in Figure EP.5.

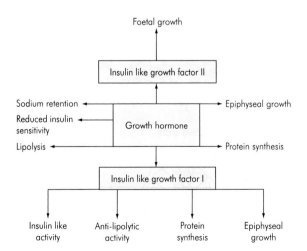

Figure EP.3 Actions of growth hormones and somatomedins

- Stimulation of calcium release from bone
- Stimulation of the rate of calcium reabsorption from the renal tubules
- Increased urinary phosphate excretion
- Acceleration of the rate at which vitamin D is converted to its active form (1,25 dihydroxycholecalciferol) within the kidneys

Vitamin D

Vitamin D is a fat-soluble vitamin, which is derived from either dietary sources (vitamin D_2) or by UV radiation from sunlight stimulating the production of vitamin D_3 (cholecalciferol) in the skin. Once in the circulation cholecalciferol is converted to 25-hydroxycholecaliferol in the liver and then 1,25-dihydroxycholecaliferol in the kidneys (Figure EP.15). The formation of this active metabolite is stimulated by PTH, low plasma calcium and low plasma phosphate levels.

Vitamin D elevates plasma levels of both calcium and phosphate by increasing the rate of calcium uptake from the gut, stimulating phosphate absorption from the gut stimulating osteoclastic bone reabsorption

Calcitonin

Calcitonin is secreted by the C cells of the thyroid gland. It acts on bone to reduce the rate of calcium release and therefore tends to lower plasma calcium levels.

ABNORMALITIES OF CALCIUM CONTROL

Deficient secretion

Hypoparathyroidism may be due to autoimmune disease or secondary to accidental damage during thyroid surgery. A low PTH level results in hypocalcaemia and hyperphosphataemia. The hyperexcitability of nerves and muscles causes tetany, laryngeal spasm or even convulsions.

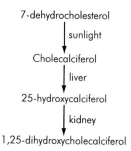

7-dehydrocholesterol

↓ sunlight

Cholecalciferol

↓ liver

25-hydroxycalciferol

↓ kidney

1,25-dihydroxycholecalciferol

Figure EP.15 Hydroxylation of vitamin D

Deficient vitamin D activity may be a result of reduced dietary intake (or malabsorption) in associated with low levels of UV exposure. Failure of Vitamin D activation may also be a problem in patients with chronic renal failure. The most obvious effects are demineralisation of bone leading to osteomalacia in adults and rickets in children.

Excess secretion

Primary hyperparathyroidism, usually due to a PTH secreting tumour (often bronchogenic oat cell) results in hypercalcaemia and a low plasma phosphate. Bone reabsorption causes cyst formation whilst calcium is deposited elsewhere in the body e.g. renal calculi.

Hypervitaminosis D is a consequence of excessive vitamin D supplements in the diet. In this case, both plasma calcium and phosphate levels are high.

THE PANCREAS

STRUCTURE

The pancreas is divided by connective tissue septa into lobules, each of which contains a secretory unit, the acinus. Lying between the pancreatic acini and ducts involved in the production and release of digestive enzymes are groups of cells known as the islets of Langerhans, which are responsible for the endocrine functions of the pancreas. They account for approximately 2% of the volume of the pancreas, compared to the exocrine part, which occupies 80%, the remainder being ducts and blood vessels. There are four cell types within these islets each producing a different hormone.

- Insulin is secreted by B cells
- Glucagon is secreted by A cells
- Somatostatin is secreted by D cells
- Pancreatic polypeptide is secreted by F cells

Insulin

STRUCTURE AND BIOSYNTHESIS

Insulin is a polypeptide containing two chains of amino acids linked by disulphide bridges. In humans, its gene is situated on the short arm of chromosome 11. The precise amino-acid sequence of insulin shows slight variations between species, which are not sufficient to affect biological activity of a particular insulin in a different species, but enough to cause the formation of antibodies, which inhibit the injected insulin. Human insulin prepared in bacteria by recombinant DNA techniques is now widely used to counteract this problem.

Like other polypeptide hormones, insulin is synthesised as part of a larger preprohormone. The leader sequence is removed as it enters the endoplasmic reticulum of the B cell. The molecule then folds, and disulphide bridges form to make proinsulin. The A and B chains of the insulin molecule are connected by C-peptide, which is detached before secretion.

Insulin stimulates a wide variety of responses in its target tissues: skeletal muscle, fat and liver, which appear to be initiated by the interaction of insulin and a protein receptor in the cell membranes of these tissues.

The core of the insulin receptor consists of four polypeptide chains, joined in a cylindrical shape. When insulin binds, a structural change occurs, creating a tunnel through which molecules such as glucose can enter the cell. In addition, binding of insulin activates an enzyme component of the receptor located on the inside of the cell (tyrosine kinase), and this enzyme stimulates production of a second messenger that leads to promotion of the other metabolic effects associated with insulin, such as fat, protein and glycogen synthesis.

Cells can alter the input of glucose by regulating the number of receptors present on the cell surface.

REGULATION OF INSULIN SECRETION

There are several agents regulating the secretion of insulin (Figure EP.16) but the major factors are:

- Elevation of plasma glucose concentration stimulating a rapid rise in insulin secretion. This negative feedback system maintains blood glucose concentration within a narrow range. As glucose levels decline, so insulin levels fall 3–4 hours after a meal
- Increased amino acid concentrations stimulating insulin secretion and therefore promoting their cellular uptake and use for protein synthesis.
- Somatostatin secretion, which inhibits insulin release

CONTROLLING FACTORS IN INSULIN SECRETION

Stimulation	Inhibition
Hyperglycaemia	Hypoglycaemia
Beta agonists	Beta-blockers
Acetylcholine	Alpha agonists
Glucagon	Somatostatin
	Diazoxide
	Thiazides
	Volatile agents

Figure EP.16

Metabolic actions of insulin

Insulin is an anabolic hormone affecting carbohydrate, protein and lipid metabolism in the following manner.

Carbohydrate metabolism
Insulin promotes:

- Glucose uptake in most body tissues particularly in both the liver and skeletal muscle (as cerebral metabolism is highly dependent on glucose brain cells are freely permeable to glucose even in the absence of insulin).
- Glycogen storage
- The use of glucose for energy

Protein metabolism
Insulin promotes protein accumulation within cells by:

- Stimulating amino acid uptake
- Stimulating protein synthesis
- Inhibiting conversion of amino acids to glucose (gluconeogenesis)

Lipid metabolism
Insulin promotes the deposition of triglycerides in body lipid stores by:

- Inhibiting the breakdown of lipids by lipase
- Stimulating fatty acid synthesis from glucose
- Promoting glycerol synthesis in lipid cells
- Promoting carbohydrate metabolism so that fat is spared

Glucagon

Glucagon is a catabolic hormone, which tends to raise blood glucose levels. The secretion of glucagon from the cells of the pancreatic islets is regulated by numerous factors (Figure EP.17) but chiefly influenced by low plasma glucose concentrations and high levels of circulating amino acids.

CONTROL OF GLUCAGON SECRETION

Stimulation	Inhibition
Hypoglycaemia	Hyperglycaemia
Stress	Somatostatin
Sepsis	Insulin
Trauma	Free fatty acids
Beta agonists	Alpha agonists

Figure EP.17

METABOLIC ACTIONS OF GLUCAGON

Glucagon effects tend to oppose those of insulin and have effects on carbohydrate and lipid metabolism as detailed below.

PREGNANCY

Normal pregnancy involves major physiological and anatomical adaptations by maternal organs. It is important that anaesthetists involved in the care of the pregnant woman understand these changes to provide anaesthetic care which is compatible with safe delivery of the baby.

CARDIOVASCULAR SYSTEM

There are multiple changes in the cardiovascular system many of which are compensatory changes designed to cope with the growing foetus, uterus and placenta. These are summarised in Figure PN.1. Although the majority of changes occur during pregnancy, significant changes also occur during labour and immediately following delivery of the baby.

CHANGES IN HAEMODYNAMIC PARAMETERS DURING PREGNANCY

	Parameter	Change
Heart	Cardiac Output	↑ by 50%
	Stroke volume	↑ by 30%
	Heart rate	↑ by 25%
	Ejection Fraction	↑ by 20%
	Left ventricle mass	↑ by 50%
	Left ventricular end diastolic volume	↑ by 10%
Systemic circulation	Systemic vascular resistance	↓ by 20%
	Pulmonary vascular resistance	↓ by 34%
	Systolic blood pressure	↓ by 6–8%
	Diastolic blood pressure	↓ by 20–25%

Figure PN.1

Cardiac output

Patient posture has been found to influence cardiac output measurements significantly during pregnancy (Figure PN.2). Measurements performed in the lateral position to avoid aorto caval compression, demonstrate an increase in cardiac output by 5 weeks gestation. Cardiac output continues to increase from this time,

THE EFFECT OF POSITION ON CARDIAC OUTPUT DURING PREGNANCY

Position	Change in cardiac output
Supine	Baseline
Left lateral	↑ by 13.5%
Lithotomy	↓ by 17%
Steep Trendelenberg	↓ by 18%

Figure PN.2

resulting in a rise of 35–40% by the end of the first trimester, increasing to 50% by the end of the second trimester (Figure PN.3). Cardiac output then remains at 50% above non pregnant levels throughout the third trimester.

A further transient rise in cardiac output occurs at delivery, as a result of labour and uteroplacental transfusion into the maternal intravascular volume.

HEART RATE AND STROKE VOLUME

The increase in cardiac output in pregnancy is produced by a combination of increased heart rate, reduced systemic vascular resistance (SVR) and increased stroke volume. Heart rate is increased above non pregnant values by 15% at the end of the first trimester. This increases to 25% by the end of the second trimester, but there is no further change in the third trimester.

Stroke volume is increased by about 20% at 8 weeks and up to 30% by the end of the second trimester, then remaining level until term (Figure PN.3)

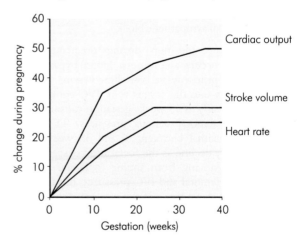

Figure PN.3 Cardiovascular changes during pregnancy

Systemic vascular resistance

SVR is reduced during pregnancy. The average SVR in pregnancy is 979 compared with 1700 dyn.s/cm^5 in non pregnant women. The decrease in the SVR results from the development of a low-resistance vascular bed (the intervillous space) and vasodilatory effects of oestrogens, prostacyclin and progesterone.

Distribution of the cardiac output during pregnancy is different from the non pregnant state with increased blood flow to the uterus, kidneys and skin. Uterine blood flow varies from 500 to 700 ml/min (about 10–12% of the cardiac output) at term, of which > 80% perfuses the placenta. The flow to the kidneys is increased and so is the flow to the skin due to peripheral vasodilatation. Flow to the liver and brain remains unchanged.

Blood pressure

Blood pressure falls during pregnancy. Systolic blood pressure is minimally affected with a maximum decline of 8% during early and mid-gestation, returning to non pregnant levels at term. Diastolic blood pressure falls to a greater extent with early and mid-gestational decreases of 20–25%, and returns to normal at term. In the supine position, 70% of mothers have a fall in blood pressure of at least 10%, and 8% have decreases between 30 and 50%.

Aorto caval compression

Compression of the inferior vena cava (IVC) and aorta by the gravid uterus occurs during pregnancy and reduces cardiac output. The severity of this effect is dependent on:

- Patient position
- Gestation
- Systemic blood pressure
- Presence of sympathetic block

In the supine position during pregnancy, IVC obstruction occurs and venous blood bypasses this obstruction primarily via vertebral venous plexuses which empty into the azygos vein. IVC compression develops as early as 13 weeks gestation causing a 50% increase in femoral venous pressures. This effect becomes maximal between 36 and 38 weeks, after which it may decline as the foetal head descends into the pelvis. Moving from supine to lateral position reduces the femoral and IVC pressures, but these are still elevated above those of the non pregnant woman indicating that the compression of the IVC is not completely relieved by lateral positioning. In the supine position, 5–8% of pregnant women experience a substantial drop in blood pressure (supine hypotension

syndrome), and the patients develop systemic signs of shock, i.e. pallor, sweating, nausea, vomiting and syncope.

Obstruction of the aorta in the supine position has been demonstrated angiographically but the higher pressures in the aorta prevent total obstruction. This does not cause maternal hypotension but causes arterial hypotension in the lower extremities and in the uterine arteries, which can lead to inadequate uterine blood flow resulting in foetal asphyxia and bradycardia.

Electrocardiogam (ECG) and echocardiogram

The ECG in pregnancy may show the following changes:

- Sinus tachycardia
- Rotation of the electrical axis of the heart to the left
- ST segment depression
- T-wave flattening

However, these changes are thought to be of no clinical significance.

Echocardiographic studies during pregnancy have shown:

- Left ventricular hypertrophy by 12 weeks gestation
- A 50% increase in left ventricular mass at term
- A 12–14% increase in aortic, pulmonary and mitral valve sizes

HEART SOUNDS

The apical impulse moves to the fourth intercostal space and mid-clavicular line. Most pregnant women develop a loud and sometimes split first heart sound. A third heart sound is common, and 16% of women have a fourth heart sound. A grade I–II early to mid-systolic heart murmur is commonly heard at the left sternal edge. This may be due to tricuspid re-gurgitation resulting from dilatation of the tricuspid valve.

Venous pressure

In the absence of IVC compression by the uterus, central venous pressure (CVP) and pressure in the upper limbs is normal. However, during late pregnancy when in the supine position, IVC compression occurs and CVP may decrease dramatically. IVC compression can also cause increased venous pressure in the lower limbs.

During labour various factors can cause an increase in CVP, including:

- Contractions that can increase CVP by about 5 cmH$_2$O

- Expulsive efforts of the second stage can create a major rise in CVP by up to 50 cmH$_2$O
- IV ergometrine 0.25 mg after delivery of the baby can produce a rise in CVP of 8 cmH$_2$O, which can last up to 60 min

There are no observed changes in pulmonary capillary wedge and pulmonary artery pressures during pregnancy. Recent non invasive studies have demonstrated a high incidence of asymptomatic pericardial effusion during normal pregnancy.

HAEMATOLOGY

Blood volume

Plasma volume, total blood volume and red blood cell (RBC) volume all increase during pregnancy (Figure PN.4). Plasma volume rises by 15% during the first trimester and can reach 50% above non pregnant values by 32 weeks; it then remains at this level unchanged. Plasma volume returns to non pregnant levels by 6 days post delivery. There is often a sharp rise of up to 1 litre in plasma volume 24 H after delivery. This is of significant importance in patients with cardiac disease such as those with fixed cardiac output. Such patients may develop pulmonary oedema during this period.

RBC volume falls during the first 8 weeks of pregnancy, increasing back to non pregnant levels by 16 weeks and then rising to 30% above non pregnant levels by term. This increase in RBC volume is due to raised erythropoietin levels that occur from 12 weeks gestation. The lesser increase in RBC volume relative to the increase in plasma volume results in overall reductions of about 15% in haemoglobin (Hb) and haematocrit.

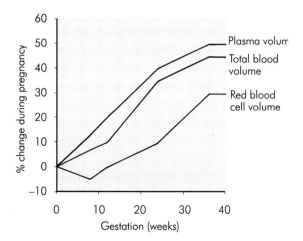

Figure PN.4 Percentage changes in plasma volume, total blood volume and red blood cell volume during pregnancy

The above changes combine to give total blood volume increases of 10, 30 and 45% at the end of the first, second and third trimester respectively (Figure PN.4). Oestrogens and progesterone appear responsible for the increase in plasma volume through their effect on the renin angiotensin aldosterone systems.

White cell count (WCC)

The blood WCC rises progressively during pregnancy from non pregnant levels to 9–11 $\times$ 10^9/l. This is predominantly an increase in polymorphonuclear cells. There is a further leucocytosis to about 15 $\times$ 10^9/l during labour. White cell count returns to normal by 6 days post delivery.

Coagulation

Pregnancy is associated with enhanced platelet turnover, clotting and fibrinolysis (Figure PN.5). Thrombocytopenia (platelets < 100 $\times$ 10^9/l) occurs in 0.8–0.9% of normal pregnant women, while increases in platelet factor and β thromboglobulin suggest elevated platelet activation and consumption. Since there is no change in platelet count in the majority of women during pregnancy, there is probably an increase in platelet production to compensate for the increased consumption.

The concentrations of most coagulation factors (I, VII–X and XII) are increased and a few (XI and XIII) are reduced. The levels of Factors II and V remain the same during pregnancy. There are increases in fibrinogen degradation products (FDP) and plasminogen concentrations which indicate increased fibrinolytic activity during pregnancy.

Plasma proteins

The plasma concentration of albumin is reduced to 34–39 g/l, but globulin and fibrinogen levels are increased. Overall, the total plasma protein concentration falls to 65–70 g/l. These reductions in plasma proteins are associated with the following changes:

- Total colloid osmotic pressure is reduced by 5 mmHg
- Drug-binding capacity of the plasma is altered with consequent changes in pharmacokinetics and dynamics (e.g. a reduction in plasma α acid glycoprotein concentration reduces the lignocaine binding capacity)
- Plasma concentration of pseudocholinesterase is reduced by 20–25% at term
- Erythrocyte sedimentation rate (ESR) and blood viscosity are increased

HAEMATOLOGICAL CHANGES DURING PREGNANCY

	Parameter	Change
Blood volumes	Total blood volume	↑ by 45%
	Plasma volume	↑ by 50%
Blood cells	Red blood cell volume	↑ by 30%
	White cell count	↑
	Haematocrit	↓ by 15%
	Haemoglobin	↓ by 15%
Plasma proteins	Total plasma protein	↓ by 18%
	Albumen	↓ by 14%
	Globulin	↑ or ↓
	Plasma cholinesterase	↓ by 20–25%
	Colloid osmotic pressure	↓ by 18%
Coagulation	Platelets	↓ by 0–5%
	Prothrombin time	↓ by 20%
	Bleeding time	↓ by 10%
	Partial thromboplastin time	↓ by 20%
	Antithrombin III	↓ by 10%
	Fibrin degradation products	↑ by 100%
	Plasminogen	↑
	Fibrinolysis	↑
Clotting factors	I	↑ by 100%
	II	↑ or nil
	V	↑ or nil
	VII	↑ by 100%
	VIII	↑ by 150%
	IX	↑ by 100%
	X	↑ by 30%
	XI	↓ by 40–50%
	XII	↑ by 30%
	XIII	↓ by 50%

Figure PN.5

Fluid compartments

Both extravascular and intravascular water content increases during pregnancy. The increase in extravascular water varies from 1.7 litres in women without oedema to 5 litres in women with oedema.

The above haematological changes are summarised in Figure PN.5.

RESPIRATORY SYSTEM

Anatomical changes

Capillary engorgement of the nasal, pharyngeal mucosa and larynx begins early in the first trimester. This may explain why many pregnant women complain of difficulty in nasal breathing, experience more episodes of epistaxis and experience voice changes. The thoracic cage increases in circumference by 5–7 cm because of the increase in both the antero posterior and transverse diameters from flaring of the ribs. Flaring of the ribs begins early in pregnancy and is, therefore, not entirely due to pressure from the enlarging uterus. The enlarging uterus displaces the diaphragm upwards in the later weeks of pregnancy, but the internal volume of the thoracic cavity remains unchanged.

Lung mechanics and volumes

Inspiration is mainly as a result of diaphragmatic movement since flaring of the ribs reduces chest wall movement. Bronchial smooth muscle relaxation decreases airway resistance but lung compliance remains unchanged. Factors contributing to airway dilatation include direct effects of progesterone, cortisone and relaxin.

Forced expiratory volume at one second (FEV_1), the ratio of FEV_1 to forced vital capacity (FVC), and the flow volume loop remain unchanged demonstrating that large airway function is not impaired during pregnancy.

The following changes in lung volumes occur during pregnancy, relative to non pregnant values:

- Tidal volume increases steadily from the first trimester by up to 45% at term (Figure PN.6)
- Functional residual capacity (FRC) is decreased by 20–30% at term due to reductions of 25% in expiratory reserve volume (ERV) and 15% in residual volume
- Closing capacity can encroach on FRC, increasing ventilation–perfusion mismatch and leading to the ready occurrence of hypoxia, particularly in supine and Trendelenberg positions

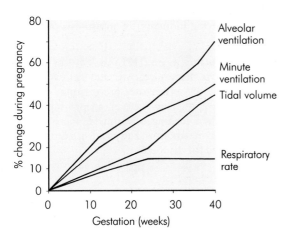

Figure PN.6 Respiratory changes (%) during pregnancy

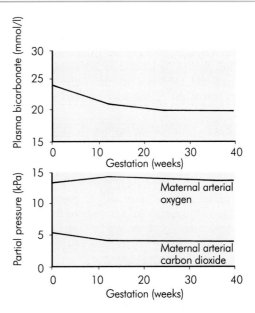

Figure PN.7 Changes in arterial bicarbonate, oxygen and carbon dioxide during pregnancy

- Inspiratory capacity increases by 15% at term due to increases in inspiratory reserve and tidal volumes

MINUTE VENTILATION (MV)

MV is increased by up to 50% above non pregnant values at term. Since respiratory rate remains unaltered, this increase is due to larger tidal volumes. The increased MV levels are stimulated by the high progesterone levels and increased carbon dioxide production occurring during pregnancy.

Dead space is greater by 45% due to dilatation of large airways, however, the concomitant increase in tidal volume leaves the ratio of dead space to tidal volume unchanged.

DIFFUSING CAPACITY

Diffusing capacity of the lungs for carbon monoxide (DLCO) is increased during the first trimester, but then decreases until 24–27 weeks gestation, when it remains unchanged until term.

Blood gases

$PaCO_2$ decreases to 3.7–4.2 kPa by the end of the first trimester and remains at this level until term (Figure PN.7). This is due to alveolar hyperventilation and gives rise to various compensatory mechanisms in an attempt to maintain normal pH. Metabolic compensation for the respiratory alkalosis reduces the serum bicarbonate concentration to about 18–21 mmol/l, the base excess (BE) by 2–3 mmol/l and the total buffer base by about 5 mmol/l. Metabolic compensation is not complete, which explains the elevation of maternal blood pH by 0.04 units.

PaO_2 in upright pregnant women is in the region of 14.0 kPa, higher than that in non pregnant women (Figure PN.7). This is due to lower $PaCO_2$ levels, a reduced arterio venous oxygen difference and a reduction in physiological shunt. The small progressive decline in the PaO_2 during the second and third trimesters is due to an increase in arterio venous oxygen difference.

When PaO_2 is determined in the supine position, the values after mid-gestation are often < 13.3 kPa. This occurs because:

- FRC is less than the closing volume in up to 50% of supine pregnant patients
- Aorto caval compression reduces cardiac output which increases arterio venous oxygen difference and reduces mixed venous oxygen content

DYSPNOEA DURING PREGNANCY

About 60% of normal pregnant women with no history of cardiorespiratory disease experience dyspnoea. Dyspnoea during pregnancy is, therefore, not always an indication of organic disease. It commonly occurs in the first and second trimesters and is probably a result of lowered $PaCO_2$ levels.

Pulmonary circulation

Pulmonary vascular resistance is reduced from 119 dyn.s/cm⁵ in the non pregnant woman to 78 dyn.s/cm⁵ in the pregnant woman at term. Pulmonary blood flow is increased in pregnancy due to increased cardiac output, and pulmonary blood volume is also greater as demonstrated by increased vascular markings on chest X-ray. The normal woman can cope with these changes and the pressures in the right ventricle, pulmonary artery and pulmonary capillaries are not raised.

The above respiratory system changes are summarised in Figure PN.8.

OXYGEN CONSUMPTION

Oxygen consumption is increased in pregnancy by 30–60% due to the metabolic demands of the foetus, uterus and placenta. The decreased FRC and increased metabolic rate predispose the mother to the rapid onset of hypoxia during induction of anaesthesia or airway obstruction.

Human placental lactogen (HPL) and cortisol increase the tendency to hyperglycaemia and ketosis, which may unmask or exacerbate pre-existing diabetes mellitus. The pregnant woman adapts rapidly to starvation. When feeding is withheld, there is early activation of fat metabolism. Fatty acids are utilised and glucose is saved for the foetus.

GASTRO-INTESTINAL SYSTEM

Pregnant women have been regarded for many years as

RESPIRATORY CHANGES DURING PREGNANCY COMPARED WITH NON PREGNANT PATIENTS

	Parameter	Change
Anatomy	Capillary engorgement of URT	↑
	Upper airway	Dilated
	Diaphragm	Elevated
	Thoracic circumference	↑ by 5–7 cm
Lung volumes	Tidal volume	↑ by 45%
	Inspiratory reserve volume	↑ by 5%
	Expiratory reserve volume	↓ by 25%
	Residual volume	↓ by 20%
	Functional reserve capacity	↓ by 30%
	Vital capacity	nil
	Total lung capacity	↓ by 0–5%
	Closing capacity	nil
Ventilation	Minute ventilation	↑ by 50%
	Alveolar ventilation	↑ by 70%
	Respiratory rate	↑ by 0–15%
	Dead space	↑ by 45%
Lung mechanics	Diaphragm movement	↑
	Chest wall movement	↓
	Total pulmonary resistance	↓ by 50%
	Lung compliance	nil
	FEV_1	nil
	FEV_1/VC	nil
	Flow volume loop	nil
Arterial blood gases	$PaCO_2$	↓ to 3.7–4.2 kPa
	PaO_2	↑ to 13.3–14.6 kPa
	pH	↑ to 7.44
	HCO_3^-	↓ to 18–21 mmol/l
Oxygen consumption		↑ by 30–60%

Figure PN.8

being at higher risk of acid aspiration because of the reduction in barrier pressure, increased gastric secretion, reduced gastric pH and delayed gastric emptying.

Barrier pressure

Barrier pressure (lower oesophageal sphincter [LOS] pressure minus gastric pressure) is reduced significantly during pregnancy compared with the non pregnant state, due to increased intragastric pressure and reduced LOS pressure (Figure PN.9). LOS pressure appears to return to normal by 48 h post delivery.

Heartburn occurs in 55–80% of pregnant women and may occur at < 20 weeks gestation. This is thought to be due to gastro-oesophageal reflux that occurs when barrier pressure is reduced. Lowered barrier pressure can be asymptomatic.

Causes of reduced barrier pressure include:

- The altered position of the stomach that displaces the intra-abdominal part of the oesophagus into the thorax and lowers LOS pressure
- The relaxant effect of progesterone
- Elevation of intragastric pressure in the last trimester in both standing and supine positions
- Intragastric pressure is raised in lithotomy position (increased by 5.6 cmH$_2$O) and Trendelenberg position (increased by 8.8 cmH$_2$O)

Gastric secretion

The total acid content of the stomach and pepsin secretion are reduced during pregnancy. This may be due to decreased plasma gastrin levels. Commonly used criteria assess the risk of acid aspiration as high, when gastric pH is < 2.5, and gastric volume is > 25 ml. During early gestation (< 15 weeks), 37% of women have been found to fulfil these criteria, but this percentage was comparable with that in non pregnant controls. In patients at term undergoing elective Caesarean section, 49% are at risk of acid aspiration, compared with 42% of controls. Approximately 50% of women in labour have gastric pH < 2.5.

Gastric emptying

Gastric emptying is not delayed during pregnancy but becomes delayed during labour, particularly if opioids are administered. When labour is conducted with epidural or no analgesia, gastric emptying is only slightly reduced. The use of epidural opioids as a bolus appear to reduce gastric emptying compared with patients with no epidural opioids, but the effect of low dose opioid infusions is less clear. Provided that opioids have not been used during labour, gastric emptying returns to normal within 24–48 H post delivery.

CENTRAL NERVOUS SYSTEM

There are substantial pressure and volume changes in the epidural and subarachnoid spaces which have important effects upon the spread of solutions within these compartments (Figure PN.10).

Epidural space

Compression of the IVC by the gravid uterus results in

GASTRO-INTESTINAL TRACT CHANGES DURING PREGNANCY COMPARED TO NON PREGNANT PATIENTS (NON PREGNANT VALUES IN BRACKETS)

Parameter	Value
LOS pressure	15.7 cmH$_2$O) (15.2)
Gastric pressure (supine)	11.1 cmH$_2$O (5.7)
Barrier pressure	4.6 cmH$_2$O (9.5)
Heartburn	↑
Gastric acid secretion	↓
Gastric emptying	nil or ↓

Figure PN.9

CNS CHANGES DURING PREGNANCY

Parameter	Change
MAC of volatile anaesthetic agents	↓
Beta endorphins	↑
Epidural space volume	↓
Epidural space pressure	↑
Cerebrospinal fluid pressure	↑
Cerebrospinal fluid volume	↓
Cerebrospinal fluid composition	nil
Cerebrospinal fluid pH	↑
Sensitivity to local anaesthetics	↑
Local anaesthetic dose requirements	↓

Figure PN.10

increased venous pressure below the level of the obstruction. Venous blood is then diverted through vertebral plexuses within the epidural space and this causes epidural veins to become engorged. Consequently, the epidural volume is reduced and any solutions injected into the lumbar epidural space will spread more extensively.

Pressure in the epidural space of non pregnant patients is usually negative (-1 cmH$_2$O), but in the pregnant woman, it is slightly positive. During contractions, the epidural pressure rises by 2–8 cmH$_2$O, while during expulsion, it ranges between 20 and 60 cmH$_2$O.

Subarachnoid space

There are no changes in the constituents or the specific gravity of cerebral spinal fluid (CSF) during pregnancy. CSF pressure is increased by aorto caval compression and by uterine contractions during labour. Baseline pressure in labour in between contractions is 28 cmH$_2$O. It is 22 cmH$_2$O when the uterus is displaced laterally to relieve aorto caval compression. During painful contractions, the pressure is increased and it may reach 70 cmH$_2$O in the second stage.

Sympathetic nervous system

There is increased sympathetic nervous system activity throughout pregnancy and it is maximal at term. The effect is primarily on the venous capacitance system of the lower extremities which counteracts the adverse effects of uterine compression of the IVC. Hence, sympathetic block due to either epidural or spinal anaesthesia can result in marked decrease in blood pressure in pregnant women compared with non pregnant patients.

Drugs and the nervous system

There are reduced requirements for local anaesthetics when administering spinal or epidural anaesthesia during pregnancy. This may be due to decreased volumes of the epidural and subarachnoid spaces, or increased nerve fibre sensitivity to local anaesthetics.

The minimal alveolar concentration (MAC) of inhalational anaesthetic agents is reduced by 40%, which may be related to gestational increase in progesterone levels. β endorphin levels in the mother are increased during gestation, labour and delivery.

ENDOCRINE SYSTEM

Thyroid gland

The thyroid gland increases in size during pregnancy.

A goitre may develop as a result of increased blood flow and follicular hyperplasia. Iodine uptake by the thyroid gland increases. Thyroid binding globulin levels double, but free plasma tri-iodothyronine and thyroxine remain at the non pregnant level or fall so that the mother remains euthyroid.

Adrenal gland

The maternal adrenal gland remains the same size but the width and secretion of the zona fasciculata are increased. Plasma cortisol and other corticosteroids increase to three-to-five times the non pregnant level by term. The half-life of cortisol is prolonged.

Pituitary gland

The pituitary gland increases in weight making the anterior pituitary very sensitive to haemorrhage and hypotension because its blood supply does not come directly from arterial vessels, but from a portal system whose pressure is below that of the systemic arteries.

Pancreas

The islets of Langerhans and the number of β cells increase during pregnancy as does the number of receptor sites for insulin. However, there is a resistance to the action of insulin, possibly due to the presence of human placental lactogen, prolactin and other pregnancy hormones. The upper limit of normal blood glucose in the glucose tolerance test is 7.5 mmol/l in the second trimester and this rises to 9.6 mmol/l in the third trimester.

RENAL FUNCTION

Renal function changes from early pregnancy (Figure PN.11). Renal plasma flow increases to 30–50% above the non pregnant level by 30 weeks, then declines gradually. The glomerular filtration rate (GFR) increases to about 150 ml/min in the second trimester and falls towards term. As a result the plasma concentrations of urea and creatinine decrease.

The tubules are presented with more urine volume due to the increase in GFR and they loose some of their re-absorptive capacity. Glucose, uric acid and amino acids are not completely re-absorbed and there is an increased loss of protein of up to 300 mg a day.

Renal sodium retention and, therefore, water retention are increased in pregnancy. Progesterone helps to conserve potassium during pregnancy.

MUSCULO SKELETAL SYSTEM

Placental production of the hormone relaxin stimulates

RENAL CHANGES DURING PREGNANCY

Parameter	Change
Renal plasma flow	↑
Glomerular filtration rate	↑
Urine volume	↑
Renal tubular re-absorption	↓
Glycosuria	↑
Proteinuria	↑
Creatinine clearance	↑
Plasma urea concentration	↓
Plasma creatinine concentration	↓

Figure PN.11

generalised ligamentous relaxation. This results in widening of the pubic symphysis, increased mobility of the sacroiliac, sacrococcygeal and pubic joints. As the uterus enlarges, lumbar lordosis is enhanced to maintain the woman's centre of gravity over the lower extremity. As a result, most pregnant women experience low back pain.

Hyperpigmentation of the face, neck and abdominal midline (linea nigra) are due to the effects of increased levels of melanocyte stimulating hormone (MSH).

WEIGHT GAIN

Weight increases by 10–12 kg due to increases in maternal body water and fat, the foetus, placenta, amniotic fluid and the uterus. At term, 40% of the weight gained is often in the foetus, amniotic fluid, placenta and uterus. Breast enlargement is typical in normal pregnancy due to human placental lactogen secretion. Enlarged breasts may be a cause of difficult intubation and the use of a short handle laryngoscope or polio blade may help to overcome this problem.

THE PLACENTA

Although the placenta appears as a physical barrier between maternal and foetal tissues, it brings the maternal and foetal circulation into close apposition for physiological exchange across a large area. Foetal well-being depends on good placental function for the supply of nutrients and the removal of waste products.

EMBRYOLOGY AND ANATOMY

The ovum is fertilised in the Fallopian tube and it enters the uterine cavity where it rapidly converts to a blastocyst with an inner and outer cell mass. The outer cell layer of the blastocyst then proliferates to form the trophoblastic cell mass. At implantation, the trophoblast erodes into the surrounding decidua of the endometrium and its associated capillaries until the blastocyst is surrounded by circulating maternal blood (trophoblastic lacunae).

The placental tissue develops from the chorion that consists of the trophoblast and mesoderm of the developing blastocyst. The trophoblast differentiates into two layers, the thick outer syncytiotrophoblast and the thin inner layer, cytotrophoblast. In the second week of development, the (inner) cytotrophoblast layer begins to proliferate and extend cellular fingers into the (outer) syncytiotrophoblast (Figure PN.12). The cytotrophoblast cell columns and their covering syncytiotrophoblast extend as villous stems into the lacunae of maternal blood within the decidua. A mesodermal core appears within the villous stems. These villous stems form the framework from which the villous tree will later develop. Cellular differentiation of the villous mesoderm results in the formation of blood cells and blood vessels and form the villous vascular network. With development, the villi branch out extensively into the lacunae (intervillous spaces) forming the villous tree and thereby increasing their surface area (Figure PN.13).

Cytotrophoblastic cells grow into the lumens of the maternal spiral vessels within the decidua where they replace the endothelial cells, invade and destroy the musculo elastic medial tissue. As a result of the destruction of the smooth muscle, the walls of the spiral vessels in the decidua become thin and their vasoconstrictor activity is reduced. This wave of trophoblastic invasion starts at 10 weeks and is complete by 16 weeks. A second wave of vascular trophoblastic invasion occurs from 16 to 22 weeks and extends more deeply into the myometrial portions of the spiral arteries. These vessels are easily dilated as maternal flow to the placenta increases. Failure of this physiological change is found in pre-eclampsia and intra-uterine growth retardation. This means that these vessels still respond to vasoconstrictor stimulation and there is reduced flow to the intervillous space. Further maturation of the villi result in a marked reduction in the cytotrophoblast component and decrease the diffusional distance between the foetal villi and maternal intervillous blood. At term in humans, only a single layer of foetal chorionic tissue (syncytiotrophoblast) separates maternal blood and

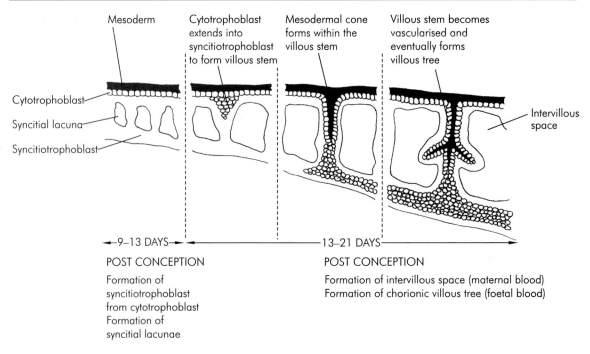

Figure PN.12 Early development of the placenta showing formation of the villous tree and the intervillous space

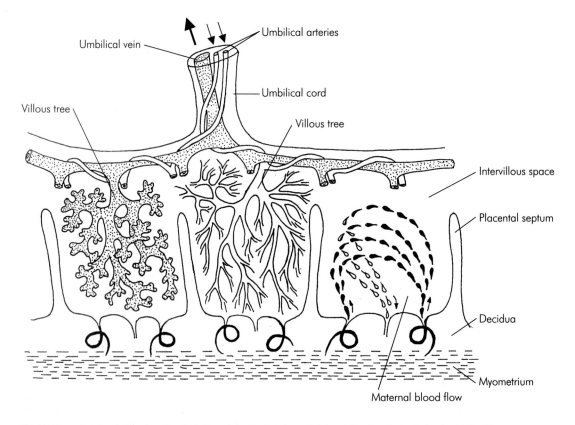

Figure PN.13 Placental circulation showing the villous tree (foetal placental circulation), spiral arteries and intervillous space (maternal placental circulation)

foetal capillary endothelium. Hence, the human placenta is classified as a haemo monochorial villous placenta.

The placenta is connected to the developing embryo by a connecting stalk that subsequently becomes the umbilical cord containing the umbilical vessels. The placenta is supplied with maternal blood from the uterine blood vessels. Blood enters the intervillous space from the open ends of the uterine spiral arteries (Figure PN.13). The intervillous space is a large cavernous expanse into which the villous trees reach. Blood enters the intervillous spaces and flows into loosely packed areas, then into densely packed intermediate and terminal villi. It then empties into collecting veins. However, the relative direction of the blood flow is haphazard and behaves like a concurrent system, but with maternal blood flow exceeding foetal blood flow. The area of densely packed terminal villi is where placental exchange occurs. Maternal placental blood flow is a low pressure system; the pressure in the intervillous space is on average 10 mmHg. The increasing demands of the growing foetus require 100–150 spiral arteries to feed directly to the placenta. The maternal circulation through the intervillous space is fully developed by 20 weeks. Blood flow will increase from 50 ml/min at 10 weeks to between 500 and 800 ml/min at term.

Two umbilical arteries arising from the foetal internal iliac arteries carry de-oxygenated foetal blood via the umbilical cord to the placenta and a single umbilical vein returns oxygenated blood to the foetus. The umbilical arteries divide into chorionic arteries that feed the multiple placental lobules and these in turn subdivide into the villous tree which end as capillaries in the terminal villi (Figure PN.13). Foetal sinusoids formed within the terminal villi provide a large endothelial surface area and make it the ideal region for maternal foetal exchange. Each villous tree drains into a large vein that perforates the chorionic plate to become chorionic veins. Each of the venous tributaries course towards the umbilical cord attachment site where they empty into one umbilical vein.

The placenta grows dramatically from the third month of gestation until term. There is direct correlation between growth of the foetus and that of the placenta. By term, the mature placenta is oval and flat with an average weight of 500 g, average diameter of 20 cm and thickness of 3 cm.

Uterine blood flow

Uterine blood flow is influenced by intrinsic and extrinsic factors. Chronic regulation of uterine blood flow occurs mainly through intrinsic factors. These include prostaglandins (prostacyclin), nitric oxide and oestrogens. Extrinsic factors are more involved in the acute changes of uterine perfusion.

In general, uterine blood flow (UBF) is related to perfusion pressure and vascular resistance according to the following formula:

$$UBF = \frac{\text{Uterine arterial pressure} - \text{Uterine venous pressure}}{\text{Uterine vascular resistance}}$$

Any factors that alter uterine perfusion will affect placental perfusion. Uterine arterial pressure is reduced by systemic hypotension. Uterine venous pressure is increased by IVC compression, uterine contractions and valsava manoeuvre (i.e. pushing in the second stage of labour).

Uterine vascular resistance is affected by endogenous and exogenous vasoconstrictors. Endogenous vasoconstrictors such as catecholamines are increased by stress and pain during labour.

FUNCTIONS OF THE PLACENTA

The placenta is a foetal organ with the following functions:

- Placental transfer of products between maternal and foetal blood
- Transfer of immunity by transfer of immunoglobins from the mother
- Endocrine function
- Detoxification of drugs and substances transferred from the mother

PLACENTAL TRANSPORT

Mechanisms of placental transport

These are discussed in further detail on page 228 and include:

- Simple diffusion
- Facilitated transport
- Secondary active transport
- Active transport
- Pinocytosis
- Bulk transport

Placental transport of substances

The placenta acts as a barrier between maternal and foetal tissues. However, it is an imperfect barrier and most substances will cross the placenta as detailed below.

OXYGEN

Oxygen crosses the placenta by simple diffusion that depends mainly on the difference between the oxygen tension of the maternal blood in the intervillous space and the foetal blood in the umbilical artery. The PO_2 of blood in the intervillous space varies greatly but will be dependent on maternal arterial PO_2 (Figure PN.14).

BLOOD GAS TENSIONS IN MATERNO FOETAL TRANSFER

Location	PO_2 (kPa)	PCO_2 (kPa)
Maternal artery	13.3	3.9
Foetal umbilical artery	2.0	5.9
Foetal umbilical vein	3.9	4.7

Figure PN.14

Other factors affecting oxygen transfer include the shape of the foetal oxyhemoglobin dissociation curve and the Bohr effect. The foetal oxyheamoglobin dissociation curve (P_{50} = 2.5–2.8 kPa) lies to the left of the maternal curve(P_{50} = 3.6 kPa). This favours the transfer of oxygen from the mother to the foetus. A rise or fall in CO_2 tension (with corresponding fall or rise in pH) leads to right or left shift response in the dissociation curve and also affects oxygen transfer (the Bohr effect). At the gas exchange interface, foetal blood gives up carbon dioxide, becomes more alkaline (left shift) and develops a greater affinity for oxygen. The maternal blood on the other hand takes up carbon dioxide, becomes more acidic (right shift) and promotes release of oxygen. This is referred to as the double Bohr effect and it accounts for 2–8% of the transplacental transfer of oxygen. Factors determining oxygen transfer across the placenta are summarised in Figure PN.15.

- High materno-foetal oxygen concentration gradient
- Double Bohr effect
- Shape of the foetal oxyheamoglobin dissociation curve
- High foetal haemoglobin concentration
- Functional status of the placenta
- Uterine blood flow and placental perfusion

The placenta is a metabolically active organ using 30% of the total oxygen delivered to it.

CARBON DIOXIDE

CO_2 crosses the placenta by simple diffusion. It is

FACTORS DETERMINING TRANSPORT OF OXYGEN FROM THE MOTHER TO THE FOETUS

- High materno-foetal oxygen concentration gradient
- Double Bohr effect
- The shape of the foetal oxyhaemoglobin dissociation curve
- High foetal hemoglobin concentration
- Functional status of the placenta
- Uterine blood flow and placental perfusion

Figure PN.15

present as dissolved CO_2 (8%), bicarbonate ion (62%), and carbamino haemoglobin (30%), with very small quantities as carbonic acid (H_2CO_3) and carbonate ion (CO_3^{2-}). Dissolved CO_2 is the form that crosses the placenta. The placental membrane is highly permeable to CO_2, which is 20 times more diffusible than oxygen.

A rise or fall in oxygen tension leads to a reduced or increased affinity for CO_2 (Haldane effect) and this affects the transport of CO_2. The materno-foetal transfer of oxygen produces de-oxyhaemoglobin in the maternal blood that has a greater affinity for CO_2 than oxyhaemoglobin. As the foetal blood takes up oxygen, it enhances CO_2 release. This is known as the double Haldane effect and it may account for as much as 46% of the transplacental transfer of CO_2. HCO_3^- is not a major contributor to this process because of its ionised form, but it does act as a source of CO_2 through the carbonic anhydrase reaction that keeps CO_2 and HCO_3^- in equilibrium.

GLUCOSE

Glucose crosses the placenta by facilitated transport, which is stereospecific for the D-isomer. The placenta uses most of the glucose absorbed from the maternal surface.

AMINO ACIDS

Amino acids cross the placenta by means of secondary active transport. Much of the transplacental transfer of amino acids occurs by way of linked carriers for both amino acids and sodium. The transport of sodium down its concentration gradient drags amino acids into the cells. The process is stereospecific.

FATTY ACIDS

Fatty acids probably cross the placenta by simple diffusion.

ELECTROLYTES AND WATER

Sodium and water cross the placenta by simple diffusion and bulk transport. Iron, iodine, calcium and phosphate require active transport.

PROTEINS

The placenta is relatively impermeable to plasma proteins. However, some immunoglobulins particularly IgG crosses the placenta by pinocytosis.

HORMONE SECRETION

The placenta produces the following hormones:

- Human chorionic gonadotrophin (HCG)
- Human placental lactogen (HPL)
- Hypothalamic-releasing factors
- Hypothalamic inhibitory factors
- Oestrogens
- Progesterone
- Thyroid-stimulating hormone (TSH)
- Prostaglandins

Human chorionic gonadotrophin

A rapid rise in HCG production in early pregnancy stimulates the corpus luteum to secrete progesterone which is required to maintain the viability of the pregnancy. The role of HCG in late pregnancy is not clear. The presence of HCG in urine forms the basis of the routine urine test for pregnancy.

Until the end of the eighth week, the corpus luteum continues to secrete progesterone. The placenta gradually takes over this role and becomes responsible for the secretion of progesterone which reaches a peak just before labour.

It is likely that the interaction between these placental peptides is important in the control of growth and development of the foetus.

PLACENTAL TRANSFER OF DRUGS

Measurement of placental drug transfer

Foeto-maternal (F/M) concentration ratios of drugs are frequently used as an index of placental transfer of drugs but are influenced by several factors such as:

- Site of foetal sampling
- Time interval between drug administration and sampling
- Whether drug is given as bolus or infusion

Factors affecting placental drug transfer

Most drugs given enough time will cross the placenta. The rate of transfer is dependent on:

- Lipid solubility
- Degree of ionisation
- pH of maternal blood
- Protein binding
- Materno foetal concentration gradient
- Placental blood flow

LIPID SOLUBILITY

Lipophilic molecules diffuse readily across lipid membranes, of which the placenta is one.

DEGREE OF IONISATION

Only the non ionised fraction of a partly ionised drug crosses the placental membrane. Most drugs used in anaesthesia, analgesia and sedation are poorly ionised in the blood and their placental transfer is almost unrestricted. Muscle relaxants are highly ionised and, therefore, their transfer is almost negligible.

pH OF MATERNAL BLOOD

The pH of maternal blood can alter the degree of ionisation of a drug. This effect is dependent on the pKa of the drug. If the pKa is near the pH of blood, then small changes (such as may occur during labour) in blood pH produce large changes in drug ionisation.

PROTEIN BINDING

The diffusibility of a protein-bound drug is negligible compared with that of free drug. Protein binding is influenced by blood pH and concentration of plasma proteins. Acidosis reduces the protein binding of local anaesthetic and low serum albumin in pre-eclampsia will cause a higher proportion of unbound drug and, therefore, promote transfer of drugs across the placenta.

MOLECULAR WEIGHT OF DRUG

Drugs with molecular weight of 600 Daltons or less readily diffuse across the placenta. Most drugs used in anaesthetic practice have molecular weights < 600 and, therefore, diffuse readily.

MATERNO-FOETAL CONCENTRATION GRADIENT

When a drug is transferred by simple diffusion, its rate

of transfer is determined by Fick's law of diffusion, which states that:

$$\dot{Q} = kA\frac{(C_m - C_f)}{D}$$

where:

$\dot{Q}$ = rate of diffusion per unit time
k = diffusion constant
A = surface area available for exchange
C_m = maternal concentration of free drug
C_f = foetal concentration of free drug
D = thickness of diffusion membrane

The diffusion constant depends on physicochemical properties of the substance such as molecular size, lipid solubility and degree of ionisation.

PLACENTAL BLOOD FLOW

With poorly diffusible drugs, the concentration in maternal and foetal blood changes little during placental transit, hence blood flow has little impact on transplacental gradient. With highly diffusible drugs, concentration gradient falls significantly as a result of transfer, hence blood flow has a marked effect on gradient.

Placental transfer of individual drugs

OPIOIDS

All opioids cross the placenta in significant amounts. Pethidine is commonly used during labour. It is about 50% plasma protein-bound and has almost unrestricted placental transfer. Maximum uptake by foetal tissue occurs 2–3 H after a maternal IM dose, which is when neonatal respiratory depression is most likely to occur. Longer half lives for pethidine and its active metabolite norpethidine, in the neonate compared with the mother, mean that there is a risk from cumulative side effects in the neonate (Figure PN.16).

HALF LIVES FOR PETHIDINE AND NORPETHIDINE FOR MOTHER AND NEONATE

Half lives (hours)	Pethidine	Norpethidine
Mother	4	21
Neonate	19	62

Figure PN.16

Morphine is poorly lipid-soluble and weakly plasma protein-bound, but readily crosses the placenta. Fentanyl is highly lipid-soluble, crossing the placental membrane rapidly but is largely albumen-bound (74%). Alfentanil is less lipophilic than fentanyl but is more highly bound to plasma protein.

LOCAL ANAESTHETIC AGENTS

Local anaesthetic agents cross the placenta by simple diffusion. Commonly used local anaesthetics have molecular weights ranging from 234 Daltons (lidocaine) to 288 (bupivacaine). They are weak bases and have relatively low degrees of ionisation and high lipid solubility at normal pH. Local anaesthetic accumulation in the foetus can occur if the foetus is acidotic, due to 'ion trapping'. This occurs when reduced pH in the foetus produces increased ionisation of the local anaesthetic and resultant lower diffusibility.

Drugs that are highly plasma protein-bound (bupivicaine, etidocaine) will have reduced placental transfer and lower F/M ratios compared with those with lower plasma protein binding (lidocaine, mepivicaine).

Transfer to the foetus is also affected by other factors, which include dose, site of administration and effects of adjuvants such as epinephrine. Higher doses result generally in higher maternal and foetal blood concentrations. The vascularity of the site of injection will determine the rate of absorption of the drug. For example, absorption from the paracervical injection is greater than epidural injection. Addition of epinephrine to local anaesthetic solutions affects the rate of absorption from the site of injection but the true effect of epinephrine on the various local anaesthetics is still unclear. The addition of epinephrine is thought to reduce absorption of lidocaine but not bupivacaine.

INHALATIONAL AGENTS

The high lipid solubility and low molecular weight of these agents facilitate rapid transfer across the placenta. Halothane rapidly crosses the placenta (F/M ratio = 0.87) and can be detected in umbilical venous and arterial blood within 1 min. Enflurane and nitrous oxide also cross rapidly (F/M ratio = 0.6 and 0.83 respectively) but there is limited information on isoflurane. Diffusion hypoxia may occur in a neonate exposed to nitrous oxide immediately before delivery. Therefore, it is advisable to administer supplementary oxygen to these neonates.

INDUCTION AGENTS

Sodium thiopentone is a highly lipophilic weak acid and it is 75% bound to plasma albumin. It rapidly crosses the placenta (F/M ratio = 0.4–1.1) and so do methohexitone and ketamine. However, the pharmacokinetics of propofol are yet to be investigated fully. Foeto maternal concentration ratios of 0.65–0.85 have been reported.

MUSCLE RELAXANTS

These drugs are fully ionised and poorly lipid-soluble and, therefore, do not readily cross the placenta.

ANTI-CHOLINERGICS

The placental transfer rates of anti-cholinergic drugs correlate directly with their ability to cross the blood-brain barrier. Atropine is detected in umbilical circulation within 1–2 min of maternal IV injection. In contrast, glycopyrrolate is poorly transferred.

VASOPRESSORS

Vasopressors are often used to treat hypotension secondary to regional anaesthesia. Ephedrine appears to cross the placenta easily.

BENZODIAZEPINES

Diazepam readily crosses the placenta. It is highly non ionised and very lipophilic. The F/M ratio reaches 1 within minutes of injection and reaches 2 an hour after injection. Midazolam has a F/M ratio = 0.76 but it has a short half-life.

SECTION 2: 14
FOETAL AND NEWBORN PHYSIOLOGY

A. R. Wolf

FOETAL CIRCULATION

PULMONARY FUNCTION

RENAL FUNCTION

HEPATIC FUNCTION

THERMOREGULATION

NOCICEPTION

As the foetus develops from a single dependent cell into a fully formed neonate capable of sustained life outside the womb, the physiology of individual organs and the integrated systems of the body undergo substantial developmental changes. Although physiology in the early stages may be crude and significantly different from that observed in maturity, it usually reflects functional differences that allow the foetus to cope with the challenges of the intrauterine environment, and also with the sudden, extreme changes needed for adaptation to extra-uterine life. For example, the presence of foetal haemoglobin in utero allows oxygen to be extracted from the placenta in a very low oxygen environment compared to after birth. In considering developmental physiology (ontogeny) it is necessary to see foetus, pre-term newborn, neonate, infant, child and adolescent as stages of development that merge into each other.

FOETAL CIRCULATION

The foetus and placenta encompass a unit in which the placenta enables the foetus to eliminate carbon dioxide and metabolic waste products in exchange for oxygen and nutrients from the maternal circulation. Blood leaves the placenta in the single umbilical vein with an oxygen saturation of approximately 80%. The ductus venosus, shunts half of the oxygenated umbilical venous blood through the liver to enter the Inferior vena cava (IVC). This mixed IVC blood with a saturation of 65% enters the right atrium, but only 1/3 passes into the right ventricle. The majority is directed through the foramen ovale to the left atrium and left ventricle to supply the heart, brain and upper body with relatively oxygenated blood. Venous blood from the superior vena cava with low saturation (25%) is directed preferentially to the right ventricle and pulmonary artery. In the foetus, pulmonary vascular resistance is high and less than 10% of cardiac output passes through the lungs. This is achieved by intense vasoconstriction in the pulmonary arterioles and patency of the ductus arteriosus which allows the majority of blood passing into the pulmonary artery to join the aorta. This mixed aortic and ductal blood flow supplies the lower body with blood with a saturation of approximately 55%. Blood returns to the placenta via two umbilical arteries arising from the internal iliac arteries. Placental blood flow is large: comprising 60% of the foetal cardiac output. See Figure FP.1.

At birth, with onset of spontaneous ventilation in the lungs and loss of the placenta, the circulation changes dramatically. The first breath generates a negative pressure of approximately 50 cmH$_2$O, drawing in about 80 ml of air and expanding the functional residual capacity. Pulmonary vascular resistance falls rapidly, allowing blood to flow from the right ventricle through the lungs. As placental flow ceases with clamping of the umbilical cord, systemic vascular resistance rises. The result is a reversal of right to left flow through the ductus arteriosus. Exposure to oxygenated blood and reduced prostaglandin-E$_2$ production stimulates ductal constriction, with functional closure in the majority of newborns by 24 hours. A shunt murmur may be audible prior to closure. Histological obliteration occurs by 3 weeks in most normal term infants. Preterm babies have a higher incidence of patent ductus arteriosus, and may require medical treatment with indomethacin, or surgical ligation. The ductus venosus closes passively due to absent blood flow.

After the first breath, pulmonary venous blood returns to the left atrium, causing pressure in the left atrium to exceed that in the right. This effect on raised left atrial pressure is enhanced by the sudden rise in systemic vascular resistance from loss of the placental blood flow. The valve-like foramen ovale closes, thus preventing de-oxygenated blood from the right atrium crossing to the left.

Although the pulmonary vascular resistance is reduced after birth it continues to fall for several days after birth and the pulmonary arteriolar medial walls remain very muscular. This muscle layer reduces considerably over the first few months and becomes thin walled and elastic with little muscle by 6 months. However, immediately after birth resistance in the pulmonary circuit is higher than in adults and the pulmonary arterioles remains very reactive. If the neonate becomes hypoxic, hypercapnic or acidotic, pulmonary vasoconstriction can lead to raised right-sided pressures and significant shunting through the foramen ovale and reversion to a foetal-type circulation. This condition is called persistent pulmonary hypertension of the newborn (PPHN). Oxygen, hyperventilation or nitric oxide may be needed to reverse the condition, and extracorporeal membrane oxygenation (ECMO) has been successfully used in severe and persistent cases.

THE HEART

The newborn heart consists of cardiac myofibrils that are poorly organised and lacking the structured architecture of the mature heart. The increased ratio of connective tissue to contractile tissue compared to adults results in limitation in myocyte contractility and ventricular compliance. In addition calcium

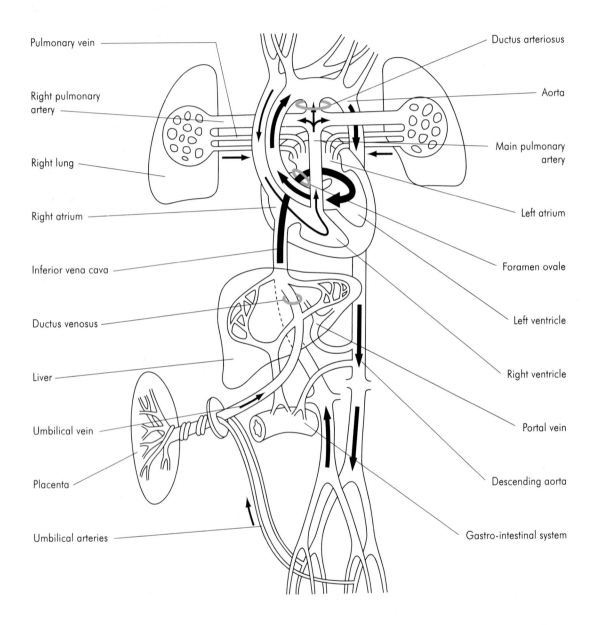

Figure FP.1 – Foetal Circulation

metabolism is immature in neonatal myocytes. Consequently there is a relatively flat Starling curve, and while inadequate pre load is poorly tolerated, overloading results in early cardiac failure. The stroke volume is relatively fixed, and increases in cardiac output are achieved largely by increases in heart rate. Ventricular end-diastolic volume increases from 40ml/m^2 body surface area at birth to 70 ml/m^2 in children over 2 years of age. Normal heart rate at birth ranges from 100–170 beats/min, decreases with age and reaches adult values by puberty. (See Figure FP.2). The pre-term neonate has significantly lower blood pressure than the term infant and adult levels are not reached until adolescence.

Autonomic innervation of the heart and blood vessels is incomplete in the newborn, with a relative lack of sympathetic supply. This is highlighted by the relatively small falls in blood pressure associated with high spinal blockade when using regional anaesthesia. Moreover, neonates are also less sensitive to the effects of catecholamines, needing much larger doses than older children or adults to achieve an increase in blood pressure and heart rate. Note the following facts:

- Both ventricles weigh the same at birth, although the right ventricle is the dominant ventricle in foetal life, possessing a thicker wall at the time of delivery
- In the foetus, the 2 ventricles are effectively in parallel, with the dominant right ventricle pumping approximately 2/3 of the combined ventricular output via the pulmonary artery, through the ductus arteriosus and into the aorta
- The left ventricle enlarges rapidly after birth, and by age 6 months reflects the adult ratio. This change is mirrored in the ECG, which shows right axis deviation at birth with an axis of up to +180 degrees, and changes to +90 degrees by 6 months.

PULMONARY FUNCTION

The foetal lung is filled with fluid essential for lung maturation and development. Irregular breathing movements are made in utero, which helps development of respiratory muscles, including the diaphragm and intercostal muscles. As full term approaches, catecholamines and tri-iodothyronine (T3) stimulate the reabsorption of pulmonary fluid by reversal of the chloride pump mechanism. Final reabsorption is stimulated by the physical passage through the birth canal. This stage is less effective in babies born by Caesarian section, and can lead to a condition called transient tachypnoea of the newborn (TTN). Type II pneumocytes produce surfactant under hormonal stimulation (cortisol) from 26 weeks gestation. Surfactant stabilises alveoli by reducing surface tension and artificial surfactant administration may be needed in preterm infants to prevent them developing Respiratory Distress Syndrome (RDS), Term babies may also be surfactant deficient if they

NORMAL CARDIOVASCULAR VALUES IN CHILDHOOD

AGE (mmHg)	SYSTOLIC BP (mmHg)	DIASTOLIC BP (beats/min)	HEART RATE
Preterm 750g *	45	25	>120
Birth	60	35	>120
Neonate	70 – 80	40 – 50	120 – 150
3 – 6 months	80 – 90	50 – 60	120 —140
1 year	90 – 100	60 – 80	110 —130
5 years	95 – 100	50 —80	90 – 100
12 years	110 – 120	60 —70	80 – 100

Note*: Mean arterial BP less than or equal to gestational age in weeks is a good rule of thumb for preterm infants.

Figure FP.2

suffer severe acidosis or hypoxia, or if they are born from mothers with diabetes mellitus.

The bronchial tree is fully developed at birth, in contrast to the alveoli, which continue to expand in both size and number, thus increasing the surface area of the lung by up to 25 times. Newborn infants, have extremely compliant chest walls with compressible, horizontally-aligned ribs. The diaphragm is the major muscle of ventilation in infancy, but can fatigue more easily in the neonate. In the first year of life, the percentage of type 1, slow-twitch muscle fibres, which fatigue more slowly, increase from 10% to 25% (the adult level).

Newborn infants show ventilatory responses to changes in PaO_2 and $PaCO_2$, but these are less responsive and affected by other factors such as gestational and postnatal age, temperature, wake-sleep cycles and drugs. Neonates react to hypoxia with a brief period of hyperpnoea followed by centrally mediated respiratory depression. In the weeks that follow, as chemoreceptors mature, the infant develops a predominantly hyperpnoeic response to hypoxia. In sleeping infants the arousal response to hypoxia (normal in adults) is much diminished, and often completely absent during rapid-eye movement (REM) sleep. Intercostal muscle activity is inhibited during REM sleep, and can lead inefficient ventilation as the chest wall recesses on inspiration. Periodic respiration, where rapid shallow breathing alternates with apnoeas of up to 10 seconds, is normal in many infants.

RENAL FUNCTION

In the developing embryo, the first nephrons form during week 5, are functional from week 8 and have reached their full complement by week 36. After this there is merely growth in size and number of cells in existing nephrons rather than new nephron formation. Renal blood flow comprises 5% of cardiac output at birth, but with reduced renal vascular resistance, this increases to 20% by 1 month of age, with increasing flow to cortical areas. The glomerular filtration rate (GFR) is correspondingly low at birth (30ml/min), and is even lower in preterm infants (3 ml/min). By 2 years GFR has increased to near adult levels (110 ml/min). Low GFR and immature tubular function limits the neonates ability to deal with water and solute loads notably sodium and glucose and they are unable to effectively excrete hydrogen ions or retain bicarbonate as a compensation for acidosis.

HEPATIC FUNCTION

During intrauterine life, the foetus excretes fat-soluble unconjugated bilirubin via the placenta and maternal liver. There is a physiological rise in bilirubin soon after birth, due to both an increased bilirubin load and immaturity of neonatal hepatic enzymes. The peak occurs on day 3–4 of life, due to immature oxidation–reduction reactions (phase I), with levels dropping in the second week of life as conjugating enzymes needed for glucuronidation mature (phase II). This drop takes longer in preterm babies and the risk of kernicterus (damage to basal ganglia and auditory pathways) from unconjugated bilirubin entering the brain via an immature blood-brain barrier is significant. Infants handle hepatically excreted drugs differently to older children and adults. Immature enzyme systems play a role, but so does the difference in blood supply to the liver. Infants receive a higher proportion of their hepatic blood supply via the portal vein than via the hepatic artery. Any increase in intra-abdominal pressure, e.g. post-abdominal surgery, reduces clearance of hepatically excreted drugs such as fentanyl.

THERMOREGULATION

Neonates lose heat readily because of their higher surface area to body weight ratio and relative paucity of subcutaneous fat. Pre-term infants have particularly thin skins, needing higher ambient temperatures and humidity. Heat loss occurs by evaporation, radiation, convection and to a lesser extent, conduction, as well as by insensible losses such as through respiration. Infants are seldom able to increase heat production enough to compensate for heat loss, and newborns need to be nursed in a thermoneutral environment (at an ambient temperature that minimises oxygen consumption and heat loss).

Unlike older children and adults who generate heat involuntarily by shivering, newborns rely on non-shivering thermogenesis to increase their basal metabolic rate and thereby retain heat. This is a function of their unique brown fat, present in the first few weeks of life as an adaptive, protective entity. These specialised adipose cells are situated around the kidneys and adrenals, in the mediastinum and around the scapulae. They are abundant in mitochondria and have a rich blood and autonomic nerve supply. Norepinephrine in sympathetic nerve endings stimulates the hydrolysis of triglycerides to fatty acids and glycerol, resulting in oxygen consumption and heat production.

NOCICEPTION

Circumstantially, even the most preterm neonates have similar types of responses to painful stimuli in terms of cardiovascular, stress and behavioural responses as the adult, but the presence or absence of pain as a conscious event can never be proven. Little can be inferred on the actual experience of pain or the attendant emotions, if any relating to it in the neonate. Much depends on the nature of self awareness, consciousness and the development of "self" in foetal life. Given the impossible task of making judgements on the nature of pain perception in the foetus and neonate, the term nociception is more appropriate.

Nociceptive pathways develop early in gestation and even in early development and they can produce complex protective responses to painful stimuli. Dorsal horn cells in the spinal cord have formed synapses with developing sensory neurones by 6 weeks gestation, and peripheral nerves migrate to the skin of the limbs by 11 weeks achieving a similar density of nociceptive nerve endings as the adult by birth. The first appearance of transmitter vesicles is seen at 13 weeks gestation and further synaptic connections and organisation of the dorsal horn structure continues up to 30 weeks.

The foetal neocortex has a full complement of cells by 20 weeks and thalamo-cortical tracts can be shown to synapse with dendritic processes of the cells in the neocortex by 24 weeks gestation. Myelination of some ascending nociceptive tracts are seen by 30 weeks but thalamo-cortical radiations are not myelinated until 37 weeks and some nociceptive tracts are myelinated much later. However, lack of myelination does not imply lack of function: transmission of nerve impulses within the central nervous system still takes place in unmyelinated nerves albeit at a reduced velocity. Noxious stimuli can produce both haemodynamic and stress responses in a human fetus as young as 18 weeks gestation and these responses can be reduced by pre-treatment with analgesic drugs. Visual and auditory evoked potentials are present by 30 weeks gestation and a complex EEG reactive to external influences has developed.

Overall, even the very preterm infant has complex interneuronal connections capable of integrated responses to tactile or nociceptive input. These infants show inconsistent responses to external stimuli, which may reflect the late functional connections of sensory afferents (particularly C-fibres) within the spinal cord. However, the combination of larger receptive fields, recruitment of non-nociceptive afferents and reduced inhibitory controls result in "underdamped" responses (long lasting, exaggerated and poorly localised) once afferent stimuli have achieved central activation above a threshold level. Inconsistency of response to more complex noxious stimuli may also reflect the profound effects that conscious state and other external responses have on behaviour.

Although new-born infants often have short lived behavioural and stress responses to noxious stimuli, there is evidence in this age group that surgical trauma or injury can have long term consequences for sensory and pain behaviour in infancy. It is clear that in neonates repeated noxious stimuli produce hypersensitivity to further stimulation and that poor operative analgesia can be associated with long lasting hyperalgesia and behavioural changes such as irritability, reduced attentiveness and poor orientation which may continue long after the expected duration of pain.

References and further reading

Steward DJ. Outline of Pediatric Anatomy and Physiology in Relation to Anesthesia in: Manual of Pediatric Anaesthesia. Churchill Livingstone. 5th edition, 2000

Wolf A. Fetal and neonatal physiology and pharmacology: relevance to anaesthesia and intensive care. Chapter In General Anaesthesia (6th edition) Browne BR, Prys-Roberts C (eds), Butterworth Heinmann (Oxford) 1996

Duncan H. Physiology of Fetal Adaptation at Birth. Current Paediatrics (1999) 9, 118—122

SECTION 3: 1
PHYSICAL CHEMISTRY

T. C. Smith

INTERMOLECULAR AND INTERATOMIC BONDS

> Atomic structure
> Valency
> Ionic bonds
> Covalent bonds
> Dative bonds
> van der Waals forces
> Hydrogen bonds
> Hydrophobic bonds
> Strength of intermolecular bonds

DIFFUSION

> Simple diffusion
> Non ionic diffusion

SOLUBILITY AND PARTITION COEFFICIENTS

OSMOSIS

> Pharmacological aspects of osmosis

DRUG ISOMERISM

> Structural isomerism
> Dynamic isomerism
> Stereoisomerism

PROTEIN BINDING

INTERMOLECULAR AND INTERATOMIC BONDS

The two main types of intermolecular bond are ionic and covalent although weaker bonds, essential for intermolecular interactions, also exist. The structure of the component atoms determines the type of bonds within the molecule.

ATOMIC STRUCTURE

When considering atomic structure, certain definitions aid understanding:

- Atom – the smallest part of an element that can take part in chemical reactions
- Element – a group of atoms all having the same atomic number
- Molecule – a combination of atoms which is the smallest unit of a chemical substance that can exist while still retaining the properties of the original substance
- Atomic number – the number of protons in each atom of an element

Knowledge of the basic structure of atoms is important in understanding the types of intermolecular bond and their functions. A schematic view of atomic structure is shown in Figure PC.1.

An atom consists of a nucleus (central core) of neutrons and protons, surrounded by a cloud of negatively charged electrons. Figure PC.2 shows the properties of these components. The charge of an atom is the number of protons minus the number of electrons. It is clear that almost all the mass of an atom is in the nucleus. The number of protons (atomic number) defines the element and the atomic mass is close to the combined masses of protons and neutrons

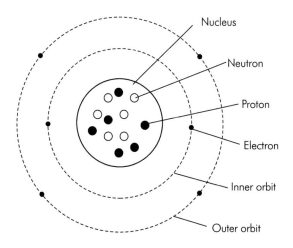

Figure PC.1 Schematic view of atomic structure

PROPERTIES OF ATOMIC PARTICLES

| | Nucleus | | |
	Proton	Neutron	Electron
Mass number	1	1	1/1836
Charge	+1	0	−1

Figure PC.2

in the atom. Elements may exist with different numbers of neutrons in the nucleus while having the same atomic number. These are called isotopes and those that release particles (radio-active) are called radio-isotopes. Carbon provides an example: it has atomic number 6 though ^{12}C (carbon 12) has six protons and six neutrons, while ^{14}C (carbon 14) has six protons and eight neutrons (radio-active). Conventionally, the mass number is shown as a prefix superscript and the atomic number is shown as prefix subscript, for example $^{12}_{6}Na$ for sodium.

Electrons are arranged in orbital shells around the nucleus, from the innermost K shell outwards to L, M, N, O, P and Q shells (Figure PC.3). These are not precise concentric rings, but the conceptual model helps to predict molecular behaviour. Shells are filled in their alphabetical order. Complete electron shells, pairs and octets of electrons confer stability. Each orbital shell has a maximum number of electrons that confer some stability when achieved.

CAPACITY OF ELECTRON SHELLS

Shell	Maximum number of electrons
K	2
L	8
M	18
N	32

Figure PC.3

VALENCY

Valency may be defined as 'The number of atoms of hydrogen that one atom of an element can combine with or replace'.

Each element has at least one valency state and the valency is used to establish possible intermolecular bonds. Each group in the Periodic table has a characteristic valency. For example, Group IA elements have a valency of +1. The valency can be predicted from the electron shell configuration as shown in Figure PC.4. Atoms of a particular element lose or gain electrons to achieve the stability described

ELECTRON PROPERTIES OF ELEMENTS

Element	Protons	Neutrons	Electrons in shell					Valency
			K	L	M	N	O	
Hydrogen	1	0	1					1
Helium	2	2	2					0
Carbon	6	6	2	4				4
Nitrogen	7	7	2	5				3
Oxygen	8	8	2	6				2
Sodium	11	12	2	8	1			1
Magnesium	12	12	2	8	2			2
Chlorine	17	18	2	8	7			1
Argon	18	18	2	8	8			0
Potassium	19	20	2	8	8	1		1
Calcium	20	20	2	8	8	2		2
Xenon	54	77	2	8	18	18	8	0

Figure PC.4

above. This loss or gain of electrons may be complete (in ionic bond) or by sharing with other atoms (in covalent bond). In this way, they adopt the electron configuration of the closest (by atomic number) rare or inert gas (for example helium, neon, argon). The inert gases are already at their most stable and do not gain or lose electrons. Consequently, they have minimal interaction with other atoms and exist as gases. Carbon is the single most important element in organic chemistry because it is chemically versatile – it can either lose or gain electrons to achieve electron stability.

IONIC BONDS

The ionic bond (also termed electrostatic) relies on the fact that certain elements (termed electrovalent) have a tendency to lose or gain electrons to form charged atoms or molecules called ions. Like charges repel, but opposite charges attract and, therefore, create a bond.

2.8.1   2.8.7   2.8   2.8.8
Electron orbital configuration

Figure PC.5 Ionic bonding illustrated by the formation of sodium chloride

This is illustrated by the formation of sodium chloride in Figure PC.5. (In Figures PC.5, 6, 7 and 9 the shading of electrons enables identification of any one electron's origin when considering the end result.)

With respect to the process shown in Figure PC.5, the movement of an electron from the sodium atom to the chlorine atom results in both ions having stable outermost shells. The sodium ion now has the electron configuration of neon, and chloride that of argon. The resultant change in charge causes a strong attraction between the sodium and chloride ions (the ionic bond) which is sufficient to maintain the precise crystalline structure of solid sodium chloride. Figure PC.6 shows another example of ionic bonding with the relevant electron configurations.

1   2.8.7   0   2.8.8
Electron orbital configuration

Figure PC.6 An ionic bond illustrated by the formation of hydrochloric acid

COVALENT BONDS

Covalent bonds have similarities with ionic bonds in that they depend on forming stable electron shells. In

Carbon atom   Hydrogen atom

Methane molecule

2.4   1

Electron orbital configuration

Figure PC.7 Covalent bonding illustrated by the formation of methane

contrast with ionic bonding, the atoms share electrons rather than donate them completely. Carbon, nitrogen, hydrogen and oxygen frequently behave in this way. The electron configuration of carbon is 2.4. Stability is achieved either by losing four electrons or by gaining four electrons resulting in a pair or an octet of electrons in the outer shells respectively. Covalent bonds may be single, double or triple, depending on the number of electron pairs that are shared. Methane (Figure PC.7) is an example of covalent bonding having four single covalent bonds. The carbon atom of methane adopts the electron configuration of neon (2.8) while hydrogen adopts the configuration of helium, both being inert gases with stable atomic configurations.

A comparison of the properties of ionic and covalent bonds is given in Figure PC.8.

DATIVE BONDS

The dative bond is a type of covalent bond in which both electrons of the shared pair are from the same atom. This bond is a feature of atoms that have complete pairs of electrons in their outer shells in the non combined state. Typical examples are oxygen, nitrogen, phosphorus and sulphur. The formation of ammonium chloride from ammonia and hydrogen chloride (Figure PC.9) illustrates this bond as well as ionic and covalent bonds.

van der WAALS FORCES

Because electrons are not rigidly fixed relative to the nucleus but move in characteristic orbitals, the resulting electron cloud has a characteristic shape. Highly electronegative atoms such as oxygen attract electrons so that the distribution of the electron cloud of the molecule is uneven. This produces dipoles where component atoms of a molecule are not electrostatically neutral. The value of these charges is much less than the $+1$ or -1 of ions and the molecule may have a polarity. van der Waals forces are the attraction and repulsion of these weakly charged areas to similar areas in neighbouring molecules. Graphite is in an example of sheets of covalently bonded carbon in which the layers are held together by van der Waals forces which are essential in receptor and enzyme bonding.

HYDROGEN BONDS

A hydrogen bond is a weak electrostatic bond between the positive nucleus of a covalently bonded hydrogen atom in one molecule and the unshared pair of electrons of a highly electronegative atom of another molecule. Oxygen, sulphur and nitrogen are highly electronegative atoms and water provides an example of hydrogen bonding (Figure PC.10). The hydrogen

Ionic	Covalent
No sharing of electrons, therefore non directional bond, therefore no particular shape	Electrons shared, therefore directional bond, therefore definite shape, so isomerism and stereo-isomerism possible
Usually solid (crystalline)	Usually highly volatile liquids or gases
Not easily vaporised	Easily vaporised
Fused state	
Melt form is a conductor	Poor conductor
Readily dissolves in water	Not readily soluble in water
Forms electrolyte in water	

Figure PC.8 A comparison of the properties of ionic and covalent bonds

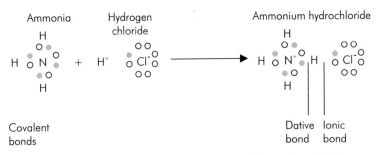

Figure PC.9. Mixed bonds illustrated by the formation of ammonium chloride

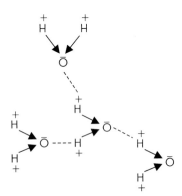

Figure PC.10 Hydrogen bonding in water (dotted lines)

bonding in water is responsible for the relatively high boiling point (compared with non polar liquids) and the structure of ice crystals.

HYDROPHOBIC BONDS

In water, individual molecules are attracted to each other by hydrogen bonds. Any molecules added to the water will disrupt this loosely held 'structure'. If the electron distribution of the additive is not uniform (it has polarity) or if it is readily ionised, then it too will form bonds with the water molecules. This will allow it to spread readily and evenly throughout the containing vessel. If, however, the electron distribution is even, then the energy required to break the hydrogen bonds of water will be greater than that released by the formation of the new bonds. In this case, the most stable arrangement exists when the additive collects together leaving as much of the water together as possible. This is easily seen when oil is added to water, and is a feature of lipids. Its density relative to water determines where the oil subsequently distributes. Vigorous mixing will provide the energy to break the hydrogen bonds and disperse the fat molecules, temporarily. This is the basis of the hydrophobic bond, which is very important physiologically, occurring at a

local level around proteins and other molecules. Areas of membranes and proteins that do not have polarity do not attract water molecules. The water molecules, therefore, tend to maintain bonds with other water molecules leaving these hydrophobic areas vacant. This promotes the movement of non polar hydrophobic molecules to these sites. Looking at this situation in overview gives the impression that the hydrophobic areas and molecules are attracted to each other but in fact there is little or no attraction at all between the two. It is, in effect, the result of displacement of the hydrophobic molecules by the attraction of water and other hydrophilic molecules.

STRENGTH OF INTERMOLECULAR BONDS

The strengths of the main intermolecular bonds are shown in Figure PC.11. The stronger the bond the higher the energy required to break it. Covalent bonds are, therefore, very difficult to break without a catalyst or enzyme to facilitate. Therefore, in physiological and pharmacological systems covalent bonds are effectively irreversible. They are 'reversed' by metabolism of the receptor–agonist or enzyme–substrate complex and replacement of the enzyme or receptor. Examples of pharmacological covalent bonding include phenoxybenzamine to alpha-adrenergic receptors, organophosphates to acetyl cholinesterase and monoamine oxidase inhibitors to monoamine oxidase.

THE STRENGTH OF INTERMOLECULAR BONDS	
Bond	**Bond energy (kcal/mol)**
Covalent	50–150
Ionic	5–10
Hydrogen	2–5
van der Waals	0.5

Figure PC.11

The strength of ionic and other bonds decreases with the distance between the molecules such that the force of attraction is given by the following formulae:

Ionic bonds: $\text{force} \propto \dfrac{1}{\text{distance}^2}$

van der Waals forces: $\text{force} \propto \dfrac{1}{\text{distance}^7}$

In the latter, neighbouring groups of electrons cause repulsion once the distance decreases below a critical level.

DIFFUSION

SIMPLE DIFFUSION

Diffusion is a property of gas mixtures and solutions. Molecules of gases can move freely and tend to distribute themselves equally within the limits of the containing vessel (Figure PC.12). In a similar way molecules and ions in solution move freely throughout the solvent, so that the distribution (and, therefore, the concentration) becomes uniform throughout the solution. Ions and molecules, therefore, move down the concentration gradient and any electrical gradient until those gradients disappear. The result is an even distribution of all the ions and molecules in the container so that any selected volume regardless of shape, size or location will have identical composition.

Graham's Law describes gaseous diffusion as follows:

$$\text{Rate} \propto \frac{1}{\sqrt{\text{density}}}$$

The rate of diffusion of a gas at a given temperature and pressure is inversely proportional to the square root of its density. Thus, the rate of diffusion increases with rising temperature as the speed of molecular movement increases.

NON IONIC DIFFUSION

Of drugs, the majority is categorised as weak acids or weak bases, which implies that they are encountered in a partly ionised form. A higher degree of ionisation confers water solubility and, thus, is desirable for admixture, for example. In contrast, the unionised form of a drug is required for lipid membrane penetration and, hence, delivery to the target. The proportion of a drug present in ionised from is dependent on environmental pH. A drug that is a weak acid will dissociate in the following way:

$HA \rightleftharpoons H^+ + A^-$

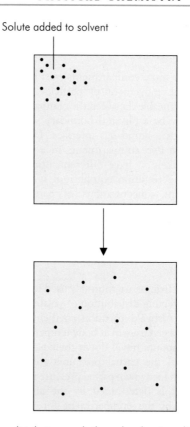

Solute added to solvent

Solute redistributes evenly through solvent resulting in uniform concentration throughout

Figure PC.12. Effect of diffusion on gas molecule distribution

The relationship between dissociation and pH can be obtained by applying the Henderson–Hasselbach equation:

$$pH = pKa + \log_{10} \frac{[A^-]}{[HA]}$$

pKa is the negative logarithm of the dissociation constant and is the pH at which the drug is 50% ionised. As a practical application of this concept consider thiopentone (pKa 7.8) which is deliberately made up in an alkaline solution, pH about 11, to render it more ionised and, therefore, water soluble. After injection parenterally, into an environment of pH 7.4, the proportion of unionised drug form will become greater enabling membrane penetration of the CNS.

SOLUBILITY AND PARTITION COEFFICIENTS

The partition coefficient of a substance can be defined as a numerical constant that defines the ratio at equilibrium of the concentrations in two adjacent compartments of that substance which readily passes through the interface.

When two or more compartments exist together then there will be movement of particles through the interface (permeable) between the compartments. The interface may be a physical boundary such as a cell membrane, or a liquid–gas interface. Unlike simple diffusion, the two compartments in a physiological system are likely to have different affinities for the particles. The resulting equilibrium will, therefore, have different concentrations of particles in the compartments. Solubility and partition coefficients can be determined for a pair of compartments for a given diffusing molecule. The coefficient is a dimensionless ratio describing the relative concentrations at equilibrium.

Partition coefficients are routinely used to describe the properties affecting distribution of volatile anaesthetic agents. The Ostwald partition coefficients used are specified for a given agent at body temperature (37°C). Gases and vapours travel down their partial pressure gradient until the partial pressures are equal. The concentration for a given partial pressure in a particular compartment is determined by the affinity of the constituents of the compartment for the specified molecule. The total amount of the molecule in any compartment will also depend on the volume of the compartment. At equilibrium, the partial pressures will be equal but the concentrations will not. Figure PC.13 shows these features using sevoflurane as an example. Sevoflurane has a blood/gas partition coefficient = 0.69. This means that at equilibrium the ratio of sevoflurane concentration in the two compartments is 0.69 in the blood for every 1.00 in the gas phase. Solubility coefficients may also be between different solvents, such as oil and water. A highly oil soluble molecule such as halothane will have a high oil/water solubility coefficient (220). A highly water soluble molecule such as sodium chloride will have a low oil/water solubility coefficient. In general, ions are more soluble in water while iso-electric and non polar molecules are more soluble in oils.

OSMOSIS

Osmosis is the passage of a solvent through a semipermeable membrane that separates two compartments having different concentrations of a solute (or solutes) to which the membrane is impermeable. A pure semipermeable membrane is one that is freely permeable to the solvent but impermeable to the solute. The glomerular membrane is an example of a functional semipermeable membrane and is freely

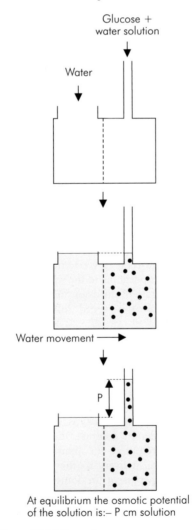

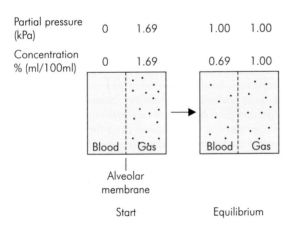

Figure PC.13 Distribution of sevoflurane between the blood and gas

Figure PC.14 Osmosis

permeable to water and smaller molecules but impermeable to larger molecules (molecular weight > 69 000 Daltons).

In osmosis, an imbalance in the concentration of non permeable molecules on two sides of a semipermeable membrane causes movement of the freely permeable solute towards the side of higher concentration. The solute tends to move, equalising concentration gradients. The osmotic pressure or potential is the pressure required to prevent this passage of solvent. Figure PC.14 shows the effect of osmosis on fluid distribution. Osmotic activity continues until the hydrostatic pressure balances the osmotic potential. All solutions have an osmotic potential for a given semipermeable membrane and concentration. The solvent (e.g. water) moves towards the compartment with the highest concentration of solute and the pressure is, by definition, negative.

Osmotic potential may be the result of a single solute, but is usually due to many different molecules. Osmotically active particles in a solution are those to which the membrane is impermeable. Cell membranes are semipermeable although ionic transport systems make this picture rather complex.

The difference between osmolarity and osmolality is:

Osmolarity – concentration by volume of solution (in mosm/l)

Osmolality – concentration by mass of solvent (in mosm/kg H_2O)

PHARMACOLOGICAL ASPECTS OF OSMOSIS

Drugs affecting the distribution of solutes between compartments will have an osmotic effect. Diuretics interfere with membrane transport of ions and other solutes through the renal cells and in the renal lumen and renal circulation. This manipulates the ionic concentrations in the medulla and, therefore, water follows ionic concentrations in the tubules and urine output is increased. Mannitol is a drug used specifically for its osmotic effects. It is a high molecular weight alcohol that remains extracellular and this produces a negative osmotic potential in the extracellular space that pulls water out of the intracellular space. It is also an osmotic diuretic because it passes readily through the glomerular membrane but is not re-absorbed.

DRUG ISOMERISM

Isomers are chemical compounds that have the same empirical molecular formula (and so the same molecular weight) but differing physical or chemical properties.

STRUCTURAL ISOMERISM

Structural isomerism is the presence of different structures with the same empirical molecular formula.

Chain isomerism

In chain isomerism the carbon skeleton varies between isomers whilst retaining the same functional group. Example: butane $CH_3CH_2CH_2CH_3$ and isobutane (2-methyl butane) $CH_3CH(CH_3)CH_3$.

Position isomerism

In position isomerism the component atoms or functional group are in different positions on an identical carbon skeleton. Example: enflurane and isoflurane (Figure PC.15).

Functional group isomerism

The functional group in this form of isomerism changes. For example the movement of the oxygen of an alcohol into the carbon chain produces an ether. Example: propanol $CH_3CH_2CH_2OH$ and methyl ethyl ether $CH_3OCH_2CH_3$.

DYNAMIC ISOMERISM

Dynamic isomerism (tautomerism) is a variant of functional group isomerism in which two isomers exist in dynamic equilibrium obeying the Law of Mass Action. The barbiturates, thiopentone and methohexitone exist in two forms (keto and enol). =S/-SH and =O/-OH groups in thiopentone and methohexitone respectively are in a dynamic equilibrium, the relative proportions of each being determined by the pH of the solution (p 604). Nitrous oxide is another tautomer.

Figure PC.15 Isomerism of enflurane and isoflurane

STEREOISOMERISM

Stereoisomerism is another form of molecular rearrangement. Stereoisomers have the same molecular formula, carbon skeleton and structure but the arrangement of the component atoms in space differs. Each atom in the molecule bonds to the same atoms as in the other stereoisomers. There are two types: optical and geometric.

Optical isomerism

Optical stereoisomerism requires atoms which are at least tetravalent (having the potential for four bonds) and different groups of molecules on each bond. Carbon is the most important tetravalent atom and has four hybridised covalent links with neighbouring molecules. Figure PC.16 shows the principles of optical stereoisomerism. The carbon atom in the chiral centre has four different groups attached to it. It can be seen that if two of these groups are interchanged then the resulting arrangement is a non-superimposable mirror image of the original. These are optical stereoisomers (enantiomers).

PROPERTIES

Enantiomers often have different crystalline structures. Characteristically, they rotate polarised light in opposite directions. The amount of rotation is a feature of the molecular structure.

CLASSIFICATION

Several methods exist for classifying enantiomers and can seem confusing. Simply put they may be described according to the actual molecular configuration about the chiral centre(s) and also by the direction in which polarised light is rotated.

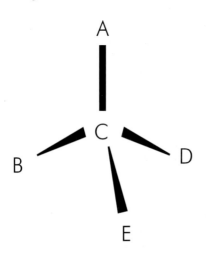

Figure PC.16 Asymmetry about a single carbon atom

The molecular arrangement is described as either right- or left-handed, based on prioritising the groups attached to the chiral atom by atomic number of the attached atoms and molecules. The details of this are beyond the scope of Fundamentals. Right-handed isomers are classified as D (from the Latin *dexter*) or R (from the Latin *rectus*), both terms referring to the right. Left-handed isomers are classified as L (from the Latin *laevus*) or S (from the Latin *sinister*), both terms referring to the left.

The optical rotation may be clockwise (to the right) or anticlockwise (to the left). Clockwise rotation is said to be dextrorotatory and is represented by (+) or *d*. Anticlockwise rotation is said to be laevorotatory and is represented by (-) or *l*.

Chiral molecules are variously classified in texts with a mixture of the above terms. It is sufficient to use either handedness or optical rotation to define the enantiomer, however for completeness both terms are often used especially with drugs. *d* and *l* have largely been superseded by (+) and (-). D and L are still used for physiological components, but R and S are usually used for drugs.

PHYSIOLOGICAL ENANTIOMERS

Glucose exists naturally as D (+) glucose (which is why it is also referred to as **dex**trose). Its right-handedness is by comparing carbon-5 with the configuration of D-glyceraldehyde. The mirror image is L (-) glucose, and is a mirror image of all the chiral carbons of glucose. Most naturally occurring carbohydrates are right-handed. Alterations in the chirality about carbon atoms (2, 3, 4) within the carbohydrate ring (interchanging hydrogen and hydroxyl group) result in epimers. Examples include D-galactose and D-mannose. D (-) fructose has the same configuration but in fructose this rotates light to the left as denoted by the (-).

Conversely, the amino acids in proteins (except glycine which has no chiral atom) all have an absolute configuration similar to that of L-glyceraldehyde. They rotate light in different directions (for example: L (+) alanine and L (-)leucine. Some D-amino acids do occur naturally for example in bacterial cell walls.

PHARMACOLOGICAL CONSIDERATIONS

Different enantiomers often have different potencies (stereoselectivity), and may be responsible for different side effects. The manufacture of most stereoisomeric drugs results in equal amounts of each stereoisomer. This is called a racemic mixture, and the rotational effects on light cancel out. Where multiple chiral atoms exist the number of stereoisomers increase greatly.

The naturally occurring receptors are often stereospecific and will interact mainly or entirely with one racemate (e.g. R(+) etomidate). The rest of the drug may be redundant. As the chemical properties are usually identical, the measurement of drug levels will not distinguish between the species. This affects pharmacokinetic calculations. The elimination of the drug may also be different for each racemate, as will be the activity of any metabolites, so each racemate will have a different pharmacokinetic profile. Unfortunately the redundant stereoisomer may be responsible for unwanted effects, and may preclude the drugs use and further development unless the desired stereoisomer can be isolated. This requires special techniques that are costly. Specific manufacture of stereoisomers is advantageous.

Geometric isomerism

Geometric (or *cis-trans*) isomerism refers to the possible atomic orientational variants about a double bond. Figure PC.17 shows an example of this. The main parts of each half are in the same plane in the *cis* (Latin - same side) isomers and in opposite planes in *trans* (Latin - other side).

Mivacurium contains two such bonds and the resultant isomers (*cis-cis*, *cis-trans* and *trans-trans*) have different pharmacokinetic profiles (p 647). *Cis*-atracurium is now available to minimise the undesirable effects such as histamine release thought to be caused by the *trans* isomers.

$$H - C - COOH$$
$$\parallel$$
$$H - C - COOH$$

cis form (maleic acid)

$$H - C - COOH$$
$$\parallel$$
$$COOH - C - H$$

trans form (fumaric acid)

Figure PC.17 An example of *cis–trans* isomerism

PROTEIN BINDING

Protein binding depends on the structure of the protein. A protein may have up to four levels of structure:

Primary structure – the chemical formula of the protein, which is usually simplified by using the component amino acids to describe it. It concerns the covalent bonds excluding cross-linking disulphide and hydrogen bonds

Secondary structure – the relative spatial positions of neighbouring covalently bonded molecules to each other. Free rotation occurs about single covalent bonds (but not double bonds). This rotation allows the molecule to settle into its most stable orientation resulting in a specific coiled protein layout held in place by disulphide bridges. This basic coil is often an alpha-helix

Tertiary structure – the shape in which the alpha-helix is subsequently arranged, which may be long and straight but usually it curls around itself

Quaternary structure – the inter-relationship between individual protein molecule subunits when more than one subunit constitutes the protein. Subunits are held together by weak bonds such as hydrogen bonds and van der Waals forces

Proteins are highly complex molecules and potentially have multiple areas or sites with individual properties. These sites vary in size, shape, electrostatic charge and their relationship to other sites. They have the potential to attract molecules of a suitable size, shape and charge in a similar manner to a three-dimensional jigsaw or key. Plasma proteins act in this way to transport poorly soluble molecules to other locations in the body. The bound molecules are generally in equilibrium with their unbound molecules, and are released as the free concentration falls.

Enzymes are specific proteins that bind molecules and then facilitate the formation or destruction of covalent bonds within molecules allowing synthesis of new molecules and destruction of other molecules. Receptors are usually proteins or glycoproteins that bind or receive specific molecules (agonists and antagonists) producing a conformational change in the receptor that is responsible for the effect. The effect of agonist–receptor complex may be to open an ion channel in a membrane, for example.

Drugs may interact with binding sites in the following ways:

- Agonist drugs have a similar structure to the intended molecule, bind to the receptor site and mimic the endogenous agonist
- Antagonist drugs have a similar structure to the

intended molecule, bind to the receptor site without causing any change but prevent the endogenous agonist binding to the receptor

- Drugs may bind to another part of the protein causing a configuration change that prevents the receptor site from binding to the agonist
- Drugs may bind to another part of the protein preventing the configuration change necessary for the physiological effect
- Drugs may bind to the protein and prevent ions reaching the opened channel

PLASMA PROTEIN BINDING

The degree of drug binding to plasma proteins is relevant to the transport of poorly soluble drugs and also in determining dose requirements.

Features of plasma proteins

The main plasma proteins involved in drug transport are albumin and globulin. Other molecules such as alpha$_1$ acid glycoprotein, which binds basic drugs, and specific carriers for cortisol and thyroxine contribute to the transport system. These molecules are large (albumin has a molecular weight of 69 000 Daltons) and have multiple, relatively non specific binding sites. As with all binding sites, the shape and charge of the site are important. The bonds are a combination of any of the relatively weak bonds (hydrogen bonds, hydrophilic bonds and van der Waals forces), which allows rapid dissociation of drugs (determined by concentration) at the site of action and for elimination. A drug will bind to a protein binding site to produce a complex in the following manner:

Drug + protein binding site $\rightleftharpoons$ Drug–protein complex.

According to the Law of Mass Action, as the concentration of free drug falls due to diffusion at locations with a low drug concentration, so the balance of the equation will shift to the left. Figure PC.18 shows the different protein binding affinities of some important drugs.

Factors affecting binding

Changes in drug or protein nature alter the amount of protein binding. The amount of protein in the plasma will alter the number of available binding sites, as will abnormalities in the protein structure. Surgery and other trauma, myocardial infarction, carcinoma and rheumatoid arthritis increase the concentration of alpha$_1$ acid glycoprotein. Changes in pH may alter the ionisation of some groups on the protein and drug resulting in either increased or decreased attraction between the molecules as well as the activity of the drug. The presence of other drugs having an affinity for

DRUG AFFINITY FOR PLASMA PROTEINS

	Predominantly bound to:	
	Albumin	**Globulin**
Basic	Bilirubin	Chlorpromazine
	Fatty acids	Lidocaine
	Tryptophan	Bupivacaine
		Propranolol
		Opioids
Acidic or neutral	Salicylates	
	Warfarin	

Figure PC.18

the same binding sites on the protein creates competition and displacement so that less of each drug will be bound. This is particularly relevant when a new drug is added after a patient has been stabilised on the first drug, and can cause toxicity from excessive plasma levels of the first drug.

Effects of changes in binding

Changes in binding alter the amount of free drug. There is considerable interpatient variation in the degree of protein binding for a given drug. Only the unbound drug is available to diffuse and attach to a site of action for pharmacological effect, and the bound portion is effectively inactive. If protein binding for a particular drug is low then the majority of the drug is free to have its effect. Any change in protein binding will need to be large before any significant change in plasma levels of free drug is seen. If, however, the proportion of bound drug is high then even small changes in the proportion of drug bound will have a pronounced effect. Depending on the direction of the effect, these changes can reduce or enhance the therapeutic effect but, more importantly, may permit toxic effects of overdose to develop. Protein binding might appear from this to be a disadvantage. In fact, it is particularly important for the transport of lipophilic drugs that may not dissolve in aqueous media in sufficient concentration to provide an effective concentration at the target site. There is also a degree of 'buffering' of the administered dose.

Protein binding affects the pharmacokinetic properties of a drug. The greater the degree of binding, the less drug there is available for diffusion into other tissues and more remains in the plasma. This shows as a low volume of distribution. A low volume of distribution results in higher elimination of the drug.

SECTION 3: 2
MECHANISMS OF DRUG ACTION

T. C. Smith

PHYSICOCHEMICAL MECHANISMS OF ACTION
  Osmotic effects
  pH effects
  Adsorption and chelation
  Radio-opacity

STRUCTURAL MECHANISMS OF ACTION
  Receptors
  Enzymes
  Ion channels
  Transmembrane transport systems

MECHANISM OF ACTION OF ANAESTHETIC AGENTS
  Physicochemical theories
  Structural theories

EFFECTS OF METABOLITES AND OTHER DEGRADATION PRODUCTS
  Pro-drugs
  Active metabolites
  Toxic products

MECHANISMS OF DRUG INTERACTIONS
  Physicochemical
  Pharmacodynamic
  Pharmacokinetic

A multitude of different mechanisms exists to explain the complex pharmacological effects of drugs. A single drug or group of drugs often acts by several mechanisms, using different mechanisms at different target sites. The various mechanisms are often interlinked so that a single drug acting on different receptors can trigger ion channel opening and enzyme activation. This chapter considers the possible mechanisms of drug action and interaction whereas Chapter 3 considers the qualitative drug–concentration related aspects of drug–receptor and drug–enzyme activity. Mechanisms of drug action are classified in Figure MD.1.

PHYSICOCHEMICAL MECHANISMS OF ACTION

OSMOTIC EFFECTS

Drugs that do not penetrate membranes or tissue barriers develop osmotic or oncotic potentials within the fluid compartment into which they are introduced or within which they are distributed. This potential then draws water into the compartment from neighbouring compartments. Mannitol (administered IV) initially increases plasma osmolarity and draws water out of the tissues. This effect can be used to reduce intracranial pressure but leakage into the brain means that this effect is temporary. Mannitol freely passes through the glomerulus but is not re-absorbed thus it carries water with it (osmotic diuresis).

MECHANISMS OF DRUG ACTION

Physicochemical (drug activity related to the physicochemical properties of the drug)
- Physical volume
- Lipid solubility
- Osmotic
- pH
- Adsorption and chelation
- Oxidation and reduction
- Radio-opacity

Structural (drug activity related to the specific conformation of the drug)
- Receptor
- Enzyme
- Ion channel

Figure MD.1

---

pH EFFECTS

Acids and bases directly affect the pH of their environment. Alteration of pH may be the primary aim of treatment or the changed pH may facilitate other actions. For example, antacids such as sodium citrate are used to neutralise gastric acid as a premedication and in the treatment of peptic ulceration. Severe metabolic acidosis can be corrected using IV sodium bicarbonate.

In some cases of drug overdose and poisoning, manipulating plasma pH facilitates the excretion of the drug. The excretion of acidic drugs such as salicylates and barbiturates can be increased by forced **alkaline** diuresis which is achieved by administering 1.26% sodium bicarbonate IV (in addition to other IV fluids). Ammonium chloride, given orally, will instead produce a forced **acid** diuresis and has been used in amphetamine overdose. Haemofiltration and haemodialysis have largely superseded these methods.

ADSORPTION AND CHELATION

Adsorption and chelation are methods of 'mopping up' ions and molecules so that they are prevented from having toxic effects. These effects are primarily used in the treatment of poisoning.

Adsorption is the process of concentrating molecules on the surface of a large molecule using weak bonds and is relatively non specific. Activated charcoal is an example, and achieves this capacity by having a large surface area for a given mass of charcoal. It is administered orally to adsorb ingested poisons and drugs which, once adsorbed onto the charcoal, are effectively too large to pass through the gut mucosa.

Chelation is the formation of a ring of atoms by the attachment of compounds or radicals to a central polyvalent metal ion – usually involving shared pairs of electrons. The porphyrin ring around iron found in myoglobin and haemoglobin is an example of a chelate. Pharmacologically, the main use of chelates is to prevent the metal ion from chemically reacting within the body, and is used in the treatment of metal poisoning. Desferrioxamine may be used to chelate iron.

RADIO-OPACITY

Contrast media rely on the property of absorption of X-rays for their function. Ideal contrast media are otherwise inert but may be selected to possess other properties to ensure that they are concentrated in specific areas such as the urinary system.

STRUCTURAL MECHANISMS OF ACTION

RECEPTORS

The specific features of receptor physiology are discussed on pages 235–238 and their pharmacodynamics on page 561. Drugs interact with receptors either to activate a response (agonist effect) or to prevent other agonists from activating a response (antagonist effect). The types of receptor effect include:

- Receptor-operated ion channels (ROC)
- G protein-coupled mediation
    Ion channels
    Second messenger systems
- Receptor-activated protein phosphorylation
- Receptor-mediated DNA transcription

The complex structural form of the receptor is responsible for the specificity that enables receptors and their mediated actions to be activated only by certain endogenous ligands specific for that receptor. Part of the structure of these proteins and glycoproteins is concerned with mediating the action, part may be responsible for keeping the molecule orientated and anchored to a membrane and part binds the agonist. The important properties of the agonist-binding site of the receptor are as follows:

- Accessibility to the agonist(s) (e.g. intra- or extracellular)
- Low energy forces bind the agonist(s)
- Occupation by the agonist produces a conformational change in receptor structure

If a drug is to mimic the effect of an endogenous agonist then it too must reach the binding site, be attracted to it and produce a conformational change. For this reason, the drugs will usually have marked structural similarities to the endogenous agonist. Sometimes the drugs are synthetic reproductions of the endogenous agonist (e.g. epinephrine), and once at the receptor site, they, therefore, have identical actions. More often, drugs are modifications of the endogenous agonist so that their pharmacokinetic profile is different. Such differences are necessary to avoid destruction in the gut, to facilitate absorption and to increase the duration of effect by reducing metabolism. Such modifications for pharmacokinetic reasons often also alter the pharmacodynamic profile. Many drugs with receptor agonist activity were found before the discovery of receptors, often from naturally occurring chemicals (e.g. morphine). Trial and error modifications of these drugs were used to alter pharmacokinetic profiles, and the balance of clinical effects was altered as a result of the drugs affecting more than one receptor. The structure–activity relationship of an agonist at a receptor is an acknowledgement of the importance of the structure in determining what activity occurs. Changes in structure are used in pharmaceutical development to alter the receptor affinity, efficacy and metabolism of drugs. With respect to the structure–activity relationship for catecholamines, the removal of key chemical groups on the molecule affects receptor affinity and specificity for subtypes of catecholamine receptors and alters re-uptake into the nerve terminal, and metabolism (by COMT and MAO).

Antagonists may be competitive or non-competitive. The competitive antagonists are attracted to the binding site but do not produce the necessary change in the receptor to produce an effect. They have structural similarities to the agonist but these are not close enough to effect a response. They are in competition for the binding sites with the agonist and act by preventing the endogenous agonist binding to the already occupied receptors. Their effects can, therefore, be overcome by increasing the concentration of agonist.

Non competitive antagonists act at different sites on the receptor or further down the chain of response and do not, therefore, directly compete with the endogenous agonist. They may change the shape of the agonist binding site, prevent the conformational change in the receptor or interfere with its mediation of an effect. In effect, they are blocking the agonist response further down the activation chain and this effect cannot be overcome by increasing the concentration of agonist. As they act at a different site their structure is unrelated to that of the agonist.

The type of bonding is important as this alters the reversibility of the antagonist. Weak forces such as van der Waals, and hydrogen bonding tend to be reversible as sufficient energy exists to break these bonds continually once formed. Irreversible bonds are usually the result of covalent bonding between receptor and drug. These are 'reversed' by metabolism of the whole drug–receptor complex.

Some receptors have multiple binding sites with specificity for different molecules. These may produce different agonist actions. An example is the $GABA_A$ receptor, which has binding sites for GABA, benzodiazepines and picrotoxin. These are all agonists at their respective binding sites as they produce an effect when they bind rather than prevent the binding of another molecule to the receptor. GABA opens the chloride channel causing hyperpolarisation of the membrane so making it less excitable (an inhibitory effect). Benzodiazepines facilitate this inhibitory effect of GABA whereas picrotoxin inhibits the effect of GABA and is, therefore, excitatory.

ENZYMES

Enzymes function by facilitating organic chemical reactions. Typically, these involve synthesis and degradation reactions but may also facilitate conformational changes. Enzymes are frequently components of receptor systems. Drugs acting via enzyme systems include:

* False substrates (dopa decarboxylase by methyldopa)
* Inhibition of enzyme function to reduce synthesis of endogenous product (ACE inhibitor)
* Inhibition of enzyme function to reduce metabolism of endogenous substrate (acetylcholinesterase by neostigmine)
* Inhibition of enzyme function to reduce metabolism of another administered drug (dopa decarboxylase by carbidopa to prevent systemic conversion of administered levodopa to dopamine)

ION CHANNELS

Ion channels may be receptor operated or electrically gated. Agonists and antagonists may affect receptor-operated channels. They may also be blocked directly by physical plugging of the channel which is the mode of action of local anaesthetics on the fast sodium channel.

TRANSMEMBRANE TRANSPORT SYSTEMS

Many molecules require a specific, usually active, transport system to transport them through a membrane. Inhibition of this process is one mode of drug action. An example is the re-uptake of norepinephrine released by neuronal discharge back into the nerve terminal (uptake 1). The tricyclic anti-depressants inhibit this process and increase the catecholamine levels in the synaptic cleft. Some drugs, e.g. methyldopa, have a similar structure to the endogenous carrier substrate (dopa) and are also carried across the membrane. Methyldopa is also a substrate for the enzymes responsible for catecholamine synthesis and the end result is the production of false transmitters. Specific pumps exist in many tissues, in particular the renal tubules.

MECHANISM OF ACTION OF ANAESTHETIC AGENTS

In general, anaesthetic agents (IV and volatile) reduce

excitatory activity and increase inhibitory activity, although there are some excitatory effects and reduction of some inhibitory effects. General anaesthesia reduces neuronal activity in the brain, especially in the ascending reticular system, reticular formation, cerebral cortex, olfactory cortex and the hippocampus. In the spinal cord, general anaesthesia suppresses both excitatory and inhibitory activity especially in lamina V of Rexed. The peripheral nervous system is, however, relatively unaffected.

The numerous theories on the mechanisms of action of anaesthetic agents can be classified according to whether they involve complex structural properties (Figure MD.2).

THEORIES OF ANAESTHETIC ACTION

Physicochemical

Lipid solubility (Meyer-Overton)
Critical volume hypothesis
Hydrate microcrystal theory
Inert gas effect
Physicochemical effects on cellular function
Membrane structure
Thermodynamic
Cell polarity
Proton pump leak theory
Microtubule dispersion
Membrane lipid phase change
Multi-site expansion hypothesis

Structural

Intracellular oxidation
Protein binding
Receptor mediated

Figure MD.2

PHYSICOCHEMICAL THEORIES

Originally, it was thought that all volatile anaesthetic agents had a common mode of action working on a specific molecular component (the unitary theory of narcosis). This fuelled the search for a physicochemical feature that would correlate with potency. Most of the physicochemical theories are derived from this quest but there is an overlap between many of these theories. The major theories are summarised below.

Lipid solubility (Meyer–Overton)

The brain has a high level of lipid. Membranes

comprise large amounts of phospholipid and dissolved anaesthetic agents might, therefore, interfere with cell membrane function. Figure MD.3 is a plot of potency (MAC) of inhaled anaesthetic agents against oil/gas partition coefficient. This shows a very close correlation in the following manner:

$$MAC (ATM) \times oil/gas = 2.1$$

Note, however, that the correlation between solubility and potency is not perfect, and it is unlikely that this alone explains the action of anaesthetic agents. The original work used olive oil and it was hoped that a better mimic of membrane solubility (e.g. lecithin) might provide better correlation.

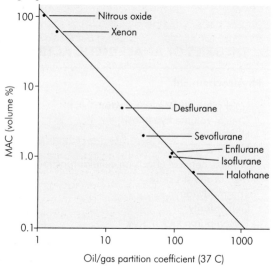

Figure MD.3 Meyer–Overton plot

Critical volume hypothesis

This is based on the experimental finding of reversal of anaesthesia by substantially increasing the ambient pressure without affecting the partial pressure of oxygen or anaesthetic agent. To demonstrate this, mice are anaesthetised with halothane in oxygen at 1 atm. Helium, having no anaesthetic properties, is pumped into the chamber at 200 atm and this reverses the anaesthesia. There is a linear relationship between increased pressure and percentage reduction in potency, and this slope is the same for all anaesthetic agents. The theory is that the absorption of inert anaesthetic molecules causes expansion of hydrophobic sites beyond a critical volume and so causes anaesthesia. Anaesthetic agents expand the membrane by about 0.5%, and the theory also works for some IV anaesthetics, narcotics and sedatives. However, at very high pressures this relationship is lost and differences between agents become apparent.

Hydrate microcrystal (aqueous) theory

There is a correlation between the partial pressure of anaesthetic gas and the decomposition pressure of gas hydrates which applies to non hydrogen-bonding molecules. The theory is that anaesthetic agents form a centre for water crystallisation (clathrates), and this in turn expands the cell membrane and occludes ionic channels. However, many agents do not form clathrates.

Inert gas effect

The potency of inert gases and vapours is inversely proportional to their vapour pressure. The correlation is not as good as that for lipid solubility.

Physicochemical effects on cellular function

These theories suggest that anaesthetic agents alter surface tension, precipitate proteins and alter membrane permeability.

Membrane structure

Anaesthetic agents may interfere with the structure of the lipid of the membrane or proteins within the membrane. They may act within the ion channels or alter the protein shape externally. In either case, fast sodium channels could be inhibited and re-polarisation by potassium flux could also be inhibited. It is thought that the membrane may be expanded so that the ion channel cannot bridge the distance. The lipid structure of the membrane normally facilitates micropore opening. Anaesthetic agents allow more fluid movement of the lipids and this may reduce the opening potential of the channels.

Thermodynamic theory

Within the temperature range 26–41°C the MAC for volatile agents falls with reducing temperature. The strength of this effect is agent dependent. For example, the MAC of halothane falls by 5% of MAC for each degree of temperature drop.

Against this theory is the finding that a temperature change of less than 1°C will mimic the cell membrane changes caused by anaesthetic agents.

Cell polarity

This theory suggests that anaesthetic agents cause changes in polarity with a reduction in electronegativity of the inside of cells. The brain is typically more electronegative than the rest of the body, but during anaesthesia this situation is reversed.

Proton pump leak theory

Pre synaptic vesicles leak more under anaesthesia. This reduces pH gradients and so neurotransmitter release is reduced. Cooling and high pressure reduce proton pump activity and neurotransmitter release.

Microtubule function

Intracellular microtubules are important in cellular activity and may be affected by anaesthetic agents.

Membrane lipid phase change

The lipids in membranes exist in either a gel phase or a fluid phase. The change in phase from fluid to gel phase entails a reduction in volume. When protein ion channels open, the increase in overall volume of the protein complex is facilitated by conversion of some lipid from fluid to gel. Anaesthetic agents lower the transition temperature at which this phase change occurs and may affect channel opening. This effect is reversible by hydrostatic pressure.

Multisite expansion hypothesis

This theory is born out of the misfits of the unitary theories. General anaesthesia may be the result of expansion of different molecular sites that are of a finite size and ultimately reach saturation. Both pressure and anaesthesia may affect these sites. The membrane changes induced by anaesthetic agents are similar to those seen with temperature fluctuations.

STRUCTURAL THEORIES

The existence of stereo-specificity for the effects of anaesthetic agents is strong evidence that interactions with protein molecules are involved in the mechanism of action (rather than lipids). General anaesthesia affects synaptic transmission much more than neuronal transmission. Possible sites of action include voltage gated ion channels and the receptor-operated ion channels. Anaesthetic agents may interfere with cellular oxygenation by enzyme binding. The more important structural theories are summarised below.

Protein binding

Anaesthetic agents bind to hydrophobic sites within proteins causing changes in the conformation of the protein. This often involves multiple molecules of agent in a given protein. Characteristic conformational changes have been identified for an individual protein which differ with different anaesthetic agents. Binding to proteins may alter membrane permeability, enzyme functions and receptor-mediated functions.

Pre synaptic effects

Anaesthetic agents may cause changes in synaptic levels of neurotransmitter by altering release and re-uptake. Raised levels of norepinephrine in the central nervous system (CNS) reduce anaesthetic potency. α_2 agonists such as clonidine reduce catecholamine release and increase anaesthetic potency. The volatile agents do not appear to affect norepinephrine levels directly.

Voltage gated ion channel effects

Changes in brain ion concentrations alter anaesthetic potency. Increases in extracellular sodium ion concentration reduce volatile anaesthetic potency, and increases in extracellular magnesium ion concentration increase potency. Increases in extracellular calcium have no effect, but the calcium antagonists verapamil and nifedipine increase potency. The effects on sodium, potassium and calcium channels tend to be inhibitory (due to hyperpolarisation of the membrane) but the effects are only seen at high concentrations which are well above those encountered clinically.

Receptor operated ion channel effects

Ion channels may be controlled by the occupancy of specific receptors for glutamate, acetylcholine, 5-HT, GABA and glycine. Receptor-operated ion channels (also called ligand-gated) are thought likely to be sites of anaesthetic action a theory which is supported by the stereospecificity of several anaesthetic agents (isoflurane, ketamine and etomidate, for example). Ligand-gated ion channels comprise glycopoprotein subunits arranged as a transmembrane cylinder. As an example, glutamate is excitatory in the central nervous system and acts on ionotropic glutamine receptor channels (iGluR's) which mediate fast excitatory neurotransmission (there are several subtypes). Ketamine is a stereospecific antagonist at the N-methyl-D-aspartate (NMDA) subtype iGluR and nitrous oxide and xenon also act on the NMDA receptor. There are nicotinic acetylcholinergic receptors in the central nervous system (structurally similar to those of the periphery) which are markedly inhibited by volatile anaesthetic agents.

GABA receptors have 5 subunits and may be A or B subtypes. $GABA_A$ type appear particularly sensitive to both intravenous and volatile anaesthetics. As a neurotransmitter, GABA is generally inhibitory and receptor binding causes an increase in cellular chloride influx with hyperpolarisation of the cell membrane. The receptor subunit composition varies between sites in the CNS and the composition alters the pharmacodynamic profile for a given drug. Benzodiazepines, for example, are only active at $GABA_A$ receptors (which possess at least one α and one γ subunit).

Barbiturates, propofol, etomidate and volatile agents increase chloride currents across the cell membrane, effects which are seen at low ambient levels of GABA only. It is unclear whether the chloride current changes seen affect synaptic transmission but a similar effect on inhibitory glycine channels is seen in the presence of volatile anaesthetic agents. Oleamide, an unsaturated fatty acid amide present in cell membranes has been suggested as an endogenous ligand for G-protein coupled receptors (5-HT and cannabinoid, for example).

Second messenger systems

There is no convincing evidence for the interference with second messenger systems by anaesthetic agents. However, volatile agents reduce cGMP levels, increase adenyl cyclase activity and reduce phosphodiesterase activity so increasing brain cAMP.

To summarise, there are many diverse theories, none of which entirely explains the mode of action of anaesthetic agents. It is likely, therefore, that anaesthesia is produced by a range of these effects and that the precise balance of the mechanisms is specific to the agent used. It is likely that the lipid solubility is important and that this influences the agents' affinity for the cell membrane. Within the cell membrane a number of affects have been postulated based on interference with the ion channels. This leads to suppression of ionic flux and so reduces neuronal activity. Synaptic transmission is also reduced probably from similar effects both pre and post synaptically. It is likely that many agents, especially the IV agents have specific sites on receptor proteins that mediate ionic channel interference and modulate neuronal activity. Anaesthetic potency is increased by:

- Increases in age, oil/gas solubility coefficient, opioids, GABA
- Decreases in sodium and magnesium ions, hydrostatic pressure, temperature
- Calcium antagonists

The overall balance is moving away from the physicochemical mechanisms towards the structural mechanisms, strongly supported by the stereo-specificity exhibited by many anaesthetic agents.

EFFECTS OF METABOLITES AND OTHER DEGRADATION PRODUCTS
PRO-DRUGS

Pro-drugs are pharmacologically inactive precursors that are metabolised within the body to produce the active drug compound. Examples of pro-drugs include L-dopa and enalapril. L-dopa is the substrate of dopa decarboxylase, which produces the active compound dopamine. It is a means of increasing brain dopamine levels as dopamine does not cross the blood-brain barrier readily and circulating dopamine is rapidly metabolised. Enalapril is hydrolysed to enalaprilat, which is the active angiotensin converting enzyme inhibitor.

ACTIVE METABOLITES

Many drugs have metabolites that are also active. The activity is usually similar to that of the parent drug. The level of activity may be greater or less than the initial drug. Examples include diazepam, which is demethylated to nordiazepam, and propranolol, which is hydroxylated to 4-hydroxypropranolol.

TOXIC PRODUCTS

Some drug metabolites have toxic effects with activity different from the parent drug rather than simply the effect of excess dose. Examples include sodium nitroprusside releasing the cyanide ion (CN^-) and, controversially, sevoflurane producing Compound A.

MECHANISMS OF DRUG INTERACTIONS

There are numerous types of drug interaction that are classified in Figure MD.4. They may be desirable (the reversal of neuromuscular blockade by anti-cholinesterases) or undesirable. Two drugs may cause the same effect and the outcome may be simply additive (summation) or synergistic. Synergism is when the combined activity of two or more drugs (or other agents) acting on the same process is such that the effect produced is greater than the sum of the effects of each drug acting alone. Conversely, drugs may reduce the desired effect either by acting in opposite ways or by preventing the other drug from acting. Drugs do not necessarily interact to increase or decrease the therapeutic effect but may cause entirely different effects or may alter the levels of the other agent. Many drugs are given in combination to make use of their interactions.

PHYSICOCHEMICAL

These are simple chemical interactions between drugs. Examples include acidic and alkaline drugs reacting to form an inactive salt, and two volume expanders having an additive effect. The combination of iron and

CLASSIFICATION OF DRUG INTERACTIONS

Physicochemical

Pharmacodynamic

Receptor based
Enzyme based

Pharmacokinetic

Absorption
Metabolism
Excretion
Protein binding

Figure MD.4

tetracyclines in the stomach significantly impair absorption of both drugs.

PHARMACODYNAMIC

These are interactions occurring as a result of competition for the binding site of an enzyme or receptor. At a receptor, there may be any combination of agonists, partial agonists and antagonists interacting with predictable effects from the competition. The overall balance of effect depends upon the affinities of each ligand for the receptor and its efficacy. There may also be interference of the one drug with the actions of the other drug further down the chain of reactions or by an action which is the opposite of the other drug. These may be additive, synergistic or antagonistic.

PHARMACOKINETIC

Pharmacokinetic interactions may alter the amount of active drug in the body. The principal effects are detailed as follows:

Absorption

Physicochemical reactions (see iron and tetracyclines above) are the simplest interference. In local anaesthesia, the vasoconstrictive properties of epinephrine and felypressin are used to slow the systemic absorption of local anaesthetic agents.

Metabolism

Many drugs interfere with common metabolic pathways affecting other drugs. This may be simple competition for a single common metabolic pathway, or may involve the induction or inhibition of the enzymatic process.

COMPETITION

Competition involves rivalry for the same binding site on the enzyme (or transport process). Many agents compete for the inducible hepatic enzymes. Other examples include the competition of ester local anaesthetic agents, mivacurium and suxamethonium for plasma cholinesterase.

ENZYME INHIBITION

Cimetidine provides an example of an enzyme inhibitor affecting the hepatic oxidation. Drugs whose metabolism is inhibited include diazepam, lidocaine, phenytoin, propranolol, theophylline and warfarin.

ENZYME INDUCTION

Repeated administration of some drugs such as barbiturates, ethanol, rifampicin and phenytoin induces higher levels of hepatic microsomal enzyme activity which accelerates their metabolism.

Renal excretion

This may be affected by mechanical means such as increased or reduced urinary output or by shared active transport secretion mechanisms (e.g. penicillins and probenecid). Drugs affecting plasma pH will alter the ability of the kidney to excrete acidic and basic drugs. Increased urine output may also enhance drug excretion.

Protein binding

Competition for protein binding sites on plasma proteins may result in displacement of the initial drug by the new drug. This increases the levels of both drugs above the expected level but this in turn increases the amount subject to elimination that offsets this effect.

SECTION 3: 3
PHARMACODYNAMICS

T. C. Smith

CONCENTRATION–EFFECT RELATIONSHIPS
Drug receptor kinetics
Important equations and their derivation

EFFICACY AND DRUG RECEPTOR INTERACTIONS
Agonists
Partial agonists
Reversible competitive antagonists
Irreversible antagonists
Lineweaver–Burk plot

VARIATIONS FROM PREDICTIONS
Occupancy response inconsistencies
Hysteresis
General variation
Pharmacogenetics

ENZYMES

Pharmacodynamics is the study of the quantitative effects of drug concentration on the activity and response at specific receptor sites. In simple terms, this is often expressed by the phrase 'what the drug does to the body'.

Both endogenous ligands and exogenously administered drugs interact with receptor sites to produce an effect. Drugs can act in a number of different ways depending on their characteristics (Figure PD.1).

The important equations concerning drug receptor interactions are explained below aided by graphical representations of these interactions. Although 'drug' is often used to describe the receptor interaction, **endogenous** agonists of the receptor act in exactly the same way.

DRUG PROPERTIES

Agonism – drug binds to the receptor and can produce a maximal response

Partial agonism – drug binds to the receptor and causes a similar but less than maximal response

Antagonism – drug may prevent binding by the agonist or interfere with the response outcome

---

Figure PD.1

CONCENTRATION–EFFECT RELATIONSHIPS

DRUG–RECEPTOR KINETICS

Key equations in pharmacodynamics describe drug–receptor interactions. The basic equations are the fundamental relationships from which the key equations are built. The following explains the mathematical features of the equations and introduces new terms sequentially. The key equations are displayed graphically to illustrate important comparisons between various drug–receptor interactions.

IMPORTANT EQUATIONS AND THEIR DERIVATION

The following conventions will be used:

=> implies that

∝ proportional to

Consider the basic chemical interaction of an agonist drug with a receptor to form a drug–receptor complex. This interaction is reversible and note that endogenous agonists act in exactly the same way.

The receptor can be considered to have two states, active and inactive. When unoccupied by an agonist the receptor is predominantly in the inactive state, but when occupied it is predominantly in the active state. The active state tends to increase the strength of the drug–receptor intermolecular bonds. So, in general, the receptor can be considered to be either unoccupied and inactive, or occupied and active.

Derivation of key equation 1

Key equation 1 is built from basic equations 1 and 2, which are detailed below. Terms used are defined as follows:

$[D]$ – concentration of free drug

$[R]$ – concentration of unoccupied receptors

$[DR]$ – concentration of drug-occupied receptors

k_1 – constant that defines the rate of the association (forward) reaction

k_2 – constant that defines the rate of the dissociation (backward) reaction

K_D – constant (the dissociation constant) that defines the equilibrium point of the whole interaction

BASIC EQUATION 1

$$\text{Drug} + \text{Receptor} \rightleftharpoons \text{Drug–Receptor complex}$$

$$D + R \underset{k_2}{\overset{k_1}{\rightleftharpoons}} DR$$

The law of mass action states that the velocity of a chemical interaction is proportional to the molecular concentrations of the reacting components. Therefore:

Forward (association) reaction $\propto [D]$
and also $\propto [R]$, so
Forward (association) reaction $\propto [D] \times [R]$, and
Backward (dissociation) reaction $\propto [DR]$

For clarity the multiplication sign is usually omitted, thus ($[D] \times [R] = [D][R]$).

The next step is to insert the constants to convert '∝' to '=', which results in the two terms:

Forward reaction $= k_1 [D][R]$
Backward reaction $= k_2 [DR]$

At equilibrium, there is no net change in the balance of concentrations and the rate of association reaction equals the rate of the dissociation reaction, so generating basic equation 2.

BASIC EQUATION 2

$$k_1 [D][R] = k_2 [DR]$$

This can also be expressed as:

$$\frac{k_2}{k_1} = \frac{[D][R]}{[DR]}$$

In any equation, constants can be combined as a single constant. In this case, the ratio of the two constants k_1 and k_2 is called the equilibrium or dissociation constant, which is termed K_D.

The final step is to substitute one constant for two, which leads to key equation 1.

Key equation 1

$$K_D = \frac{[D][R]}{[DR]}$$

K_D is a constant for a particular drug–receptor interaction. The dissociation constant is a useful value in pharmacodynamics as it permits quantitative comparisons of the equilibrium points of different drug–receptor combinations. The reciprocal of the dissociation constant represents the affinity of the drug for the receptor. In other words:

$$\text{Affinity} = \frac{1}{K_D}$$

Derivation of key equation 2

Key equation 2 is built from basic equations 3–5. The following definitions are used:

r – receptor occupancy
R_T – total number of receptors

To provide useful information it is necessary to relate receptor occupancy (r) to agonist concentration [D]. To derive key equation 2 the receptor term **not** featuring in occupancy, [R], must be substituted in key equation 1.

Occupancy is the proportion of receptors occupied by the agonist and this is described by basic equation 3.

BASIC EQUATION 3

$$r = \frac{[DR]}{[R_T]}$$

In other words, the total number of receptors is the sum of free and drug-bound receptors as given in basic equation 4.

BASIC EQUATION 4

$$[R_T] = [R] + [DR]$$

This can also be expressed as $[R] = [R_T] - [DR]$.

Substituting [R] from basic equation 4 in key equation 1 gives:

$$K_D = \frac{[D] ([R_T] - [DR])}{[DR]}$$

$\Downarrow$ rearrange

$$\frac{K_D[DR]}{[D]} = [R_T] - [DR]$$

$\Downarrow$ divide both sides by [DR]

$$\frac{K_D [DR]}{[D][DR]} = \frac{[R_T] - [DR]}{[DR]}$$

$\Downarrow$ simplify

$$\frac{K_D}{[D]} = \frac{[R_T]}{[DR]} - 1$$

Finally, rearrange to produce basic equation 5 (below).

BASIC EQUATION 5

$$\frac{K_D}{[D]} + 1 = \frac{[R_T]}{[DR]} = \frac{K_D + [D]}{[D]}$$

When basic equation 3 is substituted in basic equation 5 as follows:

$$\frac{1}{r} = \frac{K_D + [D]}{[D]}$$

and this is shown as a reciprocal, key equation 2 is obtained.

Key equation 2

$$r = \frac{[D]}{K_D + [D]}$$

Key equation 2 shows that when the drug concentration is equal to the dissociation constant the occupancy is 0.5. Therefore, the dissociation or equilibrium constant for a reversible drug–receptor interaction is the concentration of that agent that results in half the receptors being occupied.

Derivation of key equation 3

Derivation of key equation 3 requires basic equation 6. The following definitions are used:

R – response (not the same as [R] in earlier equations)

E – efficacy (a constant for a drug-receptor complex)

The receptor response produced by an agonist binding with the receptor is a function of the occupancy and the effect (efficacy) of the agonist on that receptor. For the purpose of this derivation, response is proportional to both occupancy and to the efficacy of the drug–receptor complex (basic equation 6).

BASIC EQUATION 6

$$R = E\,r$$

Substituting r from key equation 2 into basic equation 6 creates key equation 3.

Key equation 3

$$R = \frac{E\,[D]}{K_D + [D]}$$

This equation shows that when the drug concentration is equal to the dissociation constant then the response is 0.5 times the maximum, as determined by the efficacy. In other words, the dissociation constant is the concentration of drug producing a half-maximal response.

Response can be determined from any of the subsequent equations describing occupancy by multiplying by 'E'. Deviations from this model are discussed later.

EFFICACY AND DRUG RECEPTOR INTERACTIONS

Graphical plots based on key equation 3 are used to demonstrate and explain the features of the

DRUG RECEPTOR INTERACTIONS

Agonist
Partial agonist
Antagonist
    Competitive – reversible or irreversible
    Non competitive

Figure PD.2

drug–receptor interactions. These are classified in Figure PD.2.

Figure PD.3 lists the values used in the graphical examples that follow. Note that the values for equilibrium constants are not actual ones but represent concentrations for the purposes of illustration. **The equilibrium (and dissociation) constants are represented hereon by the terms K_A for agonists and K_B for antagonists.** Do not confuse these with the terms K_a and K_b used in acid–base calculations.

AGONISTS

An agonist is an agent that reversibly binds to a receptor site to produce a conformational change in the receptor that mediates a response. A pure agonist produces the maximum response that the receptor is capable of mediating and is, therefore, said to have an efficacy of 1 ($E = 1$).

Figure PD.4 plots receptor occupancy (r) against drug concentration and demonstrates the characteristic rectangular hyperbola. This shows that as the drug concentration increases so the initially high increase in occupancy reduces progressively as more receptors

TABLE SHOWING THE VALUES USED FOR THE VARIOUS LIGANDS IN THE ENSUING GRAPHS

Ligand	Abbreviation	Dissociation constant	Efficacy
Agonist 1	A_1	50	1
Agonist 2	A_2	25	1
Agonist 3	A_3	100	1
Partial agonist 1	P_1	50	0.75
Partial agonist 2	P_2	500	0.75
Reversible competitive antagonist	B	450	0
Irreversible competitive antagonist	I		0

Figure PD.3

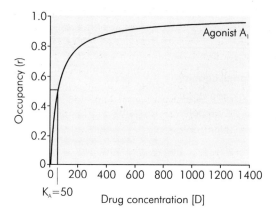

Figure PD.4 Plot of occupancy against drug concentration

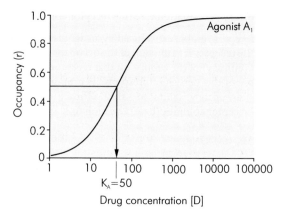

Figure PD.5 Semilogarithmic plot of occupancy against drug concentration

become occupied. The most rapid increase in occupancy occurs when the concentration is low and the number of unoccupied receptors is at its highest. The rate of increase in occupancy rapidly falls off as the agonist concentration rises and unoccupied receptors fall in number. A working model of the mechanics of this may be thought of as a decrease in opportunity for binding as fewer free receptors are left. However, it is important to remember that drug–receptor bonds are constantly being made and broken. The important points to identify on the graph are:

- Zero occupancy with zero agonist concentration
- Maximal occupancy (always 1 with competitive binding)
- Concentration at 0.5 (50%) occupancy (this is K_A)

For a pure agonist (efficacy = 1) the y-axis can also be labelled as response. At this point maximal occupancy and response are by definition both 1, but antagonists and partial agonists alter this finding and thus identifying the maximal response becomes important.

The shape of the plot makes it difficult to identify the maximum or the equilibrium constant accurately using a single plot even if a relatively small concentration range is used. The plot is useful to demonstrate the pharmacodynamic basis of the drug–receptor interaction but does not lend itself easily to comparisons and predictions with other agonists and antagonists or their interactions.

To address these problems the semilogarithmic plot is used. This plots occupancy on a linear scale against drug concentration on a logarithmic scale. This is the basis of Figures PD.5–10. Figure PD.5 uses the same agonist profile (A_1) as Figure PD.4 and shows the characteristic sigmoid shape. The occupancy is plotted as a proportion of full receptor occupancy and for a pure agonist this equates with response. The 0.5

occupancy point that determines the concentration value for K_A ($K_A = [D]$) is on the 'straight' part of the plot where the direction of curvature changes from upwards to downwards.

Figure PD.6 shows two more full agonists (A_2 and A_3) with K_A that are half and double that of the original example ($K_A = 50$). Changing K_A has the following effects:

- Parallel shift to right or left
- No change in maximal occupancy

K_A defines the affinity of the ligand for the receptor (= 1/affinity), so the lower the affinity the higher the equilibrium constant. When the affinity is doubled the K_A is halved and vice versa. The occupancy profiles for pure agonists, partial agonists and reversible competitive antagonists with identical K_A's are identical

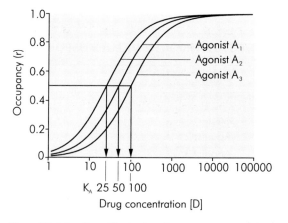

Figure PD.6 Semilogarithmic plot of occupancy against drug concentration showing the effect of changes in equilibrium constant

but variations in efficacy alter the responses proportionally.

Molecular binding of drugs

Consider 'n' to represent the number of molecules that must bind to each receptor to mediate a response. Frequently each receptor has one binding site for a particular molecule but this is not always so. The nicotinic acetylcholine receptor has two binding sites for acetylcholine one on each α subunit. For a response both sites must be occupied by the agonist simultaneously for an effect to occur. Key equation 4 shows this relationship.

Derivation of key equation 4

Key equation 4 is derived using basic equation 1.

$$nD + R \rightleftharpoons D_nR.$$

From this modification of basic equation 1 it follows that the forward reaction $\propto [D]^n \times [R]$,

$$\text{therefore } K_D = \frac{[D]^n [R]}{[D_nR]}$$

This may be rearranged to produce an expression for $[D]^n$ as follows:

$$[D]^n = \frac{[D_nR]}{[R]} K_A$$

If top and bottom of the resulting fraction are divided by the total number of receptors, key equation 4 is obtained.

Key equation 4

$$[D]^n = \frac{r}{1-r} K_A$$

If the logarithm of the whole equation is taken the formula below results:

$$n \log [D] = \log \left(\frac{r}{1-r} \right) + \log K_A$$

This formula provides a means of determining 'n'.

PARTIAL AGONISTS

A partial agonist is an agent that reversibly binds to a receptor site to produce a conformational change in the receptor that mediates a response which is less than the maximum possible. It is, therefore, said to have an efficacy of between 0 and 1.

Figure PD.7 shows a comparison of the drug–response

profile of partial agonists (P_1 and P_2) with the standard agonist (A_1). A partial agonist is one that does not elucidate a maximal response regardless of concentration and, therefore, has an efficacy (E) of < 1 but > 0. A partial agonist with the same affinity for the receptor (P_1) has the same K_A as the agonist (A_1). Characteristically, however, partial agonists also have a lower affinity for the receptor (K_D higher) as demonstrated by P_2.

The following features are apparent:

- Sigmoid-shaped curve
- Response curve shifts downwards
- Shift not parallel
- Maximal response < 1
- Response maximum = efficacy (E)

A partial agonist has the same occupancy profile for a given K_A as a full agonist. The K_A of the partial agonist is a feature of **occupancy** and not response. It is calculated by appreciating that the point of half-maximal occupancy is achieved at half maximal response. In Figure PD.7 the maximal response of each partial agonist is 0.75 of the pure agonist so the K_A

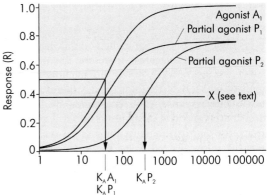

Key
$K_A A_1 = K_A$ of A_1
$K_A P_1 = K_A$ of P_1
$K_A P_2 = K_A$ of P_2

Figure PD.7 Semilogarithmic plot of response against drug concentration showing the effect of the reduction in efficacy which a partial agonist displays

concentration is read off at a response (R) of 0.375 as indicated by the line labelled X.

Figure PD.8 shows the effect on response of the addition of a partial agonist in the presence of various constant concentrations of agonist. For a given concentration of a pure agonist, addition of increasing amounts of partial agonist will eventually result in the observed effect approaching that of the partial agonist alone. At receptor level, competition ensures that the

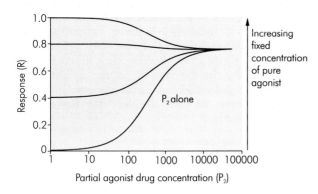

Figure PD.8 Semilogarithmic plot of combined response against partial agonist drug concentration. Each line represents the response in the presence of a fixed concentration of pure agonist

partial agonist displaces the pure agonist from an increasing proportion of the receptor pool until it occupies (almost) all receptors.

REVERSIBLE COMPETITIVE ANTAGONISTS

A reversible competitive antagonist is an agent that reversibly binds to a receptor site without mediating a response. A pure antagonist, therefore, has an efficacy = 0. These agents act by preventing the bonding of an agonist with the receptor and, therefore, any subsequent response. The occupancy profile of a reversible competitive antagonist is the same as that for an agonist or partial agonist for a given dissociation constant. However, as $E = 0$ for the antagonist, response will be zero **irrespective of drug concentration**.

Figure PD.9 shows the effect of adding fixed concentrations of a reversible competitive antagonist on the agonist dose response plot. Occupancy is similarly affected. The important features are:

- A parallel shift to the right
- Antagonist overcome by increasing agonist concentration
- No change in maximal response

The effect of the reversible competitive antagonist can always be overcome by increasing the concentration of the agonist. K_A does not change, but the effect is similar to that of a change in agonist affinity. The dose ratio is the quantitative measure of this effect. This is the ratio of the concentration of agonist in the presence of the antagonist at a given level of response (usually 0.5) to the concentration of agonist alone that produces the same response. In other words, the dose ratio is the

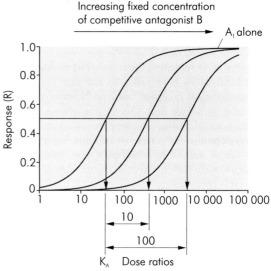

Figure PD.9 Semilogarithmic plot of response against drug concentration showing the effect of introducing increasing doses of competitive antagonist possessing no intrinsic activity

factor by which the agonist concentration must be increased to achieve the same effect as in the absence of the antagonist. Using Figure PD.9 as an example, $K_A = 50$ and the concentration with drug B is 500, producing a dose ratio of 10.

The dose ratio is dependent on antagonist concentration and antagonist receptor affinity, but independent of agonist affinity. The antagonist binds with the receptor in a similar manner to the agonists and the equations for occupancy derived above apply. Thus for a competitive antagonist:

Antagonist + Receptor ⇌ Antagonist–Receptor complex
  [B]   +   [R]   ⇌   [BR]

where:

[BR] = concentration of occupied receptors

K_B = constant that defines the equilibrium point of the whole interaction

r_B = antagonist occupancy of receptor

In a similar manner to the agonist binding, this produces the following definition of antagonist affinity for the receptor,

$$\text{Antagonist affinity} = \frac{1}{(K_B)}$$

The antagonist is only effective in the presence of the agonist with which it competes for the binding sites.

Derivation of key equation 5

Key equation 5 is a simple modification of key equation 1 in which the concentrations are represented by their ratio to the equilibrium constant (K_A). A similar ratio for the antagonist, relative to its own equilibrium constant with the receptor (K_B), may be added. This will have the same effect as increasing K_A because of its mathematical position in the equation. Dividing the terms of key equation 1 by K_A gives:

$$r_A = \frac{[D_A]/K_A}{[D_A]/K_A + K_A/K_A} = \frac{[D_A]/K_A}{[D_A]/K_A + 1}$$

and adding the ratio for the antagonist B gives key equation 5.

Key equation 5

$$r_A = \frac{[D_A]/K_A}{[D_A]/K_A + [D_B]/K_B + 1}$$

This predicts that the addition of antagonist B necessitates an increase in the concentration of drug A to achieve the same receptor occupancy with drug A as in the absence of the antagonist. Taking the term that has replaced K_A/K_A in the equation provides a ratio relative to this which describes the effect of the antagonist on the agonist–receptor interaction. This is the dose ratio:

$$\text{Dose ratio} = [D_B]/K_B + 1$$

This is not constant but is proportional to antagonist concentration and increases linearly. The affinity of the antagonist is defined by the K_B and the potency pA_2 is derived from this. In a similar way to pH, pA_2 is the negative logarithm of the concentration of reversible competitive antagonist that has a dose ratio of 2. pA_2 is constant for a particular antagonist–receptor interaction. Substituting '2' for dose ratio enables calculation of pA_2, thus:

$$2 = [D_B]/K_B + 1$$

$\Downarrow$ rearrange

$$1 = [D_B]/K_B$$

$\Downarrow$ take logarithms

$$\log 1 = 0 = \log [D_B] - \log K_B$$

$\Downarrow$ rearrange

$$-\log [D_B] = -\log K_B = pA_2 \text{ (as dose ratio is 2)}$$

Therefore, potency as an antagonist is defined by receptor affinity (K_B). Competitive antagonism involves direct competition for the receptor in exactly the same way as the pure agonist and partial agonists.

The competition exists between agonist and antagonist or partial agonist and there is only space for one drug molecule at each receptor-binding site at any time. The balance of this competition is determined by the relative affinities of the competing molecules.

IRREVERSIBLE COMPETITIVE ANTAGONISTS

The irreversible competitive antagonist competes with the agonist for receptor sites but once attached it dissociates only very slowly or not at all because of the strength of the bond which is usually covalent. There is no change in agonist affinity, and the equilibrium constant for the agonist in the presence of antagonist is unchanged, so the concept of pA_2 is inappropriate.

Figure PD.10 shows the effect of adding fixed concentrations of an irreversible competitive antagonist with zero efficacy on the dose–response plot. Occupancy is similarly affected. The important features are:

- A downward shift
- Antagonism is not overcome by increasing agonist concentration
- Reduced maximal response

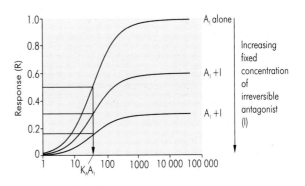

KEY

$K_A A_1 = K_A$ of A_1

Figure PD.10 Semilogarithmic plot of response against drug concentration showing the effect of introducing increasing doses of an irreversible competitive antagonist possessing no intrinsic activity

The maximal response is reduced in proportion to the reduction in receptors not occupied by the antagonist represented by r_B. A simple modification to key equation 1 to produce basic equation 7 is all that is required to illustrate this point.

Basic equation 7

$$r_A = \frac{D_A}{D_A + K_A}(1-r_B)$$

Key equation 2 states that the maximum occupancy (and response) cannot be > 1. Basic equation 7 predicts the maximum occupancy and, therefore, the maximum response to be $1 - r_B$. In receptor terms the concentration–effect relationship is based on the interaction of the agonist with the remaining unoccupied receptors. Therefore, at any given concentration the effect will be a constant proportion of the maximal response with that level of antagonist. The equation predicts that the overall effect is similar to that of a partial agonist alone.

LINEWEAVER–BURK PLOT

The double reciprocal plot in Figure PD.11 is a form of concentration–effect graph to convert a sigmoid curve into a straight line. It is used to determine the type of drug–receptor interaction and the equilibrium constants. The intersection with the Y-axis (1/R) gives the reciprocal of efficacy. The intersection with the X-axis gives the negative reciprocal K_A for a single drug.

VARIATIONS FROM PREDICTIONS

OCCUPANCY RESPONSE INCONSISTENCIES

Receptor occupancy produces a response at the receptor (R = E r) However, the response is not necessarily identical to the occupancy even for a pure agonist because many receptor systems have silent receptors. Silent receptors represent a proportion of the total receptor pool that must be occupied before there is any response at all. This is a conceptual model and the silent receptors are not a discrete subgroup. Interactions between receptors can also alter the shape of the plots from the theoretical.

HYSTERESIS

Hysteresis is a feature of changes in a dynamic system in which the response to a stimulus in one direction does not follow the same path when in the opposing direction. The binding of a drug to a receptor confers a degree of stability and energy must be supplied to break this bond. A rise in drug concentration results in diffusion of drug towards receptors which facilitates binding. During decreases in drug concentration, there is a lag phase before which drug–receptor bonds will break and thus the system demonstrates 'hysteresis'.

GENERAL VARIATION

Within biological systems there is variation between individuals that usually has a normal distribution.

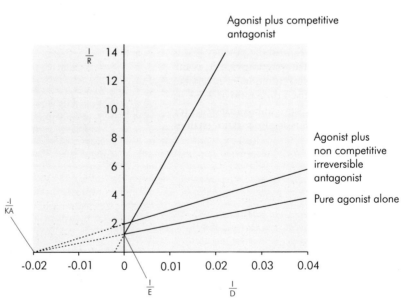

Figure PD.11 Lineweaver–Burk or double reciprocal plot

A single individual may exhibit temporal variation. There are a number of pharmacological terms that use a representative sample of the total population to describe the response. For example:

- ED_{50} – dose causing the specified effect in 50% of the sample population
- LD_{50} – dose causing a lethal effect in 50% of the sample population
- Ratio of $ED_{50}:LD_{50}$ – therapeutic index

Some of these variations originate from identifiable physiological differences such as age, gender and race but most are the result of pharmacokinetic differences.

PHARMACOGENETICS

Genetic variation can alter drug metabolism. For example, the metabolism of warfarin and phenylbutazone varies much less between identical twins than in the rest of the population. Specifically, the drug suxamethonium is metabolised by plasma cholinesterase. Abnormal and deficient plasma cholinesterase result from abnormalities in the gene responsible for transcription of this enzyme leading to inherited deficiencies which are described in more detail on page 57–58.

Fast and slow acetylators exist for the metabolism of such drugs as hydralazine, procainamide and isoniazid. Slow acetylators may show a higher incidence of unwanted effects for a given dose. Slow acetylators receiving hydralazine are more likely to develop SLE syndrome, for example.

ENZYMES

Enzymes are closely related to receptors in their structure and related functional properties. Many receptors have enzymatic actions (e.g. $Na^+K^+ATPase$ in the cell membrane). They possess binding sites that bind substrates with low energy bonds. Enzymes are proteins sometimes linked with co-enzymes such as vitamins or ions. They provide a low energy pathway that facilitates a reaction so that equilibrium is reached more rapidly. Enzymes do not alter the final product nor alter the position of the equilibrium. The effects of an enzyme are similar to that of providing energy in other ways such as thermal energy, but avoid the obvious tissue damage that this would entail. Enzymic processes may be synthetic or destructive. Enzyme kinetics, which bear a strong resemblance to receptor kinetics are outlined below.

Thus for a synthetic reaction:

$$xA + yB \rightleftharpoons A_xB_y.$$

The law of mass action indicates that the reaction rate in each direction is proportional to the product of the concentrations on each side. x and y represent numbers of substrate molecules A and B; A_xB_y is the product of the reaction. The relative concentrations at equilibrium are defined by the equilibrium constant (K_{eq}).

$$K_{eq} = \frac{A_xB_y}{[A]^x[B]^y}$$

The equilibrium constant is a feature of the reaction itself regardless of whether or not an enzyme is present. Therefore, an additional concept is required to compare enzymatic function. This is the initial velocity of the enzyme-catalysed reaction, the velocity of the reaction when negligible substrate has reacted.

The equation for initial velocity is based on the reaction:

$$\text{Substrate (S)} + \text{Enzyme} \rightleftharpoons \text{Product (P)} + \text{Enzyme}$$

which may be expressed as follows:

$$V = \frac{V_{max}[S]}{K_m + [S]}$$

where:

V = initial velocity
V_{max} = maximum initial velocity
K_m = concentration at which the initial velocity is half the maximum initial velocity

Note that this is identical in structure to key equation 3 describing receptor interactions and, therefore, describes a rectangular hyperbola (Figure PD.12).

Some caution should be exercised when alluding to the similarities. While drug and substrate concentrations are comparable terms and V_{max} and the initial velocity of the substrate–enzyme interaction might be compared with the efficacy and response of the drug–receptor interaction, K_m is not an equilibrium constant. With this in mind, the equations and plots used in the drug–receptor interactions described above can be used to understand the inhibition of enzyme reactions and their plots. Semilogarithmic plots could be used in exactly the same way as with the receptor interactions and similar features would be apparent, but by convention the double reciprocal (Lineweaver–Burk) plot is favoured.

Enzyme inhibition may be competitive (reversible) or non competitive which may be reversible or irreversible. Neostigmine provides an example of a competitive enzyme inhibitor. Ecothiopate and monoamine oxidase inhibitors are a non reversible enzyme inhibitors.

False substrates compete for the binding site and in addition have a product, so they are reversible and competitive. Methyldopa is a false substrate for the enzyme dopamine decarboxylase. Inhibition of the enzyme will be the result of more prolonged binding to the enzyme during the reaction. Although neostigmine is a competitive inhibitor of acetyl cholinesterase and is hydrolysed by plasma cholinesterase of which it is a substrate, it is also slowly hydrolysed by the acetylcholinesterase and is, therefore, a false substrate for this enzyme.

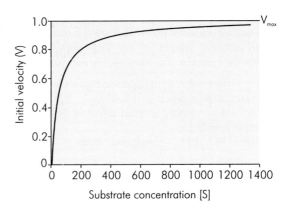

Figure PD.12 Plot of initial velocity against substrate concentration

SECTION 3: 4
PHARMACOKINETICS

T. C. Smith

DRUG ADMINISTRATION
  Absorption
  Enteral administration
  Parenteral administration

DISTRIBUTION
  Blood flow to tissues
  Drug uptake by tissue
  Active transport
  Protein binding
  Placental transfer

ELIMINATION
  Enterohepatic circulation
  Biotransformation
  Extraction ratio
  Excretion

PHARMACOKINETIC MODELS
  Compartment models
  Volume of distribution
  Elimination kinetics
  Effective levels

Pharmacokinetics is the study of the movement of a drug through the compartments of the body and the transformations (activation and metabolism) that affect it. Phamacokinetics is often referred to as 'what the body does to the drug'. Figure PK.1 shows an overview of these processes.

DRUG ADMINISTRATION

Drugs are administered by many different routes. The aim of drug administration is to achieve therapeutic levels of the drug at its site (or sites) of action. In general, this is achieved using the vascular compartment as the transport mechanism for redistribution. Drug administration is, therefore, designed to produce suitable drug levels within the blood. The choice of route for a particular drug takes into account physical properties, target site of action,

consideration of possible toxic effects and the practicalities of administration. The routes are summarised in Figure PK.2 in a practical classification. The enteral and topical routes are most easily accessible, but require absorption across a barrier or membrane to establish their effect.

ABSORPTION

Absorption is the process of taking the drug from the site of administration to the blood. This is necessary for all enteral and parenteral routes except for IV administration. Systemic absorption may occur from topically administered drugs but this is not the intended route. Absorption involves the crossing of barriers between administration site and vascular compartment with subsequent movement across the physical distance between the two. The distance within

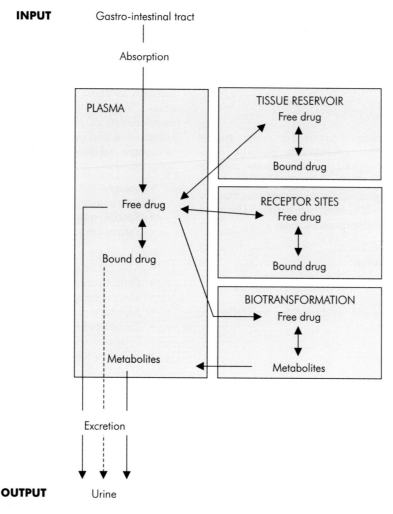

Figure PK.1 Overview of pharmacokinetic processes

ROUTES OF DRUG ADMINISTRATION

Enteral	Oral
	Buccal
	Rectal
Parenteral	Intravenous
	Intramuscular
	Subcutaneous
	Intradermal
	Transdermal
	Inhalational
	Transtracheal
Topical	Skin
	Eyes
	Ears
	Intranasal
	Vaginal
	Urethral

Figure PK.2

any local compartment is traversed by simple passive diffusion down the concentration gradient. Most barriers are made up of cells closely linked by tight junctions. The cell, thus, acts as both a filter and a device for active uptake so the drug must pass into and then out of the cell to cross the barrier. The main principles affecting absorption include:

- Simple passive diffusion
- Facilitated diffusion
- Active uptake
- Pinocytosis

The rate of diffusion is shown by the following formula:

$$\text{Rate of diffusion} \propto \frac{CAP}{T}$$

where:

C = concentration difference either side of membrane
A = area of membrane
P = membrane permeability
T = membrane thickness

The ability of a drug (or any molecule) to pass through a membrane is influenced by:

- Solubility in the membrane (lipid solubility)
- Degree of ionisation
- pH
- Size of molecule
- Carrier processes
- Pinocytosis
- Partition coefficient across the membrane

ENTERAL ADMINISTRATION

Enteral administration encompasses any route that requires the gastro-intestinal tract. Where a patient is incapacitated access to the stomach and small intestine can still be achieved using a naso-gastric tube or an endoscopically sited naso-duodenal small bore feeding tube. Most enterally administered drugs have sites of action distant from the GIT and, therefore, require absorption first. This exposes them to the first-pass effect, which is elimination during passage through the liver via the hepatic portal vein. The hepatic portal vein receives blood from the GIT from oesophagus to upper rectum. Oral and naso-gastric administrations imply that the drug enters the stomach but absorption may occur throughout the length of the GIT. Buccal administration, and to a degree rectal administration, bypass the liver and so avoid the first-pass effect. Enterally administered drugs may also be subjected to other effects before absorption, including neutralisation of alkaline drugs by gastric acid and enzymatic action in the intestinal lumen or wall. The advantages and disadvantages of enteral administration are as follows:

Advantages
- Easy to give
- Special equipment not required
- Patient can self administer

Disadvantages
- May not be appropriate route
- Patient unable to swallow
- Drug destroyed in the GIT lumen
- May have excessively high first-pass effect
- Drug may be irritant to GIT
- First-pass effect and bio-availability variable
- Effective dose unpredictable

Most drugs administered enterally require absorption followed by distribution via the blood to the effector sites. It is difficult to measure effector levels of drug but blood levels can be used as a predictor of achievement of an effective level. Absorption is, therefore, the mechanism for achieving an effective plasma level, and absorption and uptake are essential to this aim. For IV administration this stage is, however, bypassed. IV administration involves administration of a bolus of drug that rapidly becomes distributed throughout the whole circulating volume.

First-pass effect

Enterally administered drugs absorbed from the stomach, small intestine or colon enter the hepatic portal vein. The whole of the absorbed drug dose passes through the liver and, therefore, is potentially subjected to hepatic metabolism and extraction (elimination) before entering the systemic circulation. This is termed the first-pass effect.

Bio-availability

Bio-availability is the amount of drug administered by a given route that reaches the systemic circulation. IV administration, therefore, achieves 100% bio-availability. Bio-availability is usually taken to refer to oral administration (oral bio-availability) but other routes also have a bio-availability. Bio-availability is reduced by destruction in the lumen, poor absorption and metabolism. Oral bio-availability is greatly influenced by the first-pass effect so that a high first-pass effect produces a low bio-availability.

PARENTERAL ADMINISTRATION

By definition, parenteral administration uses routes other than the GIT. Following absorption, the drug is transported in the blood. This may be in the plasma or the red blood cells or both, and may involve protein binding. The absorption process is generally simpler than enteral absorption but still entails some degree of variability between patients, sites and drugs. The advantages and disadvantages of parenteral administration are as follows:

Advantages
- Unaffected by first-pass metabolism
- Plasma levels may be more predictable
- Does not require functioning GIT
- Does not require patient assistance

Disadvantages
- Administration requires training
- Not usually self administered
- Administration usually requires injection
- Requires special equipment

IM injection is one of the commonest methods of parenterally administering drugs avoiding the need to cannulate a vein and slowing the onset of the effect which may confer a safety advantage. The absorption profile means that the drug will be absorbed slowly over a period and will last longer than the same drug administered intravenously. The factors affecting absorption from an IM injection are:

- Drug solubility in blood
- Tissue binding
- Protein binding
- Blood flow to site

Transdermal

Fentanyl and glyceryl trinitrate (GTN) are examples of drugs that may be administered transdermally. The method avoids the first-pass effect and provides a slow absorption and, therefore, a prolonged effect without significant peaks and troughs in plasma levels. Transiderm-nitro® '5' comprises a reservoir of 25 mg GTN with a contact surface area of 10 cm^2 which achieves an average 24 H absorption of 5 mg. A plateau in the plasma level of glyceryl trinitrate is achieved within 2 H of application. This plateau level is directly proportional to the surface area of the permeable membrane of the patch. It is important, therefore, that the patch makes good contact with the skin. Transiderm-nitro® '10' achieves double the transfer (10 mg per 24 H) by doubling the contact surface area to 20 cm^2.

Inhaled

Inhaled anaesthetic agents are covered elsewhere (see pages 589–600). Their effect is dependent on achieving sufficient brain concentration of agent (which is produced from an alveolar concentration) secondary to an inhaled dose at the nose or mouth.

Inhaled bronchodilators act in a topical manner, but systemic absorption also occurs.

DISTRIBUTION

Once a drug is absorbed into the circulation it undergoes distribution. An overview of mass drug movement is shown in Figure PK.3.

The distribution to individual tissues depends on the solubility of the drug in those tissues and its delivery to them. The factors determining the uptake of and speed of distribution to an individual tissue are:

- Plasma protein binding
- Blood flow to tissue
- Mass of tissue to which distributed
- Tissue/blood partition coefficient
- Tissue protein binding
- Facilitated transport
- Drug ionisation
- Drug molecular size

BLOOD FLOW TO TISSUES

Blood flow determines the speed and amount of drug

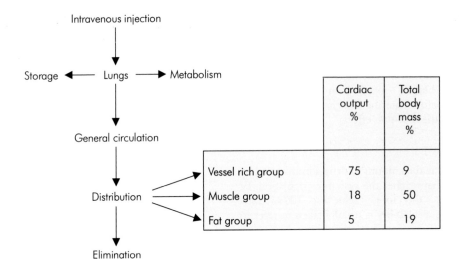

Figure PK.3. Overview of drug distribution

reaching the tissue capillaries and, therefore, the amount available for uptake into that tissue.

Three compartments are generally used to explain pharmacokinetic principles, these are the vessel rich group (VRG), muscle group (MG) and fat group (FG). The vascularity of these tissue groups varies and the proportion of cardiac output received by them is shown in Figure PK.3.

DRUG UPTAKE BY TISSUE

Uptake depends on the drug concentration in tissue and blood, and the partition co-efficient. The blood concentration will change as it flows through the capillaries provided that tissue and blood are not at equilibrium. The drug will pass into (or out of) the tissue towards equilibrium. The commonest mode of transit is diffusion but carrier-facilitated diffusion and active transport systems also occur. The partition coefficient indicates the ratio of drug concentration in neighbouring tissue compartments at equilibrium and drug movement will occur towards this equilibrium point. As blood concentration falls due to redistribution and elimination, then the balance will be restored by movement out of the tissue back into the blood. The speed of transfer to and from compartments depends on the degree of deviation from the equilibrium partition coefficient and the ease of molecular movement. The mass of tissue involved will alter the rate at which equilibrium is reached and so in turn will alter the rate of uptake. For a given partition coefficient, a large volume of tissue will increase both total uptake and rate of uptake of the drug but will reduce the speed of achievement of equilibrium.

The ease of transfer between compartments is influenced by:

- Ionisation (determined by pH and pKa)
- Membrane components
- Molecular size

Figure PK.4 shows the temporal relationship of drug distribution within various compartments following an IV bolus administration of a typical IV induction agent.

Drug distribution causes the blood concentration to fall. The VRG then has more drug than plasma so movement is reversed and the drug moves from the tissue back into the blood. At this early stage, the blood concentration is higher than that in either the muscle group or the fat group. There is a net redistribution from VRG to MG and FG. Later the same effect will occur from MG to FG, and much later the drug in FG will return to the blood and be eliminated. All redistribution processes require the blood as an intermediary phase.

ACTIVE TRANSPORT

Penicillin is a drug that is actively transported. This is a unidirectional process regardless of the concentration gradient. Probenecid blocks active transport in the liver, kidney and choroid plexus, which increases the proportion in the blood, and so the apparent volume of distribution is reduced.

PROTEIN BINDING

Protein binding alters the concentration of free drug as a proportion of the total. Different proteins have different affinities for drugs. Albumin mostly binds

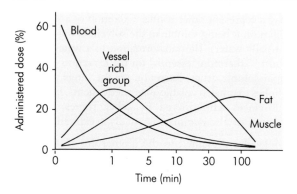

Figure PK.4. Drug distribution in various tissues against time following IV bolus administration of thiopentone

EXAMPLES OF FOETO-MATERNAL (F-M) CONCENTRATION RATIOS

Induction agents	
Propofol	0.65–0.85
Thiopentone	0.4–1.1
Volatile agents	
Isoflurane	0.7–0.91
Nitrous oxide	0.83
Opioids	
Alfentanil	0.3
Fentanyl	0.1–1
Morphine	0.92
Pethidine	1
Muscle relaxants	
Suxamethonium	0.04
Atracurium	0.05–0.2
Vecuronium	0.11–0.12
Local anaesthetics agents	
Bupivacaine	0.2–0.4
Lidocaine	0.5–0.7
Ropivacaine	0.2

Figure PK.5

acidic drugs such as aspirin, whereas α_1-glycoprotein is more important for basic drugs. The amount of drug bound is influenced by plasma pH (which alters the ionisation of the drug), age and certain disease states. Hypo-albuminaemia is a common finding in chronic disease and in hepatic (reduced synthesis) and renal (increased loss) failure in particular which reduce the amount of albumin available for drug binding and, therefore, increase the amount of free drug. Note that α_1-glycoprotein is increased in:

- Obesity
- Trauma
- Burns
- Post operative period
- Myocardial infarction
- Carcinoma
- Inflammatory diseases

PLACENTAL TRANSFER

Most drugs cross the placenta to some degree. Transfer is favoured by high lipid solubility and a high unionised proportion. Placental blood flow and metabolism also influence transfer. The ratio of concentrations in foetal and maternal placental blood is called the foeto-maternal concentration ratio (Figure PK.5).

ELIMINATION

Elimination is the removal of active drug from the body and has two components, biotransformation and excretion. It may, thus, occur simply as excretion of the unchanged active form of the drug or after inactivation. Many drugs require biotransformation to enable excretion. Alternatively, an irreversibly inactivated enzyme or receptor (e.g. inhibited monoamine

oxidase) may need to be replaced by fresh, unaffected protein.

ENTEROHEPATIC CIRCULATION

Hepatocytes possess active transport systems that concentrate certain drugs (e.g. digoxin) and conjugates (e.g. morphine) within the bile. In the gut, the glucuronide becomes hydrolysed and active drug is re-absorbed into the hepatic portal vein. Enterohepatic circulation prolongs the half-life of a drug.

BIOTRANSFORMATION

There are two basic phases of biotransformation: I and II. Phase I reactions are simple chemical reactions such as oxidation, reduction and hydrolysis that tend to be destructive. Oxidation and reduction are mainly hepatic functions where cytochrome P_{450} is particularly important. Hydrolysis is widespread and may take place in the plasma by free enzymes such as plasma cholinesterase. Phase II reactions are important for the removal of substances that are not readily water-soluble. They are more complex synthetic reactions that add molecular groups (such as acetylation or glucuronide conjugation) and biotransformation often involves several of these reactions after which final products may be excreted. Biotransformation predominantly occurs in the liver but other sites in the body such as the lungs, the plasma and the kidney are also involved.

EXTRACTION RATIO

The extraction ratio (ER) is a measure of the effectiveness of an organ to remove or process a substance. Hepatic extraction is the most useful to consider, this being the proportion of drug delivered to the liver which is extracted and does not appear in the hepatic vein. Note that this is a dimensionless ratio, which may be expressed as:

$$ER = \frac{C_a - C_v}{C_a}$$

where:

C_a = arterial concentration of a substance
C_v = venous concentration of a substance

The extraction of a drug depends on:

- ER
- Enzyme activity
- Drug–protein binding
- Red blood cell partitioning
- Perfusion

Clearance represents a volume of blood completely cleared of drug in unit time (see pages 367–368). For example, in the case of hepatic clearance:

Hepatic clearance = $\dot{Q}_{hep} \times ER$

where: $\dot{Q}_{hep}$ = hepatic blood blow

A high ER results in the hepatic clearance being highly dependent on liver blood flow because most of the delivered drug is extracted. Enzyme activity, protein binding and red cell partitioning, therefore, have less influence on hepatic extraction. A low dependence on blood flow but a high dependency on the other factors accompany a low ER.

EXCRETION

Excretion involves the removal of active drug and its metabolites from the body. The main routes of excretion are in urine and bile, but the lungs, faeces and sweat represent other routes. Excretion of a substance relies on it being soluble in the solvent being excreted (usually water). Biotransformation to a water-soluble form is, therefore, essential for the excretion of highly lipid-soluble drugs. Excretion via the lungs primarily applies to inhaled volatile anaesthetic agents. However, substances administered by other routes, such as ethanol are also eliminated partially in expired gases.

Molecules presented to the glomerulus in the renal plasma will cross the basement membrane into the renal tubules but there is a 'cut off' at a molecular weight of about 69 000 Daltons, dependent on shape and charge. In effect, this applies mainly to water-soluble compounds, because highly lipid-soluble substances will only be present free in the plasma in very low concentrations. Similarly, protein binding will reduce the amount of free drug available to cross the glomerulus. If the drug in the filtrate is not re-absorbed as much as the water in the kidney tubule then the concentration of the drug will increase by the time it reaches the renal pelvis. However, it is the amount of drug excreted that is important in elimination and not the concentration, although the two are interdependent. Tubular re-absorption occurs to a limited extent and this is affected by ionic charge that is in turn altered by pH. A high filtration rate will facilitate elimination so good renal blood flow is desirable, but the absolute volume of urine produced is less important.

Active transport systems exist for some drugs (such as penicillin), which are actively secreted into the tubules. Probenecid may be used to block this penicillin transport and, thus, prolong the half-life of the drug.

PHARMACOKINETIC MODELS

Measurement of drug levels in blood and other fluids is relatively easy when compared with the measurement of tissue drug levels. Models are created to help to describe, understand and predict the pharmacokinetic behaviour of drugs and mathematical relationships are used to describe these inter-relationships.

COMPARTMENT MODELS

Compartment models are based on the body behaving as if it is divided into a number of hypothetical interlinked spaces or compartments. Each compartment has specific properties of volume and transfer rates for a particular drug. One-, two- and three-compartment models are routinely used, but note that these compartments do not correspond precisely to anatomical structures. Consistent solubilities are assumed throughout, so the volumes are calculated based on partition coefficients = 1. The models are used mathematically to describe the changes in plasma concentration with time, and so predict and compare pharmacokinetic profiles. Figures PK.6–8 illustrate one-, two- and three-compartment models.

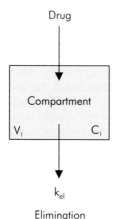

Figure PK.6 A one-compartment model

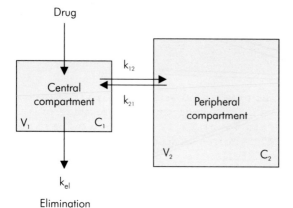

Figure PK.7 A two-compartment model

One-compartment model

The simplest model is a one-compartment model. In this, all tissues are represented as a composite, single compartment (1). A drug of dose (D) is administered to the compartment and is considered evenly distributed throughout. The plasma concentration (C) of the drug is measured to calculate the volume (V) of this hypothetical compartment, the plasma being the 'window' through which the compartment can be 'viewed'. By definition:

$$C = \frac{D}{V}$$

The elimination rate constant (k_{el}) defines the overall rate of removal of drug from this single compartment, and is a combination of all the modes of elimination for that drug.

Two-compartment model

The one-compartment model is too simple to describe accurately the behaviour of most drugs, and the single compartment is, therefore, divided into central (1) and peripheral (2) compartments. Again the plasma is the 'window' to the compartments and is not necessarily equivalent to the central compartment. The central compartment is the intermediary compartment through which the peripheral compartment is accessed. Many drugs, including thiopentone, show a good approximation to this model.

Three-compartment model

Some drugs, such as propofol, require further compartments to be added to allow accurate pharmacokinetic predictions. In this model, a third, deep peripheral compartment is added, and this communicates with the central compartment, but at a much slower rate.

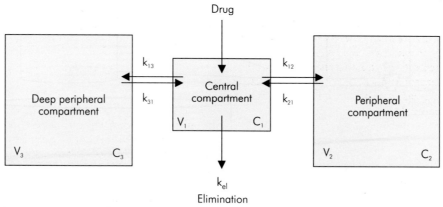

Figure PK.8 A three-compartment model

Any model is an approximation, but by increasing the number of compartments, the correlation with the real situation can be improved. However, the size of the improvements diminishes as the number of compartments increases.

Water analogue model

Mapleson described a model for the pharmacokinetic behaviour of inhaled anaesthetic agents using a series of interconnected cylinders of water (Figure PK.9). In this model, the following analogies exist. The height of the water determines the pressure and is analogous to the agent partial pressure. The cross sectional area of each cylinder is analogous to the solubility of the agent in that tissue, and the amount of agent in the tissue is represented by the volume of water in the cylinder. The resistance of the connecting pipes represents the transfer characteristics, a small bore (high resistance)

tube representing a slow transfer. The model will proceed towards the equilibrium state in which all the cylinders will have an equal volume of water.

VOLUME OF DISTRIBUTION

Volume of distribution may be explained using the models above. These model compartments are defined as having a consistent concentration throughout. Therefore, if the amount of drug in the compartment is known, measuring the concentration of the drug will enable calculation of the apparent volume through which the drug is distributed. The model works on the basis that the drug is equally distributed throughout that calculated volume. Usually, the drug dose given is known and the plasma concentration that would exist if distribution occurred without elimination can be calculated. The apparent volume of distribution does

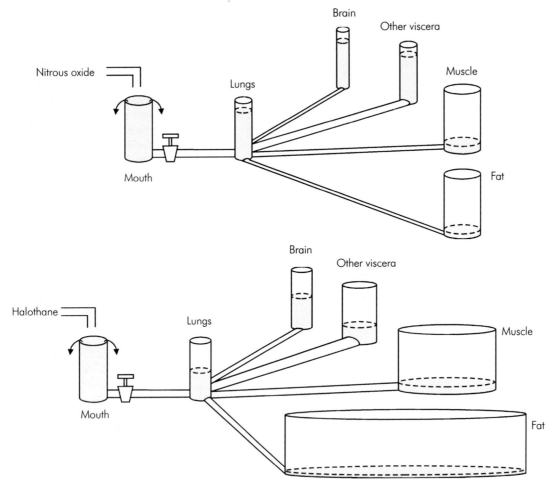

Figure PK.9. Mapleson's water analogue models. The levels illustrate the situation in the early part of maintenance
Reproduced with permission from Mapleson, Pharmacokinetics of inhaled anaesthetics. In: Prys-Roberts C, Hug CC Jr (eds). Pharmacokinetics of Anaesthesia. Oxford, Blackwell, 1984, pp 89–111.

not exist as an identifiable anatomical entity but rather is a mathematical concept representing the composite result of multiple volumes with differing solubilities for a given drug.

The apparent volume of distribution is, thus, used as a tool to describe the way in which drugs are distributed. Drugs that are mainly confined to plasma have low volumes of distribution, while drugs that are highly tissue bound have a high volume of distribution. The volume of distribution may easily exceed the total volume of the body. High tissue binding results in a low plasma concentration. This low concentration spread evenly throughout the calculated volume for a given dose results in a very large value for volume of distribution.

ELIMINATION KINETICS

Zero- and first-order kinetics are used to describe the elimination characteristics of a drug. Most drugs are eliminated with first-order kinetics.

Zero-order kinetics

In zero-order kinetics the elimination system is saturated at clinical levels and elimination is, therefore, constant and unrelated to drug concentration. A fixed mass of drug is eliminated in unit time irrespective of the blood concentration and the concentration, therefore, declines at a constant rate. This is demonstrated in Figure PK.10 in which a constant amount of drug is removed in each time interval resulting in a similar linear decline in drug concentration.

Ethanol is an example of zero-order elimination, and high levels of phenytoin, thiopentone and salicylates also show zero-order features. As the concentration falls so the elimination pathways may no longer be saturated and first-order kinetics takes over. Phenytoin exhibits first-order kinetics at low levels and zero-order at higher levels. Kinetics may also be affected by saturation of other components such as protein binding, carrier-mediated active transport mechanisms and enzyme systems.

First-order kinetics

In the first-order model, the rate of drug elimination is proportional to the plasma drug concentration such that:

$$\text{Elimination} = dC/dt \propto C$$

where:

dC = a small change in concentration
dt = a small change in time
C = concentration

The elimination pathways are not saturated but are gradually recruited as the concentration of drug increases, and vice versa. The rate of change of drug concentration is, therefore, also proportional to the drug concentration. The change in concentration is a lowering of concentration and so the formula has a minus sign. Thus, for first-order kinetics:

$$\frac{dC}{dt} = -kC$$

This can be calculated from the following derived formula called **Key equation 1**:

$$C = C_0 \, e^{-k_{el} t}$$

where:

k_{el} = elimination rate constant
C_0 = concentration (C) at time (t) = 0

Figure PK.11 demonstrates this process in which a constant volume is cleared of drug in each time interval resulting in an ever declining rate of fall in drug and drug concentration. Although the drug concentration decreases with time, it approaches but never actually reaches 'zero' drug concentration. The rate of that decrease (the gradient of the slope) also falls with time. This is an exponential decay.

HALF-LIVES AND TIME CONSTANTS (FIGURE PK.12)

In first-order kinetics, the time taken for the concentration to halve (half-life) is a feature of exponential functions of this type. Half-lives are hybrid constants that are dependent on primary constants. The time constant, another such feature, is based on the rate of change of concentration (the gradient of the plot). The time constant is the time that it would take for the drug concentration to reach zero if elimination continued at the rate of the chosen starting point. Time constants (τ) also apply to exponential functions of the form $y = 1 - e^{-x}$. Figure PK.13 shows the proportion of the initial concentration that exists after a given number of time constants. The initial concentration in this sense may be any point on the plot from which timing is started. As the time constant and half-life are constants for a given exponential function, they must have a constant relationship which is described by the formulae:

$$t_{\frac{1}{2}} = \tau \log_e 2 \text{ and } \tau = \frac{1}{k_{el}}$$

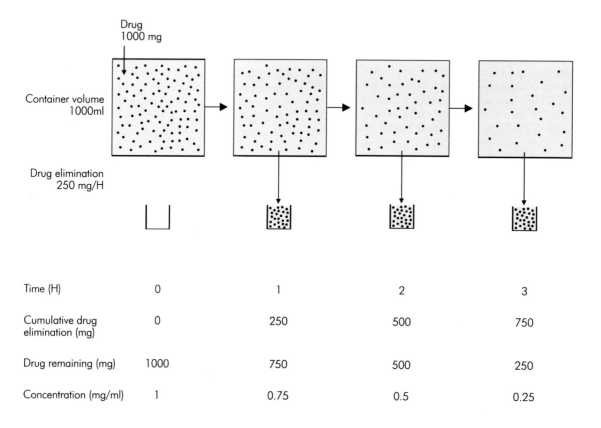

Time (H)	0	1	2	3
Cumulative drug elimination (mg)	0	250	500	750
Drug remaining (mg)	1000	750	500	250
Concentration (mg/ml)	1	0.75	0.5	0.25

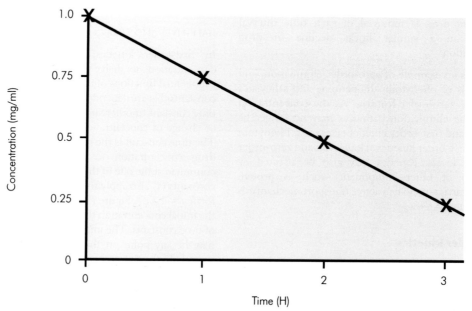

Figure PK.10. Effect of zero-order elimination on drug concentration

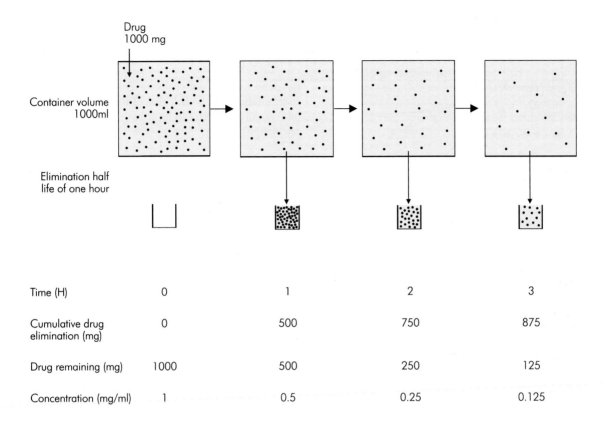

Time (H)	0	1	2	3
Cumulative drug elimination (mg)	0	500	750	875
Drug remaining (mg)	1000	500	250	125
Concentration (mg/ml)	1	0.5	0.25	0.125

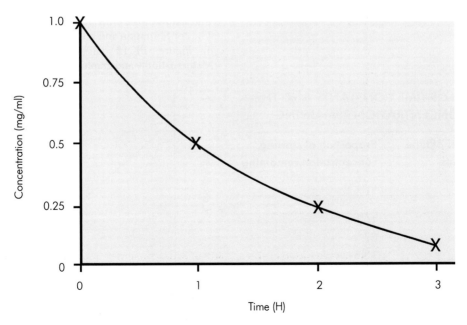

Figure PK.11. Effect of first-order elimination on drug concentration constant regardless of the concentration

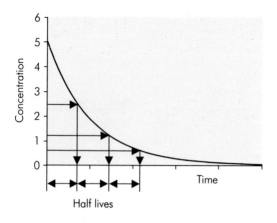

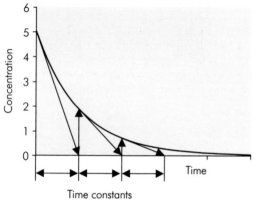

Figure PK.12. Plot of drug concentration against time showing half-lives and time constants (using linear scales)

TABLE OF TIME CONSTANTS AND THE CONCENTRATION REMAINING

Number of time constants	Proportion of starting concentration remaining
N	e^{-N} (%)
0	100
1	37
2	13.5
3	5.0
4	1.8

Figure PK.13. Time constants and the concentration remaining

Derivation of key equation 2

Using key equation 1 an expression relating the half-life and the elimination rate constant can be derived.

Key equation 1

$$C = C_0 \, e^{-k_{el} t}$$

By definition, at one half-life from time zero the concentration will be half that of the concentration at time zero (time zero can be chosen arbitrarily for this calculation).

$$\tfrac{1}{2} C_0 = C_0 \, e^{-k_{el} t_{\frac{1}{2}}}$$

⇓ divide both sides by the common factor (C_0)

$$\tfrac{1}{2} = e^{-k_{el} t_{\frac{1}{2}}}$$

⇓ take natural logarithm of both sides

$$\log_e \tfrac{1}{2} = -k_{el} t_{\frac{1}{2}}$$

⇓ rearrange

$$t_{\frac{1}{2}} = -\frac{\log_e \tfrac{1}{2}}{k_{el}}$$

⇓ as $-\log_e \tfrac{1}{2}$ equals $\log_e 2$, substitute to create key equation 2:

Key equation 2

$$t_{\frac{1}{2}} = \frac{\log_e 2}{k_{el}} = \frac{0.693}{k_{el}}$$

The natural logarithm 'log$_e$' may also be written 'ln'. The concentration and rate of decline of concentration in Figure PK.12 fall exponentially with time. Mathematically and graphically, it is easier to work with

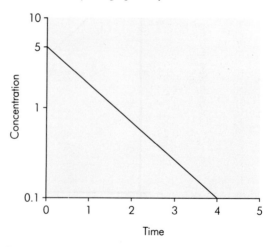

Figure PK.14. Semilogarithmic plot of concentration against time

linear relationships. Using a logarithmic scale for the concentration (or the natural logarithm of the concentration) against time on the original linear scale (Figure PK.12) produces a straight line (Figure PK.14).

The straight line can now be extrapolated to the y-axis (t = 0) to obtain a theoretical (or apparent) value for concentration at the time of injection (C_0). This is the predicted concentration if there was instantaneous uniform distribution of the drug of dose (D) throughout the compartment at the time of injection before any elimination has occurred. This single-compartment model can then be used to calculate the volume of distribution (V_d) as follows:

$$C_o = \frac{D}{V_d}$$

In practice, this simple exponential decline is masked in the clinical situation by the combined affects of absorption, distribution, redistribution and elimination. Most clinical data sets of plasma (or blood) levels of an intravenously injected drug have a pattern similar to Figure PK.15.

This two-compartment model can be seen to have two linear (graphical) components that can be separated. The initial rapid decline is the result of rapid redistribution throughout the central compartment being predominant. Later, redistribution to the peripheral compartments is predominant. Clearance is constant throughout, but elimination is proportional to concentration and is greatest earlier in the process. Each component has a half-life and volume of

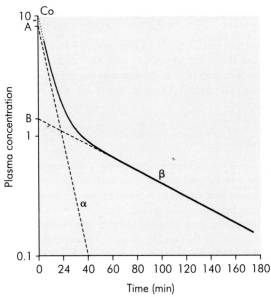

Figure PK.15. Semilogarithmic plot of plasma concentration against time

distribution. Elimination half-life ($t_{1/2\beta}$) is the usual value quoted. To calculate elimination half-life using the graph, the following steps may be followed.

STEP 1

Extrapolate the straight line of the distribution phase to the y-axis (t =0). Call this 'C_0' as before.

STEP 2

The elimination phase has a slope of β. Extrapolate the straight line of the elimination phase to the y-axis (t = 0). Call this 'B'. This is the initial concentration that would have existed if there was instantaneous distribution to equilibrium on IV injection. This can be used to calculate a value for the volume of distribution following equilibration with the tissues. This is also an approximation of the volume of distribution at steady state ($V_{d\,SS}$). However, this is calculated and defined as the volume of distribution when giving an infusion of a drug at exactly the same rate as total clearance of the drug.

STEP 3

Subtract B from C_0 to create concentration A.

STEP 4

Subtract the β slope from the concentration plot to create a new straight line of slope α (the distribution element of the graph). Although it may seem unusual that a curve appears as the result of the addition of two straight lines in part of the graph, this is because of the logarithmic scale used for concentration. Observation of this scale shows that it does not reach zero at the x-axis.

STEP 5

Use these values mathematically to calculate the following variables:

- $\alpha = \log_e 2 / t_{1/2\alpha}$
- $\beta = \log_e 2 / t_{1/2\beta}$
- $V_{d1} = dose/C_0$
- Area under the curve (AUC) = $A/\alpha + B/\beta$

CLEARANCE

Clearance (Cl) represents the volume of blood completely cleared of drug in unit time. The amount of drug eliminated is, therefore, dependent upon the drug concentration, which is a first-order process. Typical units for clearance are 'ml of blood/kg body weight/minute' (i.e. ml/kg/min). Total clearance is the sum of all the individual clearances such as hepatic

(Cl_H), renal (Cl_R) and others (Cl_X). Clearance can be calculated from a graph using AUC:

$$Cl = dose/AUC = \frac{dose}{A/\alpha + B/\beta}$$

In other words, clearance = volume of compartment $\times$ elimination rate constant.

Referring back to the two-compartment model, the volume of distribution at steady state (V_{dSS}) is the usual volume quoted as follows:

$$V_{dSS} = V_{d1}(1 + k_{12}/k_{21})$$

where:

k_{12}, k_{21} = intercompartment rate constants
V_{d1} = initial volume of distribution.

As the plasma concentration is determined by the addition of the α- and β-profiles, $C_p = Ae^{-\alpha t} + B\,e^{-\beta t}$. Note that at $t = 0$, $e^0 = 1$, so $C_0 = A + B$).

This is a 'best fit' and most drugs fit the two-compartment model; however, it should be remembered that this apparent mathematical model is derived from numerous distribution profiles and a range of tissue profiles. Some drugs such as propofol best approximate to a three-compartment model that is a tri-exponential model. Values pertaining to this are shown in Figure PK.16.

EFFECTIVE LEVELS

Effective levels of volatile agents can be monitored by measurement of the end-tidal concentration. Blood levels of IV agents are not readily monitored, but desired concentrations can be targeted using pharmacokinetic models based on patient demographic data, and compared with plasma equivalents of MAC which are:

PHARMACOKINETIC VALUES FOR PROPOFOL	
Compartment	$t_{1/2}$ (min)
Central (1)	2–3
Peripheral (2)	30–60
Deep peripheral (3)	180–480
V_{d1} 230 ml/kg	
V_{dss} 12 l/kg	

Figure PK.16

- MIR – minimum infusion rate that prevents response to surgical stimulus in 50% of patients
- ED_{50} – a general term to describe the dose that is effective in 50% of subjects
- EBC – effective blood concentration (sometimes called EC)

The strategy of a target concentration is one method of delivering the anaesthetic dose. A target concentration is chosen in a similar way to volatile agent concentration and a computer-controlled pump calculates bolus and maintenance infusion rate based on patient details. The target concentration is altered according to clinical need and the pump adjusts accordingly. The concept of an effective blood concentration of the agent depends on the following conditions:

- Intensity of drug action (predictable from concentration at the receptor site)
- Concentration at the receptor site proportional to free plasma concentration

In total IV anaesthesia (TIVA) using propofol, the aim is rapidly to achieve a blood level of propofol that will induce anaesthesia, and then maintain this state until the procedure is complete. Discontinuing the infusion will then lead to a rapid recovery of consciousness as blood (and brain) concentrations of propofol fall. A constant infusion achieves a plateau level, but this is slow. A loading dose is, therefore, used, based on the volume of distribution (V_d) and the desired concentration (C_p) in the following way:

$$Loading\ dose = V_d \times C_p$$

This may be followed by a maintenance dose calculated from the total clearance and the desired plasma concentration (this being equal to the amount of drug being eliminated in unit time) in the following manner:

$$Maintenance\ dose = Cl \times C_p$$

Another method of maintaining a therapeutic level over a prolonged period is to administer intermittent doses so that the bolus is given before the plasma level falling below the therapeutic threshold. For maximum interval, the dose used should raise the plasma level to the top of the therapeutic range without reaching toxic levels. Repetitive dosing results in a plateau once elimination (determined by concentration) equals elimination. The dosing interval is usually approximately that of the terminal elimination half-life.

SECTION 3: 5
ANAESTHETIC GASES AND VAPOURS

T. C. Smith

ADMINISTRATION

UPTAKE OF INHALED ANAESTHETIC AGENTS

Delivery phase
Pulmonary phase
Circulatory phase

MINIMUM ALVEOLAR CONCENTRATION (MAC)

THE IDEAL VOLATILE AGENT

SPECIFIC PHARMACOLOGY

Desflurane
Enflurane
Halothane
Isoflurane
Sevoflurane
Nitrous oxide
50% Nitrous oxide in oxygen (Entonox®)
Xenon

AGENTS OF HISTORIC INTEREST

Chloroform
Cyclopropane
Ether
Trichloroethylene

ADMINISTRATION

Volatile anaesthetic agents are liquids with a low boiling point (BP) and high saturated vapour pressure (SVP) so that they evaporate easily. The physical properties of each agent influence vaporisation. Volatile agents have higher saturated vapour pressures and lower boiling points than water. Most have a characteristic smell, which can also be pleasant.

Volatile agents are administered via inhalation through the lungs and so enter the circulation via the pulmonary alveolar capillaries. Intravenously administered agents are injected into a small part of the venous system and are then diluted by mixing with other sources of the venous blood. The injected agent then passes through the right heart before reaching the pulmonary circulation. Inhaled agents bypass this venous phase and are fairly evenly spread through the ventilated alveoli. However, there is some delay in achieving sufficiently high alveolar concentrations for induction of anaesthesia.

UPTAKE OF INHALED ANAESTHETIC AGENTS

The aim in using an inhaled anaesthetic agent is to achieve sufficient levels of anaesthetic agent in the brain and neuronal tissue, without a detrimental effect on other organs. The minimum alveolar concentration (MAC) is the concentration of agent in volumes % at equilibrium, which prevents the response to surgical stimulation in 50% of subjects. MAC acts as a guide to the concentration required for anaesthesia. Altitude reduces atmospheric pressure and, therefore, the concentration of anaesthetic agent for a given percentage, so minimum alveolar pressure might be a more useful concept. At equilibrium, the partial pressures of the agents will be identical throughout the body, but the concentrations in different tissues will be determined by the partition coefficients. When a difference in partial pressure exists between two compartments, there will be a movement down the pressure gradient until equilibrium is achieved.

Achievement of satisfactory brain levels of anaesthetic agent occurs in three stages:

- Delivery phase
- Pulmonary phase
- Circulatory phase

DELIVERY PHASE

The delivery phase involves the introduction of the anaesthetic agents into the gas to be inspired. The fresh gas mixture produced by the anaesthetic machine is passed into the anaesthetic breathing system. This is not usually modified further but when a circle breathing system is used a vaporiser may be placed within this circuit. While the details of vaporiser and breathing systems are covered elsewhere; within this chapter it is important to appreciate that the settings dialled up on the anaesthetic machine do not guarantee the same levels in the inspired gas because anaesthetic agent is lost in several ways:

- Dilution with existing gas in the breathing system
- Uptake by CO_2 absorbers
- Uptake by rubber and plastic components of the circuit

Inspired and expired concentrations of anaesthetic agents should be monitored, whenever possible, at the closest point to the patient.

PULMONARY PHASE

The following factors influence the uptake of anaesthetic agents from inhaled gas to the blood:

- Inhaled concentration
- Alveolar ventilation
- Diffusion
- Blood/gas partition coefficient
- Partial pressure of agent in the pulmonary artery
- Pulmonary blood flow
- Ventilation/perfusion distribution
- Concentration effect
- Second gas effect

Inhaled concentration

The inhaled concentration directly affects the inhaled partial pressure or tension. The higher the tension the higher the levels achieved in the blood. Levels above the desired maintenance tension for the brain (over-pressure) are often used to speed up arrival at these maintenance levels.

Alveolar ventilation

Ventilation of the lungs carries the volatile agent into the alveoli and the pre-existing gas mixture is gradually replaced. Contemporaneously, vapour is diffusing into the blood so depleting its concentration in the alveoli. Increasing alveolar minute volume speeds up the approximation of alveolar to inspired levels. Increases in physiological deadspace constitute wasted ventilation in terms of supplying vapour to the blood. In general, volatile anaesthetic agents depress respiration so as anaesthetic depth increases alveolar ventilation falls. This is one reason for a reduction in the rate of uptake of volatile agents as anaesthesia progresses.

Diffusion

The small molecules of volatile agents pass easily through the pulmonary membrane and in health diffusion is not a limiting factor. However, disease processes may reduce the surface area and increase the thickness of the alveolar membrane. For example, emphysema reduces the available area and pulmonary fibrosis increases the thickness of the membrane, so transfer of inhaled agents into the capillary blood may be delayed.

Blood/gas partition coefficient

The blood/gas partition coefficient determines the amount of agent that must be transferred to the blood to achieve equilibrium for a given tension, assuming that the blood volume is known and that there is no transfer to other tissues. This is an important point because it is this tension that drives the agent into the brain and other tissues. A low blood/gas partition coefficient indicates low solubility in blood so equilibrium will be reached with relatively small transfers of gas and, therefore, equilibrium will be rapid. Conversely, a high coefficient indicates high solubility and equilibrium will be slow. Nitrous oxide and desflurane, which have low blood/gas solubility coefficients, illustrate this point, and blood levels rapidly approximate to inspired levels. Diethyl ether, methoxyflurane and trichlorethylene are much more soluble in blood and take considerably longer. Halothane, enflurane and isoflurane lie in the middle, with isoflurane the quickest of these three. In practice, equilibration is affected by distribution to other tissues

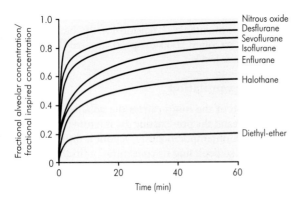

Figure V.1 Wash-in curves for volatile anaesthetic agents

and the process is slower than the simple model above, and other factors influence the relationship between individual agents. Figure V.1 shows wash-in characteristics for selected volatile agents obtained by plotting the fractional alveolar-inspired concentration as a ratio against time.

Partial pressure of volatile agent in the pulmonary artery

The rate of uptake of volatile agent from each alveolus is dependent on the tension difference between the alveolus and the capillary blood. As the concentration and tension in the blood rises the rate of uptake is reduced and so the rate of tension rise decreases.

Pulmonary blood flow

As blood passes through the pulmonary capillaries the tension of volatile agent in the capillary will increase and so reduce the rate of transfer in the latter part of the capillary. Therefore, increasing the blood flow will increase uptake.

Ventilation/perfusion distribution

Ventilation/perfusion mismatch will reduce perfusion of well-ventilated areas of lung and increase perfusion of alveoli poorly supplied with volatile agent.

Concentration effect

The uptake of volatile agent from the alveolus, during a small part of the respiratory cycle, reduces the amount left in the alveolus for subsequent parts of the cycle. Rate of uptake is proportional to the tension, which is the direct result of the concentration. Assuming that a smaller proportion of the other constituents of alveolar gas (e.g. nitrogen and oxygen) is absorbed, then the concentration of the anaesthetic agent will fall. The degree of fall will be influenced by its concentration, agents in low concentrations suffering a greater proportional loss than those in high concentrations. This means that the uptake of agents inhaled in high concentrations will be better maintained over the respiratory cycle than those administered at lower concentrations.

Second gas effect

The second gas effect embodies the same principles as the concentration effect. However, in this case the administration of a rapidly absorbed gas given in high concentration (typically nitrous oxide) together with a volatile agent of lower solubility, produces an increasing alveolar concentration of the second agent thus promoting its absorption.

CIRCULATORY PHASE

The following factors influence the transport of the volatile agent dissolved to the brain:

- Cardiac output
- Cerebral blood flow
- Distribution to other tissues

The distribution of blood to various tissues and compartments is described elsewhere (p575–577). While these principles apply to drugs that are intravenously administered, volatile agents behave in a similar fashion with the driving force of partial pressure (tension), tending toward equilibrium. The uptake of agent by the tissues is proportional to tissue perfusion, solubility and arteriovenous tension difference. The formula is:

Uptake = tissue blood flow × tissue/blood solubility × arteriovenous tension difference.

The formula produces time constants for the exponential function of tissue anaesthetic tension against time. High cardiac output and low tissue solubility produce a low time constant.

Cardiac output

Of cardiac output, 70–80% is distributed to the vessel-rich organs (brain, heart, liver, kidney) that constitute about 9% of body mass. Of the total, 14% goes to the brain (2.2% of body mass). A large proportion of the absorbed anaesthetic is thus directed to the brain. By virtue of their high lipid solubility, the brain has a relatively high affinity for anaesthetic agents.

Cerebral blood flow (CBF)

Factors affecting the proportion of cardiac output going to the brain will influence cerebral uptake of volatile agents. In shock, CBF is relatively well preserved; hence, more agent will go to the brain and equilibrium will be reached more rapidly. Increasing depth of anaesthesia during spontaneous ventilation increases CO_2 and secondarily CBF. Hyperventilation during induction of anaesthesia will reduce CO_2 and CBF and delay equilibrium.

Distribution to other tissues

Distribution of volatile agent to other tissues (dependent on the factors above) slows the initial rate of uptake by the brain. Later, these depots of anaesthetic agent act to maintain the blood and so brain levels and they act as a damper to any changes in alveolar and blood levels. This is something of an advantage, but slows recovery as much as it does induction.

MINIMUM ALVEOLAR CONCENTRATION (MAC)

This is the concentration of anaesthetic agent, which at equilibrium will prevent a reflex response to skin incision in 50% of subjects. It is a form of ED_{50} (effective dose). Other measures of potency include AD_{95} (anaesthetic dose), which is the dose required to prevent response to surgical stimulus in 95% of subjects. Various factors affect MAC for a particular agent, e.g. age, species and concomitant drugs.

THE IDEAL VOLATILE AGENT

Although the ideal volatile agent does not exist, nonetheless it remains a useful concept. The characteristics of an ideal agent are given in Figure V.2.

CHARACTERISTICS OF AN IDEAL VOLATILE AGENT

Physical

Liquid at room temperature
Low latent heat of vaporisation
Low specific heat capacity
SVP sufficiently high to allow for easy vaporisation
Stable in light
Stable at room temperature
Non flammable
Inexpensive
Environmentally safe (locally and globally)

Pharmacological

Pleasant smell
Low blood/gas solubility
Potent enough to provide surgical anaesthesia without supplement (low MAC)
High oil/water solubility
Analgesic effect
Non epileptogenic
No cardiac irritability
No cardiovascular depression
No respiratory depression
Non irritant to airways
Muscle relaxation
No increase in intracranial pressure (ICP)
Unaffected by renal failure
Unaffected by hepatic failure
Minimal metabolism

Figure V.2

BARBITURATES

Examples – methohexitone, pentobarbitone, phenobarbitone, thiopentone

CHEMICAL STRUCTURE

Barbiturates are based on barbituric acid, which contains the six-membered pyrimidine nucleus that is a building block of nucleosides. Oxypyrimidines may exist in two structural forms, enol and keto (Figure HY.4). Thiobarbiturates have a similar pair of structural forms. Chemically, barbituric acid is a condensation product (formation of the chemical bonds involves the removal of water molecules) of malonic acid and urea. Substitutions on atoms at positions 1, 2 and 5 confer and modulate hypnotic activity.

Figure HY.4 Basic chemical structure of barbiturates showing enol and keto forms

STRUCTURE–ACTIVITY RELATIONSHIP

Barbituric acid has no hypnotic activity. Clinically active barbiturates are created by the addition of various alkyl groups to C_5. Oxybarbiturates (e.g. phenobarbitone) are the basic form of barbiturate. It is thought that the $GABA_A$ receptor has a binding site for these barbiturates which have a slow onset of action

and a long duration. They function well as basal hypnotics and sedatives but are too slow for use as anaesthetic agents. Replacing the oxygen on C_2 with sulphur produces a thiobarbiturate (e.g. thiopentone) which has a rapid onset of action and a relatively short duration of action and recovery period. Replacing the hydrogen on N_1 of the basic oxybarbiturate with a methyl group produces a methylbarbiturate (e.g. methohexitone). Methylbarbiturates also have a rapid onset and short duration of action plus a short recovery. However, they also produce some excitatory activity that takes the form of sporadic uncoordinated movements during induction of anaesthesia. These may be mild or vigorous, but are usually distinguishable from the repetitive jerking of epileptiform convulsions, or the diffuse muscular shimmering (fasciculation) seen with suxamethonium. Modification of the alkyl groups on C_5 alters the potency of the drug. Oxy-, methyl-, and thiobarbiturates are clinically useful but the addition of both sulphur and a methyl group (methylthiobarbiturates) results in excessive excitatory activity precluding its use in the clinical setting.

The structural classification of barbiturates is shown in Figure HY.5.

CLINICAL EFFECTS

Phenobarbitone and pentobarbitone have a slow onset of action, and provide anxiolysis and anti-convulsant activity. The intravenously administered induction agents methohexitone and thiopentone are the most relevant to anaesthetic practice both of which are water-soluble barbiturate induction agents that induce anaesthesia within one arm brain circulation time of IV injection. They are highly lipophilic and easily and rapidly cross the blood brain barrier to penetrate the brain.

STRUCTURAL CLASSIFICATION OF BARBITURATES

		Position 2	
		Oxygen	Sulphur
Position 1	Hydrogen	Oxybarbiturate (phenobarbitone)	Thiobarbiturate (thiopentone)
	Methyl group	Methylbarbiturate (methohexitone)	Methylthiobarbiturate (no clinical use)

Figure HY.5

COMPLICATIONS ASSOCIATED WITH BARBITURATE USAGE

Porphyria

The porphyrias are a group of diverse diseases of inborn or acquired errors of metabolism that result in the secretion of excessive amounts of porphyrins and precursors (Figure HY.6).

Porphyrins comprise four pyrrole rings linked together to form a larger ring. They are fundamental constituents of haemoglobin, myoglobin, cytochromes and catalases and all contain iron. Porphyria is very rare in the UK. While still rare, **acute intermittent porphyria** is more common in South Africa, Sweden and Finland; **variegate porphyria** is more common in Sweden and Finland. Both are inherited by autosomal dominance and are the most relevant to anaesthesia. They affect the liver where haem is produced as a component of the cytochrome P_{450} enzyme, and therefore affect drug metabolism. Many drugs increase porphyrin production and administration may result in neurotoxic porphyrin levels. Drugs to avoid include barbiturates, benzodiazepines and steroids, but propofol is thought to be safe.

Subcutaneous extravasation

Extravasation of thiopentone, and to a lesser extent methohexitone, causes localised pain and tissue damage due to the highly alkaline medium in which is mixed. It does not usually cause major sequelae, but injection in proximity to a nerve may cause damage. The pain and bruising can be reduced by dilution with a small dose (10 ml) of saline, or 10 ml 1% procaine which vasodilates as well as diluting the thiopentone. The damage is due to the high pH and is immediate so any damage limitation measures should be performed as quickly as possible.

CLASSIFICATION OF PORPHYRIAS

Erythropoietic – congenital erythropoietic
porphyria
Hepatic   –   acute intermittent porphyria
hereditary coproporphyria
variegate porphyria
porphyria cutanea tarda
toxic porphyria
Erythropoietic and hepatic – protoporphyria

Figure HY.6

INTRA-ARTERIAL INJECTION

Intra-arterial injection of methohexitone and thiopentone are potentially serious complications, causing endothelial damage. This is related to the change in pH of the solution as it is diluted in the blood which results in a precipitation of insoluble micro-crystals that block the narrowing arterial tree whereas in veins any such crystals are carried away and diluted so that they dissolve before causing any problems. The precipitate causes arterial intimal damage, local release of norepinephrine and the release of ATP from damaged red cells and platelets, which initiates vascular thrombosis. Clinically there is pain with delayed or absent onset of sleep. Blanching or cyanosis of the affected area, loss of the peripheral pulse of the injected limb and gangrene may occur. Arterial thrombosis may gradually develop progressing for up to 15 days. The treatment is as follows:

- Stop the injection, but leave the needle or cannula in place
- Dilute immediately by injecting normal saline into the artery
- Administer local anaesthetic and/or vasodilator directly into the artery
    Lidocaine 50 mg (5 ml 1% solution)
    Procaine hydrochloride 50–100 mg (10–20 ml 0.5% solution)
    Phenoxybenzamine (α-adrenergic antagonist) 0.5 mg or infuse 50–200 mcg/min
- Administer papaverine systemically 40–80 mg (10–20 ml 0.4% solution)
- Consider sympathetic neural blockade (stellate ganglion or brachial plexus block). This produces prolonged vasodilatation to improve circulation and tissue oxygenation while improving clearance of the crystals
- Start IV heparin
- Consider intra-arterial injection of hydrocortisone
- Postpone non urgent surgery

THIOPENTONE

Physical

Sodium thiopentone is a thiobarbiturate. It is supplied in a rubber-topped bottle, as a pale yellow powder containing 6% anhydrous sodium carbonate (a base). The gaseous environment within the bottle is nitrogen. The sodium carbonate prevents CO_2 in the air from forming free acid that would react with the thiopentone. The sodium ion replaces the hydrogen ion that associates with C_1 and C_2 of the base compound as shown on Figure HY.7.

Figure HY.7 Structure of thiopentone

The powder is readily soluble in water producing a 2.5% (2.5 g/100 ml) solution with pH 11. At pH 11, having a pKa = 7.6 it is almost entirely (99.9%) ionised. However, once in the blood the pH falls towards 7.4 at which 61% of the drug is non ionised. This non ionised portion is the more lipid-soluble and readily crosses the blood brain barrier into the lipid-rich brain tissue. Of the drug, 60–80% is reversibly bound to protein (mainly to albumin) and is therefore non diffusible and inactive.

Clinical

IV injection of thiopentone rarely causes pain, and venous thrombosis occurs in only 3–4% of patients. Characteristically, the subject may be aware of a taste of onions or garlic before the onset of sleep. The rapid distribution half-life of 4 min leads to rapid recovery.

CENTRAL NERVOUS SYSTEM

Thiopentone causes cortical depression with a plasma level of 40 mcg/ml being typical for sleep. Rapid and smooth induction of anaesthesia occurs within one arm brain circulation time with a low incidence (4%) of minor excitatory movements. Thiopentone has no analgesic activity and may be antanalgesic. It is an anti-convulsant agent. During induction, the EEG shows the onset of high amplitude waves of 10–30 Hz, followed by depression of cortical activity with an iso-electric picture accompanied by occasional bursts of 10 Hz activity.

Cerebral metabolic rate of oxygen consumption (CMRO$_2$) is reduced, which leads to cerebral vasoconstriction with a concomitant fall in cerebral blood flow (CBF) and ICP. The fall in blood pressure that also occurs leads to a fall in CBF with an opposite effect on cerebral vascular resistance. The reduction in ICP and CMRO$_2$ are useful properties of thiopentone for use in cerebral protection for situations such as cardiopulmonary bypass or standstill, and the prevention of secondary brain damage in trauma.

A single, large dose results in the return of wakefulness when the plasma level is higher than if smaller doses are used. This is termed acute tolerance. The technique of injecting a pre determined dose without slowly titrating it to effect allows the use of lower doses while still achieving satisfactory peak concentrations in the cerebral circulation and therefore the brain. A more rapid recovery results from a correspondingly more rapid fall in cerebral plasma thiopentone concentration. Late recovery is also improved as the total dose is lower.

CARDIOVASCULAR SYSTEM

Thiopentone causes a dose-dependent reduction in vascular tone with a reduction in SVR, CVP and PCWP. Therefore, pre load and after-load are both reduced resulting in a decrease in mean arterial blood pressure and in left and right ventricular work. There is a slight compensatory increase in heart rate. High doses given rapidly can cause severe myocardial depression and hypotension particularly in hypovolaemic patients or those receiving anti-hypertensive medication. Extreme caution should be exercised if thiopentone is to be used in patients who cannot increase their cardiac output to compensate for a drop in vascular resistance such as those with valvular stenosis or cardiac tamponade. Gradual administration can produce an iso-electric EEG without any significant effect on blood pressure or heart rate. Cardiac oxygen consumption is increased in normal individuals but in ischaemic hearts, the requirement is reduced.

RESPIRATORY SYSTEM

Thiopentone causes a dose-dependent reduction in both respiratory rate and tidal volume. Manifestations of irritation such as cough and hiccup are uncommon, although it is less effective at depressing the laryngeal reflexes than propofol.

OTHER EFFECTS

Thiopentone is not emetic. It has minimal effect on hepatic, renal or adrenal function. Uterine tone is unaffected, but it readily crosses the placenta also diffusing back into the maternal circulation as plasma levels fall so this is of little practical significance.

Metabolism

Metabolism occurs in the liver with an extraction ratio of 0.1 to 0.4. Phase I mechanisms result in oxidation of the C$_5$ side chains, replacement of the sulphur with oxygen to produce pentobarbitone and cleavage of the barbiturate ring into urea and a three carbon portion. These actions are robust enough to cope with major liver dysfunction so thiopentone may still be suitable in hepatic failure. Clearance is insufficient to deal with repeated doses and cumulation therefore occurs.

Complications

Extravasation causes local damage and intra-arterial injection may cause serious damage distal to injection. Avoid in porphyria.

METHOHEXITONE

Physical

Sodium methohexitone is a methylbarbiturate (Figure HY.8), which exists as four stereo-isomers αD, αL, βD and βL. The commercial preparation is no longer available but contained only the α isomers as the β isomers cause excessive motor activity. It was supplied as a white, crystalline powder containing 6% anhydrous sodium carbonate (a base). The sodium ion replaces the hydrogen ion that associates with C_1 and C_2 of the base compound as with thiopentone.

The powder is readily soluble in water to form a 1% (1 g/100 ml) solution. It may also be reconstituted using saline or dextrose. The resulting pH ranges between 10 and 11. At this pH, having a pKa = 7.9 it is almost entirely (99%) ionised. However, once in the blood the pH falls towards 7.4 at which 76% of the drug is non ionised and can therefore cross the blood brain barrier. Of the drug, 50–65% is protein-bound (mainly to albumin).

Clinical

Methohexitone provides rapid induction of anaesthesia (within one arm brain circulation time), but often (80%) causes pain on injection. It is less cumulative than thiopentone and before the introduction of propofol, it was used in the maintenance of short procedures by intermittent bolus. It still enjoys some popularity for ECT and may be useful in patients with hypersensitivity to propofol. Pain on injection may be less when reconstituted with saline. The rapid distribution half-life is greater than that of thiopentone (6 min) resulting in a slightly slower immediate recovery of wakefulness, but elimination is faster so that overall recovery is quicker.

Figure HY.8. Structure of methohexitone

CENTRAL NERVOUS SYSTEM

Methohexitone causes cortical depression. It is a hypnotic and so provides anxiolysis, sedation and sleep. It is an anti-convulsant, although excitatory muscle movements occur in 20% of patients in a dose-related manner. The EEG is affected similarly to thiopentone but, in addition, epileptiform spikes may be present. Increasing the peak concentration by more rapid administration of the dose and the concomitant use of hyoscine or droperidol also increase the chance of excitatory movement. Opioids inhibit this movement. It has no analgesic activity. Cerebral blood flow and ICP are both reduced.

CARDIOVASCULAR SYSTEM

Methohexitone causes a dose-dependent reduction in vascular tone with a reduction in SVR, CVP and PAWP. This results in a decrease in mean arterial blood pressure that is less than with thiopentone as there is a greater increase in heart rate.

RESPIRATORY SYSTEM

There is a dose-dependent reduction in both respiratory rate and tidal volume greater than that of thiopentone. The responses to CO_2 and to hypoxia are both reduced.

OTHER EFFECTS

Methohexitone reduces renal blood flow and increases ADH secretion resulting in a fall in urine output. Splanchnic vascular resistance is increased and intestinal activity reduced. Uterine tone is unaffected, but the drug readily crosses the placenta.

Complications

Extravasation causes less damage than thiopentone. Intra-arterial injection may cause similar damage to that of thiopentone but the effects are much less pronounced. Avoid in porphyria.

STEROIDS

Examples – eltanolone, pregnenolone, pregnanolone, minaxolone

Physical

The steroid anaesthetic agents are based on the familiar steroid nucleus. Note that oxy- and hydroxy-substitutions at 3 and 20 appear to be associated with anaesthetic activity. Eltanolone is dissolved in soya bean oil.

Clinical

CENTRAL NERVOUS SYSTEM

Most of the steroid agents produce a rapid onset of action (within one arm brain circulation time) with smooth induction of anaesthesia, and a rapid recovery.

CARDIOVASCULAR SYSTEM

The steroids are less depressant to the cardiovascular system than barbiturates and propofol.

RESPIRATORY SYSTEM

The steroids are less depressant to tidal volume and respiratory rate than the barbiturates or propofol.

OTHER EFFECTS

Anaesthetic and endocrine activities appear to have no structural relationship. There is a low incidence of post operative nausea and vomiting.

Complications

Toxicity is generally low with a high therapeutic index.

PREGNANOLONE

Pregnanolone produces rapid induction and recovery of anaesthesia. It is insoluble and an emulsion must be used. It has a terminal half-life of about 50–80 min.

HYDROXYDIONE

Hydroxydione is a water-soluble steroid anaesthetic. It has little effect on cardiorespiratory physiology, some neuromuscular blockade with a low incidence of coughing and a very low incidence of nausea and vomiting. However, slow onset of action (several minutes), pain on injection and localised venous irritation have prevented its success.

MINAXOLONE

Minaxolone is a water-soluble steroid anaesthetic. It has a slower onset of action than althesin, and causes more excitatory activity. Clinical usefulness of minaxolone has been limited by associated convulsions and abnormal liver function tests.

ORG 20599 AND ORG 21465

These two water-soluble aminosteroid anaesthetic agents, which have a high therapeutic index (about 13) in animals, have been blighted by excessive excitatory movements and stability problems which limit human application.

In summary, at present there are no steroid anaesthetic agents available for clinical use.

BUTYROPHENONES

Butyrophenones are covered in detail on page 671.

PHENCYCLIDINE DERIVATIVES

Example – ketamine

Physical

Ketamine is a derivative of phencyclidine and cyclohexamine. It is supplied as an aqueous solution in several concentrations, formulated as a weak acid with a pH between 3.5 and 5.5. Ketamine has a single chiral carbon atom. It is supplied as a racemic mixture of the two stereo-isomers.

Pharmacodynamics

Ketamine is a non competitive antagonist of the calcium ion channel operated by the excitatory NMDA glutamate receptor that is likely to be responsible for anaesthesia, analgesia and neurotoxicity. Ketamine also inhibits the NMDA receptor by stereoselectively binding to the phencyclidine (PCP) binding site. Ketamine interacts with the μ, δ and κ opioid receptors. S(+) ketamine provides more potent analgesia than R(–) ketamine. There is stereoselectivity for μ and κ receptors but not δ opioid receptors. Evidence suggests that ketamine may be an antagonist at the μ receptor and that analgesia is not μ-mediated. Ketamine, especially R(–) ketamine, also interacts weakly with the σ-receptor (formerly classified as an opioid receptor). The potency of ketamine at the receptors is in the order $\mu > \kappa > \sigma > \delta$.

High doses of ketamine have a local anaesthetic action, and there is supportive evidence of fast sodium channel blockade.

Ketamine also acts stereoselectively at muscarinic acetylcholine receptors. This action is likely to be antagonist as ketamine produces anti-cholinergic effects such as bronchodilatation, delirium and a sympathomimetic action. Ketamine anaesthesia is antagonised by anti-cholinesterases. It is thought that ketamine may also have an effect on voltage-sensitive Ca^{2+} channels.

Clinical

Ketamine has a slow onset of action taking about 1 min

after IV injection to achieve an effect. Ketamine can be administered intramuscularly with an onset of sleep in 2–5 min and duration of 12–25 min. The role of extradurally and intrathecally administered ketamine has yet to be established but, in brief, it causes segmental blockade, and affects the receptors located in the spinal cord as described above.

CENTRAL NERVOUS SYSTEM

Ketamine produces sleep, analgesia and dissociation (a psychological detachment from the surrounding environment). The eyes frequently remain open and eyelash, corneal and laryngeal reflexes are preserved to a variable extent. Muscle tone is increased and marked involuntary movements are common.

Unlike other typical induction agents, it affects the limbic system rather than the thalamocortical axis. Analgesia is effected by inhibition of the affective, emotional component of pain mediated by the thalamic reticular system rather than the transmission of the nociceptive signals. As well as a slow onset time, the duration of action is much longer than that of the faster induction agents. The recovery may be associated with hallucinations, diplopia or temporary blindness. These effects are a particular problem with short procedures but those lasting beyond an hour when anaesthesia has been maintained with other agents are less of a problem.

Dissociative side effects are less in males and children, and can be reduced by the concomitant use of opioids, benzodiazepine, droperidol or thiopentone. There is no retrograde amnesia.

A significant rise (80%) in CBF, ICP, intra-ocular pressure (IOP) and $CMRO_2$ may persist for 30 min. The onset of effect is associated with a loss of α waves followed by a dominant θ wave on the EEG.

The (+) isomer is more potent than the (–) isomer for hypnosis, analgesia and dissociative effects, supporting the hypothesis that ketamine acts via receptor interaction.

CARDIOVASCULAR SYSTEM

Ketamine increases heart rate, blood pressure and catecholamine levels by a generalised increase in central nervous system (CNS) activity. These changes are marked with 30–100% increases. Direct myocardial depression counteracts the increased sympathetic activity and may leave stroke volume unaffected. Arrhythmias are not common.

RESPIRATORY SYSTEM

Ketamine has the advantage that, in the absence of opioid, it does not depress respiration greatly. It is a bronchodilator and protective reflexes are preserved to some extent. Preserved airway maintenance is particularly useful, but reflex protection of the airway from aspiration cannot be guaranteed. Because of the sparing of these reflexes and an increase in secretions coughing, hiccup and laryngospasm are more prevalent than with thiopentone.

OTHER EFFECTS

In both parturient and non parturient patients, uterine tone is increased. This is a particular problem in the presence of placental abruption or umbilical cord prolapse.

Metabolism

The pharmacokinetic profiles of both stereo-isomers are identical. Ketamine is metabolised in the liver by N-desmethylation to norketamine. Norketamine has a half to a third of the potency of ketamine and is subsequently hydroxylated. Hydroxylation of the ketamine ring plays a minor role in its metabolism.

Most appears in the bile with 20% as metabolites in the urine but some appears unchanged in urine and faeces.

IMIDAZOLES

Example – etomidate

Physical

Etomidate is a carboxylated imidazole. It is soluble in water but is unstable so it is formulated in a mixture of water and propylene glycol (pH 8.1). Etomidate has two stereo-isomers **dextro** and **laevo**, the dextro-isomer demonstrating the hypnotic effect. Figure HY.9 shows the chiral carbon atom, and the ester linkage which is hydrolysed in its metabolism.

Clinical

Etomidate is a rapidly acting induction agent. It sometimes causes pain on injection, probably caused by the propylene glycol solvent.

CENTRAL NERVOUS SYSTEM

There is rapid induction of anaesthesia within one arm brain circulation time. Excitatory muscle movements are much more frequent than with thiopentone or methohexitone. The EEG frequently shows

Figure HY.9 Chemical structure of etomidate

epileptiform activity. Cerebral blood flow, ICP, $CMRO_2$ and IOP are reduced.

CARDIOVASCULAR SYSTEM

Etomidate causes less cardiovascular depression than the barbiturates and is indicated when the cardiovascular status is delicate. It has relatively minor effects resulting in a fall in SVR, blood pressure and heart rate. There is a slight increase in contractility and cardiac output but oxygen delivery and utilisation are preserved.

RESPIRATORY SYSTEM

Etomidate reduces both tidal volume and rate. Depression is much less than that of the barbiturates.

OTHER EFFECTS

Histamine release is minimal. Etomidate has been used by infusion for ITU sedation. Unfortunately, it inhibits 11-β-hydroxylase and cholesterol cleavage, which results in inhibition of corticosteroid and mineralocorticoid synthesis. The suppression of steroid synthesis (part of the stress response to surgery) lasts for 3–6 H after a single dose, but it is only of clinical significance when infused. It is no longer licensed for use by infusion.

Metabolism

Etomidate is metabolised by esterases in the plasma and liver to produce inactive metabolites that are excreted in the urine and bile. A small amount is excreted unchanged.

PHENOLS

Example – propofol

Physical

Propofol is an alkyl phenol (2,6-di-isopropyl phenol), having minimal solubility in water. It is formulated as an isotonic 1% emulsion in a mixture of soya bean oil, purified egg phosphatide, glycerol and sodium hydroxide. This has pH 6–8.5. It has a pKa in water of 11 so at this pH it is almost entirely (> 99%) non ionised. Of the drug, 98% is protein-bound.

Propofol may be diluted using 5% dextrose to a lower limit of 2 mg/ml (0.2%) for infusion. Of 0.5% or 1% preservative-free lidocaine, 1 ml may be added to 20 ml propofol to reduce the incidence of injection pain.

Clinical

Propofol provides a rapid and smooth induction of anaesthesia (within one arm brain circulation time) and attenuates laryngeal reflexes better than the barbiturates.

CENTRAL NERVOUS SYSTEM

Propofol causes dose-dependent cortical depression. The EEG shows the development of α waves followed by slower δ waves as anaesthesia deepens. There is no epileptiform activity although in common with methohexitone, excitatory movements are seen particularly with larger doses. Propofol is an anti-convulsant, and reports of epileptic fits following prolonged propofol infusion are now thought to be due to the rapid clearance of the anti-convulsant propofol from the body with a rebound excitation. Arguably, it may not be the first choice for electro-convulsive therapy as recovery is no better than with other agents and it reduces convulsion duration (although the efficacy may be unaffected). However, with the loss of methohexitone from general availability it is becoming the prevalent option. It may have some limited anti-emetic activity.

The incidence of excitation, cough and hiccup are similar to those of thiopentone. At equi-anaesthetic doses, laryngeal reflexes are attenuated more than with barbiturates thus facilitating laryngeal mask insertion.

CARDIOVASCULAR SYSTEM

Propofol causes a dose-dependent reduction in vascular tone that reduces systemic vascular resistance and central venous pressure. The reduction in pre load together with a fall in contractility contributes to the fall in cardiac output and subsequent hypotension. Heart rate remains relatively unchanged. The reductions in systemic vascular resistance, blood pressure and cardiac output are more pronounced than with methohexitone or thiopentone. Propofol produces a variable but mild effect on heart rate.

RESPIRATORY SYSTEM

There is a fall in tidal volume with an increase in rate. The response to CO_2 is attenuated. Propofol is more depressant than thiopentone. The response to intubation is suppressed more by propofol than thiopentone.

OTHER EFFECTS

The fat emulsion of propofol can produce hyperlipidaemia. The association of hepatomegaly, metabolic acidosis and mortality with propofol sedation in intensive care has led to the CSM advice that the use of propofol by infusion is contraindicated in children of 16 years and below. In adults, it is widely used by infusion without apparent problem.

Metabolism

Propofol is conjugated in the liver by glucuronidation to make it water-soluble with 88% appearing in the urine and 2% in the faeces. Renal and hepatic failure have little effect on propofol metabolism.

Complications

Complications include excitation, and pain on injection, the incidence of which is affected by:

- Site of injection
- Speed of injection
- Concentration of propofol in the aqueous phase
- Buffering effect of blood
- Speed of IV carrier fluid
- Temperature of the propofol
- Concomitant use of adjunct drugs

Immediate pain is probably due to a direct irritant effect while delayed pain occurring 10–20 s after the start of injection is probably the result of activation of the kinin system.

Pain on injection can be reduced by the following measures:

- Using large veins
- Slow administration so that dilution of the injectate occurs
- 1 ml of 0.5 or 1% preservative-free lidocaine added to 20 ml propofol
- Administration of 2 ml lidocaine 1% into the vein prior to propofol injection

Extravasation causes no major damage. Intra-arterial injection results in some pain, loss of the pulse and some blanching but long-term there is no damage. The solvent is non irritant and there is a low incidence of hypersensitivity but note that the solvent is a good bacterial culture medium.

Propofol occasionally results in green urine.

BENZODIAZEPINES

Examples – diazepam, lorazepam, midazolam, temazepam

Chemical

The benzodiazepine skeleton is a set of two rings (benzene and diazepine; Figure HY.10), but most benzodiazepines also have a third ring at the R_5 position.

Structure–activity relationships are not clear but modifications to the basic structure primarily affect the

Figure HY.10 General structure of the benzodiazepine skeleton

pharmacokinetic profile of the drug. Benzodiazepines may be classified as in Figure HY.11.

STRUCTURAL CLASSIFICATION OF BENZODIAZEPINES

Structure	Examples
1,4-Benzodiazepine	Diazepam, Temazepam, Lorazepam
Substituted 1,4-benzodiazepine	Triazolam
1,5-Benzodiazepine	Clobazepam
Imidazobenzodiazepine	Midazolam, Flumazenil

Figure HY.11

Pharmacokinetics

The benzodiazepines act on specific receptors, which are mainly in the grey matter of the CNS where the majority of synapses is located. The greatest number of receptors is in the cerebral cortex, followed by the cerebellar cortex, thalamus, hypothalamus and limbic system, with the lowest numbers in the brainstem and spinal cord. There are three subtypes of benzodiazepine receptor represented by the abbreviation BDZ or ω. The properties of these are shown in Figure HY.12.

The clinical effects appear to be due to agonism at BDZ receptors attached to the $GABA_A$ receptor complex on the post synaptic membrane. This facilitates the action of GABA that opens the inhibitory chloride channel, and hyperpolarises the membrane. Therefore, benzodiazepines do not act directly on the chloride channels so the maximum effect is determined by the prevailing levels of GABA which should ensure a high therapeutic index.

The search for endogenous ligands of the benzodiazepine receptors has not been conclusive. There are agonists at the benzodiazepine receptors (β-carbolines), which have the opposite effect by preventing the binding of GABA to its receptor site. This is called inverse agonism. It is different from antagonism as, rather than acting by preventing the binding of benzodiazepines with no intrinsic activity of its own, the inverse agonist causes a conformational change but it is the opposite to that of the agonist. Efficacy is, in effect, negative.

All the benzodiazepines are highly lipid-soluble and cross the blood brain barrier readily. Used intravenously, the onset of effect usually takes longer than one arm brain circulation time. Brain levels follow plasma levels closely. Orally administered benzodiazepines are readily absorbed as a result of the lipid solubility.

Drugs with a low lipophilicity have a lower transfer to brain and more drug is distributed peripherally (to vessel rich tissues). This results in increased persistence of some drugs (although the elimination half-life is shorter) with a prolongation of recovery. For example, lorazepam has a short half-life but is less lipophilic compared with diazepam, so the effects may last less with the latter.

In rank order of lipid solubility: midazolam > diazepam > temazepam > lorazepam but onset of action is much the same. The benzodiazepines are bound to albumin in the plasma.

Clinical

CENTRAL NERVOUS SYSTEM

The benzodiazepine family shares the following central effects:

- Anxiolysis
- Sedation
- Hypnosis
- Anterograde amnesia
- Anti-convulsant activity
- Skeletal muscle relaxation

Benzodiazepines reduce both rapid eye movement (REM) and slow wave sleep, which in the short-term may result in a deficit of REM sleep, during treatment. Chronic administration results in tolerance, and withdrawal may result in rebound. The benzodiazepines are slow acting induction agents with a prolonged recovery.

CARDIOVASCULAR SYSTEM

Benzodiazepines administered intravenously have only minor depressant effects on the cardiovascular system in general. There is a slight reduction in SVR, pre load, cardiac output and blood pressure. However, elderly and hypovolaemic patients may be particularly sensitive to IV midazolam and this should be used with caution.

PROPERTIES OF BENZODIAZEPINE RECEPTORS

Receptor		Location	On GABA receptor	Postulated clinical effect
BDZ_1	ω_1	Central	yes	Sedation and hypnosis
BDZ_2	ω_2	Central	yes	Anticonvulsant
BDZ_3	ω_3	Central and peripheral	no	Not known

Figure HY.12

RESPIRATORY SYSTEM

Oral benzodiazepines have minimal effects on respiration. However, IV benzodiazepines have a very variable although usually slight effect on breathing. Airway maintenance is impaired, and tidal volume is reduced, with reduced sensitivity to CO_2. Respiratory rate usually increases slightly. Depression is especially likely with the concomitant use of opioids and other central depressants.

OTHER EFFECTS

Benzodiazepines reduce skeletal muscle tone via an effect on the dorsal horn of the spinal cord.

Metabolism

A number of benzodiazepines have active metabolites

METABOLISM OF BENZODIAZEPINES

Drug	Extraction ratio	Metabolism
Diazepam	Low	Oxidation
Lorazepam	Low	Conjugation
Midazolam	High	Oxidation
Nitrazepam	Low	Nitro-reduction
Temazepam	Low	Conjugation

Figure HY.13

resulting in prolonged duration of action (Figure HY.13). These may have longer half-lives than the parent compound.

The metabolism of benzodiazepines produces metabolites that are also administered in their own right. Figure HY.14 shows the important inter-relationships.

DIAZEPAM

Diazepam is a 1,4-benzodiazepine that is insoluble in water. For IV administration, it is therefore solubilised either in buffered propylene glycol and ethanol to a pH of 6.4–6.9 or in a soya bean lipid emulsion that does cause thrombophlebitis and later thrombosis.

It may be administered orally or intravenously. Diazepam is metabolised to N-desmethyldiazepam.

MIDAZOLAM

Midazolam is an imidazobenzodiazepine. This results in the ability of a water molecule to open the diazepine

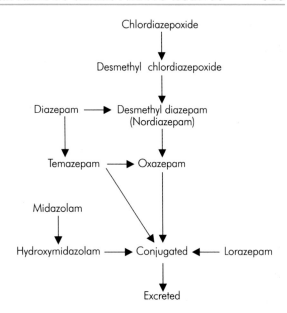

Figure HY.14 Metabolic inter-relationships of the benzodiazepine family

Figure HY.15 Structural equilibrium of midazolam

ring (Figure HY.15) thus encouraging aqueous solubility.

The equilibrium between the two forms of midazolam is determined by pH. The change from the one form to the other is relatively slow having a half-life of 10 min. The pH in the ampoule containing midazolam hydrochloride is 3.0 and so the ring is open and it is soluble. Once subjected to body pH 7.4, the diazepine ring closes and the midazolam becomes lipid-soluble allowing it readily to cross the blood brain barrier. In the plasma most of the midazolam (95%) is protein-bound. Midazolam is redistributed more rapidly than diazepam and so its duration of action is much shorter than that of diazepam.

Midazolam is hydroxylated in the liver to 4-hydroxymidazolam, which has minimal clinical activity. In the elderly, the lower hepatic blood flow and metabolic activity result in a significantly higher elimination half-life.

Diazepam and midazolam are compared Figure HY.16.

COMPARISON OF DIAZEPAM WITH MIDAZOLAM

	Diazepam	Midazolam
Physical	No imidazole ring	Imidazole ring
	Insoluble in water	Soluble in water
	Lipid emulsion	Aqueous
Chemical	Consistent structure	Structural change
	High F/M ratio	Low F/M ratio
Clinical	Anti-epileptic	Anti-epileptic
	Longer duration	Shorter duration

Figure HY.16

LORAZEPAM

Lorazepam is a 1,4-benzodiazepine used in the alleviation of anxiety and for sedation. It is used as a premedicant. It is available for oral, sublingual, IM and IV administration. The oral dose is 2–4 mg, and IV is 50 mcg/kg. Oral bio-availability is 90%, with 90% protein-bound and a volume of distribution of 1 l/kg. It is predominantly eliminated by glucuronide conjugation followed by urinary excretion, with an elimination half-life of 10–20 H.

TEMAZEPAM

Temazepam is an orally administered 1,4-benzodiazepine used in the alleviation of anxiety and for sedation. It is used as a premedicant, typically in doses of 10–40 mg (1 mg/kg up to 30 mg syrup in children). Bio-availability is high, 76% is protein-bound and the volume of distribution is 0.8 l/kg. It is predominantly eliminated by glucuronide conjugation followed by urinary excretion, with an elimination half-life of 8 H.

FLUMAZENIL

Flumazenil is an imidazobenzodiazepine and a competitive benzodiazepine receptor antagonist, bearing the closest resemblance to the structure of midazolam. It is administered intravenously to antagonise the clinical effects of agonist benzodiazepines. It also antagonises inverse benzodiazepine receptor agonists.

Flumazenil is 40–50% protein-bound to albumin and rapidly redistributed with a volume of distribution of 0.9 l/kg. Flumazenil has a high hepatic extraction ratio with a total clearance of 15 ml/kg/min. Elimination half-life is about 50 min. Flumazenil is metabolised to a carboxylic acid derivative and a glucuronide, which are both inactive.

Cautions

Flumazenil has a short duration of action. It is important to realise that its effects may wear off before the benzodiazepine agonist has been cleared with a re-emergence of the agonist effects. In addition, rapid antagonism of benzodiazepine sedation in a head-injured patient may precipitate an excessive rise in ICP. After chronic administration of benzodiazepines, flumazenil may provoke abrupt withdrawal effects.

INDUCTION AGENTS OF HISTORIC INTEREST

Examples – althesin, propanidid

Althesin is a mixture of two steroid induction agents, alphaxolone and alphadolone, solubilised in Cremophor EL. It provides a rapid onset of action and rapid recovery. It was withdrawn because of a strong suspicion of adverse reactions, probably to the Cremophor EL, a derivative of castor oil. It was never reformulated with an alternative solubilising agent.

Propanidid is a eugenol derived from oil of cloves also solubilised in Cremophor EL. It produces a rapid onset of action with a very short duration of action and rapid recovery (6 min). It is metabolised by plasma cholinesterase. A possible connection with sudden death led to its withdrawal from use.

OTHER HYPNOTIC AGENTS

Examples – buspirone, chloral hydrate, meprobamate, zolpidem, zopiclone

BUSPIRONE

Buspirone is an azaspirodecanedione used for anxiolysis. It does not appear to act on benzodiazepine receptors and the most likely mode of action is antagonism at $5HT_{1A}$ receptors. It may also reduce acetylcholine activity and increase catecholamine activity. There is marked first-pass metabolism with peak levels after 60 min. It is 95% protein-bound in the plasma. Buspirone is metabolised in the liver and has a half-life of 2–11 H.

CHLORAL AND RELATED DRUGS

Chloral, chloral hydrate, triclofos and dichloraphenazone are inter-related metabolically. These drugs are administered orally as either tablets or elixir. Triclofos is said to cause less gastric irritation than chloral hydrate. Chloral hydrate is useful for premedication of small children. A dose of 50 mg/kg (up to 1 g) acts within 45 min. Doses from 6 mg/kg in adults will produce sedation.

Clinical effects

CENTRAL NERVOUS SYSTEM

The chloral derivatives cause central depression with a mild anti-convulsant activity. There is little interference with EEG sleep patterns. They have no analgesic activity.

CARDIOVASCULAR SYSTEM

In normal dosage, there is minimal cardiovascular depression, but overdose causes profound depression with supra-ventricular tachycardia a feature.

RESPIRATORY SYSTEM

In normal dosage, there is minimal cardiovascular depression, but overdose causes profound depression.

Metabolism

Alcohol dehydrogenase present in the liver, red blood cells and other sites plays a major role in the inactivation of these drugs. Trichlorethanol is conjugated with glucuronide.

Cautions

Problems include gastric irritation, hepatic enzyme induction or inhibition and the displacement of drugs such as warfarin from plasma proteins.

MEPROBAMATE

Meprobamate is a carbamate tranquiliser having anxiolytic, anti-convulsant and muscle-relaxant properties. It acts by inhibiting adenosine uptake. It is less effective than benzodiazepines and has a lower therapeutic index. Rapid absorption follows oral administration. 90% is excreted in the urine (mainly as the hydroxy metabolite and its glucuronide conjugate). It may precipitate convulsions in susceptible patients particularly following withdrawal of the drug. Meprobamate is contra-indicated in acute intermittent porphyria.

ZOLPIDEM

Zolpidem is an imidazopyrine that acts at the benzodiazepine receptor complex of the $GABA_A$ receptor, to produce anxiolysis and sedation. It is selective for ω_1 receptor subtype producing hypnosis without the ataxia or other ω_2 effects. The effects are reversed by flumazenil. Zolpidem is rapidly absorbed with a bio-availability of 70%. Concentrations peak at about 1–3 h and it is 93% protein-bound. Zolpidem is metabolised to inactive metabolites in the liver with a half-life of 2.4 H.

ZOPICLONE

Zopiclone is a cyclopyrrolone with anxiolytic and sedative properties. It acts at the GABA–benzodiazepine receptor complex but appears to act at a different site from that affected by benzodiazepines. The overall effect is to enhance the action of GABA in promoting opening of the chloride channel. It does not reduce the amount of REM sleep. Zolpidone is well absorbed following oral administration and has a short elimination half-life of 5 H.

SPECIFIC PHARMACOLOGY

Here, molecular weight (MW) is given in Daltons, volume of distribution (V_d) in litres, clearance (Cl) in ml/kg/min and half lives ($t_{1/2}$) in minutes (unless stated otherwise).

DIAZEPAM

Structure – 1,4-benzodiazepine
Presentation
Oral – 2, 5, 10 mg tablets; 2 mg in 5 ml solution
IV – 5 mg/ml clear, yellow solution of diazepam (osmolality 7775 mosm/kg) in a mixture of solvents (propylene glycol (40%), ethanol (10%), benzoic

acid/sodium benzoate (5%), benzyl alcohol (1.5%), pH 6.2–6.9); or white opaque oil-in-water emulsion (osmolality 349 mosm/kg) using soya bean oil similar to intralipid (pH 6.0)

May also be administered rectally and intramuscularly

Storage – room temperature

Dose – IV bolus 0.1–0.3 mg/kg

Pharmacokinetics

MW	bio-availability	pH
285	Oral: 86–100%	6.2–6.9

protein binding	V_d	Cl	$t_{1/2\alpha}$	$t_{1/2\beta}$
99%	1.2	0.4	70	30 H

CNS – anxiolysis, hypnosis, sedation, anterograde amnesia; anti-convulsant; CBF, ICP and $CMRO_2$ reduced

CVS – blood pressure, cardiac output decreased; coronary vasodilation increases coronary blood flow; myocardial oxygen consumption decreased

RS – respiratory depression; hypoxic drive reduced more than response to CO_2

Other – clearance reduced by concomitant cimetidine treatment

Elimination – hepatic metabolism to desmethyl-diazepam (active $t_{1/2}$ at least 100 H), oxazepam and temazepam; oxidised and glucuronide derivatives excreted in urine; <1% unchanged

ETOMIDATE

Structure – imidazole

Presentation: IV – clear, colourless solution of 20 mg etomidate in 10 ml 35% propylene glycol in water

Storage – room temperature

Dose – IV bolus 0.15–0.30 mg/kg (maximum 60 mg)

Pharmacokinetics

MW	pH	protein binding	V_d	Cl
342	8.1	76%	3.5	11.7

$t_{1/2\alpha 1}$	$t_{1/2\alpha 2}$	$t_{1/2\beta}$
2.6	27	75

CNS – rapid induction of anaesthesia (one arm brain circulation time); excitatory phenomena common, reduced by opioids; recovery is dose-related; IOP, ICP, CBF and brain oxygen consumption ($CMRO_2$) reduced; epileptiform EEG features

CVS – systemic vascular resistance, mean arterial blood pressure fall; cardiac index and heart rate decrease slightly; atrial muscle function or contraction, ventricular dp/dt_{max}, mean aortic pressure, coronary blood flow are unchanged; myocardial oxygen delivery and consumption are preserved

RS – dose-dependent depression of tidal volume and rate; at a given CO_2 level ventilation is greater than with methohexitone; cough and hiccup common

Other – relatively high emesis rate (2–14%); pain on injection; venous thrombosis. There is no effect on renal or hepatic function. Steroid synthesis is inhibited, so infusions should not be used

Elimination – ester hydrolysis in plasma and liver, inactive metabolites; 87% in urine, 3% unchanged, rest in bile

Toxicity – adrenocortical suppression when infused over a long period; suppression direct and via ACTH

Contra-indications – porphyria

FLUMAZENIL

Structure – imdazo benzodiazepine, BDZ receptor antagonist

Presentation – clear, colourless solution of 500 mcg flumazenil in 5 ml

Dose

IV bolus – 100 mcg increments up to 2 mg

IV infusion – 100–400 mcg/H

Pharmacokinetics

protein binding	V_d	Cl	$t_{1/2}$
50%	0.9	15	60

Clinical – antagonises the effects of central benzodiazepines; benzodiazepine withdrawal effects may occur

Elimination – almost entirely metabolised in the liver, to the inactive carboxylate, which is excreted in the urine

KETAMINE HYDROCHLORIDE

Structure – phencyclidine derivative

Presentation – white, crystalline powder, for dilution with water forming clear, colourless, aqueous solutions of 10, 50 and 100 mg/ml; 10 mg/ml isotonic with normal saline; 50 and 100 mg/ml contain 1:10 000 benzethonium chloride as preservative

Dose

IV – 1–4.5 mg/kg

IM – 4–13 mg/kg

Pharmacokinetics

MW	pH	protein binding	V_d	Cl
237.5	3.5–5.5	20–50%	3	17

$t_{1/2\alpha}$	$t_{1/2\beta}$
10	120-180

CNS – slow onset of dissociative anaesthesia, light sleep, analgesia, amnesia; the EEG shows θ activity; ICP, CBF and IOP are increased; analgesia is good for burns and fractures but poor for visceral pain

CVS – increases sympathetic tone leading to increases in heart rate, cardiac output, blood pressure, and central venous pressure; baroreceptor function is maintained; and there are few arrhythmias

RS – protective respiratory reflexes are usually preserved, but cannot be relied upon; bronchodilation

Other – nausea and vomiting are common; salivation is increased; uterine tone is increased; levels of epinephrine and norepinephrine are increased

Elimination – N-demethylation and hydroxylation to produce metabolites with reduced activity; metabolites then conjugated and excreted in the urine

Toxicity – rashes 15%; emergence delirium, hallucinations; pain on injection particularly with IM injection

METHOHEXITONE SODIUM

Structure – methylbarbiturate
Dose: IV – 1–1.5 mg/kg
Pharmacokinetics

MW	pH	pKa	protein binding	V_d	Cl
284	10–11	7.9	50 – 60%	1.1	11

$t_{\frac{1}{2}\alpha1}$	$t_{\frac{1}{2}\alpha2}$	$t_{\frac{1}{2}\beta}$
6	59	4 H

CNS – rapid induction of anaesthesia (one arm brain circulation time); excitatory phenomena common, reduced by opioids; recovery is dose-related; IOP, ICP, **CBF** and brain oxygen consumption ($CMRO_2$) reduced; epileptiform features on EEG but anti-convulsant

CVS – negative inotrope; cardiac output, sympathetic tone, systemic vascular resistance, and blood pressure reduced

RS – progressive depression of tidal volume and minute volume; protective reflexes attenuated (more depression than thiopentone); cough and hiccup may occur

Renal – ADH levels increased; renal plasma flow decreased; urine output decreased

Other – post operative nausea and vomiting may occur; causes splanchnic vasoconstriction; pregnant uterus and hepatic function are unaffected; less pain on injection if saline diluent used

Elimination – 20% is located in the red blood cells; metabolised in the liver and excreted in urine; < 1% excreted unchanged

Toxicity – intra-arterial may cause constriction and thrombosis but less risk than thiopentone
Contra-indications – porphyria

MIDAZOLAM HYDROCHLORIDE

Structure – imidazo benzodiazepine
Presentation – 10 mg midazolam in both 2 and 5 ml; colourless, aqueous solution of midazolam hydrochloride. Stable in water by virtue of opening of diazepine ring
Dose
IV – 0.03–3 mg/kg depending on effect (sedation/anaesthesia) required; elderly are particularly sensitive
IM – 0.07–0.1 mg/kg for premedication
Pharmacokinetics

MW	bio-availability Oral: 44% IM: 80–100%	pH	protein binding
326		3	96%

V_d	Cl	$t_{\frac{1}{2}\beta}$
1.1	7	5 H

CNS – slow onset of action; anxiolysis, sedation, hypnosis, anterograde amnesia; anti-convulsant; CBF and $CMRO_2$ reduced

CVS – heart rate, systemic vascular resistance and blood pressure reduced

RS – tidal volume and minute volume reduced; rate increased but may cause apnoea; response to CO_2 impaired

Other – catecholamine levels reduced; renin, angiotensin and corticosteroid levels unaffected; skeletal muscle tone reduced; renal and hepatic blood flow reduced

Elimination – hydroxylated and conjugated with glucuronide in the liver, and is then excreted in urine
Toxicity – occasional pain on injection

PROPOFOL

Structure – alkyl phenol derivative, 2,6-di-isopropyl phenol
Presentation – white, isotonic, neutral, aqueous emulsion 10 mg/ml; 10% soya bean oil, 1.2% purified egg phosphatitide, 2.25% glycerol, sodium hydroxide, water
Dose
Anaesthesia
IV bolus 2–2.5 mg/kg
IV infusion 4–12 mg/kg/H
Sedation – IV infusion 0.3–4 mg/kg
Pharmacokinetics

MW	pH	pKa	protein binding
178	6–8.5	11	98%

V_d	Cl	$t_{\frac{1}{2}\alpha1}$	$t_{\frac{1}{2}\alpha2}$	$t_{\frac{1}{2}\beta}$
15	20	2.5	45	3–8 H

CNS – rapid onset (one arm brain circulation) of anaesthesia; excitatory movements common; ICP, cerebral perfusion pressure and $CMRO_2$ reduced; anti-convulsant

CVS – systemic vascular resistance, cardiac output and blood pressure reduced; variable effect on heart rate, usually a slight increase

RS – tidal volume reduced, rate increased; response to CO_2 reduced; greater suppression of laryngeal reflexes than thiopentone

Others – possible anti-emetic effect; pain on injection; excitatory movements; renal and hepatic function are unaffected

Elimination – liver and extrahepatic, unaffected by renal or hepatic disease; excreted in urine, 0.3% unchanged; non cumulative when infused

Toxicity – a small risk of convulsions in epileptic patients; may cause bradycardia or asystole, possibly due to emulsion. It is not licensed for use in pregnancy

THIOPENTONE SODIUM

Structure – thiobarbiturate

Presentation – hygroscopic yellow powder of sodium thiopentone with 6% sodium carbonate; reconstituted with water to 2.5% solution. Reconstituted solution must not be used after 24 H

Dose – IV bolus 4–6 mg/kg

Pharmacokinetics

MW	pH	pKa	protein binding
264	10.8	7.6	75%

V_d	Cl	$t_{\frac{1}{2}\alpha 1}$	$t_{\frac{1}{2}\alpha 2}$	$t_{\frac{1}{2}\beta}$
1.96	3.4	2-6	30-60	5-10 H

CNS – smooth, rapid (one arm brain circulation) induction of anaesthesia; CBF, ICP, IOP, $CMRO_2$ reduced; anti-convulsant, antanalgaesia.

CVS – negative inotropy; cardiac output, systemic vascular resistance and blood pressure reduced

RS – dose-dependant respiratory depression; response to CO_2 reduced; may cause laryngeal spasm or bronchoconstriction

Other – splanchnic vasoconstriction; no effect on pregnant uterus

Renal – ADH, renal plasma flow, urine output reduced

Hepatic – no effect, used in hepatic encephalopathy

Elimination – metabolised in the liver at 15% per h; 30% remains by 24 H; excreted in urine, 0.5% unchanged

Toxicity – tissue damage with extravasation; arterial constriction and thrombosis with intra-arterial injection

Contra-indications – porphyria

SECTION 3: 7
ANALGESIC DRUGS

K. E. Lewis

OPIOIDS

ORPHANIN-FQ SYSTEM

PERIPHERAL INFLAMMATORY MEDIATORS

NON STEROIDAL ANTI-INFLAMMATORY DRUGS (NSAIDS)

OTHER ANALGESIC AGENTS
Paracetamol
Meptazinol
Tramadol
Clonidine

FUTURE DEVELOPMENTS
Cannabinoids
Nicotinic acetylcholine receptor agonists
Tachykinins
Other centrally mediated contenders
Peripherally mediated contenders

SPECIFIC PHARMACOLOGY
Alfentanil
Codeine
Fentanyl
Morphine
Remifentanil
Naloxone
Diclofenac
Ibuprofen
Ketorolac

OPIOIDS

'Opiate' is a specific term to describe drugs derived from the opium poppy (*Papaver somniferum*). 'Opioid' describes naturally occurring, semisynthetic and synthetic compounds that produce analgesic effects by combining with opioid receptors and that are, therefore, antagonised by naloxone.

STRUCTURE

The opioids have a variety of structural bases. Morphine is a phenanthrene derivative having four rings (Figure AN.1). Rings **A** and **B** are coplanar; rings **C** and **D** are perpendicular to the **A–B** plane. Many opioids are analogues of morphine either occurring naturally or synthesised from them.

Figure AN.1 Chemical structure of morphine

The other opioid structures are based on phenylpiperidine, methadone, benzomorphan and thebaine. Examples of these are shown in Figure AN.2.

Opioids may also be classified by their activity, affinity and efficacy at opioid receptors (Figure AN.3).

MECHANISM OF ACTION

Opioids act at opioid receptors in the central nervous system (CNS), which are stereo-specific for the

STRUCTURAL CLASSIFICATION OF OPIOID DRUGS

Naturally occurring
    Morphine analogues
        morphine
        codeine

Semisynthetic
    Morphine analogues
        diamorphine
        dihydrocodeine
        naloxone

Synthetic
    Phenylpiperidines
        pethidine
    Anilino piperidines
        phenoperidine
        fentanyl
        alfentanil
        sufentanil
        remifentanil
    Diphenylheptanes
        methadone
        dextropropoxyphene
    Benzomorphan derivatives
        pentazocine
        levorphanol
    Thebaine derivatives
        buprenorphine

Figure AN.2

laevorotatory isomer. Opioid receptors exist throughout the CNS, with particularly high concentrations in the peri-aqueductal grey area and the

FUNCTIONAL CLASSIFICATION OF OPIOID DRUGS

Classification	Example	Affinity	Efficacy
Pure agonists	Morphine	High	100%
Partial agonists	Buprenorphine	Medium	Medium
Mixed agonist-antagonists	Pentazocine	Medium	Predominantly agonist
	Nalbuphine	Medium	Predominantly agonist
	Nalorphine	Medium	Predominantly antagonist
Pure antagonists	Naloxone	High	Zero

Figure AN.3

substantia gelatinosa of the spinal cord. They are also present outside the CNS and this may account for some of the other opioid effects such as gastro-intestinal effects. There are three distinct opioid receptors identified by their prototype agonists – OP_3 (μ), OP_2 (κ) and OP_1 (δ). All three receptors have now been successfully cloned and their amino acid sequence defined. The OP classification is the most recent classification scheme for opioid receptors.

A fourth variant, σ, was originally classified as an opioid receptor. The selective agonist, N-allyl normetazocine (SKF 10047) produces mydriasis, tachypnoea, tachycardia and delirium. The σ receptor is no longer classified as an opioid receptor as it does not meet the full criteria, notably:

- It has a high affinity binding for phencyclidine and related compounds
- The σ mediated effects are not reversed by naloxone
- σ receptors are stereo-specific for dextro-rotatory isomers

In common with many receptors, a number of sub-types of opioid receptors (two OP_3 (μ), three OP_2 (κ) and two OP_1 (δ)) have been identified. Initially it appeared that μ_1 was responsible for supraspinal analgesia, and μ_2 for spinal analgesia, respiratory depression and constipation, but this distinction is now in doubt. The clinical effects attributed to the receptors are shown in Figure AN.4.

Opioid analgesics act at both supraspinal and spinal levels. Supraspinal action may activate descending inhibitory pathways. In the spinal cord, the primary site for nociceptive input is the dorsal horn. The greatest abundance of opioid receptors is in the substantia gelatinosa, where they are on the pre-synaptic terminals of primary afferent sensory neurones and on the dendrites of the post synaptic inter-neurones that modulate spinothalamic transmission. These pre synaptic receptors inhibit the release of substance P, glutamate and other neurotransmitters and post synaptic receptors decrease the evoked excitatory post synaptic potential (EPSP).

Opioid receptors are all G-protein coupled receptors. μ and δ opioid receptors open potassium ion channels causing hyper-polarisation and reduced neuronal firing. At the nerve terminal the action potential plateau will shorten and so reduce calcium ion influx and neurotransmitter release. In contrast, κ receptors close calcium channels.

Natural ligands for the opioid receptors include neuropeptides such as enkephalins, endorphins and dynorphins. These exist in the CNS, and in peripheral sites such as the gastro-intestinal tract.

PHARMACOKINETICS

Figure AN.5 shows pharmacokinetic data for a selection of opioids.

DISTRIBUTION AND ACTIONS AT OPIOID RECEPTORS

Actions	Receptors		
	OP$_3$ (mu)	OP$_1$ (delta)	OP$_2$ (kappa)
Prototype against	Morphine	D-Ala, D-Leu enkephalin	Ketocyclazocine
Analgesia			
Supraspinal	++	++	++
Spinal	++	++	++
Respiratory depression	++	++	+
Miosis	++	++	++
Gastro-intestinal motility decreased	++	++	0
Smooth muscle	++	++	0
Behaviour	Euphoria	Euphoria	Dysphoria
Sedation	++	++	+
Physical dependence	++	++	+
Other			Diuresis

Figure AN.4

PHARMACOKINETIC DATA FOR OPIOIDS

	Bio-availability (%)	Protein binding (%)	pKa	V_d (l/kg)	Cl (ml/kg/min)	$t_{\frac{1}{2}\beta}$ (min)
Alfentanil	N/A	92	6.5	0.8	6	100
Codeine	60–70	7		5.4	11	168
Fentanyl	N/A	85	8.4	4	13	96
Morphine	15–50	35	7.9	3.5	15	180
Remifentanil	N/A	70	7.1	0.35	50	15
Naloxone	2	45		2	25	70

Figure AN.5

Opioids are generally well absorbed from the gastro-intestinal tract. The majority are weak bases (pKa 6.5–9.3). They are highly ionised in the acid environment of the stomach and, therefore, poorly absorbed. Conversely, in the alkaline small intestine they are predominantly unionised and readily absorbed. Following absorption, many opioids undergo considerable first-pass metabolism in the intestinal wall and liver, resulting in low bio-availability. Alternative routes of administration may be used to improve bio-availability.

Distribution depends on lipid solubility, the degree of ionisation and plasma protein binding. The lipid solubility is the main determinant of the speed of onset of action, because it determines the rate of entry into the CNS. Fentanyl is highly lipophilic and has a faster onset of action than the less lipophilic morphine. The degree of ionisation depends on plasma pH and affects lipid solubility, plasma protein binding and distribution in tissue compartments. Most opioids have a volume of distribution several times greater than total body water and a total clearance similar to hepatic blood flow.

Opioids are predominantly inactivated in the liver, by conjugation to active or inactive metabolites. The metabolites are excreted in urine and bile. Morphine glucuronide is hydrolysed in the gastro-intestinal tract and most is reabsorbed (entero-hepatic circulation). Caution is required in patients with poor renal function because active metabolites, such as morphine 6-glucuronide, may accumulate and cause respiratory depression. Accumulation of norpethidine, a metabolite of pethidine with a half-life five times that of the parent drug, causes agitation and convulsions. Diamorphine and codeine are also metabolised to morphine, which accounts for some of their pharmacological effects.

CLINICAL EFFECTS

Central nervous system

Opioids cause:

- Analgesia
- Euphoria and dysphoria
- Nausea and vomiting
- Miosis

Opioids act against continuous, dull, poorly localised pain resulting from stimulation of supraspinal and spinal pathways. Morphine and other potent opioids cause a sense of contentment and well-being (euphoria) and allay anxiety. This is mediated by stimulation of OP_3 (μ) receptors. Occasionally dysphoria may occur and this is due to stimulation of OP_2 (κ) receptors. If there is no pain morphine may cause dysphoria, manifest as restlessness and agitation. These, and nausea, are potential problems if given alone as a premedicant. Nausea and vomiting are associated with dopamine and $5HT_3$ receptor stimulation in the chemo-receptor trigger zone of the area postrema. Nausea is dose-dependent but tolerance soon develops with repeated doses. Stimulation of OP_3 (μ) and OP_2 (κ) receptors in the Edinger–Westphal nucleus causes miosis (pupillary constriction with pinpoint pupils).

Respiratory system

Opioids cause:

- Respiratory depression
- Suppression of protective reflexes

Dose-related respiratory depression is mediated via OP_3 (μ) receptors. Opioids reduce both the rate and the depth of breathing. Rate is most affected resulting in irregular, gasping respiration and apnoea with

morphine. Diamorphine, therefore, has more analgesic potency (1.5 times), more sedation and a more rapid onset of action than morphine, but it has a shorter duration of action. It has a high potential for addiction.

PAPAVERETUM

Papaveretum is based on a naturally occurring mixture of water soluble alkaloids of opium including morphine (50%), codeine (5%), noscapine (20%), papaverine, a smooth muscle relaxant (5%). Originally, 20 mg papaveretum contained 10 mg anhydrous morphine hydrochloride (equivalent to 13.3 mg morphine sulphate). However, noscapine (also called narcotine) was found to have teratogenic effects in animals and is unsuitable for females of child-bearing potential. Therefore, papaveretum has been reformulated by removal of the noscapine while keeping the remaining alkaloids in the same proportions and concentrations as in the original ampoule. Morphine hydrochloride (10 mg) is now present in 15.4 mg papaveretum rather than 20 mg, together with about 1 mg codeine hydrochloride and 1 mg papaverine hydrochloride.

Papaveretum, being predominantly composed of morphine, behaves very similarly to morphine alone. It is well absorbed orally but can also be administered by IM, IV or sub-cutaneous injection. The overall clinical effect is similar to morphine but it may be more sedative, possibly due to the non morphine alkaloids. However, the picture is unclear, with little convincing evidence that it has any advantage over morphine.

PETHIDINE

Pethidine is a phenylpiperidine opioid synthesised for anti-cholinergic properties. Pethidine is a pure OP$_3$ (μ) agonist. In equi-analgesic doses it causes less sedation than morphine and may cause less miosis due to atropine like effects on the sphincter pupillae. Euphoria is similar to morphine, and pethidine can cause dependence. Pethidine is more lipid-soluble than morphine and, therefore, penetrates the blood-brain barrier more readily. In contrast with morphine, there is a clear relationship between plasma concentration and effect. Pethidine is well absorbed from the gastro-intestinal tract but bio-availability is low (47–73%) due to the first-pass effect. Its action lasts for 2–3 H. Pethidine is metabolised in the liver by N-demethylation to norpethidine and hydrolysis to pethinic acid. Norpethidine is pharmacologically active and may cause hallucinations and convulsions. The elimination half-life of norpethidine is 14–21 H but

may increase to 13–62 H with renal dysfunction. Norpethidine toxicity may occur after prolonged courses of pethidine, large oral doses or in renal failure.

Pethidine is indicated in labour because it does not rely completely on conjugation for inactivation, a process that is underdeveloped in neonates. However, it does readily cross the placenta and the half-life is prolonged in the neonate.

Pethidine is contra-indicated in patients who are on or have been taking monoamine oxidase inhibitors in the previous 2 weeks. This delay results from the non reversible nature of the enzyme inhibition. The interactions of pethidine with monoamine oxidase inhibitors are classified as either excitatory or inhibitory. The excitatory form is characterised by agitation, delirium, headache, hyper- or hypo-tension, rigidity, hyperpyrexia and coma. This is probably due to increased concentrations of 5-HT in the CNS resulting from inhibition of 5-HT degradation by monoamine oxidase inhibitors and blockade of its re-uptake by pethidine. The depressive form causes severe respiratory and cardiovascular depression and coma. This form is probably due to inhibition of hepatic microsomal enzymes by monoamine oxidase inhibitors resulting in accumulation of pethidine.

FENTANYL

Fentanyl is an anilino-piperidine opioid. It is a potent OP$_3$ (mu) agonist with an analgesic potency 100 times that of morphine. Fentanyl is highly lipophylic (500 times more than morphine) and is, therefore, rapidly and extensively distributed (high volume of distribution of 4 l/kg). Its peak effect occurs 5 min after IV injection and its effects last for about 30 min. It is a basic amine with a pKa = 8.4 so that only 9% is in the unionised form at physiological pH. However, transfer across the blood-brain barrier is rapid due to the high lipid solubility. It is metabolised in the liver to the inactive metabolite norfentanyl. In equi-analgesic doses, it is less sedative than morphine, but large doses (50–150 mcg/kg) produce unconsciousness. Fentanyl has minimal effects on the cardiovascular system even at high doses, although bradycardia can occur. Respiratory depression occurs as with morphine in a dose-dependent manner and delayed depression has been reported. This is probably due to secondary peaks in plasma concentration during the elimination phase due to release of fentanyl from body stores. A possible explanation is that fentanyl is sequestered in the acidic environment of the stomach and subsequently reabsorbed in the small intestine. However, as there is only a small quantity in the gastric volume, which is then subject to first-pass metabolism, then the amount reaching the systemic circulation must be negligible.

Fentanyl is commonly used by the epidural or intrathecal route in combination with local anaesthetics. A single epidural bolus lasts for 1.5–3 H. It is also available in 'patch' formulation for chronic pain and has been administered as 'lollipops' to premedicate children.

ALFENTANIL

Alfentanil is a synthetic anilino-piperidine derivative and analogue of fentanyl that has 10–20% the potency of fentanyl and is an OP_3 (μ) agonist. Alfentanil is highly lipophilic but it is less lipid-soluble than fentanyl. It has a faster onset and shorter duration of action than fentanyl due to the high percentage of the unionised form in the plasma at physiological pH (89% alfentanil versus 9% fentanyl). The clearance is less than half that of fentanyl but it has a shorter terminal half-life. This is due to the lower volume of distribution (0.8 l/kg alfentanil versus 4 l/kg fentanyl) that results from the lower lipid solubility. It has similar cardiovascular and respiratory effects to fentanyl. Metabolism by N-dealkylation to noralfentanil occurs in the liver. Clearance is unaffected by renal disease but prolonged in cirrhosis. Alfentanil is a useful agent for short procedures or may be used as an infusion for longer procedures and in intensive care patients. It effectively attenuates the response to laryngoscopy.

REMIFENTANIL

Remifentanil is a synthetic anilino-piperidine. Remifentanil is structurally unique with an ester linkage (Figure AN.6), which undergoes rapid hydrolysis by non specific plasma and tissue esterases. It has a pKa of 7.07.

It is a potent OP_3 (μ) agonist with a more rapid onset and shorter duration than alfentanil and a similar potency to fentanyl. It is antagonised by naloxone.

Figure AN.6 Chemical structure of remifentanil

Remifentanil is administered as an infusion with or without an initial bolus. Of it, 70% is bound to α_1 acid-glycoprotein, which explains the relatively low volume of distribution (0.35 l/kg). It is not a good substrate for plasma cholinesterase and the clearance is unaffected by deficiencies of this enzyme or by the administration of anti-cholinesterases. The short distribution and elimination half-lives lead to a rapid recovery. The main metabolite is a very weak OP_3 (μ) antagonist with an activity of 0.02% that of the parent molecule. There is also a minor N-demethylation pathway in the liver. The dosage and duration of an infusion have almost no effect on the subsequent rate of fall of plasma concentrations. The clearance is independent of renal or hepatic function. It is formulated in glycine and, therefore, is not suitable for epidural or intrathecal administration.

SUFENTANIL

Sufentanil is an anilino-piperidine similar to fentanyl. It is a synthetic OP_3 (μ) receptor agonist with 5–10 times the analgesic potency of fentanyl and has a shorter duration of action. Sufentanil is very lipid-soluble and is 20% unionised at physiological pH. It is rapidly distributed with a volume of distribution (V_d) of 4.8 l/kg, a clearance of 13 ml/kg/min and an elimination half-life of 770 min. 90% is protein-bound. Sufentanil is widely used in the USA specifically for cardiac anaesthesia as it has minimal cardiovascular effects.

CODEINE

Codeine is a natural opioid and one of the principal alkaloids of opium. It has a 3-methyl morphine structure that is less polar than morphine and, therefore, less lipid-soluble. Codeine has 20% the potency of morphine due to a low affinity for opioid receptors. It causes little euphoria and has a low abuse potential. Codeine is less sedative than morphine and large doses may even cause excitement. Oral bio-availability is 60–70% due to methylation of the phenyl ring that protects it from the conjugating enzymes and the first-pass effect. Of codeine, 10% is metabolised to morphine, which contributes to its analgesic effect. Codeine is often combined with other preparations such as NSAIDs (aspirin and paracetamol) and used for the treatment of mild-to-moderate pain. It is commonly used in anti-diarrhoeal preparations and as an anti-tussive in cough mixtures. Codeine has traditionally been used in the management of analgesia in head injuries and neurosurgery but there are no published data to support its use. It is thought to be beneficial due to its low potency and relative lack of respiratory depression and pupillary signs.

DIHYDROCODEINE

Dihydrocodeine is a semisynthetic derivative of codeine with similar pharmacological effects. It is well absorbed orally and may cause confusion, disorientation and constipation.

BUPRENORPHINE

Buprenorphine is a semisynthetic derivative of thebaine that acts as a partial agonist at OP_3 (μ) receptors with a high affinity but low intrinsic activity. It has 30 times the analgesic potency of morphine. Buprenorphine has a high first-pass metabolism and, consequently, oral bio-availability is only 15% but it is highly lipophilic and if given by the sublingual route, bio-availability is 55%. The terminal half-life is similar to pethidine, but the duration of action is much longer (up to 8 H) due to the slow dissociation from the OP_3 (μ) receptor. Side effects are similar to morphine but it does not produce euphoria and has a low abuse potential. The respiratory depressant effects reach a ceiling or plateau level but this can become clinically significant and is not fully reversed by naloxone except in high doses due to its high affinity for the μ receptor.

NALOXONE

Naloxone is an N-allyl derivative of oxymorphone. It is a pure opioid antagonist having no intrinsic pharmacological activity. It has a high affinity for OP_3 (μ) receptors but also blocks other opioid receptors. Naloxone reverses the respiratory depression and analgesia of opioids and precipitates withdrawal in opioid addicts. It may also block the actions of endogenous opioids. IV administration of 200–400 mg naloxone will reverse the respiratory depressant effects of opioids but incremental titration (1.5–3 µg/kg) is preferable to minimise the reversal of the analgesic effects of the opioids. Naloxone acts for about 30 min so further doses or an infusion may be necessary to avoid the return of the respiratory depressant effects of any agonist that outlasts the effects of naloxone. Naloxone is also effective in alleviating the pruritis and urinary retention of intrathecal and epidural opioids. Naloxone has an oral bio-availability of only 2% because of extensive first-pass metabolism.

NALTREXONE

Naltrexone is an analogue of naloxone that has a longer duration of action (elimination half-life of 8 H). It is effective orally because it has a low first-pass effect. It is used as maintenance therapy in the management of detoxified addicts because it blocks the euphoria of high doses of opioids in relapsing cases.

ORPHANIN-FQ SYSTEM

A new G-protein-coupled receptor has been identified, which has structural similarities to the opioid receptors. However, it has a low affinity for opioids and is not an opioid receptor. It is called the opioid like orphan receptor. A possible endogenous ligand, orphanin-FQ, which is similar to dynorphin, has been identified. This is a heptapeptide and because it is relatively large and positively charged it does not readily cross the blood-brain barrier, but is present in high concentration in the brain and spinal cord. The effects of orphanin-FQ appear to be spinal analgesia but supraspinal hyperalgesia and opioid antagonism. The search for a selective antagonist of this receptor is underway and may result in new analgesic drugs in the future.

PERIPHERAL INFLAMMATORY MEDIATORS

Pharmacological manipulation of some inflammatory mediators in the periphery shows potential for future analgesic methods. Fig AN.7 shows a simple classification of the important peripheral mediators.

PERIPHERAL INFLAMMATORY MEDIATORS

- Histamine
- Tryptase
- Kinins
    Bradykinin
    Kallidin
- Eicosanoids
    Prostanoids
    Leukotreines
        Leuktriene A4
        Leuktriene B4
        SRS-A   Leuktriene C4
                Leuktriene D4
                Leuktriene E4
- Cytokines
    Interleukins
        IL-1β
        IL-8
    Tumour necrosis factor (TNF)
        TNF-α
        lymphotoxin (TNF-β)
    Nerve growth factor (NGF)
    Interferon (IFN-α, β and γ)

Fig AN.7

HISTAMINE

Histamine is located mainly bound to protein and heparin complexes within granules in mast cells and basophils. It is released in response to allergy and local inflammation. Histamine acts on histamine receptors (H_1, H_2 and H_3). H_1 agonism causes smooth muscle contraction, vasodilatation and increased vascular permeability. H_2 agonism causes gastric acid secretion and increases heart rate. Histamine is also a neurotransmitter. Histamine receptor antagonists are used to suppress inflammatory actions, for sedation, for antiemesis and in the control of gastric acid secretion. No specific analgesic properties have been identified.

TRYPTASE

The enzyme tryptase, also released from mast cells, is involved in triggering the inflammatory response. It is an agonist of the proteinase activated 2 receptors (PAR2) on sensory neurones triggering the release of neuropeptides including substance P and CGRP (calcitonin gene related peptide). Antagonists at the PAR2 receptor might inhibit inflammation.

KININS

Kinins are vasodilator peptides formed from kininogens by kallirein and include bradykinin and kallidin. Both are mediators of inflammation and are metabolised by kininogens (for example angiotensin converting enzyme (ACE). Kinins cause mast cells to degranulate, directly stimulate nociceptors and act stimulate sympathetic nerves. Two bradykinin receptors have been identified (B_1 and B_2), both of which appear to be involved in the mediation of inflammation. Sensitisation of primary afferent nociceptors is predominantly mediated via B_2 receptors. Experimental B_1 and B_2 receptors now exist and are potential anti-inflammatory and analgesics for the future.

PROSTANOIDS

Prostanoids, derived from the polyunsaturated fatty acid arachidonic acid, include the prostaglandins and thromboxanes. The synthesis of prostanoids by cyclo-oxygenase is inhibited by the NSAID's and COX_2-inhibitors (see pp 629–632). At present, there are no analgesic drugs specifically targeting the inflammatory actions of the prostanoids themselves.

LEUKOTRIENES

Leukotriene receptor antagonists are used as adjunct therapy in the control of asthma. They are discussed in Chapter 13 (pages 715–717).

CYTOKINES

These include the interleukins, interferon (antiviral), tumour necrosis factor (TNF) and nerve growth factor (NGF). Cytokines are released from immune cells as part of the inflammatory response. Interleukins (IL-1β and IL-8) are released from activated macrophages (the tissue equivalent of leukocytes – white blood cells) and cause inflammation and hyperalgesia. TNF-α is particularly prevalent in rheumatoid arthritis, septic shock, inflammatory bowel disease and autoimmune disease.

TNF-α blocking drugs

Etanercept and infliximab are TNF- blocking drugs that are licensed for use in the treatment of rheumatoid arthritis. They bind to TNF- and so inactivate it. Etanercept also inactivates lymphotoxin (TNF-β).

NON STEROIDAL ANTI-INFLAMMATORY DRUGS (NSAIDS)

The NSAIDs are a heterogeneous class of drugs grouped together by their common anti-inflammatory, analgesic and anti-pyretic properties. They are used for the treatment of mild-to-moderate pain, the treatment of chronic inflammatory conditions and in the management of post operative pain where they have an opioid sparing effect.

MECHANISMS OF ACTION

The NSAIDs primarily mediate their effects by inhibition of the enzyme cyclo-oxygenase, which reduces prostaglandin synthesis. Prostaglandins are part of a large family of unsaturated fatty acids present in all organs. They are involved in the modulation of pain both at peripheral and central sites. Prostaglandins sensitise primary nerve endings in the periphery to the algesic action of agents (such as bradykinin, histamine and serotonin) produced as part of the inflammatory response to tissue injury.

Arachidonic acid is a major component of cell membrane phospholipids and the enzyme cyclo-oxygenase (COX) converts arachidonic acid to the cyclic-endoperoxides, PGG_2 and PGH_2 (prostaglandin precursors). The spectrum of prostaglandins formed is a property of that tissue. In most tissues, cyclic endoperoxides are converted to prostaglandins E_2, D_2 and F_2 in response to tissue injury. They have a variety of effects on glandular secretion, renal function, peripheral blood vessels and the action of smooth muscle. In platelets, the cyclic endoperoxides form thromboxane A_2, which induces platelet aggregation and adhesion, and vasoconstriction. In vascular endothelial cells the cyclic endoperoxides form prostacyclin, which inhibits platelet aggregation and causes vasodilatation. The balance between these two mechanisms is important to prevent thrombosis and probably changes in the presence of endothelial damage.

Leukotrienes are also formed from arachidonic acid, under the influence of the enzyme lipoxygenase. They play an important role in mediating bronchoconstriction in allergic conditions and anaphylaxis.

The correlation between the anti-inflammatory and analgesic effects of the NSAIDs is not strong. There is evidence of a distinction between analgesic efficacy and COX inhibition. Evidence exists for spinal and supraspinal analgesic actions of NSAIDs that may involve modulation of the spinal actions of NMDA and substance P. NSAIDs may also have direct inhibitory effects on neutrophil activation and function in inflamed tissues.

The effects on prostaglandin synthesis are not restricted to inflamed tissue and this accounts for the adverse effects of NSAIDs. Cyclo-oxygenase is thought to exist as at least two isoenzymes. Cyclo-oxygenase-1 (COX_1) is important for physiological homeostasis of several systems such as the maintenance of renal blood flow, endothelial thrombogenicity and gastric cytoprotection. Cyclo-oxygenase-2 (COX_2) is induced when tissues are exposed to inflammatory stimuli. Inhibition of COX_2 produces the therapeutic effects, and inhibition of COX_1 the adverse effects of NSAIDs. Different drugs have a different selectivity

for each isoenzyme. This can explain the difference in analgesic efficacy and the propensity for adverse effects.

PHARMACOKINETICS

Figure AN.8 shows pharmacokinetic data for the NSAIDs.

NSAIDs are weak organic acids (pKa = 3–5) and are thus rapidly absorbed in the acid environment of the stomach. In general, NSAIDs have a low first-pass metabolism and, therefore, a high oral bio-availability. However, diclofenac has a high hepatic metabolism resulting in a bio-availability of 60%. NSAIDs are highly protein-bound and have the potential to displace other drugs from plasma proteins so potentiating the effects of these drugs (e.g. oral anti-coagulants, anti-convulsants, lithium and oral hypo-glycaemic agents).

In general, NSAIDs are eliminated by hepatic biotransformation followed by renal excretion.

CLINICAL EFFECTS

The ubiquitous nature of prostaglandins in the maintenance of normal homeostasis explains their diverse range of effects.

Central nervous system

NSAIDs provide analgesia for moderate-to-severe pain and in combination with opioids they have been shown to have a variable opioid sparing effect of up to 60%. This may result in improved analgesia and a reduction in opioid-related side effects.

Adverse effects include dizziness, depression, confusion and seizures.

Respiratory system

NSAIDs cause bronchospasm in susceptible individuals. 'Aspirin-induced asthma' affects between

PHARMACOKINETIC DATA FOR NSAIDS					
	Bio-availability (%)	Protein binding (%)	V_d (l/kg)	Cl (ml/kg/min)	$t_{1/2}$ (min)
Diclofenac	60	99.5	0.17	4.2	90
Ibuprofen	78	99	0.15	0.75	120
Ketorolac	85	99	0.15	0.35	300

Figure AN.8

10 and 20% of adults with asthma, and the bronchospasm can be severe and fatal.

Various hyper-sensitivity reactions, urticaria, rashes and angio-oedema have been reported. These reactions are due to COX inhibition which increases arachidonic acid levels and increases metabolism through the alternative lipoxygenase pathway to form an abundance of leukotrienes.

Gastro-intestinal system

NSAIDs cause dyspepsia, gastro-duodenal erosions, ulceration, perforation and diarrhoea. Prostaglandins play an important part in the prevention of gastro-duodenal injury by reducing gastric acid secretion, by providing gastric cytoprotection and by modulating mucosal blood flow. The decrease in the production of prostaglandins from NSAID therapy removes this gastric protection. These effects still occur with parenteral administration. Gastro-intestinal damage is more common in:

- Women
- Age > 60 years
- Previous history of peptic ulceration
- Smokers
- Alcohol ingestion

Conventional anti-ulcer therapy is relatively ineffective in preventing NSAID ulceration but co-administration of a prostaglandin analogue, misoprostol, may be effective.

Renal

NSAIDs impair renal function and may cause acute renal failure.

Prostaglandins normally play a minor role in renal blood flow by directly altering vascular tone in afferent arterioles and by indirectly altering efferent arteriolar tone via the renin angiotensin system. Renal prostaglandins are important in the maintenance of renal blood flow and glomerular filtration when blood flow is borderline. It is in these situations that NSAIDs can cause renal ischaemia leading to acute tubular necrosis and renal failure. During the peri-operative period renal blood flow may be compromised in the presence of NSAIDs and other risk factors such as the elderly, dehydration and hypo-volaemia, hypo-tension, cardiac failure, cirrhosis and co-administration of ACE inhibitors or diuretics.

'Analgesic nephropathy' is a severe and often irreversible form of NSAID induced renal toxicity recognised to be associated with long-term consumption of NSAIDs leading to chronic nephritis and renal papillary necrosis.

Haematological

NSAIDs interfere with platelet aggregation resulting in an increase in bleeding time towards the upper limit of the normal range. The inhibition of COX disturbs the balance of prostacyclin and thromboxane A_2, leading to abnormal platelet function which may disturb haemostasis. Aspirin irreversibly inhibits the enzyme so the effect lasts for the life-time of the platelets (7–10 days). Other NSAIDs have a reversible action and so only affect the platelets while the drug is present. Clinically, coagulation is not affected and the bleeding time remains within the normal range. The affect may become important with haemorrhagic disorders. Bone marrow dyscrasias have been reported with the use of NSAIDs.

Anti-pyretic

The anti-pyretic effect of NSAIDs is a consequence of central prostaglandin inhibition in the hypothalamus.

Other effects

NSAIDs delay the closure of the ductus arteriosus in the neonate if used in pregnancy. This is used therapeutically in some congenital heart defects to buy time before surgical correction.

DICLOFENAC

This is a phenylacetic acid derivative with potent anti-inflammatory and analgesic properties. It has a greater affinity for COX than other NSAIDs and is a potent inhibitor of prostaglandin synthesis. A central analgesic action of diclofenac mediated by endogenous opioid peptides has been demonstrated. It has a higher therapeutic ratio than most NSAIDs, however gastric irritation and occult blood loss are problems.

KETOROLAC

Ketorolac is a pyrroleacetic acid derivative that appears to be more effective as an analgesic than as an anti-inflammatory or anti-pyretic drug. The trimethamine salt possesses sufficient water solubility to allow it to be given parenterally. It is available in tablet form and as an aqueous solution for IV or IM injection. The original dose recommended was 30 mg IV or IM. However, there is little evidence that 30 mg provides better analgesia than 10 mg and the Committee on Safety of Medicines has recommended a starting dose of 10 mg.

IBUPROFEN

Ibuprofen is a propionic acid derivative with analgesic properties similar to aspirin. It has a low affinity for the COX enzyme and acts as a mild anti-inflammatory. Side effects are relatively few compared with other NSAIDs and it causes fewer gastro-intestinal disturbances (10–15% of patients).

There have been a few reports of toxic amblyopia. If a patient develops ocular symptoms, it should be discontinued.

ASPIRIN (ACETYLSALICYLIC ACID)

Pharmacokinetics

Aspirin is a derivative of salicylic acid obtained from willow bark. It is a simple, weak organic acid (pKa = 3.5) and, therefore, rapid absorption is facilitated in the acid environment of the stomach where it is mainly in the unionised form. However, salicylate anion trapping can occur in the alkaline environment of the gastric mucosal cells and absorption may be more effective in the larger surface area of the small intestine. The recommended dose is 300–600 mg, 6–8 hourly. After absorption, it is rapidly hydrolysed to salicylate ions by esterase enzymes in the plasma and liver. Salicylates are mainly metabolised in the liver to salicyluric acid and glucuronides and some of the steps in their metabolism may become saturated. The unchanged drug and the metabolites are excreted in the urine and their excretion is enhanced by alkaline urine. The terminal half-life, in normal therapeutic doses, is 2–3 H. However, larger doses saturate the liver enzymes and typically increase the half-life up to 30 H.

Clinical effects

Most of the analgesic effects of aspirin are related to the inhibition of prostaglandin synthesis in the periphery but it also has some central action. Relatively high doses are required to produce the anti-inflammatory effects.

Side effects

The side effects of gastric irritation, ulceration and perforation are significant. About 70% of patients on aspirin lose 5–10 ml blood daily.

Hypersensitivity reactions may occur particularly in atopic individuals causing bronchospasm, angio-oedema, skin rashes and rhinitis.

Aspirin reduces platelet adhesion and aggregation by reducing the formation of thromboxane A_2. This effect lasts for the life of the platelet as it irreversibly inhibits COX and new platelets must be formed to restore normal clotting function. This is clinically useful as low dose aspirin (75 mg/day) has been shown to reduce the risk of transient ischaemic attacks, secondary myocardial infarction and it has been used following coronary angioplasty and bypass grafting.

'Salicylism' may occur after chronic ingestion of large doses. This is a syndrome of tinnitus, dizziness, deafness, sweating, hyper-ventilation and nausea and vomiting.

Aspirin is contra-indicated in children < 12 years of age (except for specific indications such as juvenile arthritis) as it has been associated with Reyes syndrome. This is a combination of liver dysfunction and encephalopathy following an acute viral illness which has a mortality rate of 20–40%.

Drug interactions

Owing to the high plasma protein binding aspirin can displace oral anti-coagulants and sulphonylureas and increase their effects. Aspirin also interacts with uricosuric agents as it acts as a uricosuric in high doses and paradoxically decreases urate excretion in low doses.

Overdose of aspirin produces complex effects on acid–base balance. High levels of aspirin stimulate hyper-ventilation due to increased CO_2 production and oxygen consumption because of uncoupling of oxidative phosphorylation. In addition, high concentrations of salicylates directly stimulate the respiratory centre causing a respiratory alkalosis that is normally compensated for by renal mechanisms. Larger doses of aspirin can cause depression of the respiratory centre that leads to uncompensated respiratory acidosis. This is further complicated by metabolic acidosis due to the accumulation of metabolites and salicylate derivatives. This progresses to dehydration, hyper-pyrexia and coma. Treatment involves gastric lavage, forced alkaline diuresis, haemodialysis and charcoal haemoperfusion. In children, a different picture occurs during aspirin overdose. Hyperventilation is rare and the rise in plasma salicylates usually depresses the respiratory centre, leading to a mixed picture of respiratory and metabolic acidosis.

COX-2 selective NSAID's

Examples: refocoxib, celecoxib

NSAID's selective for the (inducible) COX-2 enzyme are now available.

OTHER ANALGESIC AGENTS

PARACETAMOL

Paracetamol is a para-aminophenol derivative and is an active metabolite of phenacetin (which was withdrawn because of its renal toxicity). It is an analgesic and anti-pyretic used to treat mild-to-moderate pain. Paracetamol inhibits prostaglandin synthesis but this activity is predominantly within the CNS and results in relatively little anti-inflammatory action.

Paracetamol is supplied as tablets, oral solution, suppository and in combination with codeine, dihydrocodeine, dextropropoxyphene and aspirin. It is well absorbed orally, with a bio-availability of 70–90%. Paracetamol is not significantly protein-bound. The recommended dose is 500 mg to 1 g 4–6 hourly (maximum 4 g/day) and in children 10–15 mg/kg (not advised < 3 months of age). Paracetamol is eliminated by hepatic conjugation, 60% is eliminated as glucuronide and the remainder as cystine and sulphate conjugates.

The lack of gastro-intestinal side effects with paracetamol is probably due to the action on cyclo-oxygenase and prostaglandin synthesis being mainly in the CNS.

Chronic consumption of paracetamol may lead to 'analgesic nephropathy', a chronic nephritis and renal papillary necrosis. Other side effects include skin rashes, blood dyscrasias and, rarely, haemolytic anaemia related to erythrocytic glucose 6-phosphate dehydrogenase deficiency.

Overdose of paracetamol can cause fatal hepatic necrosis. This is due to the toxic metabolite, N-acetyl-p-benzoquinone, which has a high affinity for sulphydryl groups. Normally this toxic metabolite is produced in negligible amounts (about 1%) that are inactivated by conjugation with the sulphur containing amino acids, glutathione and methionine in the liver. In overdose, the hepatic reserves of glutathione are depleted and the toxic metabolite combines with sulphydryl groups in the liver cell proteins leading to sub-acute hepatic necrosis.

Symptoms of nausea, vomiting and abdominal pain are delayed for 24–48 H. Paracetamol levels are useful as a guide to treatment while liver function tests are a poor prognostic indicator. However, a bilirubin level > 4 mg/100 ml and an INR > 2.2 are associated with a poor outcome.

Treatment involves gastric lavage, IV fluids and N-acetylcystine (a sulphydryl donor), infused within 12–15 H.

MEPTAZINOL

Meptazinol is a synthetic opioid structurally related to pethidine, with 10% the potency of morphine. It is suitable for the treatment of moderate-to-severe pain and has been used as an alternative to pethidine in labour. Meptazinol can be administered orally (200 mg 3–6 hourly), but as the bio-availability by this route is only 10%, it is often administered intramuscularly or intravenously (50–100 mg 2–4 hourly).

Meptazinol is a partial agonist at OP_3 (μ) opioid receptors and has low affinity for OP_2 (κ) receptors. Its affect on central cholinergic transmission may also contribute to its analgesic activity. Unlike many racemic opioids, both enantiomers possess analgesic activity, but the cholinergic mediated analgesia is stereo-specific.

Meptazinol appears almost devoid of respiratory depression at clinically effective doses but there is a higher incidence of nausea and vomiting than with other opioids, this may be central cholinergic in origin. It rarely causes dysphoria and has minimal cardiovascular effects.

Naloxone almost completely reverses the effects of meptazinol, although higher doses are required than for pure opioid agonists. Meptazinol also has opioid antagonist effects in opioid-dependent subjects and can be shown to precipitate withdrawal in morphine-dependent animals.

TRAMADOL

Tramadol is a phenylpiperidine analogue of codeine. Tramadol acts as a weak agonist at all types of opioid receptor with some selectivity for the μ receptor. It has 10% the potency of morphine. Tramadol also blocks the re-uptake of norepinephrine and 5-HT (serotonin) and facilitates release of the latter, to modify nociceptive transmission by activation of the descending inhibitory pathways in the CNS. Naloxone, therefore, only partially reverses the analgesic effects of tramadol. Tramadol is a racemic mixture of (+) and (–) tramadol and it appears that the two enantiomers have separate effects at opioid and non opioid sites. (+) Tramadol affects μ receptors and 5-HT re-uptake and release; (–) tramadol inhibits norepinephrine release. Effects on α_2 adrenergic, NMDA and benzodiazepine receptors may be due to indirect effects secondary to noradrenergic effects.

Tramadol is used in the treatment of moderate-to-severe pain. It is available in capsules for oral administration and as a 50 mg/ml aqueous solution for

IV or IM injection. The dose is 50–100 mg 4–6 hourly (maximum 600 mg/day) and 1–2 mg/kg for children although it is not recommended for children < 12 years old. Tramadol is well absorbed orally with a bio-availability of 68% (which rises to 90–100% with multiple doses). Only 20% is protein-bound. The volume of distribution is 200–300 litres.

Tramadol is extensively (86%) metabolised in the liver by N-desmethylation, O-desmethylation and conjugation, with 90% being excreted in the urine. The elimination half-life is 4–6 H. The metabolite, O-desmethyltramadol (half-life 9 H) has two-to-four times greater analgesic potency than tramadol and caution should be used with hepatic and renal impairment.

Tramadol exhibits little respiratory depression when compared with equi-analgesic doses of morphine. Cardiovascular effects are minimal. Other reported side effects include dizziness, sedation, nausea, dry mouth, sweating and skin rashes. There is a low potential for abuse and physical dependence although abuse has been reported. At present, it is not subject to controlled drug restrictions.

Concomitant use of monoamine oxidase inhibitors is contra-indicated. Co-administration with carbamazepine may decrease the concentration and effect of tramadol.

CLONIDINE

Clonidine is an α_2 adrenergic receptor agonist, acting pre synaptically to produce analgesia. The unwanted side effects of sedation and hypotension have led to interest in more direct administration such as epidural and intrathecal routes.

FUTURE DEVELOPMENTS

CANNABINOIDS

Δ^9-tetrahydrocannabinol (Δ^9-THC) is the main active constituent of the cannabis plant, *Cannabis sativa*, used as a recreational drug but is generating interest as an analgesic and anti-emetic in cancer treatment.

Two cannabinoid receptors have been identified, CB1 and CB2. These are both G-protein-coupled receptor complexes. CB1 is the neuronal receptor found in the brain and spinal cord. Relatively few receptors are in the brain stem. CB2 is found predominantly peripherally.

Δ^9-THC is highly lipophilic but has a low potency. Nabilone is a non selective cannabinoid receptor agonist that is less lipophilic and a more potent agonist. Anandamide, a derivative of phospholipase D, has been identified as an endogenous ligand for CB1. The breakdown pathway for this is inhibited by NSAIDs. The precise role of this in vivo is yet unclear.

Δ^9-THC causes:

- Anti-emesis
- Analgesia
- Increased pulse rate
- Decreased blood pressure
- Muscle weakness
- Increased appetite
- Euphoria then drowsiness
- Psychological interference

The main use of cannabinoids at present is in anti-emesis. Nabilone is a synthetic dibenzopyran cannabinol that acts on the vomiting centre. It is licensed for use for the antagonism of resistant cytotoxic induced nausea. It has largely been superseded by ondansetron. Δ^9-THC may have a future role in analgesia, as it appears to cause less dysphoria and drowsiness than nabilone. The route of administration (Δ^9-THC is typically obtained by smoking) may also affect the spectrum of effects.

NICOTINIC ACETYLCHOLINE RECEPTOR AGONISTS

Epibatidine from the skin of an Equadorian frog (*Epipedobates tricolour*) used as an arrow poison, has potent analgesic properties, and is an agonist of nicotinic acetylcholine receptors (nAChR). There are two enantiomers of epibatidine, R(+)-epibatidine being the naturally occurring agent. Pharmacologically their activity is similar. Nicotinic acetylcholine receptors have five sub-units (see page 292), but it is now known that there is considerable diversity in the amino acid composition of a particular sub-unit. For example, there are at least nine variants of α and four variants of β sub-unit, and this may explain the differing affinities for various agonists in different locations. In the CNS, nAChR has a higher affinity for epibatidine than for acetylcholine or nicotine. Currently, however, epibatidine has numerous nicotinic agonist effects that make it unsuitable as a pure analgesic. If drugs with a high affinity for specific central nAChR groups involved in nociception can be developed without the multitude of other effects then this may be a future method of analgesia.

TACHYKININS

Tachykinins are a group of neuropeptides including substance P and neurokinins A and B. Substance P and Neurokinin A (NKA) are released in the spinal cord in response to peripheral noxious stimuli. Three tachykinin receptors (NK-1, NK-2, NK-3) have been identified. They enhance neurotransmission in the pain pathways. In acute nociception NKA is the main mediator acting on NK-2 receptors. In pathological pain such as inflammatory hyperalgesia NK-1 receptors are more important. Substance P is more active at NK-1, and in addition stimulates the release of peripheral inflammatory mediators such as bradykinin. NK-1 receptor antagonists inhibit pain transmission and appear to reduce inflammatory vasodilatation and plasma protein leakage.

OTHER CENTRALLY MEDIATED CONTENDERS

Calcitonin gene-related peptide (CGRP) is released in the dorsal horn by afferent fibres in response to noxious stimuli. The neuropeptides somatostatin and galanin cause analgesia, while cholecystokinin inhibits opioid mediated analgesia.

Galanin is another neuropeptide released from afferent nociceptive neurones. It appears to inhibit nociceptive dorsal horn transmission.

The amino acid, glutamine released by C fibres is agonist at NMDA receptors and may be responsible (in conjunction with substance P) for 'wind-up'. Ketamine blocks the NMDA ion channel and this probably effects analgesia.

Adenosine acts on A_1 (inhibitory) and A_2 (excitatory) receptors to influence synaptic transmission. Both receptor types are found within the CNS including the dorsal horn. Intrathecal administration of adenosine analogues produces anti-nociception.

Agonists and antagonist of these neurological systems may provide future advances in analgesia.

SPECIFIC PHARMACOLOGY

In this section bio-availability applies to oral administration. Units (unless stated otherwise) are as follows:

Volume of distribution at steady state (V_d) (l/kg)
Clearance (Cl) (ml/kg/min)
Terminal half-life ($t_{1/2}$) (min)

ALFENTANIL

Structure – anilino-piperidine opioid analogue of fentanyl
Presentation: IV – colourless, aqueous solution (500 mcg/ml, 2 and 10 ml ampoules, 5 mg/ml ampoules also available)
Dose: IV
Bolus 10–50 mcg/kg
Infusion 0.5–1 mcg/kg/min
Pharmacokinetics

Protein binding	V_d	Cl	$t_{1/2}$	pKa
92%	0.8	6	100	6.5

Peak effect within 90 s, duration 5–10 min
CNS – potent OP_3 (μ) opioid receptor agonist, 10–20 times more potent analgesic than morphine
CVS – bradycardia, hypotension may occur. Obtunds cardiovascular responses to laryngoscopy and intubation in doses of 30–50 mcg/kg
RS – potent respiratory depressant; chest wall rigidity may occur
Other – nausea and vomiting; no histamine release
Elimination – predominantly hepatic metabolism by N-dealkylation to noralfentanil, < 1% excreted unchanged via kidneys
Contra-indications – concurrent administration with monoamine oxidase inhibitors

CODEINE

Structure – a morphine analogue (3-methyl morphine); a principal alkaloid of opium
Presentation
Oral – tablets 15, 30 and 60 mg; syrup 5 mg/ml
IV – colourless, aqueous solution 60 mg/ml (1 ml ampoules). Often combined with non opioid analgesics such as paracetamol as tablets (co-codamol containing 8 or 30 mg of codeine)
Dose – oral/IM 30–60 mg, 4–6 hourly.
Pharmacokinetics

Protein binding	V_d	Cl	$t_{1/2}$	Bio-availability
97%	5.4	11	168	60–70%

CNS – < 20% analgesic potency of morphine, low affinity for opioid receptors, low euphoria, rarely addictive, and low abuse potential
RS – produces some respiratory depression but not severe even in high doses, anti-tussive
Other – constipation (used as anti-diarrhoeal), mild nausea and vomiting
Elimination – 10% metabolised to morphine in liver by demethylation, remainder metabolised to norcodeine or conjugated to glucuronides. Excretion in urine as free and conjugated codeine, norcodeine and morphine. Less than 17% excreted unchanged

FENTANYL

Structure – synthetic anilino-piperidine opioid

Presentation – colourless, aqueous solution of citrate salt (preservative free). 50 mcg/ml (2 and 10 ml ampoules)

Dose IV – 0.5–3 mcg/kg for spontaneous ventilation, 1–50 mcg/kg for assisted ventilation. Peak effects in 5 min, duration of 30 min for smaller doses

Epidural – 50–100 mcg bolus, infusion 1 mcg/kg/H

Pharmacokinetics

Protein binding	V_d	Cl	$t_{1/2}$	pKa
85%	4	13	350	8.4

CNS – potent μ opioid receptor agonist, 60–80 times more potent analgesia than morphine; sedation

CVS – minimal effects even in higher doses, use in cardiac anaesthesia well established. Hypotension and bradycardia may occur particularly in hypovolaemic patients because of reduced sympathetic tone

RS – respiratory depression and reports of delayed respiratory depression probably as a result of entero-hepatic circulation; high doses may increase chest and abdominal muscle tone so impairing ventilation

Other – nausea and vomiting, decreased gastro-intestinal motility, negligible histamine release

Elimination – predominantly metabolised in liver by dealkylation to norfentanyl, an inactive metabolite; norfentanyl and fentanyl then hydroxylated and excreted in the urine.(elimination half-life increased in liver disease and elderly)

Contra-indications – concurrent administration with monoamine oxidase inhibitors

MORPHINE

Structure – a phenanthrene; a principal alkaloid of opium

Presentation

Oral – tablets 10, 20 mg; modified release tablets 5, 10, 15, 30, 60, 100, 200 mg

– solution of 10 mg/5 ml, 30 mg/5 ml; suppositories 10, 15, 20, 30 mg

IV – clear, colourless, aqueous solution of morphine sulphate 10, 15, 20, 30 mg/ml (1 and 2 ml ampoules containing preservative 0.1% sodium metabisulphate)

Dose

SC/IM – 0.1–0.3 mg/kg, peak effect after 30 min, duration 3–4 H
Rectal – 15–30 mg 4 hourly
Intrathecal – 0.2–1 mg
IV – 0.05–0.1 mg/kg
Epidural – 2.5–10 mg

Pharmacokinetics

Protein binding	Bio-availability	pKa
99%	15–50%	7.9

V_d	Cl	$t_{1/2}$
3.5	15	180

CNS – potent analgesic, agonist at μ, δ, and κ opioid receptors; sedation, drowsiness, euphoria, dysphoria, miosis (stimulation of Edinger–Westphal nucleus); tolerance and dependence

CVS – heart rate, systemic vascular resistance and blood pressure reduced

RS – respiratory rate and volume reduced, response to hypercarbia reduced; bronchoconstriction, anti-tussive, muscle rigidity

GIT – nausea and vomiting, delayed gastric emptying, constipation, contraction of gall bladder and constriction of sphincter of Oddi causing reflux into pancreatic duct and an increase in serum amylase or lipase

Other – histamine release, itching, urticaria, increased tone of ureters, bladder and sphincter leading to urinary retention, increased ADH secretion, transient decrease in adrenal steroid secretion

Elimination – extensive first-pass metabolism; therefore, oral dose 50% higher than IM dose. Conjugated in liver to morphine 3-glucuronide (70%) and morphine 6-glucuronide (5–10%), an active metabolite more potent than morphine, the remainder demethylated to normorphine. Excreted predominantly in urine as conjugated metabolites; < 10% excreted unchanged. Accumulation of morphine 6-glucuronide may occur in renal failure

REMIFENTANIL

Structure – synthetic anilino-piperidine opioid with a methyl ester linkage

Presentation – lyophilised, white powder as 1, 2 or 5 mg vials for reconstitution, which forms a clear, colourless solution, containing 1 mg/ml remifentanil hydrochloride. Further dilution to a concentration of 50 mg/ml recommended for general anaesthesia. Reconstituted solution is stable for 24 H at room temperature

Dose – IV – bolus at induction 1 mcg/kg over not < 30 s, maintenance infusion 0.05–2 mcg/kg/min titrated to desired level. For spontaneous ventilation, starting dose 0.04 mcg/kg/min, with range of 0.025–0.1 mg/kg/min titrated to effect

Pharmacokinetics

Protein binding	V_d	Cl	$t_{1/2}$
70%	0.35	50	15

CNS – potent μ opioid receptor agonist; analgesic potency comparable to fentanyl; rapid onset and recovery even after several hours' infusion

CVS – haemodynamically very stable; rarely bradycardia and hypotension

RS – respiratory rate and volume reduced, response to hypercarbia reduced; muscle rigidity, related to dose and rate of administration

Other – nausea and vomiting, no histamine release

Elimination – independent of hepatic and renal function, metabolised by de-esterification by non specific plasma and tissue esterases to inactive metabolites that are excreted in urine. Unlike suxamethonium it is not a substrate for plasma cholinesterase and clearance is unaffected by cholinesterase deficiency or the administration of anti-cholinesterases. It is not recommended for intrathecal or epidural use

Contra-indications – concurrent administration with monoamine oxidase inhibitors

NALOXONE

Structure – N-allyl oxymorphone opioid antagonist

Presentation – clear, colourless, aqueous solution containing 400 mcg in 1 ml, or 20 mcg in 2 ml naloxone hydrochloride

Dose – IV – increments 1.5–3 mcg/kg peak effect in 2 min; bolus 0.4–2 mg for suspected overdose repeated up to 10 mg lasts 20 min; may need to follow with infusion. Also administered SC and IM

Pharmacokinetics

Protein binding	V_d	Cl	$t_{1/2}$
45%	2	25	70

Clinical effects – pure opioid receptor antagonist acting at all opioid receptors; effects are related to withdrawal of the effects of any opioids and antagonism of endogenous opioids

Elimination – primarily by hepatic glucuronide conjugation followed by urinary excretion

DICLOFENAC

Structure – phenylacetic acid derivative, NSAID; potent inhibitor of cyclo-oxygenase enzyme (COX_1 and COX_2)

Presentation

Oral – enteric-coated tablets 25, 50 mg; sustained release tablets 75, 100 mg; dispersible tablets 46.5 mg; suppositories 12.5, 25, 50, 100 mg

IM – aqueous solution in 3 ml ampoules containing 75 mg diclofenac sodium, sodium metabisulphate, benzyl alcohol, propylene glycol and mannitol

Dose

Oral – 75–150 mg/day in 2–3 divided doses, children 1–3 mg/kg/day

Rectal – 100 mg 18 hourly; maximum daily dose 150 mg

Deep IM – 75 mg once or twice daily.

Pharmacokinetics

Protein binding	V_d	Cl	$t_{1/2}$	Bio-availability
99.5%	0.17	4.2	90	60%

CNS – analgesic and anti-inflammatory; dizziness; vertigo

RS – bronchospasm in atopic and asthmatic individuals

GIT – gastric irritation, dyspepsia, peptic ulceration; nausea and vomiting; diarrhoea; local irritation from suppositories

Other – renal impairment or failure; decreased renin activity and aldosterone concentrations by 60–70%; platelet aggregation inhibited; pain and local induration with IM injection; rashes and skin eruptions; transaminases raised and hepatic function impaired; blood dyscrasias; increases plasma concentrations of co-administered digoxin, lithium, anticoagulants and sulphonylureas

Elimination – significant first-pass metabolism in liver by hydroxylation then conjugation with glucuronide and sulphate; followed by excretion in the urine (60%) and bile (40%); < 1% unchanged in urine

Contra-indications – asthma, gastro-intestinal ulceration, hepatic and renal insufficiency, bleeding diathesis, haematological abnormalities, pregnancy and porphyria

IBUPROFEN

Structure – propionic acid derivative, NSAID; potent inhibitor of cyclo-oxygenase enzyme (COX_1 and COX_2)

Presentation – coated tablets 200, 400, 600 mg; slow release tablets 800 mg; capsules 300 mg; syrup 100 mg/5 ml; compound preparations with codeine (8 mg codeine/300 mg ibuprofen)

Dose – oral – 1.2–1.8 g/day in 3–4 divided doses (maximum 2.4 g/day); children 20 mg/kg in divided doses (maximum 40 mg/kg/day) not recommended in children < 7 kg

Pharmacokinetics

Protein binding	V_d	Cl	$t_{1/2}$	Bio-availability
99%	0.15	0.75	120	78%

CNS – mild analgesic and anti-inflammatory properties; malaise; dizziness; vertigo; tinnitus

RS – bronchospasm in asthmatics

GIT – dyspepsia; gastic irritation; nausea and vomiting; diarrhoea

GUT – renal insufficiency and acute, reversible renal failure

Other – rashes and hypersensitivity reactions; a few reports of toxic amblyopia

Excretion – metabolised in liver to two inactive metabolites and excreted in urine; < 1% excreted unchanged

Contra-indications – asthma; history of peptic ulceration; renal insufficiency; haemorrhagic tendencies

KETOROLAC

Structure – a pyrroleacetic acid, NSAID; potent inhibitor of cyclo-oxygenase enzyme (COX$_1$ and COX$_2$)

Presentation

Tablets – 10 mg ketorolac trometamol

IV/IM – clear, slightly yellow solution I ml ampoules containing 10 and 30 mg ketorolac trometamol

Dose

Oral – 10 mg 4–6 hourly (6–8 hourly in elderly), maximum 40 mg/day for 2 days

IV/IM – 10–30 mg 4–6 hourly, maximum daily dose 90 mg in non elderly, 60 mg in elderly, renally impaired and patients < 50 kg, for not > 2 days

Pharmacokinetics

Protein binding	V_d	Cl	$t_{1/2}$	Bio-availablity
99%	0.15	0.35	300	85%

CNS – dizziness; tinnitus

RS – dyspnoea; asthma; pulmonary oedema

GIT – dyspepsia; gastro-intestinal irritation; peptic ulceration; nausea, vomiting and diarrhoea

Other – minimal anti-inflammatory effect at its analgesic dose; renal insufficiency; acute renal failure; hyponatraemia; hyperkalaemia; interstitial nephritis; thrombocytopenia and platelet dysfunction; rashes; pruritis and hypersensitivity reactions; flushing; pain at site of injection; increased risk of renal impairment with ACE inhibitors; reduced clearance of methotrexate and lithium; increased levels of ketorolac with probenecid

Elimination – mainly metabolised to inactive metabolite acyl glucuronide, about 25% metabolised to para-hydroxyketorolac, which has 20% of anti-inflammatory and 1% of the analgesic activity of the parent drug. Excretion is primarily renal (92%), the remainder in bile (6%) and < 1% is unchanged

Contra-indications – history of peptic ulcer disease; asthma and atopic tendencies; haemorrhagic diatheses; renal insufficiency; hypovolaemia and dehydration; pregnancy; children < 16 years

REFERENCES AND FURTHER READING

Rang HP, Urban L. *BJA* 1995;**75**:145-156

Steinhoff, M. *Nature Medicine* 2000;**6**:151-158 (from BMJ 2000;**320**:334)

SECTION 3: 8
NEUROMUSCULAR BLOCKING AGENTS

T. C. Smith

MECHANISM OF NEUROMUSCULAR BLOCKADE
Monitoring neuromuscular blockade

DEPOLARISING BLOCKADE
Mechanism of action
Clinical features
Inherited Plasma Cholinesterase Abnormalities
Phase I and II blockade

NON DEPOLARISING BLOCKADE
Mechanism of action
Clinical features
Elimination

ANTI-CHOLINESTERASES
Mechanism of action
Reversible anti-cholinesterases
Organophosphorus compounds

SPECIFIC PHARMACOLOGY
Atracurium dibesylate
Cis-atracurium dibesylate
Doxacurium chloride
Mivacurium chloride
Rapacuronium
Pancuronium bromide
Pipecuronium bromide
Rocuronium bromide
D-Tubocurarine chloride
Vecuronium bromide
Suxamethonium chloride (succinyl choline)
Neostigmine bromide

Stimulation can be performed simply using a single pulse lasting 0.2 ms. However, a train of four such pulses produces more information. A train of four stimulation is defined as a sequence of four supramaximal, square-wave, electrical pulses each lasting 0.2 ms given at 2 Hz. There must be a gap of at least 10 s between each train of four to ensure reliable results. The use of electrical stimulation in the awake person, especially tetanic, is unpleasant and may be painful.

MEASUREMENT OF RESPONSE

Assessment of neuromuscular blockade can be made by the observed or palpated strength of twitch, measurement of evoked tension in a certain muscle (e.g. adductor pollicis, which should be pre loaded to give an isometric measure). Alternatively, automated Double Burst Stimulation (DBS) electromyography (e.g. Relaxograph®) can be used in which case the response from the abductor digiti minimi muscle is recorded following electrical stimulation of the ulnar nerve.

The train of four shows the following correlations:

- At 75% depression of T1, T4 is lost (a count of three twitches)
- At 80% depression of T1, T3 is lost (a count of two twitches)
- At 90% depression of T1, T2 is lost (a count of one twitch)
- When T4:T1 > 60% the patient is clinically recovered

Other indices of neuromuscular blockade include tetanic fade post-tetanic facilitation. Tetanic stimulation is electrical stimulation at 50–100 Hz. The stimulation used to produce post-tetanic facilitation is:

- Single twitch 0.2 ms – measure response
- Delay 5 s
- Tetanic burst 50 Hz for 5 s
- Delay 3 s
- Single twitch 0.2 ms – measure response

During a tetanic stimulation, the presence of a non depolarising neuromuscular blocking agent is indicated by an exponential decline in muscle response. This is the result of decreasing amounts of acetyl choline being released with subsequent action potentials. In the presence of blockade more acetyl choline is required to achieve a muscle action potential, and the repeated stimulation unmasks this decline in acetyl choline release. Post-tetanic facilitation is the augmentation of muscle response to a single twitch brought about by using a tetanic stimulation in between. This only occurs in the presence of non

depolarising blockade, and is probably the result of stimulation of pre synaptic acetyl choline receptors that enhance the subsequent release of acetyl choline from the nerve terminal.

DBS involves administering two short 50 Hz bursts (each containing 3 stimuli) separated by 750 msec. At T4/T1 of 0.5 the second burst shows a 50% reduction in force.

DEPOLARISING BLOCKADE

Examples – suxamethonium, decamethonium

Suxamethonium is the only current therapeutic example of a depolarising blocking drug. However, any agonist of nicotinic acetylcholine receptors can also cause blockade if not rapidly cleared from the neuromuscular junction. Examples include nicotine and acetylcholine in the presence of excess anti-cholinesterase.

MECHANISM OF ACTION

A depolarising block occurs when the agent stimulates the acetyl choline receptor and causes depolarisation. Persistence of the agonist at the receptor prevents re-polarisation of the end plate and so it is refractory to further stimulation. As the agent diffuses away from the junctional cleft, repolarisation occurs and muscle action potentials are once more possible. The block is reversible and attachment to the receptors is competitive. The block may be enhanced by a local increase in acetylcholine as produced by anti-cholinesterases.

CLINICAL FEATURES

Depolarising blockade is characterised by rapid onset with muscle fasciculation, as groups of muscle fibres are depolarised, which is subsequently followed by a prolonged refractory period, which constitutes the blockade.

Neuromuscular test stimulation results in:

- Reduced single-twitch height
- Reduced train of four, all of equal amplitude
- No tetanic fade
- No post tetanic facilitation

After suxamethonium administration there may be widespread muscular pains, which are worse on movement. They are particularly common in muscular, young males after early ambulation. Muscle pains may persist for several days. Pre treatment with benzodiazepines, lidocaine or small doses of non depolarising agents may help. Dantrolene has also been used with some success.

PLASMA CHOLINESTERASE ABNORMALITIES

Plasma cholinesterase is a lipoprotein enzyme comprising four polypetide chains responsible for hydolysing esters in many tissues. It is synthesised in the liver and is present in the liver, kidneys, pancreas, brain and plasma but not erythrocytes. The normal range in plasma is 4000-12000 IU/L and a fall of 700 U/L or more is significant (Plasma cholinesterase (also known as butyryl or pseudocholinesterase) is responsible for the metabolism of suxamethonium by hydrolysis of the two ester links of choline to succinic acid (Figure NJ.9). Suxamethonium is also metabolised, slowly, by acetyl cholinesterase.

A reduction in cholinesterase activity may either be due to a deficiency of cholinesterase molecules or an abnormality of the enzyme. The causes of cholinesterase deficiency are listed in Figure NJ.3. Levels fall to 75% of normal during pregnancy and to 67% of normal during the first 7 days postpartum. Patients with pre-existing genetic deficiencies are more prone to problems if acquired forms of deficiency coexist.

Plasma cholinesterase synthesis is controlled by a pair of autosomal recessive genes. Figure NJ.4 shows possible genetic configurations, their incidence and dibucaine numbers. Assessment of plasma cholinesterase activity includes global plasma cholinesterase activity levels, and dibucaine and fluoride numbers. The dibucaine number quantifies the inhibition, by a 10-5 molar solution of dibucaine

CAUSES OF PLASMA CHOLINESTERASE DEFICIENCY

Pregnancy, third trimester
Collagen disorders
Carcinomatosis
Myocardial infarction
Liver disease
Hypothyroidism
Blood dyscrasias
Amethocaine
Ketamine
Pancuronium
Anticholinesterases
Oral contraceptives
Propranolol
Cytotoxic agents
Ecothiopate eye drops

Figure NJ.3

(a local anaesthetic previously available as cinchocaine), of the activity of plasma cholinesterase in the sample on benzoyl choline. It is expressed as a percentage. The fluoride number is similar but uses 5 x 10-5 molar sodium fluoride.

Plasma cholinesterase may also exist in excess as a genetic variant or particularly in the presence of obesity or alcoholism. The result is a shortened duration of action of suxamethonium.

Plasma cholinesterase is also responsible for the metabolism of mivacurium and the concomitant use of these drugs in susceptible patients may exaggerate problems

INHERITANCE OF ABNORMAL PLASMA CHOLINESTERASE

Type	Genotype		Dibucaine number	Fluoride number	Typical apnoea	Incidence
Normal	$E_1^u E_1^u$	homozyous	80	60	1-5min	94%
Atypical	$E_1^u E_1^a$	heterozyous	60	50	10 min	1:25
Atypical	$E_1^a E_1^a$	homozyous	20	20	2 hours	1:3000
Silent	$E_1^u E_1^s$	heterozyous	80	60	10 min	1:25
Silent	$E_1^s E_1^s$	homozyous	minimal activity		2 hours	1:100,000
Fluoride resistant	$E_1^u E_1^f$	heterozyous	75	50	10 min	1:300,000
Fluoride resistant	$E_1^f E_1^f$	homozyous	65	40	2 hours	1:150,000

Note: u, a, s and f are the 4 commonest of 25 possible gene variants for plasma cholinesterase

Figure NJ.4.

Two distinct types of neuromuscular blockade (termed phase I and II blockade respectively), may result after the administration of suxamethonium. Figure NJ.5 lists the features of each type.

NON DEPOLARISING BLOCKADE

Examples – atracurium, mivacurium, pancuronium, rocuronium, vecuronium

MECHANISM OF ACTION

Non depolarising neuromuscular blockade is the result of competitive occupancy of the post-junctional receptors preventing acetyl choline from reaching one or both α sub-units of the receptor. This is probably a dynamic process with both acetyl choline and the blocking agent in equilibrium with the receptors. At least 75% of receptors must be blocked before contraction fails. The process is competitive and reversible. The block can be antagonised by a local increase in acetyl choline as produced by anti-cholinesterases. These muscle relaxants have no intrinsic activity at the neuromuscular end plate. Each has one or more quaternary ammonium groups. In the bisquaternary agents, these are usually 140 nm apart. This was thought essential for neuromuscular blocking agents, but monoquaternary agents such as d-tubocurarine are also effective.

PHASE I AND II BLOCKADE AFTER SUXAMETHONIUM ADMINISTRATION

Phase I blockade

   Well sustained response to tetanic
      stimulation
   No post tetanic facilitation
   Train of four ratio > 0.7
   Potentiated by the effect of
      anticholinesterases

Phase II blockade

   Tetanic fade
   Post tetanic facilitation
   Train of four ratio < 0.3
   Antagonised by the effect of
      anticholinesterases
   Tachyphylaxis

Figure NJ.5

A graphic illustration of the process by which depolarising and non depolarising drugs have their effects is shown in Figure NJ.6.

CLINICAL FEATURES

The predominant effect of neuromuscular blocking agents is a reversible paralysis of skeletal muscle. This reduction in skeletal muscle activity reduces venous return and, therefore, reduces cardiac output and blood pressure.

Neuromuscular test stimulation results in:

- Reduced single-twitch height
- Reduced train of four, with amplitude – twitch 1 > 2 > 3 > 4
- Tetanic fade
- Post tetanic facilitation

Aminosteroids

The acetylcholine type fragment associated with the 'D' ring of steroid nucleus is probably responsible for most of the neuromuscular antagonism. The acetylcholine type fragment associated with the 'A' ring is probably responsible for the cardiovascular effects especially the vagolytic aspects. Histamine release is not expected with the aminosteroid structure. In general, the aminosteroids are more slowly metabolised than the benzylisoquiniliniums. For the structure of the commonly used agents, see page 651.

Benzylisoquinolinium compounds

The chemical structure of benzylisoquinolinium is associated with histamine release. In general, the presence of an ester link promotes rapid degradation and metabolism leading to a short half-life and rapid transition to complete recovery.

The relative strengths of cardiovascular effects and histamine release by the non depolarising muscle relaxant drugs are shown in Figure NJ.7.

The neuromuscular blocking agents also have anti-cholinesterase activity (Figure NJ.8). The effect of pancuronium on plasma cholinesterase is clinically important and should, therefore, be particularly noted.

ELIMINATION

The non depolarising agents are usually metabolised in the liver. Other pathways exist including spontaneous degradation and enzymatic hydrolysis within the plasma. These pathways are covered under the specific drug details.

Sequence 1: Normal depolarisation

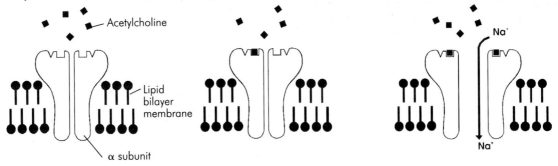

Acetylcholine released into the junctional cleft binds reversibly to receptor sites on the alpha subunits of the sodium ionophore. When the alpha site on each of the two subunits is occupied, the channel opens and allows depolarisation. Rapid metabolism enables rapid dissociation of receptor and agonist and the channel closes.

Sequence 2: Depolarising blockade

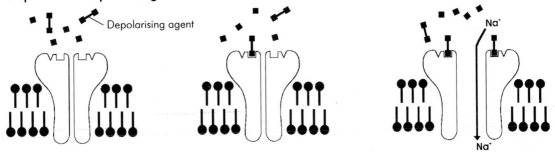

Suxamethonium and the released acetyl choline are both agonists of the receptor. When both receptors are occupied by any combination of these molecules the channel opens. However, the persistence of suxamethonium causes the channel to remain open long after the acetyl choline has been destroyed, maintaining a depolarised refractory end plate.

Sequence 3: Non depolarising blockade

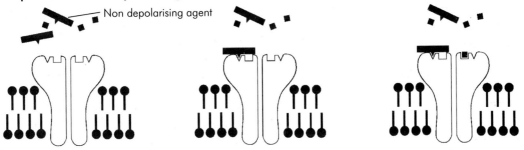

Non depolarising drugs are antagonists and bind to the receptor without opening the channel. They subsequently prevent acetylcholine from binding and as two acetyl choline molecules are required for depolarisation only one receptor needs to be occupied by the antagonist to be effective.

Figure NJ.6 Action of depolarising and non depolarising muscle relaxants

RELATIVE POTENCIES OF ADDITIONAL EFFECTS OF NON DEPOLARISING RELAXANTS

	Ganglion blockade	Vagal blockade	Histamine release	Sympathetic stimulation
Atracurium	0	0	++	0
Cis-atracurium	0	0	0	0
Doxacurium	0	0	0	0
D-Tubocurarine	+++++	0	+++++	0
Mivacurium	0	0	+	0
Pancuronium	0	+++	0	++++
Pipecuronium	0	0	0	0
Rocuronium	0	+	0	0
Vecuronium	0	0	0	0

Figure NJ.7

The non depolarising blocking agents may be potentiated by suxamethonium, IV and volatile anaesthetic agents, opioids, aminoglycosides, tetracyclines, metronidazole, lincosamides, polymixins, magnesium, verapamil and nifedipine, protamine, diuretics and catecholamine antagonists. The blockade is prolonged by hypothermia.

ANTI-CHOLINESTERASES

MECHANISM OF ACTION

The anti-cholinesterases inhibit the breakdown of acetylcholine by binding to the acetylcholinesterase enzyme in a competitive manner. This raises the background concentration of acetylcholine near the neuromuscular junction, which in turn overcomes the reduced number of functional nicotinic receptors on the muscle end plate whether due to a reduced number of receptors (myasthenia gravis) or due to blockade of existing receptors (non depolarising muscle relaxants). They can be classified as either reversible anti-cholinesterases or organophosphorus compounds. While all anti-cholinesterases act on acetyl and plasma cholinesterase the specific interaction with the enzyme varies between individual drugs.

The development of specific antibodies for steroid neuromuscular blocking agents is currently underway. These may replace the anti-cholinesterases as reversal agents in the future.

ANTICHOLINESTERASE ACTIVITY OF NEUROMUSCULAR BLOCKING AGENTS

Drug	Concentration to produce 50% inhibition of enzymatic acetyl choline breakdown (μmol/l) in the presence of various neuromuscular blocking drugs	
	Acetyl cholinesterase	Plasma cholinesterase
Suxamethonium	1300	640
Atracurium	340	420
Vecuronium	66	0.62

Figure NJ.8

REVERSIBLE ANTI-CHOLINESTERASES

Examples – distigmine, edrophonium, neostigmine, pyridostigmine

Acetyl cholinesterase has an esteratic site and an anionic site in close proximity. Physiologically, the positively charged quaternary amine of acetyl choline binds to the anionic site. The acetyl ester combines with the esteratic site and the acetylcholine is hydrolysed. The anti-cholinesterases competitively occupy these sites and prevent acetylcholine access. The anti-cholinesterases have a quaternary amine group that is attracted to the anionic site and a carbamyl ester that binds covalently to the serine amino acid of the esteratic site. The quaternary amine group is not essential for activity but when present it conveys enhanced potency and stability. The quaternary group also results in poor absorption following oral administration and a minimal transfer of the drug across the blood-brain barrier. Neostigmine is absorbed poorly from the gut as compared with the IV route. When neostigmine is used orally for the treatment of myasthenia gravis larger doses are, therefore, necessary. Equivalent doses of neostigmine are as follows: IV 0.5 mg; IM 1–1.5 mg; oral 15 mg.

Anti-cholinesterases also have some direct cholinergic agonist activity.

Physostigmine (no longer available) is an example of an anti-cholinesterase with several tertiary amine groups rather than the quaternary amine of the others. Consequently it is readily absorbed topically and orally and crosses the blood-brain barrier, but has no cholinergic agonist activity.

Edrophonium is only clinically effective for 5 min and is used in the diagnosis of myasthenia gravis. Longer acting agents are needed for treatment of the disease. Neostigmine is the only anti-cholinesterase routinely used to reverse planned neuromuscular blockade in clinical practice. Anti-cholinesterases have widespread effects subsequent to the stimulation of increased cholinergic muscarinic and nicotinic activity. Heart rate, vasomotor tone and blood pressure are reduced. At high dose levels sympathetic ganglion stimulation may predominate. Excess acetyl choline causes bronchoconstriction and increased bronchial secretion. Increased gastro-intestinal tone and secretion occurs. Secretions of saliva, sweat and tears are also stimulated. These problems are prevented by the concomitant use of muscarinic anti-cholinergic drugs such as atropine or glycopyrrolate. Anti-cholinesterases can also cause a depolarising neuromuscular blockade when used in excess or in the absence of non depolarising blockade.

Neuromuscular blockade is terminated either by endogenous elimination of the drug and diffusion of the blocking agent away from the neuromuscular junction, or, in the case of non depolarising agents, the effects can be overcome, in part, by inhibiting the metabolism of acetyl choline. If a long-acting muscle relaxant is used, it is possible for the blockade to re-establish if the effects of the anti-cholinesterase wear off before the neuromuscular blocking agent has left the receptors.

ORGANOPHOSPHORUS COMPOUNDS

Example – ecothiopate

These are primarily used as nerve gases and pesticides and may feature in cases of poisoning. In general, they have no ionic binding component but bind covalently and irreversibly to the esteratic site of the cholinesterase enzyme by the release of a relatively weakly bound component of the drug. Consequently, the enzyme is not readily reactivated. Organophosphates tend to be highly lipid soluble and readily cross the blood-brain barrier causing central nervous system toxicity. Ecothiopate differs from the general features of this group. It is the only organophosphate in clinical use, and is used in the treatment of glaucoma. It too binds covalently to the esteratic site of the enzyme but also has a positively charged quaternary ammonium group that helps binding. This positive charge means that ecothiopate does not readily cross the blood-brain barrier in contrast with other organophosphorous compounds. Although it is slowly hydrolysed it may nonetheless prolong the action of suxamethonium and mivacurium.

SPECIFIC PHARMACOLOGY

Here, units used (unless stated separately) are:

Volume of distribution at steady state (V_d) (ml/kg)
Clearance (Cl) (ml/kg/min)
Terminal half-life ($t_{1/2}$) (min)

NON DEPOLARISING DRUGS

ATRACURIUM DIBESYLATE

Structure – bisquaternary benzylisoquinolinium diester. A plant derivative
Presentation – clear, colourless, aqueous solution of pH 3.5 (10 mg/ml, 2.5, 5, 25 ml ampoules). Storage – in fridge at 2–8°C, protect from light
Dose – IV bolus 0.3–0.6 mg/kg, infusion 0.3–0.6 mg/kg/h. Initial dose lasts 30 min, $ED_{95} = 0.2$ mg/kg

Pharmacokinetics

Protein binding	V_d	Cl	$t_{1/2}$
82%	170	5.5	20

CNS – no increase in intra-ocular pressure (IOP) or intracranial pressure (ICP). Laudanosine, a metabolite and stimulant crosses the blood-brain barrier and can cause convulsions if plasma concentration > 20 pg/ml

CVS – the small amount of histamine release may lower systemic vascular resistance, central venous pressure and pulmonary capillary wedge pressure

RS – paralysis of respiratory muscles; small risk of bronchospasm due to histamine release

Other – no effect on lower oesophageal sphincter pressure; placental transfer insufficient to cause an effect in the foetus

Elimination – non cumulative. Hofmann elimination is the spontaneous fragmentation of atracurium at the bond between the quaternary nitrogen and the central chain. This occurs at body temperature and pH, producing inactive products – laudanosine ($t_{1/2}$ = 234 min) and a quaternary monoacrylate ($t_{1/2}$ = 39 min). Atracurium is also metabolised by ester hydrolysis producing a quaternary alcohol and a quaternary acid. These two mechanisms account for 40% of the elimination of atracurium, the remainder being by a variety of other mechanisms

Metabolites – 55% excreted in the bile within 7 H, 35% excreted in the urine within 7 H

Side effects – histamine release may cause bronchospasm, hypotension, and erythema and wheals generally or along the vein of injection

CIS-ATRACURIUM DIBESYLATE

Atracurium contains a mixture of ten isomers. One of these, cis–cis-atracurium is marketed as Cis-atracurium. The features are as for atracurium except:

Presentation – clear, colourless, aqueous solution of pH 3.5 (2 mg/ml in 2.5, 5, 10, 25 ml ampoules, and 5 mg/ml in 30 ml vial). Store in fridge at 2-8°C, protect from light

Dose – IV bolus 0.15 mg/kg; infusion 0.18 mg/kg/h

ED_{95} = 0.05 mg/kg

This single isomer of atracurium avoids the histamine release but is similar to atracurium in other respects.

DOXACURIUM CHLORIDE

Structure – bisquaternary benzylisoquinolinium diester

Presentation – not available in the UK

Dose – IV bolus 0.05 mg/kg. Initial dose lasts 80–90 min. Can be antagonised within 10 min. ED_{95} 30 mcg/kg

Pharmacokinetics

V_d	Cl	$t_{1/2}$
220	2.7	99

CNS – no effect

CVS – minimal effect, slight decrease in heart rate

RS – paralysis of respiratory muscles

Other – no histamine release

Elimination – doxacurium is non cumulative. Elimination is mainly renal with some hepatic excretion (unchanged) in the bile. Of it, 31% is excreted unchanged in the urine by 12 H. Doxacurium is also slowly hydrolysed by plasma cholinesterase

MIVACURIUM CHLORIDE

Structure – bisquaternary benzylisoquinolinium diester

Presentation – clear, colourless, aqueous solution of pH 4.5 (2 mg/ml, 5 and 10 ml ampoules) containing three stereoisomers – *trans–trans* (57%), *cis–trans* (36%), *cis–cis* (6%)

Dose – IV bolus 0.07–0.25 mg/kg; children 0.1–0.2 mg/kg; infusion 0.06 mg/kg/h. ED_{95} = 0.08 mg/kg (children 0.1 mg/kg)

Pharmacokinetics

Isomer	V_d	Cl	$t_{1/2}$
trans–trans	150-267	51-63	1.9-3.6
cis–trans	290-382	93-106	1.8-2.9
cis–cis	175-340	3.7-4.6	34.7-52.9

CNS – no effect

CVS – no effect

RS – respiratory muscle paralysis

Other – minimal placental transfer

Elimination – trans–trans and cis–trans isomers hydrolysed by plasma cholinesterase. The cis–cis isomer may be metabolised in part by the liver. Lasts twice as long as suxamethonium (24 min)

Toxicity – block antagonised by neostigmine. Block prolonged by reduced or atypical plasma cholinesterase as with suxamethonium. Block also prolonged if factors interfering with plasma cholinesterase are present. Heterozygotes for atypical plasma cholinesterase show a prolongation of effect of about 10 min

RAPACURONIUM

Structure – monoquaternary aminosteroid

Presentation – not available in the UK

Dose – IV bolus 1.5–2.5 mg/kg, duration 8 min

Pharmacokinetics

V_d	Cl	$t_{1/2}$
293	8.5	74

Clinical features are similar to vecuronium

Elimination – 22% of the drug appears in the urine within 24 H. Very low levels of the 3-hydroxy metabolite are produced

PANCURONIUM BROMIDE

Structure – bisquaternary aminosteroid
Presentation – clear, colourless, aqueous solution (4 mg in 2 ml)
Dose – IV bolus 0.05–0.1 mg/kg. Initial dose lasts 45–60 min; ED_{95} = 60 mcg/kg
Pharmacokinetics

Protein binding	V_d	Cl	$t_{1/2}$
15–87%	200	1.8	115

(albumin, γ-globulin)
CNS – does not cross blood-brain barrier. No increase in IOP and ICP
CVS – increase heart rate, cardiac output and blood pressure due to vagolytic action. Systemic vascular resistance unchanged
RS – respiratory muscle paralysis; some bronchodilatation
Other – increase in lower oesophageal sphincter pressure; may increase prothrombin time and partial thromboplastin time; small amount of placental transfer but no clinical effect on foetus
Elimination – 50% excreted unchanged of which 80% appears in the urine. Of it, 40% is de-acetylated in the liver to 3-hydroxy, 17-hydroxy and 3,17-dihydroxy derivatives which are eliminated in the bile. The 3-hydroxy compound has some neuromuscular antagonist activity

Note that pancuronium has some pre-junctional activity.

PIPECURONIUM BROMIDE

Structure – bisquaternary aminosteroid
Presentation – not available in the UK
Dose – IV bolus 70 mcg/kg for intubation in 3 min (up to a maximum of 100 mcg/kg). Initial dose lasts 100 min; ED_{95} = 49 mcg/kg
Pharmacokinetics

Protein binding	V_d	Cl	$t_{1/2}$
2%	309	2.4	137

CNS – no effect
CVS – no effect on the cardiovascular system
RS – paralysis of respiratory muscles
Other – does not cause histamine release

Elimination – 40% excreted unchanged in the urine by 24 H, 4% metabolised by the liver to 3-desacetylpipecuronium, 2% is excreted in the bile

ROCURONIUM BROMIDE

Structure – monoquaternary aminosteroid
Presentation – aqueous solution (10 mg/ml, 5 and 10 ml ampoules)
Storage – in fridge at 2–8°C; protect from light
Dose – IV bolus 0.6 mg/kg, infusion 0.3–0.6 mg/kg/h, initial dose lasts 38–150 min, ED_{95} = 0.3 mg/kg. Onset time of 1.5 min using $2 \times ED_{95}$ that may be shortened to 55 s using $4 \times ED_{95}$
Pharmacokinetics

V_d	Cl	$t_{1/2}$
270	4.0	131

CNS – no effect
CVS – increases heart rate, cardiac output and blood pressure slightly due to vagal blockade
RS – respiratory muscle paralysis
Other – no histamine release
Elimination – predominantly hepatic but also some renal elimination. Hepatic or renal failure can cause prolongation of effect

D-TUBOCURARINE CHLORIDE

Structure – monoquaternary alkaloid derivative of isoquinoline. Only becomes bisquaternary at very low pH
Presentation – clear, colourless, aqueous solution of pH 4–6 (10 mg/ml 1.5 ml ampoule). Recently withdrawn from the UK
Dose – IV bolus 0.3–0.5 mg/kg. Initial dose lasts 25 min
Pharmacokinetics

Protein binding	V_d	Cl	$t_{1/2}$
50%	450	2	120

(mainly albumin)
CNS – increases IOP and ICP. Does not cross blood-brain barrier
CVS – no direct effect on heart; histamine release and sympathetic ganglia blockade lowers systemic vascular resistance and heart rate
RS – paralysis of respiratory muscles; can cause of bronchospasm secondary to histamine release
Other – histamine release may cause wheals; increases saliva; reduced gastro-intestinal tone and motility; minimal placental transfer
Elimination – unchanged 44% in urine, 12% in bile at 24 H, 1% demethylated in liver

D-Tubocurarine has been superseded by newer agents. It was formerly popular during controlled hypotension as the ganglion blockade contributed to deliberately induced hypotension by inducing vasodilatation without causing a reflex tachycardia.

VECURONIUM BROMIDE

Structure – monoquaternary aminosteroid, becomes bisquaternary at pH 7.4

Presentation – freeze-dried, buffered, lyophilised cake for reconstitution, containing vecuronium bromide, citric acid monohydrate, disodium hydrogen phosphate dihydrate and mannitol

Storage – avoid light and temperatures in excess of 45°C. Reconstitution with water for injections produces clear, colourless solution of pH 4.0

Dose – IV bolus 0.05–0.1 mg/kg, infusion 0.05–0.1 mg/kg/h, ED_{95} = 0.046 mg/kg. Initial dose lasts 30 min

Pharmacokinetics

V_d	Cl	$t_{1/2}$
0.26	4.6	62

CNS – no increase in ICP

CVS – no effect

RS – respiratory muscle paralysis

Other – no increase in IOP; minimal placental transfer; no histamine release

Elimination – spontaneous de-acetylation and hepatic metabolism. Of total dose, 10–25% is excreted in urine; the rest in the bile. Most excreted unchanged. Suitable in patients with absent renal function. Hepatic failure may prolong clinical effect whereas chronic phenytoin therapy reduces the efficacy of vecuronium. There are three potential metabolites 3-hydroxy, 17-hydroxy and 3,17-dihydroxy. These have minimal neuromuscular and vagolytic activity; only 3-hydroxy is found in any significant quantity and it has 50% of the neuromuscular blocking potency of vecuronium. Vecuronium is more stable in acidic solutions and is, therefore, potentiated by respiratory acidosis

DEPOLARISING AGENTS

SUXAMETHONIUM CHLORIDE (SUCCINYL CHOLINE)

Structure – dicholine ester of acetyl choline

Presentation – clear, colourless, aqueous solution of pH 3.0–5.0 with a shelf life of 2 years (100 mg in 2 ml)

Storage – in fridge at 4°C; spontaneous hydrolysis occurs in warm or alkaline conditions

Dose – IV bolus 0.3–1.1 mg/kg; children 1–2 mg/kg. Infusion 0.1% solution at 2–15 mg/min. It is effective within 30 s and lasts for several minutes

Pharmacokinetics $t_{1/2}$ 3.5

Protein binding occurs but the extent is not known because of the transient nature of the drug

CNS – small increase in ICP which may be of relevance in the head injured patient.

CVS – increased blood pressure, bradycardia

RS – paralysis of respiratory muscles

Other – increases IOP, intragastric pressure and lowers oesophageal sphincter pressure (barrier pressure is increased). Increases gastric secretion and salivary production

Elimination – metabolised by plasma cholinesterase – complete recovery in 10–12 min. Of it, 2–20% is unchanged in urine. The elimination pathway is shown in Figure NJ.9.

Side effects – muscle pains especially muscular, young, male and after early ambulation, malignant hyperthermia trigger. May result in trismus, histamine release and hyperkalaemia – especially if denervation, burns, trauma or renal failure co-exist.

Contra-indications – malignant hyperthermia susceptibility, burns, myotonia.

Suxamethonium is a short-acting depolarising neuromuscular blocking agent. It is rapidly acting by virtue of rapid distribution to the neuromuscular junction and its depolarising mode of action. Its effect is terminated by diffusion away from the neuromuscular junction followed by rapid redistribution and hydrolysis. Hydrolysis occurs in two stages each removing choline. 80% is metabolised before reaching the neuromuscular junction.

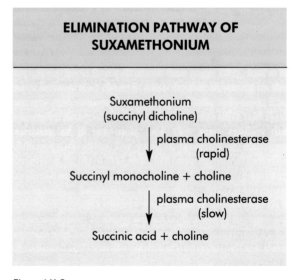

ELIMINATION PATHWAY OF SUXAMETHONIUM

Suxamethonium
(succinyl dicholine)

↓ plasma cholinesterase (rapid)

Succinyl monocholine + choline

↓ plasma cholinesterase (slow)

Succinic acid + choline

Figure NJ.9

ANTI-CHOLINESTERASES

NEOSTIGMINE BROMIDE

Structure – quaternary amine, alkylcarbamic acid ester

Presentation – clear, very pale yellow, aqueous solution in brown ampoule (2.5 mg in 1 ml)

Storage – protect from light

Dose – IV bolus 0.05–0.08 mg/kg. Peak effect 7–11 min; duration 40 min

Pharmacokinetics

V_d	Cl	$t_{1/2}$
700	8	40

Bio-availability after oral administration < 1%

CNS – central hypotensive effect at high dose; miosis, blurred vision

CVS – causes bradycardia and decreases cardiac output

RS – bronchconstriction and reduces anatomical deadspace

Other – increases in all the following: ureteric peristalsis, gastro-intestinal peristalsis, sweating, lacrimation, gastric tone and lower oesophageal sphincter pressure

↑s ACh

Elimination – hydrolysed by the acetyl cholinesterase that it antagonises and by plasma cholinesterase to a quaternary alcohol. Some hepatic metabolism occurs with biliary excretion. Of it, 50–67% is excreted in the urine

Side effects – concomitant administration of anti-cholinergics is essential when used for reversal of neuromuscular blockade. The increased gastro-intestinal tone may promote anastomotic breakdown. Neostigmine inhibits the hydrolysis of suxamethonium and mivacurium and other drugs metabolised by plasma cholinesterase. High levels of neostigmine at the neuromuscular junction causes a direct blockade of the acetyl choline receptor and the raised levels of acetyl choline have a depolarising blocking effect

Pharmacokinetic data for specific drugs are summarised in Figure NJ.10 and the chemical structures of atracurium, vecuronium, suxamethonium and neostigmine are shown in Figure NJ.11.

PHARMACOKINETIC DATA FOR NON DEPOLARISING NEUROMUSCULAR BLOCKING AGENTS

	ED_{95}	Dose	V_d	Clearance	Elimination $t_{1/2}$
	mg/kg	mg/kg	ml/kg	ml/kg/min	min
Atracurium	0.2	0.3–0.6	170	5.5	20
Doxacurium	0.025		220	2.7	99
Mivacurium	0.08	0.07–0.25			
trans-trans isomer			150–267	51–63	1.9–3.6
cis-trans isomer			290–382	93–106	1.8–2.9
cis-cis isomer			175–340	3.7–4.6	34.7–52.9
Org 9487	1.15*	1.5–2.0	293	8.5	74
Pancuronium	0.06	0.05–0.1	200	1.8	115
Pipecuronium	0.049	0.07	309	2.4	137
Rocuronium	0.3	0.6	270	4.0	131
D-Tubocurarine	0.5	0.3–0.5	450	2	120
Vecuronium	0.046	0.05–0.1	260	4.6	62

*Value quoted for ED_{90}

Figure NJ.10

Figure NJ.11 Chemical structures of commonly used neuromuscular drugs. The arrows indicate sites of cleavage (Atracurium – Hofmann degradation; Suxamethonium – ester hydrolysis).

SECTION 3: 9
LOCAL ANAESTHETIC AGENTS

T. C. Smith

STRUCTURE

MECHANISM OF ACTION

FACTORS INFLUENCING ACTIVITY
Molecular weight
Lipid solubility
pKa
pH
Protein binding

CLINICAL EFFECTS
Systemic effects

TOXICITY
Factors affecting local anaesthetic toxicity

ESTER-LINKED AGENTS
Amethocaine
Benzocaine
Cocaine

AMIDE-LINKED AGENTS
Bupivacaine
Levobupivacaine
Lidocaine
Prilocaine
Ropivacaine
EMLA

ADDITIVES
Glucose
Vasoconstrictors
Hyaluronidase
pH Manipulation
Additives with analgesic activity

SPECIFIC PHARMACOLOGY
Bupivacaine hydrochloride
Levobupivacaine
Lidocaine hydrochloride
Prilocaine hydrochloride
Ropivacaine hydrochloride

Local anaesthetic agents are used directly to block neuronal transmission. They also stabilise other electrically excitable membranes, and some examples, such as lidocaine, have clinically useful anti-arrhythmic activity.

STRUCTURE

Local anaesthetic agents comprise a hydrophilic tertiary amine group linked to a lipophilic aromatic group. They are divided into esters and amides based on the linking group. Figure LA.1 shows examples of these two types of local anaesthetic agent. Protonation of the highlighted amine nitrogen atom confers activity on the molecule once it is inside the cell.

Figure LA.1 Chemical structure of an ester (procaine) and an amide (lidocaine)

Local anaesthetic agents exist in two states, acid (protonated) and basic (non-ionised) in equilibrium according to their pKa and ambient pH, as determined by the Henderson–Hasselbach equation (Figure LA.2).

Local anaesthetic agents are weak bases. At physiological pH, there exists a mixture of non-ionised and ionised drug. This is important as only the non-ionised drug passes through the membrane, yet it is only the ionised drug that is active. Small changes in pH have marked effects on the proportion of drug that is ionised and, therefore, markedly influence the effect.

HENDERSON–HASSELBACH EQUATION FOR LOCAL ANAESTHETIC AGENTS (LA)

$$pH = pK_a + \log_{10} \frac{LA \text{ (base)}}{LA-H^+ \text{ (acid)}}$$

Figure LA.2

MECHANISM OF ACTION

Injectable local anaesthetics must be soluble and stable in water. This is achieved by creating hydrochlorides of the drug. These drugs exist within ampoules in acid solution with a high degree of ionisation that maintains solubility.

Local anaesthetic agents act by blocking the fast sodium channel in neuronal membranes. To do so the drug must be in the protonated form and the ion channel must be in the open state. The drug enters the ion channel from the intracellular direction. This process is illustrated in Figure LA.3.

Here, lidocaine is introduced extracellularly. The circled numbers below refer to Figure LA.3.

The pKa of lidocaine is 7.9, so extracellularly (at pH 7.4) 24% is in the non-ionised state and 76% in the ionised state ①. The non-ionised drug is, therefore, relatively lipophilic and passes passively down the concentration gradient through the membrane into the cell ②. Intracellularly, pH is about 7.1 and this shifts the balance of ionisation of the intracellular portion of drug towards the ionised state (86%) ③. The ionised drug, attracted by the negative charge of membrane protein then passes into the open ion channel ④, which remains open but is blocked to further transmission of sodium ⑤. Blockade by this route is use-dependent, because ionophores are only blocked while open.

Another mechanism of action may contribute to the anaesthetic activity. This involves the passage of non-ionised drug through the membrane directly blocking the sodium channel, an effect that does not rely on the sodium channel being open.

FACTORS INFLUENCING ACTIVITY

Figure LA.4 shows the pharmacological properties of important local anaesthetic agents.

MOLECULAR WEIGHT

Molecular weight itself does not affect the pharmacological properties. However, increases in molecular weight tend to be indicative of increased side chain size and, therefore, increased lipid solubility.

LIPID SOLUBILITY

The higher the lipid solubility the greater the penetration of the nerve membrane by the agent, so

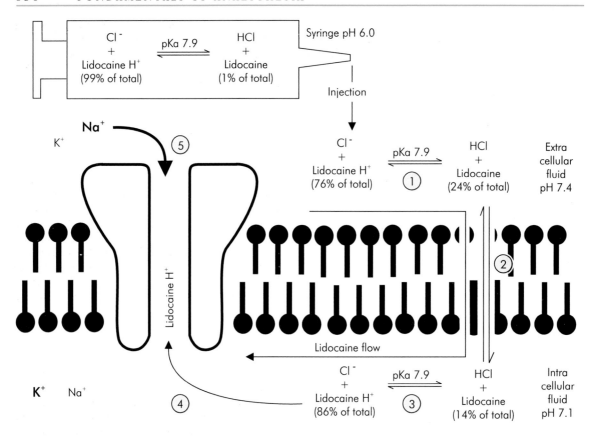

Figure LA.3 Mechanism of action of local anaesthetic agents using lidocaine as an example

PHYSICOCHEMICAL AND PHARMACOKINETIC PROPERTIES OF LOCAL ANAESTHETIC AGENTS

	Molecular weight	pKa (25°C)	Partition coefficient (heptane buffer)	Protein binding (%)	Onset	Potency (relative to lidocaine)	Duration
Esters							
Amethocaine	264	8.5	4.1	76	Slow	4	Long
Procaine	236	8.9	0.02	6	Slow	½	Short
Amides							
Bupivacaine	288	8.1	27.5	96	Medium	4	Long
Lidocaine	234	7.9	2.9	64	Rapid	1	Medium
Prilocaine	220	7.9	0.9	55	Rapid	1	Medium
Ropivacaine	274	8.1	6.1	95	Medium	4	Long

Figure LA.4

that higher lipid solubility results in greater potency. It also results in more toxicity and local irritancy. High lipid solubility also increases the rate of onset and duration of action of local anaesthetic agents.

pKa

The lower the pKa, the lower the degree of ionisation for any given pH and so the more rapid the speed of onset of the block. Increasing pKa increases the ionised proportion of the drug so that intracellularly a higher proportion is in the active state. However, this also means that less is in the non-ionised, diffusible state so the onset and offset of action are also slower. Figure LA.5 shows the effect of differences in pH and pKa on the proportion of ionised and non-ionised local anaesthetic agents.

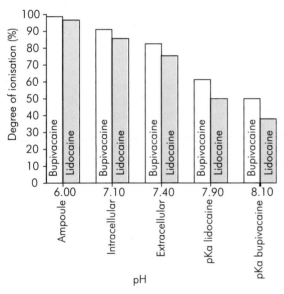

Figure LA.5 Effect of pH on the ionisation of local anaesthetic agents

pH

Acidosis (low pH) increases the proportion of ionised drug in the interstitium and, therefore, reduces the amount of drug able to cross the neuronal membrane. The local anaesthetic is, therefore, reduced in potency. Manipulation of the pH of the local anaesthetic solution by addition of alkali, buffers or carbonation may be used to alter the proportion of non-ionised drug.

PROTEIN BINDING

The degree of protein binding reflects the ability of the drug to bind to membrane proteins; the greater the binding, the longer the duration of action. Increased binding to tissue protein correlates with an increase in the duration of action and probably indicates a higher affinity for membrane proteins (for example, the fast sodium ionophore).

CLINICAL EFFECTS

The opening of the fast sodium channels in neuronal membranes and the passage of sodium through them are essential for the development and propagation of the action potential. The sharp upstroke of the action potential is gradually attenuated as more sodium channels become blocked. When the depolarisation is insufficient to generate the currents required to depolarise neighbouring membrane, then action potential propagation and neuronal transmission cease.

SYSTEMIC EFFECTS

Central nervous system

Central toxicity results from high levels of local anaesthetic agent within the brain. This may be due to direct spread from subarachnoid injection or by excessive systemic absorption. Transfer across the blood-brain barrier is influenced by lipid solubility and ionisation. The toxic CNS effects of local anaesthetic agents are as follows:

- Numbness and paraesthesiae of tongue, mouth and lips
- Metallic taste
- Light-headedness
- Tinnitus
- Slurred speech
- Muscle twitching
- Grand mal convulsions
- Coma
- Apnoea

Apnoea and convulsions result in hypoxia, hypercapnia and metabolic acidosis. The acidosis increases the proportion of ionised local anaesthetic agent. Toxicity results from the presence of ionised drug within the cell blocking the ion channel. Acidosis effectively reduces the proportion of diffusible drug within the cells, and slows clearance.

Cardiovascular system

Most local anaesthetic agents (except cocaine) relax vascular smooth muscle causing vasodilatation. In addition, centrally administered drugs cause vasodilatation by sympathetic blockade. Direct cardiovascular toxicity occurs due to the membrane stabilising activity of the drugs on myocardial muscle, by blocking voltage-gated fast sodium channels. This reduces the maximum rate of rise of the cardiac action potential and reduces the duration of the action potential. Conduction of the action potential through the myocardium is slowed. Cardiac toxicity may result in any of the following effects:

- Prolongation of PR interval
- Supraventricular tachycardia
- Decreased automaticity
- Widening of QRS complex
- Ventricular ectopic beats
- Prolongation of ST interval
- T wave changes

Note that bupivacaine decreases the baseline cardiac membrane potential.

Respiratory system

The respiratory effects of local anaesthetic agents are due to a combination of peripheral neuronal blockade and systemic toxicity. The following effects may be seen:

- Apnoea with systemic toxicity affecting the respiratory centre
- Bronchodilatation secondary to relaxation of bronchial smooth muscle

Other effects

Local anaesthetic drugs have a weak neuromuscular blocking action. Amides block plasma cholinesterase. A direct anti-platelet effect (probably due to membrane stabilisation) reduces platelet aggregation and blood viscosity. These effects are of minor clinical significance.

Anaphylactoid reactions

Anaphylactoid reactions are very rare with amide local anaesthetics, and some of those reported have been due to preservatives (such as metabisulphite and methylparaben). Effects range from local erythema and swelling to systemic hypotension and bronchospasm. More commonly, the reactions are due to co-administration of epinephrine, intravascular injection or psychological effects (vaso-vagal episodes). Reactions are relatively common with esters and cross sensitivity may occur. The metabolism of procaine produces para-amino benzoic acid (PABA) which may be allergenic.

TOXICITY

Effects resulting from systemic absorption of local anaesthetic agent are dependent on the concentration of drug within the plasma. Following an accidental IV bolus the plasma concentration will fall as redistribution and elimination occur, exactly as with other intravenously administered drugs. Slow absorption from a tissue plane (correctly administered drug) will result in much slower rise and lower peak of plasma concentration. The speed of absorption, and

MAXIMUM RECOMMENDED DOSES (and their mg/kg equivalents)				
	Adult dose (mg)		mg/kg equivalent	
	Plain	With epinephrine	Plain	With epinephrine
Ester				
Cocaine	100	*	1.5	*
Amide				
Bupivacaine	150	150	2	2
Levobupivacaine	150	150	2	2
Lidocaine	200	500	3	7
Prilocaine	400	600 (felypressin)	6	8.5 (felypressin)
Ropivacaine**	250	N/A	3.5	N/A

*Unnecessary and contraindicated
**150 mg (2 mg/kg) for epidural Caesarean section

Figure LA.6

elimination rate will determine the maximum plasma concentration which occurs. The maximum recommended doses for various local anaesthetic agents are shown in Figure LA.6.

Toxicity is influenced by:

- Potency of the drug
- Fraction of unbound drug within the plasma
- Peak plasma concentration
- Rate of rise of plasma concentration
- Plasma clearance

Figure LA.7 shows how increasing plasma concentrations of lidocaine produce increasing severity of central nervous and cardiovascular toxicity.

The pattern of toxicity is broadly similar for all local anaesthetic agents but variations exist in the relative severity of the cardiovascular and neurological effects. Bupivacaine has a narrower safety margin between central nervous system and cardiovascular toxicity and is particularly dangerous if cardiac effects do occur, as dissociation from the myocardium is slow, and successful resuscitation following cardiac arrest is

unlikely unless prolonged CPR is instituted. Bupivacaine should not be used for IVRA (Bier's block).

FACTORS AFFECTING LOCAL ANAESTHETIC TOXICITY

Cardiovascular and central nervous system toxicity depend on the mass of drug reaching the systemic circulation. The transfer of drug (by diffusion) from the circulation to organs is determined by the Fick principle. The mass of drug reaching the circulation after peripheral administration is influenced by the following factors:

- Mass of drug administered
- Site of injection
- Tissue protein binding and metabolism
- Vascularity of the injection site

Dose

The volume and concentration of local anaesthetic agents, considered individually, have little influence on systemic spread. Systemically the mass of drug rather than its administered concentration is more important.

Absorption

Absorption from different sites is influenced by the blood flow to the tissue and the uptake of the drug into the vascular compartment, which is a function of solubility. Absorption is in the order of magnitude:

intercostal > epidural > plexus > peripheral > subcutaneous.

Absorption is particularly high when agents are applied topically to mucosa (such as lidocaine spray in the oropharynx). A vasoconstrictor may be added to reduce absorption. Cocaine produces vasoconstriction in its own right and is used on the nasal mucosa to reduce vascularity before some ENT procedures.

Accidental IV injection bypasses the absorption process and subjects the patient to potentially toxic levels of drug. IV regional anaesthesia involves the deliberate introduction of local anaesthetic into the venous system of a limb isolated by tourniquet. The safety of this procedure is dependent on the drug becoming predominantly tissue-bound by the time the tourniquet is released which should not be < 20 min. Further improvements in safety can be achieved by using relatively non cardiotoxic drugs, typically prilocaine.

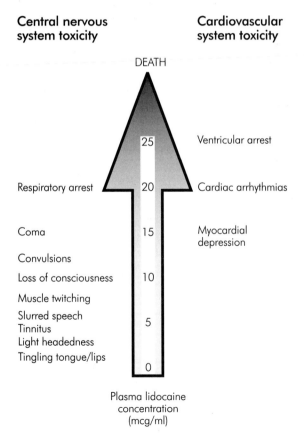

Figure LA.7 Lidocaine toxicity

Distribution

Absorbed drug passes through the lungs where a large amount of the local anaesthetic agent may become tissue-bound and in some cases metabolised. However, this ability is soon saturated by direct IV injection. After passing through the lungs, local anaesthetic drugs reach vessel rich tissues which have a high affinity. Some is distributed to muscle and fat, and later gradually released for subsequent metabolism.

Metabolism

Ester local anaesthetics are rapidly metabolised by plasma cholinesterase and systemic toxicity is rarely a problem. Amide local anaesthetics are metabolised by the liver but hepatic failure must be very severe before local anaesthetic breakdown is compromised. Lidocaine has a high extraction ratio and metabolism is, therefore, dependent on hepatic blood flow, which may be particularly relevant when IV lidocaine is used to stabilise ventricular myocardium in low cardiac output states.

Plasma protein binding

α_1 acid glycoprotein and albumin are the main sites for local anaesthetic binding within the plasma. α_1 acid glycoprotein has a high affinity but a low capacity while albumin has a low affinity but a high capacity for local anaesthetics. Figure LA.8 shows the plasma protein binding of drugs at different plasma concentrations.

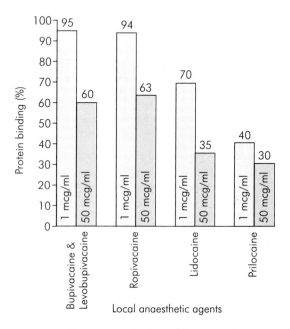

Figure LA.8 Plasma protein binding of drugs at different plasma concentrations

Protein binding acts as a buffer to changes in plasma concentration. The chemical bonds are weak and the protein readily releases the local anaesthetic as concentration falls. Toxicity is, therefore, not directly linked to plasma protein binding, tissue binding is the more important factor.

Pregnancy

Foetal blood rapidly equilibrates with maternal blood levels of free local anaesthetic agent, but as there is more α_1 acid glycoprotein in foetal blood, the overall concentration will be higher. Metabolism is less well developed in the foetus but the drug rapidly passes back to the mother as maternal levels decline; therefore, this does not present a problem. The pH of the foetal fluids is lower than maternal which acts to increase the proportion of ionised local anaesthetic agent.

ESTER LINKED AGENTS

AMETHOCAINE

Amethocaine (tetracaine) is an ester local anaesthetic agent used for topical anaesthesia. It is available as a gel (4%) for local anaesthesia of the skin before intravascular cannulation. Applied to the skin it is effective within 45 min. It can then be removed, and remains active for 4–6 hours. The preparation should not be applied to inflamed or damaged skin or highly vascular tissues as it is rapidly absorbed through mucosal surfaces. More dilute solutions (0.5 and 1%) are available for topical anaesthesia of the conjunctiva. Amethocaine is potent and readily absorbed but in common with other ester local anaesthetics, it may cause hypersensitivity.

BENZOCAINE

Benzocaine is an unusual ester local anaesthetic agent in that the side chain is an ethyl group with no amine component and, therefore, remains unionised. Benzocaine has a low potency but it may cause methaemoglobinaemia. It is a component of some throat lozenges, and may be applied directly to painful skin ulcers.

COCAINE

Cocaine is a naturally occurring ester derived from benzoic acid, and extracted from the leaves of *Erythroxylum coca*. It is available in solution and pastes in concentrations ranging from 1 to 10%. It is mainly used for topical anaesthesia and to reduce bleeding during nasal surgery. Cocaine is rapidly taken up into mucous membranes to provide anaesthesia and intense vasoconstriction. This vasoconstriction limits systemic absorption resulting in a bio-availability by this route of 0.5%. It is well known as a drug of abuse with high addictive potential, and in this role is taken by chewing, inhaling nasally, smoking or intravenously. It causes marked sympathomimetic activity and arrhythmias are a definite risk. Systemic injection must be avoided. Systemically absorbed cocaine has a volume of distribution of 2 l/kg with 98% being protein-bound. It is eliminated by plasma and liver esterases, having a clearance of 35 ml/kg/min and a half-life of 45 min.

Cocaine shares the same mechanism of action as the other local anaesthetic agents (pKa = 8.7) and also inhibits catecholamine neuronal uptake-1. Synaptic levels of dopamine and norepinephrine increase resulting in the central stimulation and euphoria, and vasoconstriction. Cocaine initially blocks the inhibitory pathways resulting in euphoria, hyperthermia, altered vision and hearing, nausea and eventually convulsions. Higher levels of cocaine also block the excitatory pathways resulting in central nervous depression leading to sedation and unconsciousness, with respiratory depression. Cocaine causes mydriasis and raised intra-ocular pressure. It is no longer used for local anaesthesia of the eye. The central stimulation increases respiratory rate and volume. A rise in sympathetic tone leads to tachycardia and hypertension, the latter being exacerbated by peripherally mediated vasoconstriction. High doses depress the myocardium. The general excitation also increases metabolic rate, which contributes to the hyperthermia and raises oxygen consumption and CO_2 production. The recommended maximum dose is 1.5 mg/kg. Cocaine should be avoided in porphyria.

AMIDE LINKED AGENTS

BUPIVACAINE

Bupivacaine is a long-acting local anaesthetic agent with a slow onset of action. Blockade of a large peripheral nerve such as the sciatic nerve may take 60 min depending on the approach but may last up to 48 H. Intrathecal injection in contrast produces an acceptable block within a few minutes. Bupivacaine is particularly prone to causing myocardial depression and, once compromised, reversal may be slow and difficult. In part this is due to the relatively high pKa but an affinity for cardiac proteins is probably more important. Recommendations to minimise systemic toxicity specific to bupivacaine include:

- Avoid bupivacaine for IVRA

- Avoid 0.75% bupivacaine in obstetric practice
- Limit dose to 2 mg/kg

Bupivacaine is predominantly metabolised by N-dealkylation to pipecolyloxylidine. N-desbutyl bupivacaine, and hydroxybupivacaine are also produced. The metabolites are excreted in the urine.

LEVOBUPIVACAINE

Levobupivacaine is the laevorotatory (l or -) enantiomer of racemic bupivacaine. It is clinically similar to racemic bupivacaine. The important differences are dose terminology and toxicity. Levobupivacaine is expressed as milligrams of base rather than of hydrochloride salt so for a given (mg) dose there is 13% more activity. Animal studies demonstrate lower cardiotoxicity but at present the maximum recommended dose remains at 2 mg/kg, and it is contraindicated for IVRA (Bier's block). Lower CNS toxicity is also apparent.

LIDOCAINE (LIGNOCAINE)

Lidocaine is primarily classified as a local anaesthetic agent but is also a Class IB anti-arrhythmic. It has a relatively rapid onset of action and intermediate duration. Combination with a longer acting agent such as bupivacaine may produce a balance of onset and duration between the two component agents alone. The cardiotoxic potential of lidocaine at equivalent levels of central nervous toxicity is about one-ninth that of bupivacaine.

Lidocaine is metabolised in the liver by microsomal oxidases and amidases. N-dealkylation followed by hydrolysis produces ethylglycine, xylidide and other derivatives that are excreted in the urine.

PRILOCAINE

Prilocaine is closely related to lidocaine in terms of pharmacological activity. It has the same pKa (7.9) but is less lipid-soluble. Speed of onset and duration are similar. It is less toxic than lidocaine, due to high tissue fixation, and rapid metabolism of systemically absorbed drug. Prilocaine is the drug of choice for IVRA.

Prilocaine is metabolised in the liver, lungs and kidney to O-toluidine, and then hydroxytoluidine, leaving less than 1% unchanged. O-toluidine is responsible for methaemoglobinaemia.

Methaemoglobinaemia

Metabolism of prilocaine following significant absorption (say after 600 mg), to O-toluidine results in the oxidation of the ferrous ion (Fe^{2+}) of the haem in haemoglobin to ferric (Fe^{3+}) to produce methaemoglobinaemia. This results in cyanosis and the abnormal haemoglobin shifts pulse oximeter **readings** towards 85%. Methaemoglobinaemia is not usually clinically detrimental but when the patient becomes compromised, methylene blue (1–2 mg/kg) may be used as a treatment. Excess methylene blue (> 7 mg/kg) may also cause methaemoglobinaemia, and as the dye has a distinctive spectral absorption it also affects pulse oximeter accuracy.

Children (especially infants) are more susceptible to methaemoglobinaemia because they have under developed metabolic processes and foetal haemoglobin is more easily oxidised. Methaemoglobinaemia also occurs occasionally after application of EMLA cream.

ROPIVACAINE

Ropivacaine is closely related to bupivacaine in terms of pharmacological activity as both drugs are pipecoloxylidides. Ropivacaine is produced as a single enantiomer which has an enantiomeric purity of 99.5% for S-ropivacaine. As ropivacaine is less lipid soluble than bupivacaine and less readily penetrates the neuronal myelin sheaths, C fibres are blocked more readily than A fibres. At high concentrations, the blocking effect is similar for both drugs but at lower concentrations ropivacaine preferentially blocks C fibres over faster than A fibres. Ropivacaine has a potential advantage that motor function can be spared (or show earlier recovery) while still achieving sensory blockade, if a suitable concentration of drug is used. Complete motor and sensory blockade can still be achieved if desired. In summary, ropivacaine provides sensory blockade similar to that of bupivacaine but motor blockade is slower in onset, less pronounced and shorter in duration. Ropivacaine is half as cardiotoxic as bupivacaine. It is mainly bound to α_1 acid glycoprotein in plasma.

EMLA

Eutectic mixture of local anaesthetic (EMLA) is a mixture of 2.5% prilocaine and 2.5% lidocaine used for topical anaesthesia of undamaged skin before intravascular cannulation and minor, superficial dermal and aural surgery. A eutectic mixture is one in which the constituents are in such proportions that the freezing (or melting) point is as low as possible, with the constituents freezing (or melting) simultaneously. The preparation is, therefore, unusual, as the local anaesthetics are not in aqueous solution, and both agents are in their pure form rather than the hydrochloride preparations used in the solutions. In theory, this means that both drugs are in the non-ionised state in EMLA. Once absorbed into the tissues, ionisation will occur. The commercial preparation (EMLA cream 5%) contains carboxypolymethylene and sodium hydroxide resulting in an oil–water emulsion.

ADDITIVES

GLUCOSE

Standard solutions of local anaesthetic agents are slightly hypobaric at body temperature and pH and, therefore, tend to move upwards in the cerebrospinal fluid away from the gravitational pull. Dextrose (glucose) is added to bupivacaine to increase the density of the solution. The specific gravity of hyperbaric (or 'heavy') bupivacaine is 1.026 at 20°C. The specific gravity of cerebrospinal fluid is 1.005 at 37°C, so the injected bupivacaine solution will sink due to gravity. This helps to control the distribution of the local anaesthetic using knowledge of the spinal curves and by manipulating the position of the patient. Note that the specific gravity of a substance or solution is the density of that solution relative to the maximum density of water, which occurs at a temperature of 4°C.

VASOCONSTRICTORS

Epinephrine

Epinephrine is added to local anaesthetic solutions to reduce vascularity of the area by direct vasoconstriction and in turn reduce the systemic uptake of the drug. This has the following effects:

- Increased duration of nerve blockade
- Greater margin of safety for systemic toxicity
- Reduced surgical bleeding

Care must be taken to avoid the systemic effects of epinephrine due to systemic uptake. For example, combination with halothane anaesthesia may result in cardiac arrhythmias, especially ventricular excitation and fibrillation. Epinephrine containing solutions should not be injected in the proximity of end-arteries such as the penile, ophthalmic (central artery of the retina), or digital arteries as there is no collateral circulation to supplement the supply if vasoconstriction is severe. To minimise the risk of serious systemic actions consider the following:

- Avoid hypoxia and hypercarbia
- Use dilute solutions (< 1:200 000)
- Limit of 100 mcg per 10 min
- Limit of 300 mcg per H

Felypressin

Felypressin is an octapeptide derived from vasopressin (ADH). In common with vasopressin, felypressin is a powerful direct acting vasopressor, but it is safe to use with halothane and has no anti-diuretic or oxytocic activity. It may however cause coronary vasoconstriction.

HYALURONIDASE

Hyaluronidase, supplied as a white, fluffy powder, is used to facilitate the spread through connective tissues following subcutaneous or IM injection. In addition to promoting the spread of local anaesthetics and other injections, it is also used to promote re-absorption of fluids and blood from extravascular tissues. Its effect is dependent on the temporary depolymerisation of hyaluronic acid. Hyaluronidase is stable in solution for 24 h at room temperature.

pH MANIPULATION

Alkalination of solutions by addition of bicarbonate increases tissue pH. This results in a higher proportion of non-ionised drug, which diffuses into the neurone more rapidly. Preparation and storage is awkward and the preparations are not widely available.

ADDITIVES WITH ANALGESIC ACTIVITY

Other agents developing roles in central and peripheral nerve blockade are shown in Figure LA.9. These additives are used to provide a synergistic effect on pain

Figure LA.10. Structures of common local anaesthetic drugs
The chiral carbon of bupivacaine (levobupivacaine) is shown in bold (**C**)

perception by interaction with specific receptors in the afferent pathways.

SPECIFIC PHARMACOLOGY

n-Heptane/aqueous phosphate buffer partition coefficient indicates lipid solubility.

N.B: The use of octanol as lipid results in different figures.

Units (unless stated otherwise) are:

Volume of distribution at steady state (V_d) (l/kg)
Clearance (Cl) (ml/kg/min)
Terminal half-life ($t_{1/2}$) (min)

Figure LA.10 shows the chemical formulae of the commonly used local anaesthetic agents.

EVOLVING LOCAL ANAESTHETIC ADDITIVES USED FOR RECEPTOR-MEDIATED ANALGESIC EFFECT

Drug	Receptor	Uses
Opioids	mu/kappa	Central and peripheral
Clonidine	alpha$_2$ adrenergic	Central and peripheral
Ketamine	NMDA	Central

Figure LA.9

BUPIVACAINE HYDROCHLORIDE

Structure – amide local anaesthetic agent, pipecoloxylidide
Presentation – clear, colourless, aqueous solutions include:
Plain solutions (0.25%, 0.5%, 0.75%)
Solutions with 1:200 000 (5 mcg/ml) epinephrine (0.25%, 0.5%)
'Heavy' 0.5% with 80 mg/ml dextrose (specific gravity 1.026) for spinal anaesthesia
Recommended maximum dose – 2 mg/kg (150 mg plus up to 50 mg 2 hourly subsequently)
0.75% is contraindicated in obstetric practise.
Pharmacokinetics

MW	pKa	partition coefficient	protein binding	V_d	Cl	$t_{1/2}$
288	8.1	27.5	96%	1	7	30

Clinical – intermediate speed of onset, long action, four times as potent as lidocaine; propensity to cardiotoxicity
Elimination – 5% excreted as pipecoloxylidine after de-alkylation in the liver, 16% excreted unchanged in urine

LEVOBUPIVACAINE HYDROCHLORIDE

As for Bupivacaine hydrochloride except:
Structure – Levorotatory enantiomer of racemic bupivacaine
Presentation – Plain solutions (2.5 mg/ml, 5.0 mg/ml, 7.5 mg/ml)
Recommended maximum dose – 150 mg (2 mg/kg), total 400 mg in 24 h
7.5 mg/ml contraindicated in obstetric practise.
Pharmacokinetics

MW	pKa	partition coefficient	protein binding	V_d	Cl	$t_{1/2}$
288	8.1	27.5	97%	1	9	80

Clinical – Levobupivacaine doses are expressed as mg of base compound whereas racemic bupivacaine is expressed as the hydrochloride salt. Levobupivacaine therefore has 13% more activity than the same dose of racemic bupivacaine.
Animal studies indicate lower CNS toxicity than bupivacaine.
Elimination – Extensive metabolism with no unchanged levobupivacaine in urine or faeces. The major metabolite is 3-hydroxylevobupivacaine excreted in urine as sulphate and glucuronate conjugates (71% of dose in urine and 24% in faeces by 48 hours).

LIDOCAINE HYDROCHLORIDE

Structure – amide local anaesthetic agent, derivative of diethylaminoacetic acid
Preparation – clear, aqueous solutions include:
Plain solutions (0.5%, 1%, 2%)
Solutions with 1:200 000 (5 mcg/ml) epinephrine (0.5%, 1%, 2%)
Gel (2%) with or without chlorhexidine for urethral instillation
Solutions for surface application to pharynx, larynx and trachea (4%) (coloured pink)
Spray for anaesthesia of the oral cavity and upper respiratory tract (10%)
Dose – topical, infiltration, nerve blocks, epidural and spinal; 0.5–10% available; 100 mg bolus then 1–4 mg/min for ventricular arrhythmias
Recommended maximum dose – 200 mg (3 mg/kg); with epinephrine 500 mg (7 mg/kg)
Pharmacokinetics

MW	pKa	partition coefficient	protein binding	V_d	Cl	$t_{1/2}$
234	7.9	2.9	64%	1	9	100

Clinical – rapid speed of onset, intermediate action; Class IB anti-arrhythmic
Elimination – 70% by de-alkylation in liver, < 10% excreted unchanged in urine

PRILOCAINE HYDROCHLORIDE

Structure – amide local anaesthetic agent, secondary amine derived from toluidine
Preparation – clear, colourless, aqueous solutions include:
Plain solutions (1%, 4%)
Solutions with 0.03 unit/ml felypressin (3%)
Recommended maximum dose – 400 mg (= 6 mg/kg); with felypressin 600 mg (= 8.5 mg/kg)
Pharmacokinetics

MW	pKa	partition coefficient	protein binding	V_d	Cl	$t_{1/2}$
220	7.9	0.9	55%	3.7	40	261

Clinical – rapid speed of onset, intermediate duration of action between lidocaine and bupivacaine, potency similar to lidocaine; may result in methaemoglobinaemia
Elimination – rapidly metabolised to O-toluidine by liver, < 1% excreted unchanged

ROPIVACAINE HYDROCHLORIDE

Structure – amide local anaesthetic agent, pipecoloxylidide

Presentation – clear, colourless, aqueous solutions of S-ropivacaine enantiomer include:

Plain solutions in 10 and 20 ml ampoules (2, 7.5, 10 mg/ml)

Plain solution in 100 and 200 ml bags (2 mg/ml) for epidural infusion

Recommended maximum dose – 250 mg (150 mg for Caesarean section under epidural); cumulative dose of 675 mg over 24 H according to data so far

Pharmacokinetics

MW	pKa	partition coefficient	protein binding	V_d	Cl	$t_{1/2}$
274	8.1	6.1	94%	0.8	10	110

Clinical – intermediate onset, long duration of action between lidocaine and bupivacaine, potency similar to lidocaine; greater separation of sensory and motor blockade, and lower cardiotoxicity than bupivacaine may be advantages

Elimination – aromatic hydroxylation to 3- (and 4-) hydroxy-ropivacaine, and N-dealkylation. 86% (mostly conjugated) excreted in the urine, of which 1% unchanged. 3- and 4-hydroxy-bupivacaine have reduced local anaesthetic activity

Contra-indication – IVRA, obstetric para-cervical block; not yet recommended in children < 12 years of age

SECTION 3: 10
CENTRAL NERVOUS SYSTEM PHARMACOLOGY

T. C. Smith

ANTI-EMETIC AGENTS

Anti-cholinergic drugs
Phenothiazines
Butyrophenones
Anti-histamines
5-Hydroxytryptamine (5-HT$_3$) receptor antagonists
Cannabinoids
Neurokinin receptor antagonists
Peripherally acting anti-emetic agents

SPECIFIC PHARMACOLOGY

ANTI-CONVULSANT DRUGS

Benzodiazepines
Barbiturates
Phenytoin
Carbamazepine
Gabapentin

ANTI-DEPRESSANT DRUGS

Tricyclic anti-depressants
Monoamine oxidase inhibitors (MAOI)
Selective serotonin re-uptake inhibitors (SSRI)
Other anti-depressants
Lithium

ANTI-PSYCHOTIC DRUGS

Phenothiazines
Thioxanthines

ANTI-PARKINSONIAN DRUGS

Levodopa
Carbidopa
Domperidone
Selegiline
Bromocriptine
Amantadine
Acetyl choline antagonists

Many drugs act on the central nervous system (CNS), with specific aims in mind. While certain categories of drugs are considered elsewhere (anaesthetic gases and vapours in Chapter 5, induction agents in Chapter 6) other drugs acting on the CNS have been grouped here. Anti-emetic agents are considered in detail, with specific pharmacology of individual agents to reflect their direct relevance to the practice of anaesthesia.

ANTI-EMETIC AGENTS

The causes of nausea and vomiting (NV) are legion. Anti-emetic therapy is most effective when directed at the likely origin. Figure CN.1 lists the more common causes of NV.

Post operative nausea and vomiting (PONV) is a specific entity. Its treatment is more appropriately directed when other risk factors are considered, and these are summarised in Figure CN.2.

Two distinct sites in the CNS, the vomiting centre and the chemoreceptor trigger zone, are implicated in the causes of NV. The chemoreceptor trigger zone lies in the area postrema outside the blood-brain barrier and possesses dopaminergic (D_2) and serotonergic (5-hydroxytryptamine, 5-HT_3) receptors. In contrast, the vomiting centre is a complex entity located in the dorsolateral reticular formation of the brainstem that possesses 5-HT_3, D_2 and muscarinic (M_3) receptors.

CAUSES OF NAUSEA AND VOMITING

Drug induced
　　Central effect – opioids, nitrous oxide
　　Local effect – poisons, copper, sodium chloride
　　Systemic effect – cytotoxic drugs
Pregnancy
Radiotherapy
Psychogenic
Vestibular
　　Labyrinthitis
　　Ménière's disease
　　Motion sickness

Stimulation of vagal afferents in the pharynx
Hypotension
Migraine
Abdominal pathology
Raised intracranial pressure

Figure CN.1

FACTORS AFFECTING THE INCIDENCE OF POST OPERATIVE NAUSEA AND VOMITING

Female > male
Children > adults > elderly
Increased if pathology is:　　gynaecological
　　　　　　　　　　　　　　intractable
　　　　　　　　　　　　　　intra-oral
Increased by gastro-intestinal stasis

Figure CN.2

Histaminic H_1 and neurokinin (NK_1) receptors are located in the nucleus of the tractus solitarius which integrates afferent signals associated with emesis. The interaction of various drugs with these sites is displayed graphically in Figure CN.3.

The major classes of drug used to combat NV possess receptor antagonism at D_2, M_3, histaminic (H_1) and 5-HT_3 receptors. The more common agents and their receptor specificity are shown in Figure CN.4.

Anti-emetic activity is ascribed to the following categories of drug – anti-cholinergic agents, phenothiazines, butyrophenones, anti-histamines, 5-HT_3 receptor antagonists, neurokinin receptor antagonists and cannabinoids. Additionally, metoclopramide and domperidone are two peripherally acting anti-emetic agents of importance.

ANTI-CHOLINERGIC DRUGS

Examples – atropine, hyoscine

Atropine and hyoscine cross the blood-brain barrier (unlike glycopyrollate, another commonly used anti-cholinergic drug) and act on muscarinic cholinergic receptors in the vomiting centre and in the gastro-intestinal tract. Anti-cholinergic agents are anti-spasmodic, reducing intestinal tone and inhibiting sphincter relaxation. They also reduce salivary and gastric secretions and so reduce gastric distension. These are the drugs of choice for the treatment of motion sickness and opioid induced nausea. Hyoscine has been popular for premedication in conjunction with opioids for this reason, and because it possesses a sedative effect. The side effects of anti-cholinergic drugs are predictable from the known effects of muscarinic cholinergic receptors. In particular, dry mouth and blurred vision can be a problem, and drowsiness is not uncommon. Bronchial secretions are rendered more viscid, but a degree of bronchodilatation

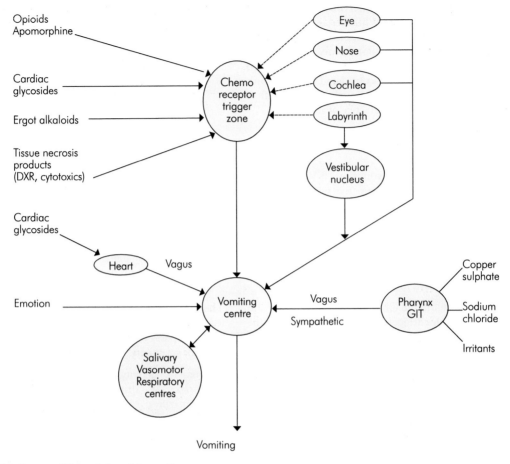

Figure CN.3. Causes of NV and sites of drug action

FREQUENTLY USED DRUGS AND THEIR RECEPTOR ANTAGONISM

	D_2	M_3	H_1	$5\text{-}HT_3$
Hyoscine	0	++++	+	0
Promethazine	+	++	+++	0
Chlorpromazine	++	+	++	+
Metoclopramide	+	0	+	++
Droperidol	+++	0	+	+
Ondansetron	0	0	0	++++
Prochlorperazine	++++	+	+	0

Figure CN.4

THE CENTRAL ANTICHOLINERGIC SYNDROME

Causes

Muscarinic anticholinergic drugs which cross the blood-brain barrier (typically atropine and hyoscine).

Risk Factors

Elderly patients most at risk

Features

Excitement
Drowsiness
Ataxia
Coma

Figure CN.5

is seen (increasing anatomical dead space). Pupillary constriction may be abolished, which removes a useful indicator of depth of anaesthesia. Anti-cholinergic agents that cross the blood-brain barrier are implicated in the development of the central anti-cholinergic syndrome, which is detailed in Figure CN.5.

Treatment of the central anti-cholinergic syndrome is accomplished by the use of an anti-cholinesterase that can cross the blood-brain barrier. In practice, this requires a tertiary amine structure and, thus, physostigmine is the drug of choice, although availability may be a problem.

PHENOTHIAZINES

Examples – prochlorperazine, perphenazine, promethazine

Phenothiazines have a variety of effects including anti-emesis. Trifluoperazine is a potent anti-emetic, but its anti-psychotic effects preclude its use as a routine anti-emetic. Phenothiazines act on the D_2 receptors in the chemoreceptor trigger zone in the area postrema, and on M_3 receptors in the same way as anti-cholinergic agents. The major effect of promethazine is anti-histaminic, although it has anti-dopaminergic and anti-muscarinic activity that contribute to the anti-emetic effect. Sedation may limit the usefulness of promethazine as an anti-emetic agent. 6 mg of buccal prochlorperazine may be a useful alternative to im injection.

BUTYROPHENONES

Examples – benperidol, droperidol, haloperidol

Droperidol is an antagonist of D_2 receptors in the chemoreceptor trigger zone. It has potent anti-emetic activity but can cause a dissociative phenomena even in relatively small doses, when the patient appears outwardly content but experiences an unpleasant feeling of helplessness and vulnerability.

Haloperidol and benperidol are primarily used as anti-psychotic agents but haloperidol possesses substantial anti-convulsant activity. It causes α_1 adrenoreceptor blockade which may result in postural hypotension.

Butyrophenones are metabolised in the liver. Side effects include extrapyramidal phenomena, neuroleptic malignant syndrome and hyperprolactinaemia with gynaecomastia.

ANTI-HISTAMINES

Examples – diphenhydramine, cyclizine, buclizine, cinnarizine

Several categories of drug may show anti-histaminic activity. Figure CN.6 lists the main categories.

ANTI-EMETIC DRUGS WITH ANTIHISTAMINE ACTIVITY	
Ethanolamines	Diphenhydramine
	Dimenhydrinate
Piperazines	Cyclizine
	Buclizine
	Cinnarizine
Phenothiazines	Promethazine

Figure CN.6

'Anti-histamine' is a term used for a group of chemically different agents that are antagonists at histaminergic receptors. Despite the discovery of a second type of histamine receptor (H_2 in gastric mucosa), the general term 'anti-histamine' is used to describe anti-H_1 drugs alone. These are particularly effective in the treatment and prevention of motion sickness. The anti-emetic action is centrally mediated, but H_1 antagonism may not be the sole mechanism of anti-emesis. The sedative effects of anti-histamines contribute to the treatment of nausea.

Ethanolamines (such as diphenhydramine) are potent anti-histamines with some anti-cholinergic activity, which are thought to work at the labyrinth and the neural interface between the labyrinth and the vomiting centre.

Cyclizine is used for motion sickness and for PONV. It has anti-cholinergic activity resulting in dry mouth and can cause tachycardia if given intravenously. Cinnarizine is almost insoluble in water and only available in the tablet form. Buclizine has a long duration of action but is only available in combined formulation with other drugs.

5-HYDROXYTRYPTAMINE (5-HT_3) RECEPTOR ANTAGONISTS

Examples – granisetron, ondansetron, tropisetron

There are four basic types of serotonergic (5-HT) receptors (5-HT_{1-4}). 5-HT_1 receptors are subdivided further (5-HT_{1A}, etc.). An especially high density of 5-HT_3 receptors is found in the area postrema and nucleus tractus solitarius where they are probably on the vagus nerve terminals. Receptors have also been identified on peripheral sections of the vagus nerve in the gastro-intestinal tract and the emetogenic effect of 5HT release can also be blocked here.

CANNABINOIDS

Example – nabilone

Cannabis is derived from the plant *Cannabis sativa*. The active constituents of cannabis are called cannabinoids. Δ-9-tetrahydrocannibol is the major active cannabinoid. A specific cannabinoid receptor has been identified in the CNS and it is thought that cannabinoids act at the chemoreceptor trigger zone. Naloxone may be used to overcome their effects. Nabilone is a synthetic derivative of the naturally occurring tetrahydrocannibol. It is effective against NV induced by opioids, cytotoxic and radiotherapy. Taken orally it is well absorbed and has a half-life of 120 min. Indications for cannabinoid therapy are limited by the side effects of hallucinations, psychosis, dizziness and dry mouth.

NEUROKININ RECEPTOR ANTAGONISTS

Example – GR205171

Selective neurokinin (NK_1) receptor antagonists have been shown to have anti-emetic activity via the nucleus of the tractus solitarius and dorsal motor nucleus of the vagus nerve. GR205171 has a broader spectrum of anti-emetic activity than 5-HT_3 antagonists. It has a half-life of 8H.

PERIPHERALLY ACTING ANTI-EMETIC AGENTS

Examples – metoclopramide, domperidone

Metoclopramide and domperidone are chemically unrelated yet functionally similar. Metoclopramide hydrochloride is a white crystalline salt that is chemically related to procaine. It is readily soluble and stable in water. It has anti-dopaminergic (D_2) activity in the chemoreceptor trigger zone and also inhibits the emetic effects of gastric irritants. It also antagonises H_1 and 5-HT_3 receptors and promotes gastric emptying through the pylorus. Extrapyramidal effects (such as oculogyric crisis) are the major potential side effects. Metoclopramide is indicated for PONV, opioid-induced nausea and NV related to cytotoxic drug treatment and radiotherapy.

Domperidone is a benzimidazole derivative that has both centrally and peripherally mediated effects. Peripherally domperidone promotes gastric emptying and increases lower oesophageal sphincter tone. It crosses the blood-brain barrier (but only slowly) and then acts on dopamine receptors in the chemoreceptor trigger zone. This impaired transit across the blood-brain barrier reduces the incidence of extrapyramidal side effects. Domperidone is indicated for the treatment of PONV and opioid-induced NV but it is limited in its application as it cannot be given parenterally. The major application of the drug is in the treatment of cytotoxic and radiotherapy-induced NV.

Miscellaneous anti-emetics

Sedatives and anxiolytics often have an anti-emetic effect by reducing the psychological component of the nausea. Propofol appears to reduce PONV.

Betahistine is a histamine analogue used for the treatment of Ménière's disease and its associated NV.

High doses of methylprednisolone or dexamethasone (glucocorticoids) are useful against the nausea of cytotoxic agents. Their mode of action is not known.

SPECIFIC PHARMACOLOGY

Here, the units (unless stated) are:

Volume of distribution at steady state (V_d) (l/kg)
Clearance (Cl) (ml/kg/min)
Terminal half-life ($t_{1/2}$) (H)

CYCLIZINE HYDROCHLORIDE AND LACTATE

Structure – piperazine
Presentation – tablet 50 mg, IV/IM 50 mg in 1 ml, and in combination with morphine
Pharmacokinetics

Bio-availability	$t_{1/2}$
80%	10

Blood-brain barrier – crossed
CNS – anti-emetic, with some sedation
CVS – slight tachycardia
RS – minimal effect
Other – increase in lower oesophageal sphincter pressure
Elimination – N-demethylation to norcyclizine (half-life 20 H, minimal activity), and also some to the oxide
Side effects – anti-cholinergic; dry mouth, blurred vision, drowsiness

DOMPERIDONE

Structure – butyrophenone derivative
Presentation – tablets 10 mg, suppositories 30 mg
Pharmacokinetics

Bio-availability	protein binding	$t_{1/2}$	V_d
15%	92%	7.5	5.7

Blood-brain barrier – poorly crossed
CNS – anti-emetic, acting predominantly outside the brain, but some antagonism of D_2 receptors in the chemoreceptor trigger zone
CVS – minimal effect
RS – minimal effect
Others – acts on peripheral dopaminergic (D_2) neurones. Increased lower oesophageal sphincter tone, increased gastric emptying, increased prolactin secretion
Elimination – metabolised by hydroxylation and oxidative N-dealkylation (90%); 30% in urine, 60% in faeces
Side effects – galactorrhoea, gynaecomastia

DROPERIDOL

Structure – butyrophenone
Presentation – tablets 10 mg, IV/IM 10 mg in 2 ml clear colourless solution. No longer available in UK.
Phamacokinetics

Protein binding	$t_{1/2}$	V_d	Cl
90%	12	2	15

Blood-brain barrier – crossed
CNS – anxiolysis, placid state, indifference to environment, may be unpleasant feelings of helplessness not outwardly expressed; anti-emesis via central D_2 antagonism in the chemoreceptor trigger zone
CVS – vasodilation and decreased arterial pressure due to α-adrenergic blockade may occur when given intravenously
RS – minute volume, functional residual capacity and airway resistance all slightly decreased
Elimination – oxidative N-dealkylation in the liver
Side effects – extrapyramidal effects, gastro-intestinal dysfunction

METOCLOPRAMIDE HYDROCHLORIDE

Structure – chlorinated procainamide derivative
Presentation – tablets 10 mg, syrup 1 mg/ml; IV 10 mg in 2 ml
Pharmacokinetics

Protein binding	$t_{1/2}$	V_d	Cl
18%	4	2.8	10

CNS – anti-emetic via chemoreceptor trigger zone, and by decreasing afferent activity from viscera to vomiting centre

CVS – some reports of hypotension, dysrrythmias and cardiac arrest
RS – minimal effects
Others – lower oesophageal sphincter pressure increased, gastric contractility and emptying increased, small intestine transport time accelerated; prolactin and aldosterone secretion increased; may increase ureteric peristalsis
Elimination – 80% in urine within 24 H of which 20% unchanged, the rest conjugated or as sulphated metabolite
Side effects – drowsiness, dizziness, extrapyramidal effects

ONDANSETRON HYDROCHLORIDE

Structure – 5-HT_3 receptor antagonist
Presentation – tablets 4 mg; IV 4 mg in 2 ml (protect from light)
Pharmacokinetics

Bio-availability	$t_{1/2}$	V_d	Cl
60%	3	1.8	6

CNS – anti-emetic
CVS – no effect with therapeutic doses
RS – no effect on respiratory regulation
Others – antagonises $5HT_3$ receptors on vagal afferents in small intestine, no effect on platelet function, or prolactin secretion
Elimination – extensively metabolised in liver, main metabolite 8-hydroxyondansetron; metabolites conjugated; <5% unchanged via urine
Side effects – constipation, headache, flushing

PROCHLORPERAZINE

Structure – piperazine phenothiazine
Presentation – tablets 5 or 25 mg, buccal tablets 3 mg, suppositories 5 or 25 mg, IM clear colourless solution 12.5 mg in 1 ml
Pharmacokinetics

$t_{1/2}$	V_d
6	20

Blood-brain barrier – crossed
CNS – anti-emetic with neuroleptic effects, acting via dopaminergic (D_2) receptors
CVS – α blockade occasionally causes postural hypotension; QT increased, ST depressed, T and U wave changes on ECG
RS – mild respiratory depressant effect
Other – lower oesophageal sphincter tone increased, anti-adrenergic activity, anti-histaminic and anti-cholinergic effects
Elimination – S-oxidation to a sulphoxide by the liver
Side effects – extrapyramidal effects

MODES OF ACTION OF ANTICONVULSANTS

GABA facilitation	Benzodiazepines
	Barbiturates
GABA agonism	Progabide
GABA transaminase inactivation	Valproate Vigabatrin
Fast sodium channel blockade	Phenytoin
Presynaptic sodium channel stabilisation	Lamotrigine Valproate

Figure CN.7

ANTICONVULSANT DRUGS

Epileptic events are the result of repetitive neuronal discharges in the CNS involving many neurones. Anticonvulsant drugs act by breaking these propagating and recycling currents either by increasing inhibitory neurotransmitter levels or by facilitating their action by modulating the γ-amino butyric acid (GABA) receptor function. There is the potential for new drugs to be developed that would inhibit excitatory neurotransmitters and their receptors (the N-methyl-D-aspartate agonist-receptor interaction is a likely target). The modes of action of anticonvulsants are listed in Figure CN.7.

The drug chosen for treatment of epilepsy depends greatly on the type of fits. Figure CN.8 shows treatment guidelines for different types of epilepsy.

In pregnancy, most anticonvulsant drugs carry a risk of causing neural tube defects, teratogenicity and coagulation disorders in the newborn. Counselling, antenatal screening, folate supplements and pre delivery vitamin K should be considered. The greatest risk to mother and baby, however, is that of the re-emergence of convulsions. Fears about the drugs may lead to poor compliance in the complacent patient. In addition, the increase in body water during pregnancy will dilute the concentration of the anticonvulsant agent thereby reducing its clinical effect.

BENZODIAZEPINES

Examples – clobazam, clonazepam, diazepam

Benzodiazepines act by attaching to a specific area of the GABA–receptor complex. The benzodiazepine has an agonist activity at this site that facilitates the opening of the chloride channel by GABA. Chloride ions then flow down the concentration gradient into the cell making it hyperpolarised (more negative) and so less excitable.

Diazepam is primarily used for the acute treatment of convulsions. It has the disadvantage of pronounced sedation, long half-life and active metabolite. Other benzodiazepines may be used prophylactically.

BARBITURATES

Examples – phenobarbitone, primidone

All barbiturates possess anticonvulsant activity but phenobarbitone is less sedative for a given anticonvulsant activity. It binds to the GABA receptor at a site distinct from the benzodiazepine receptor area, and facilitates the chloride channel opening. It is inhibitory at some excitatory synapses.

The barbiturate primidone acts by being converted to phenobarbitone.

PHENYTOIN

Phenytoin is a hydantoin that also has local anaesthetic and anti-arrhythmic properties. It has structural similarities with the barbiturates. The site of action of phenytoin is the fast sodium channel responsible for depolarisation during an action potential. It binds to the channel when it is refractory following opening and is, therefore, most effective when repetitive discharges occur. It may also interfere with calcium entry and with calmodulin protein kinases. Phenytoin can cause hirsuitism, gum hyperplasia, megaloblastic anaemia and foetal malformations.

There is the potential for interaction with other drugs including other anticonvulsants. The high degree of protein binding (85% bound to albumin) results in competition for the binding site with salicylates, phenylbutazone and valproate. Phenytoin metabolism is competitively inhibited by phenobarbitone due to enzyme induction in the liver. The same hepatic microsomal enzymes are induced by phenytoin, phenobarbitone, steroids, oestrogens and coumarins. In the same manner as for ethanol the enzyme system is readily saturated so that as doses increase the metabolism changes from first-order kinetics (metabolism proportional to concentration) to zero-order kinetics (metabolism constant and maximal), thus, 'half-life' subsequently increases with dose.

TYPES OF EPILEPSY AND DRUG CHOICE

Status epilepticus

First line	IV diazepam
Subsequently	Phenytoin or Phenobarbitone or Chlormethiazole or Paraldehyde

Prevention

Absences (petit mal)	Ethosuximide or Valproate
Tonic-clonic	Carbamazepine or Phenytoin or Valproate or Phenobarbitone
Myoclonic	Valproate or Clonazepam or Ethosuximide
Atypical (Usually childhood especially if any cerebral damage)	Clonazepam or Ethosuximide or Lamotrigine or Phenobarbitone or Phenytoin or Valproate

Figure CN.8

CARBAMAZEPINE

Carbamazepine is structurally similar to the tricyclic anti-depressants and has pharmacological similarities with phenytoin but the precise mode of action is not known. With chronic usage, the half-life decreases from 30 to 15 H due to enzyme induction.

GABAPENTIN

Gabapentin is an amino-acid. The postulated mechanisms of action are listed in Figure CN.9.

Gabapentin is used as adjunct treatment for partial seizures. It is also used to treat neuropathic pain, trigeminal neuralgia and post-herpetic neuralgia.

VALPROATE

Sodium valproate is a monocarboxylic acid that increases brain levels of GABA by inhibiting GABA-transaminase and inactive pre-synaptic Na^+ channels. It is used for petit mal, myoclonic epilepsy and infantile spasms. It also has a role in the management of chronic pain especially trigeminal neuralgia. It interferes with platelet numbers and function, and can cause neural tube defects.

LAMOTRIGINE

Lamotrigine stabilises inactive presynaptic sodium channels and so reduces neurotransmitter release. It is used to treat partial seizures, tonic-clonic and myoclonic seizures. Concentrations are increased by carbamazepine and phenytoin (enzyme inducers) and reduced by valproate.

VIGABACTRIN

Vigabactrin binds to and inhibits GABA transaminase resulting in increased GABA levels. It is used for partial epilepsy in combination therapy and as a sole agent for the treatment of the brief infantile spasms of West syndrome. Particular concerns are that a third of patients develop visual field defects and it may cause behavioural problems.

ANTIDEPRESSANT AGENTS

There are several different classes of antidepressant agents. The classic groups of tricyclic agents and inhibitors of monoamine oxidase have recently been

POSTULATED MECHANISMS OF ACTION FOR GABAPENTIN

Competes with Leu, Ile, Val, Phe for specific amino acid transmembrane transporter
Increases concentration and synthesis of brain GABA
Binds to and modulates voltage sensitive Ca^{++} channels
Reduces release of monoamine transmitter (norepinephrine, dopamine and 5-HT)
Inhibits voltage sensitive Na channels
Increases 5-HT
Prevents neuronal death by inhibition of glutamate synthesis

Figure CN.9

joined by the serotonin re-uptake inhibitors, and norepinephrine re-uptake inhibitors. The major categories of antidepressant drugs are listed in Figure CN.10.

Miscellaneous agents unrelated either structurally or functionally may also show antidepressant activity. Among these are nomifensine, maprotiline, venlafaxine, nefazodone, flupenthixol and L-tryptophan.

TRICYCLIC ANTIDEPRESSANTS

Examples – dibenzazepines (clomipramine, imipramine), dibenzcycloheptenes (amitriptyline, nortriptyline)

Tricyclic antidepressants are chemically related to the phenothiazines, but differ in that the central ring has an additional carbon atom. This changes the shape of the molecule from the planar phenothiazine molecule to a three-dimensional skeleton. Tricyclic antidepressants act by preventing re-uptake of neurotransmitter (norepinephrine primarily) into the nerve terminal of monoaminergic neurones. This action is stronger at noradrenergic and serotinergic sites than dopaminergic sites. Some drugs also act on presynaptic α_2 receptors to increase neurotransmitter release. Tricyclic agents also antagonise muscarinic cholinergic (amitriptyline is used in the treatment of nocturnal enuresis), H_1 histaminergic, and α_1 adrenergic receptors. In addition to the antidepressant effects, they cause sedation, weakness and fatigue. Cardiac effects include postural hypotension, sinus tachycardia and cardiac arrhythmias. Amitriptyline prolongs the PR and QT intervals on the ECG. In the plasma tricyclic antidepressants are 90–95% bound to albumin, and may become displaced by drugs such as aspirin which compete for the same binding sites.

While re-uptake blockade occurs soon after administration, the onset of antidepressant action takes several weeks to develop. It is not clear why this is so but it may be due to down-regulation of adrenergic and 5-HT receptors.

Tricyclic agents are metabolised by hepatic microsomal enzymes, and are, therefore, competitively antagonised by some neuroleptic drugs which share the same route of excretion. There are two main methods of metabolism; either N-demethylation converting the tertiary amine to a secondary amine, or ring hydroxylation.

MONOAMINE OXIDASE INHIBITORS (MAOI)

Examples – hydrazines (iproniazid, phenelzine), propargylamines (pargyline, selegiline), cyclopropylamines (tranylcypromine)

Two variants of monoamine oxidase have been described (MAO-A and -B). MAO-A is more effective at oxidising norepinephrine and 5-HT than MAO-B, but types A and B are equally effective in the metabolism of dopamine and tyramine. Antidepressant activity is conferred by inhibition of MAO-A. MAOI's act by antagonising the breakdown of monoamine neurotransmitters after uptake into the nerve terminal.

The classical MAOIs are irreversible (although a new class of reversible MAOIs now exists). Pargyline, phenelzine, tranylcypromine and iproniazid non-selectively inhibit both MAO-A and MAO-B, while clorygyline is selective for MAO-A. Selegiline is selective for MAO-B and is, therefore, not antidepressant but is used in Parkinsonism acting by inhibition of dopamine oxidation. Re-uptake blockade occurs soon after administration, but the onset of antidepressant action takes several weeks to develop. In a similar fashion to the tricyclic antidepressants, this may be due to down-regulation of adrenergic and 5-HT receptors. Patients being treated with MAOI drugs also become compromised in their ability to metabolise exogenously administered amines. The pressor effect of tyramine (which is found in cheese, broad beans, red wine and marmite) is greatly enhanced. Indirect sympathomimetic drugs such as those found in cough medicines will show enhanced effects. A specific

CLASSES OF ANTIDEPRESSANTS

Tricyclic antidepressants	Dibenzazepines
	Bibenzcycloheptenes
Monoamine oxidase inhibitors	Hydrazines
	Propargylamines
	Cyclopropylamines
	Reversible MAOI (RIMA)

Selective serotonin re-uptake inhibitors (SSRI)
Serotonin/norepinephrine reuptake inhibitor (SNRI)
Selective norepinephrine reuptake inhibitor (NARI)
Noradrenergic and specific serotonergic antidepressants (NaSSA)

Other antidepressants	Lithium

Figure CN.10

interaction with pethidine may result in profound coma.

Reversible MAOIs

Example – moclobemide

These drugs reversibly inhibit MAO-A (also called RIMA – reversible inhibition of MAO-A). Caution should still be exercised with foods rich in tyramine and sympathomimetic agents but the problem is likely to be less marked. The advantage of RIMAs is that they can be stopped and another antidepressant started without the need to wait several weeks for MAO enzyme regeneration.

SELECTIVE SEROTONIN RE-UPTAKE INHIBITORS (SSRI)

Examples – fluoxetine, paroxetine, sertraline

SSRIs act by increasing the level of 5-HT at the neuronal receptors. The specificity for 5-HT results in fewer anti-muscarinic and cardiac side effects than other antidepressants. Sedation is less marked than with the tricyclic antidepressants. Diarrhoea and NV are more common, and headache, restlessness and anxiety may occur. Withdrawal should be slow, over several weeks, and MAOI therapy should not be started until 2–5 weeks after stopping the SSRI treatment (dependent on which drug was being taken). SSRI should not be started until 2 weeks after stopping MAOI therapy.

SEROTONIN/NOREPINEPHRINE REUPTAKE INHIBITOR

Example – venlafaxine

Serotonin/norepinephrine reuptake inhibitors (SNRI) inhibit both norepinephrine and serotonin (5-HT) neuronal reuptake. Venlafaxine is a bicyclic phenylethylamine antidepressant that inhibits presynaptic reuptake of 5-HT, norepinephrine and to a much lesser extent dopamine. There is no effect on adrenergic, cholinergic or histaminergic **receptors**. The specificity results in lower adverse effects than with the tricyclic antidepressants

SELECTIVE NOREPINEPHRINE REUPTAKE INHIBITOR

Example – reboxetine

Reboxetine is a selective inhibitor of norepinephrine reuptake. Again the specificity results in lower adverse effects than with the tricyclic antidepressants

NORADRENERGIC AND SPECIFIC SEROTONERGIC ANTIDEPRESSANTS

Example – mirtazapine

Mirtazapine increases norepinephrine and 5-HT neurotransmission by blockade of α_2 adrenoceptors and also blocks 5-HT$_2$ and 5-HT$_3$ receptors. The 5-HT$_3$ blockade reduces the incidence of nausea. The specificity results in lower adverse effects than the tricyclic antidepressants

LITHIUM

Lithium is used prophylactically to suppress the manic element of bipolar depression (manic depressive psychosis). It is unclear how the pharmacological activity of lithium produces the clinical effect. The active component of lithium carbonate is the lithium cation (Li$^+$). Chemically lithium is the first element in group IA of the periodic table (same group as sodium and potassium). It has the atomic number 3 and a molecular weight of 7. It mimics cations, especially sodium. It passes through the fast sodium channels easily being smaller, but the Na$^+$K$^+$ATPase pump does not readily extract lithium from the cells, and it, therefore, tends to accumulate intracellularly, which in turn displaces potassium and reduces the outward leakage of potassium responsible for maintaining the negative intracellular potential. In this way, the transmembrane potential becomes reduced and neuronal depolarisation is facilitated. Lithium also reduces brain levels of norepinephrine and 5-HT acutely, reduces cyclic AMP production, and reduces inositol triphosphate.

Lithium has a low therapeutic index and plasma levels should, therefore, be maintained between 0.4–1.0 mmol/l. Toxicity occurs with levels of over 2.0 mmol/l. The half-life of the extracellular ion is about 12 H and lithium should be stopped 2–3 days before using a muscle-relaxant drug. This is particularly important for non depolarising relaxants that are potentiated. It may also delay the onset and prolong relaxation with suxamethonium. The intracellular lithium takes a further 1–2 weeks to excrete. Lithium inhibits anti-diuretic hormone (ADH) activity in the kidney via cyclic AMP and increases aldosterone secretion which can result in renal tubular damage. Lithium inhibits thyroid hormone release and thyroid hypertrophy and hypothyroidism may occur. Neurological effects include thirst, tremor, muscle weakness, confusion and seizures. Cardiac arrhythmias may be induced and all toxic effects are enhanced if dehydration occurs. Close monitoring of clinical state, lithium levels and renal function is essential to minimise toxicity.

ANTI-PSYCHOTIC DRUGS

A wide variety of drugs has anti-psychotic activity. These have been variously referred to as neuroleptics, major tranquillisers and anti-schizophrenia drugs. Specific categories of drug that have anti-psychotic activity include:

- Phenothiazines
- Butyrophenones
- Thioxanthines
- Benzamide
- Diphenylbutylpiperazine
- Dibenzodiazepines

The mode of action of these drugs in the treatment of psychosis is not precisely known. Various receptor systems have been implicated including dopaminergic, noradrenergic and 5-hydroxytryptaminergic (serotonergic). It is likely that many different receptors are affected, but D_2 dopaminergic receptors are currently thought to be the most important. While D_1 receptors increase adenylate cyclase activity generally, D_2 receptors are found both pre- and post-synaptically and blocking potency at these receptors correlates closely with clinical potency. The delay in onset of a therapeutic effect from these drugs may in part be explained by a slow increase in the numbers of D_2 receptors over several weeks. Some anti-psychotic drugs are formulated so that they may be administered by deep IM injection given at intervals of 1–4 weeks.

As anti-psychotic agents affect so many receptors, a wide diversity of adverse effects results. These are listed in Figure CN.11.

PHENOTHIAZINES

Phenothiazines may be classified chemically by the side chain on the nitrogen atom of the phenothiazine base as follows:

- Aliphatic – chlorpromazine
- Piperazine – fluphenazine
- Piperidine – thioridazine

The side chains alter the potency and specificity for the receptor types and in turn alter the clinical features (Figure CN.12).

THIOXANTHINES

Examples – flupenthixol, zuclopenthixol

Thioxanthines are similar in structure and function to the aliphatic phenothiazines and, therefore, block D_2 receptors more than D_1. Flupenthixol is also employed clinically as an antidepressant agent.

ADVERSE EFFECTS OF ANTIPSYCHOTIC DRUGS

Anti dopaminergic
    Antiemesis
    Extrapyramidal features
        Facial grimacing
        Involuntary movements of tongue and limbs
        Oculogyric crises
        Torsion spasms
    Tasikinesia
    Akithisia
    Parkinsonism
    Tardive dyskinesia
    Increased prolactin secretion

Anti muscarinic
    Dry mouth
    Constipation
    Urinary retention
    Blurred vision
    Precipitation of glaucoma

Anti alpha adrenergic
    Postural hypotension

Anti histaminergic
    Sedation

Figure CN.11

Other miscellaneous anti-psychotic drugs include: sulpiride, which has a greater affinity for D_2 than D_1 receptors; pimozide, which may prolong QT interval on the ECG; and clozapine, which has been associated with agranulocytosis.

ANTI-PARKINSONIAN DRUGS

Parkinson's disease is caused by a dysfunction within the basal ganglia. The predominant change is a deficit of dopamine with an increase in dopamine D_2 receptors but other neurotransmitters are also implicated in the pathology of the disease. Drugs that affect Parkinson's disease may act in any of the following ways:

- Increased dopamine synthesis (levodopa)
- Decreased peripheral conversion of L-DOPA (carbidopa)
- Decreased dopamine breakdown (selegiline)
- Dopamine receptor antagonists (bromocriptine)
- Dopamine receptor facilitators (amantadine)
- Acetyl choline antagonists (benztropine)

RECEPTOR SENSITIVITY OF PHENOTHIAZINES

Chain		Receptor blockade		Clinical effect	
	D_2	Alpha adrenergic	Muscarinic	Extrapyramidal	Sedation
Aliphatic	+	+++	++	++	+++
Piperidine	++	++	+++	+	++
Piperazine	+++	+	+	+++	+

Figure CN.12

LEVODOPA

Levodopa is used to increase brain levels of dopamine. Dopamine does not cross the blood-brain barrier, and racemic DOPA produces numerous systemic side effects without being effective. DOPA is well absorbed orally and 95% is converted into dopamine by DOPA-decarboxylase. This is then metabolised by monoamine oxidase and catechol o-methyl transferase (COMT). About 1% of the drug enters the brain where it is converted into its active form, dopamine. Levodopa causes an increase in the number of dopamine (D_2) receptors in the brain.

CARBIDOPA

Used in conjunction with levodopa, carbidopa increases the proportion of the oral dose of levodopa entering the brain by inhibiting its peripheral conversion to dopamine. Carbidopa itself does not cross the blood-brain barrier and, therefore, does not interfere with subsequent conversion in the brain

DOMPERIDONE

Used in conjunction with levodopa, this dopamine antagonist only crosses the blood-brain barrier slowly and is used to reduce the peripheral effects of dopamine. It has important anti-emetic activity peripherally and also at the chemoreceptor trigger zone. Domperidone permits the use of larger doses of levodopa than would otherwise be possible without gross unwanted effects.

SELEGILINE

Selegiline is a selective MAO-B inhibitor. This selectivity reduces the peripheral effects of conventional MAO inhibitors that are largely due to MAO-A inhibition. There is no effect from tyramine containing foods and drug interactions are less severe and less common.

BROMOCRIPTINE

Bromocriptine acts by direct stimulation of central dopamine (D_2) receptors. They are reserved for patients in whom levodopa is ineffective. Predictably, these drugs inhibit prolactin secretion. Bromocriptine is chemically related to the ergot alkaloids. It is often referred to as a 'dopamine facilitator'.

AMANTADINE

The mode of action of amantadine remains obscure. Possibilities include facilitation of dopamine release, inhibition of dopamine metabolism and direct D_2 agonist activity.

ACETYL CHOLINE ANTAGONISTS

Examples – benzhexol, benztropine, orphenadrine, procyclidine

Certain muscarinic antagonists can cross the blood-brain barrier having a preferential action on central muscarinic receptors, thus minimising their peripheral side effects. The central excitatory effects of acetyl choline are inhibited and this may restore the imbalance between cholinergic and dopaminergic activity that occurs in Parkinson's disease. Cholinergic antagonists also antagonise presynaptic inhibition of dopaminergic neurones so increasing dopamine release, which may prove therapeutic.

REFERENCES AND FURTHER READING

Williams PT, Smith M. An assessment of prochlorperazine buccal for the prevention of nausea & vomiting during intravenous patient controlled analgesia with morphine following abdominal hysterectomy. *European Journal of Anaesthesia*, 1999; **16:** 638–645.

Diemunsch P, Schoeffler P, Bryssine B, Cheli-Muller LE, Lees J, McQuade BA, Spraggs CF. Antiemetic activity of the NK_1 receptor antagonist GR205171 in the treatment of post operative nausea and vomiting after major gynaecological surgery. *Brit J Anaes*, 1999; **82:** 274–276.

Taylor CP, Gee NS, Su T, Kocsis JD, Welty DF, Brown JP, Dooley DJ, Boden P, Singh L. A summary of the mechanistic hypotheses of gabapentin pharmacology. *Epilepsy Research.* 1998; **29:** 233–249.

SECTION 3: 11
AUTONOMIC NERVOUS SYSTEM PHARMACOLOGY

T. C. Smith

CHOLINERGIC SYSTEM

Muscarinic receptors
Muscarinic agonists
Muscarinic antagonists
Nicotinic receptors
Nicotinic agonists
Nicotinic antagonists

ADRENERGIC SYSTEM

Adrenergic receptors
Adrenergic agonists
α-adrenergic receptor antagonists
β-adrenergic receptor antagonists

DIRECT-ACTING VASODILATING AGENTS

Calcium channel antagonists
Organic nitrates, nitrites and related drugs
Potassium channel activators
Other agents of importance

SPECIFIC PHARMACOLOGY

Epinephrine
Dobutamine
Dopamine
Dopexamine
Ephedrine
Isoprenaline
Norepinephrine
Clonidine
Esmolol
Labetalol
Propranolol
Atropine
Glycopyrrolate
Hyoscine
Glyceryl trinitrate
Sodium nitroprusside

The autonomic nervous system (ANS) comprises the sympathetic and parasympathetic nervous systems. Ganglionic synaptic transmission in the ANS is mediated by the release of acetylcholine from the pre ganglionic neurone. Both muscarinic and nicotinic receptors are involved in mediation of the post ganglionic response, as are inhibitory dopaminergic interneurones. In general, sympathetic post ganglionic neurones are noradrenergic, and parasympathetic post ganglionic neurones are muscarinic (cholinergic). The two systems tend to have opposite actions. Deliberate pharmacological manipulation of the ANS is therefore aimed at sites where physiological or anatomical differences exist between the two systems.

CHOLINERGIC SYSTEM

The important structural features of the neurotransmitter acetylcholine are the strongly positive quaternary amine in the choline part of the molecule and the partial negatively charged ester component. Choline receptor antagonists have either a tertiary or a quaternary amine (or both). Acetylcholine receptors are classified as either muscarinic or nicotinic. Nicotinic receptors are widespread in the body and are found in both sympathetic and parasympathic nervous systems. Drug actions at the nicotinic receptors of the neuromuscular junction, which is not part of the ANS, are covered on pages 641–651.

MUSCARINIC RECEPTORS

The muscarinic receptors are G-protein coupled receptors. Five subtypes have been identified (M_{1-5}) but the most important ones are M_1, M_2 and M_3, which are all antagonised by atropine. M_1 receptors are found in the central nervous system (CNS), autonomic ganglia and gastric parietal cells, M_2 receptors are found in the heart and at pre synaptic sites, and M_3 receptors are found in smooth muscle, vascular endothelium (causing vasodilatation) and in exocrine glands.

MUSCARINIC AGONISTS

Examples – carbachol, pilocarpine

Pharmacological features

In common with other agonists, these drugs bear a structural relationship to the relevant endogenous agonist (acetylcholine). Pharmacological activity is reduced by changing the nitrogen unit from quaternary to tertiary, by removing the ester and by increasing the length of the aliphatic component on the quaternary nitrogen. Such changes also reduce hydrolysis and increase the half-life. This is essential to enable the drug to be given by conventional intermittent doses.

Carbachol has a quaternary amino group with the acetyl component changed to a carbamyl group so that it produces both nicotinic and muscarinic effects. Pilocarpine has a tertiary amino group and possesses muscarinic effects only.

Clinical effects

Muscarinic agonists are used to constrict the pupil to reduce intra-ocular pressure in glaucoma, and to improve micturition by increasing detrusor muscle contraction.

The muscarinic agonists are often referred to as parasympathomimetics because the peripheral muscarinic receptors are predominantly located in the parasympathetic system. Their effects are predictable from this knowledge and are summarised in Figure AS.1.

CLINICAL EFFECTS OF MUSCARINIC AGONISTS

Cardiovascular system

Atrial contractility decreased
Heart rate decreased
Blood pressure decreased
Systemic vascular resistance decreased (via nitric oxide in the endothelium)

Respiratory system

Mucous secretion stimulated
Bronchoconstriction with increased resistance and decreased deadspace

Gastro-intestinal system

Propulsive activity increased
Salivary, exocrine pancreatic, gastric and intestinal secretions stimulated

Urogenital system

Sphincter tone decreased
Detrusor tone increased

Eye

Miosis
Ciliary muscle stimulated (poor focusing on far objects)
Lacrimation increased

Figure AS.1

MUSCARINIC ANTAGONISTS

Examples – atropine, glycopyrrolate, hyoscine

Pharmacological features

Muscarinic antagonists compete with acetylcholine in the end effector organs of the parasympathetic system, and in the sweat glands which are also muscarinic yet innervated by the sympathetic system. Atropine and hyoscine are naturally occurring agents formed from esters of tropic acid and either tropine or scopine. The tertiary amines such as atropine and hyoscine cross the blood-brain barrier whereas quaternary amines such as glycopyrrolate and ipratropium do not.

Clinical effects

Muscarinic antagonists increase cardiac activity by increasing heart rate (blood pressure often rises as a result). They inhibit most secretions and sweating. In the gastro-intestinal and urinary systems there is increased sphincter tone and reduced motility. The pupils are dilated and accommodation is blocked causing blurred vision. The clinical effects of the muscarinic antagonists are the opposite of those of the agonists and are shown in Figure AS.2.

Atropine

Atropine is initially synthesised in the levo (L) form by plants but it spontaneously racemes so that the commercial preparation contains a mixture of dextro (D) and L-hyoscyamine. There is an aromatic group in place of the acetyl group of acetylcholine and there is a tertiary amino group in place of the quaternary one. The muscarinic effects are mainly due to the L form. Atropine is chemically related to cocaine and consequently it has a weak local anaesthetic effect. Atropine readily crosses the blood-brain barrier and the placenta. Initially the drug causes CNS excitation followed by depression.

Glycopyrrolate

Glycopyrrolate has a quaternary ammonium group and does not readily cross the blood-brain barrier therefore central anti-cholinergic effects are minimal. It also has the advantage that its duration of effect is similar to that of neostigmine with which it is given concomitantly for the reversal of neuromuscular blockade.

Hyoscine

The muscarinic effects of hyoscine are mainly due to the L form. Hyoscine causes CNS depression and has a useful role as a sedative and anti-emetic in premedication.

CLINICAL EFFECTS OF MUSCARINIC ANTAGONISTS

Peripheral

Cardiovascular system

    SA node and atria hypopolarised

    Refractory period of SA node and atria increased

    Refractory period of AV node decreased

    Conduction velocity in SA node, atria and AV node increased

    Atrial contractility increased

    Heart rate increased

    Systemic vascular resistance increased (vascular receptors not innervated)

    Salivary gland arterioles vasoconstricted

Respiratory system

    Mucous secretion inhibited

    Bronchodilatation

Gastro-intestinal system

    Sphincter activity increased

    Propulsion reduced

    Biliary tree constricted

    Salivary, exocrine pancreatic, gastric and intestinal secretions inhibited

Urogenital system

    Sphincter tone increased

    Detrusor tone reduced

    Erectile tissue vasoconstricts

Eye

    Mydriasis

    Ciliary muscle relaxed

    Lacrimal secretions reduced

Central

    Sedation

    Anti-emesis

    Anti Parkinsonian

Figure AS.2

NICOTINIC RECEPTORS

The nicotinic acetylcholine receptors are part of a transmembrane protein ion channel. In the ANS, they are located in the ganglia. The pharmacology of the nicotinic receptors at the neuromuscular junction is discussed in detail on pages 641–651.

NICOTINIC AGONISTS

Nicotine is the most prevalent exogenous agent active at the nicotinic receptors. It preferentially affects autonomic ganglia rather than the neuromuscular junction, and causes central stimulation. When an excess of acetylcholine occurs such as when acetylcholinesterase is blocked by an anti-cholinesterase (for example, neostigmine or an organophosphorus compound) there will be nicotinic stimulation of the ganglia. Stimulation of autonomic ganglia has no clinical application but the following effects will be seen: vasoconstriction, hypertension, sweating and salivation. Gut motility may increase or decrease.

NICOTINIC ANTAGONISTS

Example – trimetaphan

Mode of action

Mechanisms for blockade of cholinergic neuro-transmission include receptor antagonism, depolarising blockade, and inhibition of synthesis, storage and release of acetylcholine. Nicotinic antagonists cause blockade of autonomic ganglia. Ganglion blocking agents include hemicholinium, hexamethonium, and trimetaphan. The neuromuscular blocking agents d-tubocurarine and gallamine also cause ganglion blockade. Hexamethonium and trimetaphan prevent nicotinic transmission by blockade of the open ionophore. Moreover, blockade is therefore use-dependent. Channel blocking agents are attracted to the negative membrane because they have a positive charge. Hyperpolarisation increases the attraction and consequently the effect of the block.

Clinical effects

Drugs causing ganglion blockade reduce blood pressure by a combination of vasodilatation and inhibition of compensatory effects such as tachycardia. The vasodilatation affects both arterioles (after-load) and venules (pre load). The effect on the capacitance vessels reduces venous pressure and consequently intra-operative venous oozing. In general, use, ganglion blockade causes postural hypotension as the venous tone does not increase to compensate for the upright position. Ganglion blocking drugs also reduce sweating, secretions and gut motility. They interfere with bladder emptying and may cause urinary retention.

Trimetaphan camsylate

Trimetaphan is a monoquaternary sulphonium compound that competitively antagonises acetylcholine at the post synaptic nicotinic receptors. It also has a direct relaxant action on vascular smooth muscle and causes histamine release, both of which induce vasodilatation.

Trimetaphan is used to induce hypotension during anaesthesia. It is administered by infusion at a rate of 3–4 mg/min titrated according to need. Tachyphylaxis occurs but only after infusing for 1–3 days.

Trimetaphan reduces systemic vascular resistance and may sensitise the myocardium to catecholamines. It reduces the blood pressure and inhibits any compensatory tachycardia. Trimetaphan reduces splanchnic and renal blood flow. It also slightly reduces cerebral blood flow but intracranial pressure is unaffected. Pupillary dilatation occurs and there is a small effect on skeletal muscle nicotinic receptors that may therefore impair respiratory function. In the abdomen, it enhances gastric emptying and gastro-intestinal motility while reducing secretions. Bladder detrusor tone is reduced and this may cause retention. The inhibition of sweating may cause hyperthermia.

Trimetaphan is excreted unchanged in the urine, and lasts for 10–30 min after discontinuing the infusion.

DRUGS INTERFERING WITH SYNTHESIS, RELEASE AND METABOLISM OF ACETYL CHOLINE

Hemicholinium is an example of a drug preventing acetylcholine synthesis. It does so by preventing the uptake of choline into the nerve terminal. It is not taken up and does not produce a false transmitter effect.

Magnesium ions and aminoglycosides inhibit calcium entry into the synaptic terminal, and so prevent neurotransmitter release. Botulinum toxin and β-bungarotoxin bind irreversibly to nicotinic nerve terminals and prevent neurotransmitter release (α-bungarotoxin blocks post synaptic acetyl choline receptors). The main effect of these compounds is that of muscle paralysis. However, if ventilation support is instituted then the excessive parasympathetic blockade is still a serious problem.

Metabolism of acetyl choline is inhibited by anti-cholinesterases and organophosphorus compounds, resulting in excess levels of acetylcholine. Initially, these cause increasing levels of stimulation of the parasympathetic system, but further rises cause depolarising blockade of the post synaptic membrane with muscle paralysis.

ADRENERGIC SYSTEM

The post ganglionic neurones of the sympathetic

nervous system provide the adrenergic component of the ANS. The adrenergic receptors are located on the post synaptic membrane of the end organ. Catecholamines are the agonists at these receptors. Circulating catecholamines and circulating adrenergic drugs readily affect these receptors. The ubiquity of the sympathetic nervous system results in diverse effects when drugs interfering with adrenergic neurotransmission are used.

ADRENERGIC RECEPTORS

The adrenergic receptors are structurally similar. They are G-protein coupled receptors with seven transmembrane α-helical segments. Drugs affecting the adrenergic system work either by being structurally similar to the neurotransmitter, or by interfering with storage, release or metabolism. Drugs with a structural similarity take the place of the endogenous agonist and either mimic (agonism) or block (antagonism) the effect on the receptor. The endogenous neurotransmitters and hormones norepinephrine, epinephrine and dopamine are used pharmacologically. The two basic divisions of adrenergic receptors (α and β) are affected to different degrees by various drugs. They were originally defined by their responses to norepinephrine, epinephrine, and isoprenaline in the following manner:

Agonist responses of adrenergic receptors

- α receptor:
  norepinephrine $\geq$ epinephrine $>$ isoprenaline
- β receptor:
  isoprenaline $\geq$ epinephrine $\geq$ norepinephrine

The subclassifications are now performed using selective antagonists. α and β receptors are further subdivided into α_1 and α_2 and β_1, β_2 and β_3. They may be located at different sites or at the same synapses, and drugs may have specificity for one subtype over another, although this is not usually exclusive. Figure AS.3 details the receptor sub types and their characteristics.

Clinical effects

The clinical effects of the adrenergic receptors are as follows:

- α_1 – vasoconstriction, gut smooth muscle relaxation, increased saliva secretion, and hepatic glycogenolysis
- α_2 – inhibition of autonomic neurotransmitter (norepinephrine and acetylcholine) release, stimulation of platelet aggregation
- β_1 – increased heart rate, increased myocardial contractility, gut smooth muscle relaxation, lipolysis
- β_2 – vasodilatation, bronchiole dilatation, visceral smooth muscle relaxation, hepatic glycogenolysis, muscle tremor
- β_3 – lipolysis, thermogenesis

Drugs acting on the adrenergic receptors may cause agonism, antagonism or partial agonism and often have a mixture of effects at different receptor types. Figure AS.4 shows the relative agonism and antagonism of various drugs on the adrenergic receptor subtypes.

Adrenergic drugs will be considered further according to their primary effect in the clinical setting.

Pharmacological features

The structure–activity relationship of adrenergic drugs is marked. The basic catecholamine structure consists of an organic ring and side chain. Increasing the size of the attachment to the amino group of the side chain increases the affinity for β receptors which increases the effect of both agonists and antagonists, and reduces the effect of monoamine oxidase and the uptake 1 mechanism (U1) which removes catecholamines from the synaptic cleft. The β-hydroxy group is important for α agonist activity and β antagonism, while removal reduces receptor affinity. Substitution or repositioning of the catechol hydroxyl groups results in resistance to catechol-O-methyl transferase (COMT) and uptake 1. Removal of one or both catechol hydroxyl groups reduces or obliterates receptor affinity but leaves uptake 1 intact. The structure of the more common catecholamines is shown in Figure AS.5.

CHARACTERISTICS OF THE ADRENORECEPTOR SUB TYPES		
Receptor	Location	Effect on neurotransmission
Alpha$_1$	Post synaptic	Excitatory
Alpha$_2$	Pre synaptic	Inhibitory
Beta$_1$	Post synpatic	Excitatory
Beta$_2$	Post synaptic	Inhibitory
Beta$_3$	Post synaptic	–

Figure AS.3

DRUG-RECEPTOR INTERACTIONS AT ADRENERGIC RECEPTORS

	Alpha$_1$	Alpha$_2$	Beta$_1$	Beta$_2$
Agonists				
Norepinephrine	+++	+++	++	+
Phenylephrine	++	0	0	0
Clonidine	0	+++	0	0
Dopamine	+	0	++	++
Epinephrine	++	++	+++	+++
Dobutamine	0	0	+++	+
Salbutamol	0	0	+	+++
Isoprenaline	0	0	+++	+++
Antagonists				
Phentolamine	− − −	− − −	0	0
Phenoxybenzamine	− − −	− − −	0	0
Prazocin	− − −	−	0	0
Indoramin	− − −	−	0	0
Ergotamine	pa	− −	0	0
Labetalol	− − −	−	− −	− −
Propranolol	0	0	− − −	− − −
Atenolol	0	0	− − −	−

+, Agonist activity
−, Antagonist activity
pa, Partial agonist activity

Figure AS.4

Dopamine

Norepinephrine

Epinephrine

Isoprenaline

Figure AS.5. Catecholamine structures

ADRENERGIC AGONISTS

Examples – clonidine, epinephrine, dobutamine, dopamine, dopexamine, norepinephrine, isoprenaline

Note that β adrenergic receptor agonists are covered in more detail on pages 715–716.

Clinical uses

Adrenergic receptor agonists are administered systemically for myocardial failure (inotropic), sepsis (vasoconstriction and inotropy), anaphylaxis, nasal congestion, and bronchospasm. They may be administered peripherally to cause local vasoconstriction and prolong the effects of local anaesthetics or reduce bleeding in the operative field. Inhaled β$_2$ agonists are effective in the treatment of asthma when inhaled which reduces systemic effects.

Epinephrine

Epinephrine has both α and β agonist effects and many applications. It is an inotrope and chronotrope but sensitises the myocardium to arrhythmias. The ventricles in particular become hyperexcitable. There is generalised vasoconstriction but dilatation of skeletal muscle arterioles.

Dobutamine

Dobutamine is a non selective β agonist and has both chronotropic and inotropic effects. It is usually used for its inotropic effect but tachycardia may limit the dose. It causes some vasodilatation and this may require concurrent treatment with an α agonist such as norepinephrine.

Dopamine

Dopamine is an agonist at α_1, β and dopamine receptors. The balance of these effects is dose-related. Initially only dopamine receptors are affected, but with increasing doses, β receptors and then α receptors are also affected. Peripheral dopamine receptors are located in the renal arterioles and are responsible for vasodilatation. Dopamine is often used to maintain renal perfusion when this may be compromised. Increasing the dose recruits the β receptors with their positive inotropic effect. This is limited by the onset of a tachycardia. Vasoconstriction (α_1) may become a problem as the drug dose increases.

Dopexamine

Dopexamine is an agonist of β_2 and dopaminergic (D_1 and D_2) receptors in the periphery. It also inhibits neuronal norepinephrine re-uptake (uptake 1), so enhancing the β effects. It is a positive inotrope but has the principal effect of peripheral vasodilatation especially of the splanchnic and renal arterioles. The resulting reduction in afterload improves cardiac output.

Isoprenaline

Isoprenaline is used in the treatment of bronchospasm, bradycardia and heart block. It is used to increase heart rate in complete heart block while electrical pacing is instituted. It is agonist at β_1 and β_2 receptors.

Norepinephrine

Norepinephrine is primarily an α_1 agonist and causes vasoconstriction (although it does have some β agonist effects). It is particularly useful in patients with septicaemic shock as they have a pathological reduction in systemic vascular resistance resulting in hypotension and hypoperfusion due to diversion of blood away from essential organs. The inotropic effect although small may also help. It may cause a reflex bradycardia if hypotension is overcorrected.

Salbutamol

Salbutamol is an effective bronchodilator, used in both the treatment and prophylaxis of obstructive airway disease. It is a selective β_2 agonist and this minimises the undesirable effects such as tachycardia, although this β_1 effect does still occur with higher doses. It also has a role as a uterine relaxant for the treatment of premature labour and before delivery during Caesarean section.

Clonidine

Clonidine is an α_2 agonist used as a centrally acting anti-hypertensive agent that works by reducing norepinephrine release. Its role in preventing migraine is controversial. α_2 receptors are located on the pre synaptic membrane of noradrenergic neurones and α_2 receptors have also been found in the spinal cord and at peripheral nerve endings. Clonidine may prolong the effect of epidurally administered local anaesthetic agents although it is not licensed for this route.

Metaraminol

Metaraminol tartrate has both α and β agonist effects with the α effect predominating. It increases systemic and pulmonary vascular resistance and causes increased systolic and diastolic blood pressures. Heart rate decreases in response and some inotropy occurs, although overall cardiac output may fall or may not change. Cerebral and renal blood flow are reduced by the vasoconstriction and during pregnancy uterine tone is increased. β effects increase blood glucose levels.

Methoxamine

Methoxamine hydrochloride is an α_1 agonist with similar cardiovascular effects to metaraminol. Cardiac output is unaffected but atrioventricular conduction slows. Renal and uterine blood flow are reduced and the pregnant uterus contracts.

α-ADRENERGIC RECEPTOR ANTAGONISTS

Examples – indoramin, phenoxybenzamine, phentolamine

Uses

α_1 adrenergic receptor antagonists are used as anti-hypertensives and in benign prostatic hyperplasia.

Clinical effects

α blockade causes vasodilatation with reduced systemic vascular resistance and lowered blood pressure. There is a reflex increase in heart rate and cardiac output.

Indoramin

Indoramin is an α_1 antagonist. It should be avoided in patients receiving monoamine oxidase inhibitors.

Phenoxybenzamine

Phenoxybenzamine is a haloalkylamine. The N-chloroethyl group binds covalently to part of the receptor. It therefore detaches from the receptor very slowly and behaves like a competitive irreversible antagonist. The recovery half-life is about 24 H. Phenoxybenzamine is also an antagonist of acetylcholinergic, 5-hydroxytryptaminergic and histaminic receptors. Its primary effect is that of vasodilatation.

Phentolamine

Phentolamine affects both α_1 and α_2. It does not bind covalently and so is reversible.

Labetalol

Labetalol is an antagonist at both α_1 and β receptors. The reflex tachycardia from the α blockade is antagonised by the β blockade. α blockade is more prominent when used intravenously whereas β blockade is the main effect when used orally.

Droperidol

Droperidol is an anti-psychotic and anti-emetic with an α adrenergic antagonist component. There may be some peripherally mediated hypotension especially when given intravenously.

β-ADRENERGIC RECEPTOR ANTAGONISTS

Examples: acebutolol, atenolol, metoprolol, nadolol, oxprenolol, pindolol, propanolol, sotalol

Mode of action

β receptors activate adenyl cyclase. There are two subtypes of β receptor (β_1 and β_2). In general, β_1 receptors tend to be excitatory and β_2 inhibitory. β adrenergic receptor antagonists with a specific affinity for β_1 receptors alone are called selective and those also affecting β_2 receptors are called non selective. Even those classified as selective still have some β_2 antagonism. Some β blockers are partial agonists (intrinsic sympathomimetic activity) so that at low dose there is increasing agonism as the dose increases but a plateau is reached and there is antagonism of circulating catecholamines. They may have an advantage over the others in minimising bradycardia,

PARTIAL AGONISM AND SELECTIVITY OF BETA BLOCKERS

	Antagonist	Partial agonist
Selective	Atenolol	Acebutalol
	Betaxolol	Alprenolol
	Bisoprolol	
	Esmolol	
	Metoprolol	
	Nadolol	
Non selective	Propanolol	Celiprolol
	Sotalol	Oxprenolol
	Timolol	Pindolol

Figure AS.6

reducing heart failure and maintaining perfusion to the extremities. The membrane stabilising effect that some β blockers have is, however, of little clinical importance. Figure AS.6 shows the selectivity and partial agonist properties of the β blockers.

Uses

β blockers are used in the treatment of angina, hypertension, tachyarrhythmias, anxiety, glaucoma, migraine, phaeochromocytoma and thyrotoxicosis.

Clinical effects

The clinical effects are predictable from knowledge of receptor locations. The important effects for clinical use are those of negative inotropy and negative chronotropy which reduce blood pressure and myocardial work. Coronary blood flow is reduced but this effect is less than the reduction in myocardial work. These drugs are particularly effective when sympathetic tone is increased, for example, following myocardial infarction, however care must be taken not to block a protective inotropic effect in incipient heart failure. The undesirable effects include bradycardia, bronchoconstriction, sleep disturbance, hypoglycaemia (especially with exercise) and cold extremities.

β blockers (whether selective or not) should be avoided in asthmatic patients. They should be used with caution in diabetes, peripheral vascular disease and heart failure. Calcium antagonists with negative inotropic effects (verapamil and diltiazem) act synergistically with β blockers to cause hypotension,

CLINICAL EFFECTS OF BETA BLOCKADE

Peripheral

Cardiovascular system

    Conduction velocity in SA node, atria, AV node
       and ventricles reduced (β_1)

    Atrial contractility reduced (β_1)

    Heart rate reduced (β_1)

    Blood pressure reduced (β_1)

    Class II antiarrhythmic activity (β_1)

    Skeletal muscle (β_2) and coronary vasomotor
       tone increased

    Coronary blood flow reduced

    Cardiac oxygen demand reduced

Respiratory system

    Bronchoconstriction with increased resistance
       and reduced deadspace (β_2)

Renal system

    Renin secretion inhibited (β_1)

Metabolic

    Less free fatty acid release (β_1)

    Glycogenolysis reduced (β_2)

    Insulin release reduced (β_2)

    Lipolysis (β_3)

    Thermogenesis (β_3)

Eye

    Reduced production of aqueous humour

    Constriction of ciliary muscle (β_2)

Central

    Reduced sympathetic tone

    Anxiolysis

    Tiredness

    Nightmares

    Sleep disturbance

Figure AS.7

bradycardia and conduction defects and they should not be administered contemporaneously.

Atenolol, celiprolol, nadolol and sotalol are very water soluble and therefore penetrate the brain poorly and are primarily excreted in the urine. In general, the β blockers are well absorbed orally but the first-pass effect is particularly high with alprenolol, propranolol, metoprolol, oxprenolol and timolol. Bisoprolol and sotalol have a high bio-availability.

Atenolol

Atenolol is a popular selective β blocker for the control of essential hypertension. In the clinical setting, patient compliance with the treatment is often apparent from their relatively slow heart rate. Bio-availability is 50% and protein binding is low. Atenolol is highly water soluble and is largely excreted unchanged in the urine.

Esmolol

Esmolol hydrochloride is a short acting β_1 adrenergic antagonist, and class II anti-arrhythmic. This aryloxypropanolamine is rapidly hydrolysed to a low activity acid by red cell esterases and has a half-life of only 9 min. It is used in the acute management of supraventricular tachycardias, hypertension and myocardial infarction, and is an option for suppression of the hypertensive response to laryngoscopy and intubation.

Propranolol

Propranolol is a non selective β blocker with no intrinsic sympathomimetic activity. It has been largely superseded by selective antagonists but still has a role in the management of phaeochromocytoma (in conjunction with α blockade), thyrotoxicosis and crisis, acute hypertension and tachyarrhythmias. Propranolol has a high first-pass with a bio-availability of only 10–30%. It is lipid soluble and highly protein bound (90–95%).

DRUGS INTERFERING WITH SYNTHESIS, STORAGE, RELEASE AND METABOLISM OF CATECHOLAMINES

Examples – α methyltyrosine, carbidopa, reserpine, bethanidine, bretylium, debrisoquine, guanethidine

A few drugs act by interfering with the metabolic elements of the catecholamines rather than with receptor interactions. While not widely used now as they lack specificity these agents merit brief consideration.

Synthesis

α methyltyrosine inhibits tyrosine hydroxylase and carbidopa inhibits dopa decarboxylase. Both therefore prevent the formation of dopamine, the first catecholamine in the chain of synthesis. α methyltyrosine has been used in the management of phaeochromocytoma. Carbidopa does not cross the blood-brain barrier and is therefore used to minimise the peripheral effects of L-dopa used in the treatment of Parkinsonism. The anti-hypertensive agent methyldopa is a false substrate for dopa decarboxylase and dopamine hydroxylase and results in the synthesis of a false transmitter – methyl norepinephrine. This is ineffective and as it is not metabolised by monoamine oxidase it accumulates within the nerve terminal and displaces the true neurotransmitter, which becomes depleted.

Storage

Reserpine blocks the uptake and re-uptake of norepinephrine, dopamine and 5-hydroxy tryptamine in the neuronal terminals. The neurotransmitter accumulates within the cytoplasm where MAO inactivates it and transmitter levels fall. It affects both the sympathetic and CNS but has been superseded by drugs that are more specific.

Release

Guanethidine was originally used as an anti-hypertensive but is now mainly used in the management of chronic pain. It is transported by the uptake 1 mechanism and accumulates in the nerve terminals. Initially it causes release of norepinephrine from the vesicles and then inhibits release of the diminishing levels of norepinephrine. Debrisoquine, bretylium and bethanidine have a similar mode of action. Guanethidine is used to treat reflex sympathetic dystrophy by IV regional sympathetic block (chemical sympathectomy) in which guanethidine is injected intravenously into an isolated limb.

DIRECT-ACTING VASODILATINGAGENTS

CALCIUM CHANNEL ANTAGONISTS

Examples – amlodipine, felodipine, nicardipine, nifedipine, nimodipine, nisoldipine

The calcium channel antagonists are covered in detail on pages 705–706. The calcium channel antagonists are a mixed group of drugs having in common the blockade of various calcium ionophores in cell and intracellular membranes. These vasodilators relax vascular smooth muscle preferentially and dilate coronary and other arterial smooth muscle. They can be used in conjunction with β blockers. Amlodipine, felodipine, nicardipine and nifedipine are used to treat both hypertension and angina. Isradipine and lacidipine are only useful in the treatment of hypertension. Nimodipine has a specificity for cerebral arterioles and is used to treat vascular spasm following subarachnoid haemorrhage or neuroradiological instrumentation.

ORGANIC NITRATES, NITRITES AND RELATED DRUGS

Examples – glyceryl trinitrate, isosorbide di- and mono-nitrate, nitric oxide, nitroprusside

Uses

These are direct acting vascular smooth muscle relaxants that are used to control and reduce blood pressure and to alleviate angina.

Mode of action

Both organic nitrates (NO_3^-) and sodium nitro-prusside act in a similar way. Having diffused from the vascular lumen through to the smooth muscle they are converted to nitrites (NO_2^-) by reacting with –SH groups (thiols) in the tissues. Hydrogen ions within the cells then react with the nitrite to produce nitric oxide (NO). This in turn reacts with more thiols in the muscle cell to produce nitrosothiols. These stimulate guanylate cyclase to convert guanosine triphosphate (GTP) to cyclic guanosine monophosphate (cGMP) in a comparable way to adenyl cyclase. The cGMP then relaxes the smooth muscle. Nitric oxide may be administered by inhalation to dilate selectively pulmonary arterioles. It mimics the physiological mediation by the vascular endothelial cells of a number of circulating autacoids such as bradykinin which stimulate nitric oxide synthase to convert arginine to citrulline and nitric oxide. This nitric oxide (formerly identified as endothelium dependent relaxing factor-EDRF), diffuses into the muscle cell where it has its effect.

Clinical effects

The predominant effect is that of vasodilatation affecting the venous system (pre load) in particular. The reduction in pre load reduces cardiac output, cardiac work and myocardial oxygen demand, and so these drugs are used to treat angina. Higher or more prolonged doses also dilate arterioles including the coronary vessels, and therefore reduce after-load. In the ischaemic heart, these drugs may increase the blood flow to ischaemic myocardium by dilating collaterals that bypass partial vessel occlusions.

Flushing and headaches are common and a reflex tachycardia develops, putting a practical upper limit on the degree of vasodilatation. All smooth muscle is affected somewhat but the clinically important effect is confined to the cardiovascular system.

Patients using isosorbide dinitrate and other longer acting nitrates may develop tolerance perhaps because of depletion of the tissue thiols. Excessive levels of nitrates convert haemoglobin to methaemoglobin.

Glyceryl trinitrate

Glyceryl trinitrate reduces blood pressure and coronary vascular resistance and increases subendocardial coronary blood flow by decreasing left ventricular end diastolic pressure. It may be administered by infusion, by transdermal absorption using a skin patch, or by sublingual absorption using a spray or a tablet. Gastric acid rapidly inactivates glyceryl trinitrate and once the desired effect is achieved, it may be swallowed. Within the body, it is rapidly hydrolysed in the liver producing inorganic nitrite. Some is also converted to glyceryl dinitrate and glyceryl trinitrate which have a small amount of activity and a half-life of 2 H.

Isosorbide dinitrate

Isosorbide dinitrate is usually given orally by a slow release preparation and so its effect is delayed compared with glyceryl trinitrate. It may also be given sublingually for rapid onset and by infusion for precision control of symptoms or blood pressure. The effects are similar. It is converted to isosorbide mononitrate in the liver with a half-life of 4 H.

Isosorbide mononitrate

Isosorbide mononitrate, the active metabolite of isosorbide dinitrate is given orally and is similar to its precursor.

Nitric oxide

Inhaled nitric oxide (in concentrations of about 40 ppm) is used to treat pulmonary hypertension in the intensive care setting. It diffuses through to the pulmonary vascular smooth muscle where it interacts to cause cGMP mediated relaxation. Further diffusion to the vascular lumen results in rapid inactivation as it combines with haemoglobin to form methaemoglobin.

Nitroprusside

Sodium nitroprusside is used in the control of hypertension and for induced hypotension during surgery. It affects both arterial and venous systems to cause a reduction in systemic vascular resistance followed by a compensatory tachycardia. It is administered by infusion in systems protected from light (brown syringes and yellow infusion lines are available). Nitroprusside metabolism produces the highly toxic cyanide ion (CN^-) some of which combines with haemoglobin to produce methaemoglobin, and the rest is converted to thiocyanate by rhodonase in the liver and subsequently excreted in the urine. Thiocyanate levels can be measured to monitor toxicity. A small amount combines with vitamin B_{12} to form cyanocobalamin. In excess the cyanide ion saturates these elimination processes and damages the cytochrome oxidase chain (fundamental for aerobic cellular energy production).

POTASSIUM CHANNEL ACTIVATORS

Example – nicorandil

Potassium channel activators act by opening potassium channels resulting in hyperpolarisation of the cell membrane with a reduction in electrical activity. ATP has the opposite effect, closing the channels and depolarising the membrane. Nicorandil relaxes arterial smooth muscle and reduces systemic vascular resistance. The nitrate component of the drug causes venous smooth muscle relaxation with a fall in pre load. It also has a direct dilating affect on coronary arterioles to improve perfusion of ischaemic myocardium. The intended role for nocorandil is in the treatment of angina.

OTHER AGENTS OF IMPORTANCE

Diazoxide

Diazoxide is a thiazide but unlike its diuretic counterparts it causes sodium and water retention. Diazoxide antagonises the effect of ATP on potassium channels. It has a direct effect on arteriolar smooth muscle and given intravenously causes marked hypotension and a reflex increase in heart rate and cardiac output. The increased sympathetic outflow also increases free fatty acids and blood glucose.

Hydrallazine

Hydrallazine acts both centrally and peripherally. The peripheral effect causes direct vascular smooth muscle relaxation. There is also a mild α blocking action. The drop in blood pressure causes a reflex increase in sympathetic tone. Renal blood flow is increased. Headache, dizziness, nausea and vomiting are common side effects.

SPECIFIC PHARMACOLOGY

Units (unless stated otherwise) are:

Volume of distribution at steady state (V_d) (l/kg)
Clearance (Cl) (ml/kg/min)
Terminal half-life ($t_{1/2}$) (min)

EPINEPHRINE

Structure – catecholamine; α and β agonist

Preparation – IV/subcutaneous – 1 mg in 1 ml (1:1000) and 1 mg in 10 ml (1:10 000) also added to local anaesthetics 1:200 000 (1 mg in 200 ml)

Dose – highly variable depending upon indication and route

CNS – limited crossing of the blood-brain barrier but does cause excitation. Neuromuscular transmission facilitated

CVS – heart rate increased (may be reflexly reduced); contractility, stroke volume and cardiac oxygen consumption increased; systemic vasoconstriction but vasodilatation in skeletal muscle; mean arterial pressure, systolic and pulse pressure increased, diastolic decreased; coronary blood flow increased

RS – bronchodilatation; respiratory rate and tidal volume increased; secretions more tenacious

Other – gastro-intestinal tract tone and secretions decreased, splanchnic blood flow decreased; renal blood flow increased; bladder tone reduced but sphincter tone increased; clotting factor V increased leading to enhanced platelet aggregation and coagulation; metabolic effects to increase gluconeogenesis and increase metabolic rate

Metabolism – by catechol O-methyl transferease (COMT) in the liver and monoamine oxidase (MAO) in adrenergic neurones to inactive metabolites 3-methoxy-4-hydroxy phenylethylene and 3-methoxy-4-hydroxy mandelic acid

Contra-indications – beware arrhythmias with halothane; caution with MAO inhibitors

Toxicity – there are many adverse effects but the major ones are cardiac; increases cardiac sensitivity and irritability so arrhythmias including VF and asystole are likely if given too quickly.

DOBUTAMINE HYDROCHLORIDE

Structure – catecholamine; β_1 and β_2 (and α_1) agonist

Preparation – 250 mg dobutamine and 4.8 mg sodium metabisulphite in 20 ml for further dilution prior to administration

Dose – infusion 0.5–40 mcg/kg/min

CNS – stimulant at high dose

CVS – heart rate, stroke volume, cardiac output increased, atrioventricular node conduction enhanced; vasodilatation; systemic vascular resistance and left ventricular end-diastolic pressure (LVEDP) reduced; coronary perfusion may increase

RS – no effect

Other – β_1 effect increases renin output; urine output increases secondary to increased cardiac output

Metabolism – converted to 3-O-methyldobutamine

by COMT; this is conjugated and excreted in urine (80%) and faeces (20%)

Contra-indications – increasing doses cause tachycardia, hypertension, and arrhythmias; angina may occur in susceptible patients; allergic reactions to the metabisulphite preservative have occurred

DOPAMINE HYDROCHLORIDE

Structure – catecholamine; β and α agonist

Preparation – 400 mg (1600 mcg/ml) and 800 mg (3200 mcg/ml) in 250 ml 5% dextrose (other mixtures available)

Dose – IV infusion
  1–20 mcg/kg/min
  1–5 mcg/kg/min increases renal blood flow
  5–15 mcg/kg/min inotropic
  15–20 mcg/kg/min vasoconstricts

CVS – contractility, stroke volume increased; little effect on heart rate; systemic vascular resistance, systolic, mean and diastolic blood pressures decreased; coronary blood flow increased

RS – carotid bodies stimulated leading to reduced respiratory response to hypoxia

Other – splanchnic (including renal) vasodilatation; renal blood flow, glomerular filtrate, urine (volume and sodium content) increased; prolactin secretion inhibited (also known as prolactin inhibiting hormone (PIH) secreted by the posterior pituitary)

Metabolism – by COMT and MAO to homovanillic acid and 3,4-dihydroxyphenylacetic acid. Predominantly excreted in urine conjugated and unconjugated; 25% of the dopamine is taken up into adrenergic nerve endings and is converted to norepinephrine

Contra-indications – nausea, tachycardia and arrhythmias; caution with MAO inhibitors

DOPEXAMINE HYDROCHLORIDE

Structure – catecholamine; dopamine (D_1 and D_2) and β_2 agonist

Preparation – colourless, aqueous solution adjusted to a pH of 2.5, containing 50 mg dopexamine hydrochloride in 5 ml, and 0.01% disodium edetate; requires dilution prior to use

Dose – IV infusion – 0.5–6 mcg/kg/min (start at 0.5 and increase by 0.5–1 mcg/kg/min increments with at least 15-min intervals according to need

CNS – cerebral blood flow increased; dopexamine causes nausea by its action on D_2 receptors in the chemoreceptor trigger zone

CVS – stroke volume, heart rate and cardiac output increased; systolic blood pressure increased; systemic and pulmonary vascular resistance, diastolic blood pressure, LVEDP, pulmonary artery pressure reduced; coronary blood flow increased

RS – bronchodilatation

Other – mesenteric and renal vasodilation with increased blood flow, diuresis and natriuresis; hyperglycaemia, hypokalaemia; splenic platelet sequestration; 40% of dose is bound to red cells

Metabolism – rapid tissue uptake, methylation and conjugation eliminate the drug

Contra-indications – caution with MAO inhibitors

EPHEDRINE

Structure – sympathomimetic amine; α and β agonist

Preparation

Oral, tablets 15, 30 and 60 mg, elixir 15 mg/5 ml

IV clear, colourless, aqueous solution containing 30 mg ephedrine in 1 ml

Dose – IV – 3, 6 or 9 mg increments at minimal interval of 3–4 min. Maximum of 30 mg as tachyphylaxis ensues

CNS – stimulant effect (drug of abuse)

CVS – heart rate, stroke volume, cardiac output, myocardial oxygen consumption increased; SVR, diastolic, systolic and pulmonary pressures increased; coronary blood flow increased; splanchnic and renal vasoconstriction

RS – bronchodilator; respiratory rate and tidal volume increased; irritant to mucous membranes

Other – uterine, bladder and gastro-intestinal smooth muscle relaxation; bladder sphincter tone increased; gluconeogenesis, metabolic rate and oxygen consumption increased; irritant to mucous membranes

Metabolism – up to 99% eliminated in urine unchanged; the rest by oxidation, demethylation, and hydroxylation of the aromatic part plus conjugation

Contra-indications – tachyarrhythmias (especially with halothane), nausea and central stimulation.

ISOPRENALINE

Structure – catecholamine; β agonist

Preparation – oral, tablets 30 mg; IV – colourless, aqueous solution adjusted to a pH of 2.5–2.8, containing 2 mg isoprenaline hydrochloride in 2 ml, with ascorbic acid and disodium edetate; requires dilution prior to use

Dose – IV infusion – 0.02–0.4 mcg/kg/min

CNS – stimulant

CVS – heart rate, stroke volume and cardiac output increased; SA node automaticity and AV nodal conduction increased; systemic vascular resistance and diastolic blood pressure reduced; coronary blood flow

increased; splanchnic and renal vasoconstriction, but flow may improve if treating low cardiac output

RS – bronchodilation

Other – uterine and gastro-intestinal smooth muscle relaxation; gluconeogenesis increased; antigen-induced histamine release is inhibited

Metabolism – extensive first-pass effect if taken orally. 15–75% unchanged in the urine; the rest by COMT then conjugated

NOREPINEPHRINE ACID TARTRATE

Structure – catecholamine; α (and β) agonist

Preparation – clear, colourless, aqueous solution containing 0.2 mg/ml (in 2, 4 and 20 ml ampoules) or 2 mg/ml (2 ml ampoule) with sodium metabisulphite and sodium chloride. 1 mg Norepinephrine acid tartrate (1 ml) contains 0.5 mg norepinephrine base, so the preparations contain 0.1 and 1 mg norepinephrine base/ml respectively

Dose – IV infusion 0.05–0.2 mcg/kg/min

CNS – cerebral oxygen consumption reduced

CVS – generalised peripheral vasoconstriction, systolic and diastolic blood pressure increased; a reflex fall in heart rate occurs; cardiac output may fall slightly; coronary vasodilatation causes coronary blood flow to increase; ventricular rhythm disturbances may occur

RS – mild bronchodilatation, minute volume increases

Other – hepatic, renal and splanchnic blood flow reduced; pregnant uterus contractility increased and this may compromise foetal oxygen supply; insulin secretion reduced; renin secretion increased; mydriasis; plasma water reduced by contraction of vascular space and this increases haematocrit and plasma protein concentration

Metabolism – by MAO and COMT, which in combination produce 3-methoxy-4-hydroxy mandelic acid (VMA) in the urine. 5% excreted unchanged

Contra-indications – caution with MAO inhibitors

CLONIDINE HYDROCHLORIDE

Structure – imidazoline-aniline derivative

Preparation – oral, tablets/capsules 25, 100, 250 and 300 mcg

IV – clear, colourless, aqueous solution containing 150 mcg in 1 ml

Dose – oral migraine/flushing 50–75 mcg twice daily
oral anti-hypertensive 50–600 mcg three times daily
Slow IV – 150–300 mcg for control of hypertensive crisis

Pharmacokinetics: IV dose

onset	peak	duration	V_d	Cl	$t_{\frac{1}{2}}$
10 min	30–60 min	3–7 H	2	3	6–23 H

CNS – analgesia

CVS – transient α_1 effect causes increased systemic vascular resistance and blood pressure; α_2 agonism produces pre synaptic inhibition of sympathetic norepinephrine release with reductions in SVR, blood pressure, venous return and heart rate; cardiac contractility and output are preserved; coronary blood flow increased; renal blood flow increased; rebound tachycardia and hypertension can result from sudden withdrawal

RS – no effect

Other – plasma catecholamine and renin reduced; blood glucose increased; reduction of MAC; may cause dizziness, drowsiness, headache, dry mouth and impotence

Metabolism – 65% unchanged in urine, 20% in faeces, 15% inactivated in liver

ESMOLOL HYDROCHLORIDE (SEE PAGE 711)

LABETALOL HYDROCHLORIDE

Structure – 2-hydroxy-5-[1-hydroxy-2-(1-methyl-3-phenyl-propylamino) ethyl] benzamide hydrochloride; combined α_1 and β_1 and β_2 adrenergic antagonist

Preparation – tablets 50, 100, 200, 400 mg; IV – clear, colourless, aqueous solution containing 100 mg in 20 ml

Dose – oral 100–1200 mg twice daily; IV slow bolus of 50 mg at 5-min intervals until blood pressure is controlled (duration 6–18 h, maximum dose 200 mg); IV infusion 15–160 mg/h

Pharmacokinetics

V_d	Cl	$t_{1/2}$
10	23	6 H

CNS – fatigue, confusion

CVS – heart rate, contractility, stroke volume, cardiac output, systemic vascular resistance, systolic and diastolic blood pressure decrease; coronary and renal blood flow increased

RS – potential risk of bronchoconstriction in asthmatics

Other – with IV use there is a compensatory increase in endogenous catecholamines; renin and angiotensin II reduced; platelet aggregation may be reduced

Metabolism – hepatic

Contra-indications – as for other β blockers; may interact with anti-arrhythmics of Class I and IV; crosses the placenta and causes clinical effects in the foetus including bradycardia, hypotension, respiratory depression, hypoglycaemia and hypothermia in the neonate

PROPRANOLOL

Structure – 1-isopropylamino-3-(1-naphthyloxy) propan-2-ol hydrochloride

Preparation – tablets 10, 40, 80, 160 mg; IV – clear, colourless, aqueous solution containing 1 mg propranolol in 1 ml

Dose – IV – 1–10 mg in increments

Pharmacokinetics

V_d	Cl	$t_{1/2}$
3.6	7	3 H

CNS – anxiolysis, tremor reduced, intra-ocular pressure reduced; anti-hypertensive effect may have a central component

CVS – negative inotrope and chronotrope; stroke volume, heart rate, cardiac output and blood pressure reduced

RS – bronchoconstriction, airways resistance and response to hypercapnia reduced

Other – uterine tone (especially during pregnancy) reduced

Metabolism – high first-pass effect and < 1% excreted unchanged; oxidative deamination and dealkylation with subsequent glucuronidation

Contra-indications – bronchospasm in asthmatics, masks hypoglycaemia in diabetics, exacerbates peripheral vascular disease

ATROPINE SULPHATE

Structure – tertiary amine; muscarinic, anti-cholinergic antagonist

Preparation – oral, tablets 600 mcg; IV/IM – clear, colourless, aqueous solution containing a racemic mixture of 600 mcg atropine in 1 ml

Dose – 10–20 mcg/kg

Pharmacokinetics

Bio-availability	Protein binding	pKa	V_d	Cl	$t_{1/2}$
10–25%	50%	9.8	3	17	150

CNS – variable stimulation or depression, anti-emetic, anti-Parkinsonian; competitive antagonism of muscarinic receptors cause blockade of para-sympathetic system and sweating

CVS; heart rate, AV nodal transmission and cardiac output increase (initial, temporary bradycardia with low doses due to centrally mediated increase in vagal tone); blood pressure may increase; tachyarrhythmias

RS – bronchodilator with increased anatomical dead space; respiratory rate increased; secretions reduced

Other – gastro-intestinal motility and secretions reduced; biliary anti-spasmodic effect; lower oesophageal sphincter pressure reduced; urinary tract tone and peristalsis reduced, bladder sphincter tone increased and retention may result; pupillary dilatation, inability to accommodate for near objects (may persist for several days) and raised intra-ocular pressure occur; metabolic rate increased

Metabolism –atropine ester hydrolysed into its component parts tropine and tropic acid by the liver, 94% of the dose appearing in the urine in 24 H

Contra-indications – beware glaucoma, hyperpyrexia especially in children; central anti-cholinergic syndrome

GLYCOPYRROLATE

Structure – quaternary amine; muscarinic anti-cholinergic antagonist

Preparation – IV – clear, colourless, aqueous solution containing 200 mcg/ml, 1 and 3 ml ampoules

Dose:
IV – 4–5 mcg/kg (10–15 mcg/kg in conjunction with neostigmine)

Children – 4–8 mcg/kg (10 mcg/kg in conjunction with neostigmine 50 mcg/kg)

Pharmacokinetics

Bio-availability	V_d	Cl	$t_{1/2}$
5%	0.4	13	50

CNS – does not cross the blood-brain barrier so there is no effect on the eye; competitive antagonism of muscarinic receptors cause blockade of parasympathetic system and sweating

CVS – heart rate, AV nodal transmission and cardiac output increase, blood pressure may increase; tachyarrhythmias less common than with atropine

RS – bronchodilatation with increased anatomical dead space; secretions reduced

Other – gastro-intestinal motility and secretions reduced; lower oesophageal sphincter pressure reduced; urinary tract tone and peristalsis reduced, bladder sphincter tone increased and retention may result; metabolic rate increased

Metabolism – excreted unchanged in the urine (85%) and faeces (15%)

Contra-indications – in high doses the quaternary ammonium has a nicotinic antagonist effect of significance in myasthenia gravis; limited crossing of the placenta but can still cause foetal tachycardia

HYOSCINE HYDROBROMIDE OR BUTYLBROMIDE

Structure – tertiary amine, muscarinic anti-cholinergic antagonist laevo isomer used – hyoscine-1 (scopolamine)

Presentation – hyoscine-N-butylbromide; tablets 10 mg, IV – clear colourless solution, 20 mg in 1 ml – hyoscine hydrobromide 20 mg in 5 ml

Pharmacokinetics

Bio-availability	Protein binding	V_d	Cl	$t_{1/2}$
10%	11%	2	10	150

CNS – sedation, anti-emesis, anti-Parkinsonian

CVS – initial tachycardia given IV, but may later cause bradycardia due to central effect

RS – decreases secretions, bronchodilatation, slight ventilatory stimulation

Others – anti-sialagogue, anti-spasmodic for biliary tree, and uterus; marked decrease in tear and sweat formation; decreases bladder and ureteric tone

Elimination – metabolised in the liver to scopine and scopic acid; unchanged, urine 2%, bile 5%

Toxicity – potential problem in patients with porphyria

GLYCERYL TRINITRATE

Structure – organic nitrate ester of nitric acid and glycerol (glycerine)

Preparation – sublingual tablets and oral spray, transdermal patches (5 and 10 mg), IV – clear colourless, aqueous solution containing 1 mg glyceryl trinitrate per ml with polyethylene glycol and dextrose; stored in amber ampoules with 5 and 50 ml solution

Dose – SL, 300 mcg; TD, 5 or 10 mg per 24 H; IV, 0.2–3 mcg/kg/min

Pharmacokinetics

V_d	Cl	$t_{1/2}$
0.04–2.9	600	2

CNS – intracranial pressure increased as a result of vasodilatation and headache ensues if sublingual dose continues beyond desired anti-anginal effect

CVS – venodilator with arterial dilatation as dose increases; SVR, systolic, diastolic, venous and pulmonary artery pressures reduced, myocardial oxygen demand reduced; cardiac output and coronary blood flow little effected; heart rate is unchanged in failure but increased reflexly in normal state

RS – bronchodilatation and may increase shunt

Other – relaxes other smooth muscle such as biliary and gut

Metabolism – hydrolysis of the ester bonds by red cells and the liver, and 80% of the dose is excreted in the urine

Contra-indications – substantial amount of intravenously administered GTN binds to the plastic of giving sets and syringes, therefore reduced availability

SODIUM NITROPRUSSIDE

Structure – inorganic complex

Preparation – red-brown powder containing 50 mg sodium nitroprusside in a brown glass ampoule which is reconstituted in 2 ml 5% dextrose before further dilution. It should be protected from light and yellow and brown giving sets and syringes are available for this purpose

Dose – IV infusion 0.1–1.5 mcg/kg/min (maximum of up to 8 mcg/kg/min)

Maximum dose 1.5 mg/kg; starts to accumulates once rate > 2 mcg/kg/min

Pharmacokinetics

V_d	Elimination	nitroprusside $t_{1/2}$	thiocyanate $t_{1/2}$
0.2	1 mcg/kg/min	very short	2.7 days

CNS – cerebral vasodilatation increases intracranial pressure

CVS – dilates arterioles and venules with reduced blood pressure, reduced LVEDP, reduced myocardial oxygen demand; heart rate increases but contractility is unaffected

RS – hypoxic pulmonary vasoconstriction is impaired and arterial oxygen tension may fall

Other – gastro-intestinal motility and lower oesophageal sphincter pressure are reduced; metabolic acidosis may occur

Metabolism – reacts with sulphydryl groups of plasma amino acids; higher concentrations cause non enzymatic hydrolysis in red blood cells to produce five cyanide ions from each nitroprusside molecule. One of these combines with haemoglobin (iron in ferrous state) to form methaemoglobin (iron in ferric state); most of the rest is converted to thiocyanate by rhodonase in the liver and is then excreted in the urine; small amount of thiocyanate combines with vitamin B_{12} to form cyanocobalamin

Toxicity – cyanide ions inhibit the cytochrome oxidase chain; plasma levels of > 80 mcg/l produce tachycardia, sweating, hyperventilation, cardiac arrhythmias and retrosternal pain

SECTION 3: 12
CARDIOVASCULAR PHARMACOLOGY

T. C. Smith

ANTI-ARRHYTHMICS

ADENOSINE

CARDIAC GLYCOSIDES

MAGNESIUM

CALCIUM ANTAGONISTS
Papaverines
Dihydropyridines
Benzothiazepines

PHOSPHODIESTERASE INHIBITORS
Mode of action
Clinical effects
Bipyridines
Imidazolines

SELECTIVE IMIDAZOLINE RECEPTOR AGONISTS (SIRA)

RENIN ANGIOTENSIN SYSTEM
Angiotensin-converting enzyme inhibitors
Angiotensin$_1$ inhibitors

DIURETICS
Loop diuretics
Thiazide diuretics
Potassium sparing diuretics
Osmotic diuretics
Carbonic anhydrase inhibitors

SPECIFIC PHARMACOLOGY

ANTI-ARRHYTHMIC AGENTS

Anti-arrhythmic agents are usually classified according to their effect on the electrophysiology of cardiac myofibrils. Figure CV.1 shows the different sites in the heart on which these drugs act. There are four basic classes of anti-arrhythmic agent with considerable variation in the chemical structure of the drugs within each functional class (Vaughan Williams 1970). Examples of the drugs by class are shown in Figure CV.2.

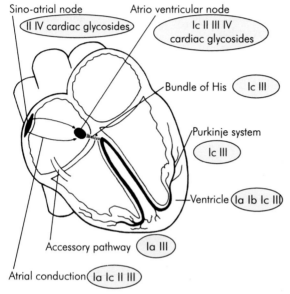

Figure CV.1 Sites of action of anti-arrhythmic agents

CLASS I

Class I drugs work in a similar way to local anaesthetic agents (lidocaine is used for both roles). They act by slowing sodium entry into cells through the fast, voltage-gated sodium channels that primarily affect the non nodal areas characterised by a fast depolarisation action potential. They reduce the maximum rate of rise of phase 0 depolarisation. The rate of phase 4 sino-atrial node depolarisation may also be reduced and with it spontaneous automaticity.

Fast, voltage-gated sodium channels may exist in three states – resting, open and refractory. In normal myocardium, their state switches between resting and open but ischaemia results in prolonged depolarisation and the channel becomes refractory. The class I anti-arrhythmics block open channels so that the more frequent the action potentials the more ionophores become blocked. The first action potential shows a slight reduction in phase 0 depolarisation. Subsequent action potentials show a progressive reduction in the rate of depolarisation as more channels are blocked. The block is, therefore, use-dependent.

Class I has three subdivisions based on the effect on the action potential duration. The effect on action potential duration is related to the type of sodium channel affected as follows:

- Class IA (e.g. quinidine) – action potential duration increased
- Class IB (e.g. lidocaine) – action potential duration decreased

ANTI-ARRHYTHMIC DRUGS BY CLASS			
I	II	III	IV
IA	Propranolol	Amiodarone	Verapamil
Quinidine	Esmolol	Bretylium	Dilitiazem
Procainamide	Sotalol	Sotalol	
Disopyramide		n-acetyl procainamide	
Cibenzoline			
IB			
Lidocaine			
Phenytoin			
Mexiletine			
Tocainide			
Ethmozine			
IC			
Flecainide			
Lorcainide			
Propafenone			
Indecainide			
Encainide			

Figure CV.2

- Class IC (e.g. flecainide) – action potential duration unaffected

The key features of the subdivisions of class I anti-arrhythmics are shown in Figure CV.3.

Class IB anti-arrhythmics have a receptor association/dissociation cycle shorter than the cardiac cycle. The initial drug effect causes gradual blockade of the ionophores to develop during the action potential depolarisation. By the time the next action potential occurs, however, the drug will have dissociated from its receptor again. If a premature depolarisation (e.g. a ventricular premature beat) occurs then the myofibril will still be blocked. Class IB anti-arrhythmics bind preferentially to refractory channels and are, therefore, selective for ischaemic myocardium. Class IB drugs also elevate the fibrillation threshold. Lidocaine is discussed on page 661. Mexiletine is similar but also has anti-convulsant properties possibly due to GABA re-uptake inhibition.

Class IC have a much slower association/dissociation cycle lasting longer than the cardiac cycle so the block is relatively constant from cycle to cycle. The overall effect is a general reduction in excitability and this is, therefore, more suitable for re-entrant type rhythms. There is little selectivity for the refractory channels of ischaemic myocardium.

Class IA drugs have features midway between those of IB and IC. Figure CV.4 shows the ECG effects of the class I anti-arrhythmics.

Class IA drugs are primarily used for supraventricular tachycardias and Class IB and C for ventricular tachycardias.

CLASS II

Class II anti-arrhythmics (β blockers) competitively block the effects of circulating and neurotransmitter catecholamines, reducing arrhythmogenicity, heart rate and contractility. This slows and so lengthens

FEATURES OF THE SUBDIVISIONS OF CLASS I ANTI-ARRHYTHMIC DRUGS

Class	Example	dV/dt of phase 0	Repolarisation	PR	QRS	QT
IA	Quinidine	Slowed	Prolonged	↑	↑	↑
IB	Lidocaine	Little effect	Shortened	0	0	↓
IC	Flecainide	Marked slowing	Little effect	↑↑	↑↑	0

Figure CV.3

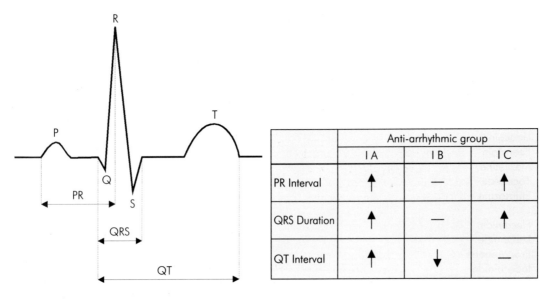

Figure CV.4 ECG effects of anti-arrhythmic drugs

phase 4 depolarisation, the phase which is shortened by catecholamines. The action potential is shortened and the refractory period of the AV node is prolonged. It is likely that these effects are mediated by a slow calcium influx that may be particularly useful in preventing post myocardial infarction ventricular arrhythmias, when catecholamine levels may be high. β blockers are covered in detail on page 689–690.

CLASS III

Class III drugs (amiodarone, bretilium, sotalol) prolong repolarisation and, therefore, the action potential, and increase the effective refractory period. Their principal uses are for the following arrhythmias:

- Atrial tachycardia
- Atrial flutter and fibrillation
- Re-entrant junctional tachycardia
- Ventricular tachycardia

Amiodarone is particularly effective for the treatment of atrial tachyarrhythmias when Wolff–Parkinson–White syndrome is also present. At higher doses, the effect may be similar to β blockade and there is a quinidine-like action. Marked hypotension may result from IV administration.

Bretylium tosylate is reserved for use in resuscitation. It is given intravenously or intramuscularly in the treatment of ventricular fibrillation after DC shock and lidocaine have been tried. It accumulates in sympathetic ganglia and reduces norepinephrine release. There is an initial post ganglionic discharge. It may cause hypotension, nausea and vomiting and should be used with caution when a cardiac glycoside has been previously administered.

Sotalol is a β-adrenergic antagonist and is classified as both a Class II and a Class III anti-arrhythmic. It is indicated for the treatment of paroxysmal supraventricular tachycardia, ventricular premature beats and ventricular tachycardia. It is more suitable than lidocaine for the treatment of spontaneous sustained ventricular tachycardia secondary to coronary disease or cardiomyopathy. The usual precautions for β blocker therapy apply. Use with caution when there is hypokalaemia and when other agents that prolong the QT interval are concurrently administered.

CLASS IV

There are numerous calcium antagonists (page 705–706), having different sites of action. Verapamil and diltiazem have anti-arrhythmic activity but nifedipine does not. Slowing of calcium influx reduces the duration of phases 2 and 3 of the action potential. At the atrioventricular node, this action is particularly beneficial in preventing re-entry rhythm problems.

ADENOSINE

Adenosine is used for rapid conversion of paroxysmal supraventricular tachycardias back to sinus rhythm (including Wolff–Parkinson–White syndrome). It may also be used in the diagnosis of conduction defects. Adenosine is ubiquitous in the body, in combination with phosphate (e.g. cyclic AMP). There are two specific types of adenosine receptor, A_1 and A_2, the effects of which are detailed in Figure CV.5.

RECEPTOR EFFECTS OF ADENOSINE

A_1

Inhibition of AV nodal conduction
Reduction of contractility
Inhibition of neurotransmitter release in CNS and PNS
Renal vasoconstriction
Bronchoconstriction

A_2

Vasodilatation (including coronary)
Inhibition of platelet aggregation
Stimulation of nociceptive neurones

Figure CV.5

The effect of adenosine in causing transient slowing of AV nodal conduction allows normal sinus nodal discharge to initiate a normal pattern of electrical depolarisation throughout the heart, and so normal sinus rhythm resumes, before the drug has been eliminated. It is an unusual drug in that a key to successful use is that its IV injection must be rapid. This is because it is metabolised rapidly with a half-life of only 8–10 s. Unlike verapamil it can be used safely in conjunction with β blockers.

CARDIAC GLYCOSIDES

The cardiac glycosides are a group of naturally occurring compounds used to improve myocardial contractility and reduce cardiac conductivity. Cardiac glycosides are found mainly in three botanical species, white foxglove (*Digitalis lanata*), purple foxglove (*D. purpurea*) and climbing oleander (*Strophanthus gratus*).

CHEMISTRY

The cardiac glycosides share the same basic structure:

- Steroid nucleus (cyclopentanophenanthrene)
- Lactone ring (five- or six-membered) – the aglycone
- Carbohydrate (up to four monosaccharide units)

The carbohydrate moiety is responsible for solubility, and the lactone ring confers pharmacological activity. Saturation of the lactone rings reduces potency, and opening of the ring abolishes the pharmacological activity. Only rings A and D of the steroid nucleus are coplanar, whereas in adrenal steroids rings A and C, and B and D are coplanar.

PHARMACOLOGICAL EFFECTS

Cardiac glycosides increase myocardial contractility and slow conduction at the atrioventricular node Isometric and isotonic contraction of both atrial and ventricular muscle is improved. Cardiac glycosides cause directly mediated vasoconstriction.

CLINICAL USES

Cardiac glycosides are used to improve contractility in hypervolaemic myocardial failure. In chronic atrial fibrillation ventricular rate becomes slower due to a direct reduction in AV nodal conduction and by a secondary reduction in vagal tone.

MECHANISMS OF ACTION

Sodium-potassium adenosine triphosphatase ($Na^+K^+ATPase$)

Cardiac glycosides specifically and reversibly bind to cardiac cell membrane $Na^+K^+ATPase$ that alters the electrolyte balance inside the myocardial fibres with more sodium and less potassium intracellularly. This results in a reduction of the transport of sodium into the cell using the Na^+Ca^{2+} ion exchange system, and intracellular calcium is better maintained and increased. The increased calcium may be responsible for the positive inotropy. However, at higher doses this interference with an essential membrane pump may be responsible for toxicity.

Interference with neuronal catecholamine re-uptake

At low biophase concentrations, there is an increase in local catecholamine levels due to interference with neuronal catecholamine re-uptake. This has positive inotropic and chronotropic effects, and may in fact increase overall $Na^+K^+ATPase$ activity. There is also an increase in local acetyl choline levels, resulting in negative inotropic and chronotropic effects.

ELIMINATION

The glycosides are highly bound to cardiac muscle, and, therefore, have very high volumes of distribution. This slows elimination considerably as most are excreted unchanged in the urine, by both simple filtration, and also by tubular secretion. Digitoxin is the exception being primarily metabolised by hepatic microsomal enzymes.

TOXICITY

The cardiac glycosides have a very low therapeutic index. Most of the toxic effects are due to potassium loss. It is, therefore, particularly important to consider potassium-sparing diuretics when diuretics are needed in conjunction with cardiac glycosides. Side effects of the cardiac glycosides are listed in Figure CV.6.

SIDE EFFECTS OF CARDIAC GLYCOSIDES
Heart block
Cardiac arrhythmias
Fatigue
Nausea
Anorexia
Xanthopsia
Confusion
Neuralgia
Gynaecomastia

Figure CV.6

CONTRA-INDICATIONS

Digoxin is contra-indicated in hypertrophic cardiomyopathy as it may increase outflow obstruction and cause sudden failure. It is also contra-indicated in cardiac amyloid.

MAGNESIUM

Magnesium is the fourth most prevalent cation in the body and the second intracellularly. Of total body magnesium, 53% is in bone, 27% in muscle and only 0.3% in plasma. Its physiological roles include incorporation as a cofactor in over 300 enzyme systems, inhibition of IP_3-gated calcium channels, muscle contraction, neuronal activity, neurotransmitter release and adenyl cyclase regulation.

USES (See Figure CV.7)

Pharmacologically magnesium is used as replacement therapy. It is recognised now that magnesium deficiency is not uncommon in hospital patients and in particular two thirds of intensive care patients may be magnesium depleted. There is now good evidence that magnesium is effective in the treatment of eclampsia and some evidence to support its use in pre-eclampsia and in preventing the hypertensive response to intubation. The treatment of cardiac dysrrhythmias is particularly indicated if hypokalaemia coexists.

CALCIUM ANTAGONISTS

Calcium is involved not only in muscle contraction but also in neurotransmitter release, hormone secretion, platelet aggregation and enzyme function. There are numerous calcium channels across cell and other membranes. These may be active or passive, triggered by chemical mediators or voltage changes, and may be coupled with other ionic exchange. The term calcium antagonist is generally used to describe those agents with a role in cardiovascular manipulation. These act primarily on the voltage gated (L-type) calcium channels, preventing opening of the ionophore. There are three main groups (papaverines, dihydropyridines, benzothiazepines) each having characteristic actions. However, even within these groups, there is considerable difference between the individual chemical structures of the drugs, and in their calcium channel specificity. The myocardial depression caused

POSSIBLE PHARMACOLOGICAL USES OF MAGNESIUM THERAPY

Correction of magnesium deficiency

Control of eclampsia and pre-eclampsia

Inhibition of premature labour

Improvement of cardiac contractility

Limitation of myocardial infarct size

Component of cardioplegia (a mixture to arrest the heart during cardiac surgery)

Correction of cardiac dysrrhythmias

Emergency treatment of torsades de pointes, digoxin toxicity, life threatening atrial and ventricular dysrhythmias

Prevention of hypertensive response to intubation

Pre-eclampsia

Reduction of catecholamine release in phaeochromocytoma surgery

Treatment of asthma

Figure CV.7

by the volatile anaesthetic agents halothane, enflurane and isoflurane is also the result of an alteration in calcium flux. Figure CV.8 shows the relative potencies of the three representative calcium antagonists.

All three groups of calcium antagonist reduce systemic vascular resistance and central venous pressure by vasodilatation. This vasodilatation is more pronounced in the arterial system and as it is combined with a slight negative inotropic effect blood pressure falls. The

RELATIVE CLINICAL EFFECTS OF CALCIUM ANTAGONISTS

	Verapamil	Diltiazem	Nifedipine
Reduction in SVR	++	+	+++
Coronary vasodilatation	++	++	++
Reduction in contractility	++	0	+
Reduction in blood pressure	+	0	++
Reflex increase in sympathetic tone	+	0	++
Slowing of AV nodal conduction	+++	++	0

Figure CV.8

reduction in after-load and contractility reduces myocardial workload and oxygen requirement. All calcium antagonists cause coronary vasodilatation but this is only of clinical relevance in coronary artery spasm.

Calcium antagonists may also interfere with non cardiac calcium channels affecting, for example, neuromuscular blockade and insulin secretion.

PAPAVERINES

Examples – methoxyverapamil, teapamil, verapamil

Papaverines predominantly act on cardiac muscle, by inhibiting the slow calcium entry during phases 2 and 3 of the cardiac muscle action potential. This lengthening of the action potential makes them appropriate for tachyarrhythmias especially re-entry supraventricular tachycardias and others of atrial origin. They also slow AV conduction giving them a role in the management of atrial flutter and tachycardia. Papaverines have relatively little effect on vasomotor tone, but the reduction in contractility is more marked than the calcium channel blockers.

DIHYDROPYRIDINES

Examples – amlodipine, nicardipine, nifedipine, nimodipine

The dihydropyridines predominantly act on smooth muscle. Clinically this mainly affects vascular tone causing peripheral vasodilatation primarily on the arterial side and so reduces after-load. This reduces cardiac workload and may improve peripheral perfusion. The resultant drop in blood pressure results in a partial compensatory increase in heart rate and cardiac output. They also cause coronary vasodilatation, but this is not generally of clinical benefit. Dihydropyridines are used to treat hypertension, angina and heart failure. Nimodipine acts preferentially on cerebral arteries and is used to prevent vascular spasm after subarachnoid haemorrhage.

BENZOTHIAZEPINES

Example – diltiazem

Diltiazem affects both cardiac and smooth muscle causing relatively mild reductions in systemic vascular resistance, blood pressure and cardiac output. It is used as an anti-arrhythmic agent and for the treatment of angina and hypertension.

PHOSPHODIESTERASE INHIBITORS

Selective phosphodiesterase inhibitors are used for their inotropic and vasodilator properties. They selectively inhibit the phosphodiesterase III isoenzyme (PDE III) responsible for the breakdown of cAMP in myocardial muscle and vascular smooth muscle. This is in contrast with the methylxanthines such as theophylline (see page 716–717) that non-specifically inhibit all five phosphodiesterase isoenzymes. There are two chemical types of PDE III inhibitors, bipyridines and imidazolines.

MODE OF ACTION

Inhibition of PDE III causes an increase in intracellular cAMP and, to a lesser extent, cGMP in myocardial and vascular smooth muscle cells. The cAMP is responsible for phosphorylation of protein kinases in the cell. In the myocardium, this increases the influx of calcium through the slow calcium channels of the sarcolemma by increasing both the number of channels open and the duration of the open state. The sarcoplasmic reticulum is also affected facilitating faster calcium release. The net effect is an increase in calcium ion availability in the cell for contraction. The raised level of cAMP is also responsible for improved re-uptake of calcium into the sarcoplasmic reticulum so active myocardial relaxation is also improved leading to an overall improvement in myocardial function.

In smooth muscle, the cAMP causes phosphorylation of the myosin light chain kinase which reduces the affinity for the calmodulin complex and dephosphorylates the myosin light chains. This results in relaxation and secondary vasodilatation. The increase in cGMP also mediates smooth muscle relaxation.

CLINICAL EFFECTS

PDE III inhibitors improve contractility in the failing heart without increasing the myocardial oxygen utilisation. The positive inotropic effect is greater than that of the cardiac glycosides and there is little chronotropic activity. Conduction in the atrium and AV node is increased, with little effect on the His–Purkinje system. PDE inhibitors cause vasodilatation and, therefore, reduce pre load and after-load. Coronary vascular resistance is also reduced but this does not appear to cause coronary steal. PDE III inhibitors also cause some bronchodilatation but this is not a major feature. These agents are used in the short-term treatment of severe congestive cardiac failure when other measures have failed. They work synergistically with β-adrenoceptor agonists and can work when these alone have failed.

BIPYRIDINES

Example – milrinone

Milrinone is supplied as a pale yellow solution of the lactate salt. It is administered as a loading dose followed by infusion. It may potentially cause hypotension because of vasodilatation, necessitating close monitoring. Of it, 80% is eliminated unchanged in the urine and it is, therefore, greatly influenced by decreases in renal function. In severe myocardial failure, glomerular filtration rate is often reduced and so half-life is increased from the normal 1 hour to several hours.

IMIDAZOLINES

Example – enoximone

Enoximone is supplied as a pale yellow solution in ethanol, propylene glycol and sodium hydroxide and has pH 12. It is administered as a loading dose followed by infusion. Enoximone reduces the refractoriness of the atrium and AV node and shortens the ventricular refractory period. Ventricular tachycardias and ectopic beats have been observed in some patients who have received enoximone. The propensity to cause hypotension (due to vasodilatation) necessitates monitoring of blood pressure. Enoximone is metabolised in the liver producing a mixture of active and inactive metabolites, and has a half-life of about 4 H.

SELECTIVE IMIDAZOLINE RECEPTOR AGONISTS (SIRA)

Example – moxonidine

Selective imidazoline receptor agonists are used for anti-hypertensive therapy. These drugs act by selective agonism at the imidazoline subtype 1 receptor (I_1) in the rostral-ventrolateral pressor area and ventromedial depressor areas of the medulla oblongata. This area is responsible for sympathetic activity and an agonist effect at I_1 receptors results in a reduction of general sympathetic nervous system activity which produces the desired effect. SIRAs have a minor effect at the α_2 receptor which might potentially result in sedation but in practice this is not seen, the commonest side effect being dry mouth

An example from this group is moxonidine, a centrally acting anti-hypertensive agent for mild to moderate hypertension. It may exacerbate cardiac conduction defects and should be withdrawn slowly over a two week period. Caution is necessary when administering moxonidine with benzodiazepines, as the sedative effects of the latter become enhanced.

RENIN-ANGIOTENSIN SYSTEM

Antagonism of the renin-angiotensin system at various levels is used to control hypertension by reducing vasomotor tone and by reducing salt and fluid retention. The first site of interference in this cascade is by antagonism of the β adrenoreceptors responsible for renin secretion. Next in line are the angiotensin converting enzyme (ACE) inhibitors then the angiotensin II receptor antagonists.

ANGIOTENSIN-CONVERTING ENZYME INHIBITORS

Examples – captopril, enalapril, lisinopril, perindropril, ramipril

Mechanism of action

ACE inhibitors block the action of the carboxypeptidase, angiotensin converting enzyme (ACE) in the lungs which converts the inactive angiotensin I (Ang I) into the active angiotensin II (Ang II) an octapeptide). Angiotensin II causes profound vasoconstriction and causes release of aldosterone resulting in sodium and water conservation. ACE is relatively non specific and also inactivates bradykinin (a vasodilator) and other kinins. These three activities produce a rise in intravascular volume and vasomotor tone with the resultant increase in blood pressure. ACE inhibitors antagonise these effects. ACE inhibitors may also cause specific renal vasodilatation, and so further enhance sodium and water excretion. The reduced breakdown of bradykinin is responsible for the side effect of dry cough experienced with ACE inhibitors. The effects of ACE inhibitors include a reduction in:

* Sodium and water retention
* Vasomotor tone
* Pre load
* After-load,
* Myocardial work

ACE inhibitors are indicated in hypertension, congestive cardiac failure, myocardial infarction and diabetic nephropathy. They are particularly effective when renin levels are raised such as when sympathetic tone is increased. Myocardial infarction and congestive cardiac failure may show such increases. In anti-hypertensive therapy the ACE inhibitors may be used alone or in conjunction with other agents using different systems such as diuretics and calcium antagonists. β blockers reduce renin secretion so the benefit of adding an ACE inhibitor will be limited.

ANGIOTENSIN₁ INHIBITORS

Examples – losartan, valsartan

Mechanism of action

The classification of the AT_1 receptor deserves further clarification. ACE converts Ang I to Ang II. Ang I is inactive and does not have identified receptors whereas in contrast Ang II is highly active. Two receptor subtypes for Ang II (roman numerals) have been identified and numbered (with arabic numerals) AT_1 and AT_2. AT_1 receptors are G-protein coupled receptors responsible for vasoconstricton and aldosterone secretion. The role of the AT_2 receptors is less clear but they are thought to be anti-proliferative for endothelial cells and to be involved in smooth muscle proliferation and differentiation.

Uses

The AT_1 inhibitors are used as anti-hypertensive agents and have clinical effects similar to the ACE inhibitors. Their main advantage is the absence of an effect on kinins so the persistent dry cough of ACE inhibitors is not seen.

Features

The clinical features of AT_1 inhibitors are very varied. The main effects are shown in Figure CV.9.

CLINICAL EFFECTS OF AT₁ INHIBITORS

Reduced sodium and water retention
Reduced vasomotor tone
Reduced pre load
Reduced afterload
Reduced blood pressure especially if sodium depletion
Reduced myocardial work
Variable reduction in aldosterone levels
Blockade of negative feedback produces a rise in renin, Ang I and Ang II
Increased insulin sensitivity and reduced catecholamines and anti-natriuretic factor (ANF)
Increased plasma potassium concentration

Figure CV.9

DIURETICS

Diuretics promote the loss of water and sodium via the urine. Interference with sodium re-absorption in the renal tubule causes increased sodium loss and the sodium takes water with it. Their precise effect is determined by which part of the renal tubule they affect. Other drugs may also indirectly increase renal water loss. The sites of action of the various diuretics are shown in Figure CV.10.

LOOP DIURETICS

Example – frusemide

These act on the thick (upper) part of the ascending loop of Henle by reducing sodium and chloride re-absorption. This interferes with the generation of the interstitial hypertonicity which is used by the collecting duct to re-absorb water. A smaller effect is due to the increased delivery of filtrate to the distal tubule. These are the most efficacious diuretics causing up to 25% of sodium and water in the filtrate to be excreted. Loop diuretics also cause vasodilatation either directly or indirectly. This increases renal blood flow without affecting the glomerular filtration rate. The protein left in the efferent capillaries supplying the remainder of the nephron is, therefore, more dilute and has a lower oncotic pressure that reduces re-absorption from the nephron. Subsequently more filtrate enters the loop of Henle, which is the primary site of action of the loop diuretics. In congestive cardiac failure, the venodilatation reduces pre load before any diuretic effect is seen.

Loop diuretics work as anti-hypertensives by reducing both blood volume and vascular tone.

The vascular effects may be mediated by interference with prostaglandin E_2 and I_2 degradation.

Loop diuretics present more filtrate to the distal convoluted tubule. The sodium–potassium exchange pump re-absorbs more sodium and, therefore, more potassium is excreted. Hydrogen ions are also excreted in exchange for some of the potassium, and bicarbonate concentration increases. Patients on loop diuretics are, therefore, at risk of hypokalaemia and metabolic alkalosis. Calcium and magnesium loss also occurs. Uric acid secretion is reduced.

Loop diuretics are highly protein bound and, therefore, do not readily pass through the glomerular membrane. They are actively secreted into the proximal convoluted tubule (via the organic acid transport system) and then travel along the tubule to the luminal membrane of the loop of Henle. Excretion occurs via the urine and they are non cumulative.

THIAZIDE DIURETICS

Example – bendrofluazide

Thiazides act on the luminal membrane pump of the distal convoluted tubule by inhibiting active sodium and chloride re-absorption. They are medium efficacy diuretics causing up to 10% of sodium and water in the filtrate to be excreted. More sodium reaches the distal tubules and results in high potassium loss in the same way as the loop diuretics, but because this is the main mode of thiazide action potassium loss is a much greater problem. Magnesium excretion is increased, but calcium and uric acid excretion are reduced.

Thiazides also cause direct vasodilation. Owing to the ability to cause hyperglycaemia they are best avoided in diabetics. Excretion is by glomerular filtration and by tubular secretion using the uric acid secretion mechanism which reduces uric acid excretion.

POTASSIUM SPARING DIURETICS

Examples – amiloride, spironolactone

Potassium sparing diuretics act on the distal convoluted tubule and collecting duct. They are low efficacy diuretics causing only 5% of sodium and water in the filtrate to be excreted, but have the advantage that they conserve potassium and are mainly used to minimise potassium loss caused by more effective diuretics. The decrease in potassium secretion

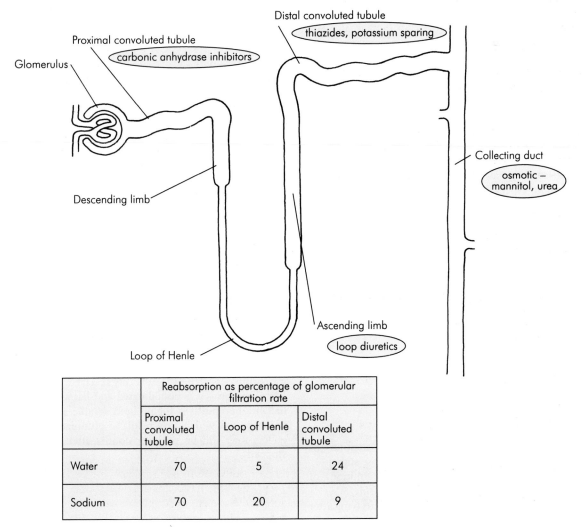

	Reabsorption as percentage of glomerular filtration rate		
	Proximal convoluted tubule	Loop of Henle	Distal convoluted tubule
Water	70	5	24
Sodium	70	20	9

Figure CV.10 Sites of action of diuretics

increases the hydrogen ion secretion and thus reduces bicarbonate excretion. They also reduce uric acid excretion. Spironolactone inhibits the sodium potassium exchange pump of the extraluminal membrane of collecting duct cells. Triamterene and amiloride interfere with the sodium channels through which the effects of aldosterone are mediated. Amiloride also inhibits sodium potassium exchange in the proximal tubule.

OSMOTIC DIURETICS

Examples – mannitol, glucose, urea

Osmotic diuretics (such as mannitol and glucose) act by passing freely through the glomerular basement membrane, but being non re-absorbable once in the tubule. The resultant effect is dependent directly upon the number of molecules and so a large number of molecules is required to produce a clinical effect. They must usually be given intravenously. Urea is classified as an osmotic diuretic but is actively secreted into the tubule as well.

CARBONIC ANHYDRASE INHIBITORS

Example – acetazolamide

Carbonic anhydrase inhibitors inhibit the enzymatic breakdown of carbonic acid, and so interfere with the re-absorption of sodium in exchange for hydrogen ion secretion especially in the proximal tubule. Their diuretic effect is mild. Their use is now mainly reserved for treatment of glaucoma and epilepsy. Other examples of carbonic anhydrase inhibitors are methazolamide, and dichlorphenamide.

SPECIFIC PHARMACOLOGY

Here, bio-availability applies to oral administration. Units (unless stated otherwise) are:

Volume of distribution at steady state (V_d) (l/kg)
Clearance (Cl) (ml/kg/min)
Terminal half-life ($t_{1/2}$) (H)

ADENOSINE

Structure – a nucleoside comprising adenine (6-amino purine) and D-ribofuranose (pentose sugar)
Presentation – IV clear, aqueous solution of adenosine 6 mg in 2 ml 0.9% sodium chloride
Dose – IV – bolus 3 mg over 2 s, then bolus 6 mg after 1–2 min if necessary, then bolus 12 mg after 1–2 min if necessary; stop if high nodal block develops

Pharmacokinetics
$t_{1/2}$
8–10 s
CNS – rare occurrence of blurred vision, headache, dizziness
CVS – inhibits AV nodal conduction, reduces contractility, vasodilatation; palpitations, flushing, hypotension, severe bradycardia may occur
RS – dyspnoea, bronchospasm may occur
Other effects – nausea
Elimination – rapid cellular uptake, adenosine deaminase, phosphorylation to nucleotide
Contra-indications – second and third degree heart block and sick sinus syndrome unless artificial pacemaker functioning; asthma
Interactions – dipyridamole inhibits adenosine uptake (if essential, use 0.5–1 mg dose); xanthines (caffeine, aminophylline) are potent inhibitors of adenosine; drugs slowing AV nodal conduction

AMIODARONE HYDROCHLORIDE

Structure – iodinated benzofuran derivative – class III anti-arrhythmic
Presentation – tablets 200 mg, 100 mg; IV – clear, pale yellow solution 150 mg in 3 ml
Dose – oral loading regimen then 200 mg/day; IV 5 mg/kg over 20 min to 2 H; onset of action by oral route is 6 days
Pharmacokinetics

Bio-availability	Protein binding	$t_{1/2}$
22–86%	97%	1300

CNS – peripheral neuropathy rare; nightmares, tremor, ataxia; corneal microdeposits (benign and reversible)
CVS – slows heart rate and may cause bradycardia, and AV block
RS – may rarely cause diffuse pulmonary alveolitis and fibrosis
Other effects – metabolite blocks conversion of T3 to thyroxine and may, therefore, cause hypo- or hyperthyroidism. Thyroid function should be monitored. It may cause chronic liver disease, and transaminases often rise, especially at start of treatment
Elimination – it is de-iodinated and has a very long half-life because it is highly lipid soluble and highly tissue bound which may result in cumulation; toxic effects may still be present months after treatment stopped

DIGOXIN

Structure – sterol lactone with sugar moiety – cardiac glycoside

Presentation – tablets 62.5, 125 and 250 mcg, elixir. IV, clear, colourless, aqueous solution, 125 mcg/ml
Dose: IV – up to 1 mg loading dose by slow (25 mcg/min) injection; typically 10 mcg/kg once daily oral or IV, monitor levels, plasma concentrations (nmol/l) – therapeutic 1.3–1.5; toxic 3.5

Pharmacokinetics

Bio-availability	Protein binding	V_d	$t_{1/2}$
75%	25%	8	35

Clearance = $0.88 \times$ creatinine clearance + 0.33

CNS – nausea, vomiting, dizziness, anorexia, fatigue, apathy, malaise, visual disturbance, depression and psychosis
CVS – positive inotropy, especially in hypervolaemic failure; negative chronotropy; slowing of AV conduction; in excess may cause complete heart block, and most rhythm disturbances especially bradycardias
Other effects – mild intrinsic diuretic affect; abdominal pain, diarrhoea; gynaecomastia (steroid related); intestinal necrosis (oral route); skin rashes; thrombocytopoenia
Elimination – 10% metabolised in the liver by progressive removal of the sugar moieties; 60% excreted unchanged in the urine by glomerular filtration and active tubular secretion

Toxicity increased by low potassium, low magnesium, high sodium, high calcium, acid–base disturbance and hypoxaemia. Poorly removed by dialysis as highly tissue bound; digoxin specific antibody fragments available for treatment of poisoning

DILTIAZEM

Structure – benzothiapine calcium antagonist – class IV anti-arrhythmic
Presentation – tablets 60 mg
Dose – 60–120 mg, 6–8 hourly
Pharmacokinetics

Bio-availability	Protein binding	V_d	Cl	$t_{1/2}$
35%	80%	5.3	15	5

CNS – no effect
CVS – causes peripheral and coronary arterial vasodilatation; decreases systemic and peripheral resistance; slows AV nodal conduction; exacerbates the negative inotropic effects of volatile agents
RS – anti-histamine effect
Other effects – renal artery dilatation increases renal plasma flow; local anaesthetic effect; reduced lower oesophageal sphincter pressure in achalasia; may inhibit platelet aggregation
Elimination – 2% is excreted unchanged in the urine; deacetylation and demethylation produce active metabolites which are conjugated with glucuronides and sulphates; renal failure has no effect on elimination

ESMOLOL HYDROCHLORIDE

Structure – aryloxypropanolamine – β blocker – class II anti-arrhythmic
Presentation – IV, clear, aqueous solution 10 ml of 250 mg/ml for dilution and infusion; 10 ml of 100 mg/ml for undiluted boluses
Dose – 50–200 mcg/kg/min; a loading dose may be used
Pharmacokinetics

Protein binding	V_d	Cl	$t_{1/2}$
56%	3.43	285	9.2 minutes

CVS – mainly β_1; used for acute SVT, acute control of hypertension and myocardial infarction; negative chronotrope and inotrope, cardiac output falls by 20%
RS – selectivity minimises increases in airway resistance
Elimination – metabolised by red cell esterases producing methanol and a primary acid (70–80% as this in urine) which has weak β antagonism and half-life of 3.5 H; < 1% is excreted unchanged in the urine. Use with caution in renal failure; hepatic failure has no effect

NIFEDIPINE

Structure – dihydropyridine calcium antagonist – class IV anti-dysrrhythmic
Presentation – tablets 10 and 20 mg and capsules 5 and 10 mg; the yellow, viscous liquid in the capsules has been used sublingually for speedy control of blood pressure; a solution is available for direct intracoronary injection
Dose – oral 10–20 mg 8 hourly, 20–40 mg 12 hourly slow release formulation
Pharmacokinetics

Bio-availability	Protein binding	V_d	Cl	$t_{1/2}$
65%	95%	0.8	10	5

CNS – marginal increase in cerebral blood flow; headache, flushing, dizziness
CVS – decreases systemic and peripheral vascular resistance, decreases pulmonary artery pressure, reflex increase in heart rate and cardiac output; increases epicardial and coronary blood flow, negative inotrope
RS – no effect
Other effects – increases red cell deformability, decreases platelet aggregation, decreases thromboxane synthesis; reduces lower oesophageal sphincter pressure; increases renin, increases catecholamines; increases hepatic blood flow; oedema of legs; eye pain; gum hyperplasia
Elimination – 85% in urine; 15% in bile; non cumulative

VERAPAMIL

Structure – synthetic papaverine derivative – class IV anti-arrhythmic

Presentation – tablets 40, 80 and 120 mg. IV, 5 mg in 2 ml

Dose – oral 40–120 mg 8 hourly; IV 10 mg (0.075–0.20 mg/kg)

Pharmacokinetics

Bio-availability	Protein binding	V_d	$t_{1/2}$
20%	90%	4.5	5

CNS – dizziness, headache

CVS – slows cardiac action potential; slows AV nodal conduction; decreases systemic vascular resistance; decreases blood pressure heart rate and cardiac output; increases coronary blood flow

RS – no effect

Other effects – local anaesthetic effect; constipation

Elimination – 70% excreted in urine as conjugated metabolites, 5% unchanged; non cumulative; half-life is increased in hepatic disease

Interactions – avoid concurrent use with β blocker as it may cause asystole or hypotension

References and further reading

Vaughan Williams EM. Classification of anti-dysrrhythmic drugs. In: Sande E, Flensted-Jensen E, Oleson KH (eds). Symposium on Cardiac Dysrrhythmias. Astra, Sodertalje, 1970, pp 449–472.

Vaughan Williams EM. Electrophysiological basis for a rational approach to anti-dysrrhythmic drug therapy. *Advances in Drug Research* 1974; 9: 69–102.

Vaughan Williams EM. Some factors that influence the activity of anti-arrythmic drugs. *British Heart Journal* 1978; 40 (suppl.): 52–61.

SECTION 3: 13
RESPIRATORY PHARMACOLOGY

T. C. Smith

ADMINISTRATION AND MODES OF ACTION

CONTROL OF BRONCHIAL CALIBRE
Adrenergic agonists
Anti-cholinergics
Methylxanthines
Steroids
Cromoglycate
Leukotriene inhibitors

RESPIRATORY CENTRE STIMULANTS

MUCOLYTICS

SURFACTANT

SPECIFIC PHARMACOLOGY
Aminophylline
Beclamethasone
Budesonide
Cromoglycate disodium
Doxapram
Ipatropium bromide
Salbutamol
Zafirlukast

ADMINSTRATION AND MODES OF ACTION

Drugs acting on the airways may be administered systemically or by inhalation. The inhaled mode allows a higher concentration of agent to be delivered directly to the bronchial tree which minimises absorption and accompanying systemic effects. Some drugs are metabolised in the lungs, resulting in a non hepatic first-pass effect.

Typically, only 10% of an inhalationally administered bronchodilator reaches the lungs. Most of this is deposited in the upper airways with little benefit with about 3% reaching the alveoli. Distribution is little affected by the presence of obstructive airways disease, or particle size.

Bronchial calibre is fundamentally affected by two opposing systems. Factors that cause an increase of intracellular cyclic AMP (such as sympathetic stimulation) result in bronchodilation. The reverse of this situation is factors that raise the intracellular concentration of cyclic GMP (such as parasympathetic stimulation) cause bronchoconstriction. The physiological and pharmacological influences on bronchial calibre are summarised in Figure RP.1.

The role of the leukotrienes in the development of bronchospasm has recently been revealed. They are so-named because of their presence in white blood cells (the leuko component) and their chemical bonds (a triene system of double bonds). Leukotrienes are produced by the action of the enzyme 5-lipoxygenase, which is found in white blood cells (particularly eosinophils) and mast cells among other tissues. 5-lipoxygenase when activated binds to the cell membrane and associates with five-lipoxygenase activating protein (FLAP), the resulting complex causing change in arachidonic acid to produce leukotriene A_4 (LTA_4) This is a precursor of a whole family of leukotrienes, LTA_4-LTF_4. LTC_4, D_4 and E_4 are spasmogenic and comprise the substance formerly termed 'SRS-A' before the leukotrienes were understood (see Fig AN.7, p 628).

CONTROL OF BRONCHIAL CALIBRE

ADRENERGIC AGONISTS

β_2 agonists

Examples – salbutamol, terbutaline, fenoterol, pirbuterol, rimiterol

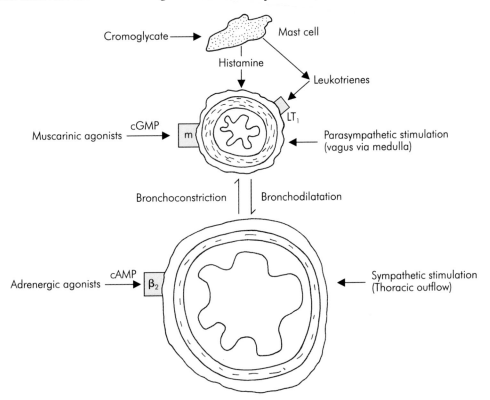

Figure RP.1 Causes of changes in bronchial calibre

Selective β_2 adrenergic receptor agonists are used in the treatment of bronchospasm and for prophylaxis. This selectivity is not absolute and high doses of these drugs will cause β_1 effects (tachycardia, tremor, hyperglycaemia, increased insulin secretion and hypokalaemia).

β_2 agonists reverse bronchospasm caused by histamine release, platelet activating factor, and members of the leukotriene family, particularly C_4, D_4 and E_4.

The β_2 agonist salbutamol is the most widely used agent in the treatment of asthma. It is conjugated in the liver and excreted in both conjugated and unchanged forms in urine and faeces. Terbutaline is a similar agent that may have advantages in some patients due to fewer sympathomimetic side effects. Terbutaline may be used antenatally to stimulate foetal lung surfactant production. Rimiterol is a short-acting β agonist of only 2 H duration.

β_2 agonists may be used as uterine relaxants for the management of premature labour, excessive contractions, or during Caesarean section to facilitate delivery. Administration for this purpose may be inhalational.

Other adrenergic agonists

Examples – epinephrine, ephedrine, isoprenaline, orciprenaline

Ephedrine, isoprenaline, orciprenaline and epinephrine are non selective sympathetic agonists with bronchodilator (β_2) actions, which are infrequently used. Epinephrine has re-emerged as an effective inhaled agent for the treatment of acute tracheolaryngobronchitis (croup) and laryngeal oedema. A dose of 0.5 ml/kg 1:1000 epinephrine up to a maximum of 5 ml may be nebulised, and given according to effect.

ANTI-CHOLINERGIC AGENTS

Examples – ipratropium and oxitropium bromide

Anti-cholinergic agents are given inhalationally and as with other inhaled bronchodilators, only 10% of the dose reaches the lungs. These drugs act at muscarinic acetyl choline receptors and so inhibit bronchoconstriction. Systemically administered anti-cholinergic drugs also affect these receptors. Anti-cholinergic agents have the following respiratory effects:
- Bronchodilatation
- Reduced airways resistance
- Increased anatomical dead space
- Increased physiological dead space

Ipratropium bromide (N-isopropylatropine) is the most widely used agent in this category. It has a rapid onset of action, but takes 2 H to peak, lasting for 4–6 H. Of the orally deposited drug, 70% passes unprocessed into the faeces. A small amount of drug is absorbed systemically from the oral mucosa and this is metabolised by the liver. Ipatropium may also block acetyl choline receptors on mast cell. It is primarily used for prophylaxis of bronchospasm, frequently in combination with other inhaled agents.

METHYLXANTHINES

Examples – caffeine, theobromine, theophylline

The methylxanthines are stimulant bronchodilators derived from plant alkaloids which have both a local effect on the bronchial tree and a general central stimulating effect which increases respiratory drive. They have a multimodal mechanism of action which includes:

- Phosphodiesterase inhibition
- Facilitation of β_2 action
- Enhanced Ca^{2+} release from sarcoplasmic reticulum in striated muscle
- Adenosine receptor antagonism

Inhibition of phosphodiesterase directly and via β_2 effects causes bronchodilatation similar to that of β_2 agonists. The enhanced release of calcium within the sarcoplasmic reticulum improves the function of the respiratory muscles. Methylxanthines are potent inhibitors of adenosine receptors and inhibit smooth muscle contraction by increasing cAMP and by direct interference with calcium entry.

Clinical effects

RESPIRATORY SYSTEM

Methylxanthines cause bronchodilatation, with increased anatomical dead space. They are effective against bronchospasm due to the release of histamine, platelet activating factor, and leukotrienes. The force of respiratory skeletal muscle contraction is increased, as is respiratory rate. Respiratory work is increased with relatively less fatigue. Methylxanthines are effective prophylactically and also indicated for the treatment of acute attacks of bronchospasm.

CARDIOVASCULAR SYSTEM

Heart rate and cardiac contractility are increased and peripheral vascular resistance is markedly reduced due to smooth muscle relaxation. This combination of effects may be helpful in the treatment of left ventricular failure.

CENTRAL NERVOUS SYSTEM

There is general stimulation which increases respiratory rate but may lead to convulsions. Although CNS excitation is relatively non specific, both vasomotor and respiratory centres are markedly affected. Convulsions are a potential hazard.

OTHER EFFECTS

These include the stimulation of gastric acid and pepsin secretion, diuresis (by dilatation of afferent glomerular arterioles) and inhibition of uterine contraction.

The methylxanthines can be considered as a family of agents with theophylline as the parent compound. Although theophylline is well absorbed orally its rapid elimination in the liver by cytochrome P_{450} and variable protein binding of about 40%, lead to unpredictable clinical effects. Theophylline levels are measured in the plasma during chronic administration to ensure adequate therapeutic concentrations. Aminophylline, the ethylene diamine salt of theophylline is more water soluble (but highly alkaline in solution) and preferred in clinical practice.

STEROIDS

Examples – beclamethasone, budesonide

Inhaled and systemic steroids may be used in the treatment and prevention of bronchospasm secondary to obstructive airways disease. Steroids act directly on intracellular receptor sites, have an anti-inflammatory action which reduces mucosal oedema and swelling and also interfere with many mediators of airways resistance. Chemical mediators suppressed by steroid treatment include prostaglandins, thromboxanes, prostacyclin, leukotrienes, platelet-activating factor and histamine. There are multiple other effects of steroids that include reductions in inflammation, smooth muscle tone, vascular permeability, pulmonary vascular resistance, all of which are useful in the treatment of bronchospasm.

The effects of inhaled steroids can be summarised as follows:

- Inhibition of arachidonic acid metabolites
- Inhibition of inflammatory response
- Stabilisation of mast cells
- Catecholamine synergism

Although inhaled steroids are used for prophylaxis, acute attacks require systemic steroids but their action by this route is slow in onset.

Beclamethasone is an inhaled steroid given in typical doses of 100–400 mcg, 2–4 times a day. Budesonide may have advantages in reaching the bronchioles in a more reliable manner, with less systemic effects.

CROMOGLYCATE

Cromoglycate, an inhaled membrane stabilising agent, is only effective in the **prevention** of bronchospasm. It inhibits the action of platelet aggregation factor on eosinophils, mast cells and platelets, suppresses axonal reflexes caused by irritants and acts as a mild mast cell stabiliser. This may be mediated by inhibition of calcium entry into the mast cell.

Bio-availability by the inhaled route is 10% (1% orally). Of the drug, 70% is protein-bound and it is excreted unchanged (50% in urine, 50% in bile). It has a half-life of 90 min but its duration of action is several hours.

LEUKOTRIENE RECEPTOR ANTAGONISTS

Examples: montelukast, zafirlukast

The release of cysteinyl leukotrienes C_4, D_4, and E_4 from eosinophils, basophils and mast cells is involved in the genesis of asthma. Leukotrienes increase mucus production, cause airway wall oedema, eosinophil migration, airway smooth muscle proliferation, bronchoconstriction and airway hyperresponsiveness. The leukotriene receptor antagonists are highly selective, and competitive. They block the effects of leukotrienes on the LT_1 receptor on bronchial smooth muscle and so antagonise the bronchoconstriction. They also reduce leukotriene production.

Montelukast and zafirlukast are indicated for the **prevention** of mild to moderate asthma as an adjunct to inhaled steroids, cromoglycate and intermittent β_2 agonists but not in the treatment of acute attacks. Exercise-induced and aspirin-induced asthma may be particularly suitable for treatment. They are administered orally with a bioavailability of 60 to 80%, although with food this drops substantially. They achieve peak plasma levels at 2 to 3H. Metabolism is hepatic.

RESPIRATORY CENTRE STIMULANTS

Examples – doxapram, ethamivan, nikethamide

Respiratory centre stimulants act by increasing respiratory drive. As their site of action is not purely the respiratory centre, increasing doses produce the effects of generalised central nervous system stimulation such as restlessness, anxiety and convulsions. These drugs are useful in the management of central respiratory depression either as a result of chronic lung disease or from drug therapy but should not be used in patients with respiratory obstruction in whom the normal central drive is preserved which may lead to further exhaustion and precipitation of respiratory collapse.

Doxapram acts via the carotid sinus chemoreceptors (and also centrally causing stimulation of the respiratory centre) to cause increased respiratory rate and tidal volume. Clinical effects last only 5–10 min and further boluses or infusion may be required for longer duration of effect. Doxapram has a higher therapeutic index than the other respiratory stimulants and has therefore found a limited niche in the recovery area because of this.

Nikethamide and ethamivan are structurally similar amines with similar effects, which act via stimulation of the respiratory centre. They have a lower therapeutic index than doxapram making central excitation more likely. These drugs are no longer available.

Other general analeptics also cause respiratory centre stimulation, but the more generalised CNS excitation precludes their use as specific respiratory stimulants.

MUCOLYTICS

Examples – carbocisteine, methylcysteine

Carbocisteine and methylcysteine (given orally) may be used to reduce the viscosity of sputum as an aid to expectoration. Dornase alpha is a specific mucolytic agent that is a genetically synthesised enzyme acting by cleavage of extracellular DNA. The specific use of dornase alpha is administration by inhalation in selected cystic fibrosis patients.

SURFACTANT

Surfactant is a physiologically occurring lipid–protein complex produced in the lung by type II alveolar cells. It lines the alveolar lung surface and has its effect by reducing surface tension which increases pulmonary compliance. Surfactant mainly comprises dipalmitoylphosphatidylcholine. Synthetic, porcine and bovine forms of surfactant have been used to treat respiratory distress in neonates, the route of administration being by direct instillation into the lungs.

SPECIFIC PHARMACOLOGY

Here, units (unless stated otherwise) are:

Volume of distribution at steady state (V_d) (l/kg)
Clearance (Cl) (ml/kg/min)
Terminal half-life ($t_{1/2}$) (H)

AMINOPHYLLINE

Structure – ethylene diamine salt of the methylxanthine theophylline
Presentation – tablets 100 mg; IV clear solution 25 mg/ml; sustained release preparations also available
Dose – oral up to 300 mg three times daily; IV cautious slow infusion 500 mcg/kg/H adjusted by serum theophylline concentrations
CNS – direct respiratory stimulant, may cause convulsions
CVS – myocardial contractility and heart rate rise, cardiac output increased; marked peripheral vasodilatation (offset slightly by vasomotor centre stimulation)
RS – bronchodilatation by β_2 action, direct respiratory centre stimulation; rise in respiratory rate
Other – general smooth muscle relaxation; renal blood flow increased
Elimination – demethylation and oxidation in the liver followed by urinary excretion
Caution – rapid IV administration may result in convulsions, tachycardia and collapse

BECLAMETHASONE

Structure – synthetic corticosteroid
Presentation – metered inhaler, 50 100 or 200 mcg per puff
Dose – up to maximum of 800 mcg daily (adult)
CNS – steroid psychosis rare but possible in high dosage
CVS – hypertension and fluid retention possible in high dosage
RS – reduction in airway sensitivity, reduction of bronchospasm; risk of *Candida albicans* infection
Other – adrenal suppression possible; osteoporosis is a risk in chronic therapy

BUDESONIDE

Structure – synthetic corticosteroid
Presentation – metered inhaler, 50 or 200 mcg per puff
Dose – 200–400 mcg twice daily

CNS – steroid psychosis rare but possible in high dosage

CVS – hypertension and fluid retention possible in high dosage

RS – reduction in airway sensitivity, reduction of bronchospasm; risk of *Candida albicans* infection

Other – adrenal suppression possible; osteoporosis a risk in chronic therapy

CROMOGLYCATE DISODIUM

Structure – organic cogener of khellin

Presentation – metered inhaler, 5 mg per puff, spincap® 20 mg, nebuliser solution 10 mg/ml (also available as eye drops)

Dose – up to 20 mg four times daily; duration of single dose 6 H

Pharmacokinetics

Bio-availability	Protein binding	$t_{1/2}$
10%	70%	90 min

CNS – no effect

CVS – no effect

RS – prophylactic against bronchospasm; may produce coughing and throat irritation

Other – used in food allergy and inflammatory eye conditions

DOXAPRAM

Structure – monohydrated pyrrolidinone

Presentation – IV clear, colourless solution 100 mg in 5 ml, or 2 mg/ml in 500 ml 5% dextrose

Dose – IV, 1–1.5 mg/kg onset 30 s, peak 2 min, lasts 10 min

Pharmacokinetics

V_d	Cl	$t_{1/2}$
1.5	5	3

CNS – carotid body chemoreceptors and respiratory centre stimulation; higher doses cause restlessness, dizziness, headache, hallucinations, convulsions

CVS – stroke volume and cardiac output increased; heart rate and blood pressure may increase

RS – tidal volume increased; rate increased with higher doses or if slow; minute volume increased. CO_2 response curve shifted to left

Others – may increase urine output, salivation, and motility of GI and urinary tracts

Elimination – 95% metabolised primarily by liver, 5% unchanged in urine

Side effects – potentiates sympathomimetic amines; increased effect if on MAOI; may cause agitation and increased skeletal muscle activity when concurrent with aminophylline therapy

Caution – if respiratory failure not due to inadequate respiratory drive, will cause agitation and convulsions

IPRATROPIUM BROMIDE

Structure – quaternary derivative of N-isopropyl atropine

Presentation – Aerocap® 40 mg dry powder formulation, metered inhaler 20 mcg per puff, nebuliser solution 250 mcg/ml also available; maximum effect 30 min after administration, duration 6 h

Dose – up to 40 mcg three times daily

CNS – no effect

CVS – no effect

RS – brochodilatation, occasional irritation and cough; paradoxical bronchospasm possible but rare

Other – may produce glaucoma and urinary retention (anti-cholinergic effects)

SALBUTAMOL

Structure – synthetic amine

Presentation – IV clear solution 5 mg in 5 ml, tablets 4 and 8 mg, syrup 2 mg in 5 ml, inhalation powder 200 and 400 mcg, nebuliser solution 5 mg/ml

Dose – IV, 250 mcg bolus; 3–20 mcg/min by infusion

Pharmacokinetics

Protein binding	V_d	Cl	$t_{1/2}$
8–64%	2.2	6.7	4

CNS – may cause excitation, anxiety, tremor

CVS – β_2 effects cause vasodilatation with decreased blood pressure; higher doses cause β_1 effects with tachycardia

RS – bronchodilator for prophylactic and therapeutic use

Other – crosses placenta and may causes foetal tachycardia

Elimination – 30% unchanged in urine; the rest unchanged in faeces, small amount of conjugated form also appears in urine and faeces

ZAFIRLUKAST

Structure - A complex cyclopentyl carbamate; a leukotriene receptor antagonist

Presentation - film-coated tablet 20 mg

Dose - 20 mg twice daily, peak 3 hours

Pharmacokinetics

bioavailability	protein binding	Cl	$t_{1/2}$
73%	99%	5	7 H

RS - Bronchodilator by inhibition of leukotriene mediated smooth muscle contraction

Elimination - hepatic by cytochrome P450

Side effects - Churge-Strauss syndrome has been reported. Look out for eosinophilia, vasculitis, rhinitis and sinusitis

Caution - It inhibits cytochrome P_{450}, so caution should be exercised with concomitant use of warfarin, phenytoin or phenobarbitone

Contraindications - Moderate to severe renal or hepatic impairment

SECTION 3: 14
ENDOCRINE PHARMACOLOGY

T. C. Smith

BLOOD SUGAR CONTROL
Insulin receptor
Glucose
Glucagon
Insulin
Oral hypoglycaemic agents

THYROID HORMONES AND ANTI-THYROID DRUGS
Hypothyroidism
Hyperthyroidism

ADRENOCORTICAL STEROIDS

OXYTOCIC DRUGS
Oxytocin
Ergometrine
Carboprost

RENAL HORMONES
Anti-diuretic hormone and analogues
ADH antagonist

SPECIFIC PHARMACOLOGY
Hydrocortisone
Dexamethasone
Insulin (soluble)
Oxytocin
Ergometrine maleate

BLOOD SUGAR CONTROL

The physiological control of blood glucose is complex. While the major role belongs to insulin, a multitude of other hormonal influences apply. It should also be remembered that insulin has other actions beyond the regulation of blood glucose. Pharmacological control of blood glucose becomes necessary in situations of elevation and depression of blood glucose beyond the homeostatic limits, in other words due to hyperglycaemia or hypoglycaemia. The causes of failure in regulation of blood glucose are given in Figure EN.1.

FAILURE OF GLUCOSE CONTROL

Hypoglycaemia

Deficiency of glucose intake and failure of
  compensatory mechanisms

Excess insulin – insulinoma
            iatrogenic

Hyperglycaemia

Deficiency of insulin

Decreased end organ sensitivity to insulin

Excess administration of glucose solutions

Figure EN.1

Treatment of hypoglycaemia is directed towards administration of glucose and removal of the root cause. Treatment of hyperglycaemia includes removal of the cause, administration of insulin in the acute phase and at a later stage augmentation of both the secretion and effect of endogenous insulin.

INSULIN RECEPTOR

The insulin receptor is a complex of 4 glycoprotein subunits ($\alpha\alpha\beta\beta$) linked by disulphide bridges to form a cylinder. The α units are entirely extracellular and contain the insulin-binding site. The β subunit spans the cell membrane and the intracellular part has tyrosine kinase activity. The α subunit has a repressive effect on this activity that is removed by the conformational change resulting from insulin binding. The tyrosine kinase acts on insulin-receptor substrate-1 (IRS-1) triggering a chain of action culminating in the activation of glycogen synthetase, phosphorylase kinase and glycogen phosphorylase. IRS-1 is also a substrate for insulin-like growth factor 1 (IGF-1) receptors. The binding of insulin to the α subunit changes the insulin receptor formation to form a transmembrane tunnel allowing glucose (and other

molecules) to pass through the membrane. The activated β subunit autophosphorylates at 6 or more tyrosine residues and these phosphorylate intracellular proteins resulting in second messenger effects on fat, protein and glycogen synthesis. Insulin has a very high affinity for the insulin receptor. This may be due to subsequent binding to the second α subunit. The interaction does not conform, to the Law of Mass Action. The insulin-receptor complex is internalised and the receptors recycled whilst the insulin itself is degrade in lysosomes.

GLUCOSE

Ideally, glucose should be administered by mouth. Its rapid absorption ensures rapid correction of limited hypoglycaemia. In more severe situations, the unconscious patient requires IV administration. Dextrose (5%) has little calorific value (840 J/l). The treatment of hypoglycaemia usually requires a 20% dextrose solution (3.36 MJ/l) or alternatively a 50% solution (8.4 MJ/l). Glucose (20%) requires a large vein but can be administered peripherally, but (50%) glucose should always be given via a central venous line. Both 20% and 50% solutions can cause damage to the blood vessels and are viscous. Extravasation of concentrated glucose solutions will cause local necrosis.

GLUCAGON

Glucagon is a polypeptide (smaller than insulin) formed in the α cells of the pancreas and also in the upper gastro-intestinal tract. Glucagon has a large number of roles in the regulation of metabolism all of which are directed to the raising of blood glucose. Although the majority of effects are physiological, glucagon has been used therapeutically in two main areas, the rapid restoration of blood glucose in severe hypoglycaemia and in cardiogenic shock, due to its positive inotropic effect.

INSULIN

Soluble (otherwise known as unmodified) insulin may be given subcutaneously or intravenously. It is short acting and has a half-life in the circulation of 5 min. Subcutaneous administration results in more gradual absorption. Administration of IV insulin allows rapid control in keto-acidotic hyperglycaemia.

Long-term control of diabetes requires a variety of preparations of insulin with differing absorption characteristics for precise control. Longer acting insulin may be obtained by the formation of insulin complexes using either zinc or protamine or both. The addition of zinc produces a crystalline insulin of intermediate action. The addition of protamine produces isophane insulin that also has an intermediate duration of action. These insulin preparations may be mixed with soluble insulin (to make 'biphasic' insulins) which will lessen temporal fluctuations in plasma insulin.

Long-acting insulin is produced by combination with both protamine and zinc (protamine zinc insulin). This preparation should not be mixed with soluble insulin because the soluble insulin will combine with any free protamine in the solution. Figure EN.2 gives a guide to the time related effects of the different categories of insulin.

Insulin may be bovine, porcine or human, the animal products being purified by crystallisation. Bovine insulin has three amino acid differences from human in its amino acid sequence and porcine one. These foreign sequences in the insulin or in impurities may be antigenic leading to insulin resistance and immuno reactivity. To overcome this the insulin is highly purified but alternatively human insulin may be used. This is the preferred choice in modern therapy. Human insulin is either synthesised by bacteria, or created by enzymic modification of porcine insulin.

Insulin is mainly used in the treatment of diabetes mellitus but may also be indicated in parenteral feeding to aid glucose utilisation.

ORAL HYPOGLYCAEMIC AGENTS

Sulphonylureas

Examples – chlorpropamide, glibenclamide, gliclazide, glipizide, tolbutamide

Sulphonylurea drugs act by augmenting endogenous insulin secretion from existing β cells within the islets of Langerhans. Sulphonylureas bind to receptors on the pancreatic β cells and increase the sensitivity of the cells to glucose. The potassium permeability of β cells is reduced by blockade of the ATP-dependent potassium channel. The membrane becomes depolarised leading to calcium influx and subsequent secretion of insulin.

In excess sulphonylureas have the propensity to cause hypoglycaemia. Most are metabolised in the liver resulting in the formation of active metabolites. The sulphonylureas and metabolites are excreted in the urine. They cross the placenta and can cause hypoglycaemia in the newborn. There is competition for albumin binding sites with sulphonamides, aspirin and other highly protein bound drugs. Factors affecting the action of the sulphonylurea family are given in Figure EN.3.

Chlorpropamide is active for 1–3 days, inactivated in the liver and excreted in the urine. It has an anti-diuretic hormone (ADH) mimicking action on renal tubules and a disulfiram-like effect in the presence of alcohol. Glibenclamide has a duration of about 24 H. Tolbutamide has a short half-life of about 5 H and may decrease thyroid iodide uptake. The third generation sulphonylureas (such as gliclazide) have a biphasic effect and are metabolised in the liver.

Biguanides

Example – metformin

Biguanides decrease hepatic gluconeogenesis and increase insulin-mediated peripheral glucose uptake They act by increasing the sensitivity of target tissues (skeletal muscle, adipose tissue and hepatocytes) to insulin. They have no effect on insulin secretion and do not require functioning β cells in the islets of Langerhans. Metformin also lowers low density lipoproteins (LDL) and very low density lipoproteins (VLDL) in the plasma.

TEMPORAL CHARACTERISTICS OF S/C INSULIN PREPARATIONS (HOURS)

	Onset	Peak	Duration
Short-acting	0.5–1	2–4	8
Intermediate-acting	1–2	4–12	12–24
Long-acting	2–4	24–40	36

Figure EN.2

EFFECT OF SULPHONYLUREAS

Augmented by:	Phenylbutazone
	Salicylates
	Alcohol
	Monoamine oxidase inhibitors
Diminished by:	Thiazides
	Corticosteroids
	Oestrogens
	Frusemide

Figure EN.3

Metformin does not bind to plasma protein and is excreted unchanged in the urine with a half-life of 3 H. All biguanides carry a risk of lactic acidosis possibly due to inhibition of oxidative phosphorylation, and are gradually falling into disuse.

Thiazolidinediones

Examples – pioglitazone, rosiglitazone, troglitazone

Thiazolidinediones are new agents intended for the treatment of type 2 diabetes mellitus. They, like the biguanides, sensitise target tissues to insulin. The thiazolidinediones activate nuclear peroxisome proliferator activated receptor γ (PPAR-γ) predominantly in adipose tissue. This increases transcription of genes in adipocyte differentiation and lipid and glucose metabolism resulting in reduced blood glucose and corresponding fall in insulin secretion. Thiazolidinediones increase high density lipoprotein cholesterol and may prove to reduce cardiovascular risk. They are to be used in conjunction with sulphonylureas or metformin. Disadvantages include weight gain and possible risks of hepatotoxicity.

Meglitinide analogues

Examples – nateglinide, repaglinide

Nateglinide and repaglinide belong to a class of oral hypoglycaemic agents structurally related to meglitinide (the non-sulphonylurea moiety of glibenclamide). They inhibit ATP-sensitive K^+ channels in pancreatic β cells in the presence of glucose. They bind to a receptor site distinct from that of the sulphonylureas and stimulate prandial insulin release. They act synergistically with metformin and thiazolidinediones by specifically targetting post-prandial hyperglycaemia. Nateglinide is a phenylalanine derivative and repaglinide is a carbamoylmethyl benzoate.

THYROID HORMONES AND ANTI-THYROID DRUGS

HYPOTHYROIDISM

Deficiency of thyroid hormones is treated with replacement therapy usually with L-thyroxine (T4). If a rapid onset of action is required (e.g. hypothyroid coma) then tri-iodothyronine (Liothyronine) is used. This is effective within a few hours and lasts up to 48 H.

HYPERTHYROIDISM

Excess of thyroid secretions may be treated in several ways. Surgical reduction of the thyroid gland, inhibition of the peripheral actions (β adrenoceptor antagonists) or specific targeting of thyroid hormone synthesis and secretion.

Specific anti-thyroid drugs have a variety of effects; the thioureylenes (such as carbimazole) block organification of iodine, potassium iodide inhibits secretion of thyroid hormones and radio-iodine causes destruction of thyroid follicle cells.

Thioureylenes

Examples – carbimazole, propylthiouracil

Thioureylenes may take 3–4 weeks to take effect. Their major action is the inhibition of iodination of thyroglobulin bound tyrosine by opposing thyroperoxidases. There is also evidence of inhibition of iodinated tyrosine coupling, and suppression of antibody synthesis in Grave's disease. The thiocarbamide group is essential for the therapeutic activity of carbimazole. Carbimazole is rapidly converted to another, active, thioureylene called methimazole. A rare but serious side effect of carbimazole therapy is the development of agranulocytosis.

Iodine/iodide mixtures

These inhibit iodine substitution on the tyrosine moieties, resulting in a decreased output of thyroid hormone by the gland.

Radio-iodine

Radio-iodine (^{131}I radio-isotope) emits β rays. These cause cellular destruction but are rapidly attenuated and have an effective penetration of only 2 mm. ^{131}I also emits γ rays that enable imaging.

ADRENOCORTICAL STEROIDS

Examples – betamethasone, cortisone, fludrocortisone, hydrocortisone, prednisolone, prednisone, triamcinolone

Hydrocortisone (cortisol) is naturally occurring whereas the other examples are synthetically derived. Cortisone has minimal activity and must be converted to hydrocortisone in the liver first. Corticosteroids are used as replacement therapy in Addison's disease and similar conditions and in higher doses for suppression of various inflammatory processes. Steroid choice is determined in part by the relative glucocorticoid and mineralocorticoid effects. Hydrocortisone is suitable for replacement therapy and short-term use. Long-term use causes excessive fluid retention compared with alternatives such as prednisolone. The relative glucocorticoid and mineralocorticoid potencies are given in Figure EN.4. The pharmacological effects of steroids are manifold, including:

- Inhibition of inflammation
- Improved transport of cellular oxygen
- Preservation of lysosome membrane integrity
- Inhibition of complement C5 activation
- Inhibition of plasminogen activator
- Negative feedback on hypothalamus and pituitary and adrenal cortex atrophy
- Inhibition of neutrophil and macrophage recruitment
- Red cell and neutrophil counts selectively increased

Corticosteroids diffuse into cells and act on specific intracellular receptors. The complex subsequently produced then moves to the nucleus and increases synthesis of certain enzymes. Glucocorticoids are lipid soluble and are transported in the plasma by corticosteroid binding globulin (CBG) and albumin. CBG is relatively specific for endogenous steroids and does not bind synthetic steroids readily. Because of its low capacity, it may become saturated when therapeutic doses of steroids are used.

The therapeutic effects of steroids are primarily a feature of the glucocorticoid effects. The side effects may be caused by either glucocorticoid or mineralocorticoid components. Mineralocorticoid side effects are seen early and mimic those of hyperaldosteronism – sodium and water retention, and

increased renal potassium and calcium excretion. Glomerular filtration rate is increased. In the gut, there is increased calcium absorption but this is insufficient to offset the renal loss. The glucocorticoid side effects tend to be seen with chronic administration and are seen relatively late on, mimicking Cushing's syndrome. The side effects of steroid therapy are listed in Figure EN.5.

OXYTOCIC DRUGS

OXYTOCIN

Oxytocin is an octapeptide similar to ADH. The pharmacological preparation is synthetic, hence the name 'syntocinon'. It binds to specific sites in the myometrium causing uterine contraction. This is probably mediated by increases in potassium permeability which reduce the membrane potential making it more excitable. Uterine sensitivity to oxytocin increases from minimal in the non pregnant to maximum at term. Oxytocin also causes contraction of breast duct smooth muscle with milk ejection.

Oxytocin causes direct vasodilatation, and a mild ADH like anti-diuretic effect, which may become significant if used for prolonged infusion. There is metabolism by both renal and hepatic routes.

ERGOMETRINE

Ergometrine stimulates uterine contraction (possibly via 5-HT receptors), and also causes vascular smooth muscle contraction although the effect is slight. It has a very mild α adrenergic blocking action. These effects are mediated via dopaminergic and 5-HT receptors. Ergometrine is a potent emetic acting on the

RELATIVE POTENCIES OF THE EFFECTS OF CORTICOSTEROIDS		
Drug	**Glucocorticoid**	**Mineralocorticoid**
Hydrocortisone	1	1
Cortisone	0.8	0.8
Prednisone	4	0.25
Prednisolone	4	0.25
Methylprednisolone	5	minimal
Dexamethasone	25	minimal
Aldosterone	0.3	400
Fludrocortisone	10	300

Figure EN.4

SIDE EFFECTS OF STEROIDS

Mineralocorticoid
Sodium retention
Potassium loss
Water retention
Renal calcium loss
Hypertension

Glucocorticoid
Muscle wasting
Fat deposition
Liver glycogen deposition
Thin, friable skin
Poor wound healing
Reduced immunity
Cataracts
Raised intra-ocular pressure
Osteoporosis
Hyperglycaemia

Figure EN.5

chemoreceptor trigger zone and vomiting centre (via D_2 receptors). After treatment with ergometrine there may occasionally be a clinical picture of hypertension with headache and blurred vision which lasts several days. Ergometrine acts within 30–60 s of IV administration (IM 2–4 min; orally 4–8 min), and lasts 3–6 H. The drug is metabolised by the liver and excreted in the bile.

CARBOPROST

Carboprost tromethamine is a prostaglandin used in the management of severe obstetric haemorrhage secondary to uterine atony that is unresponsive to oxytocin and ergometrine. It may be administered by deep intramuscular injection. Side effects include nausea and vomiting, diarrhoea, flushing and bronchospasm. There have been very rare reports of cardiovascular collapse with prostaglandin use.

RENAL HORMONES

ANTI-DIURETIC HORMONE AND ANALOGUES

Anti-diuretic hormone

ADH is an octapeptide similar to oxytocin. It may be used pharmacologically but its short half-life (10 min) is a disadvantage. ADH permits water re-absorption from the renal collecting duct and is a very potent direct acting vasoconstrictor (also known as vasopressin). ADH also increases hepatic glycogenolysis, increases factor VIII activity and encourages platelet aggregation and degranulation. It may also function as a brain neurotransmitter. An IV preparation of ADH is available but synthetic analogues last longer and are more useful.

Desmopressin (1-deamino-8-D-arginine vasopressin or DDAVP)

Desmopressin is used for the diagnosis and treatment of diabetes insipidus. It has an anti-diuretic potency about 12 times that of ADH, but it has only 0.4% the vasoconstrictor activity. Desmopressin increases factor VIII activity in the same manner as ADH and is used to cover minor surgical procedures in mild haemophilia. It may be given by oral, IV, IM, subcutaneous or nasal administration. Desmopressin is metabolised by proteases and then excreted in the urine. It has a half-life of 75 min.

Other ADH analogues include: felypressin, which has a predominantly vasoconstrictor action and is used as an adjunct for local anaesthetics in place of epinephrine; and lypressin, which is similar but shorter in duration (10 min).

The nasal route of administration is used for these agents. Terlipressin, a pro drug for ADH is used to control bleeding from oesophageal varices. Terlipressin requires IV administration.

ADH ANTAGONIST

Demeclocycline

Demeclocycline is a tetracycline derivative which opposes the effect of ADH. It has been used in cases of inappropriate ADH secretion.

Renin angiotensin system (see pages 383–384)

Inhibition of the renin–angiotensin system may be effective in the control of hypertension. Renin secretion is increased by catecholamines (β_1 effect) and reduced by β blockers. Angiotensin-converting enzyme (ACE) inhibitors inhibit the conversion of angiotensin I to angiotensin II. Angiotensin II receptor inhibiting drugs inhibit the vascular receptor for this pathway thus preventing vasoconstriction.

SPECIFIC PHARMACOLOGY

HYDROCORTISONE

Structure – glucocorticoid steroid
Presentation – IV/IM, white powder as sodium succinate for reconstitution with water for injection (many other preparations are available)
Dose – IV 100–500 mg 6–8 hourly, onset 2–4 H, lasts 8 H
CNS – mood changes
CVS – restores vasomotor tone of small blood vessels, reduces vascular permeability and resultant tissue swelling
RS – reduces bronchial wall swelling caused by asthma or anaphylaxis
Other – anti-inflammatory agent with multiple uses
Elimination – hepatic conversion to tetrahydrocrtisone
Side effects – anaphylactoid reactions have occurred
Cautions – congestive cardiac failure, hypertension, peptic ulceration, glaucoma, epilepsy, diabetes mellitus, history of tuberculosis, effect of anti-cholinesterases antagonised

DEXAMETHASONE

Structure – glucocorticoid steroid
Presentation – IV, clear, colourless solution; 8 mg dexamethasone in 2 ml
Dose – IV – 0.5–20 mg initial bolus, particularly indicated where sodium and water retention are to be avoided
CNS – may cause convulsions and increase ICP (but indicated for treatment of cerebral oedema)
CVS – minimal effect
RS – may be used for asthma and aspiration pneumonitis
Other – mineralocorticoid effects may be present to a limited extent
Elimination – liver metabolised
Side effects – as for hydrocortisone

INSULIN (SOLUBLE)

Structure – glycopeptide; formed as pro-insulin with a connecting peptide, the C fragment
Presentation – clear colourless solution of human insulin pH 6.6–8.0 (containing glycerol and m-cresol)
Dose – SC/IM/IV, typically up to 8 IU/H based on intermittent blood glucose monitoring; used as replacement for low endogenous insulin, may be necessary in total parenteral nutrition to facilitate glucose uptake into cells

OXYTOCIN

Structure – synthetic octapeptide identical to human oxytocin
Presentation – IV/IM, clear, colourless solution, 5 or 10 IU in 1 ml (available in combination with ergometrine 500 mcg in 1 ml, as syntometrine)
Dose – IV to augment labour by infusion of variable magnitude; following Caesarean delivery slow bolus of 5 or 10 IU
CNS – no effect
CVS – bolus administration causes transient hypotension with reflex tachycardia. Following term delivery usually offset by placental autotransfusion
RS – no effect
Other – breast duct smooth muscle contraction promoting milk ejection
Elimination – rapid metabolism by plasma oxytocinase (use separate line if transfusing blood or plasma)
Side effects – uterine spasm or rupture, hypotension, water intoxication (secondary to the ADH like effect)

ERGOMETRINE MALEATE

Structure – ergot alkaloid
Presentation – IV/IM, colourless solution, 500 mcg in 1 ml (available in combination with oxytocin; see above)
Dose – slow IV 125–250 mcg; IM 500 mcg
CNS – potent emetic, avoid in pre-eclampsia
CVS – direct vasoconstriction, avoid in hypertension
RS – occasional dyspnoea, chest tightness
Side effects – nausea, vomiting, vasoconstriction (potential for stroke, myocardial infaction)
Contra-indications – induction of labour, first and second stages of labour; avoid in presence of cardiac or vascular disease, or porphyria

REFERENCES AND FURTHER READING

Textbook of diabetes, volume 1, second edition. Ed: Pickup JC, Williams G, Blackwell Science Ltd 1997, Oxford. The insulin receptor and postreceptor mechanisms pp 10.1–10.14

SECTION 3: 15
GASTRO-INTESTINAL PHARMACOLOGY

T. C. Smith

REDUCTION OF GASTRIC ACIDITY
H$_2$ receptor antagonists
Proton pump inhibitors
Prostaglandins
Antacids

MUCOPROTECTIVE DRUGS
Chelates and complexes
Carbenoxolone

ANTI-SPASMODICS
Anti-cholinergics
Direct-acting smooth muscle relaxants

PROKINETIC DRUGS

LAXATIVES
Bulking agents
Faecal softeners
Osmotic laxatives
Stimulants

SPECIFIC PHARMACOLOGY
Carbenoxolone
Cimetidine
Cisapride
Omeprazole
Ranitidine

REDUCTION OF GASTRIC ACIDITY

Although gastric acidity is extremely variable, in health gastric pH may be as low as 1.0 (hydrogen ion concentration 100 mmol/l). In anaesthetic practice a pH > 3.5 (hydrogen ion concentration 300 mmol/l) is sought to minimise the risk of acid aspiration syndrome. Many drugs may be used to reduce gastric acidity, acting in a variety of ways. The sites at which agents work are detailed in Figure GP.1.

H$_2$ RECEPTOR ANTAGONISTS

Examples – cimetidine, famotidine, nizatidine, ranitidine

Histamine has two primary effects on the GI tract mediated by H$_1$ and H$_2$ receptors. H$_1$ agonism causes contraction of gut smooth muscle whereas H$_2$ agonism causes secretion of gastric acid. The H$_2$ antagonists typically resemble the imidazole ring end of histamine and are hydrophilic. The H$_2$ antagonists are competitive, reversible antagonists which each feature a five-membered ring similar to the imidazole of histamine with a specific structure as follows:

- Cimetidine – imidazole ring
- Famotidine – guanidinothiazole ring
- Nizatidine – thiazole ring
- Ranitidine – furan ring

H$_2$ antagonism inhibits both basal levels and stimulated release of gastric acid. Pepsin secretion is reduced in line with the decrease in gastric volume even though secretion of pepsin is mediated by acetyl choline. As pepsin is usually secreted in excess of requirements, this does not present a problem. H$_2$ receptors are also present in the uterus, heart, blood vessels, ductus arteriosus and the lower oesophageal sphincter. Clinically, the H$_2$ antagonists have little effect on these

THE SITES OF ACTION OF DRUGS USED TO REDUCE GASTRIC ACIDITY

Site	Example
H$_2$ receptor	Ranitidine
Proton pump	Omeprazole
Prostaglandin receptor	Misoprostol
Gastric mucosa	Aluminium hydroxide

Figure GP.1

other tissues and there are no clinical applications related to these sites.

Cimetidine

Cimetidine is an H$_2$ antagonist with slight anti-androgenic effect that may cause gynaecomastia and impotence. Peak effect is achieved 80 min after oral administration and the terminal half-life is 2 H. It is given twice daily, is metabolised in the liver and binds to cytochrome P$_{450}$ causing inhibition. It also reduces hepatic blood flow. Of cimetidine, 70% is excreted unchanged in the urine. T lymphocytes have H$_2$ receptors and blockade of these may inhibit suppressor T cell function resulting in enhanced immune system activity. This effect may be harmful in the presence of auto-immune conditions or after organ transplantation. H$_2$ receptors in the atria are responsible for atrial rhythmicicity and cimetidine may cause bradyarrhythmias, especially when given intravenously.

Famotidine

Famotidine is a recently introduced H$_2$ antagonist that may be intravenously administered twice daily. It reduces acid and pepsin content, reduces gastric volume and is about 50 times more potent than cimetidine. It is excreted in the urine having a half-life of 3 H and a duration of action of 10 H. Cytochrome P$_{450}$ is unaffected.

Nizatidine

Nizatidine is currently the H$_2$ antagonist with the shortest half-life (1.3 H). It may be given orally or intravenously. It does not affect cytochrome P$_{450.}$ In high doses, nizatidine may increase salicylate absorption. Nizatidine also causes non competitive inhibition of acetyl cholinesterase similar to that of neostigmine and so possesses prokinetic activity too.

Ranitidine

Ranitidine is the most widely used H$_2$ antagonist at present. Peak effect occurs 100 min after oral administration and the terminal half-life is 2.5 H. There is a substantial first-pass effect that is avoided by use of the IV preparation. It is metabolised in the liver and binds to cytochrome P$_{450}$ causing inhibition but this effect is only about one tenth that of cimetidine and thus rarely achieves clinical significance.

PROTON PUMP INHIBITORS

Examples – lansoprazole, omeprazole, pantoprazole

The proton pump inhibitors directly affect the acid secreting pump of the gastric parietal cells, and therefore bypass the muscarinic, gastrin and H_2 receptors. Proton pump inhibitors bind to the sulphydryl groups of cysteine amino acid residues in the $H^+K^+ATPase$ pump and prevent hydrogen ion passage. These agents are administered orally in buffered capsules to minimise the effects of gastric acid before arrival at the site of action. This allows slow release and gradual absorption of the dose. They are readily absorbed in the non ionised form. Exposure to acid conditions (pH 0.8–1.0) in the gastric parietal cell cytosol causes protonation and therefore ionisation of the drugs, and the ionised form is the active component. The active form accumulates within the parietal canaliculi near the luminal surface and binds to the target enzyme. These inhibitors are therefore very selective. The enzyme is irreversibly inhibited and reversal of effect relies on the production of replacement $H^+K^+ATPase$. The site of action of proton pump inhibitors is shown in Figure GP.2.

Omeprazole

The structure of omeprazole constitutes substituted benzimidazole and pyridine rings joined by a sulphoxide link. It is a pro drug being converted within the parietal cell to sulphenamide, the active form. It has a highly selective effect that increases over several days to a plateau probably because the reduced gastric acid reduces its degradation and increases bio-availability. Plasma distribution half-life is only 3 min but gradual absorption and accumulation in the parietal cells results in a prolonged therapeutic effect. There is

minimal crossing of the blood-brain barrier but free crossing of the placenta. Omeprazole undergoes hepatic metabolism. Untoward effects are limited although long term use may result in hypergastrinaemia, thought to be of little consequence. Cytochrome P_{450} is inhibited, leading to a prolonged half-life of benzodiazepines and phenytoin as well as other agents sharing this elimination pathway.

Pantoprazole, a second-generation agent, is similar to omeprazole although it has higher bio-availability (75%). Gradual absorption and accumulation in the parietal cells results in a prolonged therapeutic effect. The drug is conjugated in the liver and excreted in the urine (80%) and faeces.

PROSTAGLANDINS

Example – misoprostol

Prostaglandins E_2 and I_2 (PGE_2, PGI_2) inhibit gastric acid secretion and stimulate the production of mucus and bicarbonate and therefore have a protective effect on the gastric mucosa. Natural prostaglandins are rapidly eliminated and thus synthetic analogues have been developed.

Misoprostol is a synthetic prostaglandin E_2 analogue that reduces gastric acid secretion and antagonises the anti-prostaglandin effects of the NSAIDs. It is most useful when these are a factor in the causation of ulcer formation, and it can be used in conjunction with

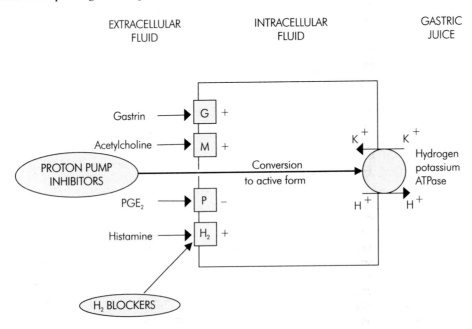

Figure GP.2. Gastric parietal cell and proton pump

NSAIDs (to prevent further ulceration) when alternatives to NSAIDs are unacceptable. The only untoward effect of note is the occurrence of diarrhoea.

ANTACIDS

Example – aluminium hydroxide

Antacids act in a simple chemical manner by neutralising acid in the stomach in the following manner:

$$acid + base \rightarrow salt + water.$$

It is important that the by products of this reaction are not toxic and cause minimal side effects. The commonest problem encountered is the production of CO_2 that causes gastric distension with discomfort, nausea and belching. Antacids are given to alleviate symptoms of dyspepsia and reflux oesophagitis, or to neutralise acid pre-operatively when a significant risk of acid aspiration exists. In the awake patient laryngeal reflexes protect the lungs from damage. In the anaesthetised patient the antacid may be aspirated and cause damage, a factor which influences antacid choice. Sodium citrate (0.3 molar) is the commonest antacid used in anaesthetic practice, because it is non particulate.

The simplest antacids are those containing the following bases either alone or in combination: magnesium carbonate, hydroxide, or trisilicate, aluminium hydroxide or glycinate. Sodium bicarbonate may also be used. Calcium and bismuth bases are no longer in general use. Solubility and speed of reaction are important in antacids suitable for clinical use; sodium and potassium hydroxide are very soluble and are therefore very basic. These readily neutralise the acid but any excess would render the stomach contents alkaline, causing potentially more damage than gastric acid. A solution is to use agents that either dissolve slowly or are less soluble. Magnesium carbonate has a crystalline structure that slows its reaction with the acid even though it is highly soluble and the hydroxides of aluminium and magnesium have a low solubility but react rapidly. The problems of antacid therapy are summarised in Figure GP.3.

A relatively large number of molecules is required for a chemical effect compared with receptor-based pharmacological methods. This can lead to excess salt and water absorption with predictable consequences. Sodium bicarbonate is so readily absorbed that it may cause iatrogenic non respiratory alkalosis. Bicarbonate and carbonate compounds release CO_2 within the stomach resulting in belching and the risk of regurgitation. Calcium compounds cause constipation

PROBLEMS OF ANTACID THERAPY

Salt and water retention
Alkalosis
Belching and regurgitation
Constipation or laxative effect
Lung damage from aspiration

Figure GP.3

and magnesium compounds have a laxative effect. Most of the antacids are suspensions and are therefore particulate in nature. Such particles if aspirated may lead to lung damage similar to acid aspiration syndrome.

MUCOPROTECTIVE DRUGS

The two main effects of mucoprotective drugs are the possession of cytoprotective activity or the enhancement of endogenous defence mechanisms. A mechanically protective barrier against acid damage to the gastric mucosa may be formed and some agents stimulate endogenous secretion of mucus from the gastric mucosa.

CHELATES AND COMPLEXES

Examples – bismuth chelate, sucralfate

Bismuth chelate

Although bismuth promotes healing of peptic ulcers, the mechanism of this action is not clear.

Sucralfate (now withdrawn)

Sucralfate is a complex of sulphated sucrose and aluminium hydroxide that, although possessing little antacid activity, has a profound cytoprotective effect. It may be used in critically ill patients unable to tolerate enteral feeding to protect the gastric mucosa and is also used in ulcer treatment to promote healing in conjunction with acid lowering drugs. It adheres to damaged gastric mucosa perhaps by virtue of its negatively charged component and forms a protective layer. It also stimulates the production of prostaglandins (particularly E_2), bicarbonate and mucus. Thromboxane release is inhibited and the production of natural sulphydryl compound is increased. Sucralfate stays in the stomach for many hours and only small amounts are absorbed. Aspiration

Dose – slow IV/IM, bolus 50 mg 6–8 hourly;. oral 150 mg twice daily

Pharmacokinetics

Bio-availability	Protein binding	V_d	Cl	$t_{\frac{1}{2}}$
50-60%	15%	1.5	10	2

CNS – no effect

CVS – no effect

RS – no effect

Other effects – placenta is readily crossed

Interactions – the increase in gastric pH increases the non ionised proportion of some drugs (such as benzodiazepines) and so increases their absorption

SECTION 3: 16
INTRAVENOUS FLUIDS

T. C. Smith

CRYSTALLOIDS

Water
Electrolytes
Solutions

COLLOIDS

Gelatins
Dextrans
Hydroxyethyl starch (HES)
Human albumin solutions (HAS)

**HAEMOGLOBIN SOLUTIONS
(EXPERIMENTAL)**

Stroma-free haemoglobin (SFH)
Micro-encapsulated haemoglobin

SYNTHETIC OXYGEN CARRIERS

Chelating agents
Perfluorocarbons

IV fluids are characterised by being given in relatively large volumes compared with other drugs. This is in part a feature of their non receptor mode of action and often there are multiple functional components in the fluid administered. The uses of IV fluids are shown in Figure IV.1.

CRYSTALLOIDS

Crystalloids are relatively small molecules that dissociate into ions and form true solutions. In clinical terms, crystalloids pass through the capillary and glomerular membranes easily, but do not readily pass through cell membranes. This situation only applies immediately after administration as metabolism and membrane pumps soon alter the distribution. The constituents of the commonly used IV fluids are shown in Figure IV. 2.

WATER

Water is the essential solvent of all the IV fluids. A figure of 1.5 ml/kg/H is a typical requirement for IV maintenance, which is the primary determinant of the

USES OF IV FLUIDS

Volume replacement	Total body water
	Extracellular water
	Intravascular (blood) volume
Provision of metabolic substrates	Electrolytes
	Carbohydrate
	Amino acids and protein
	Fatty acids
Manipulation of acid–base balance	Forced acid or alkaline diuresis
Coagulopathy correction	Platelets
	Clotting factors
Improving oxygen carriage	
Diluent for drugs	If caustic
	If low solubility
Osmotic effects	
Manipulation of blood viscosity	

Figure IV.1

TABLE OF CRYSTALLOIDS AND THEIR CONSTITUENTS

	Na^+	K^+	Ca^{2+}	Cl^-	HCO_3^-	Osmolality	pH
Sodium chloride 0.9%	150	0	0	150	0	300	5
Dextrose 5%	0	0	0	0	0	280	4
Dextrose 10%	0	0	0	0	0	560	4
Dextrose 4% Saline 0.18%	30	0	0	0	30	255	4.5
Hartmann's solution	131	5	2	111	29	278	6
Sodium bicarbonate 8.4%	1000	0	0	0	1000	2000	8

Note that ionic concentrations are in mmol/l, osmolality in mosmol/l.

Figure IV.2

volume given. The solutes determine how widely the water will be distributed in the body.

ELECTROLYTES

Cations

Sodium is primarily an extracellular ion. Typical sodium requirement is 1 mmol/kg/day. In contrast, **potassium** is primarily an intracellular ion. In concentrations similar to plasma levels, potassium solutions can be given rapidly but this will have little effect on total body potassium. Replacement of potassium by the IV route should be done slowly and requires careful monitoring when more concentrated solutions are used to avoid cardiac arrhythmias and cardiac arrest. The addition of potassium to crystalloid solutions such as Ringer's lactate (Hartmann's) is an attempt to mimic the electrolyte composition of plasma.

Calcium may be used to improve myocardial contractility when plasma levels are depleted. It is available as calcium chloride 10% ($CaCl_2$, which contains 0.68 mmol/ml = 680 mmol/l calcium ions). Note that using the combined atomic weight of calcium and two chlorine atoms (MW 111) does not provide the actual molarity of calcium. This is because calcium chloride (dihydrate) has two water molecules closely associated with it in the crystalline form in which it is weighed ($CaCl_2.2H_2O$). Calcium is also available as the gluconate 10% (0.22 mmol/ml). However, this preparation may be negatively inotropic, and can cause coronary vasoconstriction. Calcium may be useful when large amounts of blood and fresh frozen plasma have been rapidly transfused. **Magnesium** is important in enzyme systems, and in muscle and neuronal function. Magnesium can be used therapeutically for arrhythmias (especially torsades de pointes), myocardial infarction, eclampsia and pre-eclampsia.

Anions

Chloride is the predominant anion in the body and is a constituent to maintain the cationic/anionic balance of most IV fluids. **Bicarbonate** may be used to manipulate the pH of IV fluids. As heat sterilisation destroys the ion and thus produces CO_2, these solutions are sterilised by filtration and are relatively expensive. Phosphorus in the form of **phosphate** is the main intracellular anion. It is not routinely required in IV fluids but is important in long term nutrition. Phosphate buffers are an important constituent of blood cell storage solutions.

Sodium chloride 0.9% is the correct generic term for the solution isotonic with body fluids. It is also referred to as normal saline. 'Normal' in this sense is used to mean that it has the same tonicity as physiological fluids, and 'twice normal saline' refers to sodium chloride 1.8%, which is used in cases of hyponatraemia. Unfortunately, 'normal' is an imprecise term that could also be interpreted in this case as 1 molar sodium chloride.

Hartmann's solution uses lactate (another base present in the body) in place of bicarbonate and is heat sterilised. Lactate is readily metabolised in the liver.

Sodium bicarbonate 8.4% solution is used for the immediate correction of metabolic acidosis. Its alkalinity and high osmolality can easily cause tissue damage if small veins are used or if extravasation occurs. It contains 1000 mmol of sodium ions per litre and this carries a risk of fluid retention which may be a particular problem if the acidosis is the result of renal failure.

COLLOIDS

Colloids tend to be larger molecules than crystalloids and are dispersed throughout the solvent rather than forming true solutions. The component particles tend to arrange as groups of molecules and so do not readily pass through clinical semipermeable membranes. They therefore have an oncotic potential that is usually measured as colloid oncotic pressure (COP). As the number of molecules per volume of solution is usually lower than crystalloid solutions, boiling point and freezing point are less affected for a given mass of solute. Increasing the amount of colloid has little affect on osmotic pressure so electrolytes are used to achieve iso-osmolality with blood. The constituents of common colloids are shown in Figure IV. 3.

GELATINS

These are prescribed by their proprietary names as the generic term gelatin does not indicate the various component differences of the solutions. The two major gelatin solutions in widespread use are Gelofusine and Haemaccel.

Gelofusine® (Braun)

Gelofusine is a 4% solution of succinylated gelatin in saline in which the gelatin is prepared by hydroxylation and succinylation of bovine collagen. Other ions are present in negligible amounts because of the

CONSTITUENTS AND PHYSICOCHEMICAL PROPERTIES OF COLLOIDS

	Na+	K+	Ca2+	Mg2+	Cl-	Osmolality	pH
Gelofusine	154	0.4	0.4	0.4	125	279	7.4
Haemaccel	145	5.1	6.25	0	145	301	7.3
Dextran 70 (dextrose 5%)	0	0	0	0	0	287	3.5–7
HAS 4.5%	100–160	<2	0	0	100–160	270–300	6.4–7.4
HAS 20%	50–120	<10	0	0	<40	135–138	6.4–7.4

Note: Ions in mmol/l, osmolality in mosmol/l

Figure IV.3

manufacturing process. The calcium present does not warrant line flushing before giving citrated blood.

Characteristics

- Relative viscosity 1.9
- Gel point 0°C
- $t_{1/2}$ 2–4 H
- COP 35 mmHg

The majority of renal excretion occurs within 24 H and the incidence of severe anaphylaxis is about 1:13 000. The degree of frequency with which serious adverse reactions occur varies between solutions. A comparison is given in Figure IV.4.

SERIOUS ADVERSE REACTIONS FOLLOWING THE USE OF INTRAVENOUS SOLUTIONS

Solution	Frequency
Human albumin	1 : 30 000
Dextran 70	1 : 4500
Succinylated gelatin	1 : 13 000
Polygeline	1 : 2000
Hetastarch	1 : 16 000

Figure IV.4

Haemaccel® (Hoechst)

Haemaccel is a 3.5% solution of polygeline in a mixed salt solution. Polygeline is a degraded and modified gelatin with 6.3 g nitrogen equivalent per litre containing traces of phosphate and sulphate. The gelatine is cross-linked with urea, which may be released after hydrolysis, a potential problem in patients with renal failure.

Characteristics

- Relative viscosity 1.7
- Gel point <3° C
- $t_{1/2}$ 6 H
- COP 28 mmHg

DEXTRANS

The dextrans are glucose polymers that are available in several different average molecular weight preparations. Dextran 40 (average MW 40 000 Daltons) and Dextran 70 (average MW 70 000 Daltons). Dextran 110 is no longer available because of an unacceptable incidence of anaphylactoid reactions. Their main application is in the prevention of thrombo-embolism by blood volume expansion, reduction of blood viscosity and lowering of erythrocyte and platelet aggregation, although they are also used as plasma volume expanders. Dextrans are available in solution with either sodium chloride 0.9% or dextrose 5%.

HYDROXYETHYL STARCH (HES)

These are composed of at least 90% amylopectin that is etherified with hydroxyethyl groups. The degree of etherification is indicated by the prefix with hetastarch more etherified than pentastarch. The degree of substitution reflects the number of hydroxyethyl groups per glucose unit. The starch solutions have a large range of molecular weights. The polymerised glucose units are primarily joined by 1–4 linkages and the hydroxyethyl groups are attached to the 2 carbon of the glucose moiety making the resultant polymer similar to glycogen.

Hetastarch

Hespan® (Geistlich) is 6% hetastarch in sodium chloride 0.9% with pH modification by sodium hydroxide. It is almost entirely derived from amylopectin. Molecules with a molecular weight below 50 000 readily pass through the glomerular membrane and 40% is excreted by this route within 24 H. The hydroxyethyl-glucose bond remains intact and usually < 1% of the total dose remains in the body after 2 weeks. Hetastarch has a colloid oncotic pressure of 20 mmHg. Other starch solutions include hexastarch and pentastarch which have comparable characteristics.

HUMAN ALBUMIN SOLUTIONS (HAS)

Derived from human plasma by fractionation (the old term is plasma protein fraction); human albumin is heat sterilised and thus the risk of infective transmission is very low. It may be supplied as 4.5% (40–50 g/l) to reflect normal plasma or 20% (150–250 g/l) in which water is removed together with the dissolved salts. It is sometimes called 'salt poor albumin' as the sodium concentration is also lowered. At least 95% of the protein in HAS is albumin and this has been stabilised using sodium n-octanoate. HAS is used as a colloid especially if high albumin loss has been a problem (burns, for example) The 20% albumin solution will oncotically draw water from tissues and may be useful in the treatment of hypoalbuminaemia. A simple formula for calculating the amount of albumin needed in hypoalbuminaemia is:

Albumin required (g) = [desired total protein (g/l) – actual total protein (g/l)] × plasma volume (l) × 2

The use of HAS is still controversial. In addition to its colloid properties, it is involved in plasma molecular carriage, coagulation and membrane integrity. It is also a free radical scavenger. Low serum albumin is associated with poor outcome. Large volume resuscitation depletes albumin probably due to redistribution. Theoretical benefits of albumin replacement are yet to be proven in practise. At present, it is important to refrain from routine use of HAS as colloid and blind replacement, but considered use may be beneficial.

HAEMOGLOBIN SOLUTIONS (EXPERIMENTAL)

STROMA-FREE HAEMOGLOBIN (SFH)

Stroma-free haemoglobin has shown some promise experimentally as a blood substitute. The advantages and disadvantages of SFH are given in Figure IV.5.

STROMA FREE HAEMOGLOBIN

Advantages
- Effective oxygen carrier
- Passes easily into smallest capillaries
- No need for cross match
- Infection risk minimal
- Storage and transport at ambient temperature
- Long shelf life

Disadvantages
- Low P_{50}
- Poor intravascular persistence
- Nephrotoxicity
- Immunological effects
- Free radical production
- Increased nitric oxide scavenging

Figure IV.5

Oxygen affinity

The P_{50} of intracellular haemoglobin is 3.6 kPa but this drops to 1.6 kPa when free in the plasma due to loss of 2,3-DPG from the haemoglobin molecule. This very high affinity for oxygen severely reduces its release to the tissues. In the clinical setting extra-erythrocytic haemoglobin co-exists with intra-erythrocytic haemoglobin and it has been shown that intracellular haemoglobin supplies most oxygen to the tissues until very low haematocrits (< 0.2) are reached. Pyridoxylation of haemoglobin reduces the high oxygen affinity.

Intravascular persistence

Free haemoglobin dissociates to monomers and dimers with molecular weights well below the renal threshold (69 000 Daltons) and is rapidly excreted. The dimer binds to haptoglobin in plasma but within 4 H 25–40% of unmodified haemoglobin will have passed into the urine. Polymerisation of the haemoglobin produces a molecule of MW 600 000 Daltons ($t_{1/2}$ 38 H). Other methods include intramolecular cross-linking of haemoglobin and conjugation of haemoglobin with large molecules (for example dextran).

Nephrotoxicity

Red cell lysis releases haemoglobin and stroma. Minute amounts of stroma can cause renal damage so the haemoglobin solution must be washed thoroughly following lysis to produce stroma-free haemoglobin.

Haemoglobin is not nephrotoxic but severe hypovolaemia itself can cause clogging of the distal tubule.

Nitric oxide scavenging

This is increased by permeation of haemoglobin into the tissues. It results in vasoconstriction and possible neurotoxicity.

MICRO-ENCAPSULATED HAEMOGLOBIN

The physiological carriage of haemoglobin in erythrocytes avoids the problems of high oncotic pressure, prevents loss in the urine, and provides the most efficient micro-environment for the haemoglobin. Micro-encapsulated haemoglobin (non-capsule) is like an artificial red blood cell. A membrane of synthetic polymers, cross linked protein, lipid protein and lipid polymer is created with polymer haemoglobin and enzyme solution inside. The haemoglobin cannot leak out and therefore remains as a tetramer. There is no membrane antigen. Ideally the membrane is permeable to hydrophilic material but does not allow leakage of 2,3-DPG. These artificial cells are about 1 mm in diameter (compare the red cell – diameter 7 mm), which results in rapid clearance from the circulation. A less sophisticated alternative is to use a phospholipid and sterol bilayer liposome to encapsulate the haemoglobin.

SYNTHETIC OXYGEN CARRIERS

Normally only 4% of the oxygen delivered is carried in solution (0.0225 ml O_2/100 ml blood/kPa), the rest is carried as oxyhaemoglobin. To rely entirely on dissolved oxygen (if this could all be extracted) would require either an increased cardiac output to 13 l/min or an inspired oxygen pressure of 2–2.5 bar. The latter is the principle behind the treatment of carbon monoxide poisoning but requires hyperbaric equipment and risks oxygen toxicity. Therefore, an oxygen carrier is required that will carry oxygen more efficiently than plasma or plasma substitutes, and that will release it to the tissues. There are two options: perfluorocarbons and chelating agents.

CHELATING AGENTS (EXPERIMENTAL)

These are synthetic compounds based on porphyrin. They can contain iron or another metal. They need modification to avoid oxidation of the ferrous ion, a function normally carried out by the globulin, after which they may be incorporated into a membrane.

PERFLUOROCARBONS

Perfluorocarbons (PFCs) are based on a carbon skeleton with fluorine atoms, but they may also have oxygen and nitrogen atoms as part of this skeleton. PFCs absorb oxygen without having a specific binding site. This produces a linear increase in oxygen content proportional to the oxygen partial pressure. They also absorb other low polarity gases (CO_2, carbon monoxide, nitrogen) and volatile anaesthetic agents in proportion to the individual partial pressures. Fluosol-DA, is a mixture of F-decalin (FDC) and F-tripropylamine (FTPA) in a ratio of 7 FDC:3 FTPA. The only clinical use was for distal coronary perfusion during angioplasty because the maximum concentration possible did not carry sufficient oxygen. Sufficient oxygen transport is only achieved by hyperbaric partial pressures of oxygen. Second generation PFC's using egg yolk lecithin emulsions allow much higher concentrations of PFC to be used thus raising the oxygen carrying capacity to clinically useful levels for whole body perfusion at atmospheric pressure.

SECTION 3: 17
PHARMACOLOGY OF HAEMOSTASIS

T. C. Smith

ANTI-COAGULANTS

Oral anti-coagulants
Heparins
Calcium chelating drugs

FIBRINOLYTIC AGENTS

Plasminogen activators
Fibrinolytic inhibitors

ANTI-PLATELET DRUGS

Aspirin
Prostacyclin

OTHER HAEMOSTATIC MODIFIERS

Viscosity
Coagulation factors
Platelet action

The ways that haemostatic processes may be altered pharmacologically are classified in Figure CP.1.

MODE OF ACTION OF PHARMACOLOGICAL ALTERATION OF HAEMOSTASIS

Coagulation (fibrin clot formation)

Procoagulants	Desmopressin
	Vitamin K
Anticoagulants	Coumarins
	Inandiones
	Heparin
	Calcium chelating agents

Fibrinolysis

Fibrinolytic drugs	Streptokinase
	Urokinase
Antifibrinolytics	Aprotinin
	Tranexamic acid

Platelet function

Antiplatelet drugs	Aspirin
	Prostacyclin
Platelet enhancers	Ethamsylate

Figure CP.1

Figure CP.2 shows the effects of the commoner drugs on the coagulation system.

ANTI-COAGULANTS

Anti-coagulants are drugs that interfere with the process of fibrin plug formation to reduce or prevent coagulation. This effect is used to reduce the risk of thrombus formation within normal vessels and vascular grafts. The injectable anti-coagulants are also used to prevent coagulation in extracorporeal circuits and in blood product storage. There are two main types of anti-coagulants: oral anti-coagulants and injectable anti-coagulants (heparins).

ORAL ANTI-COAGULANTS

Oral anti-coagulants inhibit the reduction of vitamin K. Reduced vitamin K is required as a cofactor in γ-carboxylation of the glutamate residues of the glycoprotein clotting factors II, VII, IX and X, which are synthesised in the liver. During this γ-carboxylation process, vitamin K is oxidised to vitamin K-2,3-epoxide. The oral anti-coagulants prevent the reduction of this compound back to vitamin K. To work, coumarins must be utilised in the liver. The oral anti-coagulants do this by virtue of their structural similarity to vitamin K. Their action depends on the

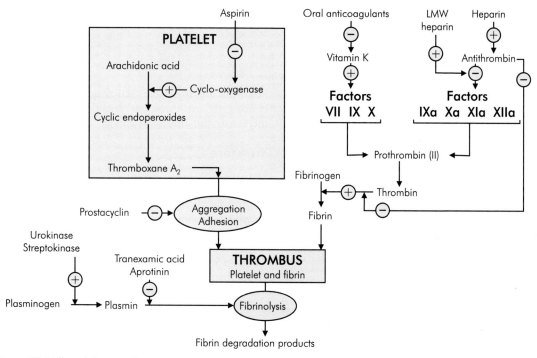

Figure CP.2 Effect of drugs on the coagulation pathway

HALF-LIVES OF VITAMIN K DEPENDENT CLOTTING FACTORS

Factor	half-life (Hours)
II	60
VII	6
IX	24
X	40

Figure CP.3

depletion of these factors, which decline according to their individual half-lives (Figure CP.3).

There are two groups of oral anti-coagulants:

- Coumarins (warfarin and nicoumalone)
- Inandiones (phenindione)

Warfarin has the most widespread use. Phenindione is more likely to cause hypersensitivity, but is useful when there is intolerance to warfarin.

Warfarin sodium

Warfarin is administered orally as a racemic mixture of D and L warfarin. It is rapidly absorbed reaching a peak plasma concentration within 1 H with a bio-availability of 100%. However, a clinical effect is not apparent until the clotting factors become depleted after 12–16 H and reaching a peak at 36–48 H. Warfarin is 99% protein-bound (to albumin) in the plasma resulting in a small volume of distribution. Warfarin is metabolised in the liver by oxidation (L-form) and reduction (D-form), followed by glucuronide conjugation, with a half-life of about 40 H.

Warfarin crosses the placenta and is teratogenic during pregnancy. In the post partum period it passes into breast milk which is a particular problem as the gut flora responsible for producing vitamin K_2 and hepatic function in the newborn are not fully developed.

Warfarin has a low therapeutic index and is particularly prone to interactions with other drugs. Interactions increasing the effect of warfarin occur in several ways:

- Competition for protein binding sites
- Increased hepatic binding
- Inhibition of hepatic microsomal enzymes
- Reduced vitamin K synthesis
- Synergistic anti-haemostatic actions

Drugs such as NSAIDs, chloral hydrate, oral hypoglycaemic agents, diuretics and amiodarone displace warfarin from albumin binding sites resulting in higher free plasma levels and greater effect. This effect is made more significant because normally only 1% of warfarin is free and a small change in protein binding has a dramatic effect on free warfarin levels. D-Thyroxine increases the potency of warfarin by increasing hepatic binding. Ethanol ingestion may inhibit liver enzymes responsible for warfarin elimination. The effect of warfarin may also be increased by acute illness, low vitamin K intake and drugs such as cimetidine, aminoglycosides and paracetamol. Broad spectrum antibiotics reduce the level of gut bacteria responsible for vitamin K_2 synthesis, and may enhance the effect of warfarin where the diet is deficient in vitamin K. Other anti-coagulants and particularly anti-platelet drugs increase the clinical effects of warfarin.

Interactions decreasing the effect of warfarin can occur in several ways, notably:

- Induction of hepatic microsomal enzymes
- Drugs that increase levels of clotting factors
- Binding of warfarin
- Increased vitamin K intake

The effect of warfarin may be reduced by induction of hepatic enzymes by barbiturates and phenytoin. Oestrogens increase the production of vitamin K dependent clotting factors (II, VII, IX, X). Cholestyramine binds warfarin reducing its effect. Carbamazepine and rifampicin reduce the effect of warfarin but the mechanism of this effect is not clear.

HEPARINS

Heparins are injectable anti-coagulants that act by binding to anti-thrombin resulting in a profound increase in anti-thrombin activity.

Structure

Heparin is a group of sulphated acid glycosaminoglycans (or mucopolysaccharides) comprising alternate monosaccharide residues of N-acetylglucosamine and glucuronic acid and their derivatives. The glucuronic acid residues are mostly in the iduronic acid form and some are ester-sulphated. The N-acetylglucosamine residues may be deacylated, N-sulphated and ester-sulphated in a random manner. This results in a chain of 45–50 sugar residues of variable composition based on the above units. The molecules are attached by the sulphated components to a protein skeleton consisting entirely of glycine and serine amino acid residues. The molecular weight of heparin ranges from 3000 to 40 000 Daltons, with a mean of 12 000–15 000. Endogenous heparin is located in the lungs, in arterial walls and in mast cells as large polymers of molecular weight 750 000. It is present in the plasma at a concentration of 1.5 mg/l.

Heparin has a strong negative charge and is a large molecule, so there is minimal absorption following oral administration. It is supplied as heparin sodium and heparin calcium.

Mechanism of action

Heparin has the following effects:

- Inhibition of coagulation by enhancing the action of anti-thrombin on the serine protease coagulation factors (IIa, Xa, XIIa, XIa and IXa)
- Reduced platelet aggregation
- Increased vascular permeability
- Release of lipoprotein lipases into plasma

The negatively charged heparin binds to the lysine residue in anti-thrombin, an α_2-globulin, which in turns increases the affinity of the arginine site of anti-thrombin for the serine site of thrombin (Factor II). This increases the inhibitory activity of anti-thrombin 2300-fold. This reversible bond is the feature of a specific anti-thrombin binding site comprising five particular residues. This particular pentasaccharide sequence is present randomly in about one-third of the heparin molecules. For full activity of heparin on thrombin (IIa) a heparin molecule must have at least 13 extra sugar residues in addition to the pentasaccharide anti-thrombin binding site sequence. The covalently bonded thrombin–anti-thrombin complex is inactive but once it is formed the heparin is released and the complex is rapidly destroyed by the liver. The active heparin section is then free to act on more anti-thrombin. Heparin acts in a similar way on the other activated serine protease coagulation factors (XIIa, Xa and IXa). The binding of heparin to both the clotting factor and anti-thrombin is important in the above enhancement of anti-thrombin. The activity of heparin on factor Xa is also mediated by increasing the affinity of anti-thrombin for the clotting factor but heparin does not bind to factor Xa. Factor Xa inhibition is enhanced with lower levels of heparin than those required for thrombin inhibition. Heparin reduces platelet aggregation secondary to the reduction in thrombin (a potent platelet aggregator). The increase in plasma lipase results in an increase in free fatty acid levels.

Low molecular weight heparins

Examples – certoparin, enoxaparin, tinzaparin)

The low molecular weight (LMW) heparins are fragments of de-polymerised heparin purified to contain the anti-thrombin specific binding site. Therefore, they all inhibit factor Xa. The molecular weight of LMW heparins ranges from 3000 to 8000 Daltons, with a mean of 4000–6500. They comprise 13–22 sugar residues. The LMW heparins have a full anti-Xa activity but much reduced anti-thrombin activity and require the presence of anti-thrombin for their effect. The reduction in interference with thrombin gives LMW heparins the following advantages:

- Minimal alteration of platelet function
- Better intra-operative haemostasis
- Possible better venous thromboembolic prophyl-axis in orthopaedic practice

Administration

Heparin is administered intravenously and subcutaneously. A typical adult dose for thrombosis prophylaxis is 5000 IU subcutaneously 8–12 hourly. For full anti-coagulation, as used during cardiopulmonary bypass, a dose of 3 mg/kg (300 IU/kg) is used to achieve 3–4 IU heparin/ml blood. Heparin has an immediate action within the plasma. Heparin has a volume of distribution of 40–100 ml/kg and is bound to anti-thrombin, albumin, fibrinogen and proteases. Increase in acute phase proteins (during acute illness) can significantly alter the clinical effect. Heparin also binds to platelet and endothelial protein, reducing bio-availability and effect. The drug is metabolised in the liver, kidney and reticulo-endothelial system by heparinases that desulphate the mucopolysaccharide residues and hydrolyse the links between them. Heparin has a half-life of 40–90 min.

LMW heparins are also administered subcutaneously and have the advantage of once daily administration. They may be used in extracorporeal dialysis circuits, and have been used in cardiopulmonary bypass. LMW heparins are much less bound to proteins in the plasma, platelets and vascular walls and bio-availability after subcutaneous administration is at least 90%. The levels of free LMW heparin are therefore much more predictable and require less monitoring. Peak anti-Xa activity is achieved within 3 to 4 H after subcutaneous injection and activity has halved after 12 H. Elimination is predominantly renal and half-life may be raised in renal failure.

Effects on coagulation studies

Heparin increases activated partial thromboplastin time (APTT), thrombin time (TT) and activated clotting time (ACT) but does not affect bleeding time.

Heparin therapy is routinely checked using the APTT and, on cardiopulmonary bypass, using ACT.

Heparin relies on the presence of anti-thrombin for its activity. Prolonged heparin therapy may lead to osteoporosis by an unknown mechanism.

Protamine

Protamine is a group of basic, cationic (positively charged) proteins of relatively LMW. Protamine is used to neutralise the effects of heparin and LMW heparins. This occurs because the negative charge of the heparin is attracted to the positive charges of the protamine. 1 mg of protamine sulphate, neutralises 1 mg (100 IU) heparin. Protamine (in excess) has anti-coagulant activity, although this effect is not as powerful as that of heparin.

CALCIUM CHELATING AGENTS

Calcium is an essential cofactor in the coagulation system. Agents that bind calcium will therefore inhibit coagulation. Citrate is used to bind calcium in stored blood to prevent its coagulation. In vivo, the citrate is metabolised by the liver reversing this inhibition. However, massive transfusion may temporarily overload the liver's capacity to metabolise citrate particularly if metabolic rate is reduced by cooling by the transfusion or by deliberate hypothermia as used in cardiac surgery. To some extent this may be overcome by administering calcium ions.

FIBRINOLYTIC AGENTS

Fibrinolysis may be **activated** or **inhibited** pharmacologically.

PLASMINOGEN ACTIVATORS

Examples – alteplase, reteplase, streptokinase, urokinase

The plasminogen activators act by catalysing the conversion of plasminogen to plasmin, the enzyme responsible for the enzymatic degradation of fibrin clot. Plasminogen activators are used to destroy clots in the following situations:

- Venous thrombosis
- Pulmonary embolus
- Retinal thrombosis
- Myocardial infarction

The drugs may also remove clot formed in response to haemorrhage, so bleeding from other sites is a risk. In some cases this can be minimised by administering the activator directly to the desired site of thrombus by catheter. However, this is technically difficult and the delay in doing so may remove any benefit. Some of these agents require heparin and or aspirin to prevent reformation of thrombus. They may reduce levels of plasminogen, α_2-anti-plasmin, α_2-macroglobulin and C_1-esterase inhibitor.

Alteplase (rt-PA) is a synthetic form of tissue type plasminogen activator (a glycoprotein). Anistreplase is a ready combined complex of plasminogen and streptokinase that is blocked by an anisoyl group. Once in the body the anisoyl group leaves the complex, which produces plasmin and so activates fibrinolysis. Reteplase is another recombinant plasminogen activator. These three agents act on fibrin bound plasminogen. Streptokinase is obtained from group C **haemolytic streptococci** cultures. Streptokinase induces an immune response that produces antibodies to the drug and limits its useful duration to 6 days. Allergy is common. Patients frequently have antibodies to protein from previous exposure to the *Streptococcus*. Urokinase is derived from human kidney cell cultures or urine and is therefore non antigenic.

FIBRINOLYTIC INHIBITORS

Examples – aprotinin, tranexamic acid

The fibrinolytic inhibitors act by inhibiting the enzymatic activity of plasmin on fibrin. They are used to prevent the breakdown of fibrin clot when excessive bleeding during surgery is a risk. Uses include the reduction of blood loss during surgery in haemophiliacs, cardiac surgery and in thrombolytic overdose.

Aprotinin is a polypeptide and inhibitor of proteolytic enzymes in general, but specifically it is used for its action on plasmin and kallikrein. It has also been tried in the treatment of acute pancreatitis. Tranexamic acid inhibits the fibrinolytic activity of both plasmin and pepsin. It is useful in upper gastro-intestinal haemorrhage and in surgery in haemophiliacs and it can be administered orally or intravenously.

ANTI-PLATELET DRUGS

ASPIRIN

Aspirin irreversibly inactivates platelet cyclo-oxygenase (COX_2) by acetylation of the terminal serine amino acid. This inhibits endoperoxide and so thromboxane (TXA_2) production within the platelets. More importantly, endothelial cells generate new cyclo-oxygenase, whereas platelets are unable to. As it is an irreversible process, the effect on an individual platelet is permanent for the 4–6-day life span of the platelet. Aspirin is not specific for platelet cyclo-oxygenase but this is more readily inactivated than endothelial cyclo-oxygenase responsible for prostacyclin production. Aspirin should be stopped 7–10 days before surgery to allow regeneration of normally functioning platelets. It may be restarted 6 H post operatively. Prolonged aspirin usage may reduce circulating levels of factors II, VII, IX and X.

Other NSAIDs also inhibit COX, but are generally less potent and the inhibition is reversible so that the overall effect on platelet function is small.

PROSTACYCLIN

Synthetic prostacyclin (epoprostenol) inhibits platelet aggregation and dissipates platelet aggregates. It can be used in haemodialysis, but must be given as an infusion because of a short half-life (about 3 min). Prostacyclin is also a potent vasodilator, so patients should be observed for hypotension, flushing and headaches.

OTHER HAEMOSTATIC MODIFIERS

VISCOSITY

Dextrans reduce the viscosity of blood and may reduce the incidence of venous thrombus formation by improving the flow characteristics of the relatively slow flowing venous circulation.

COAGULATION FACTORS

Coagulation factors may be administered as extracts (anti thrombin III and factors VIIa, VIII and IX) or as fresh frozen plasma (FFP). Vitamin K may be used to increase levels of factors II, VII and IX when there is a deficiency of vitamin K or excess of oral anti-coagulant therapy. Vitamin K_2 is produced by gut bacteria. These are reduced by broad-spectrum antibiotics and are deficient in newborn (haemorrhagic disease of the newborn). Desmopressin increases levels of Factor VIII. This may be useful to decrease surgical oozing in mild haemophilia, and in cases of massive transfusion, when clotting factors are reduced.

At present, anti-coagulants either rely on a reduction in levels of clotting factors (oral anti-coagulants) or on the enhancement of anti-thrombin. Future developments may involve the direct inhibition of specific clotting factors.

PLATELET ACTION

Ethamsylate reduces capillary bleeding probably by correcting abnormal platelet adhesion. Ethamsylate inhibits the anti-platelet action of some NSAIDs, in addition to a weak arteriolar constricting action. It is contra-indicated in porphyria.

SECTION 3: 18
ANTIMICROBIAL THERAPY

J. Stone

PRINCIPLES OF ANTIMICROBIAL THERAPY

MECHANISMS OF ACTION

β LACTAMS

PENICILLINS

CEPHALOSPORINS

CARBAPENEMS

MONOBACTAMS

GLYCOPEPTIDES

AMINOGLYCOSIDES

MACROLIDES

TETRACYCLINES

CHLORAMPHENICOL

FUSIDANES

QUINOLONES

NITRO-IMIDAZOLES

RIFAMYCINS

TRIMETHOPRIM

SULPHONAMIDES

ANTI-MYCOBACTERIALS

ANTI-VIRALS

PRINCIPLES OF ANTIMICROBIAL THERAPY

The factors that must be assessed before choosing anti microbial therapy are shown in Figure AB.1.

After treatment has commenced, the duration of therapy must be determined and regularly re-assessed, together with the need to modify the antibiotic(s) in terms of both type and dose, depending on, the clinical condition of the patient and laboratory results, e.g. sensitivity tests, plasma drug levels.

ANTIMICROBIAL THERAPY IN RENAL FAILURE

Most antibiotics or their metabolites are renally

FACTORS INFLUENCING ANTIMICROBIAL THERAPY

Patient factors

> Age
> Weight
> Renal function
> Hepatic function
> Anti-microbial allergy
> Immune deficiency or suppression
> Pregnant
> Significant medical conditions
> Site of infection
> Severity of infection
> Prophylaxis or treatment required

Organism factors

> Virulence
> Predicted microbe population
> Predicted anti-microbial susceptibility

Drug factors

> Spectrum of anti-microbial activity
> Route of administration
> Pharmacokinetics
> Synergy or antagonism with other anti microbial agents
> Toxicity profile
> Interactions with non anti microbial compounds
> Local antibiotic prescribing policies

Figure AB.1

excreted. Accumulation of potentially toxic compounds may therefore arise unless careful monitoring and dose adjustments are performed. Some antimicrobials are nephrotoxic while others should be avoided if there is pre-existing renal disease and different methods of dialysis have differing abilities to clear certain compounds.

MECHANISMS OF ACTION

Antimicrobials work by interfering with cellular functions. They target structures and functions specific to the target microbe or those that have an alternative metabolic pathway in human cells. These mechanisms target four groups of microbial sites:

- Cell wall
- Cell membrane
- Protein synthesis
- Nucleic acid synthesis

CELL WALL SYNTHESIS

Bacteria have a cell wall to prevent swelling and lysis in hypotonic environments. The cell wall comprises N-acetyl glucosamine, acetyl muramic acid and a polypeptide, which that form multiple cross links. This maintains the three dimensional integrity of the structure. The cell wall can range from several molecular layers thick in gram-negative bacteria to 100 layers in the gram-positive organisms. Anti-microbials that inhibit cell wall synthesis cause the cell to burst, and so are bacteriocidal. Antibacterial drugs targeting the cell wall cannot affect eukaryotic cells by this mechanism.

CELL MEMBRANE PERMEABILITY

Drugs that selectively interfere with cell membrane permeability are active against bacterial and fungal cells. Selectivity is conferred by targeting components of bacterial or fungal cell membranes that are not found in the host. Negatively charged lipids are abundant in the cell membranes of gram-negative bacteria and are the target of polymyxins such as colistin and polymyxin B. Sterols are present in both fungal and human cell membranes. Imidazoles and triazoles interfere with sterol synthesis and toxicity occurs with higher doses. Polyenes such as amphotericin and nystatin bind to the fungal sterols and open pores in the membrane leading to destruction of the molecular composition of the cytoplasm.

PROTEIN SYNTHESIS

Where bacterial and human ribosomes differ, they can be targeted by antibiotics. Those agents that reversibly inhibit protein synthesis are bacteriostatic. Those that bind to the 30 S subunit of the bacterial ribosome are bactericidal.

NUCLEIC ACID SYNTHESIS

Rifampicin inhibits DNA dependent RNA polymerase. The quinolones inhibit DNA synthesis and disrupt the final coiling of the DNA helix essential for its transcription. Nucleic acid analogues such as acyclovir attach to the active site of the enzymes of DNA synthesis and so block DNA synthesis.

BETA LACTAMS

This is the single largest group of anti-microbial agents presently available, and includes penicillins, cephalosporins, monobactams and carbapenems.

MECHANISM OF ACTION

The β-lactam antibiotics target the penicillin binding proteins (PBPs). These are cell wall synthesising enzymes located in the cytoplasmic membrane. PBPs are not present in mammalian cells, which accounts for the low toxicity of these drugs. The bacterial cell wall is weakened and osmotic lysis occurs. Penicillins and cephalosporins show synergy with antibiotics acting on targets within the bacterial cell because the cell wall changes increase the permeability of the cell to other compounds.

ACQUIRED RESISTANCE

Bacteria exhibit resistance to β-lactams by four mechanisms:

- Enzymatic destruction of β-lactam
- Bacterial modification of PBP target (MRSA)
- Impermeability of cell membrane to β-lactams
- Active efflux (mainly gram-negative bacteria) the bacterium excretes the drug

PENICILLINS

Examples – amoxycillin, benzylpenicillin, fluclox-acillin, piperacillin, azlocillin and mezlocillin

ADVERSE EFFECTS

These are few. Allergy is the most common problem.

True anaphylaxis is rare (0.005%) but has a mortality rate of 10%. In very high doses with meningitis and renal impairment it may cause convulsions.

BENZYLPENICILLIN

Spectrum of activity

Benzylpenicillin is active against gram-positive bacteria most anaerobes and certain gram-negative cocci (*Neisseria* sp.). Most strains of *Staphylococcus aureus* produce β-lactamase and are resistant.

Pharmacokinetics

Benzylpenicillin is unstable in acid and must be given parenterally. It is distributed widely penetrating pleural, pericardial, peritoneal and synovial spaces, but not cerebrospinal fluid in the absence of meningeal inflammation. Low levels are found in saliva. It is excreted mainly by tubular secretion in the kidney with an elimination half-life of 30 min. This process is blocked by probenecid. Aspirin and sulphonamides also prolong the half-life.

AMOXYCILLIN

Amoxycillin has a relatively broad-spectrum of activity. It is active against bacteria covered by benzylpenicillin and several gram-negative species, *Haemophilus influenzae* and most faecal streptococci. Resistance is common due to β-lactamase.

Amoxycillin is stable in gastric acid, and achieves good bio-availability after oral administration. It is otherwise very similar to benzylpenicillin. It has a half-life of 1–1.5 H. Skin rashes are more common with amoxycillin than benzylpenicillin.

Amoxycillin is the drug of choice for most acute lower respiratory tract infections acquired in the community, for *Neisseria gonorrhoeae* and for faecal streptococcal infections. It remains effective as prophylaxis for patients at risk of developing endocarditis.

FLUCLOXACILLIN

Flucloxacillin and related compounds (methicillin, cloxacillin) are unaffected by staphylococcal β-lactamase but have a narrower spectrum of activity than benzylpenicillin. Resistance to them is conferred by an altered target site (the penicillin-binding-protein). These are the 'methicillin-resistant *Staphylococcus aureus* – MRSA' based on the laboratory method of establishing sensitivity.

Flucloxacillin is well absorbed orally but high protein

binding (95%) limits its diffusion into some compartments, notably cerebrospinal fluid. It has a half-life of 45 min. Flucloxacillin remains the drug of choice for staphylococcal infections.

PIPERACILLIN, AZLOCILLIN AND MEZLOCILLIN

These drugs are distinguished from amoxycillin mainly by their activity against *Pseudomonas aeruginosa* and related species. They are destroyed by β-lactamase.

Poor absorption necessitates parenteral administration. These drugs are sodium salts and the high doses required to treat severe sepsis may cause sodium overload. They are mainly used for known or suspected Pseudomonas infections and, in combination with aminoglycosides, the treatment of febrile neutropenic patients. Most β-lactam antibiotics exhibit antibacterial synergy when given with aminoglycosides and there is some evidence that they may also be synergistic against gram-negative bacteria when given with quinolones.

Clavulanic acid

Clavulanic acid is not an antibiotic but is an inhibitor of most β-lactamases. In combination with amoxycillin it improves the spectrum of activity.

Coamoxiclav (clavulanic acid an amoxycillin combination) has been particularly successful. Pharmacokinetically the combination closely mimics that of amoxycillin alone. In addition to the side effects of amoxycillin, there is a small risk of cholestatic jaundice. Co-amoxiclav is used in the treatment of soft tissue infections, surgical prophylaxis, lower respiratory infections and urinary tract infections.

CEPHALOSPORINS

Examples – cephalexin, cefuroxime, cefotaxime, ceftazidime

These compounds are based on cephalosporin C a fermentation product of *Cephalosporium acremonium* cultivated from a Sardinian sewage outfall in 1948. They may be classified into seven groups (Figure AB.2).

CEPHALEXIN

Cephalexin is active against most gram-positive cocci, except faecal streptococci and MRSA. It is also moderately active against some enterobacteria (including *Escherischia coli*). It has negligible activity against *Haemophilus influenzae*.

Pharmacokinetics

Cephalexin is stable to gastric acid and almost completely absorbed when given by mouth and 10% is protein-bound. There is reasonable penetration into

A CLASSIFICATION OF CEPHALOSPORINS

Group	Generation	Examples	Effect of beta-lactamase	Antibacterial activity
1	1st	Cephazolin	Stable	Moderate
2	2nd	Cephalexin Cefaclor	Moderately stable	Moderate
3	2nd	Cefuroxime Cephamandole	Resistance	Moderate
4	3rd	Cefotaxime Ceftriaxone	Stable	Potent: Especially gram-negatives
5	3rd	Cefixime Cefpodoxime	Stable	Potent: Especially gram-negatives
6	3rd	Ceftazidime Cefsulodin	Stable	Potent: Especially gram-negatives and *Pseudomonas*
7	4th	Cefpirome	Stable	Enterobacteriaceae

Figure AB.2

bone and purulent sputum. It is almost entirely excreted in the urine with a half-life of 50 min.

Adverse effects

Cephalexin occasionally causes hypersensitivity, diarrhoea and abdominal discomfort, and rarely Stevens–Johnson syndrome.

CEFUROXIME

Cefuroxime is more active than cephalexin against most of the enterobacteriaceae and has useful activity against *Haemophilus influenzae*. It is similar to cephalexin against gram-positive cocci. It is not absorbed from the intestinal tract and is usually administered intravenously. It is well distributed but cerebrospinal fluid levels are not sufficient to treat bacterial meningitis. It excreted unchanged in the urine one-half being the result of tubular secretion with a half-life of 80 min.

Cefuroxime is used in the treatment of urinary, soft-tissue, bone, intra-abdominal and pulmonary infections and septicaemia. It is ineffective against faecal streptococci and most anaerobes.

CEFOTAXIME

Cefotaxime is similar to cefuroxime but with greater activity against many gram-negative bacteria (e.g. coliforms and gram-negative cocci including β-lactamase-producing strains). It is usually active against penicillin-resistant strains of *Streptococcus pneumoniae*. It has moderate activity against *Listeria monocytogenes* and limited efficacy against anaerobes. It has only slight activity against *Pseudomonas aeruginosa*.

Cefotaxime is administered intravenously. Unlike other cephalosporins, cefotaxime is metabolised in the body to desacetylcefotaxime and both the parent compound and metabolite are renally excreted. It has an elimination half-life of 80 min.

Cefotaxime has a very wide range of indications including: lower respiratory infections, septicaemia, meningitis, intra-abdominal sepsis, osteomyelitis, pyelonephritis, neonatal sepsis and gonorrhoea.

CEFTAZIDIME

Ceftazidime is similar to cefotaxime but much more active against *Pseudomonas aeruginosa*. It is less active against gram-positive cocci than other cephalosporins.

It is 17% protein-bound. Distribution of the drug around the body is similar to cefotaxime. It is mainly excreted renally with a half-life of 2 h.

CARBAPENEMS

Examples – imipenem, meropenem

Carbapenems are bicyclic β-lactam compounds with a carbapenem nucleus. Their mechanism of action is similar to other β-lactam antibiotics but they seem to have a greater affinity for penicillin-binding-protein 2 (PBP-2). This results in faster bacterial death and less endotoxin release. They are extremely broad-spectrum antibiotics, because they resistant to β-lactamase.

PHARMACOKINETICS

Carbapenems are administered intravenously. Excretion is predominantly by glomerular filtration. Carbapenems exhibit a phenomenon known as the 'post antibiotic effect'. This is a prolonged inhibition of bacterial growth for a period of time after the concentration of antibiotic has fallen below the accepted minimum inhibitory concentration (MIC). Therefore, 6, 8 and even 12 hourly dose regimes can be effective.

ADVERSE EFFECTS

Adverse effects are similar to other β-lactams. Neutropenia is a rare complication and is reversible on stopping the drug. Neurotoxicity appears to be more of a problem than with other β-lactam antibiotics but is primarily seen in patients with renal insufficiency and on high doses, particularly neonates and the elderly.

IMIPENEM

Imipenem is chemically unstable in its natural form and is supplied in crystalline form. It is highly active against virtually all gram-positive and gram-negative pathogenic bacteria, including anaerobes. Poor intracellular penetration of eukaryotic cells prevents its use against intracellular infections such as *Legionnella*. It is rapidly bactericidal against a majority of organisms but is only bacteriostatic against faecal streptococci. MRSA are not susceptible and *Pseudomonas aeruginosa* can rapidly develop resistance.

Pharmacokinetics

Imipenem is rapidly destroyed by dehydropeptidase-1 in renal tubules. It is administered with cilastatin, a selective competitive inhibitor of this enzyme. Cilastatin has similar pharmacokinetic properties to imipenem and inhibition of dehydropeptidase has no apparent adverse physiological consequences.

MEROPENEM

Meropenem is similar to imipenem but is stable to human renal dehydropeptidase, rendering the addition of cilastatin unnecessary. It is more active than imipenem against some gram-negatives but less active against gram-positives. The main benefit is that it is less neurotoxic than imipenem.

MONOBACTAMS

Example – aztreonam

Monobactams only have a single β-lactam ring while penicillins, cephalosporins and carbapenems all have two. Note that only gram-negative aerobic bacteria are sensitive. It is highly active against most of the Enterobacteriaceae, *Haemophilus influenzae* and *Neisseria* and has some activity against *Pseudomonas aeruginosa*.

PHARMACOKINETICS

Intestinal absorption is poor, so aztreonam is given by IV or IM injection. Distribution in the body is similar to other β-lactams. Elimination is renal by a combination of glomerular filtration and tubular secretion. Aztreonam has a half-life of 2 H.

ADVERSE EFFECTS

Aztreonam is similar to other β-lactams. However, as a monobactam, there appears to be very little cross-hypersensitivity with penicillins or cephalosporins. Aztreonam should still be used with caution in patients with severe penicillin allergy. Aztreonam does not seem to interfere with platelet function unlike some cephalosporins and penicillins.

GLYCOPEPTIDES

Examples – teicoplanin, vancomycin

The glycopeptides are a group of complex, high molecular weight compounds that are usually bactericidal and prevent bacterial cell wall synthesis at the substrate level. Glycopeptides are active against most gram-positive bacteria but they do not penetrate the outer membrane of gram-negative organisms because they are large polar molecules.

ACQUIRED RESISTANCE

Acquired resistance is uncommon. Gene mutations occur, which alter cell wall precursors. These precursors are called Van-A (which produces resistance to both vancomycin and teicoplanin and is inducible and present on plasmids – allowing transfer between strains), Van-B and Van-C (which produce resistance to vancomycin only and are present on bacterial chromosomes – less easy to transfer to other species). Resistance has been reported principally in various enterococcus species, which have been named vancomycin resistant enterococci (VRE).

The mechanism of resistance is not clear. The presence of mucopolysaccharide slime reduces the susceptibility of coagulase negative staphylococci. This is often present when there are microcolonies on the surfaces of joint and heart valve prostheses or on IV and peritoneal dialysis cannulae.

VANCOMYCIN

Vancomycin is used to treat difficult gram-positive bacterial infections including: MRSA, staphylococcal or streptococcal infective endocarditis, coagulase-negative staphylococci on indwelling materials and antibiotic-associated colitis (*Clostridium difficile*).

Spectrum of activity

Vancomycin is effective against: gram-positive cocci (including MRSA), coagulase-negative staphylococci (e.g. *Staphylococcus epidermidis*), streptococci, enterococci, bacillus, corynebacteria, *Listeria monocytogenes* (moderate), gram-positive anaerobes (*Clostridium perfringens* and other *Clostridia* sp.).

Pharmacokinetics

Vancomycin is administered intravenously because intestinal tract absorption is poor and IM injection causes pain and necrosis. It is widely distributed, reaching most body compartments except the cerebrospinal fluid. It may also be administered into CSF shunts and into the peritoneum, and for antibiotic associated colitis it is given orally. Vancomycin is 55% protein-bound. It is excreted, unchanged, mainly by glomerular filtration with a half-life of 6–8 H. Plasma monitoring is usually only required in those with renal impairment or those on prolonged high dose regimes. It is not removed effectively by either haemodialysis or haemofiltration.

Adverse effects

Adverse effects include hypersensitivity, nephrotoxicity, ototoxicity and occasionally neutropoenia. Chemical thrombophlebitis is relatively common when vancomycin is administered via a peripheral vein. Vancomycin induced histamine release with rapid infusion produces the 'Red man syndrome'. This comprises itching, flushing, angioedema, hypotension and tachycardia. Bronchospasm does not occur. It normally resolves within 1 H of the infusion stopping. It is prevented by anti-histamines. The hypotensive effect may be severe. Nephrotoxicity and ototoxicity may be related to impurities in earlier preparations and are now rare.

TEICOPLANIN

Teicoplanin has slightly greater activity against some streptococci and slightly less activity against staphylococci than vancomycin. It is distributed similarly to vancomycin but is more protein-bound (> 90%). The serum half-life is considerably longer (47 H) than vancomycin, partly because of the protein binding. It may be given by rapid IV infusion or intramuscularly.

AMINOGLYCOSIDES

Examples – amikacin, gentamicin, streptomycin

Aminoglycosides are naturally occurring or semisynthetic polycationic compounds with aminosugars glycosidically linked to aminocyclitols.

MECHANISM OF ACTION

Aminoglycosides bind to the 30 S subunit of the bacterial ribosome, causing inhibition of protein synthesis. It is not known why aminoglycosides are usually rapidly bactericidal but other inhibitors of protein synthesis are bacteriostatic. They cause cell membrane leakiness and consequent cell death. In general, aminoglycosides are active against *Staphylococcus aureus* and a majority of the coagulase-negative staphylococci, the enterobacteriaceae and most are effective against *Pseudomonas aeuginosa* and other *Pseudomonas* sp.

ACQUIRED RESISTANCE

There are three mechanisms of resistance to aminoglycosides:

- Altered binding site
- Reduced uptake/permeability
- Aminoglycoside modifying enzymes

ADVERSE EFFECTS

Aminoglycosides are nephrotoxic and ototoxic (vestibular and auditory). Toxicity is directly related to plasma levels, which should be monitored closely, particularly with impaired renal function. Slow IV injection will minimise the risk, but toxicity is principally associated with elevated trough levels. Ototoxicity is usually irreversible but renal function often recovers.

The ototoxicity is put to use in chemical vestibular labyrinthectomy with gentamycin delivered to the middle ear to treat Ménière's disease.

GENTAMICIN

Gentamicin is active against the enterobacteriaceae, some *Pseudomonas* sp. (e.g. *Ps. aeruginosa*) and staphylococci. It has limited activity against streptococci and *Listeria* sp. Gentamicin is used for serious gram-negative bacterial infections. It is rapidly bactericidal and has a strong synergistic effect with β-lactams. Poor tissue penetration limits its usefulness in the treatment of deep soft tissue infections and abscesses. Similarly, typhoid and other intracellular infections are relatively resistant. Selective decontamination of the intestine by oral administration may be useful but may increase bacterial resistance.

Pharmacokinetics

Gentamicin is administered parenterally because oral bio-availability is low (1%), in a dose of 1–2 mg/kg, 8 hourly. Tissue and cell penetration is poor but it crosses the placenta. Excretion is renal, mainly by glomerular filtration, with an elimination half-life of 2 H.

AMIKACIN

Amikacin has a similar anti-bacterial spectrum to gentamicin, but is less susceptible to most of the aminoglycoside modifying enzymes. It is reserved for specific sensitive strains. It is also active against *Mycobacterium tuberculosis* and other 'atypical' mycobacteria, including strains resistant to streptomycin. Any nephrotoxicity and ototoxicity that occurs is usually reversible.

STREPTOMYCIN

Streptomycin is particularly effective against *Mycobacterium tuberculosis*, but is also active against many gram-negative aerobic bacteria and staphylococci. Resistance can develop as a single step mutation that changes the structure of the ribosomal target site.

MACROLIDES

Examples – clarithromycin, erythromycin

Macrolides are naturally occurring antibiotics produced mainly by streptomyces. They comprise a macrocyclic lactone ring with two sugars attached, one being an amino sugar. They are grouped according to the number of atoms in the lactone ring, e.g. 14 for erythromycin and clarithromycin.

MECHANISM OF ACTION

Macrolides bind to the 50 S ribosome of bacteria to inhibit protein synthesis, probably by preventing the first translocation. Macrolides appear to have a therapeutic effect below their in vitro minimum inhibitory concentration. This may be achieved by inhibiting attachment and adherence by bacterial protein adhesions and by suppressing bacterial toxin and co-enzyme production. Macrolides are active against most gram-positive bacteria, gram-negative organisms some strains of Haemophilus, Legionella, *Campylobacter jejuni* and *Helicobacter pylori*. Some anaerobes are sensitive, including most gram-positive streptococci and some species of bacteroides.

ACQUIRED RESISTANCE

Acquired resistance is relatively common. There are three mechanisms of resistance to macrolides:

- Altered binding site (the ribosome)
- Drug inactivation
- Active efflux of the drug from the bacterial cell

Changing the target site results in resistance to all the macrolides and also to lincosamides and streptogramins. The resistance genes can be on either the bacterial chromosome or plasmid.

ERYTHROMYCIN

Pharmacokinetics

Erythromycin is bitter, insoluble in water and inactivated by acid. The estolate and ascitrate are the most stable in gastric acid. Enteric and film coated tablets of the base are available but incomplete absorption occurs with considerable inter-patient variation. Erythromycin is distributed widely throughout the body. It tends to be retained longer in liver and spleen. Very low levels are obtained in the cerebrospinal fluid, even in the presence of meningeal inflammation. The normal serum half-life is 1.4 H, increased to 5 H in anuric patients, so that only slight dose adjustment is required in renal failure. It accumulates with liver disease. It is eliminated primarily by hepatic inactivation and excretion in the bile, with active intestinal re-absorption. Less than 15% of active drug is excreted in the urine. It is usually given 6 hourly.

Adverse effects

Erythromycin causes gastro-intestinal upset, hepatotoxicity, ototoxicity, and cardiotoxicity. Erythromycin is a gastric irritant, and stimulant of intestinal motility (prokinetic). Nausea, vomiting and diarrhoea are common. Erythromycin may cause intrahepatic cholestasis, particularly during pregnancy. Ototoxicity is usually due to high dose erythromycin lactobionate administration in patients with renal or severe liver dysfunction. Cardiotoxicity is very rare but potentially fatal. Allergic reactions are rare (< 0.5%). Thrombophlebitis is a major problem with IV administration. Drug interactions include increased serum levels of prednisolone, theophylline, carbamazepine, cyclosporin, warfarin and terfenadine.

Clarithromycin, a derivative of erythromycin, has slightly greater activity and higher tissue levels. It requires only twice daily administration.

TETRACYCLINES

Examples – doxycycline, minocycline, tetracycline

MECHANISM OF ACTION

Tetracyclines bind to the 30 S subunit of the bacterial ribosome and prevent the binding of aminoacyl-tRNA. Protein synthesis is prevented, resulting in a bacteriostatic effect. Tetracyclines have a very broad-spectrum, including gram-positive and gram-negative bacteria, spirochaetes, some mycobacteria, mycoplasmas, Chlamydia, Rickettsia, Coxiella, and protozoa. Minocycline even shows some activity against the fungus, *Candida albicans*.

ACQUIRED RESISTANCE

Acquired resistance is very common. This is plasmid-mediated and so is easily spread between different bacterial species and is associated with multiple resistance genes. There are four mechanisms of resistance:

- Decreased cell entry
- Increased drug efflux
- Ribosomal protection by the formation of a cytoplasmic protein
- Chemical modification requiring dihydroni-cotinamide adenine di-nucleotide phosphate (NADPH) and oxygen

TETRACYCLINE

Tetracycline is particularly active against *Vibrio cholerae*, *Aeromonas hydrophila* and *Plesiomonas shigelloides*.

Pharmacokinetics

Tetracycline is less protein-bound (24%) and less lipophilic than doxycycline and minocycline. Penetration is quite good into most body tissues, although levels in tears and saliva are low. The serum half-life is about 7 H. Excretion is mainly renal (by glomerular filtration) and biliary. The bio-availability of tetracycline following oral administration is less than for minocycline and doxycycline and declines proportionally with increasing doses. Absorption is better in the fasting state but impaired by ferrous ions.

Adverse effects

Adverse effects include gastro-intestinal (nausea, epigastric pain, vomiting and diarrhoea); super infections; hyperpigmentation; photosensitivity; dental discolouration in children; hepatotoxicity; nephrotoxicity; haematological (leucopenia and thrombocytopaenia); and benign intracranial hypertension.

Bacterial and fungal super infections are particularly frequent with tetracycline. treatment. There are four types of nephrotoxicity:

- Aggravation of pre-existing renal disease
- Association with acute fatty liver
- Interstitial nephritis
- Nephrogenic diabetes insipidus and renal failure

Weak neuromuscular blockade and potentiation of non de-polarising neuromuscular blockade is seen and this is not reversed by calcium or anti-cholinesterases. Metronidazole elevates lithium and digoxin levels and interferes with the effectiveness of the contraceptive pill.

Resistance and newer, more effective antibiotics have limited the use of tetracyclines, but they remain the preferred treatment for chlamydial and rickettsial, infections, Q-fever, anthrax and plague (*Yersinia pestis*).

DOXYCYCLINE

Doxycycline is semisynthetic. It is active against some tetracycline resistant strains of *S. aureus*. It is more active than most other tetracyclines against *Streptococcus pyogenes* and *Nocardia* sp. It is strongly lipophilic, allowing widespread tissue distribution. Of it, 80–90% is protein-bound, the highest of any tetracycline. It has a long half-life of 15–25 H. Specific uses include chlamydial infection of the eye and genital tract.

CHLORAMPHENICOL

MECHANISM OF ACTION

Chloramphenicol reversibly binds to the 50 S subunit of the bacterial ribosome to inhibit bacterial protein synthesis. Chloramphenicol is therefore bacteriostatic against most organisms, but at high concentrations, it is bactericidal against *Haemophilus influenzae* and *Neisseria meningitidis* and some streptococci.

Chloramphenicol is a broad-spectrum antibiotic, active against most gram-positive bacteria, anaerobic streptococci, gram-negative bacteria, branching bacteria (*Actinomyces israeli*) and some mycobacteria.

ACQUIRED RESISTANCE

Resistance is widespread, largely plasmid mediated and readily transferred between species.

PHARMACOKINETICS

Chloramphenicol is well absorbed from the intestinal tract and IV and topical ophthalmic preparations are available. It is well distributed throughout the body, including the cerebrospinal fluid and the eye. The serum half-life is 1–3 H. It is inactivated by hepatic glucuronide conjugation, then excreted by glomerular filtration with some active tubular secretion.

ADVERSE EFFECTS

Chloramphenicol causes the following adverse effects:

- Bone marrow suppression
- Grey baby syndrome
- Optic neuritis
- Ototoxicity

Bone marrow suppression is the most important toxic effect of chloramphenicol. There are two types: an idiopathic aplastic anaemia with pancytopaenia (incidence 1 in 24 500 to 1 in 40 800) with a high mortality rate and more commonly a dose-related and reversible marrow depression.

Grey baby syndrome results from reversible myocardial dysfunction causing circulatory collapse. This is seen in premature neonates who have very high serum levels of chloramphenicol. It has a mortality rate of 50% but survivors recover 24–48 H after chloramphenicol is stopped.

Chloramphenicol inhibits the activity of several liver enzymes and concomitant administration may result in elevated levels of tolbutamide and phenytoin.

FUSIDANES

Example – fusidic acid

MECHANISM OF ACTION

Fusidanes are a group of naturally occurring antibiotics that inhibit bacterial cell protein synthesis. They are active against most gram-positive bacteria (including MRSA) and gram-negative cocci. Tolerance rapidly develops if used as monotherapy.

PHARMACOKINETICS

Fusidic acid is well absorbed following oral administration. Of it, 95% is protein-bound. It penetrates pus and wound exudates well and achieves high concentrations in brain abscess cavities, although it does not enter the cerebrospinal fluid. Levels in bone and joint are high following either IV or oral administration. It is eliminated by liver metabolism and biliary excretion with a half-life of 9 H. Fusidic acid is reserved for severe staphylococcal sepsis, in combination with a second anti-staphylococcal agent.

ADVERSE EFFECTS

Fusidic acid may cause abnormal liver function, jaundice and thrombophlebitis.

QUINOLONES

Examples – ciprofloxacin, ofloxacin

The quinolones are synthetic anti-microbials having a dual ring structure based on the 4-quinolone nucleus, and are closely related to nalidixic acid.

MECHANISM OF ACTION

Quinolones inhibit bacterial DNA-gyrase, which promotes the supercoiling of double stranded DNA. Quinolones are particularly potent against gram-negative bacteria, including the enterobacteriaceae (*E. coli*, *Klebsiella aerogenes*, *Salmonella typhimurium*, etc.), *Haemophilus influenzae* and *Neisseria* sp. Quinolones are also active against *Pseudomonas aeruginosa* and related species, *Legionella pneumophila*, *Chlamydia* sp.

ACQUIRED RESISTANCE

Acquired resistance is uncommon. Three mechanisms are known:

- Altered target site (DNA-gyrase enzyme)
- Reduced permeability of bacterial cell
- Active efflux of the quinolones from the bacterium

Reduced bacterial permeability also reduces susceptibility to β-lactams. Resistance is relatively common in *S. aureus* (including MRSA), *Pseudomonas aeruginosa*, and some enterobacteriaceae.

CIPROFLOXACIN

Ciprofloxacin is active against the vast majority of gram-negative aerobic bacteria, including *Pseudomonas*, *Legionella* sp. Aerobic gram-positive bacteria and mycobacteria are generally moderately susceptible. Ciprofloxacin is active against *Chlamydia* sp., *Rickettsia* sp., *Coxiella* sp. and *Plasmodium falciparum*. There is little activity against most spirochaetes.

Pharmacokinetics

Most quinolones have a similar pharmacokinetic profile. Ciprofloxacin is readily absorbed with a bio-availability of 80%. Tissue penetration is generally good except for cerebrospinal fluid, even with inflamed meninges. Prostatic tissue levels are approximately twice those in the plasma. Ciprofloxacin is inactivated in the liver and excreted in the urine and faeces, but 70% is excreted unchanged. There is active tubular secretion. The elimination half-life is about 4–5 H. Of ciprofloxacin, 11% is also excreted by direct transepithelial elimination into the intestinal tract.

Adverse effects

Adverse effects include gastro-intestinal symptoms; headache, dizziness, insomnia; arthralgia, acute interstitial nephritis; leucopaenia, eosinophilia, thrombocytosis and thrombocytopenia; and hypersensitivity reactions. Ciprofloxacin inhibits cytochrome P_{450}, resulting in increased serum concentrations of some drugs, including theophylline and caffeine.

OFLOXACIN

Ofloxacin has a similar activity to ciprofloxacin but the longer half-life allows once daily administration. It is mainly excreted in the urine.

NITRO-IMIDAZOLES

Example – metronidazole

MECHANISM OF ACTION

Nitro-imidazoles are synthetic anti-microbials that act by destroying DNA. They are only active when the nitro group is in the reduced form induced by the very low redox values achieved by anaerobic bacteria and some protozoa. Nitro-imidazoles are only active against anaerobes, some micro-aerophilic bacteria (*Helicobacter pylori*) and certain protozoa.

ACQUIRED RESISTANCE

Resistance in *Helicobacter pylori* is thought to be due to the redox potential internally not being low enough. Resistance in anaerobic bacteria is very rare.

METRONIDAZOLE

Spectrum of activity

Metronidazole is active against anaerobes (*Peptococcus* sp., *Clostridium* sp., *Bacteroides* sp., and *Fusobacteria*), micro-aerophilic organisms (*Helicobacter pylori*, *Gardnerella vaginalis*), protozoa (*Entamoeba histolytica*, *Giardia intestinalis* and *Trichomonas vaginalis*) and a few helminths.

Pharmacokinetics

Oral metronidazole is rapidly absorbed, almost completely. Bio-availability is 60–80% when given rectally. Only 20% is protein-bound. It is widely distributed in body tissues, including cerebrospinal fluid, pleural fluid, breast milk, saliva, vaginal secretions, abscess cavities and the prostate. The elimination half-life is 6–10 H, and 60–80% is excreted in the urine.

Adverse effects

The adverse effects of metronidazole include central nervous (headache, dizziness, confusion, depression, incoordination and peripheral neuropathy); gastro-intestinal (nausea, vomiting, abdominal discomfort and diarrhoea); haematological (neutropenia and thrombocytopenia). It has a metallic taste and may cause intra-uterine mutation. Metronidazole gives a disulfiram type reaction with alcohol, enhances warfarin anti-coagulation, and impairs phenytoin and lithium clearance. Concomitant administration of cimetidine increases plasma metronidazole

RIFAMYCINS

Example – rifampicin

MECHANISM OF ACTION

Rifampicins specifically inhibit bacterial DNA-dependent RNA polymerase, preventing the transcription of RNA from the DNA template. Eukaryotic RNA polymerase is unaffected. They have indications beyond anti-tuberculous therapy due to their wider spectrum of action than other anti-mycobacterial agents.

Rifampicins are particularly active against gram-positive bacteria, gram-negative cocci and mycobacteria. Resistance is rapid so combination therapy is essential.

PHARMACOKINETICS

Rifampicins are well absorbed following oral administration. Of them, 80% is protein-bound. Rifampicins are distributed throughout the body, including CSF, bone, tears, saliva, abscesses and ascitic fluid. The plasma half-life is 4 H. Elimination is mainly by liver metabolism, producing an active metabolite. The urine turns an orange-red colour.

ADVERSE EFFECTS

Rifampicin is well tolerated but may cause:

- Hypersensitivity reactions
- Gastro-intestinal effects
- Hepatotoxicity
- Thrombocytopenia
- Acute renal failure
- Influenza syndrome

Rifampicin induces liver microsomal enzymes, increasing the rate of metabolism of the contraceptive pill, corticosteroids, anti-coagulants, digoxin, quinidine and tolbutamide.

TRIMETHOPRIM

MECHANISM OF ACTION

Trimethoprim inhibits dihydrofolate reductase, the enzyme catalysing the conversion of folinic acid to folic acid. It therefore indirectly inhibits DNA synthesis. Trimethoprim is active against many gram-negative bacteria, including most enterobacteria, *Haemophilus influenzae* and *Bordetella*. It has moderate activity against gram-positives, including MRSA and streptococci. *Enterococcus faecalis* can utilise pre formed folinic acid and becomes relatively resistant if the patient receives supplements containing folinic acid. Anaerobes are intrinsically resistant. Trimethoprim is active against some non bacterial pathogens.

ACQUIRED RESISTANCE

Resistance is increasingly common. The mechanisms are:

- Modification of target enzyme
- Altered metabolic pathway
- Reduced cell membrane permeability

Plasmid-coded synthesis of a mutant enzyme is probably the most important mechanism and enables easy inter species transfer.

PHARMACOKINETICS

Trimethoprim is almost insoluble in water and is rapidly absorbed from the gastro-intestinal tract. Of the drug, 42% is protein-bound. Trimethoprim is extensively distributed in the body and reaches cerebrospinal fluid and prostatic tissue. Excretion is almost entirely renal with about 70% is excreted in the first 24 H. Trimethoprim is a weak base so elimination is facilitated by acidic urine.

ADVERSE EFFECTS

Adverse effects are due to folate deficiency that can be offset by giving a folate supplement, which the bacterium cannot use.

SULPHONAMIDES

Examples – sulphadiazine, sulphadimidine

MECHANISM OF ACTION

Sulphonamides inhibit folic acid synthesis (at an earlier stage than trimethoprim). Sulphonamides inhibit the incorporation of para-amino butyric acid (PABA) into folinic acid. It therefore indirectly inhibits DNA synthesis. Sulphonamides are broad-spectrum agents, active against gram-positive and gram-negative bacteria and some protozoa (*Toxoplasma gondii* and *Plasmodia*).

ACQUIRED RESISTANCE

This is very common with complete cross resistance between sulphonamides. Of *Neisseria meningitidis* in the UK, 15% is resistant and most species of enterobacteriaceae are now resistant.

PHARMACOKINETICS

Sulphonamides are well absorbed from the intestine and are widely distributed around the body, including cerebrospinal fluid and the eye. Elimination is mainly by hepatic acetylation but some oxidation and glucuronidation occurs. The parent compound and metabolites are excreted in the urine.

ADVERSE EFFECTS

Sulphonamides cause renal damage, rashes, bone marrow depression and they interfere with foetal bilirubin transport. Older sulphonamides cause crystalluria. Newer sulphonamides produce a hypersensitivity reaction resulting in tubular necrosis or vasculitis. Rarely, they may cause Stevens–Johnson syndrome, which is often fatal. Sulphonamides cross the placenta, increase free plasma bilirubin and may cause kernicterus. Sulphonamides compete for plasma protein binding sites to affect oral anti-coagulants and oral hypoglycaemic agents.

ANTI-MYCOBACTERIALS

Examples – ethambutol, isoniazid, pyrazinamide

These drugs are used specifically for their anti-mycobacterial action. Some aminoglycosides, quinolones and macrolides are also active against mycobacteria.

ETHAMBUTOL

Ethambutol inhibits the synthesis of arabinogalactan, a cell wall polysaccharide. It is employed in combination with other agents when resistance is suspected. The most important side effect is optic neuritis, which can be irreversible.

ISONIAZID

Isoniazid inhibits mycolic acid synthesis. Resistance is common but toxicity is unusual. The neurological effects can be minimised by using pyridoxine (vitamin B$_6$). Isoniazid forms part of all standard anti-tuberculous regimes.

PYRAZINAMIDE

Pyrazinamide is bactericidal and resistance is uncommon. It is particularly active against intracellular bacilli. It is usually well tolerated but uric acid excretion may be inhibited, resulting in gout. It is a component of all modern short course anti-tuberculous regimes.

ANTI-VIRALS

The main mechanisms of action of anti-viral agents are:

- Direct inactivation of virus prior to cell attachment and entry
- Blocking viral attachment to host cell membranes
- Blocking virus uncoating
- Preventing integration of virus into the host cell membrane
- Blocking transcription or translation into viral messenger RNA
- Interfering with glycosylation steps, viral assembly and release

Currently most compounds in clinical use are nucleoside analogues that block nucleic acid metabolism. They include the anti-herpes virus agents (e.g. acyclovir) a broad-spectrum anti-viral, ribavirin and the anti-HIV agents zidovudine, stavudine and didanosine.

Two agents that are active against influenza virus are amantadine and rimantadine. They appear to prevent acidification of the virus interior, required to allow fusion of the viral envelope to the endosome, which normally leads to the release of viral RNA.

Human α-interferon is produced by recombinant DNA technology using *E. coli*. It renders cells resistant to infection by a wide range of viruses. Its main clinical use is the treatment of some cases of hepatitis B and hepatitis C.

Clinical trials of many other agents and combination therapy regimes are currently underway. Recently, the results of multidrug treatment trials for HIV infection, involving at least three agents, have established this form of therapy as the gold standard for patients infected with the virus.

SECTION 3: 19
CLINICAL TRIALS –
DESIGN AND EVALUATION

L. A. G. Vries

TYPES OF TRIAL
Phased clinical trials
Cross over studies
Multi-centre trials
Meta-analysis

DESIGN OF A TRIAL
Sample size
Variability
Bias

IMPLEMENTATION OF TRIAL DESIGN
Ethics committee approval
Data collection
Data analysis
Presentation of results

A clinical trial may be defined as the process whereby the efficacy and value of treatments or interventions are compared to a control group.

This should be a prospective, rather than a retrospective process and participants, or subjects are followed in time. Investigators implement carefully defined interventions. Data are then gathered, evaluated and analysed and the results may then be published. Interventions may include treatments, screening programmes, preventative measures and diagnostic tests.

TYPES OF TRIAL

PHASED CLINICAL TRIALS

Phase I trials

In phase I trials, new treatments are administered to small groups of people. Often, useful information on safety and efficacy has been obtained from animal studies before the phase I trial. People who participate in phase I trials are often those who have failed to improve on existing, conventional therapies, or they may be healthy volunteers. One of the main purposes of this type of trial is to ascertain what the maximum safe dose of the study drug is and how it is metabolised. This maximum dose is usually referred to as the maximally tolerated dose (MTD).

Phase II trials

After the safety and maximally tolerated dose have been established, the investigators may proceed to a phase II trial. Typically, small groups of patients are started on different doses and frequencies of administration. Neither a phase I or a phase II trial is randomised. Patients may for example be given a new treatment for a certain type of cancer. If fewer people than expected die of their illness in the treatment group and side-effects or toxic effects are tolerable, then the investigators may proceed to a phase III trial. The results obtained in a phase II trial will be used to design the more comparative phase III trial.

Phase III trials

Phase III trials use the optimum treatment dose and regimen determined by the phase I and II trials to set up a randomised, controlled trial (RCT). The main aim of the phase III trial is to determine the effectiveness of the new intervention. In a RCT there is a control group receiving standard treatment, a placebo, or no treatment at all, and one or more treatment groups receiving the intervention(s) of interest. Randomisation means that all participants have the same likelihood of ending up in any of the groups.

Following phase III a drug license may be granted. The license is reviewed every five years.

Phase IV trials

Often the effectiveness referred to in phase III trials is only measured over the short term. Phase IV trials are designed to monitor the long term safety and efficacy of the new intervention. They are also called post-marketing surveillance studies and need not contain a control group.

CROSSOVER STUDIES

Crossover studies are the opposite of parallel design studies, because in the crossover model each participant will receive each of the study interventions. In effect, each participant acts as his/her own control. The main advantage of this type of controlled study is the ability to determine whether a particular patient does better on a specific treatment. The simplest cross over study design contains two periods during which the subject receives two different treatments. It is crucially important that the interventions are of rapid onset and short duration. If not then the effect of the treatment in period A may interfere with the effect of the treatment in period B. For example, if a particular disease is cured during period A, then clearly the patient will not enter period B in the same pre-treatment state as in period A. It follows that chronic, incurable conditions are better suited to a crossover study.

MULTI-CENTRE TRIALS

The multi-centre trial has gained recent popularity because it increases the power of the study by recruiting larger patient numbers. The multi-centre effort is used when a single centre cannot provide sufficient patients. The cost of a multi-centre trial is invariably higher than that of a single centre type and takes a lot more organisational effort. A universal study protocol must be devised and followed by all participants. Inter-centre differences in patient management may be difficult to eliminate as variations in working practises in the contributing sites may not be apparent to the investigators immediately and may be difficult to alter.
The need to perform a multi-centre trial arises when the variable in question occurs infrequently. For example, a study is set up to compare the incidence of neurological damage after a spinal anaesthetic with two different types of spinal needle. A large number of patients will be required to show whether or not there are any statistically significant differences because the incidence of these complications very low. An alternative to a multi-centre trial in this case would be a meta-analysis.

Fourier analysis can be used to:

- Determine the frequency spectra of electrophysiological signals (EEG, ECG, EMG)
- Determine the frequency response of electronic or mechanical systems in clinical measurement systems
- Design filters in signal processing units
- Analyse signals in cerebral function monitors
- Analyse signals in Doppler systems

CALCULUS

Calculus is based on two mathematical operations, those of 'integration' and 'differentiation'. These operations are applied to mathematical functions of the form: •

$$y = f(x)$$

If this function is plotted as a graph, then integration and differentiation can be described in relation to this curve as follows:

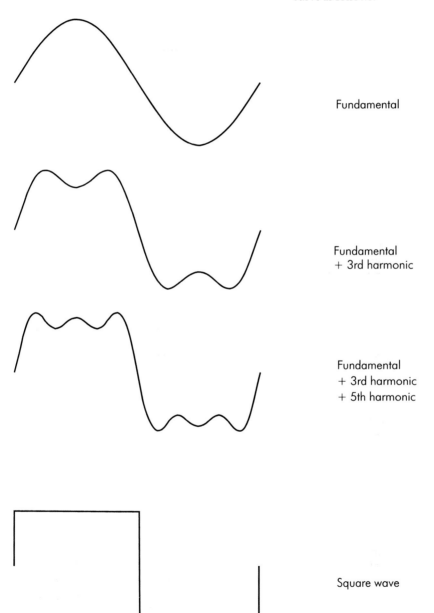

Fundamental

Fundamental
+ 3rd harmonic

Fundamental
+ 3rd harmonic
+ 5th harmonic

Square wave

Figure PH.9 Summation of fundamental and harmonics to approximate square wave

- **Differentiation** – is a mathematical operation which results in a second function (or derivative, denoted dy/dx) which defines the gradient of the curve at any point.
- **Integration** – is a mathematical operation which results in a second function (or integral, denoted ∫f(x), which can be used to determine the area under the curve between any two values of x.

Differentiation and integration are reciprocal mathematical operations. Differentiation of a mathematical function, gives a derivative function, which can be integrated to restore the original function. These basic mathematical operations are not simply tools which can calculate areas and gradients in graphs, but they define the dynamic relationship between two variables. In advanced calculus, differential equations are developed whose solutions enable the behaviour of complex systems to be modelled and predicted. This can be applied to physical, chemical and biological systems.

Integration

Integration is best described by considering an application. A useful application is provided by the calculation of volumes from a graph of gas flow against time. Consider the case of a patient blowing through a pneumotachograph (see 'Clinical measurement'). The pneumotrachograph records the expired gas flow as a function of time. If the flow were constant from the beginning to the end of expiration, the graph would look like FigurePH.10. Calculation of the expired volume is then given by:

Expired volume = flow rate × time
            = area under the flow curve.

However, in practice expiratory flow is not constant but is continuously variable, and the expiratory flow curve may be as illustrated in Figure PH.11. Here the flow rate is not constant, but varies with time and can be written as a function Q(t). In order to find the expired volume, the patient's total expiratory time is first split into small intervals of length δt (see Figure PH.12). The flow rate can be considered approximately constant over each time interval, δt. The incremental volume, δV, which flows during each δt is given by:

$$\delta V = Q(t) \times \delta t$$

The expired volume is then the sum of (Σ represents 'the sum of') these individual increments in volume.

$$\text{Expired volume} = \Sigma \, Q(t) \times \delta t$$

where Q(t) is the volume flow rate at any instant in time, and is thus the height of the rectangular strips in the Figure PH.12. Of course, the flow rate is not

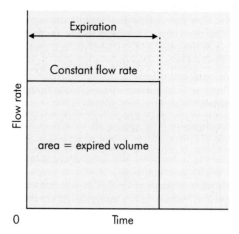

Figure PH.10 Expiratory flow curve at constant flow rate

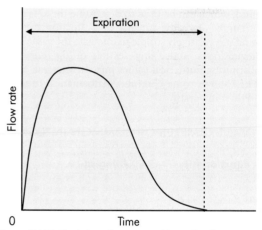

Figure PH.11 Expiratory flow curve with varying flow rate

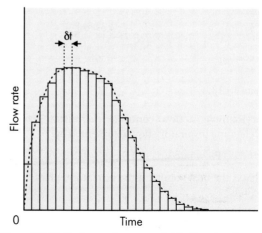

Figure PH.12 Expiratory flow curve divided into time intervals of δt

constant over each increment in time, particularly when the flow rate is changing rapidly during the rise and fall of the curve. However in the mathematical operation of integration, the width of each rectangular strip is allowed to become infinitely small. In this case the flow rate becomes effectively constant for this instant in time. The sum of instantaneous flow rates is then written:

$$\text{Expired volume} = \int_{t=t_1}^{t=t_2} Q(t) \times dt$$

The symbol '$\int$' is called the integral sign, and is a stylised 'S', indicating that we are performing a sum of infinitely narrow strips of $Q(t)$. The numbers t_1 and t_2 at the top and bottom of the integral sign are the times for starting the summing process, and finishing it.

EVALUATION OF AN INTEGRAL

If a graph can be can be described by a mathematical function, then the integral of this function can be found, which can be used to determine the area under the curve. Once the integral of a function has been found it is relatively simple to calculate the value of the integral (area under any section of the curve) by substituting numerical values into the integral. Figure PH.13 shows some common mathematical functions and their integrals.

SOME EXAMPLES OF COMMON INTEGRALS

Function f(t)	Integral
1	t
t	$t^{2}/_{2}$
t^2	$t^{3}/_{3}$
e^{at}	$\dfrac{1}{a} e^{at}$
$\sin(at)$	$-\dfrac{1}{a}\cos(at)$
$\cos(at)$	$\dfrac{1}{a}\sin(at)$

Figure PH.13

For example, a flow controlled ventilator gives an accelerating inspiratory flow represented by:

$$\text{Flow rate } V(t) = 1.4 \exp(-0.8\,t)\ \text{l/s}$$

What is the tidal volume if the inspiration phase lasts 4 seconds?

The tidal volume can be written as the integral of flow rate between the start of inspiration (t=0) and the end of inspiration (t=4):

$$\text{Tidal volume} = \int_{t=0}^{t=4} 1.4 \exp(-0.8\,t) \times dt$$

So, from the table of integrals in Figure PH.13:

$$\text{Tidal volume} = -\frac{1.4}{0.8} \exp(-0.8\,t)\ \Big|_{t=0}^{t=4}$$

The symbol $\Big|_{t=0}^{t=4}$ means that the expression to the left of the vertical bar is to be evaluated first with t = 4 and then with t = 0. The difference between these values is then the value of the integral (area under the flow curve) between 0 and 4 seconds.

$$\text{Tidal volume} = 1.75\,(e^{0} - e^{-3.2})$$
$$= 1.68\ \text{litres}$$

In practice, integration calculations can be evaluated using computers with appropriate software, or by microprocessors built into monitoring equipment or ventilators.

Differentiation

Consider the problem of determining gas flow rate, using a spirometer, which measures expired volume. The recording from the spirometer is a graph of total expired volume as a function of time. If the average flow is required, a simple ratio of total expired volume over expiratory time is taken:

$$\text{Average flow} = \frac{\text{total expired volume}}{\text{expiratory time}}$$

However, in order to determine the flow rate at each instant in time, the following approach is taken. The expiratory time is again split up into small increments, as in Figure PH.12, each of duration δt, during which the change in expire volume is δV. Then at any given time, the average flow over this small interval, δt is given by:

$$\text{Average flow} = \frac{\delta V}{\delta t}$$

This also represents the average gradient of the graph over δt.

The mathematical operation of differentiation then allows the time interval, δt, to become infinitely short, so that the above flow becomes an instantaneous flow. This is then written as:

$$\text{Instantaneous flow} = \frac{dV}{dt}$$

The letter 'd' is used to show that the intervals in V and t have become infinitely small. This mathematical process is called 'differentiation' and can be applied to any function. Differentiation of a function produces another function called the 'derivative'. This can be written as:

$$\text{Derivative of } f(t) = \frac{df(t)}{dt}$$

The derivative defines the gradient of the function at any point on its curve. Figure PH.14 shows some common mathematical functions and their derivatives.

SOME COMMON DERIVATIVES

Function f(t)	Derivative
t	1
t^2	2t
t^3	$3t^2$
exp (at)	a. exp (at)
sin (at)	a. cos (at)
cos (at)	– a. sin (at)

Figure PH.14

A comparison of the tables in Figures PH.13 and PH.14 shows that differentiation can be thought of as the inverse of integration. For example, if the function sin(t) is differentiated, the result is cos(t). Integration of cos(t) then gives sin(t), the original function. This holds true for any function.

For example, during an expiration that lasts 6 seconds, the volume, V (litres), of air expired is described by:

$$V(t) = 2.5 \sin\left(\frac{\pi}{12}t\right)$$

What is volume flow rate after 3 secs of expiration?

Differentiating the equation above gives:

$$\text{Flow} = \frac{d\,V(t)}{dt} = 2.5 \times \frac{\pi}{12} \times \cos\left(\frac{\pi}{12}t\right)$$

$$\therefore \text{ for } t=3 \text{ Flow} = 0.46 \text{ ls.}$$

SCALARS AND VECTORS

A scalar quantity is defined solely by its magnitude. Scalars include quantities such as temperature and mass.

A vector quantity requires both magnitude and direction to be defined. Vectors include quantities such as force, velocity and displacement (change in position). Simple addition or subtraction of vector quantities cannot be performed without reference to their direction. Consider the sum of a force of 1 newton added to another force of 1 newton. If the forces are in opposite directions the result is zero, if they act in the same direction the result is a force of 2 newtons.

Vector addition

Vector quantities may be added using simple geometrical rules, to give a resultant vector. If a person walks from A to B in Figure PH.15, and then from B to C, the same could have been achieved by walking directly from A to C. In other words, the resultant of the two component vectors AB and BC is the vector AC. This can be obtained graphically by simply completing a parallelogram and drawing the diagonal.

Vector resolution

The reverse of vector addition is to resolve it into a number of components. Resolving a vector into two component vectors can be performed graphically by reversing the parallelogram construction above (Figure PH. 15) If the two components required are at 90° to each other i.e. along 'x' and 'y' axes they can be calculated by simple trigonometry (Figure PH.16). The magnitude of the component in the 'x' direction can be found by dropping a perpendicular from the vector to the 'x' axis giving OB (a mathematical statement of this procedure is OB = OA cos θ). Similarly the magnitude of the 'y' component can be

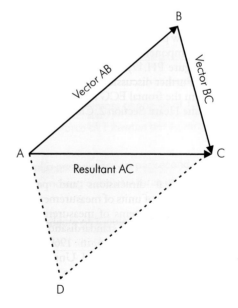

Figure PH.15 Vector addition by parallelogram construction

Critical temperature

Both pressure and temperature can change the state of a substance. Thus gases can be liquefied either by cooling or by increasing the pressure. However there is a temperature above which any gas cannot be liquefied by increasing pressure. This is the critical temperature. The critical temperature for oxygen is –119°C, and therefore oxygen in a cylinder at room temperature is always gaseous. However the critical temperature for nitrous oxide is 36.5°C. This means that at normal room temperature a cylinder of nitrous oxide contains a mixture of liquid and gas, unless the ambient temperature exceeds 36.5°C (as in a tropical country), in which case the nitrous oxide can only exist in gaseous form.

Variation of physical state with pressure and temperature

The way in which temperature and pressure determine the physical state of a substance is illustrated in Figure PH.32. This figure shows curves plotting volume against pressure for a given mass of substance. Each curve is plotted at a given temperature and is called an isotherm. The middle curve is plotted at the critical temperature (T_C), while T_H is plotted at a temperature above T_C, and T_L is less than T_C. Note the following:

T_H – at temperatures higher than the critical temperature, the substance exists only as a gas and the variation of volume with pressure at constant temperature, follows a simple hyperbolic curve or inverse relationship, according to Boyle's law.

T_C – at the critical temperature, the substance exists as a vapour at low pressures (i.e below critical pressure). However when pressure increases above critical pressure the vapour liquifies producing an inflexion point in the curve. Further increases in pressure do not then decrease the volume as the liquid state is effectively imcompressible.

T_L – at temperatures less than critical temperature, the substance exists as a liquid at high pressures. As the pressure decreases the volume remains constant until a point is reached when the liquid begins to boil (i.e at the saturated vapour pressure, SVP) and a mixture of liquid and vapour is produced. The volume of this mixture at SVP varies according to the degree of vaporisation. When complete vaporisation has occurred, volume again follows an inverse relationship with pressure.

The isotherms map out areas which define the physical state of the substance. At temperatures above T_C (plain area) the substance exists only as a gas. At temperatures below T_C the substance may be in liquid form (darker shaded area); it may exist as a vapour (lighter shaded area); or it may be a mixture of both. This diagram is representative of the behaviour of nitrous oxide, since T_C for nitrous oxide is 36.5°C.

Critical pressure

This is the minimum pressure at critical temperature, required to liquefy a gas.

Critical volume

This is the volume occupied by 1 mole of gas at critical temperature and critical pressure.

TRIPLE POINT OF WATER

Water can exist in three phases as water vapour, liquid water and ice. These phases will depend on temperature and pressure as shown in Figure PH.33. The transition between water and water vapour is demarcated by the boiling point of water (P), which is 100°C at 1 atmosphere, but which increases with increasing pressure (OA).

Water vapour and water therefore coexist along OA. Similarly the freezing point of water (0°C at 1 atmosphere) separates water and ice, but decreases with increasing pressure (OB). Ice and water thus coexist along OB. Finally OC separates ice and water vapour, and these phases coexist along this line. There is only a single point (O) at which the three phases of water coexist, at a pressure of 0.006 atmospheres and 0.01°C. This is the triple point of water.

VAPOURS AND GASES

The term 'gas' is applied to a substance which is normally in its gaseous state at room temperature and atmospheric pressure. Its critical temperature is below room temperature and therefore it cannot exist as a liquid.

The term 'vapour' refers to a gaseous substance which is normally in liquid form at room temperature and atmospheric pressure, since its critical temperature is above room temperature. Thus a vapour is a gaseous substance which is below its critical temperature under ambient conditions.

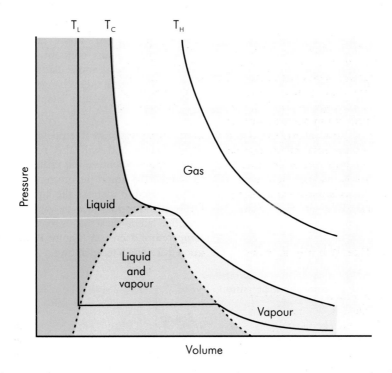

Figure PH.32 Isotherms for nitrous oxide

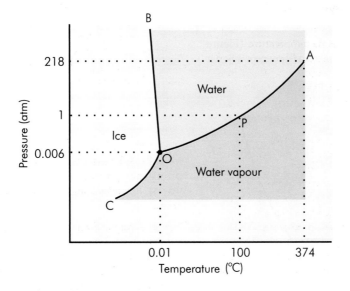

Figure PH.33 Triple point of water

Saturated vapour pressure and its relationship to boiling point

A vapour is formed from a liquid by 'evaporation', or the escape of molecules from the liquid surface. This process also occurs from the surface of solids to small extent by a process known as 'sublimation'.

When evaporation takes place from the surface of a liquid the concentration of vapor above the liquid increases. This process continues until a state of equilibrium is reached when no further increase in vapour concentration occurs. At this stage the vapour is said to be saturated, and the vapour pressure is the 'saturated vapour pressure (SVP)'

SVP can therefore be defined as the pressure exerted by a vapour when in contact and equilibrium with its liquid phase. The SVP of a liquid increases with temperature (Figure PH.34). The temperature at which the SVP becomes equal to atmospheric pressure is the boiling point of the liquid

Latent heat

When a substance changes phase from liquid to gas or from solid to liquid the molecular separation and bonding change. Water molecules in steam are about 12 times further apart than in liquid water. This increased separation of the molecules represents stored potential energy since the 'hydrogen bonding' between water molecules in liquid water are very strong. Work is therefore required to achieve this molecular separation, which is provided by the latent heat absorbed.

If ice is heated from a sub-zero temperature (Figure PH.35), its temperature will rise steadily except when it passes through the two transitions in phase from solid to liquid (freezing point) and from liquid to gas (boiling point). At these transition points the temperature remains constant while latent heat is absorbed to increase molecular separation. The latent heat associated with these changes in state, is known as 'latent heat of fusion' and 'latent heat of vaporisation' respectively.

Liquids also evaporate at temperatures lower than their boiling point and will also require latent heat of vaporisation to achieve this change in state. However the cooler the liquid the greater the amount of latent heat required to increase the liquid molecular energy levels to those possessed by vapour molecules. Thus specific latent heat of vaporisation increases as temperature decreases (Figure PH.36), and is usually quoted at a given temperature.

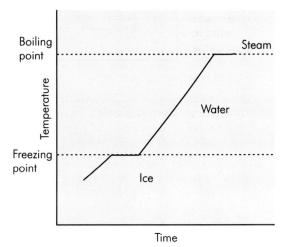

Figure PH.35 Variation of temperature of a block ice being heated

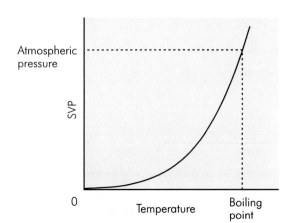

Figure PH.34 Variation of SVP with temperature

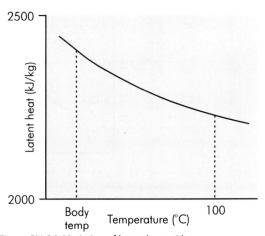

Figure PH.36 Variation of latent heat with temperature

Specific latent heat of fusion – is the energy required to change of 1 kg of substance from liquid to solid, without change in temperature. The specific latent heat of fusion for water is 334 kJ/kg.

Specific latent heat of vaporisation – is the energy required to change of 1 kg of substance from liquid to vapour, without change in temperature. The specific latent heat of vaporisation of water at 100°C is 2260 kJ/kg. At 37°C, the specific latent heat of water is 2420 kJ/kg.

Heat loss due to ventilation with cool dry gases

Poor preparation of inspired gases can cause a patient to lose body heat, because:

- The gases are not warmed and heat is lost in warming the gases to body temperature

- The gases are not humidified and heat is lost due to evaporation in order to humidify the gases in the respiratory tract

Heat loss in warming gases:

Consider ventilating with air at 20°C (body temperature = 37°C) with a minute volume of 6 l/minute . The specific heat capacity (s) of air is 998 J/kg/°C and the density of dry air at NTP is 1.29 kg/m^3

Mass (M) of air in the minute volume = volume (m^3) × density

$= 0.006 \times 1.29 = 7.74 \times 10^{-3}$ kg

Heat required to warm air to body temp = M s (37 – 20)

$$= 7.74 \times 10^{-3} \times 998 \times 17$$

$$= 131 \text{ J/min}$$

$$= 2.2 \text{ W}$$

If basal metabolic requirements are approximately 100 W this represents just over 2% of basal requirements.

Heat loss in humidifying gases

Fully saturated air at 37°C contains approximately 43 g/m^3 (0.043 kg/m^3) of water. Assume 6 l/min of ventilation with dry gases which become 100% humidified in the respiratory tract. If the specific latent heat of vaporisation of water at 37°C is 2420 kJ/kg, then the amount of water vapour required to humidify the inspired minute volume is given by:

Mass of water evaporated per minute = $6 \times 10^{-3} \times 0.043$

$$= 2.58 \times 10^{-4} \text{ kg}$$

Heat lost by evaporation per minute

$$= 2.58 \times 10^{-4} \times 2420 \times 10^3$$

$$= 624 \text{ J}$$

$$= 10.4 \text{ W}$$

Thus the total heat losses due to using cool unhumidified gases are

$$= 2.2 + 10.4$$

$$= 12.6 \text{ W}$$

Humidity is a measurement of the amount of water vapour present in the air. It may be presented in two ways, either as an 'absolute humidity' value or as a 'relative humidity' value. These are defined as:

Absolute humidity which is the mass of water vapour present in a given volume of air. The units of measurement are grams per cubic metre (g/m^3) or kilograms per cubic metre (kg/m^3). Absolute humidity value will not vary with the temperature of the air.

Relative humidity which is the ratio of the mass of water present in a given volume of air at a given temperature, to the mass of water required to saturate that given volume at the same temperature. Relative humidity is usually expressed as a percentage, and it varies with temperature.

Figure PH.37 shows how the relative humidity (RH) of a sample of air which is saturated at 20°C (RH = 100%), decreases as temperature increases. The amount of water vapour required to saturate air at 20°C is approximately 17g/m^3. However at 37°C, approximately 43 g/m^3 are required for saturation, so the RH of the given sample decreases to 39%. From this example it can be seen that humidifying inspired gases at room temperature results in only 40% RH or so at body temperature.

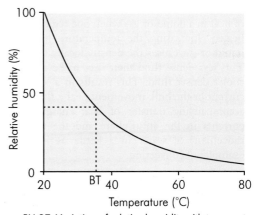

Figure PH.37 Variation of relative humidity with temperature

Calculation of RH from water vapour pressure and SVP

Since the partial pressure exerted by a gas is proportional to the mass of gas present, the relative humidity can be determined from the actual water vapour pressure and the saturated water vapour pressure at the given temperature:

$$\text{Relative humidity} = \frac{\text{actual water vapour pressure}}{\text{saturated vapour pressure}}$$

Methods of humidity measurement are discussed in Section 4 Chapter 2 'Clinical Measurement'.

HEAT TRANSFER

Heat energy can be transferred by different mechanisms these are:

- Conduction. When one end of a bar of metal is held in a fire the cool end gradually gets hotter as heat travels along the bar. This form of heat transfer is due to heat conduction. In the metal the atoms maintain a mean fixed position unlike the case of a liquid or gas. The atoms however are free to vibrate about their mean position, the amplitude of this motion being dependent on the temperature of the solid. When this vibration is increased by raising the temperature in one region, the vibration is transmitted to neighbouring atoms causing their temperature to increase and heat to be transferred. Clearly conduction requires physical continuity or contact. Gross movement of the medium transferring heat does not occur in conduction. Conduction also occurs in liquids and gases but the transfer of heat in these cases occurs mainly by convection.

- Convection. This mechanism describes the transfer of heat in a liquid or gas when one region becomes heated. Increasing the temperature locally in a liquid or gas causes the density locally to decrease. This less dense fluid then rises to be replaced by cooler denser fluid. This results in a 'convection' current or the bulk movement of the fluid with an accompanying transfer of heat energy. Hot air currents in the atmosphere and the continuous movement of water in a kettle as it boils are examples of convection.

- Radiation. Heat energy can also be transferred by electromagnetic radiation in the form of infrared radiation (see electromagnetic spectrum). This enables heat transfer to occur across a vacuum in the absence of any physical continuity or surrounding medium. Radiation is the mechanism by which heat is transferred from the sun to earth. Any object is capable of both emitting and absorbing infrared radiation with a resultant loss or gain of heat energy.

The importance of these mechanisms in anaesthesia lies in heat losses suffered by a patient during prolonged periods of anaesthesia or sedation. These mechanisms are considered together with additional factors such as losses due to evaporation from the respiratory tract and by sweating, in Section 2, Chapter 11.

GASES

Gases unlike solids and liquids, are compressible and change their volume when different pressures are applied to them. Therefore the physical behaviour of a gas can be described by three parameters, pressure (P), volume (V) and temperature (T). This is summarised by the three Gas Laws for a fixed mass of gas:

1. The relationship between volume and pressure at constant temperature is described by Boyle's law:

Pressure is inversely proportional to volume

$$P \propto \frac{1}{V}$$

or $\qquad PV = \text{constant}$

2. The relationship between volume and temperature at constant pressure is described by Charles' law:

Volume is proportional to temperature (degrees Kelvin)

$$V \propto T$$

or $\qquad \dfrac{V}{T} = \text{constant}$

3. The relationship between pressure and temperature at constant volume is described by Gay-Lussac's law:

Pressure is proportional to temperature (degrees Kelvin)

$$P \propto T$$

or $\qquad \dfrac{P}{T} = \text{constant}$

The Ideal Gas Equation

The above three laws can be summarised into a single equation, the **Ideal Gas Equation**:

$$\frac{PV}{T} = constant$$

This equation enables us to convert from one set of conditions to another when a fixed mass of gas undergoes changes in pressure, volume or temperature, since:

$$\frac{P_1 V_1}{T_1} = \frac{P_2 V_2}{T_2}$$

The Gas Constant (*R*)

The ideal gas equation may be written as:

$$PV = kT$$

where k is a constant dependent on the mass of gas present, if n = number of moles of gas present, the Ideal Gas Equation becomes:

$$PV = n\boldsymbol{R}T$$

where *R* is known as the Universal Gas Constant, and can be evaluated by considering 1 mole of gas at 273K (0°C) at a pressure of 1 atmosphere. This gives a value of *R* = 8.32 joules per °C.

Gas contents in a cylinder

From the Ideal Gas Equation, the pressure exerted by any gas is dependent on the number of moles present, therefore in a fixed volume such as a gas cylinder, the pressure in the cylinder is a measure of the amount of gas contained (e.g. in an oxygen cylinder). However this does not apply to a vapour (where liquid and gas phases are present, such as in a full nitrous oxide cylinder), since the pressure then reflects the saturated vapour pressure. However it should be noted that the critical temperature (Tc) for nitrous oxide is only 36.5°C, and if ambient temperature rises above this value nitrous oxide cannot exist in its liquid state.

AVOGADRO'S HYPOTHESIS

The above gas laws apply to any gas as long as the 'given mass' of gas remains the same, since gas behaviour is determined by the number of molecules present rather than the absolute mass present. This idea is based on a hypothesis proposed by Avogadro in 1811 which stated:

'Equal volumes of gases under the same conditions of temperature and pressure, contain equal numbers of molecules'

An important conclusion following from this hypothesis was that gaseous elements exist as molecules (O_2 and N_2) rather than as single atoms. This explained apparent anomalies in behaviour between gaseous elements and gaseous compounds.

Avogadro's number

1 mole of gas or vapour contains the same number of molecules. This is Avogadro's number:

Avogadro's number = 6.022×10^{23}

One mole of any gas or vapour occupies 22.4 litres at NTP (0°C or 273 K, and 1 atmosphere).

DALTON'S LAW OF PARTIAL PRESSURES

This states that if a mixture of gases is placed in a container then the pressure exerted by each gas (partial pressure) is equal to that which it would exert if it alone occupied the container.

Thus in any mixture of gases (e.g. alveolar gas, fresh inspired gases, air), the partial pressure exerted by each gas is proportional to its fractional concentration.

Consider a mixture of 5% carbon dioxide, 15% oxygen and 80% nitrogen. If the mixture exerts a total pressure of 100 kPa, then the partial pressures exerted by each gas are pCO_2 = 5 kPa, pO_2 = 15 kPa and pN_2 = 80 kPa.

Similarly if the total pressure exerted by the gas mixture is increased to 200 kPa, then the partial pressures become pCO_2 = 10 kPa, pO_2 = 30 kPa and pN_2 = 160 kPa.

Adiabatic compression or expansion of gases

Adiabatic when applied to the expansion or compression of a gas means that heat energy is not added or removed when the changes occur. Thus when compression of a volume of gas occurs, it is accompanied by a temperature rise, and similarly expansion of a volume of gas will produce a temperature fall. Practical consequences of this are that compression of gases will require added cooling to avoid unwanted heating of the system.

Alternatively, expansion of gases in the airway during jet ventilation can produce localised cooling which in turn can reduce the humidity of injected gases. A practical application of the adiabatic expansion of gases lies in the cryoprobe. Here expansion of gas in the probe is used to produce low temperatures in the tip for cryotherapy.

HYDRODYNAMICS

GASES, LIQUIDS AND FLUID BEHAVIOUR

Although gases and liquids differ considerably in their physical properties, they display similar behaviour under flow conditions, and can both be described as being 'fluid'. The following points are similarities in behaviour between gases and liquids:
Liquids and gases both fill the shape of their container, and are subject to constraints imposed by gravity. However because of their lower density, gases are less affected by gravity than liquids.

- The flow behaviour of gases and liquids is still largely determined by density and viscosity, although gases have much lower density and viscosity than liquids

- Flow is produced in both gases and liquids, by the application of a pressure gradient

The similarity between gases and liquids in flow behaviour, has led to the development of 'fluid mechanics', which is the study of fluids in motion, and applies equally to both gases and liquids.

VISCOSITY

Viscosity may be thought of as the 'stickiness' of a fluid. This property of a fluid can show itself in many ways. Imagine trying to pour treacle from a bottle compared to pouring water from the same bottle. Viscosity will affect the flow of fluids through a tube, the more viscous the fluid, the slower the flow through the tube. Gases are far less viscous than liquids and viscous effects only become apparent at much higher flow velocities in gases compared to liquids.

The viscosity of a fluid can be quantified by its 'coefficient of viscosity'. In order to understand how the coefficient of viscosity for a fluid is obtained, the concepts of 'shear stress' and 'shear rate' are required.

Shear stress and shear rate

A viscous force, or drag, is felt on any object either on moving through a fluid, or if the fluid moves past the stationary object. Figure PH.38 shows a thin, flat plate with a fluid flowing past it. Away from the plate, the fluid is flows faster, but closer towards the plate, the fluid is slowed down by the presence of the plate until at the surface the fluid is not moving. This happens at any surface because of adhesion between the fluid and the solid surface; it is known as the 'no-slip' condition. Near to the surface, the flow pattern is deformed from one of uniform flow velocity, to one in which layers of fluid parallel to the direction of flow 'slip' against each other giving rise to a drag effect or 'shearing' action. This shearing action at the surface gives a drag force per unit area of the plate, which is called the 'shear stress'. This is illustrated in Figure PH.38. The lengths of the arrows represent the velocity of the fluid, which diminishes to zero next to the plate. The velocity of flow thus varies between these fluid layers, i.e. a velocity gradient perpendicular to the direction of flow, or 'shear rate' is produced.

Coefficient of viscosity

The coefficient of viscosity (or simply 'viscosity') of a fluid can be defined by considering laminar flow in which two parallel layers of fluid are slipping against each other. As described above this produces two effects, a shear stress between the layers, and a velocity gradient at right angles to the direction of flow (shear rate). The coefficient of viscosity (or viscosity) is defined by:

$$\text{viscosity}, \eta = \frac{\text{shear stress}}{\text{shear rate}}$$

The units of viscosity are 'poises' after Poiseuille, who discovered the laws governing the flow of fluids through tubes. Water has a viscosity of 0.0101 poises at 20°C, while air has a viscosity of 0.00017 poises at 0°C.

Viscosity varies with temperature. Liquids generally become less viscous with increasing temperature, while gases become more viscous as temperature rises.

Newtonian fluids are fluids in which viscosity, η, is constant, regardless of the velocity gradients produced during flow. Many fluids including water, are Newtonian. Some fluids however do not behave in this way, such as the shear thinning fluids whose viscosity falls as the shear rate between layers increases, and the rheotropic fluids, which become more viscous the longer the shearing persists. Blood is a well known shear-thinning fluid.

Measurement of viscosity

Viscometers are used to obtain a measurement for the coefficient of viscosity. The simplest form of viscometer allows fluid to flow under the influence of gravity down a fine bore calibrated tube. The rate of fall

(a)

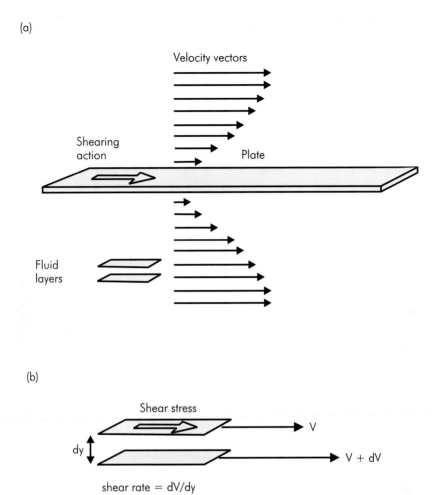

(b)

Figure PH.38 Shear stress and shear rate

of the fluid meniscus is detected by photocells from which the viscosity can be calculated.

A more complicated device uses the viscous drag created by spinning a small drum containing a sample of fluid. A pointer is mounted on a float suspended in the sample and is displaced by the torque due to the viscous drag. This records the viscosity measurement on a scale.

Viscosity and the damping of fluid flow

The viscous shearing action in a fluid flow dissipates energy as heat and is analogous to frictional effects between two solid surfaces rubbing against each other. This dissipative effect dampens the motion of fluid in a system, and thus viscous effects form a major component of 'damping' in any hydrodynamic system.

As with mechanical or electrical systems damping is an important factor in determining the behaviour of the system.

Viscous effects can also affect the pattern of flow, since fluid flow can occur with two different basic patterns laminar flow and turbulent flow. Laminar flow is smooth and streamlined while turbulent flow is rough containing eddies of swirling fluid, which disrupt the flow and create greater drag. The characteristics of these flow patterns are discussed in more detail below.

FLOW THROUGH TUBES

When a pressure difference is applied across the ends of a tube, fluid will flow from the high pressure to the low pressure. An analogy can be drawn with an electrical circuit. Fluid flow (electrical current) occurs along the tube (conductor) because of the driving pressure difference (voltage), and energy is dissipated by the viscous drag (shear stress) between the fluid and the tube (electrical resistance).

Hagen-Poiseuille law

Hagen (in 1839) and Poiseuille (in 1840) discovered the laws governing laminar flow through a tube. Consider a pressure P applied across the ends of a tube of length, l, and radius, r (Figure PH.39). Then the flow rate, Q, produced is proportional to:

- The pressure gradient (P/l)
- The fourth power of the tube radius (r^4)
- The reciprocal of fluid viscosity ($1/\eta$)

This is often combined as:

$$Q = \frac{\pi P r^4}{8 \eta l}$$

and attributed to Poiseuille, a surgeon, who verified this relationship experimentally.

Kinematic viscosity

As noted above the viscosity of a fluid influences its flow pattern by creating a damping effect. However, the inertial properties of the fluid, (dependent on fluid density), also affect the flow pattern. Thus the relative effects of inertial and viscous forces can determine the nature of fluid flow in any given situation. This is taken into account by using the kinematic viscosity (μ), which is defined as the ratio of the viscosity to the density (ρ):

$$\text{Kinematic viscosity, } \mu = \frac{\eta}{\rho}$$

If the kinematic viscosity is high, rapid irregular flow patterns in a fluid will be well damped, but if it is low then disturbances such as swirling eddies may persist for a long time.

Reynold's number

The Reynolds number (Re) is used to determine whether the flow will be laminar or turbulent in any given situation. It includes the kinematic viscosity, μ and the ratio of the inertial forces to the viscous damping forces in the fluid and is given by:

$$\text{Re} = \frac{v \, l}{\mu}$$

Where v = the mean flow velocity for flow through a tube, or the velocity a long way from an object. l = a characteristic length of the system, such as the diameter of a tube.

At low Reynolds numbers, the viscous forces dampen minor irregularities in the flow, resulting in a laminar pattern. A high Reynolds number means that the inertial forces dominate, and any eddies in the flow will be easily created and persist for a long time, creating turbulence. For flow though a tube, a Reynolds number of less than 2000 tends to give laminar flow, while between 2000 and 4000, the flow may be a mixture of laminar and turbulent depending on the smoothness of the fluid entering the tube. Above 4000, the flow will certainly be turbulent.

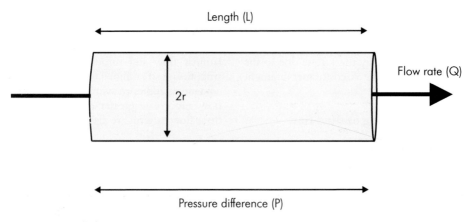

Figure PH.39 Hagen-Poiseuille law

Velocity profiles for laminar and turbulent flow in a tube

If we looked at the velocities across a tube, the velocity profile, the shapes would be different for laminar and turbulent flow, as shown in Figure PH.40.

Laminar flow. Figure PH.40a shows the profile for laminar flow. This is much more pointed than the flat central portion of turbulent flow. The arrows are flow velocity vectors and are all parallel to the axis of the tube. There is a gradual decrease in flow velocity as the walls of the tube are approached. Laminar flow tends to occur when viscous effects predominate i.e. with viscous fluids, in narrow tubes or at low flow velocities.

Turbulent flow. In turbulent flow as shown in Figure PH.40b the tube contains swirling eddies and the velocity varies continuously in time and therefore the velocity profile (broken line) is averaged in time. For the same net flow rate as in the laminar case, the flow velocity at the centre of the tube is flatter across the centre of the tube and has a lower peak value. However the velocity gradient at the walls is steeper because of an increased viscous drag associated with the turbulence. Turbulent flow tends to occur when density (inertial) effects predominate i.e. thin fluids, wide bore or uneven tubes and high flow velocities.

(a)

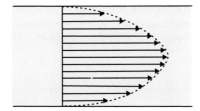

Figure PH.40a Velocity profile in laminar flow

(b)

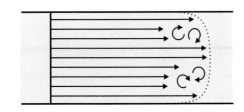

Figure PH.40b Velocity profile in turbulent flow

Transition between laminar flow and turbulence

When flow is slow it remains laminar and both viscous drag and pressure drop along the tube increase in proportion with flow velocity. As the flow velocity increases, there is an increased tendency for small eddies to disrupt the flow until at higher velocities the flow becomes turbulent. When flow is turbulent there is an abrupt change in the viscous forces, as reflected by an increased pressure drop along the tube. The slope of a graph plotting pressure drop against flow velocity becomes steeper at the laminar-turbulent transition. This transition is illustrated in Figure PH.41 and at this point the Reynolds number exceeds the threshold of approximately 2000.

A mixture of laminar and turbulent gas flow patterns is found in the airways of the lung during normal breathing. Turbulent flow occurs in the trachea and main bronchi at peak flow rates during quiet breathing, while flow in the small airways remains laminar under virtually all conditions.

Effect of varying cross section on flow velocity

In many situations flow occurs through tubes with a varying cross sectional area, as illustrated in Figure PH.42. The fluid is assumed to be incompressible, an assumption which is clearly valid for liquids, and which under normal circumstances remains surprisingly valid for gases. The volume flow rate is the product of the area of the tube and the average flow velocity, and since no fluid leaves or enters the tube, the volume flow rate must be the same at point 1 as it is at point 2. This statement can be written as:

$$A_1 v_1 = A_2 v_2$$

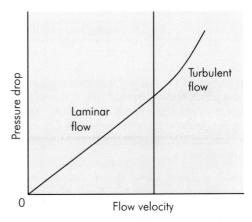

Figure PH.41 Velocity-Pressure drop curve showing transition between laminar and turbulent flow

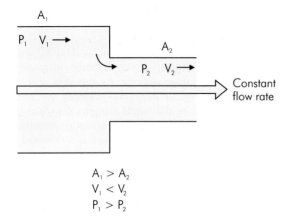

$$A_1 > A_2$$
$$V_1 < V_2$$
$$P_1 > P_2$$

Figure PH.42 Constant volume rate flow through a tube with varying cross section

As the fluid moves from a larger cross section (point 1), to a smaller cross section (point 2), the velocity increases (from v_1 to v_2). Similarly on moving from a smaller cross section to a larger cross section the velocity of flow will decrease.

Pressure and Velocity – Bernoulli's Equation

The pressure in the fluid can be related to its flow velocity by considering the balance between potential and kinetic energy for the fluid. The fluid has potential energy due to the pressure driving it in the direction of flow, and kinetic energy because it is moving. Since it is moving faster at point 2 than at point 1, its kinetic energy at point 2 is higher. For a gain in kinetic energy to occur, some potential energy must have been lost, i.e. a pressure drop occurs between point 1 and point 2. Thus the increased velocity at point 2 is accompanied by a reduced pressure. The relationship between pressure (P), and velocity (v) at any point in a fluid is given by:

$$\frac{1}{2}\rho v^2 \text{ (kinetic energy)} + P \text{ (potential energy)} = \text{constant}$$

This is Bernoulli's equation for incompressible flow, assuming no change in potential energy due to gravity (i.e. flow does not occur uphill or downhill). This is a good approximation for gases in which gravitational effects are usually negligible, or liquid flow in horizontal tubes.

Bernoulli's equation shows that as the velocity of a fluid increases, the pressure falls, or alternatively if the pressure of a gas flow falls, it gains velocity. This is illustrated by the example of gas escaping from a

cylinder at high pressure through a nozzle to the atmosphere. The gas in the cylinder acquires a high speed as it exits through the nozzle to atmospheric pressure. The potential energy initially contained in the gas due to it being compressed, has been converted to kinetic energy as the pressure falls to atmospheric pressure.

Venturi effect

The Venturi effect refers to the low pressure that is produced by a constriction in a duct with fluid flowing through it. As seen from the above discussion, this arises as a result of the Bernoulli principle. The Venturi effect is applied in devices such as the flow driven nebuliser. The Venturi flow meter (Figure PH.43) also uses the Venturi effect to estimate flow velocity from the drop in pressure at a tube constriction. However the pressure drop is not proportional to the flow velocity, and the device needs careful calibration.

INJECTION OF GAS THROUGH A JET

The use of gas injected through a narrow jet or cannula occurs in jet ventilation, the use of the Sanders injector and some types of fixed performance oxygen masks. In these devices high pressure gas is injected through a small orifice into a duct or airway open to the atmosphere. The injected gas forms a high velocity stream which drags surrounding air behind it (entrainment) due to the viscosity of the gases. This is often erroneously referred to as a 'Venturi' effect but can more accurately be attributed to viscous drag.

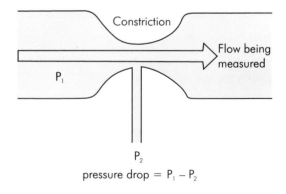

pressure drop $= P_1 - P_2$

Figure PH.43 Principle of a venturi flowmeter

ELECTRICITY

BASIC QUANTITIES AND UNITS

Electric charge

An electric charge may be positive or negative, and is produced by the accumulation of an excess or deficit of electrons in an object. Charge is measured in coulombs. Like charges tend to repel each other and opposite charges attract each other.

One coulomb is defined from the unit of current (the 'ampere' see below) as that charge which passes any point in a circuit in a second, when a steady current of one ampere is flowing.

A coulomb is equal in magnitude to the electric charge possessed by 6.24×10^{18} electrons.

Electric current

Most electrical effects are produced by the movement of charge. Any movement of electric charge forms an electric current. The current flowing in a conductor can be measured as the number of coulombs passing any given point per second. The unit of current is the ampere (amp) where

1 ampere   = 1 coulomb/s

1 milliampere   = 1×10^{-3} amp

1 microampere = 1×10^{-6} amp

When a current flows through a conductor it produces magnetic lines of force around the conductor (Figure PH.44a). This effect was discovered by Oersted and later applied by Michael Faraday to give rise to the development of electric motors and generators.

DEFINITION OF THE AMPERE

If two conducting wires are close to each other they will produce a force between them due to their magnetic fields, which depends on the size of the current in the wires. The ampere is defined as the current which, if if flowing in two parallel wires of infinite length, placed 1 metre apart in a vacuum, will produce a force on each of the wires of 2×10^{-7} $\dfrac{\text{newtons/metre}}{\text{N/m}}$ (Figure PH.44b).

Currents flow easily in conductors which commonly include metals and electrolyte solutions. Materials which do not conduct current are insulators. There are some materials with intermediate conducting properties (semiconductors) e.g. silicon, which have revolutionised electronic technology.

Electrical potential

If a positive electrical potential exists at a point, any positive charge at that point will possess potential energy and will tend to move away from it to a point at lower potential. Electrical potential is analogous to height in a gravitational field. where a mass possesses potential energy due to its height, and always tend to move downhill. The electrical potential of the earth is taken as a reference point for zero potential, and is usually referred to simply as 'earth'.

Potential is measured in volts. Charge will only move between points separated by a potential difference (also measured in volts).

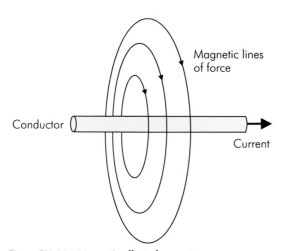

Figure PH.44a Magnetic effect of current

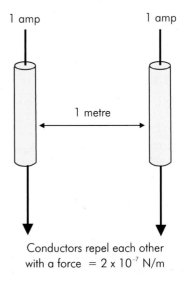

Figure PH.44b Definition of the ampère

Potential difference (Voltage)

When a potential difference (often referred to a 'voltage' since these terms have become interchangeable) is applied across a conductor it produces an electric current. A current is a flow of positive charge from the higher potential to the lower.

One volt can be defined as a potential difference producing a change in energy of 1 joule when 1 coulomb is moved across it.

ELECTRIC CIRCUITS

The flow of electric current in circuits is a critical concept. Consider a simple circuit as in Figure PH.45. An electric current flows from positive to negative and lights the lamp. However as electrons are the only mobile form of charges in a conductor, this current is actually formed by a movement of electrons in the opposite direction.

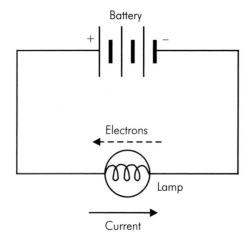

Figure PH.45 Simple circuit

Ohm's law

Electrical resistance is the electrical property of a conductor which opposes the flow of current through it. Electrical resistance is measured in ohms (Ω).

Ohm's law states that the current flowing through a resistance is proportional to the potential difference across it. In Figure PH.46, the potential difference across the resistance = V volts, the current = I amps and the resistance has a value of R Ω.

So:

$$V = IR \text{ volts}$$

The flow of current through the resistance requires the expenditure of energy, which appears as heat. The power, P, dissipated as heat is given by:

$$P = VI \text{ watts}$$

Substituting for I or V, this may become:

$$P = I^2R \text{ watts}$$
$$= \frac{V^2}{R} \text{ watts}$$

For example: Find the current flowing when a resistance of 250 Ω is connected across a 12 volt battery.

$$V = IR$$

$$I = \frac{V}{R}$$

$$= \frac{12}{250}$$

$$= 0.048 \text{ A}$$

$$= 48 \text{ mA}$$

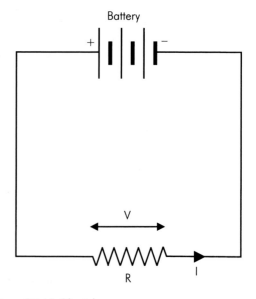

Figure PH.46 Ohm's law

Direct current (DC) and alternating current (AC)

The terms DC and AC are normally used to describe the electricity supply to a circuit or system, and are applied to either voltages or currents.

DC describes current which only flows in one direction (i.e. the polarity always remains the same). Generally DC is supplied by a battery (or power adaptor), and if the current supplied is plotted against time will give a graph as shown in Figure PH. 47a.

AC describes a supply in which the current reverses direction cyclically. If the current is plotted against time the sinusoidal curve shown in Figure PH.47b. is produced. AC is the normal mains supply and has this form because of the way in which electricity is generated and distributed. An AC voltage is described by its amplitude (peak value) and frequency. The amplitude of mains voltage is 340 V and it has a frequency of 50 Hz.

Usually mains voltage is quoted as 240 V which is the 'root mean square (RMS)' value. The RMS value for an AC voltage is the DC voltage or current, which would have the same heating effect. This is used to compare AC and DC because the heating and lighting effects (power dissipation) of a current are not dependent on the direction of flow. It is obtained mathematically by squaring the value of the voltage/current, averaging this squared value over time and then taking the square root value.

AC currents and voltages are important because they can be used to carry information. In this case they are usually referred to as signals. The properties of signals measured and generated in the body, or 'biopotentials' are discussed in more detail in Clinical Measurement. Often electrical currents and signals are a combination of DC and AC (see Figure PH.47c).

Impedance and reactance

The response of many circuit elements to DC and AC can be very different. Some devices may have a very low ability to resist the flow of AC, but offer a high resistance to DC, or vice versa (see below).

- **Resistance** is a measure of a device's ability to resist DC current. It is represented by 'R' and measured in ohms
- **Reactance** describes a device's ability to resist the flow of AC. The reactance of a device will be dependent on the frequency of AC applied. It is normally represented by 'X' and is measured in ohms

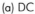
(a) DC

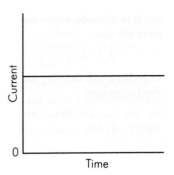

(b) AC

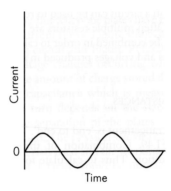

(c) DC and AC combined

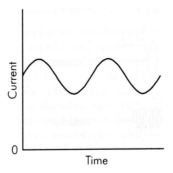

Figure PH.47(a) Direct current (DC)
(b) Alternating current (AC)
(c) DC with AC superimposed

(a)

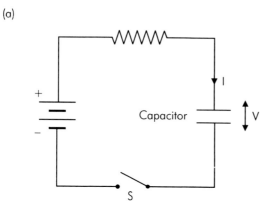

(b)

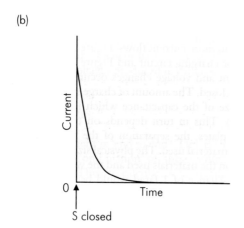

(c)

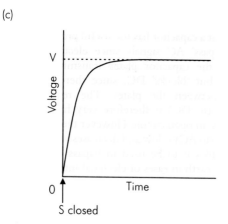

Figure PH.52 Current and voltage changes in a capacitance

PARALLEL CAPACITORS

Parallel capacitors are shown in Figure PH.53. Combination of these values is by simple addition. Thus to calculate total capacitance C_T where C_1 = 16 μF, and C2 = 32 μF:

$$C_T = C_1 + C_2$$
$$= 16 + 32$$
$$= 48\ \mu F$$

SERIES CAPACITORS

Figure PH.54 shows series capacitors of value C_1 = 16 μF and C_2 = 32 μF. To calculate the total resistance C_T:

$$\frac{1}{C_T} = \frac{1}{C^1} + \frac{1}{C_2}$$

$$\frac{1}{16} + \frac{1}{32} = \frac{3}{32}$$

Thus, C_T = 10.7 μF

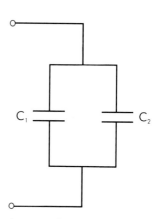

Figure PH.53 Combination of parallel capacitors

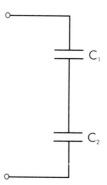

Figure PH.54 Combination of series capacitors

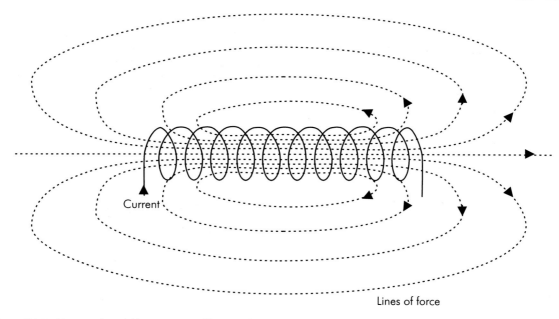

Figure PH.55 Magnetic lines of force generated by an inductance

Inductance

An inductor is made by forming a conductor into coils, which are often wound around a core (or 'former') of ferrous material. This construction has the effect of producing a concentrated magnetic field through the axis of the inductor and around it, whenever a current flows (Figure PH.55).

When a voltage is applied across the terminals of an inductor, current does not flow immediately but increases slowly in step with the build up of the magnetic lines of force. Similarly if the voltage is switched off, the current does not fall to zero immediately but dies down slowly, since as the magnetic field collapses it maintains the current flow for a while (see Figure PH.56a,b,c).

The build up and collapse of the magnetic field around an inductor tends to slow down changes in current flow, whenever the applied potential difference varies. The behaviour of inductances in an electrical circuit is thus analogous to the inertial effect of masses in a mechanical system. The unit of inductance is the henry (H).

(b)

(c)

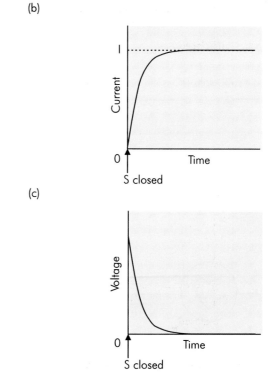

(a)

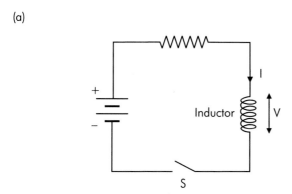

Figure PH.56 Current and voltage changes in an inductance

An inductance has a relatively low resistance to DC, simply equal to that of the coils of wire. However when AC is applied to an inductance, the continually varying current meets a comparatively high reactance. The reactance of an inductor increases with frequency. Inductors therefore tend to 'block' AC but 'pass' DC.

Inductances are therefore used as components in filters and to 'smooth out' spikes and surges in power supplies.

DEFIBRILLATOR CIRCUIT

A circuit using both capacitance and inductance is the defibrillator circuit. Its operation consists of two phases, 'charging' and 'discharging'. These phases are controlled by the switch S_1.

When charging (Figure PH.57a) S_1 connects the capacitor to the DC power supply, which charges it to deliver the required amount of energy or number of joules set by the operator. The energy stored by a charged capacitor depends on its capacitance (C) and the applied voltage (V), since

$$\text{Energy stored} = \frac{1}{2}CV^2 \text{ joules}$$

for C = 100 µF and V = 2000 V

$$\text{Energy stored} = 0.5(100 \times 10^{-6})(2000)^2$$

$$= 200 \text{ J}$$

On discharge (Figure PH.57b) S_1 connects the capacitor to the patient circuit which enables the stored charge to be delivered to the patient via the switch (S_2) on the paddles. The inductor L, in the discharge circuit has the effect of slowing down and spreading out the delivered pulse of energy to the myocardium which makes it more effective than the shorter sharper spike waveform that would be delivered without the inductance.

Transformer

A transformer consists of two inductors wound around the same form. The close physical relationship between the two coils means that current changes in one circuit (the primary winding) will induce currents in the second coil (the secondary winding) via the coupling effect of the magnetic field (Figure PH.58). The degree of coupling will depend on the number of turns in the primary winding (N_1), the secondary winding (N_2) and the quality of the former. If an AC voltage V_1 is applied across the primary, the voltage produced across the secondary (V_2) will be given by

$$V_2 = V_1 \times \frac{N_2}{N_1}$$

A transformer can thus be used to 'step up' or 'step down' AC voltages in circuits. Transformers are commonly used in distributing the electrical power supply from the national grid to domestic users. An alternative use for transformers is in transferring signals between circuits and devices such as microphones or loudspeakers.

(a) Defibrillator charging

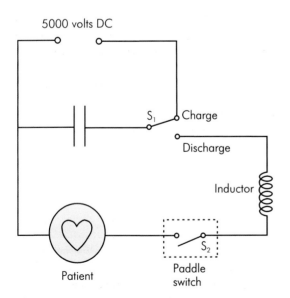

Figure PH.57a Defibrillator circuit charging

(b) Defibrillator discharging

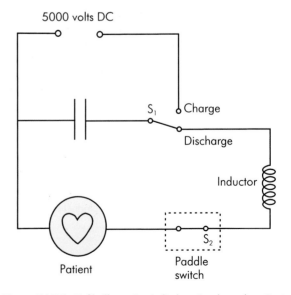

Figure PH.57b Defibrillator circuit discharging through patient

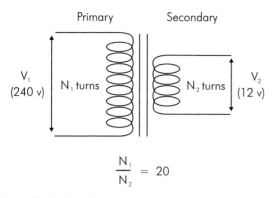

$$\frac{N_1}{N_2} = 20$$

Figure PH.58 Transformer

Diode

A diode is a semiconductor (silicon or germanium) device which only enables current to flow through it in one direction. It is often used to convert AC to DC (Figure PH.59) in order to provide a DC power supply from the AC mains. This is commonly found in the 'mains adaptors' used as a substitute for equipment batteries. Diodes are also used in protective circuits and to process signals in measurement systems.

Transistor

Transistors are also semiconductor devices. These are used to amplify small current signals, enabling small electrical signals of a few microamps to be converted to much greater signals of tens of milliamps. The basic transistor consists of a tiny slice of semiconductor material with connections to three regions the base (b), collector (c) and emittor (e). A common configuration allows a small signal fed into the base to produce an amplified signal in the collector circuit (Figure PH.60). In the early days of transistor electronics a circuit would be constructed using a few separate transistors. In modern electronics many thousands or even millions of transistors may be incorporated into a single semiconductor 'chip' which in turn is simply a single

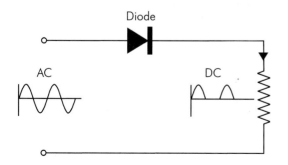

Figure PH.59 Diode circuit converting AC to DC

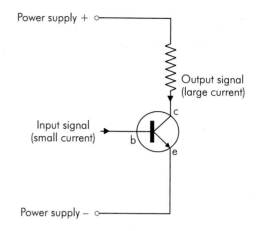

Figure PH.60 Transistor

component in a more complex device such as a personal computer.

ELECTRICAL SAFETY

The hazards associated with the use of electrical equipment are:

- Electric shock – macroshock
- Electric shock – microshock
- Burns
- Fire and explosion
- Diathermy hazards

Electric shock (macroshock)

Electric shock (macroshock) occurs with the external application of a voltage to the skin, causing an electric current to pass through the body tissues. Commonly electric shock occurs from the AC mains supply.

The mains supply in The UK consists of a 'live' line carrying the generated voltage (240 v RMS) and a 'neutral' line, which acts as a return for the current supplied. The 'neutral' line is earthed at the generator. In an intact mains circuit the current supplied in the 'live' line is equal to the return current in the 'neutral' line.

HOW ELECTRIC SHOCK OCCURS

Electric shock occurs from the mains supply, when the body forms a circuit between the live mains line, and a local earth connection or the neutral mains line.

- Earthed circuit. The local 'earth' connection may occur via the floor or ground (Figure PH.61). Alternatively earthing may take place by inadvertent contact with earthed metalwork such as an anaesthetic machine or operating table (Figure PH.62)

- Isolated circuit. In the absence of an earth connection, an individual or circuit is said to be electrically 'isolated' or 'floating'. However current can still flow if contact with an alternative return path such as the neutral supply line is made (Figure PH.63)

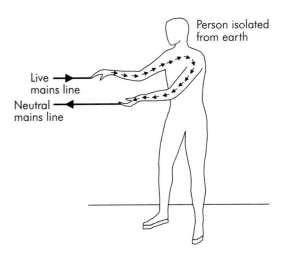

Figure PH.63 Electric shock in isolated patient by return through neutral line

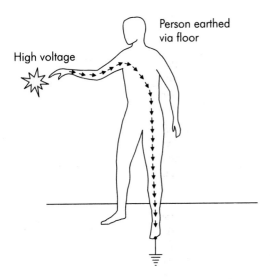

Figure PH.61 Electric shock in person earthed via floor

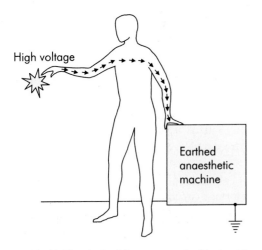

Figure PH.62 Electric shock in person earthed by touching metalwork

The effects of electric current flowing through body tissues depend on the following factors:

- Whether the current is AC or DC
- The magnitude of the current
- The tissues current passes through
- Current density
- Duration of current passage
- Pre-existing disease

AC or DC current: DC produces a single muscle spasm on contact which often throws the victim clear. Arrhythmias can be precipitated but DC shock is also used to cardiovert arrhythmias. Prolonged exposure to low DC currents can produce chemical burns. AC will cause muscle spasm due to tetanic effects which are maximal at mains frequency (50 Hz). When contact is made through the hand, muscle spasm may cause the individual to grip the contact uncontrollably, prolonging duration of the shock. AC at mains frequency is also more likely to cause arrhythmias than higher frequencies. The risk of arrhythmias decreases significantly >1 kHz, and at diathermy frequencies (>1 MHz) this risk is negligible. AC currents also cause localised sweat release which lowers skin resistance and increases tissue current (see below). AC shock is about three times as dangerous as DC for the same magnitude of current.

The magnitude of the current: When an electric shock is received from the AC mains, different physiological effects are caused as the current increases in magnitude. These are summarised opposite in Figure PH.64.

PHYSIOLOGICAL EFFECTS AT DIFFERENT CURRENT LEVELS IN AC MAINS SHOCK

Current (mA)	Effects
0 – 5	Tingling sensation
5 – 10	Pain
10 – 50	Severe pain
	Muscle spasm
50 – 100	Respiratory muscle spasm
	Ventricular fibrillation
	Myocardial failure

Figure PH.64

Currents above 100 mA may not only disturb normal function in conducting tissues, but can disrupt of epithelium and cell membranes. There may also be a direct heating effect on tissues, depending on current density (see below), duration of application and local cooling.

The main factors determining the magnitude of a current during electrocution are:

- Voltage applied to the skin
- Impedance (AC resistance) of the skin contact – location of the skin, thickness and sweating, can all affect skin contact resistance significantly. Skin contact resistance can vary between $1000 – 200\,000\,\Omega$
- Impedance of the earth connection – when the earth connection occurs via the floor the impedance of footwear becomes important
- Tissue impedance – tissue impedance is usually low ($<500\,\Omega$)

Consider an electric shock received from the live mains wire (240 v) in an individual (refer to Figure PH.61) where the skin impedance is $2000\,\Omega$, tissue impedance is $300\,\Omega$ and the earth contact resistance through shoes is $200,000\,\Omega$.

If the current pathway lies through the right hand along the right arm, through the body and then via the feet to earth:

$$\text{Total resistance} = 1000 + 300 + 200,000$$
$$= 201.3\,k\Omega$$
$$\text{Current} = \frac{240}{201300}$$
$$= 1.2\,mA$$

Normally this current would not have any harmful effects in a person, although it may be discernable as a tingling sensation.

The tissues or organs through which the current passes: Currents passing through conducting tissues can disrupt normal physiological function. Consider an individual with one hand in contact with live mains terminal and the other hand earthed through an anaesthetic machine (refer to Figure PH.62). The current pathway in this case is right hand and arm, chest, left arm and hand. The current flowing is given by:

$$\text{Total resistance} = 1000 + 300 + 1000$$
$$= 2.3\,k\Omega$$
$$\text{Current} = \frac{240}{2300}$$
$$= 104\,mA$$

This current through the chest would not only deliver a painful shock but also carries a significant risk of inducing ventricular fibrillation or other arrhythmias, since it will pass through the heart.

The current density: This is obtained by dividing the total current flowing by the cross sectional area that the current flows through. The effect of electric currents on tissues will be more dependent on current density in the tissue than on the total current passing through the tissue. If a current passes through a diathermy probe tip the current density will be much higher than in the case of the diathermy pad (Figure PH.65). Thus tissue is burnt at the probe but not at the pad. If the pad is improperly applied, the contact surface area may be reduced and unwanted burns may occur. It is therefore important to ensure that diathermy electrode plates are properly and uniformly applied to the patient in order to avoid accidental burns.

Duration of current passage: The longer the duration of current flow, the more damage is caused to tissues in the current path, since the total amount of heat dissipated in the tissues depends on time.

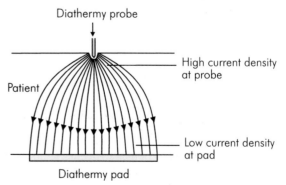

Figure PH.65 High current density at diathermy probe and low current density at diathermy pad

Power $= I^2 R$ Watts

Total heat $= I^2 R T$ Joules

Where T = time in seconds

A small DC current which may not produce excessive heating of tissues locally, can still produce 'chemical' burns by an electrolytic effect.

Pre-existing disease in a patient: The presence of ischaemic heart disease increases the likelihood of problems such as arrhythmias.

Prevention of electric shock (macroshock)

Macroshock is prevented by the following measures:

- Equipment should be designed to suitable specifications. Different classes of equipment are specified for the medical working environment.
  Various classes of equipment are specified for use in differrent applications. The safety specifications may refer to the risk of electric shock as follows:
  Class I – Earthed
  Class II – Double insulated but not earthed
  Class III – Low voltage (<24 v), battery powered

- Earth circuits. These are designed into equipment in order to reduce risk of electric shock and reduce interference.
  Earth connections reduce the risk of electric shock by maintaining exposed metalwork at zero potential. Such metal work cannot then deliver an electric shock current if inadvertently contacted.
  However such earth connections may also increase the risks shock if an individual is already in contact with a high voltage, since contact with earthed metalwork can then complete the circuit (Figure PH.62).
  Earth connections can also provide a discharge pathway for static charges or leakage currents, which reduces the risk of 'microshock'.
  Poor design of earth circuits can however, actually generate leakage currents, which can act as a source of 'microshock'. This occurs where multiple earth connections are used, each connection being at a slightly different potential causing small currents to flow through earth circuits or patient.
  The optimum earth circuit connects all earth circuits to earth at a single point via a good quality contact.
  Earth casing or shielding around conductors carrying high frequency AC reduces both the transmission and pick up of interference signals, particularly in the case of high frequencies. Co-axial cables are often used with an earthed outer conductor surrounding and screening an inner wire in sensitive circuits.

- Isolated patient circuit. An option most commonly used, is the isolated patient circuit, in which there is no earth connection to the patient. Faulty or obsolete apparatus may form an unwanted earth connection via an indifferent ECG electrode which can lead to macroshock and microshock risk (Figure PH.66).

- Leakage currents. This term refers to small electric currents (<500 μA) which arise unintentionally. These currents may originate through faulty equipment, faulty components, faulty earth connections or the accumulation of static charges. Such currents can either pass or 'leak' down to earth through a designed safety circuit (e.g. earth connection, antistatic shoes) or may flow through an unintentional pathway creating a risk of microshock.

- Isolating transformer. This system supplies all equipment attached to the patient via a transformer so that no equipment associated with the patient is directly connected to the mains.

- Circuit breaker. This is a sensitive mains switch which operates to disconnect the mains, whenever abnormal currents are detected due to dangerous equipment faults or the occurrence of electrocution.

- Suitable footwear. Footwear impedance should be designed to isolate the wearers from earth. The impedance should be high enough to prevent large current passing to earth (avoiding electric shock) in case of contact with a high voltage source, but low enough to allow a leakage current to earth to prevent the wearer and clothing from accumulating a static charge. Such shoes normally have an impedance of between 100 kΩ and 1 MΩ.

Microshock

In microshock current is delivered internally to the myocardium causing arrhythmias. The conducting pathway may be through an intravenous catheter or pulmonary artery catheter and its contained fluid. Figure PH.67 shows a patient earthed via two circuits. One (a) is via the pulmonary artery catheter monitor (E_2), and the other (b) is via an indifferent ECG electrode (E_1). If the voltage at E_2 is greater than the voltage at E_1, even by 100 millivolts, then a leakage current may be generated, great enough to cause microshock. The magnitude of currents required to produce ventricular fibrillation in microshock is in the order of 100 – 150 μA. This is much smaller than in the case of macroshock.

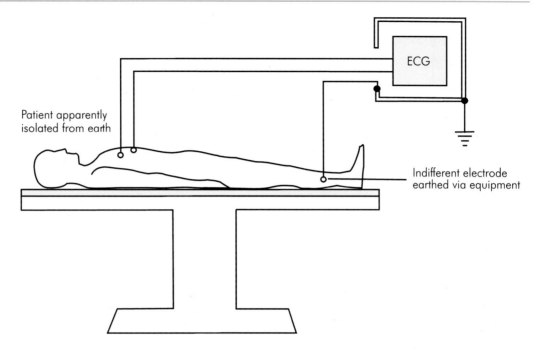

Figure PH.66 Unwanted earth connection via indifferent ECG electrode

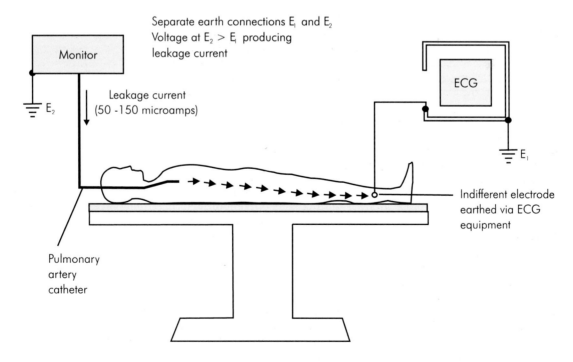

Figure PH.67a Microshock via pulmonary artery catheter

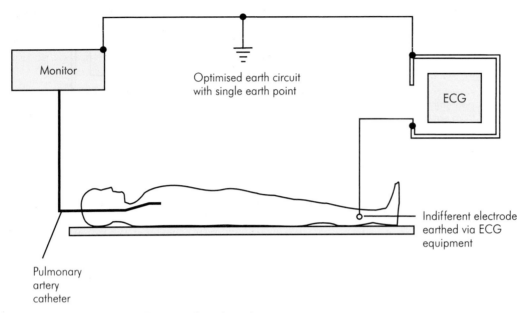

Figure PH.67b Optimised earth circuit with single earth connection

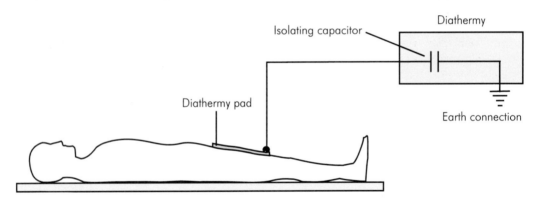

Figure PH.68 Isolating capacitor in diathermy equipment

Some potential sources of microshock:
- Central venous catheter
- Pulmonary artery catheter
- Temporary external pacemaker
- Oesophageal temperature probe in lower third of oesophagus
- Statically charged staff touching any of the above

PREVENTION OF MICROSHOCK

- Appropriate equipment in good order. Equipment specifications may refer to leakage current generation and the risk of microshock. For example: CF (Cardiac, floating) – leakage <50 μA through cardiac connection. BF (Non cardiac, floating) – leakage <500 μA through patient connection with single fault

- Suitable footwear impedance
- Antistatic flooring
- Isolated patient circuit – with no earth connection to patient
- Optimum design of earthing circuits for equipment
- Correct humidity in theatre

Diathermy hazards

Diathermy uses high frequency (0.4 – 1.5 MHz) currents to generate heat in the tissues during surgery. This is applied via a probe to produce coagulation and cutting effects. The most common risks in the use of diathermy, are of unwanted diathermy burns as well as the usual risks of electric shock associated with the use of any electrical equipment. In addition diathermy signals can cause interference in monitoring equipment and possibly indwelling pacemakers.

PREVENTION OF DIATHERMY HAZARDS

- Use of isolated patient circuit
- Use of isolating capacitor. In diathermy devices an isolating capacitor is used which effectively 'short circuits' (see reactance of capacitors) high frequency diathermy currents to earth, reducing the risk of unintentional diathermy burns. However at low frequencies (mains frequency and DC) the patient remains isolated reducing the risk of macroshock and microshock (Figure PH.68).
- Proper application of diathermy pad
- Avoiding inadvertent patient contact with earthed metalwork
- Use of bipolar diathermy. This form of diathermy uses a pair of probes, one to deliver the diathermy signal and the other to act as a return circuit. They are arranged as the arms of forceps, which restricts the current field to a small area surrounding the forcep tips. In this way no diathermy pad is required and no electric field exists in the peripheral parts of the patients body. This reduces the risk of unwanted peripheral diathermy burns, and also decreases possible inteference with monitoring equipment and pacemakers.

Electrical burns

Burns may occur during electrocution in different ways:

- Flash burns. This term describes the effect of arcing around the individual in high voltage (>1000 V) shock, when electric arcing occurs to earth from the body or clothing
- External burns. These may occur due to ignition of clothing or other inflammable materials around the individual e.g. gases or vapours
- Tissue burns. These may occur at the point of contact with the high voltage source or earthing point. They are localised and are due to the passage of high density electric currents sometimes with accompanying arcing

Explosions and fire

In an operating theatre there is a risk of fire or explosion due to the ignition of gas mixtures. The mixture usually consists of a fuel with oxygen or another oxidising agent such as nitrous oxide.

Inflammable gas mixtures may simply burn generating temperatures of several hundred degrees Celsius at atmospheric pressure.

Explosions are a much more violent reaction generating a rapid rise in temperature to several thousand degrees Celsius, and a high pressure shock wave which propagates outwards at speeds greater than the speed of sound.

For explosion or fire to occur the following are required:

- An inflammable agent. Examples include diethyl ether, cyclopropane, ethyl chloride and ethyl alcohol.
- An oxidising gas. These include oxygen, air, and nitrous oxide
- Inflammable or explosive concentrations. Inflammable agents will only burn between flammability limits in different oxidising gases e.g. the concentration flammability limits for cyclopropane in air are 2.4 to 10%, while in oxygen the limits for cyclopropane are 2.5 to 60%. Explosions occur when the mixture reaches stoichiometric proportions. Stoichiometric concentrations occur when the proportions of inflammable agent and oxidising gas are the same as the ratios required by the chemical reaction. An excess concentration of inflammable agent or oxidising gas reduce the likelihood of explosion.

The reaction for cyclopropane when it burns is:

$$2C_3H_6 + 9O_2 \rightarrow 6CO_2 + 6H_2O$$

Therefore a stoichiometric mixture consists of 2 parts cyclopropane to 9 parts oxygen, which is equivalent to an 18% concentration in oxygen or a 4.3% concentration in air.

- A source of ignition and activation energy. for example diathermy, electrostatic sparks and surgical laser use

PREVENTION OF FIRE AND EXPLOSION

- Use of non-flammable agents
- Avoiding high risk (5 cm radius) and low risk (25 cm radius) zones with electrical equipment likely to generate sparks
- Use of appropriate antistatic equipment, footwear and clothing
- Awareness of equipment specifications (Figure PH.69). The APG label refers to equipment which is safe to use within the high risk zone, where oxygen and nitrous oxide may be the oxidising agents. While the AP label is used for the low risk zone where anaesthetic gases and air mixtures provide the risk
- Adequate air conditioning with 5–10 air changes per hour
- Appropriate scavenging system
- Use of specialised equipment in the surgical field during laser surgery

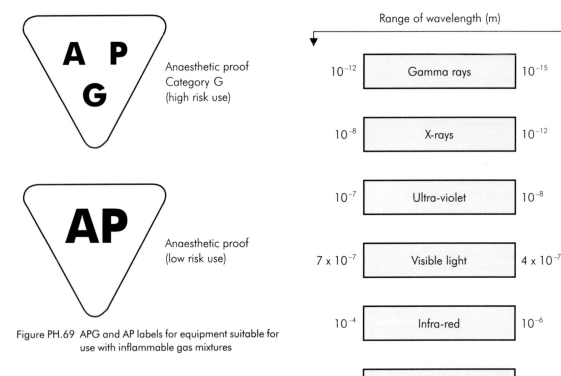

Figure PH.69 APG and AP labels for equipment suitable for use with inflammable gas mixtures

Anaesthetic proof
Category G
(high risk use)

Anaesthetic proof
(low risk use)

LIGHT

Light is a type of electromagnetic wave (EM) and forms a narrow band of frequencies in the electromagnetic spectrum (Figure PH.70), which are defined as those frequencies detectable by the human retina. The EM spectrum covers many different forms of radiation ranging from low radio frequencies at the lower end of the spectrum, to γ rays at the high frequency end of the spectrum. Wavelengths of low frequency radio signals are hundreds of metres ($>10^2$ m), while those of γ radiation are in the order of 10^{-12} m or less.

Light has a dualistic nature and in some phenomena it is best considered as a stream of discrete particles or quanta of energy called photons. These phenomena include the action of light on photocells and photomultipliers as applied in oximetry and spectrophotometry.

TRANSVERSE WAVES, LIGHT WAVES AND LIGHT RAYS

A light wave can be visualised as being analogous to a surface wave on water occurring when a stone is dropped into a pond. The surface wave is formed by water particles moving up and down and the shape of a wave as it moves across the surface is called a

Figure PH.70 Electromagnetic spectrum

wavefront. The wave moves across the surface in a plane at right angles to the particle motion. This is called a transverse wave. The direction that waves travel in is often represented by a single straight line at right angles to the plane of particle motion giving rise to the wave. This is referred to as a ray (Figure PH.71a). Light waves are also transverse waves produced by the vibration of photons emitted from the light source (Figure PH.71b).

WAVELENGTH OF LIGHT

Wavelengths of light are normally quoted in nanometres (nm, 1 nm = 10^{-9} m), which have replaced the more traditional unit of the ångström (1Å = 10^{-10} m). The lowest frequencies of visible light are dark red with wavelengths of around 700 nm, while the highest frequencies visible are violet with wavelengths of around 400 nm.

A stone dropped into water at X creates
circular waves which travel outwards

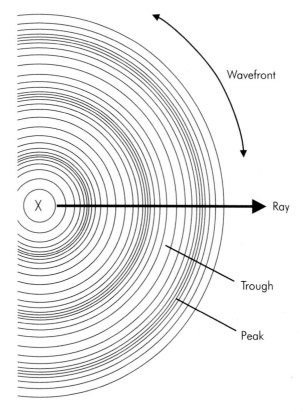

Wavefront

Ray

Trough

Peak

Transverse wave
on water surface

X

Direction of wave travel

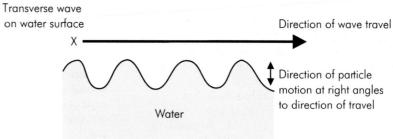

Direction of particle
motion at right angles
to direction of travel

Water

Figure PH.71a Particle motion, wavefront and ray in a transverse wave

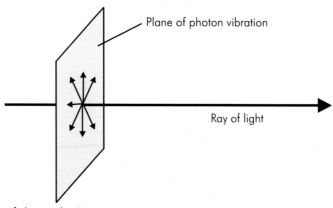

Plane of photon vibration

Ray of light

Figure PH.71b Light ray showing plane of photon vibration

SPEED OF LIGHT

The speed of light in a vacuum is a fundamental constant in physics, which has a defined value of 299 792 458 m/s. This value is now used to give the definition for the standard unit of length, the metre. The speed of light decreases with the density of the medium. Thus light travels more slowly in air and is even slower in glass.

REFRACTION OF LIGHT

A consequence of the changes in the speed of light between different media is that the path of light is 'bent' when it travels across a boundary from one medium to another. Consider light travelling from air to glass as shown in Figure PH.72. The light path is represented by a 'ray' or line drawn at right angles to the wave front. As the ray crosses the boundary from air to glass it 'bends' towards the normal. When light passes from a dense medium to a less dense medium, its path is deviated away from the normal.

The refraction of the light can be quantified using two angles, the angle of incidence (i) and the angle of refraction (r). The deviation produced is dependent on the ratio of the speeds of light in air and glass (c_1 and c_2 respectively), which will be a constant.

Snell's law, states that for light travelling between two given media

$$\frac{\sin i}{\sin r} = \frac{c_1}{c_2}$$

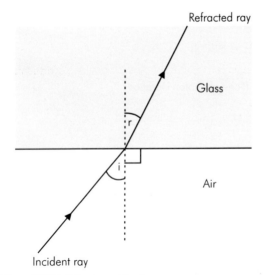

Figure PH.72 Refraction of light

The refractive properties of a medium are measured by its absolute refractive index (n), which is defined by:

$$\text{refractive index} = \frac{\text{speed of light in a vacuum}}{\text{speed of light in medium}}$$

$$n = \frac{c}{c_1}$$

When considering light passing from air to a medium the value of the refractive index relative to air is virtually the same as its absolute value because the refractive index of air is 1.0003 (i.e. the speed of light in air is almost the same as in a vacuum).

Snell's law then becomes:

$$\frac{\sin i}{\sin r} = \frac{1}{n}$$

Refraction results in the apparent distortion of images and distances, when viewing objects in one medium from another. This is why objects at the bottom of a pool of water appear to be more shallow than they actually are. Refraction is also responsible for the actions of lenses including that in the eye. The refractive index for glass is 1.5, for water n = 1.33.

REFLECTION

When a light ray is reflected from a boundary between two media or from a surface (Figure PH.73), the geometry is again defined by the angles made with the normal to the surface. In this case the angles are the angle of incidence (i) which is always equal to the angle of reflection (r). The use of reflection occurs in mirrors and the design of dish aerials or mirrors to focus light or other waves.

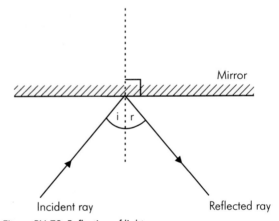

Figure PH.72 Reflection of light

Total internal reflection

When light passes from a dense medium to a less dense medium (e.g. glass to air) Snell's law will only apply over a range of angles. This is because the angle of refraction is greater than the angle of incidence, the light being deviated away from the normal (Figure PH.74a). As the angle of incidence increases, a value is reached when the angle of refraction becomes 90° (Figure PH.74b). This value of the angle of incidence is called the critical angle (C). In this case applying Snell's law:

$$\frac{\sin C}{\sin 90°} = \frac{1}{n}$$

When the angle of incidence exceeds C, total internal reflection occurs (Figure PH.74c). This is used in the construction of prisms to guide light in optical equipment, and also in the use of optical fibres to conduct light in fibreoptic equipment. The critical angle for glass is approximately 42°.

POLARISED LIGHT

All electromagnetic waves including light are transverse waves. This means that the particle movement giving rise to the wave is in a plane at right angles to the direction in which the wave is travelling. Frequently the particle movement occurs in many different directions within the plane described. This is the case in light emitted by a high temperature source such as a light filament or the sun, since it is emitted at random from the atoms in the source. This type of light is said to be 'unpolarised', and can be considered to be a mixture of vertical and horizontal components.

Unpolarised light may be filtered so that only light with particle oscillation in a single direction (vertical or horizontal), is allowed to pass. The light is then said to be polarised. Light can be polarised by passage through different crystals (e.g. quinine iodosulphate, toumaline). Vertically polarised light can only pass through a crystal with its optical axis aligned vertically (Figure PH.75). If such a crystal were then to be rotated through 90° (i.e. become horizontally aligned) it would only allow horizontally polarised light to pass.

Dextro (*d*) and laevo (*l*) rotatory substances

Many pharmacological compounds are optically active causing polarised light to rotate either to the right or to the left. The optical activity of such substances can be investigated by using a combination of a vertically aligned (polariser) and horizontally aligned (analyser)

(a) i < C

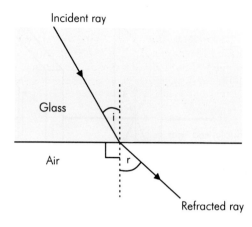

(b) i = C

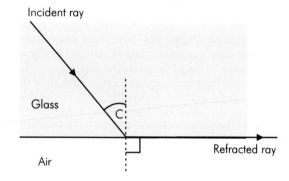

(c) i > C

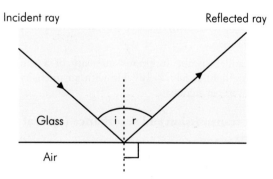

Figure PH.74 Total internal reflection

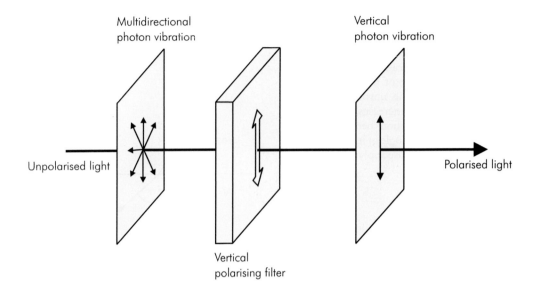

Figure PH.75 Non-polarised light filtered to give polarised light

crystal filters (Figure PH.76a). These in combination do not allow any light to pass. When an optically active substance is placed between the filters the vertically polarised light is rotated and some light then passes through the analyser (Figure PH.76b). The analyser is then rotated until the light passing through is once again extinguished (Figure PH.76c). The rotation of the analyser must then match the rotation caused by the substance under test. For detail of optical isomerism see Section 3 Chapter 3.

Luminous intensity and the candela

It is required sometimes to quantify the luminous intensity or brightness of a source. The luminous intensity of a source can be defined by the amount of light energy emitted per second (power) through unit solid angle (steradian) by the source, and is measured in candelas.

The candela is the luminous intensity of a source emitting light at 540×10^{12} Hz with an intensity of 1/630 watt per steradian.

Light transmission and absorbance (optical density)

When light passes through a substance some of the energy is absorbed. The absorption of light energy is dependent on the length of the path travelled and the absorptive properties of the substance. The absorption of monochromatic light (single wavelength) by a layer

of solution or gas, is used In absorption oximetry and spectrometry.

Consider the absorption of monochromatic radiation by a layer of substance. It is determined by a combination of two laws:

Lambert – Bouguer law: When a layer of solution of known thickness (d), is transilluminated by monochromatic light, the transmitted light (I) is related to the incident light (I_O), by:

$$I = I_O\, e^{-(ad)}$$

Where (ad) is the 'absorbance' or 'optical density' of the layer of solution. This in turn is the product of its thickness (d) and the quantity (a) known as the extinction coefficient of the solution (Figure PH.77). Thus if the absorbance of the solution layer is 1.0, only 37% of the light is transmitted, but doubling the absorbance to 2.0 reduces the transmitted light to 13.5%.

Beer's law: This states that for a solution absorbance is a linear function of molar concentration combining the above laws gives:

Lambert-Beer law which relates the transmitted light to both molar concentration and thickness of the solution layer by expressing the absorbance as:

$$Absorbance = \xi\, c\, d$$

Where ξ = molar extinction coefficient, c = molar concentration, d = thickness.

(a)

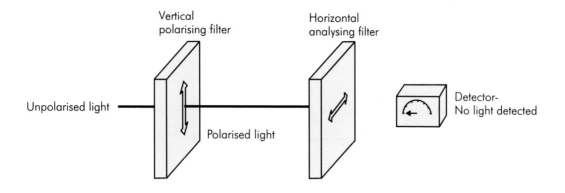

(b)

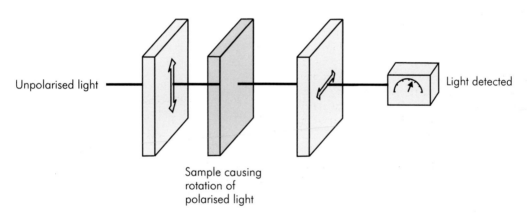

(c)

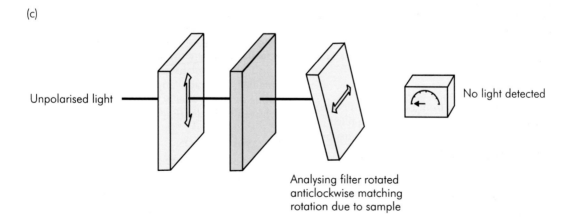

Figure PH.76a,b,c Polariser and analyser filters set up to determine rotation by D and L compounds

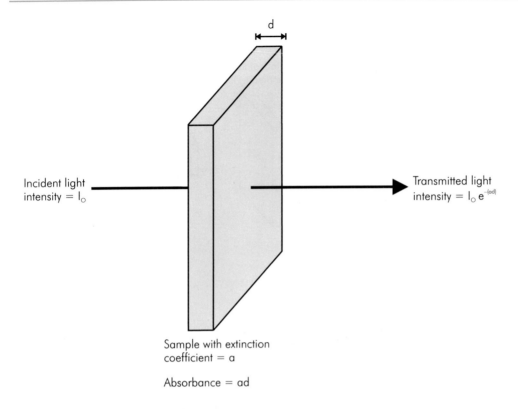

Figure PH.77 Light transmission and absorbance of a layer of material

To measure the concentration of a particular compound in a mixture, the mixture is transilluminated with monochromatic light at the wavelength where absorbance is maximal. The machine must be calibrated with a pure solution of the compound, and then the measured concentration can be calculated. Further details of this technique are given in Section 4, Chapter 2.

LASERS

Laser is an acronym derived from Light Amplification by Stimulated Emission of Radiation, and is applied to devices which emit a special form of light radiation. Laser light has the following characteristics:

- It is monochromatic
- All radiated waves are in phase
- The light waves emitted do not diverge but remain in a narrow beam
- High light energy intensities can be produced with a relatively low power source

Stimulated Emission

This describes the reaction when a high energy atom is struck by an incoming photon. The high energy state atom is 'stimulated' to lose energy by giving out two light particles with the same phase and frequency. This process is called 'stimulated emission' (Figure PH.78a). These emitted photons can then each stimulate the further emission of photons by striking two further high energy atoms. In this way provided that a suitable population of high energy atoms can be maintained, a cascade amplification process is set up resulting in a high energy light source emitting waves which are all in phase (Figure PH.78b).

LASER CONSTRUCTION

All lasers consist of three basic parts:

- A source of energy to raise the electrons from the ground state to an excited one (a process known as pumping)
- A suitable laser substance capable of stimulated emission

(a)

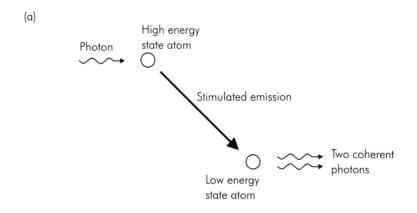

(b)

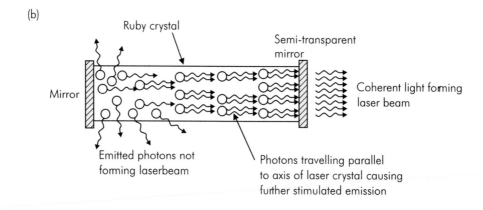

(c)

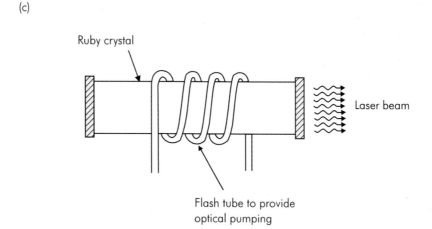

Figure PH.78a,b,c Laser system, detail of device

- A system of mirrors to reflect light repeatedly backwards and forwards through the laser substance. This process amplifies the light many times over.

Figures PH.78b and PH.78c show simplified diagrams of a ruby laser. The pumping energy source is a flash tube, which feeds continuous or pulsed energy into the laser material to produce high energy state atoms. These undergo stimulated emission producing photons which are then reflected backwards and forwards between the mirrored surfaces. The reflected photons in turn produce further stimulated emission, and an amplifying cascade is built up. At one end the mirror is partially transparent allowing light to escape as a highly parallel coherent beam. This beam can then be focused to produce extremely high light power intensities.

Many substances can act as laser materials. The properties of some commonly used lasers in surgery are summarised below.

PROPERTIES OF SOME SURGICAL LASERS

Laser material	Application	Properties
Synthetic ruby	Early use in eye surgery	
Argon	Replacement for ruby laser in eye surgery Used for retinal coagulation and repairing retinal detachment Used for removal of birthmarks	Passes through vitreous and aqueous humour. Absorbed by haemoglobin. Also absorbed by pigmented skin Can be transmitted by optical fibres for endoscopic application
Carbon dioxide	The most commonly used laser in surgery Superficial surgery removing thin layers of tissue at a time	Absorbed by water therefore low penetration to <200 μm. Cannot be used endoscopically
Nd-YAG (Neodymium-Yttrium-Aluminium-Garnet)	Coagulation and cutting	Not absorbed by water therefore good penetration of tissues. Can be used endoscopically

Figure PH.79

Laser safety

Lasers are classified according to their degree of hazard from Class 1 (the least dangerous) to Class 4 (most dangerous). Domestic lasers (CD players, laser printers) are safe either because of the wavelengths used and their low power. However all surgical lasers are Class 4, being inherently hazardous as they are specifically designed to damage tissue. Safety precautions when working with lasers include:

- Appropriate training for all staff
- A designated suitably equipped area with all exposed surfaces matt finished
- All instruments with matt finish
- No inflammable material in the vicinity of the patient or in the operating field
- All theatre staff must wear protective eye glasses, and protection for the patient's eyes and skin against stray laser light.
- The laser theatre must be well ventilated with a suitable smoke extraction system
- Precautions against use of inflammable or explosive anaesthetic gases

X RAYS

X rays are a form of EM radiation with wavelengths in the range of 10^{-8} m to 10^{-12} m. The main properties of X rays in medical applications is their ability to penetrate tissue and their ionising effect. The latter represents a hazard in their use but a property which is also used therapeutically in X radiotherapy.

X rays are generated in an X ray tube, by bombarding a high temperature anode with electrons generated by a cathode (Figure PH.80). The electrons are accelerated in the tube using a high voltage electric field. X ray machines are thus rated by the current and voltage that can be delivered e.g. a portable X ray set may deliver 100 mA at 90 kV.

RADIOACTIVE ISOTOPES AND RADIATION

An element may exist in different forms due to variations in its nuclear structure.

These different forms are called isotopes of the element. Each isotope will differ in atomic mass number but will possess the same atomic number. Some basic facts about the structure of an atom are listed below:

- The nucleus consists of neutrons and protons and is orbited by electrons
- The atomic mass number is equal to the number of neutrons plus the number of protons in the nucleus. It is the nearest integer to the atomic weight
- The atomic number is equal to the number of protons in the nucleus and determines which element is present

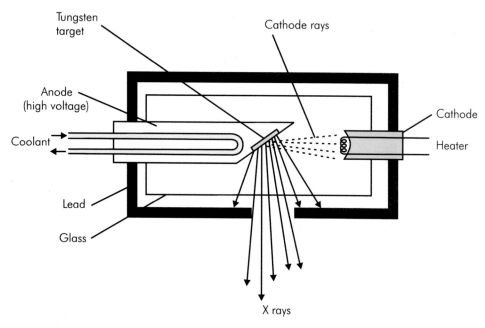

Figure PH.80 X ray tube

• Notation used to identify isotopes is as follows:

atomic mass number
        [element symbol],
atomic number

Thus $^{1}_{1}$H is the symbol for hydrogen.

Some isotopes are stable and retain their nuclear structure indefinitely, while other isotopes are unstable and decay spontaneously. Unstable isotopes are said to be radioactive, and they decay by emitting radiation. Some examples of stable and unstable isotopes are shown in Figure PH.81.

SOME OF THE STABLE AND UNSTABLE ISOTOPES OF HYDROGEN AND CARBON

Element		Atomic Number	Neutrons	Atomic mass Number	Stability
Hydrogen	$^{1}_{1}$H	1	0	1	stable
Deuterium	$^{2}_{1}$H	1	1	2	stable
Tritium	$^{3}_{1}$H	1	2	3	unstable
Carbon	$^{10}_{6}$C	6	4	10	unstable
Carbon	$^{12}_{6}$C	6	6	12	stable
Carbon	$^{14}_{6}$C	6	8	14	unstable

Figure PH.81

Radioactive decay

Decay of a radioactive isotope involves the emission of nuclear particles from the substance resulting in the formation of another isotope or another element. An example is the uranium series, which occurs when uranium decays. This series of reactions finally results in the formation of lead, but involves a chain of intermediate decay reactions. Some of these are illustrated in Figure PH.81. Each of these reactions involves the emission of a specific type of particle with a characteristic mean energy level. Each reaction also has a particular half-life (see below).

The energy possessed by elementary particles (e.g. electrons or protons) is usually measured in electronvolts (eV). The electronvolt is defined as the change of kinetic energy occurring when a particle with a charge of e (the charge on an electron) moves through a potential difference of 1 volt.

$$1 \text{ eV} = 1.602 \times 10^{-19} \text{ joules}$$

$$1 \text{ MeV} = 1.602 \times 10^{-13} \text{ joules}$$

Radiation from radioactive isotopes

The types of radiation emitted from radioactive isotopes are:

α particles: A combination of 2 protons and 2 neutrons (equivalent to a helium nucleus) e.g.

$$^{226}_{88}\text{Ra} \rightarrow \, ^{222}_{86}\text{Rn} + \, ^{4}_{2}\text{He}$$

radium   radon   helium (α particle)

β particles: An electron which is negatively charged, this is derived from a neutron splitting to give a proton and a high energy electron. The creation of another proton in the nucleus will increase the atomic number of the atom and thus change the element present.

$$^{14}_{6}\text{C} \rightarrow \, ^{14}_{7}\text{N} \quad + \text{ e}^{-}$$

carbon 14 nitrogen   electron (β particle)

Sometimes an electron may be emitted from the nucleus with a positive charge in which case it is called a positron.

γ radiation: Is electromagnetic radiation with wavelengths $< 10^{-12}$ m, which is emitted during most nuclear reactions, usually following the emission of an α or β particle.

DECAY HALF-LIFE

The decay of a radioactive element from one isotopic form to the next form in its series follows an exponential decay curve i.e.

$$N = N_0 \, e^{(-\lambda t)}$$

Where N is the number of atoms of the element present at time = t, N_0 is the number of atoms present at time = 0, and λ is the decay constant for the element. λ is related to the decay time constant (K), for the element by:

$$\lambda = \frac{1}{K}$$

The half-life for the element $(T_{1/2})$ is the time for the mass of element to decay to a half of its initial mass, and is related to the time constant, K, by:

$$T_{1/2} = 0.693 \text{ K}$$

The half-life may have a value ranging from seconds to millions of years (see Figure PH.82).

Units of radioactivity

The activity of a radioactive sample is measured by the number of disintegrations occurring per second. The SI unit of measurement used is the bequerel which is defined as,

$$1 \text{ bequerel (bec)} = 1 \text{ disintegration per second}$$

The curie is a traditional unit which is the activity of one gram of radium, where 1 curie = 3.7×10^{10} disintegrations per second = 3.7×10^{10} bec

APPLICATIONS OF RADIOACTIVE ISOTOPES

Radioactive isotopes are used in many applications clinically. These include:

- Measurements with labelled substances – Cr-51 in measurement of red cell volume
- Cancer therapy – use of yttrium-90 in pituitary tumours
- Diagnostic uses – imaging techniques with Technetium-99 as in assessment of cardiac function

MEASUREMENT OF EXPOSURE TO IONISING RADIATION

Exposure to ionising radiation can result in both short and long term sequelae.

The short term effects of radiation exposure appear as the symptoms of acute radiation sickness. These are

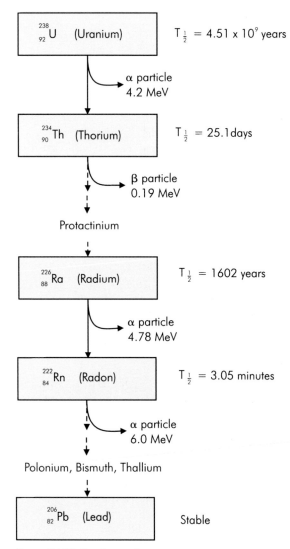

Figure PH.82 Uranium series

dose dependent and include nausea, vomiting, anorexia general lassitude, weakness and can lead to death over a period of days or less. The long term effects include an increased incidence of cancers and genetic defects in the population which occur after a period of years. A dose of radiation can be measured by the effects it produces in different ways.

- Energy absorbed by air
  A dose of radiation can be measured by the energy absorbed by the irradiated air. The röntgen is a unit used to measuring X radiation dosage and is defined as: 1 röntgen (R) is the dose of X radiation giving 83.3 ergs of energy to 1 gram of air.

- Energy absorbed by body tissue
  Radiation energy absorbed depends on the substance irradiated, and therefore the energy absorbed by body tissues will not be the same as that absorbed by air, even when exposed to the same dose of radiation. The SI unit of radiation dose absorbed by body tissues, is the gray. 1 gray (Gy) is the dose of radiation giving an absorbed energy of 1 joule per kilogram of soft tissue.

Biological effect

Different types of ionising radiation provide different levels of biological hazard when absorbed. Thus even though the same amount of energy may be absorbed from different types of radiation, different sequelae may result. For instance 200 kV X rays are less damaging than γ rays or β particles. Alpha particles are even more damaging in their ionising effect by a factor of 10 or more. Therefore to assess risk in exposure to ionising radiation a unit of biological effectiveness is used. The SI unit of biological effectiveness used is the sievert. One sievert (Sv) – is the radiation dose equivalent to 1 Gy of absorbed radiation from 200kV X rays in terms of biological damage.

Thus if 1 Gy of radiation is absorbed from 200kV X rays, the biological dose equivalent will be 1 Sv by definition. However an absorbed dose of 1Gy from α particle radiation will have a dose equivalent to 10 Sv.

Biologically significant levels of ionising radiation have been estimated in terms of their acute effects and their effect on the incidence of cancer and genetic defects in the population. These at best are an estimate since the rate of delivery of a given dose can vary as well as individual response. An average dose of 1 mSv per individual over a population is believed to increase the incidence of cancer by 13 and genetic defects by 8 per million of population during the following years. A whole life exposure of 1 Sv is thought to reduce life span by 1 year.

Some estimated doses of ionising radiation are shown below in Figure PH.83.

SOME ESTIMATED IONISING RADIATION DOSES	
Description	**Dose/time**
Max permitted dose	5 mSv per year
Natural background dose	1.25 mSv per year
Dose causing nausea	1 Sv per few hours
Dose causing death within days	10 Sv per few hours

Figure PH.83

SECTION 4: 2
CLINICAL MEASUREMENT

M. Tidmarsh
E. S. Lin

MEASUREMENT SYSTEMS

ELECTRICAL SIGNALS

PRESSURE MEASUREMENT

BLOOD PRESSURE MEASUREMENT

MEASUREMENT OF GAS FLOW

MEASUREMENT OF GAS AND VAPOUR CONCENTRATIONS

OXYGEN MEASUREMENT

CARBON DIOXIDE MEASUREMENT

MEASUREMENT OF pH

PULSE OXIMETRY

NEUROMUSCULAR MEASUREMENT

MEASUREMENT OF DEPTH OF ANAESTHESIA

TEMPERATURE MEASUREMENT

MEASUREMENT OF HUMIDITY

MEASUREMENT OF PAIN

Clinical measurement in anaesthesia is usually concerned with the direct measurement of a physical quantity such as the pressure, flow or concentration of a gas. Alternatively assessment of a physiological parameter such as neuromuscular blockade, depth of anaesthesia or pain levels may be required. In these instances measurement is made indirectly, using a related physical variable such as a stimulated muscle twitch, the electroencephalogram or a visual analogue scale.

The process of measurement is performed using apparatus that can be referred to as the measurement system. This may be as simple as a ruler with pencil and paper or as sophisticated as the integrated electronic monitoring systems available in operating theatres and intensive care units. In the final analysis data obtained must be interpreted, but note below:

> The data obtained by making measurements can only be interpreted correctly if:
>
> - The relationship between the data and the physical quantity or parameter being measured is understood.
> - The characteristics of the measurement system are known.

MEASUREMENT SYSTEMS

Measurement of a physical quantity is a process in which the quantity being measured provides an input to a measurement system, which then processes this input to yield an output in the form of a reading or display. This concept is illustrated in Figure CM.1, where a measurement system is represented as a 'black box' with an input and output.

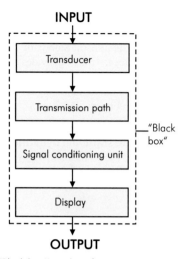

Figure CM.1 "Black box" analogy for a measurement system

The measurement system consists of component 'black boxes' representing:

- A transducer – a detecting element to convert the quantity being measured (the input) into usable data or a signal, usually an electrical signal. Examples of common transducers are:
  Microphone, which converts sound to an electrical signal
  Thermistor, which converts temperature variations into an electrical signal
  Piezoelectric crystal, which converts pressure variations into an electrical signal
- A transmission path – the means by which the transducer signal is transferred to the signal conditioning unit or the display unit. Examples include an electrical or optic cables, a length of tubing or an infrared link
- A signal-conditioning unit – processes the transducer signal to make it suitable for display or storage. Signal processing includes functions such

ANALOGUE AND DIGITAL METHODS OF SIGNAL DISPLAY AND STORAGE		
Function	**Analogue**	**Digital**
Display	Oscilloscope	Digital Voltmeter
	Moving Coil Meter	Light Emitting Diodes
	Chart Recorder	Liquid Crystal Display
Storage	Magnetic Tape	Computer Hard Disk
	Chart	Floppy Disc
		Magnetic Tape
		CD ROM

Figure CM.2

as amplification, filtering, and analogue to digital conversion. It may occur before or after the signal passes along the transmission path

- A display or storage unit – provides the output of the system as a display and also stores the signals or data. It may employ analogue or digital methods, which are detailed in Figure CM.2

The performance of a measurement system can be characterised by its **static** and **dynamic** characteristics. These determine the relationship between the quantity being measured (input) and the reading (output).

STATIC CHARACTERISTICS

Static characteristics define the performance of a measurement system when it is dealing with an input which is not changing (or changing only slowly). Under these circumstances there is enough time for the system to reach a steady-state before the measured quantity changes, so that the output follows changes in the input accurately. Static characteristics include:

- Accuracy – closeness between the measurement obtained and the 'true' value of the quantity being measured, e.g. if a pressure has a 'true' value of 10 cmH_2O, an accurate system may read 10.01 cmH_2O and may be described as having an accuracy of 0.1%. In an inaccurate system reading 11 cmH_2O the accuracy may be quoted as 10% (Figure CM.3a)
- Sensitivity – relationship between changes in the output reading of the system and changes in the measured quantity. The sensitivity of a pressure measurement system may be described as the change in output signal voltage for a given change in pressure, e.g. 1 volt per cmH_2O for a sensitive system or 100 mV per cmH_2O for a system 10 times less sensitive. Less sensitive systems will cover a wider range of pressure measurement than sensitive systems (Figure CM.3b)
- Linearity – in a linear measurement system the output reading varies in proportion to the measured quantity. Thus, in a linear pressure measurement system, if the pressure doubles the output voltage will double. When the output voltage is plotted against the input pressure, a straight line is obtained. The gradient of this line gives the sensitivity of the system. It is usually desirable for a system to be linear and any non linearity may be quoted as a percentage of the operating range of the instrument (Figure CM.3b). Some instruments may be intrinsically non linear reflecting their underlying mechanism, e.g. hot wire ammeter, or rotameter
- Hysteresis – a property of a measurement system that produces an error dependent on whether the

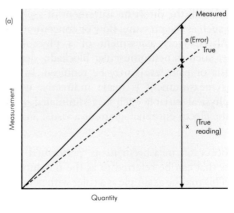

(a)

Accuracy $= \frac{e}{x} \times 100\%$

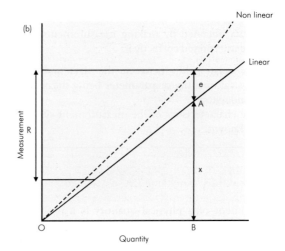

(b)

Sensitivity $= \frac{x}{OB}$

Non linearity $= \frac{e}{R} \times 100\%$

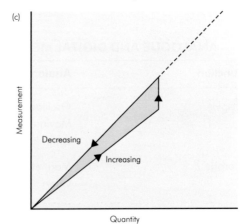

(c)

Figure CM.3. Static characteristics of a measurement system: (a) accuracy, (b) sensitivity and (c) hysteresis

measured value is decreasing or increasing. Hysteresis in a mechanical device is caused by elastic energy stored in the system, or frictional losses between moving parts. Figure CM.3c shows how hysteresis in a measurement system produces errors in the measurement of increasing and decreasing pressures

- Drift – variation in the reading from an instrument that is not caused by change in the measured quantity. It is usually caused by the effect of internal or external temperature changes on the measurement system, and unstable components in the system

DYNAMIC CHARACTERISTICS

Every system requires a certain time to settle to a steady-state when presented with a change in its input. This response time may affect the accuracy of the measurement, since if the input is changing rapidly, the measuring system may not have adequate time to reach steady-state and, thus, will not give an accurate reading. The dynamic characteristics of a system reflect its ability to respond to rapidly changing inputs.

Step response of a system

An important dynamic characteristic of any measurement system is its response to a rapid increase in input or a 'step' function (Figure CM.4). This can be simulated by dipping a thermometer at room temperature into boiling water, or rapidly opening a tap connecting a pressure gauge to a pressurised container. In a perfect measuring instrument, the output or 'step response' produced by a step input, should also be a step function occurring instantaneously to give a reading of the measured quantity.

In practice, the step response differs from the ideal due to the properties of the system, and the output only reaches a 'true' steady-state value after a finite time. The time lag for an instrument between a 'step' input and the output reaching its final value, is reflected by:

- Response time – time taken from occurrence of the 'step' input to the instrument output reaching 90% of its final value
- Rise time – time taken for the output of the instrument to rise from 10 to 90% of its final value

Damping in a measurement system

The step response of an instrument may also fall short of the ideal in the shape of the output signal produced. Some examples are shown in Figure CM.5, where in curve (a) the output overshoots and oscillates about the true value. In curve (b) the response does not reach the true value in the time plotted; in curve (c) the output reaches a steady reading of the true value within the shortest time compatible with no overshoot. The property that determines these effects in the step response is called the 'damping' of the system.

All instruments will possess damping that affects their dynamic response. This includes mechanical, hydraulic, pneumatic and electrical devices. In an electromechanical device such as a galvanometer there are mechanical moving parts such as the meter needle and bearings. Damping in these components arises from frictional effects on their movement. This may arise unintentionally or may be applied as part of the instrument design to control oscillation of the needle when it records a measurement. In a fluid- (gas or liquid) operated device, damping occurs due to viscous

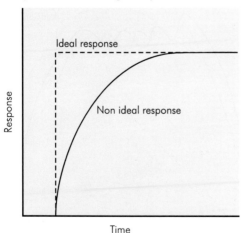

Figure CM.4 Step input to a measurement system

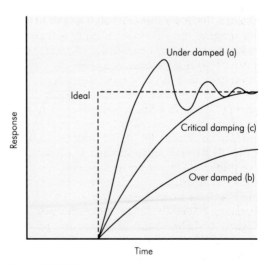

Figure CM.5 Effects of damping on the step response of a system

forces that oppose the motion of the fluid. While damping in electrical systems is provided electronically by electrical resistance which opposes the passage of electrical currents.

Note particularly that:

> Damping is an important factor in the design of any system. In a measurement system it can lead to inaccuracy of the readings or display:
> **Underdamping** can result in oscillation and overestimation of the measurement
> **Overdamping** can result in underestimation of the measurement
> **Critical damping** is usually an optimum compromise resulting in the fastest steady-state reading for a particular system, with no overshoot or oscillation

Frequency response of a measurement system

Any measurement system in practice will only respond to a restricted range of frequencies, either by design or due to the limitations of its components. Thus, if the system were to be tested with input signals of the same amplitude but different frequencies it would only produce an output over a limited range of frequencies. Within this frequency range the system may respond more sensitively to some frequencies than others. The response of the system (system gain) plotted against signal frequency is called the frequency response of the system (Figure CM.6).

BANDWIDTH

The highest frequency that a system responds to is the high 'cut-off' frequency, above which input signals will produce no output. An example of such a cut-off is in the frequency response of the human auditory system, which at best may have a high 'cut-off' frequency of 20 kHz. Similarly a system may possess a low cut-off frequency, the lowest frequency audible by the human ear being 15 Hz. The frequency range between low and high cut-off frequencies is referred to as the bandwidth.

DISTORTION DUE TO POOR FREQUENCY RESPONSE

Any input signal can be characterised by its frequency spectrum that defines the different frequency components, into which the signal can be resolved. The frequency response of a measurement system does not cover the spectrum of a signal thus blocking part of the input signal. Alternatively, an instrument may be more sensitive or attenuate certain frequencies, causing it to give falsely high or low readings, within its operating frequency range. This can occur at natural frequencies or resonances. Distortion of a signal is illustrated in Figure CM.7.

It might initially be assumed that the ideal frequency response for a system would be one with equal sensitivity at all frequencies from very low to very high frequencies (i.e. a flat response from 0 to ∞ Hz), but this would also enable 'noise' to pass through the system with the measurement signal, thus causing error and distortion.

The frequency response of a mechanical system is determined by its inertial and compliance elements (equivalent to masses and springs), while in an electrical circuit it is determined by the inductances

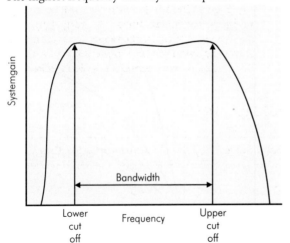

Figure CM.6. Frequency response of a system

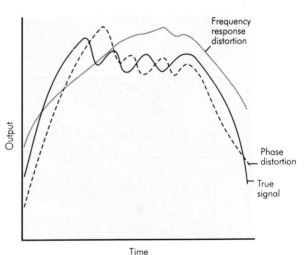

Figure CM.7. Causes of signal distortion

and capacitances. There is often a design compromise between providing accuracy and reducing noise levels.

NATURAL FREQUENCIES OR RESONANCES

A measurement system may possess natural frequencies or resonances determined by inertial and compliance elements in a mechanical system (or inductances and capacitances in an electrical circuit). These resonances appear as peaks in the systems frequency response and can produce distortion in a signal display and errors in the readings (Figure CM.8). Good design practice can ensure that these resonances do not lie in the operating frequency range of the instrument, or ensure appropriate levels of damping to smooth out these unwanted peaks.

Phase shift response

Fourier analysis demonstrates how a signal is composed of a series of component frequencies. In a signal being measured each component wave will undergo a different delay in time or phase shift (a phase shift is a time delay expressed as an angle, i.e. the units

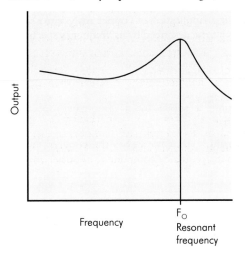

Figure CM.8 Example of a resonant frequency

are degrees or radians) introduced by its passage through the measurement system. If a measurement system significantly alters the relative phases between the components of a signal passes it can distort the signal. Any measurement system will have a 'phase shift response', consisting of the phase shift occurring at different frequencies, which can be plotted against the frequency axis. This phase shift response will be dependent on the components of the system, and can be responsible for distortion or errors in an instrument.

ELECTRICAL SIGNALS

In modern measuring instruments the transducer usually produces an electrical current or voltage, which varies according to the measured parameter. This voltage or current is a signal. Signals in clinical measurement are usually voltage signals or 'biological potentials'. Most biological potentials vary in time, many in a repetitive or cyclical fashion, e.g. electrocardiogram, airway pressure during respiration. Some signals such as the electroencephalogram and evoked potentials are not cyclical but vary irregularly.

BIOLOGICAL POTENTIALS

The characteristics of some common biological potentials are outlined in Figure CM.9.

Electrical signals can be described in the following ways:

- As a voltage (or current) varying in time – any signal can be represented as a voltage (or current) plotted along the 'time' axis, i.e. it is a 'time-variant' signal. The height of the signal above the time axis is measured in volts, millivolts or microvolts (V, mV, μV) (Figure CM.10). If a current, it will be in amps, milliamps or micro-amps (A, mA, μA). The amplitude of a signal is the range of variation (volts or amps) between maximum and minimum values
- As periodic or non periodic – a signal that varies

COMMON BIOLOGICAL SIGNALS		
Signal	Voltage range	Frequency range (Hz)
Electro-encephalogram (EEG)	1–500 μV	0–60
Electrocardiogram (ECG)	0.1–50 mV	0–100
Electromyogram (EMG)	0.01–100 mV	0–1000

Figure CM.9

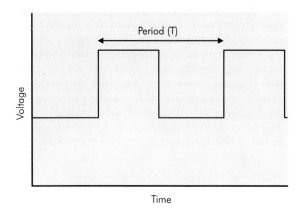

Figure CM.10 Voltage signal that varies with time – square wave

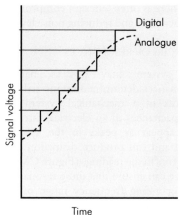

Figure CM.12 Analogue and digital signals

with a repeating pattern in time, at regular intervals is said to be periodic (Figure CM.11). Each cycle of the signal has the same shape or waveform, and possesses a period, T = duration of one cycle (s), a frequency (Hz) and an amplitude, the maximum swing in voltage or current, spanned by the signal. The simplest type of periodic signal is a sine wave

- As analogue or digital – an analogue signal is continuous in time and the magnitude of the signal varies smoothly without discernible increments. The signal is, thus, analogous to most natural varying processes. Signals produced by transducers are usually analogue signals. A digital signal is produced from an analogue signal by sampling the signal at regular intervals, and recording the magnitude with changes in fixed increments rather than on a continuous varying scale. Such a signal can be represented completely by a set of numbers. This adapts the signal for processing by digital systems and manipulation by computer, which can have significant advantages (Figure CM.12)

- As a series of frequency components – a mathematical method of analysis was invented by Jean Fourier (a French mathematician) in 1822. This has evolved both theoretically and practically to become one of the most powerful tools used in signal processing. Application of Fourier analysis to a signal enables it to be described by its 'frequency spectrum'

FREQUENCY SPECTRUM OF A SIGNAL

In describing a signal by its frequency spectrum consider that:

Fourier analysis, thus, describes the conversion of a signal into its frequency components. Fourier analysis

> - Any signal varying continuously in time can be broken down into a collection of sine and cosine waves, which if added to⌐ ⌐ther yield the original signal
> - The component waves exist as sine–cosine pairs at the same frequency
> - Each pair of components has a combined amplitude and can be plotted as a point on the 'frequency' axis giving the frequency spectrum for the signal

is most suitable for periodic signals, but can still be used for non periodic waveforms using an approximation which treats the waveform as if it were a periodic signal with a very long period.

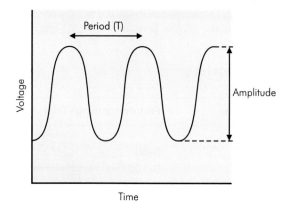

Figure CM.11 Periodic voltage signal – sine wave

ELECTRICAL 'NOISE'

A signal may be modified by any of the components of the measurement system. If the changes introduced are intentional, they represent 'signal processing' or 'signal conditioning'. Unwanted alteration of the signal by the system is distortion and introduces error. The addition of unwanted components to the signal by the system or from outside electrical interference is called 'noise'. These unwanted components can be added to a signal changing its value at any instant and its appearance on display. This may occur due to noise being generated in the measurement system itself, or due to the 'pick up' of interference from external sources such as diathermy or fluorescent lighting.

Signal-to-noise (S/N) ratio – in some cases the noise signals may be so large as to obscure the measurement signal altogether. An awareness of the magnitude of noise components in the signal is necessary to assess the accuracy of the measurements. This can be expressed by the S/N ratio, which is the ratio of signal amplitude to noise amplitude expressed in decibels (Figure CM.13).

SIGNAL PROCESSING

Signal processing modifies a measurement signal by using various functions, for example:

• Amplification, to make it suitable for display,

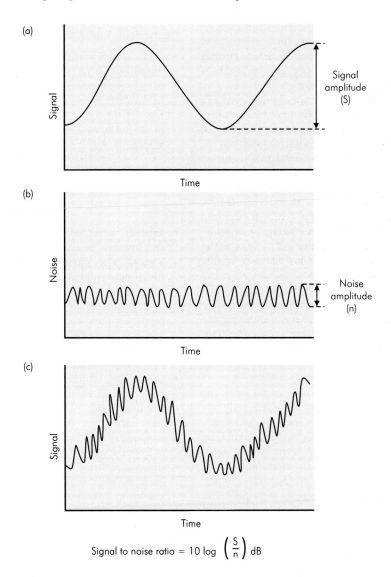

$$\text{Signal to noise ratio} = 10 \log \left(\frac{S}{n} \right) \text{ dB}$$

Figure CM.13 Illustration of signal-to-noise ratio: (a) signal, (b) noise and (c) noisy signal

storage or transmission – many biological signals are very small in amplitude (e.g. electro-encephalogram (EEG) signals may be microvolts, while ECG signals may be millivolts). Such signals are usually too small to drive display or storage units, and require amplification. Low amplitude signals are also unsuitable for transmission since noise signals picked up may be of similar or greater amplitude giving a low S/N ratio and obscuring the signal

- Filtering to remove noise – often noise signals are in a different frequency range from the wanted measurement signal. In these cases the noise can be reduced by using filters to block out the unwanted frequencies. A **low-pass** filter rejects all frequencies above a given threshold. Such a filter would be used to avoid high frequency interference from a source like diathermy. A **high-pass** filter rejects low frequencies below a set threshold, whereas a **notch** filter rejects a specific frequency, such as 50 Hz to avoid pick up from mains cables
- Spectral analysis – a signal is usually displayed as a time varying voltage or current. In some cases (e.g. cerebral function monitoring) a display of the signal frequency spectrum is required, which can be achieved using electronic processing. A common method first converts the analogue signal to a digital signal, and then applies a mathematical algorithm called the Fast Fourier Transform (FFT). Transformation of a signal to its spectral components can also make some processing functions such as filtering easier and more accurate. It also enables more complex analysis to be readily performed by computers
- Analogue to digital (A to D) conversion – often required before applying other processing functions, and is always necessary in order for the signal to be stored and analysed in a computer. This is because most electronic manipulation of signals uses digital electronics as opposed to analogue methods
- Averaging to remove noise – in some cases the amplitude of the measurement signal may only be a fraction of the noise amplitude (i.e. S/N ratio is very low), and when displayed the wanted signal may be completely obscured by noise. If the wanted signal is repetitive and the noise is random in time, multiple repetitions and summations of the combined signal, lead to an increase of the S/N ratio as the random noise cancels itself out. This is called averaging and is used in the extraction of evoked potentials, where the evoked signal is only a few millivolts in amplitude, hidden in background noise. Averaging > 2000 repetitions may be required to obtain a clear signal

AMPLIFIERS

As previously noted, the components of a measuring system can be considered as 'black boxes' in the way that the measurement system as a whole has been examined as a 'black box'. Thus, an amplifier is simply an electronic 'black box' which when presented with an electrical signal at its input produces an output which is of greater amplitude. The purpose of an amplifier in measuring systems is to increase the power of a low amplitude signal in order that it can be used to drive a display or storage unit. An amplifier contains an electronic circuit that requires a power supply, and channels power from this power supply into the signal increasing the voltage, current or both voltage and current.

Characteristics of an amplifier include:

- Gain, which is the ratio of the amplitude of the output signal (A_O) to the input signal (A_I). It is usually expressed as decibels (db). Such units may be used to express any ratio by taking 10 times the $\log_{10}$ of the ratio). Thus, if the output amplitude produced by an amplifier, A_O, is 100 times the input amplitude, A_I:

$$\text{Amplifier gain} = 10 \log (A_O/A_I)$$
$$= 10 \log 100$$
$$= 20 \text{ db}$$

- Frequency response and phase response – an amplifier will be characterised by these responses as a result of its circuit design, just as the complete instrument will have these responses dependent on the combined effects of its component parts
- Upper cut-off frequency, which is the upper frequency limit, above which signals are blocked or 'cut-off'. Measured in Hertz (Hz)
- Lower cut-off frequency, the lower frequency limit below which signals are blocked or 'cut-off'
- Bandwidth, which is the extent of the frequency range passed by a system or amplifier, i.e. the amplifier only amplifies signals within this frequency range. It, therefore, lies between upper and lower cut-off frequencies and is also measured in frequency units (Hz)
- Input impedance, which is the electrical impedance 'seen' by the transducer signal at the input of the amplifier. Maximum power transfer takes place when the input impedance of the amplifier matches the output impedance of the transducer. Measured in ohms
- Output impedance, the electrical impedance seen 'looking' back into the output terminals of the amplifier. Maximum transfer of signal power from

the amplifier requires matching of the output impedance to the input impedance of the transmission path or the display unit

PRESSURE MEASUREMENT

Pressure is defined as force per unit area and may be measured in various units in the clinical setting. Some examples are shown in Figure CM.14.

UNITS IN THE CLINICAL MEASUREMENT OF PRESSURE

Quantity measured	Unit
Blood pressure	mmHg
Airway pressure	cmH$_2$O
Partial pressure of blood gas	kPa
Gas cylinder pressure	Bar, psi

Figure CM.14

In anaesthesia, pressure measurements are usually applied to gases (cylinders, anaesthetic machines, breathing circuits) or liquids (intra-arterial pressure monitoring).

Pressures are not usually absolute measurements but are generally measured relative to atmospheric pressure. When interpreting pressure measurements various factors should be considered, such as:

- Transmission path – pressure transducers are often remote from the site at which pressure is sampled. The pressure is transmitted to the transducer by a length of tubing. The dynamic characteristics of this transmission path can significantly affect the final pressure measurements and signal displayed
- Sampling site – pressure may be sampled at a site remote from where the measurement is actually required, due to lack of access. Although static pressures may be equal throughout a closed system, pressures may differ significantly in a dynamic situation. A common example is the measurement of proximal airway pressures, which may not necessarily reflect distal airway pressures
- Static or fluctuating conditions – if the pressure is not varying rapidly it can be considered as static in which case the dynamic characteristics of the transmission path and measuring system may not affect the measurement significantly. This may not be the case when measuring a rapidly fluctuating pressure

Common types of device used to measure pressure in gases or liquids include the aneroid gauge, manometer and piezoresistive strain gauge.

ANEROID GAUGE

This type of gauge is a mechanical device that uses the pressure being measured to operate a mechanism coupled to a pointer. It can be used to measure high or low pressures, and is usually employed when measuring pressures greater than one bar.

In the Bourdon gauge the measured pressure is applied to a spiral tube which uncoils as the pressure increases. This uncoiling movement is coupled to a pointer that indicates the pressure. Another form of aneroid mechanism relies on the expansion of a capsule produced by connection to the sampled pressure. This expansion drives a pointer over a scale (Figure CM.15).

- Advantages – simple technology, mechanically robust and convenient to use. Operate in any position and do not require power supply. Suitable for high or low pressures
- Disadvantages – not suitable for very low pressures (< 5 cmH$_2$O). Not easily re-calibrated

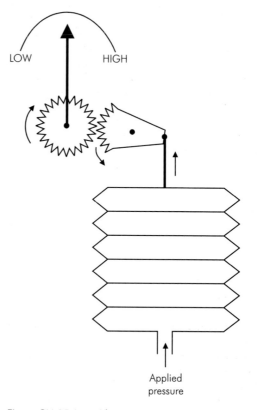

Figure CM.15 Aneroid gauge

MANOMETER

The manometer is the most basic device for measuring pressure and, because of its simplicity, represents a standard method of calibrating other devices. The unknown pressure is measured by balancing it against the pressure due to a column of a liquid (Figure CM.16). The liquids used most commonly are water for lower pressures and mercury for higher pressures. Pressure units are, thus, commonly cmH_2O and mmHg. Accuracy and sensitivity can be increased by angling the manometer tubing and using a liquid with a lower density than water (e.g. alcohol). Surface tension between the liquid and the manometer tubing can cause an error, which causes the water manometer to read too high and the mercury manometer to under read.

- Advantages – simplicity of mechanism and no need for calibration. A standard method used to calibrate other techniques of pressure measurement
- Disadvantages – bulkiness of the device and lack of a direct reading

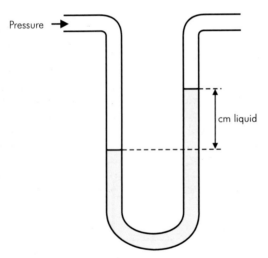

Pressure →

cm liquid

Figure CM.16 Manometer

PIEZORESISTIVE STRAIN GAUGE

This device is based on a semiconductor material with piezoresistive properties that cause it to vary in electrical resistance when subjected to a mechanical strain. The semiconductor is deposited on to the surface of a thin diaphragm that flexes when a pressure difference is applied across it. The distortion of the diaphragm produces a strain in the piezoresistive material that forms one arm of a bridge circuit etched onto the diaphragm. This results in a small signal current from the transducer that can then be amplified and processed.

- Advantages – versatility, since it can be used for measurement of high or low pressures. The electronic signal and display making it suitable for on line display, automated data logging and linking to a computer. It is also easily adaptable for measuring differential pressures since the diaphragm can be mounted with each face of the diaphragm enclosed in its own chamber and isolated from the other. Differential pressures can be used to measure gas flows, with the use of a suitable pneumotachograph head
- Disadvantages – requires power supply and signal processing unit. Susceptible to electrical interference but has to be used in electronically hostile environments (operating theatres and intensive care units)

BLOOD PRESSURE MEASUREMENT

Blood pressure is a determinant of tissue perfusion, oxygen delivery, and cardiac work. It varies between individuals and is subject to a diurnal rhythm (lowest when the subject sleeps). Note:

Recorded blood pressures not only reflect cardiovascular performance but also artefact. Factors affecting blood pressure measurement include:

- Cardiac output
- The pulsatile nature of blood flow
- Systemic vascular tone
- Hydrostatic pressure variation in the circulatory system
- The characteristics of the measurement system used

Failure to recognise this can result in errors of interpretation and inappropriate action.

For example, changing the measurement site by 10 cm in height produces an error of 7.5 mmHg in the pressure measurement. For this reason, a standard reference point is taken, usually the level of the heart.

Since blood flow is pulsatile, the blood pressure varies according to the phase of the cardiac cycle.

METHODS OF MEASURING BLOOD PRESSURE

The value of the displayed blood pressure is a function of the method used to measure it. The validity of any such measurements, is strongly influenced by the observer's familiarity with the particular strengths and weaknesses of the technique employed. These can be divided into indirect and direct methods.

Indirect methods

These are most commonly based on an occlusive cuff, which is inflated to a pressure above that of the artery and then slowly deflated. Once the cuff pressure falls below that of the artery, pressure transients begin to pass beneath the cuff and can be measured. Blood pressure values are derived from these pressure transients and can be measured manually or automatically.

MANUAL OCCLUSIVE CUFF METHODS

Manual methods rely on auscultation and palpation and are historically the earliest, but have become superseded by automated non invasive techniques, which provide a continuous display of blood pressure.

Riva-Rocci (1896) described the use of an occlusive cuff to measure systolic pressure by palpation.

Using an occlusive cuff, Korotkov (1905) first described the measurement of blood pressure by auscultation. 'Korotkov sounds' heard over the artery as the cuff pressure falls, are the result of turbulent blood flow, vibration in the arterial wall and pressure transients created as the extent of arterial occlusion decreases (Figure CM.17).

> Phase I – clear tapping synchronous with the pulse
> Phase II – sounds become softer about 5–10 mmHg below phase I
> Phase III – as the diastolic point approaches, sounds become more intense
> Phase IV – sounds suddenly become muffled
> Phase V – sounds disappear

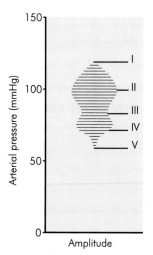

Figure CM.17 Representation of Korotkov sounds

von Recklinghausen (1931) described a dual cuff (occlusive, and sensing) technique, employing aneroid valves in series within a sealed metal block, the oscillotonometer. This provided a visual measure of systolic, diastolic, and mean arterial pressures displayed on a dial, connected by levers to an aneroid gauge.

- Advantages – simple and well-established. Do not require sophisticated equipment or power supplies. Encourage patient contact
- Disadvantages – dependent on operator technique and require manual intervention

AUTOMATED OCCLUSIVE CUFF METHODS (OSCILLOMETRY)

Oscillometry is the most common method of automatic blood pressure measurement in clinical practice. It is a development of von Recklinghausen's oscillotonometer. The accuracy of blood pressure measurement has been improved by coupling the rate of cuff deflation to heart rate. A single occlusive cuff is employed using a dual sensing connection, which replaces the double cuff of the oscillotonometer. A pneumatic pump periodically inflates the cuff to a point 25–30 mmHg above the systolic pressure and allows air to escape through a bleed valve producing controlled deflation (about 2–3 mmHg/s). Vibrations of the arterial wall produce pressure transients that are transmitted via a sensing channel to an electrical transducer in the apparatus. The data is then analysed by a microprocessor. Using algorithms that relate the rate of change of pressure transient amplitude to blood pressure, systolic, diastolic, and mean arterial pressures are calculated. The effects of electrical noise are reduced by comparing successive arterial pulsations as the cuff pressure decreases. If these do not correlate the data is rejected.

Systolic pressure corresponds to the point where the amplitude of pulsations is increasing, and is about 25–50% of maximum. Diastolic pressure, corresponds to the point where the amplitude of pulsations has declined to 80% of the maximal pulse amplitude. Mean arterial pressure is the maximum amplitude point.

- Advantages – principal advantages of these instruments is that they free the operator's hands, allowing measurements to be obtained conveniently when access to the patient is difficult, allow calculation of the mean arterial pressure, provide alarm capabilities, and the capacity for data transfer
- Disadvantages – while correlating fairly well with invasive measurements, they are less accurate at extremes of blood pressure (will over read at low pressures, and under read at high pressures), and

should not be regarded any more accurate than manual techniques. All these instruments assume the presence of a regular cardiac cycle, when absent, e.g. atrial fibrillation, blood pressure measurements become inconsistent. The automatic cuff increases the risk of underlying tissue damage (in the elderly, particularly when the frequency of measurement is high, and the instrument is used for prolonged periods). Incorrect cuff placement may be responsible for nerve entrapment injuries, i.e. the ulnar nerve at the elbow

PENAZ TECHNIQUE

In oscillometry blood pressure measurement relies on gradual deflation of a cuff, which limits the frequency of measurement. To overcome this limitation, Penaz first described a continuous non invasive technique in 1973. This monitors the diameter of the digital artery using an infrared plethysmograph, which is mounted in a pneumatic cuff. The infrared signal responds to arterial dilation and contraction during each cardiac cycle. By using a pump servo-controlled by the infrared signal, the infrared signal is maintained constant, at a value corresponding to mean arterial pressure, by inflating and deflating the cuff. Thus, as the artery dilates in systole cuff pressure is increased, and as arterial diameter reduces during diastole, cuff pressure decreases. This duplicates the arterial pressure waveform in the cuff, which is then displayed on the machine.

- Advantages – method provides a record of the changing trends in blood pressure, and in patients with normal, or vasodilated fingers, correlates well with invasive methods
- Disadvantages – results are less reliable in patients with peripheral vascular disease. Small differences in cuff positioning or tightness result in significant changes in the measured pressure. These measurements display a downward drift because of relocation of tissue fluid, necessitating repeated calibration. When used for > 20–30 min, the cuff causes discomfort. If peripheral blood flow is poor, there is the potential for vascular occlusive damage

DOPPLER ULTRASOUND

Employs an encapsulated array of transducer crystals that can transmit and receive ultrasound waves. These are coupled to the skin by a layer of silicone gel (preventing excessive reflection), and positioned directly over the artery. Movements in the arterial wall caused by pressure transients as they pass beneath the cuff cause Doppler shifts in the frequency of the transmitted ultrasound waves. The amplitude of the shift provides a measure of the systolic and diastolic pressures.

- Advantages – can be used for patients of all ages
- Disadvantages – requires the accurate positioning of the transducers, and the use of the correct ultrasound coupling medium. The signals are prone to movement artefact, and are distorted by diathermy and arrhythmias

Sources of error in indirect methods

In comparison with direct methods of blood pressure measurement (the 'Gold Standard'), indirect methods tend slightly to under read, with the diastolic pressure showing the greatest degree of variability. The sources of error include:

- Detection of Korotkov sounds, which are complex with a large proportion of the sound energy being below the audible range. This reduces sound transmission to the observer. In addition, observer detection of the sounds will be dependent on aural acuity. The generated sounds are flow dependent and, thus, factors affecting flow can introduce inaccuracy (e.g. in high output states, and post exercise, Phase V may not occur)
- Cuff size – width of the cuff effects the measured value of blood pressure; too narrow, then there is a tendency to over estimate, too wide, then there is a tendency to under estimate. As a consequence, there have been efforts to standardise the widths of blood pressure cuffs. The World Health Organisation (WHO) recommends that adult cuffs should be 14 cm wide, and should cover two-thirds of the length of the upper arm, or its width should be 20% greater than the diameter of the arm. Suggested widths are shown in Figure CM.18
- Zero and calibration errors, particularly in aneroid devices
- Pneumatic leaks

RECOMMENDED CUFF WIDTHS FOR DIFFERENT AGES

Age (years)	Cuff width (cm)
Adult	12–14
4–8	9
1–4	6
Neonate	2–5

Figure CM.18

- Speed of deflation – when too fast, then there is insufficient time to detect audible change

Direct method (intra-arterial pressure monitoring)

Provides an invasive, continuous measure of blood pressure by beat-to-beat reproduction of the arterial pressure waveform. It is particularly useful in the following situations:

- Cardiovascular instability
- Where blood pressure manipulation is required (inotropes or vasodilators)
- Where non invasive blood pressure measurement is likely to be difficult and/or inaccurate (obesity)

The method requires the insertion of a short parallel-sided cannula into an artery. A continuous flow of either saline or heparinised saline at rates between 1 and 4 ml/H is used to reduce clot formation in the cannula. The cannula is connected by a short length of narrow bore, non compliant plastic tubing containing saline to a pressure transducer, which is usually of the piezoresistive strain gauge type. More recently, catheter tip pressure transducers have been developed but remain comparatively expensive. The piezoresistive strain gauge produces a low amplitude signal requiring signal processing before analysis and display.

The design of an intra-arterial pressure monitoring system must take into account the following considerations:

- The frequency and phase shift responses of the system has to be adequate to allow good reproduction of the arterial signal. An approximate guide is that acceptable accuracy requires a frequency response extending to 8–10 times the maximum heart rate expected. In man, the most important information is contained within the frequency range 0–20 Hz. The system can, thus, be designed to have an upper cut-off frequency > 20 Hz
- The transducer and connecting tubing should be chosen to avoid natural frequencies or resonances occurring within the desired frequency response. Mechanical resonances due to the properties (compliance and inertial elements) of the transducer and column of saline in the connecting tubing, can be shifted above the desired cut-off frequency by reducing the diameter of the connecting tubing
- Components must also be chosen to provide the optimum degree of damping. Usually 'critical damping' is aimed for but since frequency response, phase shift response and damping requirements

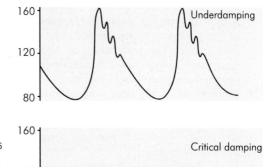
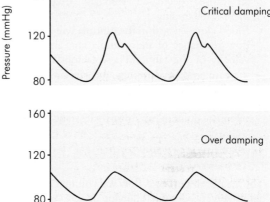

Figure CM.19 Measurement system damping

may conflict a compromise may have to be arrived at. It is important to be able to recognise abnormal levels of damping to interpret the arterial waveforms appropriately. Figure CM.19 illustrates the effect of damping on arterial pressure waveforms

- Advantages – provides a continuous display of the pressure wave form, providing an immediate assessment of blood pressure which is regarded as the 'Gold Standard'
- Disadvantages – cannulation can be difficult, particularly in low-output states, and may require consideration of multiple sites before success. Disconnection: if unrecognised this may result in serious blood loss and, in the extreme, exsanguination. Infection is particularly relevant in cases of prolonged use. Distal vascular insufficiency may result directly from cannulation, or arise from subsequent thrombosis of the cannulated artery. This risk is increased by insufficient collateral circulation, which should always be checked before cannulation. Emboli (air or thrombus) can cause distal vascular occlusion

Sources of error in arterial pressure monitoring

- Air bubbles – a recording system with a high resonant frequency and critical damping is preferable. Standard pressure transducers have a natural frequency of about 100 Hz, but the addition of the connecting tubing, tap and cannula markedly reduces this. The presence of air bubbles in the system also decreases the resonant frequency of the system and increases the damping

- Catheter wall compliance – if compliant tubing is used to connect the cannula and transducer it will distend with the pulse wave, and like the presence of air causes decreased resonant frequency and increased damping
- Blood clots – if within the cannula will increase the flow resistance of the cannula and also the flow velocity of the saline. These factors also tend to increase system damping and decrease resonant frequency
- Zero point – it is important to choose a zero reference point to minimise hydrostatic errors

MEASUREMENT OF GAS FLOW

The measurement of gas flow and volumes is applied in clinical practice for the following uses:

- To test pulmonary function in patients
- To monitor gas flows in anaesthetic machines
- To monitor respiratory flows and tidal volumes in patient breathing circuits

Devices used in pulmonary function testing are outlined below.

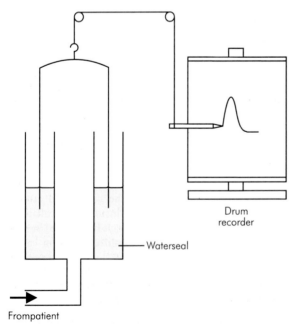

Figure CM.20 Benedict–Roth Spirometer

BENEDICT–ROTH SPIROMETER

Consists of a light bell that traps a closed volume of air over water. The subject breathes in and out of this trapped gas causing the bell to rise and fall following the inspired and expired volumes. A sensor or pen coupled to the bell, traces its movement giving a spirometric trace from which gas flow rates and lung volumes can be derived (Figure CM.20). This device is relatively large in size and not portable.

VITALOGRAPH

Records expiratory flow rates and volumes by collecting expired gas from the subject in a bellows. A recording pen is coupled to the bellows tracing an expired volume graph (Figure CM.21). It is more portable than the Benedict–Roth Spirometer but only measures forced expiratory volumes and flows. The results obtained are also very dependent on subject technique.

WRIGHT RESPIROMETER

Another continuous volume recorder that has been designed specifically for clinical application. It operates by using the gas flow to drive a spinning vane (and is, thus, a type of anemometer), which is coupled by clockwork gears to the display dials. The total volume that can be recorded is 1000 litres, and like the dry gas meter its accuracy and reliability is dependent on the mechanical quality of its clockwork mechanism. It can only measure unidirectional flow but has the advantages of being small, portable and requires no power supply. Flow rates can only be derived by averaging recorded volumes over time and, thus, the device is labelled 'inferential' (Figure CM.22).

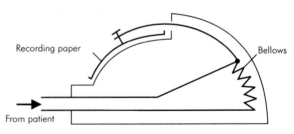

Figure CM.21 Vitalograph

DRY GAS METER

Based on the gas meters used for measuring domestic gas consumption. It measures large volumes of gas by continually feeding the gas flow into a pair of

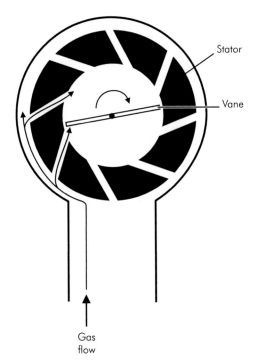

Figure CM.22 Cross section of a Wright Respirometer

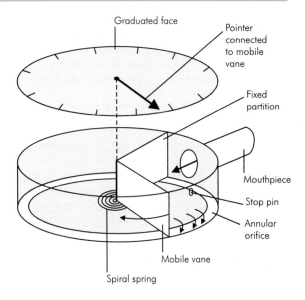

Figure CM.23 Exploded diagram of a peak flow meter

reciprocating bellows. As each bellows fills alternately, its movement records an increase in volume by a clockwork counter and operates inlet and exhaust valves to direct the gas flow through the machine. In this way the flow of very large volumes (10^6 litres) of gas can be measured, compared with the several litres capacity of the closed volume spirometers. However, average flow rates can only be estimated over time, and cannot be measured directly.

ELECTRONIC VOLUME METER

Here the spinning vane mechanism described in the Wright Respirometer is adapted to give an electronic signal. One method uses a fixed blade stator to create a spiral flow to drive the blades of the vane. The spinning blades interrupt a light signal from light-emitting diodes (LED), which is then picked up by photoelectric cells. These provide an electrical signal that can be processed and calibrated to give volume measurements. This device has the advantages of being free from the mechanical errors associated with clockwork mechanisms, and is able to measure volumes from bi-directional (inspiratory and expiratory) flow. It does, however, require a power supply, signal processing and display unit.

PEAK FLOW METER

This device records the maximum expiratory flow of a patient by using the expired gas to operate a shutter controlling a variable orifice through which the gas escapes to the atmosphere. The greater the expiratory flow the larger the orifice opened up by the shutter. The displacement of the shutter is non returnable and is recorded by a pointer which, thus, records the maximum expiratory flow reached (Figure CM.23).

GAS FLOW MEASUREMENT IN ANAESTHETIC MACHINES

Rotameter

Gas flows from an anaesthetic machine into a ventilator or patient circuit are most commonly measured using rotameters. The rotameter is a variable orifice flowmeter in which the gas flow to be measured is passed upwards through a vertically mounted glass (or plastic) tube. This tube has a tapering internal diameter, wider at the top and narrower at the bottom. Gas flow through the rotameter is controlled by a needle valve at the bottom.

A bobbin with a smaller diameter than the internal diameter of the rotameter tube, acts as a pointer, and is moved up or down the tube by the force of the gas flow as it increases or decreases. The bobbin may vary in design, but the most common type is shaped like a 'spinning top' with spiral grooves cut in the sides causing it to spin in the gas flow. The spin reduces friction and sticking of the bobbin. Readings on this type of bobbin are taken from the top edge.

When the gas flow is steady the bobbin settles at a point where the force of the gas flow acting on it and passing round it equals the bobbin weight. At high flows the bobbin is near the top of the rotameter and the cross-section of the annular space around the bobbin, is greater than at low flows, when the bobbin is near the bottom of the rotameter and the orifice cross-section is small.

GAS FLOW PATTERN IN A ROTAMETER

The pattern of gas flow through a rotameter is a mixture of turbulent and laminar flow, due to the flow conditions as the gas passes the bobbin (Figure CM.24). When the cross-sectional area open to flow is small, i.e. the bobbin is near the bottom of the rotameter, flow past the bobbin likens to flow in a 'tube'. This is because the cross-sectional area open to flow is small and a 'tube' in this context is defined by having a diameter < length. In this case flow is laminar and gas viscosity is the main determinant of flow. When the bobbin is near the top of the rotameter at high flows, the annular cross-sectional area open to flow is large. Flow here is similar to that through an 'orifice', an orifice being defined by having a diameter > length. In this case flow is turbulent and density

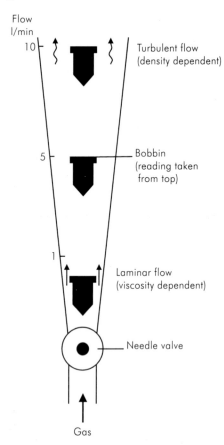

Figure CM.24 Working principles of a rotameter

becomes the most important gas property determining flow. The importance of the flow pattern is that because the viscosities and densities of gases can differ significantly (e.g. oxygen and helium have similar viscosities but their densities are 1.33 and 0.17 kg/m³), a rotameter can only be calibrated accurately for a specific gas or mixture.

- Advantages – simple design and reliable, does not require power supply, no signal transmission path, conditioning unit or display to go wrong
- Disadvantages – only calibrated for specific gas under standard pressure and temperature conditions. Actually part of the gas circuit; therefore, failure may be hazardous, and sensitive to circuit changes downstream

FEATURES OF THE ROTAMETER BLOCK

Rotameters on an anaesthetic machine are arranged in an array, a different one for each gas. Different arrangements exist, but it is desirable for oxygen to enter the common flow last. In the design of the array, certain features need to be considered for increased safety:

- If the first gas to enter the flow line is oxygen (Figure CM.25a), it can leak from the breakage of any subsequent rotameter, potentially giving rise to a hypoxic gas mixture. Thus, the order of gases entering the flow line can increase the risk of hypoxia, and theoretically the safest position for oxygen would be last in order of entering the common flow (Figure CM.25b). Changes in the rotameter order would, however, bring its own risks and, thus, internal channelling is used to separate the individual gas flows. Thus, even when the oxygen control knob is **first** in order channelling can ensure that oxygen is the **last** gas to enter the flow line (Figure CM.25c)
- The oxygen control can be mechanically linked to other gases to prevent hypoxic mixtures being selected
- Positioning vaporisers at the outlet of the rotameters can increase the pressure in the rotameters and, thus, affect their calibration since the density of the gases becomes altered

GAS FLOW MEASUREMENT IN BREATHING CIRCUITS

Pneumotachograph

The pneumotachograph obtains a signal (dependent on the gas flow) by the use of a pneumotachograph head, which is inserted into the breathing circuit, or

(a)

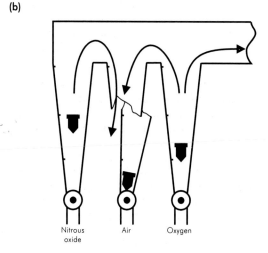

Oxygen   Air   Nitrous oxide

(b)

Nitrous oxide   Air   Oxygen

(c)

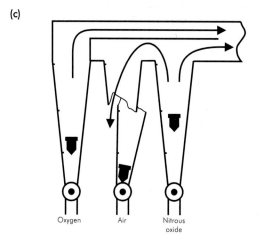

Oxygen   Air   Nitrous oxide

Figure CM.25 Rotameter block faults

through which a patient can breathe directly during pulmonary function testing. Common types of pneumotachograph heads are:

- Fixed resistance, where the signal is a differential pressure signal produced by gases flowing through a fixed flow resistance. These include the screen and Fleisch heads
- Hot wire – a low signal is produced by the gas flow cooling a heated resistance wire
- Pitot tube, in which the flow signal is dependent on the pressure difference between dynamic and static pressures in the centre of the pneumotachograph head

The flow signal is passed to a signal conditioning unit from which it can be analysed and displayed. Tidal volumes are calculated by integrating the flow signal over the duration of inspiration or expiration. Linearity of a pneumotachograph head signal is important in making calibration and calculation of volumes easier. Flow should be corrected for changes in gas mixture. Correction will include gas **viscosity** if flow is laminar, but gas **density** for turbulent flow.

SCREEN PNEUMOTACHOGRAPH

The most commonly used design consisting of a short connector with a gauze screen mounted across the middle, through which the gas flows (Figure CM.26a). The diameter of the head must be large enough to ensure laminar flow through the screen. The screen acts as a flow resistance and produces a small pressure drop across it. This pressure drop is sampled by a pair of pressure ports, one on either side of the screen, which feed the differential pressure to a differential pressure transducer. The pressure transducer produces a small electrical signal for conditioning, analysis and display. This pneumotachograph head is linear over a wide range and of a convenient size but turbulence may be produced at high flow rates.

FLEISCH PNEUMOTACHOGRAPH

The pneumotachograph head passes the flow through an array of fine bore ducts to ensure laminar flow over a wide range (Figure CM.26b). It is larger and bulkier than the screen head.

HOT WIRE PNEUMOTACHOGRAPH

In this device two 'hot' wires are used mounted at right angles to each other, across the lumen of the pneumotachograph head. The hot wires are resistive wires heated by a controlled current passing through them. The gas flow produces cooling of the wires which is dependent on the flow rate, which in turn

(a) Screen

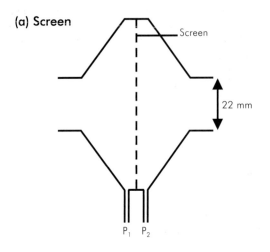

(b) Fleisch

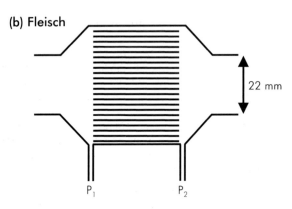

(c) Pitot

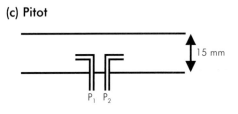

$P_1 - P_2 =$ differential pressure

Figure CM.26 Pneumotachograph heads

varies their resistance giving a small electric signal. Disadvantages are limited frequency response and the requirement for a stabilised power supply.

MODIFIED PITOT TUBE PNEUMOTACHOGRAPH

This device is based on the Pitot tube, which is used to measure local gas speed (as in an aircraft air speed gauge. It consists of a connector with two small diameter (1–2 mm) pressure sampling tubes mounted axially in the centre of the gas flow path the open ends

of these tubes acting as pressure sampling ports (Figure CM.26c). One sampling port faces downstream and one upstream. The downstream port measures the 'static' pressure. The upstream port gives a 'total' pressure reading, which is greater than the static pressure, since gas impacts on the port creating an additional pressure ('dynamic' pressure) due to its kinetic energy. The difference between the total pressure and static pressure port is measured by a differential pressure transducer and is dependent on the gas velocity[2]. The pneumotachograph is calibrated for gas flow but is non linear, requiring linearisation in the signal processing unit. It has the advantage of being simple mechanically, small in size (and dead space) and cheap to produce. The flow through this head is turbulent.

MEASUREMENT OF GAS AND VAPOUR CONCENTRATIONS

In the past the analysis of gas concentrations in gas mixtures and blood samples, relied on chemical methods. These were relatively slow, laborious and inaccurate compared with modern methods. They included:

- The Haldane apparatus – a volumetric technique based on gas absorption, which was used to measure component gases in a respiratory gas mixture. Oxygen was absorbed by passage through pyrogallol
- The van Slyke apparatus – a method for the measurement of blood gases. Haemoglobin was released from red cells by inducing rapid haemolysis with saponin. CO_2 was displaced by lactic acid and oxygen displaced by potassium ferrocyanide, enabling volumetric measurements to be made

Gas analysers based on physical principles have largely superceded these chemical methods. These have improved accuracy, they can also provide continuous breath-to-breath measurement, and by generating a proportional electrical signal they facilitate data storage and processing.

GAS ANALYSERS

All modern gas analysers generate electrical signals that are proportional to the concentration of a measured component gas. The signals are small and require signal conditioning to improve accuracy, and compensate for non linearity.

Step response of gas analysers

Gas analysers like many other instruments suffer a finite delay before registering a change in sample composition. This time lag may be measured as:

- Delay time – time from a stepped change in concentration/partial pressure at the sampling site to detection of a 10% increase at the sample chamber. Largely due to the time required for the sample to pass from sampling orifice to the measurement chamber
- Rise time – time required for the display to rise from 10 to 90% of the stepped change in gas concentration/partial pressure at the sampling site
- Response time – time from the gas reaching the sample chamber to the analyser displaying 95% of the final measurement (Figure CM.27)

Types of gas analyser

Gas and vapour analysers can be usefully divided into discrete analysers (extremely accurate), or continuous analysers (less accurate).

Discrete analysers are rarely used in clinical anaesthesia. An example of discrete analysis is provided by gas/liquid chromatography. In this method the unknown gas mixture is injected into a stream of carrier gas (e.g. nitrogen) flowing through a column of liquid coated particles, the 'stationary phase' (e.g. polyethylene glycol). As the gas mixture passes through the column the various component gases are slowed down according to their solubility in the stationary phase liquid, and, thus, appear separated out at the end of the column. On exit from the column the gases are assayed by a method such as infrared absorption, or thermal conductivity detection which yield a series of

peaks corresponding to the component gases. The gases are identified by comparison of the time lags of the different peaks with those for known gas samples, and their concentrations are given by the height of their peaks. This method is very accurate, very sensitive, but expensive, and is usually only used for research purposes.

Continuous analysers include:

- Mass spectrometers
- Infrared absorption
- Polarography
- Galvanic fuel cell
- Ultra violet absorption
- Paramagnetism
- Thermal conductivity

MASS SPECTROMETERS

These instruments can separate complex mixtures of gases. The sample is continuously drawn into the apparatus through a narrow sampling tube. Some of the sample passes into an evacuated steel ionising chamber, where it is ionised by a beam of electrons. The resulting mixture of ions then diffuses through a slit in the chamber, and a negatively charged plate accelerates them. These charged ions are then separated to give a spectrum (Figure CM.28). There are two methods of separating the ions based on magnetism and mass:

1. Magnetic sector method – the ions, once accelerated are deflected by a strong magnetic field,

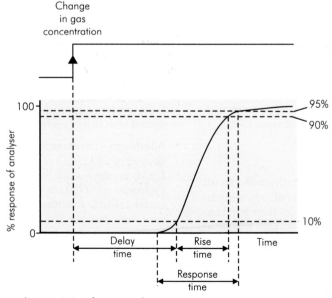

Figure CM.27 Response characteristics of a gas analyser

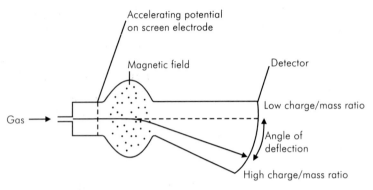

Figure CM.28 Mass spectrometer

which separates out different particle streams according to mass and charge. Each of the deflected ion streams is then measured at a different detector plate. The number of detector plates (usually four to six) determines the number of gases that can be measured. As most ions have the same charge, separation mainly depends on molecular mass

2. Quadrupole method – the spectrometer despite possessing only one detector can measure up to eight different species of particle. The ions reach the detector through a passage formed by four steel rods, the quadrupole. These rods are energised by a radio-frequency signal, which enables them selectively to allow ions with a specific mass to pass through to the detector. The quadrupole signal can be varied to scan for ions of different masses, thus producing a sequential assay for different gases. The mass range is less than that of a magnetic sector spectrometer, and the use of a single shared detector makes it less accurate

- Advantages – versatile, allowing measurement of a variety of component gases in a mixture with a rapid response time (< 0.1 s). The presence of water vapour can interfere with sample measurement and prolong the rise time. For this reason many mass spectrometers incorporate a correction for the presence of water vapour
- Disadvantages – needs complex equipment with high capital, installation and maintenance costs

INFRARED (IR) ABSORPTION

A molecule composed of two or more dissimilar atoms will absorb IR light. Absorption of wavelengths between 2.5 and 25 μm will cause covalent bonds to bend and vibrate, increasing the molecule's rotational speed. Different gas molecules absorb specific wavelengths of IR light. Thus, by detecting increased absorption at particular frequencies gases can be identified and their concentrations determined. These instruments can be classified as:

- Dispersive – usually multiple gas analysers where the radiation from the IR source is split and delivered to the sample sequentially, e.g. IR spectrophotometer
- Non dispersive – single gas analysers where only one wavelength is used, e.g. the capnograph specifically used for CO_2 (Figure CM.29)

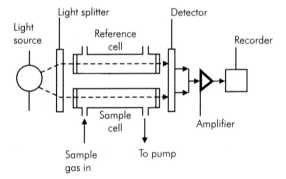

Figure CM.29 Infrared absorption gas analyser

The most frequently used IR gas analyser is the IR spectrophotometer. Modern machines use specific LED to split the IR irradiation into different wavelengths. The sample chamber is trans illuminated, and the absorption of IR radiation measured and compared with that of a reference chamber.

- Advantages – fast enough to follow breath-to-breath changes of CO_2, N_2O and volatile anaesthetics
- Disadvantages – as the response time increases with molecular size (250 ms for CO_2, increasing to 750 ms for a volatile anaesthetic agent), rapid respiratory rates may decrease the accuracy of end tidal and inspiratory volatile agent concentrations

ULTRA VIOLET (UV) ABSORPTION

Some gases composed of similar atoms will not absorb IR radiation (O_2, H_2, N_2), but will absorb UV light (as will halogenated vapours). These molecules all possess characteristic UV absorption spectra, absorbing light of very short wavelength. The only clinical analyser based on this method measures halothane, with a quoted accuracy of 0.2% over the range 0–5%.

- Advantages – acceptable accuracy
- Disadvantages – absorbed quanta are of sufficient energy as to disrupt the molecule, producing toxic breakdown products, which cannot be returned to the breathing circuit unless passed through soda-lime. The response time is slow, > 1 s

PARAMAGNETISM

Molecules can be either paramagnetic (attracted towards a magnetic field) or diamagnetic (repelled by a magnetic field). Paramagnetic molecules possess two unpaired electrons spinning in the same direction in the outer electron shell (e.g. oxygen). The Pauling analyser uses the ability of oxygen to distort a non homogeneous magnetic field as the basis to detect the presence of oxygen in a gas mixture. The analyser consists of a cell with a sealed glass dumb bell (containing nitrogen, a weakly diamagnetic gas) and a mirror, suspended by wires (but free to rotate) between the poles of a magnet. The paramagnetic effect of oxygen displaces the dumb bell causing it and the mirror to rotate. The degree of rotation of both dumb bell and mirror is proportional to the concentration of oxygen present in the mixture. By reflecting a beam of light off the suspended mirror, the degree of rotation can be detected using a photocell. The resulting electrical signal, after processing provides a measure of oxygen concentration. No other gases of clinical interest have this property (Figure CM.30).

Various modifications have been made to the basic design to compensate for external vibration, excessive gas flow rates, and pressurisation of the cell.

- Advantages – commercial versions of this type of analyser are compact, relatively cheap, and remain unaffected by other common gases
- Disadvantages – slow response times (5–20 s), mainly the result of large sample chambers

THERMAL CONDUCTIVITY

A gas with a high thermal conductivity will conduct heat more readily than one with a low conductivity (i.e. in comparison with air, CO_2 has 35% conductivity, whereas helium has 600%). This is the basis of instruments known as katharometers. When a gas is passed over a heated wire, the wire is cooled to a temperature that depends on the temperature of the gas, its flow rate and the thermal conductivity of the gas.

The fall in wire temperature causes a decrease in electrical resistance. This fall in resistance is used to produce a small signal related to gas concentration, by connecting the wire as one arm of a Wheatstone bridge circuit. These analysers have been used mainly to measure CO_2 and helium concentrations, and have also found use in gas chromatography systems.

- Advantages – relatively simple and inexpensive technology
- Disadvantages – slow response times (about 5 s) unless operated at low pressure (100 mmHg)

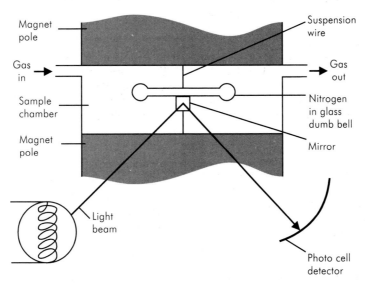

Figure CM.30 Pauling type of paramagnetic analyser

ELECTROCHEMICAL METHODS

These methods are based on an electrochemical reaction in buffer solution occurring between two electrodes and involving dissolved gas molecules. There are two main devices:

- Polarographic electrode – consists of a pair of electrodes of specific materials (depending on the gas being measured) in an electrolyte solution. When these electrodes are maintained at a potential difference, a current is produced between them through the electrolyte solution, which is dependent on the concentration of the gas in solution. In this device the reaction is driven by the voltage applied to the electrodes
- Fuel cell – effectively a primary cell (as in a battery) consisting of two electrodes of specific materials, in an electrolyte solution, that generates its own current through the solution due to the potential difference produced between the electrodes. Again the current in the solution is dependent on the dissolved gas concentration. This device drives the reaction itself, by the current it generates, but ultimately the reagents in the cell will be used up, and the reaction will cease. Hence, the name 'fuel cell'

Other methods of gas analysis

Several other physical properties have been used as the basis for analysers notably:

- Solubility – the basis of the Drager Narkotest®, which measures the effect of different concentrations of various volatile anaesthetic agents (cyclopropane, methoxyflurane, halothane, diethyl ether) on the length of four bands of silicon rubber. There is a linear relationship between the concentration of the volatile agent, and the measured length of the rubber bands. Measurements require correction for the presence of nitrous oxide
- Density – basis for the Waller chloroform balance. A sealed glass bulb filled with air is counterbalanced with a small weight in a gas tight chamber. If a gas with a density greater than air is introduced into the chamber, there is an apparent decrease in the weight of the glass bulb. This reduction in weight is proportional to the difference in densities between air, and vapour/air mixture, and can be used as the basis to calculate the amount of volatile agent present
- Refractive index – the difference in the velocity of light passing through a vacuum and through a transparent substance/gas determines the refractive index of that substance. The measured delay in the passage of light through a gas is dependent on the number of molecules present. The Rayleigh Refractometer, measures this transmission delay. If the refractive index of the gas is known, it is possible to calculate gas concentration
- Velocity of sound – when a gas oscillates at a particular frequency, its structure will begin to resonate. The resonance depends on the velocity of sound in the gas mixture, which is in turn a function of gas composition
- Raman light scattering – when a photon of light passes through a gas, it gives up a portion of its energy to the gas molecule. This is then re-emitted at a longer wavelength characteristic to that gas

Sources of error in gas and vapour measurements

Gas sampling errors can arise when sampling gases from a breathing circuit due to:

- Contamination – gas samples can become contaminated with secretions, debris, or water vapour
- Poor gas mixing – significant concentration gradients may occur in a circuit and be sustained by laminar flow conditions giving anomalous results
- Altered vapour pressure – significant temperature gradients occur between inspired and expired gases, which can alter the vapour pressure in the sampled gas
- Altered pattern of flow at the sampling point – excessive sampling rates can cause local flow and gas concentrations to change at the sampling point
- Variation in absolute pressure – pressure may vary from point to point in a circuit, which can give rise to different results depending on the location of the sample site

Instrument errors. A major source of instrument sampling error is the 'ram-gas effect'. The flow velocity of gas as it enters the sampling port can alter sample composition. This effect can be reduced by using lower sampling rates, and ensuring that the sampling port is set at right angles to the main gas flow.

Patient errors. Chronic lung disease can lead to increased non homogeneity of the alveolar time constants throughout the lung. This results in a corresponding variation of alveolar gas composition between different lung units. Thus, expiratory gas samples may not be representative of lung performance as a whole.

OXYGEN MEASUREMENT

Oxygen measurements in arterial blood can be made using various parameters including gas tension (PaO_2), blood oxygen content (CaO$_2$) and haemoglobin oxygen saturation (SaO$_2$).

These parameters are all related to each other in the oxygen dissociation curve. Current measurement techniques can be applied either 'in vitro', i.e. remote from the patient using samples of gases or blood collected from the patient; or alternatively they can be applied directly to the patient, enabling 'in vivo' measurements to be made. The 'in vivo' measurements usually employ the same basic technology as the 'in vitro' methods, but have been adapted to provide immediate bedside results.

IN VITRO MEASUREMENTS OF OXYGEN CONCENTRATIONS

Measurement in gas mixtures

Can be done using the following methods, which have been previously described:

- Paramagnetic analysers – have slow response times due to their large sample chambers which limits their practical use
- Mass spectrometers – although versatile, with a rapid response, these instruments are too complex and expensive for widespread use

Measurement in blood samples

This is almost universally done using electrochemical methods and forms the basis for both in vitro and in vivo techniques. The two most common techniques already mentioned above are the polarographic electrode and the galvanic fuel cell.

These devices are based on the electrochemical reduction of oxygen at a cathode, using electrons generated at the anode. For each molecule of O$_2$ reduced, four electrons move between the electrodes. This generates an electrical current that is proportional to the concentration of oxygen present in the sample. Application of Henry's Law (the number of molecules in solution is proportional to the partial pressure) enables the partial pressure of oxygen to be calculated from the current measured.

OXYGEN ELECTRODE (POLAROGRAPHIC ELECTRODE, CLARKE ELECTRODE)

This comprises a gold or platinum cathode and silver/silver chloride anode in a potassium chloride electrolyte solution, both covered by an oxygen permeable membrane. A polarising DC voltage of 0.6 V is applied and maintained between the electrodes (Figure CM.31). Electrons are produced by the

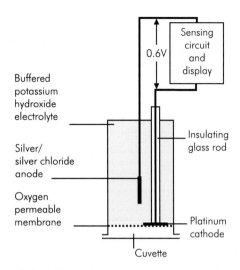

Figure CM.31 Clarke electrode

silver/silver chloride anode, and migrate to the cathode to reduce oxygen molecules as given below:

$$O_2 + 2H_2O + 4e^- \rightarrow 4(OH)^-$$

The current flow between the electrodes is measured by a galvanometer.

The membrane covering the electrodes serves to protect the cathode from protein deposition, which increases with applied voltage, reduces the available electrode surface area, and reduces the localised depletion of oxygen that can occur around the cathode. However, although this membrane prolongs electrode life it also increases response time of the electrode.

Initially the generated current increases with applied voltage until it reaches a plateau, where no further increase occurs in spite of increasing the applied voltage. The plateau value is the point where the rate of oxygen reduction has become the limiting factor, and is proportional to the oxygen concentration in the sample.

- Advantages – robust, and can be battery powered, making it portable
- Disadvantages – limited life span, the silver anode of the silver/silver chloride electrode being eventually consumed by the current

GALVANIC FUEL CELL

This is analogous to the primary cell of a battery, it is composed of a silver cathode, lead anode, and a molar potassium bicarbonate buffer solution (Figure CM.32). The electronegativity of the electrode metals produces a redox reaction at the cathode, reducing oxygen molecules in solution. This reaction is

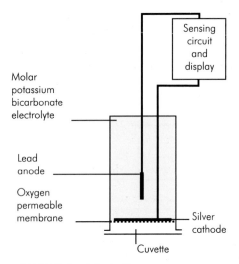

Figure CM.32 Galvanic fuel cell

essentially the same as in the oxygen electrode. Thus, a self generated current is produced in between the electrodes which is dependent on the concentration of dissolved oxygen. No polarising voltage is necessary. The redox reaction occurring at the cathode, however, is temperature-sensitive and the cell reagents will be consumed as in the Clarke electrode.

- Advantages – compact, and unaffected by the presence of N_2O, does not require a power supply
- Disadvantages – relatively slow response time, too slow to measure breath-to-breath changes. Life span of 6–12 months

Sources of error in electrochemical methods

- Blood gas factor – the measured oxygen values are lower for blood compared with gas samples. This is thought to reflect the delay caused by oxygen diffusion in blood, and the localised depletion of oxygen that occurs at the cathode; this is a consistent effect requiring mathematical correction
- Stability – as these systems utilise a two point calibration (gas containing zero oxygen, and one containing a fixed concentration); calibration drift occurs when protein and lipid deposits build up on the membrane or bubbles form in the electrolyte solution. To prevent this, a combination of regular electrode cleaning and quality control is necessary
- Interference – erroneous effects can result from substances other than oxygen being reduced at the cathode (including N_2O), which can be avoided by specific membrane selection
- Temperature – modern blood gas analysers measure at 37°C. If a patient has a temperature that differs more than 2°C mathematical correction is necessary

IN VIVO MEASUREMENT OF OXYGEN CONCENTRATION

Intravascular oxygen electrodes

This is a bipolar variant of the Clarke electrode in which both the anode and cathode are mounted within a fine tube covered by an oxygen permeable membrane. The whole assembly is small enough to pass through an 18 G cannula (response times vary between 5 and 60 s).

- Advantages – provide a continuous measurement of arterial oxygen tension
- Disadvantages – as for the monopolar variant, the electrode is temperature sensitive, and subject to calibration drift due to protein deposition. Access of oxygen to the cathode is flow dependent, which can introduce error at low blood flow states (largely overcome by using a pulsed polarising current). Rapid response times are only achieved at the expense of poor accuracy at low flow rates

Trans cutaneous oxygen electrodes

These provide a measure of the oxygen that has diffused from capillaries in the dermis of the skin. The electrode comprises a ring shaped anode, a central cathode, and electrolyte solution enclosed by an oxygen permeable membrane. The electrode housing contains a heating element and a thermistor to allow temperature compensation. The whole assembly is held in direct contact with the skin by adhesive tape. Locally heating the skin increases capillary blood flow, improving the correlation between trans cutaneous and PaO_2. Trans cutaneous PO_2 increases with local temperature up to the point where tissue damage occurs, about 44 – 46°C.

- Advantages – useful in neonatal monitoring, particularly in detecting hyperoxia. Response times are a function of diffusion distance, and vary from 10 to 15 s in infants to 45–60 s in adults
- Disadvantages – excessive heating can increase the oxygen diffusion distance (oedema) and eventually lead to burns. Heating also increases skin metabolism, and causes the ODC to shift to the right. Essentially, trans cutaneous PO_2 is a better index of skin oxygen delivery than PaO_2 (correlation between cutaneous and arterial PO_2 is best in infants). Changes in cutaneous PO_2 lag behind changes in PaO_2

Conjuctival oxygen tension electrode

The electrode consists of a ring cathode (gold or platinum), an anode (silver or silver/silver chloride), and a thermistor (for temperature compensation).

These elements are covered by a membrane composed either of silicon oxide or polyethylene, and mounted on an ophthalmic former. This is placed under the eye lid in the conjuctival fornix (local anaesthesia is necessary for the awake patient), and held in place by the orbicularis occuli. Response times are similar to those obtained with trans cutaneous electrodes.

Mass spectrometer

In addition to its in vitro application, the mass spectrometer can also be used as an 'in vivo' analyser. In vivo the mass spectrometer is in direct continuity with the patient either via a intravascular perforated metal catheter covered with a gas permeable membrane, or a trans cutaneous oxygen electrode. The estimated response time varies between 3 and 50s.

Optodes

This method is different from the others described, in that measurement does not depend on the consumption of oxygen. Oxygen will 'quench' the fluorescence of certain dyes. The magnitude of this quenching effect is a function of oxygen concentration. This provides the basis for the technique, which uses an intravascular probe, composed of an optical fibre with a dye coated tip, covered by an oxygen permeable membrane. Sequential illumination of the fibre causes the dye to fluoresce. The intensity of fluorescence is dependent on the concentration of oxygen present at the tip and is measured using a photomultiplier. The inclusion of a thermocouple allows for temperature compensation.

- Advantages – independent of blood flow. Initial results suggest favourable stability and response times
- Disadvantages – probes are expensive and subject to fibrin deposition. In addition, prolonged use may result in the deterioration of the dye making measurements invalid

CARBON DIOXIDE MEASUREMENT

CO_2 is the metabolic end product of the aerobic oxidation of glucose. It is a soluble gas and is an important determinant of tissue pH. CO_2 is transported in the blood either as carbamino-Hb compounds, bicarbonate, or dissolved in solution.

The direct measurement of the partial pressure of CO_2 in arterial blood ($PaCO_2$) can provide information regarding: pH, adequacy of ventilation and metabolic status.

While the indirect measurement of end tidal CO_2 reflects cardiac output, pulmonary blood flow, and can confirm correct endotracheal intubation.

The relationship between CO_2 and pH is described by the Henderson–Hasselbach equation:

$$pH = pKa + \log_{10} \frac{[HCO_3^-]}{[PaCO_2]}$$

An early method of measuring CO_2 levels indirectly, was the Astrup technique, which used pH measurements to derive the PCO_2 level of a sample from a Siggard–Andersen diagram, by interpolation. This technique was time consuming and inaccurate. Modern techniques, measure either arterial or end tidal CO_2 levels. These can be applied in vitro where the measurements are made on blood or gas samples remote from the subject, or in vivo, where the oxygen measurement system is in direct continuity with the patient.

The CO_2 electrode

This technique is used in modern blood gas analysers. It uses two electrodes, a glass pH electrode, and a silver/silver chloride reference electrode, both maintained at 37°C. The glass electrode is covered by a layer of cellophane or Nylon mesh with a thin layer of sodium bicarbonate between the electrode and the covering. Both electrodes are enclosed within a membrane (Teflon or silicon rubber) which while permeable to CO_2, is impermeable to blood cells, plasma, and hydrogen ions (Figure CM.33). Using a two point calibration system, buffers of known CO_2 concentration are used to establish the relationship between pH and CO_2. The system relies on the carbonic acid equilibrium:

$$H_2O + CO_2 \leftrightharpoons H_2CO_3 \leftrightharpoons H^+ + HCO_3^-$$

The diffusion of CO_2 across the membrane causes the equilibrium to shift to the right in accordance with the Law of Mass Action. This generates hydrogen ions and causes a fall in pH, which is proportional to the concentration of CO_2 (0.01 pH units for every 0.1 kPa change in CO_2).

- Advantages – generally regarded as accurate and stable
- Disadvantages – response times are governed by the permeability properties of the membrane, and the rate of conversion of CO_2 into bicarbonate (the rate of reaction can be accelerated by inclusion of the enzyme, carbonic anhydrase). Accuracy depends on membrane integrity, since it is vital to ensure that the only change in pH at the electrode results from

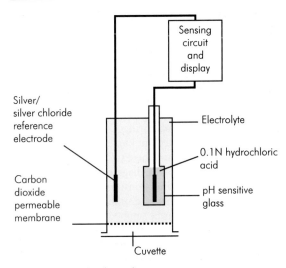

Figure CM.33 CO_2 electrode

the shift in the carbonic acid equilibrium. This can be monitored by measurement of electrical resistance across the membrane

IN VIVO MEASUREMENT OF CO_2 CONCENTRATION

Transcutaneous electrodes

The measurement of transcutaneous CO_2 requires a modification of the basic CO_2 electrode. The electrode is part of a housing, which also contains a heating element and thermistor (for temperature compensation). This is held in direct contact with the skin by adhesive tape. The skin is heated to a temperature between 42 and 44°C. This increases capillary blood flow, CO_2 production in the skin, and CO_2 solubility. As described by Severinghaus, the measured transcutaneous CO_2 is usually greater than arterial CO_2 (PaCO$_2$):

$$\text{Transcutaneous } CO_2 = 1.33 \times PaCO_2 + 0.5 \text{ kPa}$$

• Advantages – gives a continuous measurement of CO_2 concentration in capillary blood
• Disadvantages – risk of skin burns. Response times are slow, and the correlation between transcutaneous and arterial CO_2 is variable

Intravascular probes

Miniaturised versions of the CO_2 electrode have been commercially produced that are small enough to be inserted through an arterial cannula.

Optodes

Similar to the method used to measure oxygen, CO_2 is measured indirectly by recording the change in pH of a buffer, which in turn causes a change in the intensity of fluorescence of a pH-sensitive dye. The intravascular probe is composed of an optical fibre with a dye-coated tip covered by a thin layer of buffer. This is separated from the blood by a CO_2 permeable membrane. Any change in light intensity is proportional to the change in buffer pH, caused by the diffusion of CO_2 across the membrane. Changes in fluorescence are detected by a photomultiplier.

End tidal CO_2 (ETCO$_2$)

ETCO$_2$ measurement is now an established clinical tool. In normal individuals, the ETCO$_2$ usually measures 0.5–0.8 kPa less than the arterial CO_2. The magnitude of this difference increases with respiratory disease, particularly where there is significant ventilation perfusion mismatch. The capnograph provides a continuous display of repeated ETCO$_2$ estimations (Figure CM.34).

The majority of the commercial capnographs are based on infrared spectrophotometry, and can be classified as either 'sidestream' or 'mainstream' monitors according to their sampling system.

Sidestream capnograph

The most common type of capnograph are the sidestream type, where the sample gas is drawn from the main respiratory flow through a side port via a narrow tube to the sample cuvette (flow rates between 50 and 500 ml/min). Following CO_2 measurement, the gas is either returned to the expiratory limb of the breathing circuit (of particular relevance to low flow anaesthesia) or scavenged.

• Advantages – generally more convenient than mainstream monitors; the patient attachment is less bulky, and more robust
• Disadvantages – without elaborate water traps/filters to remove water vapour, the measured value of ETCO$_2$ would be invalid. A suction pump

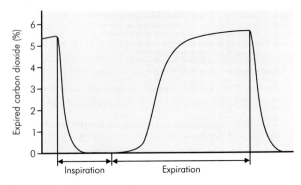

Figure CM.34 Capnograph trace

transfers the sample from the site of sampling to the measurement chamber; this sampling rate can in itself introduce error. The response time of these instruments tends to be longer than mainstream analysers

Mainstream capnograph

In the mainstream capnograph, the measuring head inserts into the breathing or ventilator circuit so that it carries the main gas flow. The capnograph head acts as the sampling chamber, and is trans illuminated by IR light through side windows.

- Advantages – the position of the probe makes removal of a sample of gas from the breathing circuit unnecessary. The system is far less complicated (no suction pump required); the errors due to gas sampling are eliminated. Response times are significantly less than the 'sidestream' type
- Disadvantages – probes are fragile, expensive, heavy, and require support and direct contact with the skin may cause a burn. The sensor window must remain clean to prevent inaccuracy and calibration problems

During anaesthesia the capnograph trace can provide immediate verification of successful tracheal intubation. However, in addition to this, both the shape of the capnogram, and the value of the $ETCO_2$ measurement can reflect clinical changes (Figure CM.35):

MEASUREMENT OF pH

In 1909 Sorenson defined pH as the log to the base 10 of the reciprocal of the hydrogen ion concentration $[H^+]$:

$$pH = -\log_{10} [H^+]$$

Under normal conditions, buffer systems within the body (bicarbonate, phosphate, haemoglobin, and protein) maintain the pH within a narrow range (7.38–7.42). The pH scale can be used as a clinical measure of acid–base status; this has both diagnostic, and therapeutic value. The SI unit of pH is the hydrogen ion concentration expressed as nmol/l.

INDIRECT ESTIMATION OF pH

Because of difficulty in measuring $[H^+]$ directly, blood pH was estimated by derivation from the Henderson–Hasselbach equation:

$$pH = pKa + \log \frac{[HCO_3^-]}{H_2CO_3}$$

or

$$pH = pKa + \log \frac{[HCO_3^-]}{\alpha.PCO_2}$$

where pKa is the equilibrium constant for the dissociation of carbonic acid, and α is the solubility coefficient for CO_2. This method is inaccurate because the values of pKa and α vary with temperature.

pH electrode

To overcome the problems of indirect estimation of pH, a glass electrode was developed to enable measurement of blood pH directly. This method is employed in most modern blood gas analysers. First

CAUSES OF CHANGES IN END TIDAL CO_2 CONCENTRATIONS		
Change	**Cause**	**Diagnosis**
↓ $ETCO_2$	↑ alveolar ventilation	↑ respiratory rate, tidal volume
	↓ CO_2 production	Hypothermia
	↑ Dead space	Pulmonary embolus, shock, hypotension
	Technical error	Calibration error, air contamination
↑ $ETCO_2$	↓ alveolar ventilation	↓ respiratory rate, ↓ tidal volume
	↑ CO_2 production	Sepsis, hyperpyrexia, thyrotoxicosis
	↑ inspired CO_2	Rebreathing, CO_2 added to inspired gases, administration of $NaHCO_3$

Figure CM.35

described in 1933, the glass electrode has been extensively modified to produce what is now a stable, sensitive instrument capable of pH measurement using increasingly smaller volumes of blood. The electrode itself is non selective and will respond to more than one particular anion or cation. Specificity is achieved by enclosing the electrode in a membrane with ion selective permeability; in this way only H^+ ions have access to the electrode.

The actual pH electrode consists of two component electrodes:

- Silver/silver chloride electrode (Ag:AgCl)
- Mercury/mercury chloride electrode ($Hg:Hg_2Cl_2$), calomel

Each component electrode consists of a metal conductor and electrolyte solution, the metal conducts electrons, the electrolyte solution conducts ions. A potential difference or electromotive force (EMF) is generated at the interface of the two electrodes (electrode potential). If the temperature remains constant, the only remaining variable is the pH difference between the inner buffer solution of the electrode, and the sample. A saturated solution of KCl provides a salt bridge that completes the circuit between the sample and second calomel electrode. To minimise diffusion of KCl into the sample, a porous plug is placed at the end of the measurement pathway (Figure CM.36).

As the pH electrode responds to the activity of H^+ rather than concentration, the electrodes must be calibrated using standard solutions of known pH. The pH scale of the electrode depends on the pH of the standard solutions rather than the absolute concentration of H^+. Modern blood gas analysers use two different buffers; the first (pH 6.841) has the same pH as the buffer inside the electrode and is taken as the arbitrary zero. The second buffer (pH 7.383), is used as a reference against which the blood pH is measured.

PULSE OXIMETRY

Oximetry is a spectrophotometric technique (trans illumination of a sample and measurement of absorbed radiation), that measures % haemoglobin saturation (SaO_2). In addition, it can also provide an indirect measure of oxygen tension and content, by use of the oxygen dissociation curve (ODC).

There are two forms of oximetry **transmission** (or absorbance) and **reflectance** oximetry. Of the two techniques, transmission oximetry is the most commonly used for both in vitro and in vivo measurements.

TRANSMISSION OXIMETRY

Basic principles

The absorption of radiation by a layer of solution is determined by a combination of two laws:

- Lambert–Bouguer Law – when a layer of solution of known thickness (d) is trans illuminated by monochromatic light, the transmitted light (I) is related to the incident light (I_O) by

$$I = I_O \, e^{-(ad)}$$

where (ad) is the 'absorbance' or 'optical density' of the layer of solution. This in turn is the product of its thickness (d) and the quantity (a) known as the extinction coefficient of the solution. Thus, if the absorbance of the solution layer is 1.0, only 37% of the light is transmitted, but doubling the absorbance to 2.0 reduces the transmitted light to 13.5%
- Beer's Law – states that for a solution, absorbance is a linear function of molar concentration

Combining the two laws gives the Lambert–Beer Law which relates the transmitted light to both molar concentration and thickness of the solution layer by expressing the absorbance as

$$\text{absorbance} = \varepsilon \, c \, d$$

where: ε is molar extinction coefficient
c is molar concentration
d is thickness.

The Lambert–Beer Law does not describe the in vivo relationship exactly and still requires the use of corrective algorithms before haemoglobin saturation

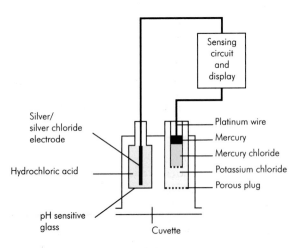

Figure CM.36 pH electrode

can be calculated. To measure the concentration of a particular compound in a mixture, the mixture is trans illuminated with monochromatic light at the wavelength where absorbance is maximal. The machine must be calibrated with a pure solution of the compound, and then the measured concentration can be calculated.

Absorbance curves for HbO_2 and Hb

Absorbance can be plotted against wavelength to give curves for HbO_2 and Hb (Figure CM.37). It can be seen that the absorbance of both compounds is high for shorter wavelengths (< 600 nm) of light since they are both basically red in colour. However, at longer wavelengths in the red region of the electromagnetic spectrum, the absorbance of HbO_2 is less than that of Hb. This gives HbO_2 a brighter red appearance than Hb. At these longer wavelengths, the curves display secondary peaks in absorbance, one at 660 nm for de-oxyhaemoglobin, and one at 940 nm for oxyhaemoglobin.

The Isobestic point is the point at which the absorbances for HbO_2 and Hb are equal, i.e. it is the point at which the absorbance curves cross. It is dependent only on haemoglobin concentration. Some earlier oximeters corrected for haemoglobin concentration using the wavelength at the isobestic points.

Functional saturation

To determine haemoglobin saturation, monochromatic light at the two secondary peak wavelengths (660 nm and 940 nm), must be used to transilluminate the sample. Measurement of the absorbances at these wavelengths enable the concentrations of HbO_2 and Hb to be calculated, and hence the haemoglobin saturation. This saturation measurement is referred to as the 'functional saturation' since it is only based on the principal form of haemoglobin and ignores the presence of minor haemoglobin species such as carboxyhaemoglobin (HbCO), methaemoglobin (HbMet), sulphaemoglobin (HbSul) and foetal haemoglobin (HbF). It is calculated by:

$$\text{functional haemoglobin saturation} = \frac{100 \times [HbO_2]}{[HbO_2] + [Hb]}\%$$

Fractional oxygen saturation

Most co-oximeters measure light absorbance at a minimum of four different wavelengths. This enables measurement of the minor haemoglobin species in addition to the principal forms, oxyhaemoglobin and deoxyhaemoglobin. The more accurate 'fractional saturation' may then be calculated by:

fractional haemoglobin saturation =

$$\frac{100 \times [HbO_2]}{[HbO_2]+[Hb]+[HbCO]+[HbMet]}\%$$

The two most commonly detected minor species of haemoglobin are HbMet, and HbCO which constitute < 1% and < 2% (in non smokers) of the total of Hb concentration respectively. This means that under normal circumstances, it is adequate to measure functional SaO_2.

CO-OXIMETER

This instrument requires haemolysis of the blood sample (either by chemical or physical means), prior to measurement of haemoglobin saturation. It is often incorporated into a blood gas machine.
- Advantages – light absorbance is measured at several different wavelengths enabling fraction saturation estimation
- Disadvantages – unable to provide continuous saturation monitoring, moderately expensive capital cost and maintenance, to obtain fractional saturation which is not normally significantly different from functional saturation

PULSE OXIMETER

A pulse oximeter consists of a peripheral probe and a processing/display unit. The probe contains two LED that trans illuminate the chosen tissue with monochromatic light at red (660 nm) and infrared (940 nm) wavelengths. A photodiode (PD), detects the transmitted light converting it to an electrical signal. The functional haemoglobin saturation (SaO_2) is then

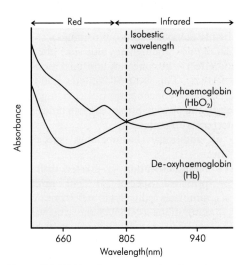

Figure CM.37 Absorbance curves in oximetry

calculated from the signal by the processing unit and displayed. One LED emits red and the other infrared light, but the PD is unable to differentiate between wavelengths. To overcome this problem only one LED trans illuminates at a time, the LED switching on and off alternately. The pulses in the PD signal are then identified in time to give separate values for red and infrared absorbances. Multiple pulses are used in each measurement cycle to minimise any motion artefact and a specific sequence is set up including a period of no trans illumination. This time period when both LED are switched off is used to provide a correction for ambient light conditions.

The trans illumination signal of the pulse oximeter can be divided into two components:

- AC component – a rapidly changing signal that corresponds to the light absorbed during the pulsatile portion of arterial blood flow
- DC component – represents the light absorbed constantly by the resting volume of tissues and arterial blood

The AC component constitutes a small proportion of the total signal, but is the major determinant of accuracy. It ranges from 1 to 5% of the DC component in a normal pulse wave. These signals are processed by the internal algorithm of the device to calculate SaO_2.

Oximeters are calibrated using data previously obtained from human volunteer studies, in which saturations were recorded while the subjects breathed various inspired oxygen concentrations, including hypoxic levels. On ethical grounds, these studies were limited to minimum measured saturations of 80%. As a result, commercial oximeters are most accurate over the saturation range 80–100%. Any saturation values below this level are obtained by extrapolation, and suffer from increasing errors. Even within the normal range, the intrinsic error of some oximeters has been estimated to vary between 0 and 13%.

The response time of the device is particularly important. Prolonged response time can be attributed to:

- Instrumental delay – relating to the averaging time used to reduce movement artefact. Increasing the averaging time prolongs the response time
- Circulatory delay – response time is the time taken for changes in central saturation to reach the peripheral circulation. It varies according to probe site (about 10–15 s for an ear probe; > 60 s for a finger probe). Both cold induced vasoconstriction and venous engorgement can increase response times 2–3-fold

REFLECTANCE OXIMETRY

Used for continuous invasive measurement, i.e. monitoring mixed venous saturation with an oximetric pulmonary artery catheter (OPAC). Light of specific wavelength passes along a fibre optic channel to the tip of the catheter, where it is reflected back up a second channel in the OPAC, by the passing blood. The intensity of the reflected light is measured by a photodiode.

Sources of error in oximetry

- LED – each emit light over narrow spectral range either side of the central or principal wavelength, i.e. 660 or 940 nm. This can vary up to ± 15 nm between LED of the same type introducing an error in the measurement of absorbance and the calculation of SaO_2. Oximeters compensate for this by using internal software
- Ambient light – can be minimised by using shielded probes, and sequential LED cycling
- Low perfusion states – amplitude of the probe signal amplitude depends on tissue perfusion (decreased perfusion reduces signal amplitude). The oximeter attempts to compensate by amplifying the total signal (AC and DC components). This has the effect of making the S/N ratio worse. Under poor conditions the noise may become the predominant signal. When this occurs, the ratio of scaled signals for both 660 and 940 nm approach unity, corresponding to a falsely displayed saturation of 85%. To prevent this happening, modern machines have S/N ratio limits, which if exceeded, will interrupt the display
- Motion artefact – can be reduced by increasing the signal averaging time, but only at the expense of response time. Alternatively some oximeters employ sophisticated internal algorithms which help identify obviously spurious readings
- External dyes – methylene blue has the most dramatic effect – as concentration increases, SaO_2 values decrease. This reduces oximeter readings by up to 65% at a concentration of 2–5 mg/kg for between 10 and 60 min. Some dark nail polishes can also interfere with oximetry
- Effect of additional haemoglobin species on absorbance:
  HbMet – light absorption is greater than both principal species at 940 nm, and simulates reduced Hb at 660 nm. At high saturations (> 85%) the true value is underestimated; at low values (< 85%) it is overestimated
  HbCO – has minimal absorption at 940 nm, but has a similar absorbance to HbO_2 at 660

nm; this results in overestimation of SaO_2

HbF – essentially the same absorption spectra as adult haemoglobin and has no effect on oximetry

HbS – no reported effect on oximetry. It should be noted that in patients with sickle disease there is a shift in the ODC to the right. Thus, for any given PaO_2, the corresponding saturation is less than expected

- Anaemia – there is a linear trend to underestimate SaO_2 as the concentration falls; at haemoglobin levels of 8 g/100 ml this can be 10–15%. Polycythaemia has no effect. Accuracy is less at low saturation levels in anaemic patients
- Diathermy – interference effect largely depends on the particular oximeter. This can be reduced by using suppression filters

NEUROMUSCULAR MEASUREMENT

Neuromuscular measurement is used in for the following applications:

- Assessment of neuromuscular blockade during surgical anaesthesia to guide the use of muscle relaxants
- Identification of the type of neuromuscular blockade present (depolarising, non depolarising, or type II block)
- Localisation of peripheral nerves for regional techniques

METHODS OF NEUROMUSCULAR MEASUREMENT

The basic technique involves two stages. First, the pulsed electrical stimulation of a peripheral motor nerve, and secondly the assessment of the muscular response.

Electrical stimulation of a peripheral nerve

Needle or surface electrodes are located over or close to a peripheral motor nerve.

A standard electrical pulse stimulates the nerve producing a measurable muscle twitch. It should be noted that muscle response is related to delivered current and not applied voltage. The electrical characteristics of the stimulator pulse should include:

- A square wave pulse with a uniform amplitude
- A pulse current amplitude appropriate for the

particular application, i.e. low amplitude (0.5–5.0 mA), for needle electrodes and higher amplitude for skin electrodes (10–40 mA)

- An optimal pulse length of 0.2 ms. This is a result of the compromise between current pulse amplitude and duration of current flow, since excessive values of either increases the risk of neural damage
- Various patterns of pulses, including single or trains of pulses at 1–2 Hz, and tetanic bursts at between 50 and 100 Hz

All currently used nerve stimulators are battery powered and are isolated electrically from all other objects. Skin electrodes are used for intra-operative neuromuscular monitoring and require relatively high current pulse amplitudes. This provides 'supramaximal' stimulation that ensures maximum recruitment of muscle fibres, thus providing a baseline for a control twitch when using relaxants. Peripheral nerve location for local anaesthetic blocks is performed using needle electrodes, insulated except for the needle tips. These stimulate with much lower currents. Dual function stimulators with controls for both neuromuscular monitoring (external mode) and nerve location (internal mode) are now commercially available.

Assessment of neuromuscular blockade

The assessment of muscular response to electrical stimulation provides the basis for neuromuscular monitoring. A variety of methods providing an indirect measure of contractile, force have been employed. These include:

- Vision and touch
- Mechanomyography
- Acceleromyography
- Electromyography

For effective clinical application of neuromuscular blockade monitoring, the method of assessment needs to combine accuracy with practical convenience. When monitoring neuromuscular blockade, it is important to realise that different muscle groups demonstrate different sensitivities to muscle relaxants.

VISION AND TOUCH

The muscle twitch that results from the electrical stimulation is assessed either by observation (i.e. either degree of contraction or a simple count of pulse when using 'train of four'), or by palpation.

- Advantages – simple and convenient
- Disadvantages – inaccurate, and provides only a gross assessment of muscle response

MECHANOMYOGRAPHY

In this method the muscle becomes a force-displacement transducer. A small preload is attached to the muscle to maintain isometric conditions. Electrical stimulation, causes the muscle to contract against the pre load, generating a tension that is proportional to the force of contraction. This 'generated' tension is converted to an electrical signal, which can then be measured. For access and convenience, adductor pollicis is the muscle normally used.

- Advantages – more accurate than 'vision and touch'
- Disadvantages – correct positioning of the transducer, selection of the preload, and immobilisation of the hand, makes this method inconvenient and difficult to maintain

ACCELEROMYOGRAPHY

This method requires careful positioning of a joint, usually a digit, such that the distal end remains free hanging. Electrical stimulation of the appropriate motor nerve causes muscle contraction and movement of the digit. The measured acceleration of the distal part is directly proportional to the force of muscle contraction. By fixing a piezoelectric wafer to the distal part of the digit, it is possible to covert the measured acceleration into an electrical signal which can then be measured.

- Advantages – more objective than 'vision and touch'
- Disadvantages – as with mechanomyography there are problems with joint positioning, which make this technique inconvenient and inconsistent

ELECTROMYOGRAPHY

This measures muscle activity by recording the magnitude of the evoked compound action potentials from either skin or needle electrodes overlying a particular muscle (adductor pollicis or the hypothenar eminence is the most commonly used site). The active electrode is placed over the motor nerve, the indifferent electrode is placed over the tendon insertion.

- Advantages – avoids the mechanical problems of using and calibrating transducers attached to joints
- Disadvantages – simple alteration in hand position can alter electrode geometry sufficiently enough to change the measured response

STIMULATION PATTERNS IN NEUROMUSCULAR MONITORING

Several patterns of current pulses for neuromuscular stimulation, have been developed to improve sensitivity in the monitoring. These are designed to exaggerate specific characteristics of non depolarising muscle blockade, e.g. 'fade' which describes decreased muscle twitch amplitude with repeat stimulation and 'post tetanic facilitation', an increase in the response following tetanic stimulation due to increased mobilisation of acetylcholine. The various stimulation patterns include:

- Single twitch
- Train of four
- Tetanic stimulation
- Post tetanic count
- Double burst

Single twitch

A supramaximal electrical stimulus is delivered at 1 Hz. At this frequency there is sufficient time for complete muscle fibre recovery between stimuli, avoiding any misinterpretation of twitch height arising from fade. The ratio of the measured twitch height after relaxant administration (T_1), to the control twitch height before relaxant (T_c), provides a measure of muscle relaxation. Normal muscle function corresponds to a $T_1:T_c$ ratio = 1.0. This falls steadily to zero as receptor occupancy increases from 75 to 100%, reflecting acetylcholine receptor occupancy at the neuromuscular junction.

- Advantages – useful for assessment of neuromuscular blockade with depolarising relaxants (suxamethonium chloride), where there is neither fade nor post tetanic facilitation
- Disadvantages – limited application due to the narrow range of receptor occupancy detected (i.e. 25%) and the requirement for a means of measuring twitch height, e.g. mechanomyography

Train of four (TOF)

This pattern consists of four identical stimuli delivered at 2 Hz. Non depolarising muscle relaxants cause a reduction in height of the first twitch compared with a pre relaxant supramaximal stimulus, and also a serial reduction in height of the four response twitches. There is a relationship between receptor occupancy and the number of visually detectable twitches (Figure CM.38).

The degree of neuromuscular blockade can be more objectively assessed by calculating the ratio of the fourth (T_4) and first (T_1) measured twitch heights (T_4/T_1). The consensus of opinion is that for adequate respiratory function, the T_4/T_1 ratio must be > 70%.

- Advantages – more sensitive than the single twitch. Gives a quantitative result with simple visual assessment

ACETYLCHOLINE RECEPTOR OCCUPANCY CORRESPONDING TO NUMBER OF TOF TWITCHES DETECTABLE	
Detectable twitches	% Receptor blockade
4	> 75
3	75
2	80
1	90
0	100

Figure CM.38

Normal neuromuscular junction

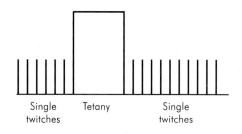

Single twitches   Tetany   Single twitches

Non depolarizing agent present

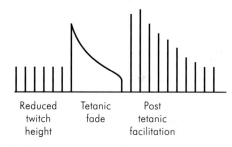

Reduced twitch height   Tetanic fade   Post tetanic facilitation

Figure CM.39 Response patterns after neuromuscular stimulation

- Disadvantages – although more sensitive than the single twitch, TOF remains a basically inaccurate method. The fade of TOF pulses on administration of relaxant does not correlate with the reappearance of TOF pulses during recovery

Tetanic stimulation

The extent of detectable fade following a tetanic stimulation depends on the degree of muscle blockade and the amplitude and duration of the tetanic burst.

By increasing the amplitude of the tetanic burst, it is possible to detect fade at much lower levels of receptor occupancy. A tetanic burst of 50 Hz for 5 s produces a muscle response comparable with a maximal voluntary effort. The absence of fade following this stimulus can be interpreted as the return to full muscle power (Figure CM.39).

- Advantages – can be used to assess neuromuscular blockade at relatively low levels of receptor occupancy
- Disadvantages – cannot quantify receptor occupancy from post tetanic fade. It is an unpleasant sensation in the conscious patient, and leaves an unpleasant sensory aftermath when applied to the unconscious patient

Post tetanic count (PTC)

This pattern is sometimes known as post tetanic potentiation or facilitation. Intense muscle blockade can completely abolish the response to a train of four. Tetanic stimulation increases the mobilisation of acetylcholine (Ach) in the pre synaptic membrane. Subsequent electrical stimulation using twitches at 1 s intervals, releases supranormal concentrations of Ach, sufficient to overcome the effect of non depolarising relaxants. The number of resultant twitches (PTC)

depends on the frequency of the tetanic burst, the amplitude and duration of the burst, and degree of neuromuscular blockade present.

This method can produce a response at relatively high levels of receptor occupancy, and a PTC < 5 indicates profound neuromuscular blockade. A PTC > 15 is at least equivalent to two twitches of a TOF, and at this level, successful pharmacological reversal of the remaining muscle blockade is possible.

Double burst

This variant pattern was introduced to improve the manual assessment of fade. This consists of two tetanic bursts of 50 Hz. Each burst is composed of three tetanic twitches (at 20 ms intervals), the bursts being separated by 750 ms. Muscle response is clinically detected as just two separate twitches (T_1 and T_2). The T_2:T_1 ratio is closely related to the TOF ratio (Figure CM.40).

MEASUREMENT OF DEPTH OF ANAESTHESIA

In 1845, Snow made the first documented attempt to assess anaesthetic depth, describing five levels of ether anaesthesia. This was refined by Guedel during the

Normal neuromuscular junction

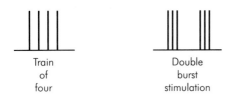

Non depolarising agent present

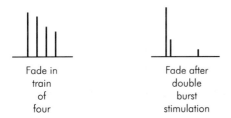

Figure CM.40 Response patterns after double burst stimulation

First World War, who developed the chart classification of ether anaesthesia based on lacrimation, pupil size and position, respiratory pattern, and peripheral movements. Advances in anaesthesia (in particular the introduction of curare soon after the Second World War) made previous classifications obsolete. As a consequence a new system was developed based on the graded assessment of autonomic activity, which includes 'lacrimation', a parameter surviving from Guedel's chart classification. The ideal measuring system for assessing anaesthetic depth would:

- Identify a universally acceptable indicator of conscious awareness
- Translate this measurement into a convenient clinical scale
- Eliminate the risk of conscious awareness

To date no system fulfils any of these criteria.

Clinically applied methods for assessment of anaesthetic depth include the following:

- Tunstall's 'isolated arm' technique – provided a gross visual indicator of inadequate anaesthesia by detecting movement in forearm muscles isolated from the effect of muscle relaxants, by a tourniquet
- Integrated clinical scores (e.g. Evan's score)
- Lower oesophageal contractility
- Frontalis electromyogram

- Electro-encephalogram
- Evoked responses – include auditory-evoked responses (AER), brain stem-evoked responses (BSER), and visual-evoked responses (VER)

INTEGRATED CLINICAL SCORES

The most commonly quoted score is the Evan's or PRST score. This scoring system was designed to assess the elements of autonomic activity; P (systolic blood pressure), R (heart rate), S (sweating) and T (tears). The scoring system is outlined in Figure CM.41.

In practice scores range from 0 to 8, the midpoint of the range is rarely exceeded, reflecting the redundancy within this scoring system.

- Advantages – simple requiring no specialised equipment
- Disadvantages – parameters are not specific for the effects of anaesthesia. Values vary widely among individuals and can be significantly effected by various drugs, and pre-existing disease states

EVAN'S SCORING SYSTEM FOR DEPTH OF ANAESTHESIA		
Parameter	**Measurement**	**Score**
P	< Control + 15	0
	< Control + 30	1
	> Control + 30	2
R	< Control + 15	0
	< Control + 30	1
	> Control + 30	2
S	Nil	0
	Skin moist to touch	1
	Visible beads of sweat	2
T	No excess tears, eye open	0
	Excess tears, eye open	1
	Tear overflow, eye closed	2

Figure CM.41

LOWER OESOPHAGEAL CONTRACTILITY

There are two types of smooth muscle contraction detectable in the lower oesophagus:

- Provoked lower oesophageal contractions (PLOC) – result from sudden distension of the oesophagus, as if due to the arrival of a food bolus. PLOC are induced by the rapid inflation of a balloon catheter in the lower oesophagus. This causes smooth muscle contraction and is detected by a more distally placed pressure transducer. The dose response curve for PLOC is more shallow than that for spontaneous lower oesophageal contractions (SLOC)

- SLOC – arise spontaneously and can be induced by emotion and stress in the awake individual. It is believed that SLOC are under the control of a central oesophageal motility centre, the activity of which is influenced by higher centres. SLOC arise spontaneously, and can be detected by the same pressure transducer

An attempt to improve the available information by combining the measurement of SLOC frequency and PLOC amplitude lead to derivation of the oesophageal contractility index (OCI):

$$OCI = 70 \times (SLOC\ rate + PLOC\ amplitude)$$

- Advantages – easy to interpret, can be used in the presence of muscle relaxants
- Disadvantages – consensus opinion is against this method being a reliable measure of anaesthetic depth

FRONTALIS ELECTROMYOGRAM (FEMG)

The frontalis muscle was chosen for this purpose because it receives both visceral and somatic fibres from the facial nerve, and it is less sensitive than other muscles to the effects of muscle relaxants. The dual nerve supply means that this muscle can be influenced by autonomic activity. Using two surface electrodes compound action potentials from this muscle are recorded.

- Advantages – non invasive, convenient and easy to apply electrodes
- Disadvantages – recording EEG signals poses technical problems due to low amplitude and interference. There is a wide inter-individual variability in measured FEMG

ELECTROENCEPHALOGRAM (EEG)

This method provides a continuous non invasive assessment of cerebral activity. The generated electrical signal is the summated product of excitatory and inhibitory post synaptic activity controlled and paced by subthalamic nuclei. To have any clinical use, these signals require extensive processing. The EEG is a varying voltage signal, with amplitudes between 1 and 500 µV. For the purposes of interpretation, the

FREQUENCY BANDS IN THE EEG SIGNAL

Band	Frequency range (Hz)
α	8–13
β	> 13
δ	< 4
θ	4–7

Figure CM.42

frequency spectrum is divided into four bands (Figure CM.42).

If the EEG frequency spectrum for a patient undergoing deepening anaesthesia is plotted, sequential changes are noted. The EEG of an awake patient has a low amplitude and high frequency. Deepening anaesthesia causes a progressive increase in signal amplitude and reduces frequency. All volatile anaesthetics induce these sequential changes in the EEG signal.

CEREBRAL FUNCTION ANALYSING MONITOR (CFAM)

This device produces a continuous display of an analysed EEG signal from two symmetrical pairs of scalp electrodes. The top trace displayed shows the mean amplitude of the signals plotted in time (within 90% confidence limits), while the bottom traces show the power amplitude in each frequency band. Thus, at any instant the CFAM display shows the overall mean amplitude and relative power in each frequency band (α, β, θ and δ).

COMPRESSED SPECTRAL ARRAY

This system plots sequential segments of the EEG power spectrum, to give a three dimensional picture of power amplitude vertically (y-axis), frequency horizontally (x-axis) and time (z-axis). This creates a three-dimensional plot of 'peaks' and 'valleys' showing how the power spectrum of the EEG changes with the course of time (Figure CM.43).

- Advantages – EEG monitoring reflects cerebral electrical activity rather than peripheral muscular or autonomic function
- Disadvantages – unreliable predictors of depth of anaesthesia. At best they provide a trend of

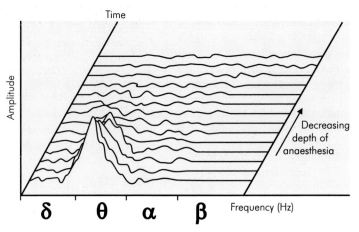

Figure CM.43 Compressed spectral array

information that needs to be combined with clinical observation

Note:

> The EEG represents a general indicator of cerebral perfusion and metabolic activity. Hypoxia, hypotension, cerebral oedema, and metabolic encephalopathy can significantly depress signal output. As such, any change in the character of the EEG signal needs to be interpreted with this in mind, and cannot be entirely attributed to anaesthesia. Interpretation is further complicated in that different anaesthetic agents have different effects on the EEG signal.

EVOKED RESPONSES

These signals are of very low amplitude (1–2 μV) compared with the EEG background trace (10–300 μV) and electrical noise due to neuromuscular activity. They are extracted from the background EEG and noise signal by computer averaging. The signals consist of a series of identifiable peaks and troughs, each with a time delay relative to the stimulus, which is referred to as the latency. The early signal (from 0 to 10 ms) is the 'brainstem response', based on its presumed origin. Signals between 10 and 100 ms are middle latency and contain the early cortical response. Signals beyond this (100–1000 ms) represent the late cortical response arising mainly from the frontal cortex and association areas.

The signal latencies are increased and the peaks and troughs are attenuated or even abolished, by anaesthesia, sedation and sleep. There is an increasing

volume of data that suggests that the early cortical waves of the AER can detect dose related changes in a range of general anaesthetic agents, respond to surgical stimulation, and correlate with the explicit and implicit memory of events during anaesthesia.

- Brain stem-evoked responses (BSER) are generated using an auditory stimulus and are sometimes referred to as auditory-evoked responses (AER). The signal has six distinguishable peaks (I–VI), the anatomical origin of which has caused much debate. It is suggested that the first is derived from the cochlear nerve, the second from the cochlear nucleus, the third from the superior olivary complex, and the fourth and fifth from the inferior colliculus. BSER are not affected significantly by IV anaesthetic agents thus limiting their usefulness in total IV anaesthesia
- Visual-evoked response (VER) arises from stimulation of the visual pathway by a pulsed flash of light. This modified flash test produces variable results, and as such is more suited to a qualitative rather than quantitative assessment. The signals represent a mainly cortical response

TEMPERATURE MEASUREMENT
TEMPERATURE SCALES

- Fahrenheit (1714) developed this temperature scale using the first mercury thermometer. The zero point was set using a mixture of sodium chloride and ice. According to this scale, ice melted at 32°F, water boiled at 212°F and body temperature was assumed to be 100°F
- Centigrade (1742) is a scale developed by Celsius having two fixed points, 0°C for the melting point of ice and 100°C for the boiling point of water

- Kelvin (absolute temperature scale) – uses absolute zero, and the triple point of water, 273.15 K. The boiling point of water according to this scale is 373 K

Conversion between temperature scales

simple conversion between temperature scales can be made as follows:

Fahrenheit to Centigrade   (°F)   =   (°C × 9/5) + 32

Centigrade to Fahrenheit   (°C)   =   (°F – 32) × 5/9

Kelvin to Centigrade   (K)   =   (°C + 273)

TEMPERATURE MEASUREMENT SITE

Small temperature gradients exist between different parts of the body in normal subjects. The ability of a measured value to reflect core temperature depends on the site chosen. This will also determine the response time, i.e. the speed with which a change in body temperature is registered. The following sites may be used:

- Oesophagus – correct probe position is in the lower 25% of the oesophagus. When correctly placed the measured values provide a good estimate of cerebral blood temperature. If placed above this level, however, the probe may under read due to the cooling effect of the inspired gases
- Nasopharynx – probe should be positioned just behind the soft palate. Compared with the oesophageal probe this provides a less accurate measure of core temperature
- Tympanic membrane – aural canal temperature provides an accurate measure of hypothalamic temperature. It has a short response time and correlates well with the results obtained from an oesophageal probe
- Blood – blood temperature can be measured using the thermistor of a pulmonary flotation catheter. This method provides the best continuous measure of core temperature
- Rectum – rectal temperature is influenced by the heat generated by gut flora, the cooling effect of blood returning from the lower limbs and the insulation of the temperature probe by faeces. The rectal temperature is normally 0.5–1.0% higher than core temperature and compared with other sites the response time is slow

THERMOMETERS

These can be classified as:

Direct-reading thermometers – where the display and site of measurement are in direct contact

Remote-reading thermometers – where the display is distant from the site of measurement

The choice of thermometer is determined by the application, the clinical environment, the required accuracy, and need for a continuous display.

Clinical measurement of temperature uses the following devices:

- Mercury glass thermometer
- Chemical thermometer
- Resistance thermometer
- Thermistors
- Thermocouples

Note that dial thermometers usually measure the environmental temperature.

Direct-reading thermometers

LIQUID EXPANSION THERMOMETERS

These consist of a glass bulb filled with either alcohol or mercury, which is connected to a narrow evacuated glass capillary tube. When warmed the liquid expands causing a column of liquid to rise up the capillary tube. The temperature corresponds to a point on a calibrated temperature scale measured by the height of the fluid column. If the cross-sectional area of the capillary tube is constant, then the relationship between expansion of the liquid and the column height will remain linear.

- Advantages – simple, no power supply required
- Disadvantages – poor visual display of temperature, slow response time, limited temperature range (requiring a low-reading thermometer for hypothermia), cannot be read remotely, easy breakage, unsuitable for insertion into cavities

CHEMICAL THERMOMETERS

Chemical thermometers consist of a series of cells, each containing a mixture of chemicals, the colour of which is temperature dependent. The particular chemical mixture is chosen to suit the required temperature range, and the colour change usually occurs within 30 s. The older single use thermometers relied on a series of dye containing crystals. The newer reusable thermometers use liquid crystal technology. In these, the solid crystals are colourless, as they melt the realignment of the composite molecules produces the change in colour.

- Advantages – fast response time, no breakage problem, disposable
- Disadvantages – usually only possible to differentiate temperature intervals of about 0.5°C

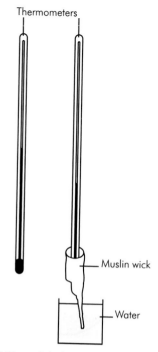

Figure CM.45 Wet and dry bulb thermometer

incorporated into a simple electrical circuit as either a resistor or capacitor, any increase in the humidity results as a detectable change in either resistance or capacitance. This method provides a rapid, sensitive measure of humidity and is often used in control systems for air conditioning systems. These transducers display hysteresis

MEASUREMENT OF PAIN

Pain is one of the most difficult physiological phenomena to quantify but its impact on the individual patient and to healthcare in general, make assessment an essential part of clinical practice. Pain has been defined by the International Association for the Study of Pain as 'An unpleasant sensory and emotional experience associated with actual or potential tissue damage'.

Pain is, thus, multidimensional and has to be assessed using both subjective and objective methods of measurement.

- An observer performs **objective** measurement. In addition to assessment of the pain dimensions outlined above, objective measurements also include measurements associated with the physical changes accompanying pain

- **Subjective** measurement is data that is self-reported by the patient

Most of the methods of assessing pain dimensions are common to both patient and observer.

DIMENSIONS CHARACTERISING PAIN

Pain can be characterised by the dimensions summarised in Figure CM.46.

DIMENSIONS CHARACTERISING PAIN

Dimension	Parameter measured or described
Physical	Location Intensity and character Frequency and duration
Functional	Aggravating and relieving factors Disability, e.g. walking distance, self care Productivity, e.g. employment, recreation
Behavioural	Rubbing, grimacing, guarding, vocalisation Gait and posture Medication frequency and dosage
Affect	Degree of depression
Cognition	Degree of understanding

Figure CM.46

ACUTE AND CHRONIC PAIN

A further dimension defining the nature of a pain condition is the classification into acute pain or chronic pain.
- Acute pain is pain occurring in the first few days following surgery or trauma
- Chronic pain is a term applied to pain persisting beyond the acute period or associated with chronic disease

These pain conditions differ in prognosis, management and outcome, but there does exist a 'grey' area between them, in cases where acute pain conditions evolve into chronic ones.

PHYSIOLOGICAL CHANGES ASSOCIATED WITH PAIN

Physiological changes are associated with both acute and chronic pain conditions. In acute pain, these signs

PHYSICAL SIGNS ASSOCIATED WITH PAIN

Pain	Signs
Acute pain	Heart rate
	Blood pressure
	Respiratory rate
	Lacrimation
	Sweating
Chronic pain	Changes in limb size and muscle bulk
	Changes in skin temperature and sweating
	Localised swelling
	Muscle spasm

Figure CM.47

are reflected by autonomic changes, which can be recorded and scored. They are particularly useful when assessing pain in unconscious or obtunded patients, but are not specifically associated with pain and are open to misinterpretation (Figure CM.47).

SINGLE-DIMENSION PAIN MEASUREMENT

Single-dimension measurements can be applied to both acute and chronic pain situations and include:

- Use of body chart for pain location – a simple diagram on which the patient or observer marks the areas corresponding to the pain
- Visual analogue scale – a straight line drawn between two extremes, e.g. 'no pain' and 'worst pain imaginable'. The patient marks a point on this line to represent their current status. It can be used for various parameters such as pain, mood, pain relief and disability. The value is taken as the distance of the mark along the scale from the origin. The validity of these scales is questioned concerning their reproducibility and reliability. Current opinion is that visual analogue scales are reliable when used with the appropriate group of patients and under controlled circumstances. These scales are not suitable for very young children, the immediate post operative period or the visually impaired
- Numerical ranking or pictorial ranking – an alternative to using visual analogue scales, and may be more suitable for some groups of patients (e.g. children). These scales are marked by numbers, or pictures of faces, to represent increasing or decreasing pain. The gradation is, thus, not

continuous, but is limited to a finite number of choices. This may make the results more reproducible in some cases and the method may be easier to use for patients, but a loss of sensitivity can result

- Word descriptor ranking – here assessment is dependent on a choice of a word descriptor from a list. The assessment is obtained by scoring for each word to give a pain rating index (PRI). Alternatively using free choice from non scored word lists, the total number of words chosen (NWC) can be recorded. Multiple word descriptor lists can be used to produce multidimensional pain assessment. This method can be adapted for visually impaired patients

MULTIDIMENSIONAL PAIN MEASUREMENT

These methods can be applied to produce a more complete assessment of a pain condition by combining assessment of multiple pain dimensions. They include:

- McGill questionnaire – first described by Melzack in 1975. It consists of a body map and word descriptor sections for evaluating the intensity and other characteristics of pain. It is a relatively involved questionnaire taking around twenty min or more to complete, depending on patient skills. This limits its application since it is not suitable for children, highly anxious patients or patients in the immediate post operative period. It is commonly used in research
- Memorial pain assessment card – a collection of linear analogue scales for different pain dimensions such as intensity, pain relief or mood. It can also include a limited set of word descriptor lists
- Pain observation chart – can be designed for patients to record a number of pain dimensions on a diary basis, e.g. pain intensity, pain relief and drug side effects to optimise drug regimes. Alternatively pain charts can be designed for observers or carers to record objective assessment data on a diary/timetable basis to optimise post operative analgesia
- Beck depression inventory – provides a self-reported index of depression that can be used to quantify changes in depression levels due to treatment of chronic pain conditions

ASSESSMENT OF PAIN IN CHILDREN

Pain assessment in children is dependent on the age and skills of the child, and is affected significantly by their interaction with their parents. Some of the methods used are summarised in Figure CM.48.

METHODS OF PAIN ASSESSMENT IN CHILDREN	
Age (years)	**Method**
Infant	Observation – crying, motor withdrawal
1–3	Observation – crying, withdrawal, facial expression, lip smacking, aggressive behaviour
3–5	Pictorial-ranking scales Colour-matching scales
5–12	Visual analogue scales Number-ranking scales
> 12	Multidimensional scales

Figure CM.48

SECTION 4: 3
ANAESTHETIC EQUIPMENT

E. S. Lin

MEDICAL GAS PIPELINE SERVICES

GAS CYLINDERS

ANAESTHETIC MACHINES

VAPORISERS

BREATHING CIRCUITS

OXYGEN DELIVERY SYSTEMS

RESUSCITATION BAGS AND VALVES

ENDOTRACHEAL TUBES

LARYNGEAL MASK AIRWAY

SCAVENGING SYSTEMS

VENTILATORS

HUMIDIFIERS

INTRAVENOUS EQUIPMENT

REGIONAL ANAESTHESIA EQUIPMENT

METHODS OF DISINFECTING AND STERILISING

MEDICAL GAS PIPELINE SERVICES

The medical gas pipeline services (MGPS) provide wall gas and vacuum supplies at working areas such as operating theatres, resuscitation and recovery areas. The MGPS consist of the following:

- Oxygen (at 420 kPa)

- Medical air (at 700 and 420 kPa)

- Nitrous oxide

- Medical vacuum

- Scavenging vacuum

The gases and services are distributed by a medical pipeline network to specialised terminal outlets. Equipment can then be connected to these outlets by non-interchangeable flexible hosing.

The MPGS distribution network consists of especially cleaned and degreased medical quality copper pipes. These are colour coded and installed to government specified standards. Different areas of the network are isolated by special valves connected into the network by non-interchangeable threaded (NIST) unions.

The pipeline terminal outlets consist of Schrader sockets which are clearly labelled and colour coded for the service or gas. They are matched for a specific connecting flexible pipeline by a collar indexing system. Each flexible pipeline is colour coded with unique terminal and equipment ends. The terminal end consists of an indexed Schrader probe that fits into its specific terminal socket. The other end of the hose is a non-interchangeable (NIST) union, which connects on to a piece of equipment. These design features of the hoses and terminal sockets ensure that the gases or services cannot be cross-connected to equipment.

OXYGEN SUPPLY

Oxygen is stored centrally in a vacuum insulated evaporator (VIE). This consists of an inner stainless steel tank with an outer steel jacket. A vacuum is maintained between the tank and jacket for insulation. The VIE has the following features:

- It contains liquid and gaseous oxygen with an inner temperature of −183°C (lower than the critical temperature of oxygen, which is −118°C).

- The pressure within the VIE is approximately 1100–1300 kPa and varies with demand of oxygen.

- There is a main outlet at the top of the VIE, for oxygen withdrawal to supply the distribution pipeline.

- Liquid oxygen may also be withdrawn via a separate outlet and fed through a superheater, in order to 'top up' the supply line and maintain pressure during periods of high demand.

- A reserve supply provided by a cylinder bank, is available in case of VIE failure.

- The VIE normally contains enough oxygen for 10 days supply, while the reserves are adequate for 24 hour use.

A schematic diagram of a VIE is shown in Figure EQ.1.

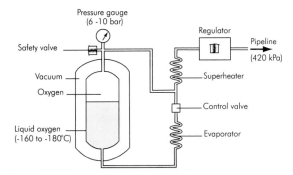

Figure EQ.1 Vacuum insulated evaporator

NITROUS OXIDE SUPPLY

Nitrous oxide is supplied from a central bank of gas cylinders, which contain a mixture of liquid and gas (critical temperature of nitrous oxide is 36.5°C). These are connected to the distribution pipeline network by a control panel, which regulates the gas pressure. The control may also provide local heating in order to avoid condensation and freezing due to the cooling caused by the evaporation of the liquid nitrous oxide. A reserve bank of cylinders is also provided.

MEDICAL COMPRESSED AIR

Compressed air for medical use must be much purer than its industrial equivalent. It is generated by compressors and will contain oil mist as well as water vapour. In a hospital two types of supply are required, a low pressure supply (420 kPa) for anaesthetic machines and ventilators, and a higher pressure supply (700 kPa) to provide power for surgical equipment. The pipeline network may be supplied either by a bank of air cylinders or by a local compressor system. If a local compressor is used care must be taken to ensure the purity of the compressed air produced.

MEDICAL VACUUM

Medical vacuum is required for suction, and BS4957 specifications suggest a vacuum level of 53 kPa (400 mmHg). Medical vacuum is also required for scavenging of anaesthetic gases but it is not recommended that the same vacuum supply is used for both purposes because:

- Suction requires relatively low flow rates but high levels of vacuum, which if applied inadvertently to a patient's airway would be harmful.

- Scavenging requires low vacuum levels with high flow rates. The high flow rates used to remove waste anaesthetic gases could reduce suction levels during surgery.

- Waste anaesthetic gases contain volatile vapours which may be absorbed by lubricants and ultimately cause system failure.

Suction vacuum systems incorporate bacterial filtration and drainage to dispose of aspirated body fluids

GAS CYLINDERS

Gases and vapours are supplied from cylinders in the absence or failure of piped gas supplies. The cylinders are made of molybdenum steel, which is stronger than carbon steel. This enables cylinders to be made lighter in weight and with thinner walls. They are used to supply the following gases and vapours (Figure EQ.2).

Gases and vapours supplied in cylinders

Content	Gas/ Vapour	Cylinder pressure kPa (psi)	BP at 1 atm (°C)	Critical Temperature (°C)
Oxygen	gas	13 700 (1980)	– 183	– 118
Air	gas	13 700 (1980)		
Nitrous oxide	vapour	4400 (640)	– 89	36.5
Carbon dioxide	vapour	5000 (723)	– 78.5	31
Entonox	mixture	13 700 (1980)	gas separation at – 6°C	
Helium	gas	13 700 (1980)	– 269	– 268

Figure EQ.2

CYLINDER IDENTIFICATION

Cylinders possess various markings on the cylinder or its label which include:

- Tare weight of cylinder

- Hydraulic test pressure of cylinder

- Identity of gas (symbol)

- Density of gas

- Serial number of cylinder

- Owner of cylinder and manufacturer of gases

The cylinders are also identified visually by a symbol and colour coding which are listed in Figure EQ.3.

Colour coding of gas cylinders (for UK and ISO)

Substance	Gas/Vapour	Symbol	Color coding Cylinder	Color coding Shoulder
Oxygen	gas	O_2	black	white
Air	gas	AIR	black	white/black
Nitrous oxide	vapour	N_2O	blue	blue
Entonox	gas and vapour	N_2O/O_2	blue	white/blue
Carbon dioxide	vapour	CO_2	grey	grey
Helium	gas	He	brown	brown

Figure EQ.3

Pin Index System (PIS)

Gas cylinders are also identified mechanically by a pin indexing system, which conforms to both British Standard (BS) and equivalent International Standards Organisation (ISO) specifications. This system prevents the wrong cylinder from being connected to an anaesthetic machine.

The pin index system is designed into the outlet valve block of the cylinder and is illustrated in Figure EQ.4. The cylinder valve block face matches up to the inlet port of the anaesthetic machine. This face contains the gas outlet from the cylinder, which is made gas tight by a metal and rubber ring seal, the Bodok seal. Beneath the outlet are six possible positions for indexing holes. Pins on the anaesthetic machine inlet fit into these holes. If the positions of these pins do not match the index holes on the valve block outlet, the cylinder cannot be fitted to that particular inlet on the anaesthetic machine. Figure EQ.4 shows PIS positions for some of the gases commonly used and detail of the cylinder head arrangement.

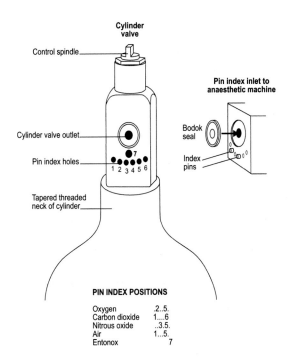

Figure EQ.4 Pin index system for gases and detail of the cylinder head

Cylinder testing

Cylinders are hydraulically tested every 5 years using water under high pressure. Water or water vapour remaining in a cylinder may represent a hazard because it may condense and freeze (affecting the operation of the outlet valve), if the cylinder empties rapidly. Random cylinders from a batch may be destructively tested by the manufacturers using water under pressure.

Cylinders may be inspected endoscopically for cracks and defects on their inner surfaces and they can also be tested ultrasonically.

Estimation of cylinder contents

The contents of a cylinder for both gases and vapours, are estimated by weighing the cylinder and subtracting the weight of the empty cylinder or 'tare' weight. The tare weight is recorded on the cylinder itself. Cylinder contents can thus be estimated by weighing a cylinder and subtracting the tare weight of the cylinder.

Gases: In the case of gases, such as oxygen and air, cylinders are initially filled to a given pressure (13 700 kPa). Since gases are not liquified in the cylinder (temperature < critical temperature), the cylinder contents can also be estimated by the cylinder pressure.

This gradually decreases as the cylinder empties. The mass of gas present is directly proportional to the pressure according to the Universal Gas law and the volume of the contents available at atmospheric pressure can be estimated using Boyle's law.

Vapours: In the case of vapours (such as nitrous oxide or carbon dioxide) the contents of the cylinders are a mixture of gas and liquid. The cylinders are initially filled to a given 'filling ratio'. The filling ratio is defined as the weight of the substance contained divided by the weight of a volume of water equal to the internal volume of the cylinder. This ratio is set at 0.75, since if the cylinders are overfilled there is a risk of rupture with increases in ambient temperature.

The cylinder pressure cannot be used to estimate cylinder contents in the case of a vapour, because it does not vary as the cylinder empties. This is because the cylinder pressure is maintained at saturated vapour pressure (SVP), while liquid is present. The cylinder pressure only falls when the cylinder is nearly empty and all of the liquid contents have evaporated. Cylinder pressure in the case of vapour content only, varies if the temperature changes. This can occur when the cylinder is emptied rapidly, due to absorption of latent heat of vaporisation causing cooling of the contents. Under these circumstances the cylinder pressure will decrease with cooling but will be restored as the cylinder warms up again. (See Figure EQ.5).

(a) Slow emptying of cylinder

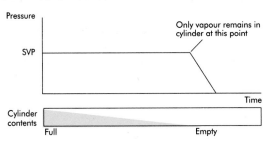

(b) Rapid emptying of cylinder

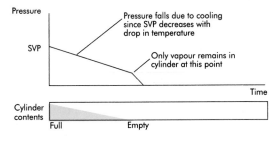

Figure EQ.5 Pressure and temperature changes in a cylinder containing vapour

PRESSURE REGULATORS

The high pressure inside gas cylinders is reduced by a pressure regulator before connection to equipment such as an anaesthetic machine. An example of a single stage regulator which might be used to reduce oxygen cylinder pressure from 13 700 kPa to 420 kPa is shown in Figure EQ.6. Cylinder pressure (P) is reduced to the supply pressure (p) as oxygen passes through the small inlet valve (area = a) into the control chamber. The pressure in the control chamber (p) is controlled by a compression spring acting on a diaphragm (area = A) which is coupled mechanically to the inlet valve. The supply pressure is thus controlled by the force (F) in the spring. This can be expressed by the following equation:

F = Force acting on conical valve + Force acting on
    diaphragm

$$= P a \quad + p A$$

It is assumed that the force in the spring remains constant i.e. the range of movement in the spring is small compared to its total length. Then any change in the supply or cylinder pressures will cause a compensating change as the diaphragm moves and varies the effective area of the inlet valve. In the above equation, if F is constant, a decrease in pA (drop in supply pressure due to increased demand) causes an increase in Pa (increased flow from cylinder). Alternatively if Pa decreases (due to cylinder pressure falling as it empties), pA will increase (increased flow from cylinder).

Thus the pressure regulator not only reduces the cylinder pressure to a suitable supply pressure but also compensates for changes in demand or cylinder pressure. The sensitivity of this control depends on the ratio of the area diaphragm to the area of the valve, which is usually (200: 1).

ANAESTHETIC MACHINES

Surgical anaesthesia is usually provided through a continuous flow anaesthetic machine which consists of the following components:

- Metal framework and pipeline circuitry
- Medical Gas Pipeline Service connections
- Connections for gas cylinders and pressure gauges for cylinder contents
- Safety mechanisms
- Back bar including vaporiser connections

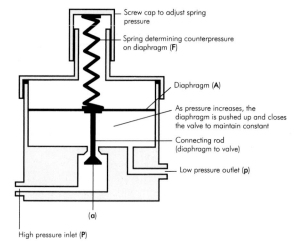

Screw cap to adjust spring pressure

Spring determining counterpressure on diaphragm (F)

Diaphragm (A)

As pressure increases, the diaphragm is pushed up and closes the valve to maintain constant

Connecting rod (diaphragm to valve)

Low pressure outlet (p)

(a)

High pressure inlet (P)

Figure EQ.6 Single stage pressure regulator (Old EQ.2)

- Common gas outlet and auxiliary gas outlets
- Vaporisers
- Rotameters (See page 807)
- Scavenging circuitry
- Suction circuitry

The basic arrangement of these components is illustrated in Figure EQ.7. Modern machines often incorporate electronic monitoring, safety features and a mechanical ventilator.

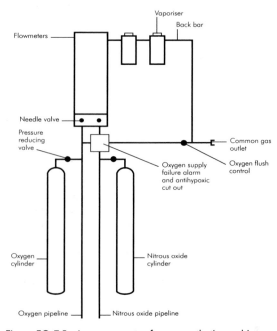

Vaporiser

Back bar

Flowmeters

Needle valve

Pressure reducing valve

Oxygen supply failure alarm and antihypoxic cut out

Common gas outlet

Oxygen flush control

Oxygen cylinder

Nitrous oxide cylinder

Oxygen pipeline

Nitrous oxide pipeline

Figure EQ.7 Basic components of an anaesthetic machine

METAL FRAMEWORK AND PIPELINE CIRCUITRY

The metal framework of the anaesthetic machine is usually made of stainless steel and is electrically earthed via anti-static wheels, which reduce risks of electric shock, interference with rotameters, and fire or explosion of inflammable agents. The frame incorporates pipeline circuitry with both fixed and detachable joints. The pipes are usually brass or copper with brazed fixed joints. More recently nylon pipes have been introduced. Detachable joints are screw threaded and sealed with a compressible washer, O-ring seal or polytetrafluoroethylene (PTFE) tape. Different diameter pipes are used for each gas to prevent cross connection.

MEDICAL PIPELINE GAS SERVICE (MPGS) CONNECTIONS

Non-interchangeable screw threaded (NIST) connections are used for MPGS supplies. Flexible colour coded hoses are used to connect to gas specific wall terminals. The machine end of these hoses is a male NIST connector which is made gas specific by:

- A non-interchangeable threaded nut
- A specific diameter shoulder with O-ring seal
- A specific diameter forward shaft

The machine MPGS connections are the female counterpart of the above hose connectors. They also incorporate metal gauze filters and one way non-return valves to prevent retrograde leakage.

PIN INDEXED SYSTEM (PIS) CONNECTIONS FOR GAS CYLINDERS

The PIS connections for the cylinder gas supplies consist of a gas inlet with the male counterpart of the PIS, i.e. pins corresponding to the indexing holes on the cylinder valve block. A yoke with arrangement secured by a screw fitting holds the cylinder valve block in place. The cylinder inlets also incorporate metal gauze filters and one way non-return valves to prevent retrograde leakage. Retrograde leakage through gas inlets, if great enough, has been known to alter the gas mixture delivered to the patient, and can lead to the delivery of a hypoxic mixture. The PIS connection is made gas tight by a metal and rubber ring seal in the cylinder valve block (Bodok seal). Pin index positions have been described in Figure EQ.4 previously.

SAFETY MECHANISMS

Several safety mechanisms are incorporated into the design of an anaesthetic machine. These include

- **Secondary pressure regulators-** Which smooth out gas pressure fluctuations within the anaesthetic machine, that occur due to changes in pipeline pressure or variations in demand from the machine. Such fluctuations in machine pressure can cause inaccuracies in the fresh gas mixture, or disturb the performance of rotameters and oxygen monitors. Secondary pressure regulators are set to pressures below the anticipated pressure fluctuations and are designed to maintain working pressures within 10% over a wide range of flow rates, from hundreds of millilitres to tens of litres.

- **Oxygen failure warning device** – Monitoring of the delivered fresh gas oxygen concentration is mandatory, but the anaesthetic machine also has a built in oxygen failure device. This is mounted upstream of the rotameter block and is designed according to BS4272 specifications, which include:

  – Audible alarm > 60db at a distance of 1 metre from the machine, for 7 seconds or more

  – Activation when the oxygen supply falls to 200 kPa

  – Power supply derived from the oxygen supply pressure

  – Alarm that cannot be switched off or reset until the oxygen supply is restored

  – Alarm coupled to a gas cut off valve which cuts off anaesthetic gases and opens the machine pipeline circuitry to air

An early oxygen failure warning device was the Ritchie whistle (1960) and many modern devices are similar in principle. A diagram showing how such a device works is shown in Figure EQ.8.

- **Oxygen bypass circuit** – Bypasses the rotameter block and back bar to provide an emergency oxygen flow of at least 30 litres/min to the common gas outlet. The control is usually a push button situated near the common gas outlet, which is recessed to prevent accidental operation, and cannot be locked to prevent barotrauma to the patient.

BACK BAR

The back bar is the horizontal part of the anaesthetic machine circuit between the rotameter block and the

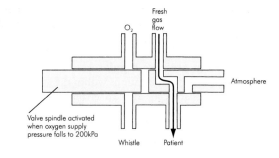

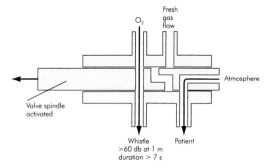

Figure EQ.8 Oxygen failure warning device (Ritchie whistle)

common gas outlet. It is downstream of the rotameter block and feeds fresh gas mixture to the common gas outlet. Vaporisers are mounted on the back bar enabling volatile agents to be added to the fresh gases. The pressure in the back bar is approximately 1 kPa at the outlet end, and may be 7–10 kPa at the rotameter end depending on:

- Total gas flow
- Circuit connection to common gas outlet
- Vaporisers used and their settings

Total occlusion of the common gas outlet produces pressures of approximately 30 kPa in the back bar. The maximum pressure that can be produced in the back bar is limited by a 'blow off', or pressure relief valve at the outlet end (threshold set to 30–40 kPa). This protects the rotameter block and vaporisers from overpressure damage, and the patient from barotrauma to a limited degree.

VAPORISER CONNECTIONS

The connection system for vaporisers (and the vaporisers themselves), are designed with the following features:

- Prevention of gas leakage from the back bar with or without a vaporiser in place

- Prevent of volatile agent leakage into the back bar circuit
- Convenient installation and removal of vaporisers
- Safety interlock mechanism to prevent use of more than one volatile agent simultaneously

Figure EQ.9 illustrates some of these design features. The potential hazards caused by poor design or usage of the vaporiser connection system include:

- Leakage of gas causing inadequate fresh gas mixtures or pressures to be delivered to the patient
- Leakage of volatile agent into the fresh gas flow
- Damage or injury caused by difficulty in attaching or detaching vaporisers
- Contamination of downstream vaporisers by upstream volatile agent, when no safety interlock mechanism is present
- Contamination of soda lime in the breathing circuit by trichlorethylene (no longer used in the UK), which produces a neurotoxin

In early machines where more than one vaporiser could be switched on at a time, a more volatile agent (e.g. halothane), if placed upstream, could be absorbed by a less volatile agent (e.g. triclorethylene). This could lead to the release of a maximal concentration (determined by the saturated vapour pressure) of the absorbed agent on subsequent use of the downstream vaporiser. In modern machines with a good safety interlock mechanism, the sequence of vaporisers on the back bar presents no significant hazard.

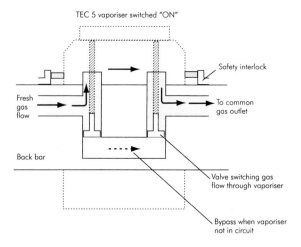

Figure EQ.9 Vaporiser backbar connections

GAS OUTLETS

The common gas outlet is a 22 mm male (external) and 15 mm female (internal) tapered outlet which supplies fresh gas mixture to the patient breathing circuit or a mechanical ventilator. It may be mounted on a swivel (Cardiff Swivel) for increased convenience. It can withstand bending moments of up to 10 Nm (equivalent approximately to 40–50 kg weight hanging from the outlet). It may be threaded to prevent accidental disconnection.

The auxiliary gas outlets are Schrader oxygen or air sockets which can be used to power devices such as a ventilator or a venturi injector.

ANAESTHETIC MACHINE MAINTENANCE

Servicing of machines should follow manufacturer's guidelines. Typically servicing is performed at 3 to 6 month intervals. Each machine should have an attached logbook to record commissioning date, servicing dates, faults, repairs and modifications.

ANAESTHETIC MACHINE CHECKLIST

The anaesthetic machine should be checked by the anaesthetist before each operating session. A checklist is published by the Association of Anaesthetists of Great Britain and Ireland (1997) as a card, which is usually attached to each machine. This is reproduced at the end of the chapter in Figure EQ.42.

VAPORISERS

The functions of a vaporiser are:

- To produce vaporisation of the volatile anaesthetic agent

- To mix the vapour with the fresh gas flow to the patient

- To control the mixture so that a given concentration of volatile agent is delivered to the patient, in spite of varying gas flow rates and ambient temperature conditions.

The design of a vaporiser is determined by the clinical application and the volatile agent being used. Choice of a vaporiser for use in the absence of compressed gas supplies will differ from that where piped supplies are available. While a vaporiser suitable for use with desflurane will be very different from one for use with

isoflurane. The important properties of volatile agents when considering vaporiser design are saturated vapour pressure (SVP), boiling point (BP) and MAC. These are shown for some commonly used agents in Figure EQ.10.

Properties of some commonly used volatile agents			
Volatile agent	SVP (kPa) at 20°C	BP (°C) at 100 kPa	MAC
Halothane	31.9	51	0.76
Enflurane	23.1	56	1.68
Isoflurane	31.5	48	1.15
Sevoflurane	21.3	58	2
Desflurane	88.5	23	6

Figure EQ.10

Two different types of vaporiser are considered here, variable bypass and measured flow.

- **Variable bypass vaporiser** – In this vaporiser the fresh gas flow to the patient circuit is split into two streams by a flow splitting valve. One stream bypasses the vaporising chamber and is free from volatile agent. The other stream passes through the vaporiser chamber and becomes saturated with vapour. This second stream then rejoins the bypass flow to give the required concentration of vapour in the fresh gas flow to the patient (see Figure EQ.11). The final vapour concentration is controlled by using the flow splitting valve to vary the fraction of the gas flow passing through the vaporiser chamber. Accuracy is therefore dependent on the flow splitting valve maintaining a constant 'flow splitting ratio' over the range of flow rates used. There are two main types of variable bypass vaporiser described below, *plenum* vaporisers and *draw over* vaporisers.

- **Measured flow vaporiser** - This vaporiser has a chamber in which the volatile agent is heated by an electrical element to produce pure vapour under pressure. The pressure produced in the chamber is equal to the saturated vapour pressure (SVP) of the volatile agent at the preset temperature. The vaporiser then controls the addition of the pressurised vapour to the fresh gas flow using pressure sensor controlled valve, to maintain a given volatile percentage in the patient's inspired gases. This type of device is used for desflurane (Figure EQ.12).

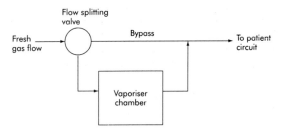

Figure EQ.11 Principles of a variable bypass vaporiser

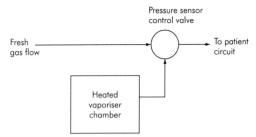

Figure EQ.12 Principles of measured flow vaporiser

PLENUM VARIABLE BY-PASS VAPORISER

(Examples: Ohmeda TEC 5, Blease Datum, Drager Vapor)

In the plenum vaporiser the inspired gases are at higher than atmospheric pressure (backbar pressure 1 – 8 kPa) and pressurise the vaporiser chamber (*plenum* – Latin for full). Pressurisation increases the density of the carrier gas in the chamber thus ensuring better mixing with the vapour at low flows. When the vaporiser chamber is at atmospheric pressure, carrier gas density is less than vapour density, and at low flow rates gas will tend to pass across the top of the chamber without mixing.

The plenum vaporiser is the most commonly used type in hospital practice and includes models such as the TEC series (Ohmeda) and Vapor series (Drager). Plenum vaporisers have a relatively high flow resistance (approximately 0.4 kPa per litre/min of flow) and are therefore unsuitable for placing 'in line' in a spontaneously breathing circuit.

To illustrate: in order to develop a peak inspiratory flow rate of 30 litres/minute through this vaporiser, a patient would need to develop a peak inspiratory pressure of 30 × 0.4 = 12 kPa (>120 cm H$_2$O), compared with a normal inspiratory pressure of< 2 kPa. Effectively the plenum vaporiser acts as a flow restrictor, and for a spontaneously breathing patient a circuit with a reservoir bag is usually needed to supply the peak inspiratory flow rates. Figure EQ.13 illustrates the design of a simple plenum vaporiser

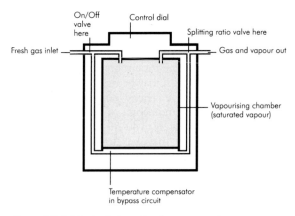

Figure EQ.13 Basic design of a plenum vaporiser

Flow splitting ratio

The performance of variable bypass vaporisers depends on the flow splitting ratio, which is the ratio of the bypass flow to the gas flow through the chamber.

For example If total gas flow through the anaesthetic machine backbar is 5 l/min and flow through the vaporiser is 0.2 l/min, what is the flow splitting ratio?

Vaporiser chamber flow = 0.2

Bypass flow = 5.0 – 0.2 = 4.8

Flow splitting ratio = 4.8/0.2 = 24

So, consider the concentration of vapour in an isoflurane vaporiser chamber at 20°C (SVP for isoflurane at 20°C = 31.5 kPa (assume ambient pressure in the vaporiser chamber to be 105 kPa).

Saturated vapour concentration in the vaporiser chamber is given by the ratio:

$$\frac{SVP}{\text{pressure in vaporiser chamber}} \times 100\%$$

$$= \frac{31.5}{105} \times 100\%$$

$$= 30\%$$

To find the flow splitting ratio required to produce a final concentration of 1% isoflurane:

$$\text{Final concentration} = \frac{\text{concentration in vaporiser chamber}}{(\text{flow splitting ratio} + 1)}$$

To obtain 1% isoflurane the vapour must be diluted by a factor of 30. Therefore a flow splitting ratio of 29 is required, i.e. 1/30 (3.3%) of the total flow must pass through the chamber.

It can be seen that the more potent the volatile agent the greater dilution of the vapour is required and the greater the flow splitting ratio.

DRAW OVER VARIABLE BYPASS VAPORISERS

(Examples: Epstein, Macintosh, Oxford (EMO), Goldman, Oxford Minature)

In the draw over vaporiser the inspiratory gases are at atmospheric pressure and are drawn through the vaporiser chamber by the inspiratory efforts of the patient. The vaporiser and flow splitting valve must therefore have low resistance. This type of vaporiser has the advantage that atmospheric air can be used as the carrier gas (supplemented by cylinder oxygen if required).

However, accuracy is poor in this type of vaporiser since flow rates vary considerably through the vaporiser with the respiratory cycle. The ability of the flow splitting valve to maintain a constant splitting ratio becomes poor over the wide range of flows. At low flow rates the resistance of the flow splitting valve will become relatively more significant and gases will tend to bypass the vaporiser causing a fall in volatile concentrations. At high flow rates there will be increased dilution of the vapour in the vaporiser chamber and again concentrations will tend to be reduced. Figure EQ.14 shows a simple draw over vaporiser.

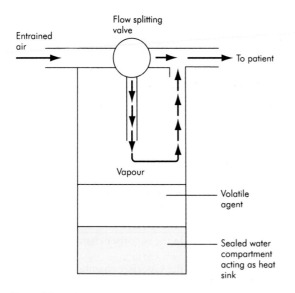

Figure EQ.14 Draw over vaporiser

MEASURED FLOW VAPORISERS

(Example: Ohmeda TEC 6 Desflurane vaporiser)

The measured flow vaporisers produce a separate independent flow of vapour or saturated carrier gas.

This flow is then metered into to the patient's fresh gas flow to produce the required concentration of volatile (Figure EQ.15). Thus no splitting of the fresh gas flow occurs. This method is used in the desflurane vaporiser (TEC 6) because the boiling point of desflurane at sea level is 23.6°C, which is approximately room temperature. In such a case, use of a plenum vaporiser with an intermittently boiling volatile agent would make its performance unpredictable. The desflurane vaporiser therefore heats the volatile agent to 39°C to produce a chamber pressure of approximately 194 kPa. A continuous flow of desflurane vapour from the chamber is then added into the fresh gas flow via the concentration control valve.

The desflurane vaporiser has features which include:

- Mains supply, with back up battery

- Three built in heaters to boil the desflurane and to prevent condensation in different parts of the vaporiser

- A warm up time of 10 minutes, during which the control dial is locked

- Electronic circuitry to indicate ' Ready for use', warn against low levels of desflurane, disconnection, and switch off when tilted.

- Supplies concentrations up to 18% (3 MAC)

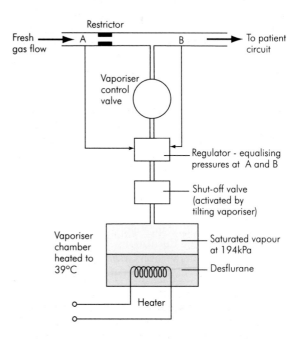

Figure EQ.15 Measured flow vaporiser

Vaporiser performance

Vaporiser performance is dependent on the range of flow rates, the ambient conditions, the carrier gas mixture used, together with the design and maintenance of the vaporiser.

- **Flow rate** of carrier gas passing through the vaporiser is important because as flow rate increases, an increasing amount of vapour is required to saturate the carrier gas. At higher flow rates the carrier gas in the vaporiser chamber may not become fully saturated and thus the concentration of the volatile agent delivered to the patient tends to fall. Figure EQ.16 shows how volatile agent concentration might vary with increasing flow rate in a plenum vaporiser. In addition high flow rates will accentuate the temperature effects in the chamber (see below). Performance of a vaporiser will therefore be more consistent if variations in flow rates are minimised. A large surface area for vaporisation in the vaporiser chamber will be able to maintain saturation of the carrier gas over a wider range of flow rates.

- **Temperature -**The concentration of vapour in the vaporiser chamber is dependent on the SVP of the volatile agent and the ambient pressure in the chamber. Temperature affects the performance of a vaporiser due to the variation of SVP with temperature. A main cause of temperature falling in the chamber is the absorption of latent heat as vaporisation occurs. This will become more marked at higher flow rates when the rate of vaporisation is increased.

Compensation to correct for such fluctuations is achieved by adjusting the gas flow through the vaporiser chamber. Temperature compensation was performed manually in early vaporisers by altering the flow splitting valve according to the temperature in the vaporiser. However this has been superseded by automatic devices, such as a bimetallic strip controlled flow valve, which is built into the chamber outlet of modern models. This valve automatically increases the flow through the vaporiser chamber should temperature in the chamber start to fall.

Further compensation is obtained by increasing the thermal capacity of the vaporiser in order to smooth out temperature fluctuations. This was achieved in the EMO draw over vaporiser by filling a compartment in the base of the vaporiser with water. Alternatively in the later plenum vaporisers a large heavy mass of copper is incorporated into the vaporiser body. This enhanced thermal capacity acts as a heat source in case of temperature falls, and a heat sink should ambient temperature rises, thus smoothing out the effects of temperature fluctuations. Figure EQ.17 shows how vaporiser performance might vary with temperature in a typical modern vaporiser.

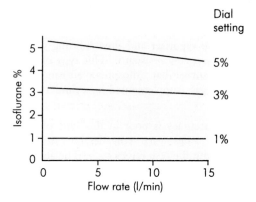

Figure EQ.16 Concentration changes with flow in a plenum vaporiser

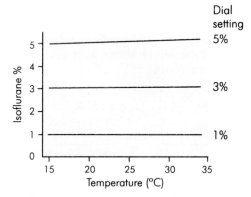

Figure EQ.17 Concentration changes with temperature in a plenum vaporiser (TEC 4) at 5 l/min oxygen flow.

- **Atmospheric pressure** – From the calculation example for plenum vaporisers given above (see 'splitting ratio'), the concentration of volatile agent in the vaporiser chamber is dependent on the ratio:

$$\frac{SVP}{\text{Pressure in the vaporiser chamber}}$$

The pressure in the vaporiser chamber is essentially atmospheric pressure, therefore if atmospheric pressure is increased the final volatile concentration delivered will be reduced. On the other hand at altitude where atmospheric pressure is reduced the volatile concentration delivered is increased. It should be noted that although the delivered concentration may increase at altitude, the partial pressure exerted by the volatile agent in the tissues will remain unchanged.

- **'Pumping effect'** – This effect is produced by repetitive changes in circuit resistance at the common gas outlet. It can be produced when the outlet is periodically obstructed by assisting ventilation or attaching a minute volume divider ventilator (e.g. Manley) to the outlet. This results in alternating compression and release of the saturated gas in the vaporiser chamber, which in turn produces surges of volatile agent concentration in the patient circuit. Mechanisms to reduce this pumping effect include increasing the flow resistance of the vaporiser and insertion of a non-return valve at the outlet of the vaporiser.

- **Carrier gas composition** – Increasing the nitrous oxide content of the carrier gas can produce a small reduction in the volatile concentration delivered. This is because the nitrous oxide reduces the viscosity and increases the density of the gas mixture, which decreases the gas flow through the vaporiser chamber due to the flow splitting valve characteristics. Nitrous oxide also has increased solubility in volatile agents, which can cause a further transient fall in volatile agent concentration when the nitrous oxide fraction is increased. This effect is not significant clinically.

- **Mechanical stability** – Poor fitting of the vaporiser to the backbar can result in gas leaks, loss of backbar pressure or tilting which can allow leakage of volatile agent into the bypass circuit. Regular checking of vaporiser seating and improvements in vaporiser and backbar design can minimise risks of these problems.

- **Overfilling** - Direct leakage of volatile agent into the patient circuit can also be caused by over filling of the vaporiser and is potentially fatal. Care should be taken in filling and checking vaporisers.

- **Vaporiser maintenance** – Vaporisers should be serviced annually and calibration should also be checked regularly. Drainage and cleaning of vaporiser chambers (two weekly intervals) can prevent the build up of unwanted substances (such as thymol, a waxy stabilising agent used in halothane), which can reduce evaporation rates in the vaporiser chamber and cause moving parts to stick if they accumulate.

DESIGN FEATURES OF A VAPORISER

The desirable features in a vaporiser depend to some extent on the specific application (portable or fixed, compressed gas supplies available or not), but some general specifications include:

- Large surface area for vaporisation in the vaporiser chamber
- Large heat sink
- Temperature compensation valve for flow through vaporiser
- Accurate flow splitting valve
- Low flow resistance for draw over vaporiser
- Stable mechanical mounting
- Safeguard against leakage into patient circuit
- Safety interlock device
- Clear liquid level gauge
- Agent specific filling port
- Easy emptying and cleaning

BREATHING SYSTEMS

'Breathing system' describes the equipment used to deliver fresh gases and volatile agents to a patient. The following general terms are used to describe breathing systems:

- **Open system.** In its simplest form a breathing system may just be a method of augmenting room air, an open hose and a cupped hand, nasal cannulae delivering oxygen or a clear plastic oxygen mask. These are referred to as 'open' breathing systems.

- **Closed system** - This controls the gas mixture delivered to the patient, using a sealed mask and circuit. Closed systems can be classified into 'rebreathing' and 'non-rebreathing' systems.

  Rebreathing – is the inhalation of previously expired gases including carbon dioxide and water vapour. Many of the breathing systems used in practice allow rebreathing, but are normally used with high enough fresh gas flow rates to prevent rebreathing. These types of system include the Bain and Magill circuits, and are described below in the Mapleson classification.

  Non- rebreathing – describes breathing systems in which rebreathing is prevented. This can be achieved by; a non-rebreathing valve, a carbon dioxide absorber or high fresh gas flow rates in a rebreathing system.

Most practical breathing systems function as semi-closed and partially rebreathing systems. They are often capable of operating as non-rebreathing systems, depending on the magnitude of fresh gas flow (FGF) used.

BREATHING SYSTEM PERFORMANCE

Breathing systems may have to work in different environments each of which may influence the design of the circuit. The optimum circuit for a given application will be a compromise between various features which include;

- Low dead space: **Apparatus dead space** is the volume between the patient and the expiratory valve. **Functional dead space** extends to all of the volume contaminated with expired gases during each ventilatory cycle. It may be greater than apparatus dead space in an inefficent circuit, or less in other cases where FGF flushes out expired gases before inspiration (Figure EQ.18).

- Efficient operation in both spontaneously breathing (SV) patients and those requiring controlled/ assisted ventilation (CV). Efficiency in this context is measured by minimum fresh gas flow (FGF) required to prevent rebreathing, expressed as a multiple of patient's minute ventilation (MV). The Magill attachment requires a FGF of greater than 0.7 MV to prevent rebreathing in a spontaneously breathing patient.

- Economical use of fresh gas supply and volatile agent. Economy of usage of anaesthetic gases is needed where supplies are restricted, or to minimise costs. In the operating theatre piped gas supplies are usually available. In other areas gas supplies may be limited and occasionally pressurised supplies may not even be available. Environmental considerations and pollution are also a concern in the work environment.

- Physical size or weight. The weight and bulk of a circuit's components may be a factor discouraging its use, as the circuit may drag on endotracheal tubes or laryngeal masks, and displace them from a patient's airway. Factors such as apparatus dead space are likely to be in proportion to the size of the circuit's components. It is not always convenient to use breathing systems via an anaesthetic machine in resuscitation areas and a simpler system such as the Waters circuit may be more practical.

BREATHING SYSTEM COMPONENTS

A breathing system may consist of all or some of the following components:

- Face mask
- Gas hoses and connectors

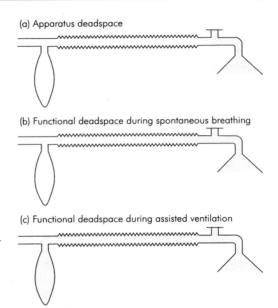

(a) Apparatus deadspace

(b) Functional deadspace during spontaneous breathing

(c) Functional deadspace during assisted ventilation

Figure EQ.18 Functional deadspace within Magill circuit

- Adjustable pressure limiting (APL) expiratory valve (Figure EQ.18)

- Reservoir bag (inflating or self inflating)

- Carbon dioxide absorber

- A valve to switch between controlled (CV) or spontaneous ventilation (MV) modes

- One way valves to prevent rebreathing

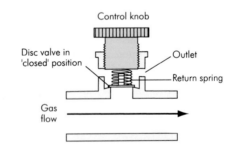

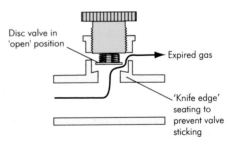

Figure EQ.19 Adjustable pressure limiting expiratory valve

Masks and hoses - Used to be made of black rubber which was antistatic and autoclavable. Modern equivalents are lightweight, disposable and transparent or semi-transparent. These features make the components easier to handle, cheaper and safer. Hoses come in three standard sizes; 22 mm diameter for adult breathing circuits, 15 mm diameter for paediatric breathing circuits and 30 mm diameter for scavenging circuits.

Hose connectors - Are of standard male and female sizes to fit the hose diameters. They are also designed with standardised tapers to allow convenient but secure push fitting between circuit components. 22 mm (15 mm for paediatric circuits) connections fit the breathing circuit hoses together and to valves, reservoir bags and masks. 15 mm connectors join the circuit to endotracheal tubes and laryngeal masks. Tapers are designed according to ISO and BS standards. Some connectors possess 22 mm external and 15 mm internal tapers to facilitate connection between the circuit hoses and an endotracheal tube or laryngeal mask.

Reservoir bags – Come in 0.5 litre, 2 litre and 4 litre sizes and are made of black rubber or distensible synthetic. The compliance of the bag is designed to be low enough to prevent development of harmful pressures if the system valves are accidentally closed.

Mapleson Classification for breathing systems

This system classifies breathing systems according to their configuration of the following components.

- Reservoir bag
- Flexible hosing
- Adustable pressure limiting expiratory valve
- Face mask

The different configurations are described and illustrated in Figure EQ.20.

PRACTICAL BREATHING SYSTEMS

Various breathing systems have been developed empirically for different applications.

Some systems consist of the basic components described in the Mapleson classification (above) and therefore fit into the system described. Other circuits such as the circle system are more complex, and do not fit into the Mapleson system. Some examples are described in Figure EQ.21.

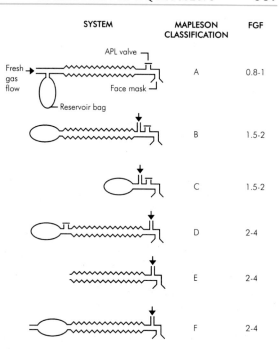

FGF is the fresh gas flow required to avoid rebreathing during spontaneous ventilation quoted as multiples of minute volume

Figure EQ. 20 Mapleson classification system for breathing systems

CIRCLE SYSTEM

A typical circle system is shown in Figure EQ.22. The system consists of a carbon dioxide absorber, a reservoir bag, one way valves to ensure unidirectional gas flow and hoses with a Y piece to connect the patient into the circuit. The circle system can be used with spontaneously breathing patient, or control/assist can be given manually using the reservoir bag.

The optimum configuration for the components is also shown in Figure EQ.21, with the FGF and reservoir bag located in between the carbon dioxide absorber and the one way inspiratory valve. This arrangement minimises the inspiratory resistance of the circuit.

The circle system has the following advantages:

- Low FGF rates can be used without causing rebreathing. This enables low FGF rates to be used and gives economy of anaesthetic gas usage.

- Recirculation of volatile agent giving economy and low pollution rates

- Low functional dead space equal to the volume of the patient Y-piece due to removal of carbon dioxide by the absorber.

Examples of commonly used circuits		
Circuit	Mapleson	Comments
Magill	A	Good for SV. May be used for CV but requires twice MV. APL valve convenient near patient, but drags on endotracheal tube or mask
Lack	A	Co-axial circuit delivering FGF via outer hose. Expiratory limb though inner with APL valve at anaesthetic machine. Disadvantages are high inspiratory resistance and large apparatus dead space. Also parallel twin hose Lack circuit offers low flow resistances but more bulky.
Bain	D	Co-axial circuit. FGF delivered through inner hose. Suitable for SV or CV less efficient for SV than Magill but more efficient for CV. Disadvantages of co-axial system are that cracks or disconnection in inner hose may go unnoticed.
Waters circuit	C	Practical circuit for resuscitation. Requires low pressure oxygen supply. Low dead space. Suitable for SV or CV.
Ayre's T- piece	E	Suitable for paediatrics. The expiratory limb forms apparatus dead space but also acts as an inspiratory reservoir. This limb should be equal to the tidal volume to prevent dilution of inspired gases by entrained air. Requires 2 – 4 times MV to avoid rebreathing.
Jackson Rees Modification of Ayre's T- piece	F	Paediatric circuit. Open ended reservoir modification of bag in expiratory limb
Humphrey	ADE	Twin hose system which switches between Mapleson A for SV, and D/E for CV.

Figure EQ.21

The disadvantages of the circle system are:

- More components than simpler systems (such as Magill or Bain) creating a bulky system requiring a separate mounting on the anaesthetic machine

- One way valves to ensure unidirectional flow which increase flow resistances and are a potential source of problems such as sticking

- Inspiratory and expiratory flow resistances are higher than in the case of the Magill or Bain systems. These higher flow resistances are dependent on FGF rates in the circle. Low FGF rates increase inspiratory resistance but decrease expiratory resistance. High FGF rates produce the opposite effect, decreasing inspiratory resistance and increasing expiratory resistance. Work of breathing is therefore lowest with high FGF rates. This effect is not significant in a fit adult, but can become important in frail patients or children.

Controlled mechanical ventilation (CMV) with the circle system

CMV can be applied using the circle system, by using a 'bag in the bottle' type of ventilator. This effectively acts as a 'bag squeezer', and the ventilator is connected into the circle system in place of the reservoir bag. In such a case the tidal volume delivered may depend on both the ventilator setting and the FGF. Modern circle systems incorporate ventilators which monitor the delivered tidal volume and compensate for changes in FGF.

An alternative arrangement is the use of a servo-type ventilator which delivers 'driving' gas (oxygen) via the reservoir bag limb and allows expiration through the same limb. In such a configuration the driving gas must not 'contaminate' the patient circuit. This means FGF must be greater than the MV, and the length of the reservoir limb tubing must have a volume greater than 1.5 times the tidal volume.

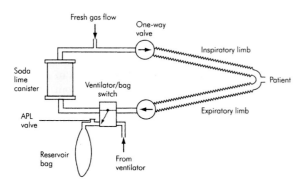

Figure EQ.22 A typical circle system

Use of volatile agents with the circle

When volatile agents are used with the circle the commonest configuration is with a plenum vaporiser located out of the circle (Vaporiser Outside Circle, VOC). The FGF thus passes through vaporiser first, and then into the circle system. In the past draw over vaporisers were used positioned in the circle system (Vaporiser Inside Circle, VIC).

Both methods have disadvantages at low FGF. In summary:

- **VOC** – Expired gas dilutes the inspired gases and reduces inspired volatile concentrations, until equilibrium is reached when end tidal volatile concentrations equal inspired concentrations. Also the performance of many plenum vaporisers may be inaccurate at low flow rates.

- **VIC** – Inspired gases are recirculated through the vaporiser resulting in continually increasing volatile concentrations, and may reach saturation levels.

Carbon dioxide absorption

Carbon dioxide absorption is used to prevent rebreathing, and is most commonly used in the circle system in combination with low FGF rates. A combination of chemical reactions is used to absorb carbon dioxide. First carbon dioxide is dissolved in water to form carbonic acid, and the carbonic acid then reacts with calcium hydroxide to form calcium carbonate and water. These reactions are shown below:

$$CO_2 + H_2O = H_2CO_3 = H^+ + HCO_3^-$$
$$Ca(OH)_2 + H^+ + HCO_3^- = CaCO_3 + 2H_2O$$

This reaction is exothermic and produces water, providing a warm moist environment in the carbon dioxide absorber for the FGF to pass through. The pH

of the reagents increases as the reaction proceeds enabling an indicator to be used to show when the calcium hydroxide is exhausted.

Some practical points concerning the use of carbon dioxide absorbers are outlined below:

- **FGF rates** – Use of carbon dioxide absorption with the circle system can reduce FGF rate to a few hundred millilitres per minute, once equilibrium has been reached. This FGF is required to replace absorbed oxygen (100 – 300 ml/min) and gases lost through leakage and the APL valve.

- **Calcium hydroxide preparation** – The most commonly used preparation is soda lime which is a mixture of 80% $Ca(OH)_2$, 4% NaOH and 16% H_2O. The soda lime is in the form of granules, which are designed to be small enough to give low spaces between granules and thus high efficiency absorption, but not too small so as to provide too high a resistance to gas flow.

- **Soda lime** – The absorption capacity of soda lime is in the order of 25 litres of carbon dioxide per 100 g of soda lime. The colour change indicating exhaustion of the granules (commonly pink to white) may occur before full capacity absorption due to surface reaction on the granules. This can lead to apparent regeneration of granules as the surface and core of the granule equilibrate when used soda lime is left standing. Soda lime dust is caustic and can cause morbidity if a soda lime canister is located too close to the patient's airway in the breathing system. This can occur in the to-and-fro configuration used with a Waters canister (Mapleson C) system. 'Channelling' may occur in soda lime canisters which are poorly packed. This is the formation of channels through the soda lime granules through which gases pass without adequate exposure to the soda lime, and results in incomplete carbon dioxide absorption

OXYGEN DELIVERY SYSTEMS

In the spontaneously breathing patient various systems exist to provide enhanced fraction of inspired oxygen (FiO_2) for the spontaneously breathing patient. These can be required in locations such as recovery areas, resuscitation areas, labour suites and ambulances. The types of device used include nasal cannulae, face masks and attachments for enhancing the FiO2 through laryngeal masks or endotracheal tubes. See Section 1 Chapter 4.

Oxygen delivery systems may be described by the following terms:

Variable performance – This term refers to the FiO2 delivered by a particular system. In a variable performance system the FiO2 delivered is dependent on the oxygen flow rate. The range of flow rates used is usually between 2 – 15 litres/minute and such devices are capable of producing FiO2 up to 0.8 – 0.9. Variable performance systems require an inspiratory oxygen reservoir in order to achieve the higher FiO2 levels, and may be classified as being of 'no capacity' if they have no reservoir capacity (nasal cannulae), 'small capacity' in the case of face masks, and 'large capacity' when a reservoir bag is included. Non-return valves are also incorporated in order to restrict entrainment in face masks and to prevent rebreathing from reservoir bags.

The FiO2 delivered in the variable performance systems depends on:

- Oxygen flow rate
- Tidal volume
- Respiratory rate
- Capacity of the system
- Use of non-return valves

Fixed performance – A fixed performance device delivers an FiO2 which is independent of the oxygen flow rate used. These systems are usually based on a venturi jet which is fed by the oxygen supply and entrains room air. They are often applied in patients with chronic respiratory disease in whom oxygen dependent respiratory drive is suspected.

Low dependency – Describes systems used to increase FiO2 in patients breathing spontaneously at atmospheric pressure

Medium dependency – Describes the use of a system which supplies a degree of positive airway pressure to a spontaneously breathing patient (e.g. a continuous positive airway pressure (CPAP) system). These systems are used in high dependency areas or intensive care units.

High dependency – Describes systems used to control the FiO2 in patients requiring mechanical ventilation

Figure EQ.23 summarises some characteristics of commonly used devices.

Figures EQ.24 and 25 show varaible and fixed performance systems respectively.

Oxygen delivery systems for spontaneously breathing patients			
Device	**Type**	**FiO2**	**Comments**
Nasal cannulae	Variable, no capacity	0.21–0.3	Alternative for patients who cannot tolerate masks. Performance unpredictable, affected by nasal obstruction and mouth breathing
Face mask	Variable, low capacity	0.21–0.5	Performance depends on entrainment through holes in mask and around mask. Enhanced by flap valves. Increases functional dead space
Face mask with reservoir and non-rebreathing valve	Variable, large capacity	0.21–0.80	Provides high FiO2. Suitable for head injury patient. Recommended by ATLS
Venturi face mask	Fixed	0.24–0.60	Performance depends on colour coded venturi jets. FiO2 determined by jet size and entrainment ratio. Requires reservoir tubing between jet and face mask. Dependent on tidal volume.
Venturi T-piece	Fixed	0.24–0.60	Used for laryngeal masks or endotracheal tubes. FiO2 determined by jet size and entrainment ratio. Requires high flow rates and reservoir tubing in expiratory limb.

Figure EQ.23

No capacity device

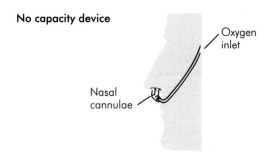

Oxygen inlet

Nasal cannulae

Small capacity device

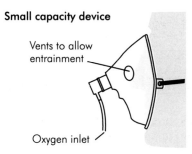

Vents to allow entrainment

Oxygen inlet

Large capacity device

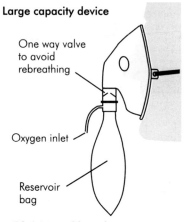

One way valve to avoid rebreathing

Oxygen inlet

Reservoir bag

Figure EQ.24. Variable performance oxygen delivery systems

RESUSCITATION BREATHING SYSTEMS

Such systems are used during resuscitation, to apply artificial ventilation to patients who are not breathing spontaneously. They also allow the patient to breathe spontaneously through them. There are two commonly used systems the Ambu system and the Laerdal system

Venturi mask

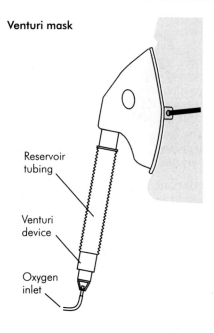

Reservoir tubing

Venturi device

Oxygen inlet

Venturi T-piece

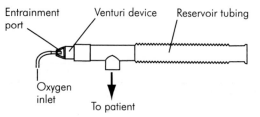

Entrainment port   Venturi device   Reservoir tubing

Oxygen inlet

To patient

Figure EQ.25 Fixed performance oxygen delivery systems

The basic components of these systems are:

- **Self-inflating bag** – This has a volume of approximately 1500 ml for the adult (500 ml for a child, 250 ml for an infant). The walls are reinforced to make the bag self inflating. One end of the bag is the inlet for fresh gas and is sealed by a flap valve. This also possesses an inlet for oxygen supplementation. The other end of the bag is connected to the patient via a non-rebreathing valve. (Figure EQ.26)

- **Non-rebreathing valve** – There are several designs for this valve in common use. These include the Rubens valve, the Laerdal valve and different types of Ambu valve. These valves open the patient's airway to the bag during inspiration, and then during expiration, close the connection to the bag and allow patient's gases to expire to the atmosphere. Figure EQ.27 and 28 show examples of some non-rebreathing valves used in resuscitation systems. The Rubens valve possesses a spring loaded bobbin which slides to open the patient's airway to the bag during inspiration (or inflation). During expiration the spring closes the airway to the bag and opens it to the atmosphere. High pressures in the bag can hold the bobbin in the inspiratory position. The Ambu valve (type E) uses a double leaf valve to produce the same reciprocal inspiratory and expiratory functions of the valve.

- **Oxygen reservoir bag** – This is fitted over the fresh gas inlet to the self inflating bag and is inflated by the supplementary oxygen supply. It also possesses an inlet flap valve to allow entrainment from the atmosphere should the demand of the patient exceed its capacity. Without the reservoir bag the delivered FiO2 is limited to less than 0.5. Using a reservoir bag can increase the FiO2 to 1.

- **Oxygen supply** – This enters the bag or reservoir via narrow bore tubing and nipple connector. The flow rate used is between 2 to 15 l/min. The final inspired oxygen concentration delivered to the patient will depend on the oxygen flow rate, respiratory rate, tidal volume and whether a reservoir is used.

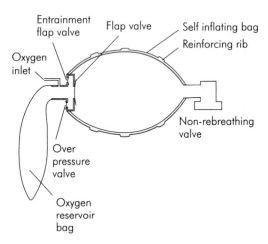

Figure EQ.26 Self inflating bag

INSPIRATION

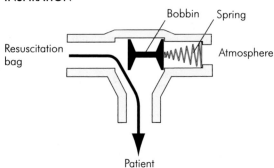

EXPIRATION

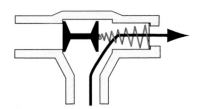

Figure EQ.27 Rubens non rebreathing valve

INSPIRATION

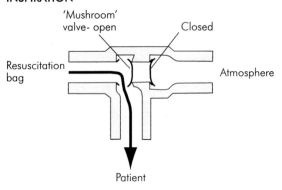

EXPIRATION

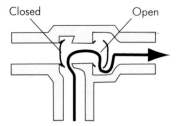

Figure EQ.28 Ambu non rebreathing valve

ENDOTRACHEAL TUBES

A plastic or rubber tube inserted into the trachea provides the definitive airway allowing positive pressure ventilation while preventing contamination of the lungs from the contents of the pharynx. The original tubes were made by Rowbotham and Magill in 1920 from rubber tubing of varying diameter and cut to the correct length by hand. Both oral and nasal tubes were designed and these were connected to the breathing circuit by a metal adapter. Later developments included the cuff with pilot balloon, double lumen tubes for thoracic surgery, and anatomically shaped tubes e.g. Oxford or RAE (Ring, Adair, Elwyn) tubes.

Red rubber produced inflammatory reactions at the site of contact and has been superseded by non-irritant transparent plastic. The tubes are often marked with the initials IT (implant tested) or Z79 (which refers to a room number related to the toxicity sub committee of ANSI) according to the American National Standards Institute. The tube is marked with the internal and external diameters in mm, the length in cm, and usually also a radio-opaque line to aid visualisation on chest X-ray. High volume cuffs when inflated are associated with a lower pressure on the tracheal mucosa and are appropriate for long operations or intensive care use. The pressure in the cuff can also increase as nitrous oxide diffuses through the thin plastic wall. While this can be prevented by filling the balloon with saline some tubes have been designed with an oversize pilot balloon (Brandt pattern) or with a cuff filled with self expanding foam and the connecting tube is left open to the atmosphere. The requirements of ENT surgery has lead to designs which minimise the obstruction to the surgeon's vision (microlaryngoscopy tubes), or which cannot be kinked (wire reinforced tubes) and tubes resistant to ignition by the operating laser.

To describe a tube, identify the following features; single or double lumen, material, the cuff and pilot balloon with self sealing valve, the bevel with or without eyes, and special features.

THE LARYNGEAL MASK AIRWAY

First produced commercially in 1986 to the design of Dr Archie Brain, the LMA offers an airway intermediate between the face mask and tracheal tube and represents arguably the most significant advance of the decade. It consists of a wide tube terminating at one end in a 15 mm connection and at the other in an inflatable cuff that is placed over the laryngeal opening. When inflated the cuff provides an airtight seal sufficient to permit gentle positive pressure ventilation if the chest compliance is normal although it does not protect the trachea from soiling by stomach contents and should not therefore be used if aspiration is a possibility. The LMA is produced in a range of sizes from #1 (neonate) to #5 for large adults. There is a standard pattern and a reinforced pattern for use in ENT surgery. The construction materials withstand repeated cleaning and autoclaving for up to 40 times and this should be noted on the record card that is supplied by the manufacturer. The intubating LMA allows for the passage of an ETT through the lumen, blindly into the trachea. The LMA is latex free in all its variants.

SCAVENGING SYSTEMS

An appropriate scavenging system is mandatory in each anaesthetic room and operating theatre in order to avoid pollution by anaesthetic gases and agents. Although there are no studies proving side effects caused by chronic exposure to low levels of anaesthetic gases or vapours, the alleged side effects include:

- Increased incidence of spontaneous abortion

- Vitamin B_{12} inactivation by nitrous oxide with neurological sequelae

- Increased incidence of female births

- Reduced fertility in females exposed to nitrous oxide

- Increased incidence of minor congenital abnormalities

- Increased incidence of leukaemia and lymphoma in exposed females

RECOMMENDED LEVELS OF POLLUTANTS

There is legal requirement under a code of practice drawn up by the Health and Safety Commission (HSC, 1996), to control exposure levels of many pollutants including anaesthetic agents. Some of the recommended maximum levels of exposure (averaged over any 8 hour time period) are listed in Figure EQ.29.

Maximum anaesthetic pollutant levels recommended by the HSC

Pollutant	Maximum level (ppm)
Nitrous oxide	100
Halothane	10
Enflurane	50
Isoflurane	50

Figure EQ.29.

TYPES OF SCAVENGING SYSTEM

Scavenging systems are designed to collect the waste gases and vapours from the anaesthetic machine and dispose of them, without affecting the breathing or ventilation of the patient, and without affecting the safe operation of the anaesthetic machine. The different types of scavenging system include, passive systems, active systems and absorber systems.

All scavenging systems require a device for collecting the waste gas from the breathing system, ventilator or patient. To cope with wide fluctuations in gas flow (from 0–130 l/min) there needs to be a reservoir to collect waste gases. The patient may either be protected by positive and negative pressure relief valves or, in an active system, an open ended reservoir. The standard size of connections is 30 mm to avoid wrong connections and the risk of obstruction of the patient's expiratory pathway must be minimised. Figure EQ.30 shows the design of scavenging systems.

Passive systems

Early scavenging systems were passive in that the patient's expiratory effort was required to propel waste gas down an additional length of tubing to the outside atmosphere. While the flow of gas could be assisted by either placing the end near the air conditioning outlet or terminating the roof vent with an extractor cowl, these systems were notably inefficient. Despite a maximal tubing resistance of 0.5 cmH$_2$O the increased resistance to expiration and the potential for complete obstruction represented a distinct hazard to the patient without measurably protecting the theatre staff.

Active systems

Modern active scavenging is usually driven by a fan unit remote to the theatre unit which produces a sub atmospheric pressure capable of large gas flows (75

l/min, peak flow 130 l/min per patient) in a piped distribution system. Distribution is terminated in each theatre where it is connected to the reservoir collection system. The reservoir usually houses a visual flow indicator which should be periodically checked to ensure the system is working. The system should operate within the pressures of -0.5 cmH$_2$O and +5 cmH$_2$O at 30 l/min flow.

Absorbers

Absorbers are usually based on activated charcoal and can, to a limited extent, absorb volatile agents (which may be released again by the use of heat).

MECHANICAL VENTILATORS

A mechanical ventilator is designed to automatically inflate the lungs when a patient is unable to breathe spontaneously. This is most commonly achieved by applying positive pressure applied to the patient's airway, as in intermittent positive pressure ventilation (IPPV). Alternative techniques also include high frequency methods such as high frequency jet ventilation (HFJV), and the use of negative pressure applied to the patient's chest wall (cuirass)

A ventilator can be described by different characteristics, which can be divided into:

- **Ventilation cycle parameters** – This term refers to the parameters (pressure, flow rate) which are defined during the inspiratory and expiratory phases of each ventilation cycle. It also defines how the ventilator switches between inspiratory and expiratory phases. Detailed discussion is presented below in 'Mapleson classification for ventilators'.

- **Mechanics** – Which describes the mechanism and power supply used to generate the ventilation cycle, e.g. minute volume divider, 'bag in the bottle'. These characteristics will often determine its physical size and power requirements.

- **Clinical features** – Which describe the features which determine its clinical field of application (operating theatre, ICU, neonatal unit). These include its ability to provide ancillary modes such as positive end expiratory pressure (PEEP), continuous positive airway pressure (CPAP), and synchronised intermittent mandatory ventilation (SIMV).

PASSIVE SCAVENGING

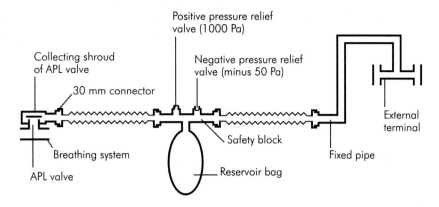

ACTIVE SCAVENGING

Figure EQ.30 Scavenging systems

IDEAL CHARACTERISTICS OF A VENTILATOR

The ideal specifications for a ventilator will vary according to its clinical application. Clearly the requirements of a ventilator for the intensive care unit will be very different from those for a ventilator to be used in an ambulance. Usually clinical application will dictate the physical parameters of the ventilation cycle and the mechanics of the ventilator.

Within the limitations of its clinical application a ventilator should:

- Provide appropriate ventilation modes for its particular application
- Have easy switching between automatic and manual functions
- Be simple and practical to use
- Be mechanically well designed and reliable
- Have appropriate, reliable and readily visible monitoring and alarms
- Be easy to clean and sterilise

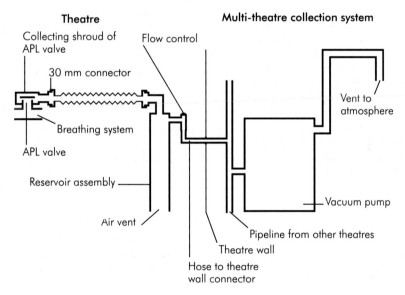

MAPLESON CLASSIFICATION FOR VENTILATORS

This scheme classifies positive pressure ventilators according to the different phases of the ventilation cycle:

- Inspiratory phase

- Cycling between inspiration and expiration (inspiratory cycling)

- Expiratory phase

- Cycling between expiration and inspiration (expiratory cycling, inspiratory triggering)

Inspiratory phase

During inspiration either pressure or flow rate can be determined by the ventilator mechanism. Thus a ventilator can be described either as a 'pressure generator' or 'flow generator'.

Flow generators and pressure generators are basically different in mechanical design. A pressure generator must be capable of providing high flow rates at the preset inspiratory pressure, which means it must have a low internal impedance to flow. In the case of the flow generator, in order for it to deliver the preset flow rate irrespective of variations in lung compliance, its internal impedance must be very high to attenuate the effect of variations in lung compliance on ventilator performance.

Some properties of pressure and flow generators are listed in Figure EQ.31.

Comparison between pressure and flow generator ventilators		
Property	**Pressure generators**	**Flow generators**
Inspiratory pressure	Inspiratory pressure and pattern (e.g constant, sinusoidal, triangular) preset on ventilator.	Inspiratory pressure will vary according to respiratory mechanics of patient. High inspiratory pressures may be produced with low lung compliance (e.g. adult respiratory distress syndrome).
Inspiratory flow rate	Inspiratory flow rate (and hence tidal volume) will vary according to respiratory mechanics of patient. High flow rates may be produced with high lung compliance (e.g. neonates)	Inspiratory flow rate and pattern (e.g. constant, ramp) preset on ventilator
Tidal volume	Tidal volume will vary according to lung compliance. Decreased lung compliance will reduce tidal volume	Preset tidal volume will be delivered at the expense of airway pressure, unless an inspiratory pressure limit is preset.
Risk of barotrauma	Low risk	High risk unless pressure limit preset on ventilator
Risk of volutrauma (Excessive tidal volumes)	High risk unless limit on tidal volume preset on ventilator	Low risk
Compensation for leakage	Some limited ability to compensate for small leaks in circuitry between ventilator and patient, since ventilator always acts to deliver preset inspiratory pressure	Any leakage from connecting circuit will be lost as it is counted by ventilator as delivered flow (tidal volume)
Clinical application	Suitable for paediatrics or neonates because of low risk of barotrauma and ability to compensate for small leaks. Requires tidal volume limit. Safer for emphysematous lungs	Appropriate for ICU because of ability to deliver flow (tidal volume) with low lung compliance. Requires inspiratory pressure limitation to reduce risk of barotrauma

Figure EQ.31

VENTILATOR PERFORMANCE AND REDUCED LUNG COMPLIANCE

As can be seen from Figure EQ.31, inspiratory pressures and flow rates are affected by both lung compliance and the type of ventilator used. The differences between pressure and flow generators when ventilating patients with normal or reduced lung compliances, can be illustrated by the pressure and flow curves during a ventilation cycle. The flow curve also gives information about the tidal volume, since volume is obtained from the area under the flow curve. The inspired tidal volume delivered is thus equal to the area under the flow curve during inspiration. Expired tidal volume is given by the area under the flow curve during expiration.

Figure EQ.32 shows a **pressure generator** delivering constant inspiratory pressure. Flow rate increases to a peak during inspiration and then decreases exponentially during expiration which is passive. The areas (tidal volumes) under the inspiratory and expiratory parts of the flow curve are approximately equal. When lung compliance is reduced the peak inspiratory flow rate reached is lower and the inspiratory and expiratory tidal volumes are reduced.

Figure EQ.33 shows a **flow generator** delivering constant flow during inspiration with a **preset tidal volume**. Inspiratory pressure will rise rapidly initially and reach a peak, which then decreases exponentially during expiration. When lung compliance is reduced the ventilator still delivers the same constant inspired flow with the same duration (preset tidal volume), peak inspiratory pressure however is increased. The lower the compliance (i.e. the stiffer the lungs), the greater the inspiratory pressures required to deliver the preset flow and tidal volume.

Figure EQ.34 shows a **flow generator** delivering constant flow with **pressure limitation** and a **preset tidal volume**. With normal lung compliance the pressure limit is not exceeded and an inspiratory pressure curve as in Figure EQ.33 is produced. When reduced lung compliance is present the inspiratory pressures are increased. If the pressure exceeds the preset limit and inspiration is cut short, and the tidal volume delivered is reduced below the preset value.

(a) Pressure generator with constant inspiratory pressure (I - inspiration, E - expiration)

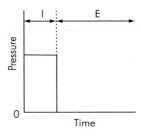
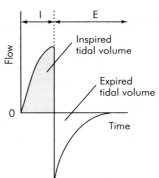

(b) Effect of reduced compliance in pressure generator

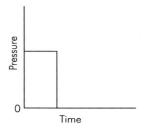
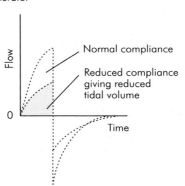

EQ.32 Inspiratory patterns from Pressure generator

(a) Flow generator with preset tidal volume (I - inspiration, E - expiration)

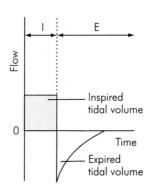

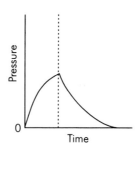

(b) Effect of reduced compliance on flow generator with preset tidal volume

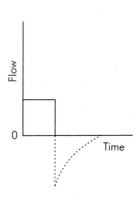

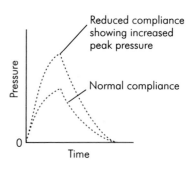

EQ.33 Inspiratory patterns from a Flow generator with preset tidal volume

Cycling between inspiration and expiration (inspiratory cycling)

The change between inspiration and expiration can be triggered by various parameters. This function is referred to as cycling and may be described as follows:

- Volume cycling. Inspiration stops and expiration begins when the preset tidal volume is delivered. An inspiratory pause may be used which prolongs the inspiratory phase.

- Pressure cycling. Inspiration occurs up to a preset inspiratory pressure at which expiration is then triggered.

- Time cycling. The inspiratory phase occurs for a fixed duration which is preset, and at the end of this time expiration is triggered. This type of cycling will effectively preset tidal volume in a flow generator.

Expiratory phase

Expiration is normally passive but during the expiratory phase, positive pressure can be applied to give Positive End Expiratory Pressure (PEEP). This technique is usually applied in the Intensive Care Unit to improve oxygenation and recruit lung volume in patients with certain lung pathologies such as Adult Respiratory Distress Syndrome. Surgical anaesthesia in the operating theatre does not usually involve the use of PEEP

Cycling between expiration and inspiration (expiratory cycling)

The change from expiration to inspiration usually occurs on a timed basis (i.e. expiratory time cycling) as determined by the preset ventilation frequency e.g. if a frequency of 12 breaths/min is preset, then expiratory

(a) Flow generator with preset tidal volume and pressure limitation

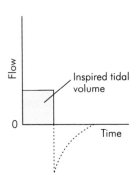

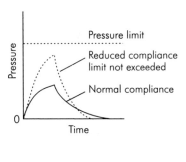

(b) Effect of reduced compliance on flow generator with pressure limitation
causing reduction of tidal volume

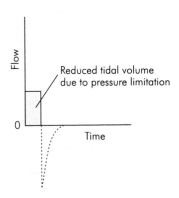

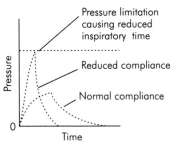

EQ.34 Inspiratory patterns from a Flow generator with pressure limitation and preset tidal volume

cycling will occur (i.e. inspiration will be triggered) every 5 seconds.

Alternatively, in supported or assisted ventilation modes (such as synchronised intermittent mandatory ventilation, SIMV) which are used to give ventilatory support to patients with some degree of spontaneous respiratory effort or who are being weaned from mechanical ventilation.

In these case inspiration may be triggered by negative pressure changes or flow rates generated by the patient's own spontaneous inspiratory efforts.

VENTILATOR MECHANICS

The mechanical design of ventilators centres around the driving mechanism which delivers fresh gas to the patient. Secondary aspects such as the power supply,

control mechanisms, monitoring and reliability, are often equally as important, in determining the ventilator's clinical performance. Some examples of the different mechanical designs used for ventilators are summarised in Figure EQ.35. A ventilator may have the advantages of simplicity and reliability, or may be very complex in design, in order to cope with more specialised clinical applications.

CLINICAL FEATURES OF VENTILATORS

Most ventilators can be used to ventilate normal lungs. For the more specialised clinical applications, for patients with respiratory pathology or for weaning from mechanical ventilation, additional clinical features or ancillary modes may be required in a ventilator. Some examples of these modes are outlined in Figure EQ.36.

Ventilator mechanics		
Ventilator	Mechanism	Comments
Minute volume divider	Driven by the fresh gas supply. The fresh gas flow passes into bellows, which divide it up into tidal volumes by filling repeatedly. The first bellows empty into second bellows, which deliver the tidal volume to the patient.	Simple reliable mechanism. No additional power supply required. Limited capability for patients with abnormal lungs. Workhorse ventilator for theatres and anaesthetic rooms.
'Bag in bottle' or 'Bag squeezer'	Fresh gas flow for the patient enters bellows (bag) mounted in a container (bottle). The ventilator compresses the bellows downwards, by pressurising the bottle during inspiration. The bag is then opened to an expiratory port during expiration. Different sizes of bellows used for adults and children. Modern versions microprocessor controlled	The patient circuit is isolated from the ventilator circuit. This means the ventilator is used as a servoventilator, to ventilate a patient through a separate breathing system such as a circle or Bain. Often incorporated into anaesthetic machines.
Microprocessor controlled electronic ventilator	Usually employs a bellows mechanism driven mechanically (e.g. spring loaded). Sophisticated electronics and monitoring to provide accurate control and triggered modes of ventilation.	Used for intensive care. Complex and software driven. Provides ancillary modes for difficult lung pathologies (ARDS, bullous lung disease) and weaning.
High frequency jet ventilator	Uses high MPGS supply (400 kPa) to inject into an endotracheal tube, tracheostomy tube, or other interface circuit, which connects to the patients airway. The ventilator – patient interface is an important factor in determining performance	Used for intensive care and thoracic surgery. Does not require a sealed airway to ventilate patient. Increased risk of barotrauma and problems with humidification when applied for prolonged periods.

Figure EQ.35

SOME EXAMPLES OF VENTILATORS

Manley MP3 (Figure EQ.37a)

- Ventilation cycle parameters: A pressure generator which is time cycled on inspiration (determined by rate of filling of first bellows) and volume cycled on expiration (preset tidal volume control on second bellows).

- Mechanics: Minute volume divider, simple, reliable, and no power supply required.

- Clinical features: Used in operating theatre, anaesthetic rooms, but not suitable for ICU.

Ohmeda 7800 (Figure EQ.37b)

- Ventilation cycle parameters: A flow generator which is time cycled.

- Mechanics: A 'bag in bottle' (bag squeezer), which is used with circle breathing system and incorporated into anaesthetic machines. It uses wall supply gas to drive the bag squeezer and has a separate microprocessor control unit.

- Clinical features: Incorporated into anaesthetic machines, therefore used in operating theatre and anaesthetic rooms.

Ancillary modes in ventilators

Mode	Description	Comments
Positive End Expiratory Pressure (PEEP)	0 – 15 cmH$_2$O of positive airway pressure maintained during expiration	Applied to improve oxygenation, recruit lung volume and prevent micro-atelectasis
Continuous Positive Airway Pressure (CPAP)	0 – 15 cmH$_2$O of positive airway pressure maintained during inspiration and expiration	Applied to assist patients' spontaneous breathing by improving oxygenation and reducing the work of breathing.
Intermittent Mandatory Ventilation (IMV)	This mode supports patients who are breathing spontaneous, but inadequately. It supplies a minimum minute volume, as a preset number of mandatory breaths per minute. The patient breathes spontaneously between mandatory breaths.	Applied to patients who are being weaned from mechanical ventilation. A disdvantage is that mandatory breaths may 'stack' on top of spontaneous breaths giving high airway pressures.
Synchronised Intermittent Mandatory Ventilation (SIMV)	This form of IMV synchronises the mandatory breaths with the patient's spontaneous breathing	Avoids 'stacking' of mandatory breaths and spontaneous breaths
Pressure Support (PS)	An 'assisted' mode in which the ventilator provides a mechanical breath when triggered by the patient's spontaneous effort. The ventilator is set to act as a pressure generator in this mode.	Used as a supporting mode in spontaneously breathing patients being weaned fron mechanical ventilation or with respiratory failure

Figure EQ.36

Drager Evita 4 (Figure EQ.37c)

- Ventilation cycle parameters: A flow or pressure generator, with multiple cycling abilities.

- Mechanics: Mechanically driven bellows with full microprocessor controls and monitoring. Software driven.

- Clinical features: ICU ventilator with multiple ancillary modes including PEEP, CPAP, SIMV and BIPAP.

Accutronic Monsoon (Figure EQ.37d)

- Ventilation cycle parameters: Effectively a pressure generator, although the airway pressure cannot be preset directly. The airway pressure generated depends on the ventilator settings of frequency, drive pressure and duty cycle. Time cycled in both 'inspiration' and 'expiration' although the terms are not directly applicable during high frequency ventilation.

- Mechanics: High frequency jet ventilator, which can operate between 1 and 20 Hz .

- Clinical features: Used in ICU and for thoracic surgery.

HUMIDIFIERS

Humidity refers to the amount of water vapour present in a gas or the atmosphere.

It is defined in two ways:

Absolute humidity (AH) is the mass of water vapour present in a given volume of air or gas (g/m^3 or kg/m^3). This value will not vary with the temperature of the air.

CHECKLIST FOR ANAESTHETIC APPARATUS

The following checks should be made prior to each operating session.

1. **Check that the anaesthetic machine is connected to the electricity supply (if appropriate) and switched on**

   - Take note of any information or labelling on the anaesthetic machine referring to the current status of the machine. Particular attention should be paid to recent servicing. Servicing labels should be fixed in the service logbook

2. **Check that an oxygen analyser is present on the anaesthetic machine**

   - Ensure that the analyser is switched on, checked and calibrated

   - The oxygen sensor should be placed where it can monitor the composition of the gases leaving the common gas outlet

3. **Identify and take note of the gases that are being supplied by pipeline, confirming with a 'tug-test' that each pipeline is correctly inserted into the appropriate gas supply terminal**

   Note that CO_2 cylinders should not be present on the anaesthetic machine unless requested by the anaesthetist. A blanking plug should be fitted to any empty cylinder yoke

   - Check that the anaesthetic machine is connected to a supply of oxygen and that an adequate supply of oxygen is available from a reserve oxygen cylinder

   - Check that adequate supplies of other gases (nitrous oxide, air) are available and connected as appropriate

   - Check that all pipeline pressure gauges in use on the anaesthetic machine indicate 400 kPa

4. **Check the operation of flowmeters**

   - Ensure that each flow control valve operates smoothly and that the bobbin moves freely throughout its range

   - Check the operation of the emergency oxygen bypass control

5. **Check the vaporiser(s):**

   - Ensure that each vaporiser is adequately but not over filled

   - Ensure that each vaporiser is correctly seated on the back bar and not tilted

   Check the vaporiser for leaks (with vaporiser on and off) by temporarily occluding the common gas outlet

   When checks have been completed turn the vaporiser(s) off

   A leak test should be performed immediately after changing any vaporiser

Continued on next page

6. Check the breathing system to be employed

- The system should be visually inspected for correct configuration. All connections should be secured by push and twist
- A pressure leak test should be performed on the breathing system by occluding the patient port and compressing the reservoir bag
- The correct operation of unidirectional valves should be carefully checked

7. Check that the ventilator is configured appropriately for its intended use

- Ensure that the ventilator tubing is correctly configured and securely attached
- Set the controls for use and ensure that an adequate pressure is generated during the inspiratory phase
- Check that the pressure relief valve functions
- Check that the disconnect alarm functions correctly
- Ensure that an alternative means to ventilate the patient's lungs is available

8. Check that the anaesthetic gas scavenging system is switched on and is functioning correctly

- Ensure that the tubing is attached to the appropriate expiratory part(s) of the breathing system or ventilator

9. Check that all ancillary equipment which may be needed is present and working

- This includes laryngoscopes, intubation aids, intubation forceps, bougies, etc. and appropriately sized face masks, airways, tracheal tubes and connectors
- Check that the suction apparatus is functioning and that all connections are secure
- Check that the patient can be tilted head-down on the trolley, operating table or bed

10. Ensure that the appropriate monitoring equipment is present, switched on and calibrated ready for use

- Set all default alarm limits as appropriate (it may be necessary to place the monitors in the stand-by mode to avoid unnecessary alarms before being connected to the patient)

Association of Anaesthetists of Great Britain and Ireland 1997

Figure EQ.42 Association of Anaesthetists checklist

SECTION 4: 4
BASIC STATISTICS

D. J. Rowbotham

TYPES OF DATA
  Qualitative
  Quantitative

DESCRIBING DATA
  Qualitative
  Quantitative

STATISTICAL TESTS
  Basic principles
  Testing qualitative data
  Testing quantitative data
  Multiple groups
  Paired data
  Study power
  Confidence intervals
  Linear correlation
  Linear regression
  Data transformation
  One and two tailed tests
  Sequential analysis

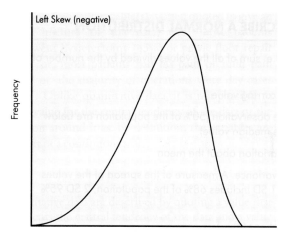

Figure ST.7 Non normally distributed data; mode, mean, median

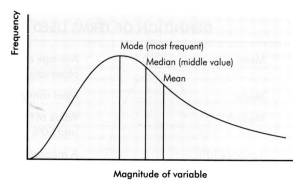

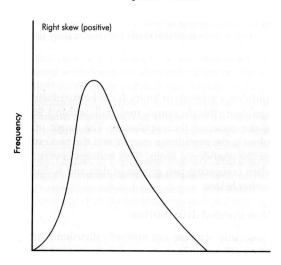

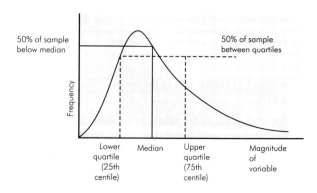

Figure ST.8 Interquartiles

STATISTICAL TESTS

The basic principles behind statistical tests and several specific tests often used in anaesthetic studies are described. Applying the correct test is important and Figure ST.9 gives a simple scheme to help this process.

BASIC PRINCIPLES

In life, and especially in medicine, nothing is certain. It is very difficult to state with absolute certainty that one population is different from another. Therefore, when testing the difference between samples the concept of probability must be embraced. P is used to denote the probability of an event occurring (event always occurs, $P = 1$; event never occurs, $P = 0$). Therefore, the probability (P) of heads on tossing a coin is 0.5 (50%). When comparing two samples, depending on how different they are and on the variability of the data, there is a definable probability that they are

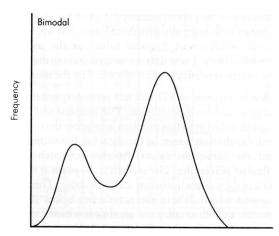

Figure ST.6 Non normally distributed data

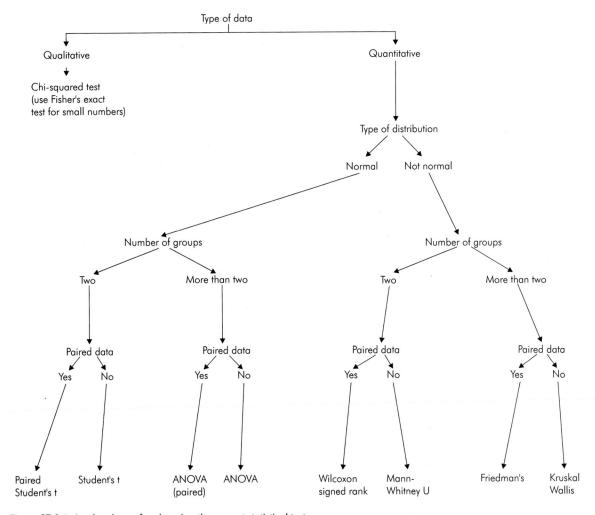

Figure ST.9 A simple scheme for choosing the correct statistical test

significantly different. Most study samples are relatively small compared with the population as a whole and it can rarely be said that one population is definitely different to anther, i.e. P = 1. Compromise, therefore, becomes necessary and it is accepted that if there is only a 1:20 probability, i.e. P = 0.05, that the difference between the samples is due to chance, then there is a statistically significant difference between them. This is the principle behind most statistical tests and each one gives a value to P. Note that in adopting this approach it is accepted that there is a 1:20 chance of making an error (type I or 'α' error) of assuming a difference when there is none. Note the probability of a type I error has been deliberately set at the 0.05 level.

Conventionally, when a statistical test is used, the null hypothesis is applied. The hypothesis states that there is no difference between means of the samples. If the test gives P > 0.05, there is no difference and the null hypothesis is accepted. If P < 0.05, the null hypothesis is rejected as there is a statistically significant difference between the samples.

TESTING QUALITATIVE DATA

Some statistical tests (see below) that perform mathematics on the values in the samples, rely on the mean reflecting the central tendency and assume a symmetrical distribution of data around the mean. Clearly, these tests are not appropriate for qualitative data as the data are not numerical or part of a continuous scale. Tests for these data derive values from the raw data and then perform mathematics on these derived data to arrive at a value of P. The chi-squared (c^2) test is the classical test for this type of data.

χ^2-test

The test compares the frequency of observed results against the frequency that would be expected if there was no difference between the groups. Imagine a study where droperidol has been compared with placebo for the prevention of post operative vomiting. In the data from the two groups are patients who vomited and those who did not ('yes' versus 'no'). The χ^2-test constructs a contingency table. As there are two treatment groups and two possible outcomes, this is called a 2 × 2 contingency table (Figure ST.10).

In the example, there were 40 patients in each group – 34 vomited in the placebo group compared with 10 in the droperidol group. The expected (E) incidence of vomiting and no vomiting, if there was no difference between the groups, are shown. For example, the number of patients who vomited should be 22 (E = 22) in each group if there was no difference. A calculation can now be performed on each of the four sets of data using:

$$\frac{[E - O]^2}{E}$$

where   E = expected frequency and
          O = observed frequency.

The results of each of the four calculations are added together to give χ^2:

$$\chi^2 = \Sigma \frac{[E-O]^2}{E}$$

P depends on χ^2 and the degrees of freedom (N) that may be calculated using:

Degrees of freedom (N) = (number of columns – 1) × (number of rows – 1).

In the example, degrees of freedom = 1; and, using χ^2 P

A 2 × 2 CONTINGENCY TABLE FOR A CHI-SQUARED TEST

	No vomit	Vomit	
Totals			
Placebo	6	34	40
	(E=18)	(E=22)	
Droperidol	30	10	40
	(E=18)	(E=22)	
Totals	36	44	80

Figure ST.10

can be gleaned from statistical tables – though automatically using computer software.

There are a few further points to be made regarding the χ^2-test:

- More than two groups and more than two outcomes measures can be dealt with by increasing the size of the contingency table, e.g. 3 × 2, 3 × 3, etc.
- In 2 × 2 tables, the calculation may be inaccurate and a correcting factor is often applied. This is the Yates' correction factor and involves subtracting 0.5 from each E – O calculation in each cell
- The results of the test are only reliable if < 20% of the expected frequencies are < 5. Under these circumstances, Fisher's exact test should be used. Manual calculation of this test is extremely difficult and is understood only by statisticians. However, many statistical computer packages include the test, often as an option with the χ^2-test when the program detects problems with the number of expected frequencies of < 5

TESTING QUANTITATIVE DATA

It is important to know the distribution of the data before applying any tests on quantitative data because tests used for normal data assume that the mean reflects the central tendency and that there is a symmetrical distribution of data around the mean. Other tests do not assume this and can be used for non normal data.

Test for normally distributed data

The Student's t-test (described by William Gosset) is most commonly used when comparing data from two normally distributed samples. It calculates 't', which depends not only on the magnitude of the absolute differences between the means, but also on the degree of confidence that the calculated mean represents the whole population (see above). The equation is as follows:

$$t = \frac{\text{Difference between the means}}{\text{Standard error of the difference}}$$

Therefore, t will increase with a large absolute difference between the means, a large sample size and a small sample variation. The latter two factors reduce the SEM and, therefore, the error of the difference. P can be read from statistical tables if t and the sample numbers are known.

Non normal data

If the data are not distributed normally, the mean and SEM cannot be relied upon and the Student's t-test may give spurious results. In this situation, the

Mann–Whitney U-test is often used. The Wilcoxon two-sample rank sum test is similar but it is important not to confuse this test with the Wilcoxon signed rank test that is used for paired data (see below). Because of this potential confusion, it is best to use the term Mann–Whitney U-test when comparing two groups of non parametric data.

The Mann–Whitney U-test ranks all the data in order of magnitude and then assigns a ranking score to each one. For example, if there are 40 variables then the largest one will be assigned the value '1' and the smallest will be ranked '40'. The test then performs mathematics on these scores – not the data – and negates the effect of a skewed distribution. U is obtained, which, along with the number in the sample, gives P.

COMPARING MORE THAN TWO GROUPS

When comparing data from three groups, a Student's t-test or Mann–Whitney U-test may be appropriate depending on the distribution of the data. The data are normally distributed so, using a t-test, group 1 is compared with group 2, group 2 with group 3, and then group 3 with group 1. Multiple t-tests are thus being applied to these data and this is not acceptable. Every time a discrete statistical test is used there is a 1:20 chance that a difference will be assumed when there is none – this is acceptable. However, it also means that if 20 comparisons are performed on the same data with the same test it is likely that a significant difference will be found in one (or more) of the tests when none exists. Multiple testing, therefore, increases the chance of finding a non existent difference and should not be performed.

If there are more than two groups, it is necessary to compare the data with analysis of variance (ANOVA). The mathematics of this are complicated but it is sufficient to understand that these techniques must be used under these circumstances. The Kruskal–Wallis test is used for non parametric data of more than two groups.

However, if the data are normally distributed a modified t-test, known as the Bonferroni test, can be used. This is similar to the Student's t-test but it applies a correction factor to allow for the error introduced by multiple testing.

TESTING PAIRED DATA

Data are considered paired if the two variables under test are from the same patient. If, for example, blood pressure is measured in two groups of patients given either etomidate or propofol for induction of anaesthesia and blood pressure is measured before and after induction, then the two measurements are paired. In this situation a paired test will examine the relationship between these measurements in each patient, i.e. the change in blood pressure. In this example, a paired students t-test is appropriate (assuming the data are normally distributed). If there are more than two groups, an ANOVA for paired data can be used.

The majority of paired data in anaesthetic studies arise from the within patient comparisons. However, it is possible to design a study where every patient in one group is paired with another. For example, if a 60 year old, 70 kg patient who smokes is entered into one treatment group, the investigators may recruit a similar patient into the other group to ensure that patients in both groups have an equivalent pair. Paired statistical tests may then be performed. Paired tests are attractive to researchers because they are more sensitive and generally require fewer patients in each group to achieve statistical significance.

Non parametric data can also be paired. Under these circumstances the Wilcoxon-signed-rank test for paired data is appropriate. If there are more than two groups, the Friedman's test is used.

STUDY POWER

This is a very important concept and should be understood by all those reading the scientific literature. Suppose the effect of a new drug on urine output in volunteers is to be tested. An IV dose of the drug is given to one group (n = 8) and placebo to another (n = 8). The mean (SEM) urine output in the next hour is placebo 103.5 (11.6) ml and drug 141.5 (20.0) ml.

There is quite an increase in the urine output in the treated group indicating that the drug may have a diuretic effect. However, a Student's t-test gives P = 0.12, i.e. there is no statistical difference. Can it now be said that this drug has no diuretic effect? The risk of assuming a difference when there is none (type I, or 'α', error) has been covered previously, but when performing statistical tests there is also a risk of assuming no difference when there may be a clinically relevant difference. This might have occurred in the example. This error is called a type II, or 'β', error. Three factors make a type II error more likely:

1. Small sample numbers
2. A large variation in the study population
3. Situations where small differences are clinically important

Conventionally, a 1:20 chance (5%) of making a type I error ($\alpha = 0.05$) is accepted. More leeway is allowable for type II errors and it is, therefore, acceptable to allow a 4:20, or 1:5, (20%) chance of making a type II error ($\beta = 0.2$). Accordingly, a study is said to have sufficient power if $\beta \leq 0.20$.

If no difference is detected between two groups in a study, it can only be concluded that there is no clinically important difference if the 'power' of the study is satisfactory. If the power is insufficient, i.e. a type II error has been made, then all that can be said is that insufficient numbers were studied. The latter outcome is a disaster for the investigators as they may have spent large amounts of time and money performing the study. It also raises ethical questions in that patients were exposed to the study and absolutely no useful information has resulted. To avoid this, the power of a proposed study should and can be calculated at the protocol stage. This ensures that, if no differences are found at the end of the study, a meaningful conclusion can still be made, i.e. there is no clinically important differences between the groups. Under these circumstances this is just as important and relevant as if a difference was found.

The numbers of patients needed to ensure sufficient power can often be calculated with ease, either with equations or nomograms. For example:

$$n > \frac{2 K \sigma^2}{d^2}$$

where:

- n = numbers needed in each group
- σ^2 = variance of the measured variable (can be acquired from a pilot study or data from other studies investigating similar patient groups)
- d = minimal clinically important difference. The investigator sets this. For example, detecting a difference in heart rate of 1 bpm is not important in most circumstances. It may be that the smallest difference that it needed to be detect is 8 bpm, i.e. if the study cannot detect a difference of 7 bpm this will not be a problem as the difference is not clinically important
- K = a constant read from a table. It depends on the 'a' and 'b' one wishes to adopt (usually a = 0.05, b = 0.20)

CONFIDENCE INTERVALS

The concept of the confidence interval of a mean taken from a study sample has previously been alluded to. Considering the data from the diuretic drug example, the 95% confidence intervals (CI) for the mean urine output is 1.96 SEM either side of the mean. The mean (95% CI) for the placebo group is, therefore, 103.5 (80.6 – 126.4) ml, and 141.5 (102.3 – 180.7) ml for the group receiving the drug. Because of the small number of patients and wide variation, it can be seen that there is very little confidence in the means of either group (in other words, the confidence intervals are wide). Mean urine output after placebo may be 80.6 ml and, after the drug, 180.7 ml. If this were the case, the study would have shown a marked diuretic effect of the test drug. Conversely, the means may be 126.4 and 102.3 ml respectively. This would indicate a small reduction in urine output associated with the drug. Therefore, the confidence intervals suggest that a t test is unlikely to give a value of $P > 0.05$, our study design is inadequate and no meaningful conclusion can be drawn from our data.

There was a mean difference between the groups of 38 ml. It is possible to calculate the 95% CI of this difference and this value is often given by computer software calculating t-tests. In this example, the interval is –87 to +11.6 ml. This information is more useful than P (i.e. = 0.12) as it gives information on the power of the study. Although there was no statistical difference, the placebo group when compared with the active group may well have produced 87 ml less urine. This is a clinically significant change in hourly urine output and, if the negative findings of the small study are accepted, an important effect may be missed. Equally, the placebo group may have produce 11.6 ml more than the active group. Therefore, the confidence intervals of the difference of the means indicates, again at a glance, whether there is any statistical difference (both limits would be negative or positive), how large any differences may be and, if there is no significant difference, what magnitude of differences could be missed.

LINEAR CORRELATION

It is often speculated whether one variable can be correlated (usually with a straight line or linear relationship) to another, for example drug clearance and renal function. If there is a good correlation between the variables it **may** be that the kidney clears the drug under investigation. However, it is important to remember that a correlation is only a mathematical relationship and that it does not imply a causal link. For example, if plotting yearly usage of the laryngeal mask against yearly subscriptions to the Internet, it is likely that a correlation will be found, i.e. both have been increasing at a similar rate in recent years. Clearly, however, use of the laryngeal mask has not caused people to surf the information highway, or vice versa.

When investigating correlation, two values need to be ascertained: the magnitude of the correlation and the statistical probability that the correlation exists.

The two variables under investigation from each patient or sample are plotted as a scatter diagram (Figure ST.11). If the points are more or less in a straight line, it cannot be concluded immediately that there is a linear correlation; the magnitude of this relationship must be known. Calculation of the correlation coefficient (r) gives this information. If r = 1 (Figure ST.11a), there is a perfect relationship. A lesser r, for example 0.7, implies a looser relationship (Figure ST.11b). If r = 0, there is no relationship (Figure ST.11c); if r = –1, there is a perfect inverse relationship (Figure ST.11d). It is important to remember that r is *not the slope of the line*; it is a measure of how close the values fit to this line. The *slope* of the line is described by the *regression* coefficient (see below).

The value r gives a measure of the magnitude of any correlation, but it is a poor measure of how confident one can be of this. For example, there is a perfect correlation (r = 1) in Figure ST.11e. However, there are only two points in this example and clearly nothing can be made of the data. Therefore, it is important to check the P of the correlation also before significance is assigned to any correlation.

The square of the correlation coefficient (r^2) is a useful term; its importance is described below under linear regression.

Calculating these values is complex but most software packages will perform them with ease. The Pearson's correlation coefficient is calculated for normal (parametric) data and the Spearman's correlation coefficient is used for non normal (non parametric) data.

LINEAR REGRESSION

It is often found that one set of variables is related or correlated to another. For example, inspired CO_2 and tidal volume. While this alone is useful, more information can be obtained by finding the exact nature of the relationship rather than simply knowing that the relationship exists. If this relationship is discovered the value of a (dependent) variable can be predicted as the other (independent) is changed. This relationship is called the regression coefficient. It is called the linear regression coefficient if the relationship is linear.

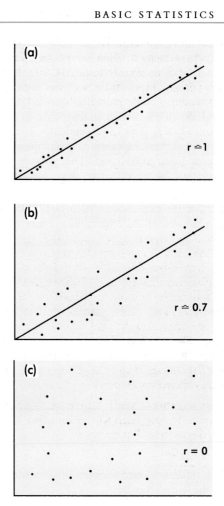
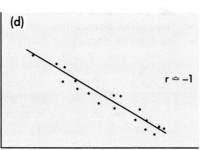
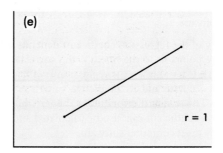

Figure ST.11 Correlation coefficients

In the example, the same inspired CO_2 could be used many times (perhaps using 20 volunteers) to get several measures of tidal volume for each inspired CO_2 and to calculate the mean. Mean tidal volumes against inspired CO_2 could then be plotted (Figure ST.12). The independent value is plotted on the x-axis. In the example, inspired CO_2 is the independent variable, tidal volume the dependent value. Clearly, there is some degree of linear correlation. The purpose of regression analysis is to calculate the *quantitative* relationship. Regression answers the question, 'To what extent does increasing the inspired CO_2 influence tidal volume', not, 'is there a relationship?'

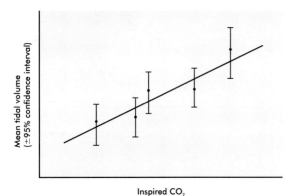

Figure ST.12 Linear regression

When a straight line is plotted between the points the equation for the line is given by:

$$y = bx + a$$

where: b = slope of the curve and
        a = intercept on the x-axis.

The slope (b) is the regression coefficient, and if it is known then it is possible to predict 'y'. This is the purpose of the regression coefficient. As can be seen from Figure ST.12, unless the correlation is perfect the points do not lie exactly on a straight line, and when calculating the regression coefficient a 'line of best fit' is derived using the 'method of least squares'. This involves complicated mathematics and is best left to computer software.

The accuracy of the regression coefficient depends on how well the points fit to the line, i.e. the correlation coefficient (r). If $r = 1$, then the regression coefficient is extremely accurate and its predictive value can be relied upon. The standard error and/or the 95% CI of the regression coefficient can also be calculated and is performed by most computer software.

The concept of r^2 (square of the correlation coefficient, or coefficient of determination) was mentioned above

and is a very useful and much quoted value. It is equal to the proportion of the total variation in the dependent variable that is explained by the regression coefficient. For example, if the correlation is perfect ($r = 1$) then $r^2 = 1$ and all the variation in the dependent variable (tidal volume in the example) can be explained by the regression coefficient. However, if $r = 0.8$, $r^2 = 0.64$ and only 64% of the variation in tidal volume can be explained by the regression line. Therefore, it can be seen immediately how inaccurate any predictions based on the regression line are likely to be and how other unmeasured factors may influence the dependent variable (in the example, this may be the variation in sensitivity of the respiratory centres to CO_2 in the volunteers).

DATA TRANSFORMATION

There are many tests that can only be performed on normally distributed data. Usually, this is not a problem as there are several tests available for non normal data (see above). However, there are some situations were no suitable tests are available, particularly for complicated designs of analysis of variance and regression analysis. Therefore, it is acceptable to manipulate the raw data to make it normally distributed.

Logarithmic transformation is performed most frequently. The log of each value is calculated and the distribution of the transformed data re-analysed. If it is now distributed normally, tests suitable for this type of data can be performed.

ONE- AND TWO-TAILED TESTS

When two means are compared, the point of interest is whether one is bigger than the other, or vice versa. However, in some situations one mean is bound to be larger or smaller than another. For example, when nitroprusside or placebo is given to patients and systolic blood pressure is measured, mean systolic pressure after nitroprusside is bound to be lower than after placebo. In this situation, when testing for statistically significant changes, one-tailed tests can be performed. In most computer software, the output from many tests, e.g. t-test and Mann–Whitney U-test, include both a two- and a one-tailed P.

SEQUENTIAL ANALYSIS

Occasionally, the results of a study are extremely important. Imagine a blinded study investigating the effect of a new drug on outcome in endotoxic shock. After considering the power of the study, it might decided that 100 patients should be enrolled. The data (survived/not survived, i.e. binary data) will be analysed only when the study has ended. However, what if the drug has a miraculous effect and, after investigating only 20 patients, there is a clear statistical improvement in survival? This would mean that about 40 more patients in the study would receive placebo and be denied life-saving therapy. (Alternatively, if the new drug had a disastrous effect, the lives of these patients would be put at risk.) To prevent this unacceptable risk to the patients in the study the technique of sequential analysis is often used. In this example, matched pairs would be entered and each patient would be given, in a randomised blinded fashion, either active treatment or placebo. A chart is then prepared upon which the outcomes of each pair of patients are plotted and the design of the chart is such that the plot crosses a predetermined line when $P = 0.05$ or 0.01, depending on the certainty required about whether there is a true difference. When the desired certainty is reached the study is stopped.

Index

A band 285, 301
'a' wave 315, 317, 340
  cannon 318
abdominal emergencies, acute 24
abdominal trauma 183
abdominal wall 214–15
abducent nerve (VI) 210, 217
ABO
  blood groups 264
  grouping and screening 266
  incompatibility reactions 266
absolute pressure 788
absorbance 822–4, 860
  curves in oximetry 861
absorption
  drug 573–4
  drug interactions 557
  gastro-intestinal 466–70
  local anaesthetic agents 659
AC see alternating current
acceleromyography 864
accessory nerve (XI) 211
acclimatisation, to high altitude 423, 424
accuracy 834
Accutronic Monsoon ventilator 903, 904
ACE inhibitors 11, 707–8
acetazolamide 710
acetyl-CoA 477, 480, 482
  in acetylcholine synthesis 292, 293
  ketone formation 488–9
  in lipid metabolism 487
  synthesis 482
acetyl-CoA carboxylase 487
acetylator status 569
acetylcholine (Ach) 429, 446
  drugs blocking synthesis, release and
      metabolism 685
  gastro-intestinal actions 462, 463
  inactivation 293
  neuromuscular blocking agents and
      641, 642, 644, 645
  in neuromuscular transmission 291,
      293
  receptors see cholinergic receptors
  synthesis and storage 292–3
acetylcholinesterase 293, 646, 647
  see also cholinesterase, plasma
acetylsalicylic acid see aspirin
acid–base balance, renal mechanisms
    387–91
acid–base disturbances
  compensation 391–2

correction 391–2
  renal pH regulation 391–4
acid diuresis, forced 551
acid-sensing ion-channel (ASIC)
    receptors 449
acidosis
  ammonia excretion 391
  in CPR 156
  see also metabolic acidosis; respiratory
    acidosis
ACTH see adrenocorticotropic hormone
actin 285
  in cardiac muscle 301
  filaments 223, 285–6
  in muscle contraction 286–8
  in smooth muscle 295
action potentials (APs)
  cardiac 301, 302–7
    atrial vs ventricular 304
    fast response 302–5
    pacemaker vs myocardial cell 305
    refractoriness 304–5
    slow response 302, 305–7
  ion channels and 305–6
  neurones 427–8
  skeletal muscle 293
  smooth muscle 295, 296
activated carriers 478, 479
activated clotting time (ACT) 749–50
activated partial thromboplastin time
    (APTT) 18, 269
  causes of prolonged 270
  heparin therapy and 749–50
active transport 230–1
  drugs 576, 578
  in kidney 370–1
  primary 230–1, 370–1
  secondary 231, 371
acupuncture, in labour 83
acute abdominal emergencies 24
acute chest syndrome, in sickle cell
    disease 262
acute lung injury (ALI) 186
  transfusion-associated (TRALI) 266
acute respiratory distress syndrome
    (ARDS) 180
acyclovir 766
AD_{50} 591
Addison's disease 505
adenoidectomy 93, 117
adenoids 194
adenosine 635

effects on blood flow 346, 358
for peri-arrest arrhythmias 157, 158,
    160, 162
peri-operative therapy 53, 69
pharmacology 703, 710
receptors 703
adenosine diphosphate (ADP) 273, 478
adenosine triphosphate see ATP
adenylyl cyclase 228, 237
ADH see anti-diuretic hormone
adhesion molecules, cell 226–7
adiabatic compression/expansion 797–8
adjustable pressure limiting (APL)
    expiratory valve 888
ADP (adenosine diphosphate) 273, 478
adrenal cortex 502, 503
  deficient secretion 505
  excess secretion 505–6
  hormones 503–5
adrenal gland 502–7
  in pregnancy 520
adrenal medulla 502, 506
  hormones 506–7
adrenaline see epinephrine
adrenergic receptor agonists 687–8,
    715–16
adrenergic receptors 446, 686
  subtypes 686
  see also α-adrenergic receptors; β-
    adrenergic receptors
adrenergic system 685–91
adrenocorticotropic hormone (ACTH)
    498, 500
  actions 503, 504
  excess secretion 505
adsorption 551
advanced life support (ALS) 152–62
  airway management 152–3
  algorithm 155
  circulation 153–4
  drug usage 156–7
  paediatric 166–8
  peri-arrest arrhythmias 157–62
  in pregnancy 164
  techniques applied 154–6
  ventilation 153
advanced trauma life support (ATLS) 173
adventitia 333
afterload 324–5
  definition 324–5
  measurement 325
age, body fluid compartments and 243

ageing 238–9
    adaptive evolution theory 239
    and dyshomeostasis 238
    non adaptive evolution theory 239
    theories 239
    'wear and tear' theory 239
    see also elderly patients
agonists 235, 547, 561
    inverse 612
    mechanism of action 552
    partial 561, 565–6
    pharmacodynamics 563–5
AIDS 105–6
    encephalopathy 106
    see also HIV
air
    compressed, for medical use 877
    cylinders 878
    embolism 55–6, 341
airway(s)
    assessment, in basic life support 150–1
    combitube 34, 152
    conducting 397
    gas flow 406–7, 801
    patency, ensuring 30–1
    pre-operative assessment 3, 35
    in pregnancy 516
    sensory receptors 420
    surgical 152–3
    trauma, post operative 79
    upper see upper airway
    see also laryngeal mask airway;
            nasopharyngeal airway;
            oropharyngeal airway
airway management
    in advanced life support 152–3
        paediatric patients 166
        in pregnancy 164
    in basic life support 150–1
        paediatric patients 164
    devices 34–5
    intra-operative 48–9
    in major trauma 175–6
    unconscious patient 62, 63
airway management device (AMD) 34
airway obstruction
    airway resistance 407
    basic life support 150
    intra-operative 54
    in major trauma 175
    upper
        by foreign body 151
        induction of anaesthesia 41
        in infant or child 164, 165
        post operative 62–3
airway pressure (P_{AW}) 50
airway resistance 406
    factors affecting 407
    location 407
    measurement 407
albumin 248, 250
    drug binding 548, 576–7
    glomerular filtration 365
    solutions, human (HAS) 740, 741
    synthesis 490–1
alcohol, breath 113
aldosterone 384, 503–4

actions 348, 385, 468, 503–4
    excess secretion 505
    pharmacology 726
    regulation of secretion 383, 503
alfentanil 627, 635
    pharmacokinetics 623, 627
algogens 449
alkaline diuresis, forced 551
alkalising agents, in CPR 156, 168
alkaptonuria 485
allergy 281
    anaesthetic drugs 28–30
    latex 107–8
    see also hypersensitivity
allodynia 450
allosteric modulation 236
α-adrenergic receptor antagonists 688–9
α-adrenergic receptors 446, 686
    drug–receptor interactions 687
    subtypes 686
α error 919, 921
α globin genes 260, 261
α particles 828
α rhythm 432, 867
α_1-adrenergic receptor antagonists 688–9
α_1-glycoprotein 577, 660
alphadolone 614
alphaxolone 614
alteplase 750
alternating current (AC) 805
    shock 812, 813
althesin 614
altitude
    acclimatisation 423, 424
    illnesses 424
    lung function 422–4
    vaporiser performance 886
    ventilatory response to oxygen 421
alveolar–capillary membrane 398, 410
alveolar cells (pneumocytes)
    type I 398
    type II 198, 398
alveolar dead space 401
alveolar ducts 397–8
alveolar gas equation 409, 423
alveolar hypoventilation, post operative
        65–7
alveolar sac 397–8
alveolar ventilation 401
    effects of varying 409, 410
    at high altitude 423
    response to $PaCO_2$ 420–1
    volatile agent uptake and 589–90
alveolar volume (VA) 401
alveoli 198, 397–8
    gas diffusion into blood from 410
    gas tensions 409–10
alverine 734
amantadine 679, 766
Ambu non-rebreathing valve 893–4
Ambu system 893–4
American Society of Anesthesiologists
        (ASA) scoring system 4
amethocaine 656, 660
amikacin 760
amiloride 709–10
amino acids 483

metabolism 484, 485, 491
    defects 484, 485
    placental transfer 524
    pool 484
    re-absorption in proximal tubule 375
    stereoisomerism 546
aminoglycoside antibiotics 102, 760–1
aminophylline 717, 718
aminosteroids 644
amiodarone 701, 703
    in CPR 154, 157
    in paediatric patients 168
    in peri-arrest arrhythmias 158, 159,
            160, 162
    pharmacology 710
amitriptyline 676
amlodipine 691, 706
ammonia
    excretion 390–1
    formation 485, 491
amniotic fluid embolism 55, 85
amoxycillin 756
AMPA receptors 451
ampere 803
AMPLE mnemonic 184
amplifiers 806, 840–1
amygdala 447
amylase
    pancreatic 464, 466
    salivary 462, 466, 475
anabolism 478
anaemia
    aplastic 17
    classification 16–17
    Cooley's 263
    oximetry and 863
    pre-operative assessment 16–18
    in renal failure 101
    in sickle cell disease 262
anaesthetic agents
    cerebral blood flow and 94
    in liver disease 100
    mechanism of action 553–6
        physicochemical theories 553–5
        structural theories 555–6
        theories 553
    in renal disease 102
    see also anaesthetic gases and vapours;
            intravenous anaesthetic
            agents; neuromuscular
            blocking agents; specific agents
anaesthetic gases and vapours 587–600
    absorbers 896
    administration 589
    chemical structures 593
    clinical properties 592–4, 595
    concentration inhaled 589
    historic 600
    ideal 591–2
    induction of anaesthesia 27–8
    in labour 83
    maintenance of anaesthesia 45–7
    maximum exposure levels 895, 896
    mechanism of action 553–6
    metabolism/toxicity 594
    minimum alveolar concentration see

minimum alveolar
concentration
  pharmacology 592–600
  physical properties 592, 883
  placental transfer 526
  in renal disease 102
  scavenging systems 895–6
  side effects 895
  uptake 589–91
  see also gas(es); *specific agents*
anaesthetic machines 880–3
  back bar 881–2
  basic components 880–2
  checklist 883, 910–11
  gas flow measurement 847–8, 849
  gas outlets 883
  maintenance 883
  safety mechanisms 881, 882
  vaporiser connections 882
analgesia
  intra-operative 48
  in labour 83–9
  in major trauma 184
  patient-controlled (PCA) 74, 84
  post operative 73–6
    in day case surgery 98
    paediatric patients 92
analgesic drugs 619–38
  see also non-steroidal anti-
      inflammatory drugs; opioids;
      specific agents
analgesic nephropathy 631, 633
analogue to digital (A to D) conversion
    840
analogue signals 833, 838
analysis of variance (ANOVA) 919, 921
anandamide 634
anaphylactoid reactions 28, 281
  local anaesthetics 658
anaphylaxis 28–30, 281
  clinical features 28–9
  follow up 29–30
  transfusion-related 266
  treatment 29, 30
anatomy, clinical 189–218
androgens
  adrenal 503, 505
  excess secretion 506
aneroid gauge 841
angina 11–12
angiotensin I 383, 707
angiotensin II 383–4, 707
  actions 383–4, 385
  GFR regulation 370
  vasoconstrictor effects 347, 348
angiotensin II receptor type 1 (AT₁)
    inhibitors 708
angiotensin converting enzyme (ACE)
    348
angiotensin converting enzyme (ACE)
    inhibitors 11, 707–8
angiotensinogen 383
†ngström 818
anistreplase 750
ankle block 141, 142
annulospiral fibres 438
Anrep effect 325

ANSI (American National Standards
    Institute) 895
antacids 39, 90, 733
antagonists 235, 547–8, 561
  competitive 552
    irreversible 567–8
    reversible 566–7
  mechanisms of action 552
  non competitive 552
  pharmacodynamics 566–8
antecubital fossa 215, 216
anterior median fissure 433
anterior spinal artery 435
  thrombosis 435
anti-arrhythmic agents 701–3
  class I 701–2
  class II 702–3
  class III 703
  class IV 703
  in CPR 154, 157
  in paediatric patients 168
  in peri-arrest arrhythmias 162
  Vaughan Williams classification 701
anti-cholinergic drugs 669–71
  anti-spasmodic 734
  placental transfer 527
  premedication 4
  and reflux 40
  respiratory actions 716
  see also muscarinic antagonists
anti-cholinesterases 646–7, 671, 685
  mechanism of action 646
  non depolarising relaxant activity 644,
    646
  pharmacology 651
  reversible 647
anti-coagulants 747–50
  central nerve blocks and 85, 134
  in deep venous thrombosis 70
  oral 747–8
  in pulmonary embolism 70
  see also heparin; warfarin
anti-D antibody prophylaxis 265
anti-diuretic hormone (ADH,
    vasopressin) 448, 499
  adrenal steroids and 382
  analogues 727
  antagonist 727
  blood flow regulation 347
  in CPR 156
  in haemorrhage 353
  inappropriate secretion 500
  osmotic and volume regulation 247,
    387
  pharmacology 727
  regulation of secretion 382
  removal from blood 382
  renal actions 380, 381–2, 383
  synthesis and storage 382
anti-emetic agents 76–7, 669–73
  mechanisms of action 669, 670
  peripherally acting 672
anti-histamines (H₁ antagonists)
  in anaphylaxis 30
  pharmacology 669, 670, 671
anti-hypertensive therapy, pre-operative
    10–11

anti-mycobacterials 765–6
anti-parkinsonian drugs 678–9
anti-platelet drugs 134, 750–1
anti-port carriers 230, 231, 372
anti-psychotic drugs 678
anti-spasmodics 734
anti-thrombin 271
anti-thyroid drugs 725
anti-virals 766
antibodies *see* immunoglobulins
antibody-dependent cell-mediated
    cytotoxicity (ADCC) 276
antibody response 275–6
anticonvulsant drugs 674–5
antidepressants 675–7
antigen presentation 274–5
antigen presenting cells (APCs) 274–5
antimicrobial therapy 753–66
  mechanisms of action 755–6
  principles 755
  in renal failure 755
anus, surgery to 111
anxiolytics, anti-emetic 672
aorta 333, 334
  baroreceptors 349, 350
  compression in pregnancy 514
  pressure curve 314, 315
  pressure wave 337
  traumatic rupture 181–2
aortic bodies 351, 419–20
aortic regurgitation 16, 316
aortic sinuses 201
aortic stenosis 15–16, 316
aortic sympathetic plexus 218
aortic valve 201, 316
  in cardiac cycle 314, 315
  sounds 317
aorto caval compression, in pregnancy
    514
AP label 817, 818
APG label 817, 818
apneustic centre 419
apnoea
  mivacurium 58
  suxamethonium 57–8, 66–7
apoproteins 488
appendicectomy 92
aprotinin 750
APTT *see* activated partial thromboplastin
    time
aquaporin-2 (AQP2) 371, 382
aquaporins (AQP) 371
aqueduct of Sylvius 441
aqueous theory, anaesthetic agent action
    554
arachidonic acid 386, 629–30
arachnoid mater 127, 204, 433
arachnoid villi 441
arcuate arteries, renal 364
area under the curve (AUC) 585, 586
argon laser 826
arrhythmias
  conduction system defects 308
  CPR 153–4
  during anaesthesia 52–3
  in electric shock 812
  life-threatening peri-arrest 157–62

physiological 312
post operative 69
pre-operative assessment 12–13
sinus 312
volatile agents and 593–4
arterial blood gases *see* blood gases,
    arterial
arterial blood pressure
    determinants 339–40
    diastolic 337
    during postural change 507
    in exercise 355
    measurement *see* blood pressure
        measurement
    newborn infant 533
    in pregnancy 514
    systolic 325, 337
    technological factors affecting 340
    Valsalva manoeuvre and 353
    volatile agent effects 593
arterial cannulation, in major trauma 177
arterial compliance (Ca) 325, 338–9
    effect on arterial pressures 339–40
    resistance–capacitance (RC) circuit
        339
arterial system 337–40
arteries 333, 334
    blood volume (ABV) 339
    elastance (Ea) 325, 328
    flow velocity 337
    pressure wave 337, 338
arterioles 333, 334, 342
    control of vascular system 345
aryepiglottic muscle 196
arytenoid cartilages 195
ascorbic acid *see* vitamin C
aspiration, pulmonary
    post operative 64
    in pregnancy 89–90, 519
    prevention 4, 31, 39–40, 731–3
    treatment 40
aspiration pneumonitis (Mendelson's
        syndrome) 4, 64, 89–90
aspirin 23, 632, 750–1
    central nerve blocks and 85, 134
    drug interactions 632
    overdose 632
    pharmacokinetics 632
    side effects 631, 632
assessment, pre-operative *see* pre-
        operative assessment
Association of Anaesthetists of Great
        Britain and Ireland
    anaesthetic apparatus checklist 910–11
    monitoring standards 50, 51
    post operative recovery
        recommendations 61
asthma 8, 715–17
Astrup technique 857
asystole 153, 154, 163
    abandoning resuscitation 169
    in paediatric patients 166
atelectasis
    absorption 64
    post operative 64
atenolol 687, 690
atheroma, in diabetes 22

ATLS (advanced trauma life support) 173
atmospheric pressure 787–8
    vaporiser performance and 886
atom 539
    structure 539
atomic mass number 539, 826
atomic number 539, 826
ATP 477, 478, 479, 486
    cycle 478
    in muscle contraction 287–8, 290, 301
    production 480, 482–3
ATPases 231
atracurium 644, 646
    chemical structure 652
    elimination 648
    isomers 547
    pharmacology 647–8, 651
atrial conduction pathways 307
atrial contraction 315
atrial ectopic beats 53, 69
atrial fibrillation (AF)
    peri-arrest 158, 160
    peri-operative 16, 53
atrial flutter 53, 158
atrial natriuretic peptide (ANP) 347, 348,
        386–7
atrial pressure 314, 315
atrial stretch receptor reflex 327, 350
atrial tachycardia with A-V block 53
atrioventricular (AV) block 158–61
    first degree 158
    second degree 158, 163
        Mobitz type I 158, 163
        Mobitz type II 158, 163
    third degree (complete) 158, 163, 308
atrioventricular (AV) junctional rhythm
        308
atrioventricular (AV) node 202, 305, 307
atrioventricular (AV) valves *see* mitral
        valve; tricuspid valve
atropine
    in CPR 154
    gastro-intestinal actions 734
    in paediatric patients 168
    in peri-arrest arrhythmias 158, 161,
        162
    pharmacology 669–71, 684, 695–6
    placental transfer 527
    in post operative arrhythmias 69
auditory-evoked responses (AER) 868
auditory nerve 210
Auerbach's plexus 456
auscultation of breath sounds 37
autocrine secretion 222
automated external defibrillators (AEDs)
        156
automaticity, cardiac pacemaker cells 305,
        306–7
autonomic nervous system (ANS) 206,
        445–7
    coronary blood flow regulation 356–7
    during awareness 48
    effects of stimulation 446–7
    heart rate control 326–7
    lungs 414
    neurotransmitters and receptors 445–6
    pharmacology 681–97

smooth muscle 295, 296
    see also parasympathetic nervous
        system; sympathetic nervous
        system
autonomic neuropathy
    diabetic 103–4
    Valsalva manoeuvre 353
autoregulation 346
    cerebral blood flow 358
    coronary blood flow 357
    renal blood flow 369–70
AV *see* atrioventricular
averaging 840
Avogadro's hypothesis 797
Avogadro's number 797
awareness 47–8
    definitions 47–8
    detection 48
    in obstetric anaesthesia 90
    prevention 48
    see also consciousness; depth of
        anaesthesia
axillary artery 138
axillary block 137–8
axon 427
Ayre's T-piece circuit 890
    Jackson Rees modification 890
azlocillin 757
aztreonam 759
azygos vein 198, 204

B-cells (lymphocytes) 275, 279
    memory (B$_M$) 275
    pulmonary 422
Bachmann bundle 307
back pain
    after epidural or spinal anaesthesia 88,
        133
    post operative 79
back surgery 114, 115
    epidural analgesia after 85
bacterial contamination, blood for
        transfusion 266
bag, self-inflating 153, 893, 894
Bain breathing circuit 887, 890
Bainbridge reflex 327, 350
bandwidth 836, 840
bar chart 915
baralyme 598
barbiturates 604–7
    anticonvulsant 674
    chemical structure 604
    clinical effects 605
    complications 605
    structure–activity relations 604
    see also methohexitone; thiopentone
barometric pressure 787–8
baroreceptor reflexes 327, 350
    afferent arteriolar 383
    cardiopulmonary 350
    carotid and aortic 350
    in haemorrhage 352
    renal 386
baroreceptors 349–50
barotrauma
    pulmonary 65, 73
    risk, ventilators 898

barrier pressure 457
  in pregnancy 519
basal ganglia 433, 439, 440
basal metabolic rate (BMR) 477
  measurement 477
base excess 9
basic life support (BLS) 150–2
  ABC 150–2
  algorithm 149
  paediatric 164–6
  in pregnancy 164
basophils 277
Bateson's venous plexus 433
Battle's sign 179
Bazett's formula 309
Beck Depression Inventory 873
beclomethasone 717, 718
Beer's law 822, 860
bendrofluazide 709
Benedict–Roth spirometer 846
benperidol 671
benzhexol 679
benzocaine 660
benzodiazepines 611–14
  antagonist see flumazenil
  anticonvulsant 674
  chemical properties 611
  clinical effects 612–13
  mechanism of action 552–3, 612
  metabolism 613
  pharmacokinetics 612
  placental transfer 527
  receptors (BDZ) 612
benzothiazepines 706
benztropine 679
benzylisoquinolinium compounds 644
benzylpenicillin 756
bequerel 828
Bernoulli's equation 802
β-adrenergic receptor antagonists (beta-blockers) 689–90
  anti-arrhythmic actions 702–3
  clinical effects 689–90
  mode of action 689
  for post operative hypertension 68
  pre-operative 10–11
  uses 689
β-adrenergic receptors 446, 686
  drug–receptor interactions 687
  subtypes 686, 689
β-endorphin 450
β error (type II error) 770, 921–2
β globin genes 260, 261
beta lactam antibiotics 756–7
β particles 828
β rhythm 432, 867
β₂-adrenergic receptor agonists (β₂ agonists) 8, 687, 715–16
betahistine 672
bethanidine 691
Bezold–Jarisch reflex 351
bias 770–1
bicarbonate (HCO₃-)
  in body fluids 249–50
  buffer system 388–9
  gastric secretion 463
  in intravenous fluids 740

pancreatic secretion 464
plasma
  in pregnancy 517
  renal regulation 389
  re-absorption 373, 375–6, 389–90
    H⁺ and 389, 391
    NaCl and 389–90
    T_m 389
  sodium see sodium bicarbonate
  standard 9
Bier's block 144–5
bigeminy, ventricular 53
biguanides 22–3, 724–5
bile 464–6
  canaliculi 490
  composition 250, 461
  control of secretion 465–6
  pigments 465
  salts 464–5
bilirubinaemia 100
binding site modulation 236
bio-availability 575
biological potentials 837–8
biotin deficiency 476
biotransformation 577–8
  see also drug metabolism
bipyridines 707
birth, circulatory changes at 360, 531
bismuth chelate 733
'black boxes' 833–4, 840
bladder emptying 394
bladder tumour, transurethral resection (TURBT) 112
blastocyst 521
bleeding diathesis, epidural analgesia and 84–5
bleeding time 272
blinding 771
blood
  bacterial contamination 266
  buffer systems 388
  CO₂ transport 412–13
  cross matching 266
  gas diffusion from alveoli to 410
  grouping and screening 266
  oxygen transport 410–12
  pH see pH, arterial blood
  products, for transfusion 55, 267, 268
  'storage lesion' 260
  temperature 869
  viscosity 336–7, 751
blood brain barrier 254, 358–9, 441
blood flow 333–6
  autoregulation 346
  drug distribution and 575–6
  local control mechanisms 346–7
  neurological control 348–51
  regional, during exercise 354
  in single vessel 336
  systemic humoral control 347–8
  turbulent 335
  velocity 335
blood gas barrier, pulmonary 398, 410
blood gases, arterial
  measurement 854–6, 857–8, 859–60
  pre-operative 9
  in pregnancy 517, 518

blood groups 264–5
  ABO system 264
  other red cell antigens 265
  Rhesus system 264–5
  testing 266
blood loss
  in haemorrhagic shock 177
  intra-operative management 52
  physiological responses 352–3
  post operative management 78–9
  see also haemorrhage
blood pressure see arterial blood pressure;
  venous pressure
blood pressure measurement 842–6
  automated occlusive cuff methods 843–4
  direct methods see intra-arterial pressure monitoring
  Doppler ultrasound 844
  factors affecting 842
  indirect methods 843–5
    sources of error 844–5
  manual occlusive cuff methods 843
  Penaz technique 844
blood transfusion see transfusion
blood vessels 333
  diameters and pressures 333, 334
  flow in see blood flow
  function 333, 334
  structure 333
  see also arteries; capillaries
blood volume 244, 351–2
  central venous pressure and 351–2
  control 352
  during exercise 355
  in pregnancy 515, 516
blood warmers 907
blood/gas partition coefficient 590
Bodok seal 878, 881
body fluids 241–55
  compartments see fluid compartments
  composition 249–50
  osmolality 247
  pH regulation 387–91
  volume regulation 382–7
  see also extracellular fluid; fluid(s);
    interstitial fluid; intracellular
    fluid; transcellular fluids
body mass index (BMI) 99, 475
body temperature 492–3
  cerebral blood flow and 94
  control 447–8
  disturbances 492–3
  measurement 868–70
  measurement sites 869
  oxyhaemoglobin dissociation curve and 260
  regulation see thermoregulation
  see also hypothermia; malignant hyperthermia
body weight
  estimation, paediatric patients 166
  gain in pregnancy 521
Bohr effect 260, 411
  double 524
Bohr's equation 401–2
boiling point 791, 794

bone marrow failure 267
Bonferroni test 921
botulinum toxin 685
bougie, gum elastic 32
Bourdon gauge 841
Bowditch phenomenon 327–8
Bowman's capsule 363, 364, 365
Boyle–Davis gag 117
Boyle's law 796
brachial artery 215, 216
brachial plexus
    anatomy 137, 205, 207, 208
    injuries 79
brachial plexus blockade 137–9
    axillary approach 137–8
    complications 139
    drug doses and volumes 138
    indications 137
    supraclavicular approach 137, 138–9
brachiocephalic vein 216
bradycardia
    cardiac output 328
    intra-operative 53
    peri-arrest 158–61
    post operative 69
    sinus 312
bradykinin 348, 451, 629
    ACE inhibitor actions 707
    receptors 629
brain 431–3
    circulation 357–9
    volatile agent transport to 591
brain-derived neurotrophic factor
        (BDNF) 449, 451
brain injury, traumatic 179
brain stem 433
    control of posture 440
    respiratory centres 419
    'vomiting centre' 471
brain stem-evoked responses (BSER) 868
Brandt pattern endotracheal tubes 895
breath sounds, auscultation 37
breathing
    in basic life support 150, 151
        paediatric patients 164
    Cheyne–Stokes 421
    failure at end of surgery 57–8
    frequency (f) 50
    in major trauma 176–7
    rescue 151
    work of 407–8, 421, 790
    see also respiration; ventilation
breathing systems 887–91
    checks 911
    circle system 889–91
    closed 887
    commonly used 889, 890
    components 888–9
    dead space 888
    gas flow measurement 848–50
    gas sampling errors 854
    in latex allergy 108
    Mapleson classification 889
    non-rebreathing 887
    open 887
    performance 888

post operative oxygen administration
        73
    rebreathing 887
    resuscitation 153, 893–4
bretylium 691, 701, 703
British Standard (BS), gas cylinders 878
Broca's speech area 431, 432
Brodmann's area 4 (primary motor
        cortex) 431, 439
Bromage motor block scale 129
bromocriptine 679
bronchi 198, 199
    control of calibre 715–17
    inadvertent intubation 36
    major 397
    small 397
    smooth muscle tone 407
bronchial arteries 414
bronchial tree 198, 199, 397
bronchioles 198, 397
    respiratory 397
bronchitis, chronic 8, 9
bronchodilators 8, 9, 715–17
bronchopleural fistula, traumatic 183
bronchopleural segments 198
bronchopneumonia, post operative 64
bronchospasm
    in anaphylaxis 28–9
    intra-operative 54
    NSAID-induced 630–1
    pharmacology 715–17
    post operative 67
Broselow tape 166
brown fat 534
Brown Sequard syndrome 434–5
bruising, post operative 80
buccal administration 574
Buck's fascia 143
buclizine 671
budesonide 717, 718–19
buffers
    definition of pK 388
    physiological 388
bulking agents, laxative 735
Bullard laryngoscope 32
bundle branch block 308
bundle branches 307
bundle of His 202, 307
bundle of Kent 307
β-bungarotoxin 685
bupivacaine 656, 661, 664
    caudal anaesthesia 136
    epidural analgesia/anaesthesia 87, 89,
        133
    hyperbaric 662
        for spinal anaesthesia 89, 128, 129,
            130
    intravascular injection 88
    maximum dose 658
    peripheral nerve blocks 138, 141, 142,
        143
    structure 663
    toxicity 659
buprenorphine 628
burns 184–5
    electrical 817
    flash 817

'rule of nines' 184, 185
buspirone 615
butyrophenones 671, 678
butyryl cholinesterase see cholinesterase,
        plasma

'c' wave 315, 317, 340
cadherins 227
Caesarean section 89, 163
caffeine 716
calcitonin 508
calcitonin gene-related peptide (CGRP)
        635
calcium (Ca^{2+}) 252
    absorption 469–70
    in cardiac action potentials 304, 305
    in cardiac muscle contraction 301–2
    homeostasis 507–8
    imbalance 252, 253, 508
        see also hypercalcaemia;
                hypocalcaemia
    intravenous therapy 7, 740
    in neuromuscular transmission 293
    second messenger function 237, 238
    in skeletal muscle contraction 286,
        287, 288–9
    in smooth muscle contraction 295–6
    in synaptic transmission 429
calcium channel antagonists 691, 705–6
    anti-arrhythmic 703
    benzothiazepine 706
    dihydropyridine 706
    papaverine 706
    pre-operative 11
calcium channels
    dihydropyridine 287, 289
    L-type 304, 306, 705
    ryanodine receptor 287, 289
    T-type 305, 306
    voltage-gated 429
calcium chelating agents 750
calcium hydroxide 891
calcium pumps (Ca^{2+}-ATPases) 231, 302,
        371
calculus 780–3
calmodulin 238, 296
calorie 791
calorimeter 477
calsequestrin 288
Camper's fascia 215
candela 822
cannabinoid receptors 634
cannabinoids 634, 672
Cannabis sativa 634
cannon 'a' waves 318
capacitance 807–8
capacitance vessels 345
capacitors 806, 807
    isolating 816, 817
    parallel 808
    series 808
capillaries 333, 334, 342–5
    exchange 342–3
    network 342
    permeability 343
capillary filtration 248, 343–5
    equilibrium 344–5

Starling forces 343–4
capillary wall 245
  diffusion across 248, 343
  transport across 248, 343
capnograph 858–9
  mainstream 859
  sidestream 858–9
  see also end tidal carbon dioxide
captopril 707
carbachol 683
carbamazepine 675
carbamino compounds 412
carbapenem antibiotics 758–9
carbenoxolone 734, 735
carbidopa 679, 690
carbimazole 725
carbocisteine 718
carbohydrate
  absorption 467
  dietary intake 475
  digestion 466, 467
  metabolism 479–83
    defects 483
    hepatic 491
    hormonal regulation 509, 510
  stereoisomerism 546
β-carbolines 612
carbon dioxide (CO₂)
  absorber 889, 891, 905
  body stores 412–13
  cylinders 878
  diffusion 410
  embolism 55–6
  end tidal expired see end tidal carbon
    dioxide
  in expired gas, detection 37–8
  measurement 857–9
    in vitro 857–8
    in vivo 858–9
  oxyhaemoglobin dissociation curve
    and 260
  placental transfer 524
  total volume expired (V T CO₂) 402
  transport 412–13
carbon dioxide (CO₂) electrodes 857–8
  intravascular 858
  transcutaneous 858
carbon dioxide (CO₂) laser 826
carbon dioxide (CO₂) tension (partial
    pressure)
  alveolar (PaCO₂) 402, 409–10
  in arterial blood (PaCO₂) 9, 54
    cerebral blood flow and 94, 358, 442
    CNS chemoreceptor response 255
    measurement 857–8
    in pregnancy 517
    raised post operative 65–7
    respiratory alkalosis and 393
    ventilatory response 420–1
  end tidal (PE'CO₂) 50
  in mixed expired gas (PçCO₂) 402
  transcutaneous 858
carbonic acid 389, 412
carbonic anhydrase 260, 389, 412
carbonic anhydrase inhibitors 710
carboprost 727

carboxyhaemoglobin (HbC), and
    oximetry 861, 862–3
carboxypeptidase 464
cardiac arrest
  advanced life support 153–4, 155
  causes 149
  diagnosis 150, 153
  drug therapy 156–7
  in paediatric patients 164
  see also cardiopulmonary arrest
cardiac arrhythmias see arrhythmias
cardiac axis 309, 310–11, 784
  calculation algorithm 311
  rapid estimation 311
cardiac contusion 180–1
cardiac cycle 313–18
  cardiac valves 314–17
  central venous pressure waveform
    317–18
  diastolic function 315
  ECG waves 308–9
  heart sounds and murmurs 317
  left vs right side 316–17
  systolic function 314–15
  ventricles 313
cardiac failure 330
  Frank–Starling curve and 320
  transfusion-associated 266
cardiac glycosides 703–4
cardiac index (CI) 322
cardiac muscle 301–2
  excitation–contraction coupling 301–2
  force–velocity curve 320–1
  structure 301, 302
  vs skeletal muscle 296–7, 301
  vs smooth muscle 296–7
cardiac muscle cells 301
  action potentials see action potentials
    (APs), cardiac
  excitability 304
  Frank curve 320
  resting membrane potential (RMP)
    303–4
cardiac output (CO) 321–3
  cardiovascular coupling 328, 329
  control 323–8
  distribution to organs 355
  effects of heart rate 327–8
  in exercise 354–5
  measurement 322–3
  in pregnancy 513
  volatile agent uptake and 591
cardiac physiology 299–330
cardiac pump 318–28
  control of function 323–8
  end diastolic pressure–volume
    relationship 319
  end systolic pressure–volume
    relationship 319–21
  ventricular pressure–volume loop 318
  see also cardiac output
cardiac tamponade 177
cardiac valves 315–17
  see also specific valves
cardiac vector 309, 310–11, 784
cardiac veins 202–3
Cardiff Swivel 883

cardiopulmonary arrest 149–50
  in paediatric patients 164
  in pregnancy 162–4
  see also cardiac arrest
cardiopulmonary bypass surgery 267, 268
cardiopulmonary resuscitation (CPR)
    150–62
  complications 157
  drug usage 156–7
  ethical aspects 168–9
  in infants and children 164–8
  peri-arrest arrhythmias 157–62
  in pregnancy 162–4
  see also advanced life support; basic life
    support
cardiovascular coupling 328–9
cardiovascular disease
  diabetic 104
  pre-operative assessment 9–16
cardiovascular system 299–330
  ageing effects 239
  barbiturate effects 606, 607
  benzodiazepine effects 612
  during exercise 353–5
  etomidate effects 610
  ketamine effects 609
  local anaesthetic effects 657–8
  in newborn infant 531–3
  opioid effects 624
  patient positioning and 45
  pharmacology 699–712
  post operative complications 67–9
  in pregnancy 513–15
  propofol effects 610
  response to Valsalva manoeuvre 353
  in spinal anaesthesia 128
  volatile agent effects 593–4, 595
  see also circulation; heart
cardioversion, direct current (DC)
  in peri-arrest arrhythmias 158, 159,
    160, 161
  in post operative arrhythmias 69
carnitine acyl-transferase 487
carnitine shuttle 487
carotid arteries 357
carotid bodies 351, 419–20
carotid canal 218
carotid sinus
  baroreceptors 349, 350
  massage 158, 350
catabolism 475, 478
cataract surgery 118
catechol-O-methyl transferase (COMT)
    686
catecholamines 506–7, 686
  abnormalities of secretion 507
  cardiac glycoside actions 704
  control of blood flow 347
  control of secretion 506–7
  drugs interfering 690–1
  in haemorrhage 352
  pharmacology 686, 687
  structure 687
  see also dopamine; epinephrine;
    norepinephrine
cauda equina 127
caudal anaesthesia 126, 135–7

factors determining 356–7
   volatile agent effects 593
coronary circulation 356–7
coronary heart disease *see* ischaemic heart
      disease
coronary perfusion pressure (CPP) 357
coronary sinus 202, 203
corpus luteum 525
correlation, linear 922–3
correlation coefficient (r) 923
   square (r²) 923, 924
corticospinal tract (pyramidal tract) 203,
      204, 435
corticosteroid binding globulin (CBG)
      726
corticosteroids 503–5
   in anaphylaxis 30
   hypothalamic-pituitary axis
         suppression 498
   pharmacology 725–6
   relative potencies 726
   in respiratory disease 8, 717
   side effects 726, 727
   surgery in patients on 23, 505
   see also glucocorticoids
corticotrophin-releasing hormone
      (CRH) 498, 504
cortisol 221, 503, 504
   see also hydrocortisone
cortisone 725, 726
cosine functions 779
cosine wave 838
cough reflex 422
coulomb 803
coumarins 747–8
countercurrent mechanism, renal 379,
      380
countercurrent multiplication 380–1
counterpulsation 356
countertransport 231, 371
covalent bonds 540–1, 542
covalent modulation 236
CPAP (continuous positive airway
      pressure) 62, 903
CPR *see* cardiopulmonary resuscitation
cranial nerves 206–11
   see also individual nerves
'crash' induction 41
creatine 485–6
creatine kinase (CK) 486
   CK-MB isoenzyme 181
creatine phosphate (CP) 290, 479, 486
creatinine 485–6
   clearance 368
   plasma 101
Cremophor EL 614
Creutzfeld–Jakob disease 107
crico-arytenoid muscles 196
crico-thyroid ligament 195
crico-thyroid muscle 196
crico-tracheal ligament 195
cricoid cartilage 193, 194, 195, 196
cricoid pressure 40
cricothyroid muscle 193
cricothyroidotomy
   in failed intubation 36
   needle 153, 176

for retrograde intubation 35
   surgical 153
crista terminalis 201
critical angle 821
critical damping 779, 836
critical incidents, intra-operative 52–7
critical pressure 792
critical temperature (T꜀) 792, 793
critical volume 792
critical volume hypothesis 554
cromoglycate 717, 719
cross matching, blood 266
crossover studies 769
cryoprecipitate 268
crystalloids 78, 739–40
CSF *see* cerebrospinal fluid
CT scan *see* computed tomography
cuffed oropharyngeal airway (COPA) 34,
      152
cuffs, blood pressure measurement 843–4
   size, WHO recommendations 844
cuneate tract 436
curie 828
Cushing reflex 351
Cushing's syndrome 381, 500, 505
cut down, peripheral 177, 186
CVP *see* central venous pressure
cyanide ions 692
cyanocobalamin *see* vitamin B₁₂
cyanosis
   intra-operative 52
   in oesophageal intubation 37
   post operative 64
cyclic AMP 228, 237, 238
   phosphodiesterase III inhibition and
         706
cyclic GMP 228, 237, 238
cyclizine 77, 671, 672
cyclo-oxygenase (COX) 386, 488, 629–30
   aspirin actions 750–1
   type 2 (COX₂) 630, 632
cyclopropane 592, 600
   explosion/fire risks 817
cylinders 878–80
   colour coding 878
   connection to anaesthetic machines
         881
   estimation of contents 797, 879
   filling ratio 879
   identification 878
   pin index system (PIS) 878, 879, 881
   pressure regulators 880
   tare weight 879
   testing 879
cystic hygroma 3
cytochrome oxidase 692
cytochrome P₄₅₀ 491, 577, 605
cytokines 276, 281, 629
cytoplasm 223
cytoskeleton 223–4
cytosol 223
cytotoxic cells 276
cytotoxic T-cells (T꜀) 276
cytotrophoblast 521, 522

D-dimers 272
dacrocystorhinostomy (DCR) 119

Dalton's law 797
damped oscillation 779
damping 835–6
   arterial pressure waveforms 845
   critical 779, 836
   fluid flow 799
dantrolene, in malignant hyperthermia
      56, 57
data 915
   attribute 915
   categorical 915
   collection 772
   continuous 915
   describing 915–17
   discrete 915
   interval 915
   nominal 915
   ordinal 915
   paired 921
   qualitative 915–16, 919–20
   quantitative 915, 916–17, 920–1
   ratio 915
   transformation 924
dative bonds 541
day case surgery 97–9
   admission facilities 98–9
   anaesthetic technique 98
   medical fitness 98
   social circumstances 97–8
   suitable operations 97, 98
DC *see* direct current
DDAVP (desmopressin) 727, 751
dead space 401–2
   alveolar 401
   anatomical 401
   apparatus 888
   functional 888
   physiological 401–2
   in pregnancy 517
deamination 484
debrisoquine 691
decay half life 828
decerebration 440
decibels (db) 840
decortication 440
deep peroneal nerve 141
   block 142
deep venous thrombosis (DVT)
   intra-operative 55
   post operative 69–70
   prophylaxis 70
   risk group classification 70
defibrillation 154–6
   early 152
   in paediatric patients 166
   in pregnancy 164
   in VF/VT 153–4
defibrillators
   automated external (AEDs) 156
   circuits 810
   DC 154–6
degrees of freedom 917, 920
dehydration 251
delay time 851
δ rhythm 432, 867
demeclocycline 727
dental anaesthesia

paediatric patients 92–3
see also oral surgery
dental extraction 119–20
　paediatric patients 92–3
　wisdom teeth 120
dental trauma 79
deoxyribonuclease 464
deoxyribonucleic acid (DNA) 232–3
dependence, opioid 624
depolarising neuromuscular blockers
　　642–4
　clinical features 642–3
　mechanism of action 642, 645
　pharmacology 650, 651
　see also suxamethonium
depth of anaesthesia 47–8
　integrated clinical scores 866
　measurement 865–8
derivative 783
dermatomes 205
desferrioxamine 551
desflurane 594–5
　chemical structure 593
　clinical properties 592–4, 595
　physical properties 592, 594, 883
　vaporiser 885
desmopressin (DDAVP) 727, 751
desmosomes 225
detoxification 491–2
'dew point' 871
dexamethasone 726, 728
dextrans 741, 751
dextro (d) rotatory substances 546, 821–2,
　　823
dextrose 546, 723
　solutions 78, 104, 739
diabetes insipidus 381, 500, 727
diabetes mellitus 102–5, 510
　blood sugar control 723–5
　cataract surgery 118
　complications 22, 102–4
　diet controlled 103, 104
　insulin controlled 23, 103, 104
　insulin-dependent (IDDM)/type
　　　I/juvenile onset 20–2, 23, 510
　management 103, 104, 105
　non-insulin-dependent
　　　(NIDDM)/type II/maturity
　　　onset 20–2, 23, 510
　osmotic diuresis 375
　post operative hypoglycaemia 71
　pre-operative management 20–3
　pregnancy 104–5
　tablet controlled 22–3, 103, 104
diabetic nephropathy 103
diabetic neuropathy 103–4
diacetylmorphine 625–6
diacylglycerol (DAG) 228, 237
dialysis 20, 102
diamorphine 625–6
diaphragm 200–1, 402
　orifices 200
　traumatic rupture 182
diaphragmatic splinting 67
diastole 313, 314, 315
diathermy
　bipolar 817

electrodes, current density 813
　hazards 816–17
　oximetry and 863
　pacemakers and 14–15
　safety precautions 817
diazepam 611, 613, 615–16
　anticonvulsant action 674
　placental transfer 527
　vs midazolam 614
diazoxide 692
dibucaine number 643
dichloraphenazone 615
diclofenac 631, 637
　pharmacokinetics 630
dicrotic notch 314, 315
dicyclomine 734
didanosine 766
dielectric 807
diethyl ether 592, 600
differentiation 781, 782–3
diffusing capacity of lungs for carbon
　　　monoxide (DLCO), in
　　　pregnancy 517
diffusion 228–9, 343, 543
　across capillary wall 248, 343
　across cell membrane 228–9
　anaesthetic gases and vapours 590
　facilitated 231
　ion 230
　non ionic 543
　rate 574
　simple 543
diffusion hypoxia 65
digestion 466
digital signals 833, 838
digitoxin 704
digoxin
　in narrow complex tachycardia 160
　pharmacology 704, 710–11
　toxicity 158, 704
dihydrocodeine 628
dihydropyridine receptor 287, 289
dihydropyridines 706 1,25-
　　　dihydroxycholecalciferol 469–70,
　　　508
diltiazem 705, 706
　anti-arrhythmic activity 701, 703
　pharmacology 711
dilutional techniques
　cardiac output measurement 322
　fluid compartment volume
　　　measurement 244
dimensional analysis 786–7
diode 806, 811
diphenhydramine 671 2,3-
　　　diphosphoglycerate (2,3-DPG)
　　　50, 260
　in chronic anaemia 17
　HbF affinity 410
　in stored blood 260
direct current (DC) 805
　shock 812
　see also cardioversion
disability, in major trauma 178
disinfection 908
disseminated intravascular coagulation
　　　(DIC) 19, 267, 268

dissociation constants
　acids and bases *see* pKa
　drug–receptor interactions 562, 563
distal tubule, renal 363, 379–80
　bicarbonate re-absorption 390
distortion, signal 836–7
distribution, drug 575–7
　see also volume of distribution
diuresis
　forced acid 551
　forced alkaline 551
　osmotic 375, 551
diuretics 708–10
　loop 708–9
　osmotic 545, 710
　potassium sparing 709–10
　thiazide 10, 709
DNA 232–3
do not attempt resuscitation (DNAR)
　　　orders 168
dobutamine 687, 688, 693
domperidone 672, 673, 679, 734
dopa decarboxylase 690–1
dopamine 429, 506, 686
　pharmacology 687, 688, 693
　renal actions 387
　structure 687
dopamine D_2 receptors 669, 670, 678
dopexamine 688, 693–4
Doppler ultrasound
　blood pressure measurement 844
　cardiac output measurement 322–3
　cerebral blood flow estimation 358
dornase alpha 718
dorsal horn 449, 450, 451
dorsal nucleus of vagus 210, 211
dorsal penile nerves 143
dose ratio 567
double-blind trial 771
double burst stimulation (DBS) 642, 865,
　　　866
double reciprocal plot 568, 569
doxacurium 646, 648, 651
doxapram 71, 717–18, 719
doxycycline 761, 762
[dp/dt max] 315
Drager Evita 4 ventilator 903, 904
Drager Narkotest 854
drift 835
driving, after day case surgery 97
droperidol 670, 671, 673, 689
drug(s)
　absorption 573–4
　administration 573–5
　distribution 575–7
　effective levels 586
　elimination *see* elimination
　excretion 578
　mechanisms of action *see* mechanisms
　　　of drug action
　placental transfer 525–7, 577
　pre-operative assessment 23
　in pregnancy 520
　protein binding *see* protein binding
drug interactions 556–7
　pharmacodynamic 557
　pharmacokinetic 557

physicochemical 556–7
  synergistic 556
drug metabolism 573
  hepatic 491–2
  interactions affecting 557
  in newborn infants 534
  phase I 491, 577–8
  phase II 491, 578
  volatile agents 594
drug metabolites
  active 556
  toxic 556
drug–receptor interactions 561–9
  agonists 563–5
  irreversible competitive antagonists
      567–8
  key equations 561–3
  molecular binding of drugs 565
  partial agonists 565–6
  reversible competitive antagonists
      566–7
  variations from predictions 568–9
dry gas meter 846–7
ductus arteriosus 359, 531
  closure 360, 531, 631
  patent 531
ductus venosus 359, 531
Duffy antigens 265
dura mater 127, 204, 433
dural tap, inadvertent 87–8, 137
DVT see deep venous thrombosis
dwarfism 500
dye dilution, cardiac output
      measurement 322
dynorphins 622
dysdiadochokinesia 439
dysfibrinogenaemia 268
dyshomeostasis 238
dysphoria, opioid-induced 623
dyspnoea, in pregnancy 517

E-selectin 277
ear, structure 444
ear, nose and throat (ENT) surgery
      117–18
  day case 97
  paediatric patients 92–3
earth circuits 811–12, 814
ECF see extracellular fluid
ECG see electrocardiogram
echocardiography
  to measure stroke volume 321
  pre-operative 13
  transoesophageal (TOE) 321
ecothiopate 647
ectopic pregnancy 116
ED_{50} 47, 569, 586
edrophonium 647
EEG see electro-encephalogram
effective blood concentration (EC, EBC)
      47, 586
effective circulating volume (ECV) 382
effective levels 586
efficacy (E) 563–8
  agonists 563–5
  irreversible competitive antagonists
      567–8

partial agonists 565–6
  reversible competitive antagonists
      566–7
egg phosphatide 610
eicosanoids 222, 488
Einthoven's triangle 309
ejection, ventricular 314
ejection fraction (EF) 321
  measurement 326
elastance
  arterial (Ea) 325, 328
  ventricular (Ees) 319, 328
elderly patients
  day case surgery 98
  spinal anaesthesia 129
  see also ageing
electric charge 803
electric circuits 804–11
  earthed 811–12, 814
  elements 806–11
  isolated 812, 814
electric current 803
  density 813
electric shock (macroshock) 811–14
  factors influencing 812–14
  prevention 814
electrical burns 817
electrical equipment
  APG and AP labels 817, 818
  classes 814
  high and low risk zones 817
  safety 814, 816, 817
electrical noise see noise, electrical
electrical potential 803
electrical safety 811–17
electrical signals 805, 837–41
  biological 837–8
  frequency spectrum 838
  sine and cosine functions 779
electrical stimulation
  patterns in neuromuscular monitoring
      642, 864–5, 866
  peripheral nerve 641–2, 863
electricity 803–17
electro-encephalogram (EEG) 432, 837
  during anaesthesia 867, 868
electrocardiogram (ECG) 307–13, 837
  anti-arrhythmic drug effects 702
  cardiac axis calculation 310–11
  in CPR 153, 154
  electrolyte disturbances and 7, 312–13
  heart rate calculation 310
  intra-operative monitoring 311
  leads 309–10, 784
  in peri-arrest arrhythmias 163
  physiological arrhythmias 312
  pre-operative 12–13
  in pregnancy 514
  in pulmonary embolism 70
  waves and cardiac cycle 308–9
electrochemical gas analysis methods 854
  for oxygen 855–6
electrolytes
  balance 249–50
  disturbances 250–2
      effects on ECG 7, 312–13
      pre-operative 5–7

problems and causes 6
  in renal disease 101, 102
  in intravenous fluids 740
  placental transfer 525
  see also calcium; chloride; magnesium;
      potassium; sodium
electromagnetic (EM) spectrum 818
electromyogram (EMG) 837
  double burst stimulation (DBS) 642,
      865, 866
  frontalis 867
  neuromuscular monitoring 864
electronic volume meter 847
electrons 539
electronvolt 828
electrostatic (ionic) bonds 540, 541, 543
element 539
elimination 577–8
  first order 581–6
  half life ($t_{\frac{1}{2}\beta}$) 585
  Hofmann 648
  kinetics 581–6
  rate constant (k_{el}) 579, 581
  zero order 581, 582
eltanolone 607
Embden–Meyerhof pathway (glycolysis)
      290, 480
embolism
  amniotic fluid 55, 85
  fat 55
  gas (air) 55–6, 341
  intra-operative 55–6
  thrombus see thrombo-embolism
emergence from anaesthesia 61, 71
emergencies
  acute abdominal 24
  intra-operative 52–7
emergency surgery, in diabetes 104
EMG see electromyogram
EMLA cream 662
emphysema 8, 9
enalapril 556, 707
enantiomers 546
end diastolic point (EDP) 318, 319
  measurement 324
end diastolic pressure–volume
      relationship (EDPVR) 319, 324
end diastolic volume (EDV) 318
  measurement 324
end plate potential 293
end systolic point (ESP) 318, 319, 328
end systolic pressure–volume
      relationship (ESPVR) 319–21
end systolic volume (ESV) 318
end tidal carbon dioxide ($ETCO_2$)
  causes of changes 859
  intra-operative monitoring 50, 54
  measurement 857, 858–9
  partial pressure ($Pe'CO_2$) 50
  post intubation checks 37–8, 153
endocrine disease 20–3
endocrine system 495–510
  ageing effects 239
  pharmacology 721–8
  in pregnancy 520
endocytosis 231

endometrium, transcervical resection
        (TCRE) 116
endomysium 285
endoplasmic reticulum (ER) 224
endorphins 450, 622
endothelial cells
    control of blood flow 346–7
    fenestrations 342
    glomerular capillaries 364
endothelins 347, 370, 414
endothelium 342–3
endothelium-derived relaxing factor
        (EDRF) see nitric oxide
endotracheal intubation 30–8, 49
    aids 32
    awake 36
    blind nasal 35
    in burns 184
    in CPR 152
    difficult
        anticipated 35–6
        management 31–5
        prediction 3
        in pregnancy 90
    failed, management 35–6
    in head injury 41, 95–6, 179
    indications 30–1, 49
    laryngoscopy technique 31
    local anaesthesia for 143–4
    in major trauma 176
    in obstetric anaesthesia 90
    paediatric patients 91, 166
    patient positioning 31
    pre-operative airway assessment 3
    retrograde 35
    sequelae 79
    in upper airway obstruction 41, 63
endotracheal tubes 895
    confirmation of correct placement
        36–8, 153
        clinical signs 36–7
        errors 37
        objective signs 37–8
    direct visualisation of position 36–7
    misplacement 36
    paediatric sizes 166
energy
    balance 475–7
    mechanical 788–91
    for muscle contraction 290
    potential 789–90
    production 477–8
    requirements 475
enflurane 595–6
    chemical structure 593
    clinical properties 592–4, 595
    isomerism 545
    physical properties 592, 595, 883
enkephalins 622
enoxaparin 749
enoximone 707
ENT surgery see ear, nose and throat
        (ENT) surgery
enteral administration 574–5
enteric nervous system 456
enterohepatic circulation 464–5, 577
Entonox 599

cylinders 878
in labour 83
see also nitrous oxide
entrainment 802
environmental control, in major trauma
        178
enzymes 547, 569–70
    drug actions via 569
    false substrates 553, 570
    induction 557
    inhibition 553, 557, 570
    kinetics 569–70
eosinophils 717
ephedrine
    bronchodilator actions 716
    for hypotension 69, 89, 126
    pharmacology 694
epibatidine 634
epidural analgesia/anaesthesia 126, 130–4
    complications 133–4
    drug doses and volumes 133
    equipment 131, 907
    indications 130–1
    in labour 84–9
        complications 87–9
        contraindications 84–6
        technique 86–7
        test doses 87
    for laparotomy 111
    in obese patients 99
    for obstetric surgery 89
    patient controlled (PCEA) 87
    physiology 131
    technique 131–2
    vs spinal anaesthesia 131
    see also combined spinal–epidural
        (CSE) anaesthesia
epidural blood patch 88, 130
epidural catheters 907
epidural haematoma
    intracranial 94
    spinal, after central nerve blocks 134
epidural needles 907
epidural space 433
    anatomy 86–7, 126
    factors affecting spread of drugs 132
    in pregnancy 519–20
epiglottis 195, 196
epilepsy
    drug treatment 674–5
    enflurane risk 596
epimers 546
epimysium 285
epinephrine (adrenaline) 429, 446, 506–7
    in anaphylaxis 29, 30
    blood flow control 347
    bronchodilator actions 716
    control of secretion 506–7
    in CPR 153, 154, 156
        in paediatric patients 166, 168
        in pregnancy 164
    for epidural anaesthesia 87, 89, 133
    excess secretion 507
    halothane anaesthesia and 596
    in local anaesthetic solutions 662–3
    metabolic actions 221, 479
    in peri-arrest arrhythmias 161, 162

in peripheral nerve blocks 142, 143
pharmacology 686, 687, 693
structure 687
synthesis 506
epoprostenol 751
equilibrium constants
    drug–receptor interactions 562, 563
    enzymes 569
equipment 875–911
    checklist 910–11
    electrical see electrical equipment
    intravenous 906–7
    in latex allergy 108
    paediatric 91
    regional anaesthesia 907
equivalent weight 245
ergometrine 515, 726–7, 728
ergotamine 687
erythrocytes see red blood cells
erythromycin 734, 761
erythropoiesis 259
erythropoietin (EPO) 259, 353
    in pregnancy 515
esmolol 68
    for peri-arrest arrhythmias 160
    pharmacology 690, 701, 711
etanercept 629
ethambutol 765–6
ethamivan 718
ethamsylate 751
ethanolamines 671
ether (diethyl ether) 592, 600
ethics, CPR 168–9
ethics committees 772
ethmoidal sinus 192
ethyl chloride 592
etomidate 609–10, 616
    adverse reactions 603
    clinical effects 609–10, 616
    metabolism 610
    physical properties 609
European Society of Regional
        Anaesthesia (ESRA),
        thromboprophylaxis and central
        neural blockade guidelines 134
Eustachian tube 444
eutectic mixture 662
evacuation of retained products of
        conception (ERPC) 116–17
Evan's score 866
evaporation 794
evoked potentials 840
evoked responses 866, 868
excitation–contraction coupling
    cardiac muscle 301–2
    skeletal muscle 288–9
excitatory postsynaptic potential (EPSP)
        430
excretion, drug 578
    interactions affecting 557
exercise 353–5
    moderate 354–5
    severe/to exhaustion 355
exocytosis 231, 293
expiration 403
expiratory cycling 900–1
expiratory neurones, medullary 419

expiratory reserve volume (ERV) 399
expired air respiration (EAR) 151, 153
  paediatric patients 164
expired volume calculation 781–2
explosions 817
exponential curves 776
exponential functions 776–7
exposure, in major trauma 178
extracellular fluid (ECF) 77, 243–4
  buffer systems 388
  volume (ECV)
    measurement 244
    reduced *see* hypovolaemia
    regulation 382–7, 448
extraction ratio (ER) 578
extradural *see* epidural
extraocular muscles 217
extravasation, barbiturates 605
extremity trauma 183
eye
  penetrating injury 119
  structure 442–3
  trauma, intra-operative 79

face masks 889, 892
  with reservoir and non-rebreathing
    valve 892
  Venturi 72, 892, 893
facial nerve (VII) 210
  palsy 79–80
facial trauma 180
factor V-Leiden 271
faecal softeners 735
Fahrenheit scale 868
family *see* relatives
famotidine 731
Faraday constant 303, 786
farads 807
fasciculus cuneatus 203, 204
fasciculus gracilis 203, 204
Fast Fourier Transform (FFT) 840
fasting, pre-operative 4, 39
fat
  brown 534
  embolism 55
fats *see* lipids
fatty acids 486–8
  β-oxidation 487
  essential 475
  free (FFA) 486, 487
  placental transfer 525
  synthesis 487–8
febrile non haemolytic transfusion
    reactions (FNHTR) 266–7
feedback systems
  negative 222–3
  positive 223
feeding centre, hypothalamic 448
felodipine 691
felypressin 663, 727
femoral nerve 206
  anatomy 140
  block 139–41
femoral vein cannulation 186
femur, fractured neck of 114–16
fentanyl 626–7

epidural 625, 627
  pharmacokinetics 623, 626
  pharmacology 636
  transdermal 575
ferritin 469
FEV$_1$ 400, 401
  pre-operative testing 8, 9
FEV$_1$/FVC ratio (FEV%) 9, 400
fever (pyrexia) 492
  epidural analgesia and 86
  see also malignant hyperthermia
fibrin degradation products (FDPs) 272,
    279
fibrinogen 273
  deficiency 270
fibrinolysis 272
fibrinolytic agents 750
fibrinolytic inhibitors 750
fibrinolytic system 272
Fick principle 322
Fick's law 343, 410, 526
filters 840
  high-pass 840
  low-pass 840
  notch 840
filtration, across capillary wall 248, 343–5
filum terminale 127, 203
fire 817
first-order kinetics 581–5
first-pass effect 574, 575
Fisher's exact test 920
flail chest 176
flavine adenine dinucleotide (FADH$_2$)
    479, 482
flecainide 701, 702
Fleisch pneumotachograph 849, 850
Flexiblade laryngoscope 34
flow 333–6
  damping 799
  laminar *see* laminar flow
  resistance 336
  through tubes 799–802
  turbulent *see* turbulent flow
  velocity 335, 801–2
  see also blood flow; gas flow
flow splitting ratio 884
flowmeters
  checks 910
  see also rotameter
flucloxacillin 756–7
fludrocortisone 726
fluid(s) 241–55
  behaviour 798–802
  flow *see* flow
  Newtonian 798
  see also water
fluid balance
  disorders 250–2
  in liver disease 100
  post operative 77–9
  pre-operative assessment 4–5
  regulation 382–7, 448
  in renal disease 101, 102
fluid compartments
  distribution of solutes 248
  membranes separating 245
  volumes 243–4

  measurement 244
  in pregnancy 516
  water movements between 245–8
fluid loss
  insensible 77
  post operative 77
    assessment 78
    management 78–9
  third space 77
fluid overload (water intoxication) 5, 251,
    252
fluid therapy
  in burns 185
  intra-operative 50–2
  in major trauma 177–8
  in obstetric anaesthesia 89
  paediatric patients 91–2
  in paediatric resuscitation 168
  post operative 69, 78–9
  pre-operative 5
  see also intravenous fluids
flumazenil 66, 71, 614, 616
fluoride number 643
fluoxetine 677
flupenthixol 678
fluphenazine 678
foetal circulation 359–60, 531–3
  changes at birth 360, 531
foetal death, intra-uterine 85
foeto-maternal (F/M) concentration
    ratios 525, 577
foetus 531–5
  neocortex 535
  nociception 535
  oxygen saturation 360
  pulmonary function 533
folate deficiency 476
folic acid, absorption 467
follicle-stimulating hormone (FSH) 498,
    500
food intake, regulation 448
footwear impedance 814
foramen of Magendie 441
foramen magnum 218
foramen ovale 218, 359, 531
  closure at birth 360, 531
foramen spinosum 218
foramina of Munro 441
force
  required to inject with a syringe 788
  work done by 789–90
force–velocity curve, cardiac muscle
    320–1
forced expiratory volume in one second
    see FEV$_1$
forced vital capacity (FVC) 9, 400, 401
forceps delivery 89
foreign body, upper airway obstruction
    151
fossa ovalis 201
Fourier analysis 779–80, 837, 838
Fowler's method, dead space
    measurement 401
fractional area change (FAC) 321, 326
Frank curve 320
Frank–Starling curve 319–20
  and cardiac failure 320

in exercise 355
FRC *see* functional residual capacity
'freezing point' 791
frequency
    lower 'cut-off' 836, 840
    natural or resonant 837
    upper 'cut-off' 836, 840
frequency response 836–7, 840
frequency spectrum of a signal 838
frequency table 915
fresh frozen plasma (FFP) 18, 268, 751
fresh gas flow (FGF) 50, 888
    breathing systems 888
    circle breathing system 889, 890, 891
Friedman's test 919, 921
frontal lobe 431
frontalis electromyogram (FEMG) 867
frusemide 708–9
fuel cell 854
    galvanic 855–6
fumarate 482
functional residual capacity (FRC)
        399–400
    measurement 400
    in pregnancy 90, 516
    respiratory system compliance and
        403, 404
    in surgical patients 45, 64
functions, mathematical 775–80
fuse 806
fusidanes 763
fusidic acid 763
FVC *see* forced vital capacity

G-cells, gastric 462
G proteins 227–8, 236, 237
    drug actions via 552
GABA receptor–benzodiazepine receptor
        complex 552–3, 612, 615
GABA receptors 555–6
    anticonvulsant actions 674
GABA$_A$ receptors 552–3, 555, 604
gabapentin 675
gain, amplifier 840
galactosaemia 483
β-galactosidase 478
galanin 635
gallbladder function 465–6
galvanic fuel cell 855–6
γ efferent system 222–3, 294
γ radiation 828
ganglion blocking drugs 685
gap junctions 225
    gastro-intestinal smooth muscle 455–6
    smooth muscle 295, 296
gas(es) 791, 792–4
    adiabatic compression/expansion
        797–8
    anaesthetic *see* anaesthetic gases and
        vapours
    analysis
        methods 850–4
        sources of error 854
    contents in a cylinder 797
    critical temperature 792
    cylinders *see* cylinders
    definition 792

density 854
diffusion 410, 543
embolism 55–6, 341
exchange 408–13
explosion/fire risks 817
fluid behaviour 798–802
injection through a jet 802
physical behaviour 796–8
piped supplies 877
refractive index 854
sampling errors 854
solubility 854
velocity of sound in 854
volumes, measurement 846–50
gas analysers 850–4
    continuous/discrete 851
    response characteristics 850–1
    sampling errors 854
    types 851–4
gas constant 797
gas flow
    in airways 406–7, 801
    fresh *see* fresh gas flow
    measurement 846–50
        in anaesthetic machines 847–8
        in breathing circuits 848–50
    rate
        calculation 782–3
        vaporiser performance and 886
gas/liquid chromatography 851
gastric acid
    aspiration *see* aspiration, pulmonary
    reduction 39, 731–3
    secretion 462
gastric emptying 40, 459
    control 459–60
    in pregnancy/labour 519
gastric inhibitory peptide 457, 459
gastric juice 462–4
    composition 250, 461
    control of secretion 463–4
    in pregnancy 519
gastric motility 458–60
    control 459
gastric tube 39, 178
gastric volume 39
    reduction 39
gastrin 457, 459, 462, 463
gastro-intestinal (GI) motility 455–61
    control 456–7
    in specific regions 457–61
gastro-intestinal (GI) tract 453–71
    afferents 471
    ageing effects 239
    digestion and absorption 466–70
    innervation 456
    muscle structure 455–6
    NSAID effects 631
    opioid effects 624
    pharmacology 729–36
    in pregnancy 518–19
    secretory functions 461–6
    in spinal anaesthesia 128
gastro-oesophageal reflux, in pregnancy
        519
gauge pressure 788
Gay–Lussac's law 796

gelatins 740–1
Gelofusine 740–1
gene 233, 234
general anaesthesia
    inhalational 45–7
    intravenous 47
    obstetric 89–90
general surgery 111–12
    day case 97
    paediatric patients 92
genetic code 232–3
genioglossus muscle 191
genito-urinary system, ageing 239
genome, human 233
gentamicin 760
GFR *see* glomerular filtration rate
Gibbs–Donnan effect 248–9
gigantism 500
Glasgow Coma Scale (GCS) 94, 95
    in major trauma 178, 179
glass
    critical angle 821
    refractive index 820
glial cell line-derived neurotrophic factor
        (GDNF) 449
glial cells 427
glibenclamide 22, 724
gliclazide 724
glipizide 724
globin genes 260, 261
globulins 491, 548
globus pallidus 439
glomerular basement membrane 365
glomerular capillaries 364
glomerular filtration 364–7
    coefficient 367
    equilibrium 367
    forces 365–7
    fraction 367
    pressure 367
    structural basis 364–5
    tubulo-glomerular feedback 367, 370
    ultrafiltrate 365
glomerular filtration rate (GFR) 365
    measurement 368
    in newborn infants 534
    peritubular fluid uptake and 377
    in pregnancy 520
    regulation 369–70
    single nephron (SNGFR) 367
glomerulus 363, 364–5
    blood supply 363, 364
    structure 364, 365
glossopharyngeal nerve (IX) 143, 192,
        194, 210
glucagon 464, 509–10
    metabolic actions 221, 479, 509–10
    therapy 723
glucocorticoids 503, 504–5
    actions 505
    ADH interactions 382
    anti-emetic action 672
    deficiency 505
    excess *see* Cushing's syndrome
    regulation of secretion 504–5
    see also corticosteroids
gluconeogenesis 480, 481–2

in starvation 489
glucose 479–80
  administration 723
  blood
    control 491, 509, 723–5
    in diabetes 22, 102
    in pregnancy 520
  in local anaesthetic solutions 662
  placental transfer 524
  re-absorption in proximal tubule 374–5
  sodium co-transport 375
  stereoisomers 546
  storage as glycogen 481
  T_m-limited transport 374–5
  transport 231
  see also dextrose
glucose-6-phosphate 480, 481
glutamate 451, 555
glutamine 635
glyceryl trinitrate (GTN) 68
  pharmacology 691, 692, 696
  transdermal 575
glycine solutions 112, 113
glycocalyx 226
glycogen 290, 480–1
glycogenesis 480, 481
glycogenolysis 480–1
glycolipids 486
glycolysis 290, 480
glycopeptide antibiotics 759–60
glycopyrrolate
  in bradycardia 53, 69, 126
  pharmacology 684, 696
glycosuria 22
gold, oral 19
golden hour 173
Goldman cardiac risk index 12
Golgi apparatus 224–5
Golgi tendon organs 294–5, 420, 438
Goodpasture's syndrome 281
Goormaghtigh cells (extraglomerular
    mesangial cells) 364, 365
gout 486
GR205171 672
gracile tract 436
Graham's law 543
granisetron 671–2
granulomatous hypersensitivity 282
gravity
  pulmonary effects 405–6, 415
  venous system and 340
gray 829
greater palatine foramen 218
greater palatine nerve 191, 193
grey baby syndrome 763
growth hormone (GH) 221, 498–9, 500
growth hormone receptor 498
guanethidine 691
guanosine triphosphate (GTP) 486
guanylyl cyclase 228, 237
Guedel, A.E. 865–6
Guedel airway 49
  see also oropharyngeal airway
gum elastic bougie 32
gynaecological surgery 97, 116–17
gyri 431

H zone 285, 286
H^+ (protons)
  concentration 387–8
  oxyhaemoglobin dissociation curve
    and 260
  renal secretion 372, 376, 391
    bicarbonate re-absorption and 389
    urinary buffering and 390
  see also pH
H^+-ATPase 231, 371
H^+-K^+-ATPase 371, 390
  in gastric acid secretion 462, 463
  inhibitors see proton pump inhibitors
H_2 receptor blockers 39, 90, 731
haem 468
Haemaccel 741
haematocrit 336, 337
haematological disease 16–19
haematology 257–82
  day case 97
  in pregnancy 515–16
haematoma, upper airway obstruction 62,
    63
haemodialysis (HD) 20
haemodynamics, in pregnancy 513–15
haemoglobin (Hb) 259–61, 410–11
  absorbance curve 861
  adult (HbA and HbA_2) 261, 410
  Barts 263
  C (HbC) 260, 261
  Chesapeake 261
  CO_2 transport 412
  concentration 16, 17
    in pregnancy 515
  D (HbD) 261
  E (HbE) 261
  embryonic 260, 261
  foetal (HbF) 260, 261, 410, 863
  Kansas 261
  M 261
  micro-encapsulated 743
  oxygen binding 259–60, 410–11
  S (HbS) 18, 261, 863
  saturation with oxygen see oxygen
    saturation
  solutions 742–3
  stroma-free (SFH) 742–3
  structure 259
  synthesis 260–1
  Zurich 261
haemoglobin Barts–hydrops syndrome
    263
haemoglobin H disease 263
haemoglobin SC disease 18
haemoglobinopathies 260–4
  see also sickle cell disease; thalassaemia
haemolytic disease of the newborn
    (HDN) 264, 265
haemophilia 268
haemopoiesis 259
haemorrhage
  in major trauma 173, 177–8, 179
  massive 54–5
  physiological response 173, 352–3
  post tonsillectomy 117–18
  shock 177–8
  see also blood loss; hypovolaemia

haemostasis 267–73
  pharmacology 745–51
haemothorax 187
  massive 176
haemotympanum 179
Hagen–Poiseuille law 336, 406, 800
hair hygrometer 871
Haldane apparatus 850
Haldane effect 411, 412, 524
  double 524
half life ($t_½$) 581–5, 776–7
  decay (radioactive) 828
  elimination ($t_{½β}$) 585
haloperidol 671
halothane 596
  chemical structure 593
  clinical properties 592–4, 595, 596
  hepatitis 101
  in obese patients 99
  physical properties 592, 596, 883
  repeat use 101
  solubility coefficient 544
  in upper airway obstruction 41
haptoglobin 491
harmonics 779, 780
Hartmann's solution 739, 740
  intra-operative use 52
  post operative use 78, 79
head injury 93–7, 179–80
  analgesia in 184
  assessment 179
  indications for CT 180
  induction of anaesthesia 41, 95, 185–6
  intubation and ventilation 95–6, 179
  management 94–5
  in maxillo facial trauma 120, 121
  pathophysiology 93–4
  patient transfer 96–7
head and neck
  blood vessels 215, 216
  surgery 111
head tilt manoeuvre 150
headache, post dural puncture see post
    dural puncture headache
Health and Safety Commission (HSC)
    895
healthcare workers
  infective risks 105–7
  latex allergy 107
hearing 444
heart 301–2
  anatomy 201–3
  blood supply 202–3
  chambers 201
  conduction system 201–2, 307
  electrical axis see cardiac axis
  nerve supply 202
  newborn infant 531–3
  physiology 299–330
  pump function see cardiac pump
heart blocks 158–61
  see also atrioventricular (AV) block
heart disease
  cardiac arrest 149
  epidural analgesia 85–6
  ischaemic see ischaemic heart disease
  valvular 15–16

heart murmurs 317
heart rate (HR) 326–8
  calculation from ECG 310
  cardiac output and 327–8
  in childhood 533
  control 326–7
  in pregnancy 513
  volatile agent effects 593
heart sounds 316, 317
  in pregnancy 514
  S1 317
  S2 317
  S3 and S4 317
  splitting 317
heartburn, in pregnancy 519
heat 791–6
  capacity 791
    specific 791
  energy, units 791
  latent 794–5
  loss
    humidifying gases 795, 904
    mechanisms 492, 493, 796
    warming gases 795
  production 492
  transfer 796
heat and moisture exchanger (HME) 871,
    905
heat sink, vaporisers 886, 887
Heimlich manoeuvre 151, 164
helium cylinders 878
helium dilution method, FRC
    measurement 400
helium–oxygen mixtures, in upper
    airway obstruction 41
HELLP syndrome 85
hemianopia
  bi-temporal 443
  homonymous 443
hemicholinium 685
Henderson–Hasselbach equation 388,
    543, 655, 857
Henle, loop of see loop of Henle
henry 810
Henry's law 855
heparin 748–50
  administration 749
  central nerve blocks and 85, 134
  for DVT prophylaxis 70
  effects on coagulation studies 749–50
  low molecular weight see low
      molecular weight heparin
  mechanism of action 749
  monitoring therapy 269
  reversal of effects 18, 750
  structure 748–9
hepatic failure 100
hepatic lobules 489
hepatitis A 105, 106
hepatitis B 105, 106
hepatitis C 105, 106
hepato-renal syndrome 101
hepatocytes 489, 490
herbal preparations 23
Hering–Breuer reflex 420
Hering's nerves 349, 419–20
hernia repair

inguinal field block 141–3
  laparoscopic 112
heroin 625–6
Hespan 742
hetastarch 742
hexamethonium 685
hexose monophosphate (HMP) shunt
    480, 481–2
high-density lipoproteins (HDL) 488
high frequency jet ventilation (HFJV)
    896
high frequency jet ventilator 117, 902
high molecular weight kininogen
    (HMWK) 269
hip
  fractures 114–16
  replacement, total 114
hippocampus 433, 447
His, bundle of 202, 307
His–Purkinje system 305, 307
histamine 277, 281, 629
  airway resistance effects 407
  control of blood flow 347, 348
  gastric actions 462, 463, 731
  non depolarising relaxants and 644,
      646
  receptor antagonists see anti-
      histamines; H$_2$ receptor
      blockers
histogram 916
HIV 105–6, 766
  needlestick injury and 105, 106–7
  precautions 106, 107
HLA molecules 274
Hofmann elimination 648
homeostasis 221
  ageing effects 238
  control mechanisms 222–3
  local cell responses 222
homocystinuria 485
homone replacement therapy 23
hormones 234, 235, 497
  cellular mechanisms of action 497
  control of secretion 497
  metabolic effects 221
  placental 525
  smooth muscle control 296
  see also individual hormones
Horner's syndrome 139
hose connectors 889
hoses, gas 889
hot wire pneumotachograph 849–50 5-
    HT see 5-hydroxytryptamine
Hudson mask 72
Huffman prism laryngoscope 32, 33
Hüfner constant 49
human albumin solutions (HAS) 741,
    742
human chorionic gonadotrophin (HCG)
    525
human genome 233
human immunodeficiency virus see HIV
human placental lactogen (HPL) 518, 525
humidification, oxygen 73
humidifiers 903–5
  bottle 905
  hot water bath 905, 906

humidity 795–6, 870–2, 903–4
  absolute (AH) 795, 871, 903
  importance of controlling 904
  measurement 871–2
  relative (RH) 795, 871, 904
    calculation 796
    temperature and 795, 871
  transducers 871–2
Humphrey breathing circuit 890
hyaluronidase 663
hydralazine 68, 692
hydrate microcrystal theory, anaesthetic
    agent action 554
hydrochloric acid 462, 540
  see also gastric acid
hydrocortisone 504, 505
  pharmacology 725–6, 728
  see also cortisol
hydrodynamics 798–802
hydrogen bonds 541–2
hydrogen ions see H$^+$
hydrophobic bonds 542
hydrostatic pressure 787
  in capillary exchange 342–3
  in glomerular filtration 365–7
  proximal tubules 377, 384–5
  pulmonary intravascular 415
hydroxydione 608
hydroxyethyl starch (HES) 741–2 5-
    hydroxytryptamine (serotonin)
    429 5-hydroxytryptamine (5-
    HT$_3$) receptor antagonists 77,
    669, 670, 671
hygrometers 871
hyo-epiglottic ligament 195
hyoglossus muscle 191, 193
hyoid 193
hyoscine 669–71, 684, 696, 734
hyperaemia
  active 346
  in inflammation 277
  reactive 346
hyperaldosteronism, primary 505
hyperalgesia 450–1
hyperbaric solutions 128
hypercalcaemia 253
hypercapnia 54, 392
hypercarbia 54, 149
hyperglycaemia 723
hyperkalaemia 6, 7, 252, 253
  ECG changes 7, 313
hypermagnesaemia 253, 313
hypernatraemia 5–7, 251
hyperparathyroidism 508
hypersensitivity 280–2
  contact 282
  granulomatous 282
  tuberculin-type 282
  type I (immediate) 281
  type II 281
  type III 281
  type IV (delayed) 281–2
  see also allergy
hypertension
  drug treatment 10–11
  during anaesthesia 52
  isolated systolic 10

post operative 67–8
pre-operative assessment 9–11
relevance to anaesthesia 11
hyperthermia, malignant (MH) 56–7,
    492
hyperthyroidism 502, 725
hypertonic solutions 229, 248
hyperuricaemia 486
hyperventilation
    at altitude 423–4
    respiratory alkalosis 392, 393
hypervolaemia 252, 387
hypnosis 45
hypnotics 601–18
hypoadrenalism 505
hypobaric solutions 127
hypocalcaemia 253, 313
hypocapnoea 54
hypocarbia 54
hypofibrinogenaemia 270
hypoglossal canal 218
hypoglossal nerve (XII) 211
hypoglycaemia 723
    in insulin excess 510
    post operative 71
hypokalaemia 6, 7, 252, 253
    ECG changes 7, 312–13
hypomagnesaemia 253, 313
hyponatraemia 6, 251–2
hypoparathyroidism 508
hypotension
    in aorto caval compression 514
    in central neural blockade 126, 128
    during anaesthesia 52
    in haemorrhagic shock 177
    for middle ear surgery 118
    in obstetric anaesthesia 89
    post operative 68–9
hypothalamic-pituitary axis 498–9
hypothalamus 447–9, 497, 499
    control of pituitary function 497–8
    functions 447–9
    thermoregulation 492
    vasomotor control 349
hypothermia 492–3
    in major trauma 178
    in surgery and anaesthesia 493
hypothyroidism 502, 725
hypotonic solutions 78, 229, 248
hypoventilation
    post operative 65–7
    respiratory acidosis 392
hypovolaemia 251, 252
    ADH response 387
    cannulation of major vessels 186–7
    clinical assessment 78
    epidural analgesia in 85
    pathophysiology 173–4
    post operative 68–9, 78–9
    see also fluid loss; haemorrhage
hypovolaemic shock 177–8
hypoxia/hypoxaemia
    blood flow changes 346
    cardiopulmonary arrest 149
    diffusion 65
    hypocapnia 393
    in newborn infants 534

post operative 64–5
    causes 64–5
    clinical features 64
    in obese patients 99
hypoxic pulmonary vasoconstriction
    (HPV) 414, 415
hypoxic ventilatory drive 8, 421
    loss of 73
hysterectomy 116
hysteresis 834–5
    in drug–receptor interactions 568
    in inspiration–expiration loops 405,
        790
    thermistors 870

I band 301
I:E ratio 50
ibuprofen 632
    pharmacokinetics 630
    pharmacology 637–8
ICAM-1 277
ICP see intracranial pressure
Ideal Gas Equation 797
ileal brake 460
ilio-inguinal nerve 214
iliohypogastric nerve 142, 214
imidazoles 609–10
    see also etomidate
imidazolines 707
imipenem 758–9
imipramine 676
'immobile needle' concept 137
immune complex-related diseases 281,
    282
immune system 273–6
    antibody-mediated response 275–6
    antigen presentation 274–5
    cell-mediated immunity 276
    mononuclear phagocyte system 273–4
    volatile agent effects 594
immunoglobulin superfamily 227
immunoglobulins 275
    in hypersensitivity reactions 281
    plasma 250
    structure 275, 276
impedance 806
    footwear 814
    input 840
    output 840–1
    systemic vascular 325
    thoracic 321
implant tested (IT) endotracheal tubes
    895
incisura 337
indoramin 687, 689
inductance 809–10
induction agents 27–8
    historic 614
    ideal 603
    pharmacokinetics 603
    placental transfer 526–7
    see also intravenous anaesthetic agents;
        specific agents
induction of anaesthesia 25–42
    anaphylactic reactions 28–30
    'crash' 41

in head injury 41, 95, 185–6
inhalational 27–8
intravenous 27
in major trauma 185–6
methods 27–8
in obstetric anaesthesia 90
paediatric dental surgery 92–3
rapid sequence (RSI) 40–1, 90
regurgitation and vomiting during
    38–40
in trismus 121
in upper airway obstruction 41
see also endotracheal intubation
inductor 806
inert gas effect 554
infections, complicating caudal
    anaesthesia 136–7
infective risk groups 105–7
inferior alveolar nerve 191
inferior epigastric artery 214, 215
inferior oblique muscle 217
inferior thyroid artery 197
inferior vena cava (IVC), compression in
    pregnancy 514
inflammatory mediators 277–9
    peripheral 628–9
inflammatory response 276–80, 451
infliximab 629
infra orbital nerve 208
infrared (IR) absorption gas analyser 852
inguinal canal 215
inguinal field block 141–3
inhaled administration 575, 715
inhaled anaesthetic agents see anaesthetic
    gases and vapours
inhibitory postsynaptic potential (IPSP)
    430
inositol triphosphate 228, 237
input impedance 840–1
INR (international normalised ratio) 18,
    269
inspiration 402–3
inspiratory cycling 900
inspiratory-expiratory loops 405, 789–90
inspiratory flow rates/patterns 898, 899,
    900
inspiratory neurones, medullary 419
inspiratory pressures 898, 899, 900
    constant 899
    limitation 899, 901
    raised, during anaesthesia 54
inspiratory reserve volume (IRV) 399
inspiratory time:expiratory time (I:E)
    ratio 50
insulators 803
insulin 508–9
    controlled diabetes 103, 104
    deficiency 510
    excess secretion 510
    in hyperkalaemia 7
    infusion regimen 104
    metabolic actions 221, 479, 509
    pharmacology 723–4, 728
    preparations 23, 723–4
    receptor 509, 723
    regulation of secretion 509
    structure and biosynthesis 508–9

insulin-like growth factor I (IGF-I) 499
insulin-like growth factor II (IGF-II) 499
insulinoma 510
integral 782
integration 781–2
intercalated disks 301
intercellular communication 234–8
intercept 775
intercostal muscles 213–14
intercostal nerves 214
intercostal spaces 213–14
interdigestive migratory motor complex
    (MMC) 459, 460
α-interferon, human 766
interferon γ 274
interleukin 1 (IL-1) 274, 275
interleukin 2 (IL-2) 274, 275
interleukins 629
intermediate filaments 223
intermittent mandatory ventilation
    (IMV) 903
intermittent positive pressure ventilation
    (IPPV) 896
    indications 49
    intra-operative 49–50
    pattern 49–50
    practical guidelines 50
intermolecular bonds 539–43
    strength 542–3
internal jugular vein 216
internal laryngeal nerve 197
international normalised ratio (INR) 18,
    269
international sensitivity index (ISI) 269
International Standards Organisation
    (ISO), gas cylinders 878
internuncial neurone 434
interquartiles 917, 918
interscalene block 137
interspinous ligament 87, 126
interstitial fluid 243, 244
    brain 254
    composition 249, 250
    re-absorption, in haemorrhage 352
intestinal obstruction 23–4
intima 333
intra-arterial injection, barbiturates 605
intra-arterial pressure monitoring 845–6
    sources of error 845–6
    system design 845
intra-ocular fluid 244, 255
intra-ocular pressure, control 118, 119
intra-operative management 43–58
    critical incidents 52–7
    failure to breathe 57–8
    maintenance of anaesthesia 45–52
    in major trauma 186
    patient positioning 45
    in regional anaesthesia 125–6
intra-osseous access
    in CPR 156, 166
    in major trauma 177
intra-uterine foetal death 85
intracellular fluid (ICF) 77, 243
    buffer systems 388
    composition 249–50
    volume measurement 244

intracranial haematoma 94, 179
intracranial pressure (ICP) 441–2
    cerebral blood flow and 94, 358
    control 441–2
    factors affecting 94, 442
    normal 358, 441
    raised 94–6, 358
    volatile agent effects 592–3, 595
intramuscular (IM) administration 575
intrapleural pressure 403, 405
intrathecal anaesthesia see spinal
    anaesthesia
intratracheal drug administration
    in anaphylaxis 29
    in CPR 156, 166–8
intravascular injection, inadvertent, local
    anaesthetic agents 88, 136, 141
intravenous access see venous access
intravenous (IV) administration 574, 575,
    603
intravenous anaesthesia, total (TIVA) 47,
    586
intravenous anaesthetic agents 601–18
    adverse reactions 603
    ideal 603
    induction of anaesthesia 27
    maintenance of anaesthesia 47
    mechanism of action 553–6
    pharmacokinetics 603
    see also specific agents
intravenous cannulae 906
intravenous equipment 906–7
intravenous fluids 737–43
    colloids 78, 740–2
    crystalloids 78, 739–40
    haemoglobin solutions 742–3
    serious adverse reactions 741
    synthetic oxygen carriers 743
    uses 739
    see also fluid therapy
intravenous giving sets 906–7
intravenous immunoglobulin (IVIg) 274
intravenous regional anaesthesia (IVRA)
    144–5, 659
intrinsic factor 463, 467
intubation see endotracheal intubation
inulin clearance 368
iodine 501, 725
iodine-131 (radio-iodine) 725
ion channels 226, 230
    action potentials and 305–6
    drug actions on 553
    G protein 236
    kidney 371
    receptor-operated see receptor-
        operated ion channels
    voltage-gated see voltage-gated ion
        channels
    see also specific types
ion conductance 427–8
ion pumps 231
ionic bonds 540, 541, 543
ionisation, drug
    diffusion and 543
    placental transfer and 525
ions
    diffusion 230

    distribution across membrane 248–9
IPPV see intermittent positive pressure
    ventilation
ipratropium bromide 716, 719
iproniazid 676
iron
    absorption 468–9, 470
    deficiency 17, 476
irritant receptors, airways 420
ischaemic heart disease (IHD)
    ECG abnormalities 12–13
    pacemakers 14
    pre-operative assessment 11–13
ISI (international sensitivity index) 269
islets of Langerhans 508
iso-shunt diagram 418
isobaric solutions 127
Isobestic point 861
isoflurane 597
    chemical structure 593
    clinical properties 592–4, 595, 597
    isomerism 545
    physical properties 592, 597, 883
isolated circuits 812
isolated patient circuit 814, 815
isomerism, drug 545–7
    chain 545
    dynamic 545
    functional group 545
    geometric 547
    optical 546–7
    position 545
    stereo– 546–7
    structural 545
isomers 545
isometric muscle contraction 289, 290
isoniazid 765–6
isoprenaline 686
    bronchodilator actions 716
    in peri-arrest arrhythmias 158–61
    pharmacology 687, 688, 694
    structure 687
isosorbide dinitrate 691, 692
isosorbide mononitrate 691, 692
isotherms 792, 793
isotonic muscle contraction 289
isotonic solutions 78, 229, 248
isotopes 539, 826
    radioactive see radioactive isotopes
    stable and unstable 827
isovolumetric ventricular contraction 314
isovolumetric ventricular relaxation 314,
    315
IT (implant tested) endotracheal tubes
    895

'J' receptors 420
Jackson Rees modification of Ayre's T-
    piece circuit 890
jaundice 100
jaw thrust manoeuvre 150, 164
jet ventilation 802
joint replacement surgery 114
joule 791
journals, scientific 772
jugular foramen 218
jugular venous pressure (JVP) 341

juxtaglomerular apparatus 383

K⁺ *see* potassium
K_A 563, 564–5, 566–7
kallikreins 269, 272, 277, 348
katharometers 853
K_B 563, 566–7
K_D 562
Kell antigens 265
Kelvin scale 791, 869
K_{eq} 569
kernicterus 534
ketamine 47, 608–9, 616–17
    clinical effects 608–9, 616–17
    in local anaesthetics 663
    metabolism 609
    pharmacodynamics 555, 608
    physical properties 608
ketoglutarate 482
ketone bodies 489
ketones 488–9
ketorolac 630, 631, 638
ketosis (ketoacidosis) 489
Kety method, cerebral blood flow
        estimation 358
Kidd antigens 265
kidney 361–94
    in acid–base disturbances 391–4
    ADH actions 381–2
    blood supply/vasculature 363–4
    control of ECF volume and Na⁺ re-
        absorption 382–7
    drug excretion 578
    drug interactions 557
    hormones 727
    lymph drainage 364
    morphology 363–4
    neurological reflexes 386
    NSAID effects 386, 631
    pH regulation 387–91
    see also glomerulus; renal
kinematic viscosity 800
kininogenase 281
kinins 277, 629
    ACE inhibitor actions 707
    control of blood flow 347, 348
    renal actions 387
K_m 569
knee arthroplasty, total 114
Kohn, pores of 398
Korotkov sounds 843, 844
Krebs' (citric acid) cycle 480, 482
Kruskal–Wallis test 919, 921
Kupffer cells 490

L-dopa (levodopa) 556, 679
labels, medical devices 909
labetalol 68
    pharmacology 687, 689, 695
labour
    analgesia 83–9
        complementary methods 84
        epidural analgesia 84–9
        psychological methods 83
        systemic analgesics 84
    pain 83
Lack breathing circuit 890

lactase 475
lactate 480, 481
lactose intolerance 483
Laerdal non-rebreathing valve 893–4
Laerdal system 893–4
laevo (*l*) rotatory substances 546, 821–2,
        823
Lambert–Beer law 822, 860
Lambert–Bouguer law 822, 860
laminar flow 801
    blood 335, 336
    gas in airway 406, 801
laminectomy 114
lamotrigine 675
language 432
lansoprazole 731–2
laparoscopic cholecystectomy 111–12
laparoscopy, gynaecological 116
laparotomy 111
Laplace's law 320, 325
large bowel
    motility 460–1
    secretion 461
laryngeal mask airway (LMA) 34, 895
    in CPR 152
    in day case surgery 98
    in failed intubation 36
    intra-operative use 49
    intubating 34
    in major trauma 176
    post operative oxygen via 72
    ProSeal 176
laryngeal spasm
    in children 91, 119
    post operative 62
laryngeal tube 34–5
laryngopharynx 194
laryngoscopes
    blades 32–4
    Macintosh 31, 32
laryngoscopy
    direct, view 195
    ENT 117
    grading of view 31, 32
    in major trauma 176
    technique 31
larynx 194–7
    cartilages 194–5
    functional anatomy 397
    ligaments 195
    muscles 196
    obstruction, post operative 62, 63
    paediatric patients 91
    traumatic injury 183
lasers 824–6
    classes 826
    construction 824–6
    safety 826
    surgical 826
latent heat 794–5
    of fusion, specific 795
    and temperature 794
    of vaporisation 794
        specific 795
lateral crico-arytenoid muscle 196
lateral cutaneous nerve of forearm 215
lateral foramina of Lushka 441

lateral intercellular spaces (LIS), proximal
        tubule 371, 376, 377, 384
lateral position
    for caudal anaesthesia 135, 136
    for spinal anaesthesia 128–9
latex allergy 107–8
Law of Mass Action 548, 723, 857
laxatives 734–5
LD_{50} 569
leakage currents 814
learning difficulties, dental anaesthesia 93
least squares method 924
left atrium (LA) 201
    pressure 315
left coronary artery 202
left ventricle (LV) 201, 313
    pressure 314
    RV interactions 329
    volumes 314–15
legal issues 79, 80
length 786
lesser palatine foramen 218
leucocytes 277
leukotriene receptor antagonists 629, 717
leukotrienes 277, 451, 488
    biosynthesis 630
    in bronchospasm 715
    mast cell 281
levobupivacaine 658, 661, 664
    for peripheral nerve blocks 141
    for spinal anaesthesia 89
levodopa (L-dopa) 556, 679
lidocaine 656, 661, 664
    anti-arrhythmic actions 53, 159, 162,
        701–2
    caudal anaesthesia 136
    in CPR 154, 157
    epidural anaesthesia 89, 133
    intratracheal 29
    maximum dose 658
    mechanism of action 655, 656
    metabolism 660, 661
    peripheral nerve blocks 138, 141
    spinal anaesthesia 130
    structure 655
    toxicity 659
    for upper airway anaesthesia 144
ligamentum denticulatum 204
ligamentum flavum 86, 87, 126
ligand-gated ion channels *see* receptor-
        operated (ligand-gated) ion
        channels
ligands 234, 235
    signal transduction 236–7
light 818–28
    polarised 821–2, 823
    rays 818, 819
    reflection 820–1
    refraction 820
    speed 820
    transmission 822–4
    wavelength 818
    waves 818, 819
lightwand 32
lignocaine *see* lidocaine
limbic system 349, 447–9
'line of best fit' 924

linea nigra 521
linear correlation 922–3
linear functions 775
linear measurement systems 834
linear regression 923–4
Lineweaver–Burk plot 568, 569
lingual nerve 191, 192, 210
lipase
    pancreatic 464, 466, 475
    salivary 462, 466
lipid solubility
    ligands 235
    local anaesthetics 655–7
    placental drug transfer and 525
    theory of anaesthetic agent action
        553–4
lipids
    dietary intake 475
    digestion and absorption 466–7, 469
    membrane, anaesthetic agent actions
        555
    metabolism 486–9, 491
        hormonal regulation 509, 510
    lipoproteins, plasma 486, 488 5-
        lipoxygenase 715
liquids 791
    hydrodynamics 798–802
lisinopril 707
lithium 23, 677
lithotomy position 46
liver 489–92
    disease 99–101, 268
    drug clearance 578
    drug extraction 578
    drug metabolism 491–2
    halothane-induced dysfunction 101
    metabolic functions 490–2
    in newborn infants 534
    physiology 99–100
    structure 489–90
LMA see laryngeal mask airway
local anaesthesia
    for cataract surgery 118
    in major trauma 184
    paediatric dental surgery 93
    post operative analgesia 75
    see also regional anaesthesia/analgesia
local anaesthetic agents 653–65
    absorption 659
    additives 662–3
    amide linked 655, 656, 661–2
    clinical effects 657–8
    distribution 660
    doses 658, 659
    for epidural analgesia 87
    ester linked 655, 656, 660–1
    factors influencing activity 655–7
    inadvertent intravascular injection 88,
        136, 141, 659
    intratracheal 29
    mechanism of action 655, 656
    pharmacokinetics 656
    physicochemical properties 655–7
    placental transfer 526
    in pregnancy 520, 660
    protein binding 656, 657, 660
    specific pharmacology 663–5

structure 655, 663
    toxicity 658–60
    see also specific agents
locus ceruleus 450
log roll 183
logarithmic transformation 924
logarithms 775
loop diuretics 708–9
loop of Henle (LOH) 363, 377–9
    control of sodium re-absorption 385–6
    countercurrent mechanism 379, 380
    long and short loops 379, 385–6
lorazepam 613, 614
losartan 708
loss of resistance (LOR) technique 132
low-density lipoproteins (LDL) 488
low molecular weight heparin (LMWH)
        70, 749
    administration 749
    central nerve blocks and 23, 134
lower motor neurone 434
lower oesophageal contractility 866–7
lower oesophageal contractions
    provoked (PLOC) 866–7
    spontaneous (SLOC) 867
lower oesophageal sphincter (LOS) 457
    in pregnancy 519
    tone 40, 458
Luer lock 906
lumbar nerve, first 214
lumbar plexus 205, 209
lumbar spine, anatomy 126
lumbar vertebrae 212
lumbosacral plexus 205, 209
luminous intensity 822
Lund and Browder chart 184–5
lung 198–9
    acute injury see acute lung injury
    blood vessels and lymphatics 398
    chemoreceptors 351
    compliance 403, 899
    contusion 180
    defence mechanisms 422
    disease see respiratory disease
    foetus and neonate 533–4
    functional anatomy 397–8
    functional zones 415–16
    at high altitude 422–4
    mechanics see respiration, mechanics
    metabolic functions 422, 423
    non-respiratory functions 422
    physiological shunting 417–18
    respiratory airways 397–8
    stretch receptors 327, 350, 420
    see also pulmonary
lung volumes 398–400
    airway resistance and 407
    dynamic 400
    measuring devices 846–50
    in pregnancy 516–17, 518
    pulmonary vascular resistance and 414
    spirometric 398–9
    see also pulmonary function testing;
        specific volumes
lusitropy 315
luteinising hormone (LH) 498, 500
lymph 252–4

lymph nodes 253
lymphatic system 252–4, 345
lymphatic vessels 253, 345
lymphocytes 277–9
lymphokine activated killer (LAK) cells
    276
lysosomes 224
lysylbradykinin 277, 348

M line 285
MAC see minimum alveolar
    concentration
Macintosh laryngoscope 31, 32, 33
macrolide antibiotics 761
macrophages 273–4, 276
    alveolar 398, 422
    in hypersensitivity reactions 282
    in inflammation 277, 279
macroshock 811–14
macula densa 383
Magill breathing circuit 887, 890
Magill endotracheal tube 895
magnesium 252
    imbalance 252, 253, 313
magnesium (sulphate) therapy 704–5,
    740
    in peri-arrest arrhythmias 159, 162
    uses 705
magnesium trisilicate 39, 90
magnetic effect, electric current 803
magnetic lines of force 809
magnetic sector method, mass
    spectrometry 851–2
maintenance of anaesthesia 45–52
    airway control 48–9
    analgesia 48
    fluid management 50–2
    monitoring 50, 51
    prevention of awareness 47–8
    self-ventilating patients 45–7, 49
    techniques 45–7
    ventilated patients 49–50
major anterior radicular artery 435
major histocompatibility complex
        (MHC) molecules 274, 275, 276
malignant hyperthermia (hyperpyrexia)
        (MH) 56–7, 492
Mallampati classification system 3
maltase 475
mandible 193
    fractures 120, 121
mandibular nerve 208–10
Manley (MP3) ventilator 789, 902, 904
Mann–Whitney U test 919, 921
mannitol 710
    in head injury 96, 180
    in liver disease 101
    mechanism of action 545, 551
manometer 842
manual in-line stabilisation (MILS) of
    neck 175–6
MAOIs see monoamine oxidase
    inhibitors
Mapleson classification
    breathing systems 889
    ventilators 898–901
Mapleson's water analogue model 580

indications 71
see also oxygen delivery systems
oxyhaemoglobin (HbO₂), absorbance
    curve 861
oxyhaemoglobin dissociation curve
    (ODC) 50, 260, 411
    factors affecting 260, 411
    foetal 524
    left shift 411
    right shift 411
oxyntic glands 462
oxytocic drugs 726–7
oxytocin 448, 499, 500
    pharmacology 726, 728

P mitrale 16
P–R interval 308
P wave 308
pacemaker cells
    cardiac 302, 305
        action potentials 305–6
        automaticity 305, 306–7
    smooth muscle 295, 296
pacemaker discharge rate, cardiac 306–7
    autonomic control 326–7
pacemaker potential 296
pacemakers, cardiac 14–15
    generic code 14
    pre-operative assessment 14, 15
    surgical diathermy and 14–15
pacing
    in advanced life support 156
    transcutaneous 158, 161–2
paediatric patients 90–3
    anaesthetic equipment 91
    caudal anaesthesia 135, 136
    CPR 164–8
    day case surgery 98
    fluid therapy 91–2
    induction of anaesthesia 27, 28
    methaemoglobinaemia 662
    ophthalmic surgery 93, 118–19
    pain assessment 873, 874
    postoperative analgesia 92
    pre-operative assessment 90–1
    sickle cell disease 262
    specialist surgery 92–3
    weight estimation 166
PAH *see* para-aminohippuric acid
pain 449–51
    acute 872
    chronic 449, 872
    descending inhibitory pathways 450
    dimensions 872
    effects on blood flow 351
    gate control theory 449
    in labour 83
    measurement 75, 872–3
        in children 873, 874
        multidimensional 873
        single-dimension 873
    neuropathic 451
    newborn infants 535
    nociceptive/inflammatory 450–1
    physiological signs 872–3
    post operative, adverse effects 73, 74

relief *see* analgesia
    service, acute 75–6
    transmission 430, 431, 449–50
palatoglossus muscle 191
pancreas
    endocrine function 508–10
    exocrine secretion 461, 464
    in pregnancy 520
    structure 508
pancuronium 644, 646
    pharmacology 649, 651
pantoprazole 732
pantothenic acid deficiency 476
papaveretum 626
papaverines 706
para-amino benzoic acid (PABA) 658
para-aminohippuric acid (PAH)
    clearance 368–9
    secretion in proximal tubule 376
    T_m-limited transport 368
paracellular movement, kidney 370, 371
paracetamol 633
    overdose 633
paracrine secretion 222
paramagnetic gas analysers 853, 855
paramedics 174
parametric (normal) distribution 916–17
paranasal sinuses 192
parasympathetic nervous system 206,
    445, 446
    effects of stimulation 447
    gut innervation 456
    heart rate control 326–7
    neurotransmitters and receptors 445–6
    vascular control 346
parasympathetic tone 445
parasympathomimetic agents 683
parathyroid glands 507–8
parathyroid hormone (parathormone,
    PTH) 507–8
parathyroidectomy 111
parenteral administration 574, 575
parietal cells 462
parietal lobe 431
Parkinson's disease 678
partial agonists 561, 565–6
partial pressures, Dalton's law 797
partition coefficient 543–4, 576
    blood/gas 590
patch clamping 305–6
patient-controlled analgesia (PCA) 74, 84
patient controlled epidural analgesia
    (PCEA) 87
Pauling analyser 853
peak expiratory flow rate (PEFR) 8, 9
peak flow meter 847
Pearson correlation coefficient 923
PEEP (positive end expiratory pressure)
    900, 903
pelvic trauma, major 178, 183
Penaz technique, blood pressure
    measurement 844
pendelluft 404
penicillamine 19
penicillins 576, 578, 756–7
penile block 143
pentobarbitone 604

pentose phosphate pathway (PPP) 480,
    481–2
peppermint oil 734
pepsin(ogen) 462, 466
peptidases 466
percentiles 917
percutaneous nephrolithotomy (PCNL)
    113
perfluorocarbons (PFCs) 743
peri-aqueductal grey (PAG) 450
pericardial fluid 244
pericardium 203
pericytes 342
perineal nerves 143
periodic functions 779
periodic signals 838
peripheral cut down 177, 186
peripheral nerve blocks 137–43
peripheral nerve stimulators 863
    needles 907
    for peripheral nerve blocks 137
    in prolonged neuromuscular blockade
        66, 67
peripheral nerves 205–6
    electrical stimulation 641–2, 863
peripheral nervous system 430
peripheral vascular system, control
    345–51
peripheral venous access, in major
    trauma 177
peritoneal dialysis, continuous
    ambulatory (CAPD) 20
peritoneal lavage, diagnostic (DPL) 183
peritubular capillaries, renal 377, 384–5
permissiveness, hormone-mediated 497
peroxisomes 224
persistent generalised lymphadenopathy
    (PGL) 106
persistent pulmonary hypertension of the
    newborn (PPHN) 531
PET scanning 358
pethidine 626
    in labour 84
    MAOI interaction 626
    metabolism 623, 626
    placental transfer 526
    in post anaesthetic shivering 71
pH
    arterial blood 9, 387–8
        cerebral blood flow and 358
        placental drug transfer and 525
        in pregnancy 517
    body fluid
        normal 387–8
        renal regulation 387–91
    dissociation and 543
    drug actions 551
    gastric 462, 731
    indirect estimation 859
    local anaesthetic potency and 657, 663
    measurement 859–60
    see also H⁺
pH electrode 859–60
phaeochromocytoma 507, 690
phagocytes 273–4
phagocytosis 274, 276
pharmacodynamics 559–70

drug interactions 557
  enzymes 569–70
  see also drug–receptor interactions
pharmacogenetics 569
pharmacokinetics 571–86
  distribution 575–7
  drug administration 573–5
  drug interactions 557
  elimination 577–8
  models 578–86
pharyngeal airways 152
pharyngeal plexus 194
pharynx
  anatomy 193–4
  constrictor muscles 193–4, 196
  functional anatomy 397
  mucosal tears, in oral surgery 120
  in swallowing 458
phase angles (shifts) 778–9, 837
phase response 840
phased clinical trials 769
phencyclidine derivatives 608–9
  see also ketamine
phenelzine 676
phenindione 748
phenobarbitone 604, 674
phenols 610–11
  see also propofol
phenothiazines 671, 678, 679
phenoxybenzamine 687, 689
phentolamine 687, 689
phenylephrine 687
phenylketonuria 485
phenytoin 674, 701
phosphate
  in intravenous fluids 740
  re-absorption in proximal tubule 375
  T_m-limited transport 375
  urinary buffering system 390
phosphodiesterase 238
  III isoenzyme 706
  non specific inhibitors 706
phosphodiesterase (PDE) III inhibitors
    706–7
phospholipase C 237
phospholipids 486
photoreceptors 443
phrenic nerves 200, 201
physical chemistry 537–48
physics, applied 773–829
physiology, organisation and control
    221–3
physostigmine 647, 671
pia mater 127, 204, 433
Pierre Robin syndrome 3
piezoresistive strain gauge 842
pilocarpine 683
pilonidal sinus 111
pimozide 678
pin index system (PIS) 878, 879, 881
pinocytosis 343
pioglitazone 725
pipecuronium 646, 649, 651
pipeline services, medical gas (MGPS)
    877–8
piperacillin 757
pirenzipine 734

piriform fossae 194
PIS (pin index system) 878, 879, 881
Pitot tube pneumotachograph 849, 850
pituitary gland 497–500
  abnormalities of function 500
  anterior 497–9
    hormones 498–9, 500
    hypothalamic control 448
  posterior 499
    hormones 499, 500
  in pregnancy 520
pKa 543
  local anaesthetics 656, 657
placenta 521–7
  abruption 85
  blood flow 526
  circulation 522, 523
  development and anatomy 521–3
  functions 523–7
  hormone secretion 525
  retained, operative removal 89
  transfer of drugs 525–7, 577
    factors affecting 525–6
    measurement 525
  transport 523–5
plasma 243, 244
  colloid osmotic pressure 248
  composition 249, 250
  fresh frozen (FFP) 18, 268, 751
  osmolality 247
    control 382, 387
plasma membrane see cell membrane
plasma proteins 248, 250
  drug binding 548
  placental transfer 525
  in pregnancy 515, 516
  see also protein binding
plasma volume 244
  measurement 244
  in pregnancy 515
plasminogen activators 750
platelet activating factor (PAF) 279, 281,
    717
platelet concentrates
  bacterial contamination 266
  indications for use 267
platelet count 17
platelets 272–3
  alpha granule contents 272
  function 272–3
  NSAID actions 631
  in pregnancy 515
plethysmography, body 400
pleura 199–200
pleural fluid 255
pneumatic compression devices 45, 70
pneumocytes see alveolar cells
pneumotachographs 848–50
  fixed resistance 849
  Fleisch 849, 850
  hot wire 849–50
  Pitot tube 849, 850
  screen 849, 850
pneumotaxic centre 419
pneumothorax
  accidental intra-operative 57
  chest drain insertion 187

open 176
  post operative 65
  tension 57, 65, 176
podocytes 365
poises 798
Poiseuille's law 336, 800
polarised light 821–2, 823
polarographic electrode 854, 855
polio laryngoscope 32, 33
polycythaemia, at high altitude 424
polygeline 741
polynomials 775
Pompe disease 483
pons, respiratory centres 419
PONV see post operative nausea and
    vomiting
porphyrias 605, 751
  acute intermittent 605
  variegate 605
porphyrin-based compounds 743
portal hypertension 100
positioning, patient 45
  for caudal anaesthesia 135, 136
  endotracheal intubation 31
  for epidural anaesthesia 132
  hazards related to 45, 46, 79–80
  in pregnancy 513, 514
  for spinal anaesthesia 128–9
positive end expiratory pressure (PEEP)
    900, 903
positive feedback 223
post antibiotic effect 758
post dural puncture headache (PDPH)
  after accidental dural puncture 88, 133
  after spinal anaesthesia 89, 128, 130
post-herpetic neuralgia 451
post-marketing surveillance 769
post operative complications 62–71
  cardiovascular 67–9
  CNS 70–1
  respiratory 62–7
  thrombo-embolism 69–70
post operative management 59–80
  analgesia 73–6
  care of unconscious patient 61
  day case surgery 97–8
  fluid balance 77–9
  oxygen therapy 71–3
  sequelae of anaesthesia 79–80
post operative nausea and vomiting
    (PONV) 76–7, 471
  prevention 76–7
  risk factors 76, 669
  treatment 77
post tetanic count (facilitation) (PTC)
    642, 644, 865
posterior crico-arytenoid muscle 196
posterior median sulcus 433–4
posterior spinal arteries 435
posture
  blood pressure regulation 507
  control of 440
Poswillow report (1990) 92
potassium (K^+)
  balance
    disorders of 252, 253
    role of aldosterone 504

see also hyperkalaemia;
    hypokalaemia
in body fluids 249–50
in cardiac action potentials 304, 305
cerebral blood flow and 358
in intravenous fluids 740
in neuromuscular transmission 293
in neuronal action potentials 428
transmembrane gradient 303, 427
potassium (K^+) channels 306
potassium channel activators 692
potassium chloride, in peri-arrest
    arrhythmias 159, 162
potassium sparing diuretics 709–10
potential difference 804
power
    mechanical 788–91
    study 770, 921–2
    used in breathing 790
powerstroke, myosin–actin 287, 301
prazosin 687
pre-eclampsia 85, 90
pre load 323–4
    definition 323–4
    measurement 324
pre-operative assessment 3–4
    concurrent medical disease 7–23
    concurrent medication 23
    concurrent surgical disease 23–4
    paediatric patients 90–1
pre-operative management 1–24
    see also pre-operative assessment
pre-operative preparation 4–7
    for regional anaesthesia 125
pre synaptic effects, anaesthetic agents
    555
precordial thump 153, 154
prednisolone 725, 726
prednisone 726
prefrontal cortex 431
pregnancy 511–27
    acid aspiration and pneumonitis
        89–90, 519
    anaesthesia in 83–90
    analgesia in labour 83–9
    anticonvulsant drugs 674
    cardiovascular changes 513–15
    central nervous system changes
        519–20
    CPR 162–4
    in diabetes 104–5
    ectopic 116
    endocrine changes 520
    gastro-intestinal changes 518–19
    haematological changes 515–16
    local anaesthetic agents 520, 660
    musculoskeletal changes 520–1
    operative anaesthesia 89–90
    renal function 520
    respiratory changes 516–18
    in sickle cell disease 263
    suction termination (STOP) 116–17
    weight gain 21
    see also placenta
pregnanolone 607, 608
premedication 4
    children 91

premotor area 439
pressure 841
    absolute 788
    critical 792
    measurement 841–2
    physical state and 792
    units
        clinical 841
        interconversions 786
    and velocity 802
pressure regulators
    cylinder 880
    secondary 881
pressure sensitive receptors, airways 420
pressure sores
    after obstetric epidural analgesia 89
    post operative 45, 80
pressure support (PS) ventilation 903
pressure–volume (PV) loops
    respiratory system 405
    ventilator 789–90
    ventricular 318, 319, 326, 790
preterm infants
    cardiovascular system 531, 533
    nociception 535
    thermoregulation 534
    see also newborn infant
prilocaine 656, 658, 661–2, 664
    for intravenous regional anaesthesia
        145
    methaemoglobinaemia 662
    structure 663
primary survey 174–8
primidone 674
prion disease 107, 117
prism laryngoscope (Huffman) 32, 33
pro-drugs 556
probability 918–19
probenecid 576, 578
procaine 655, 656
prochlorperazine 670, 671
    pharmacology 673
    in PONV 77
procyclidine 679
progesterone 525
prokinetic agents 734
prolactin 498, 500
prolactin-inhibiting hormone (PIH) 498
promethazine 670, 671
prone position
    back surgery 114, 115
    hazards 45, 46
propanidid 614
propantheline 734
propofol 610–11, 617–18
    adverse reactions 603
    bolus dose technique 47
    clinical effects 610–11, 618
    complications 611, 618
    manually controlled infusion 47
    metabolism 611
    minimum infusion rate (MIR) 47
    pharmacokinetics 586, 617
    physical properties 610
    target controlled infusion 47
    total intravenous anaesthesia 47
proportionality 775

propranolol 687, 690, 695, 701
ProSeal laryngeal mask airway 176
prostacyclin (PGI_2) 346, 386, 630
    pulmonary vascular resistance and 414
    synthetic (epoprostenol) 751
prostaglandins 451, 488, 629
    gastric actions 631, 732–3
    metabolism in platelets 273
    NASID actions 629–30
    renal 370, 386, 631
prostanoids 629
prostatectomy 112
protamine 750
protein binding 547–8
    anaesthetic agent actions 555
    drug distribution and 576–7
    effects of changes in 548
    factors affecting 548
    interactions affecting 557
    local anaesthetics 656, 657, 660
    mechanisms 547–8
    placental transfer and 525
protein C system 271
protein kinases 236, 237
proteinase activated 2 receptors (PAR2)
    629
proteins
    catabolism 491
    dietary intake 475
    digestion and absorption 466, 468
    glomerular filtration 365
    metabolism 483–6, 509
    plasma *see* plasma proteins
    primary structure 547
    quaternary structure 547
    secondary structure 547
    synthesis 233–4, 490–1
    tertiary structure 547
proteoglycan, glomerular basement
    membrane 365
prothrombin time (PT) 18, 269
proton pump *see* H^+-ATPase; H^+-K^+-
    ATPase
proton pump inhibitors 39, 731–2
proton pump leak theory 554–5
protons 539
    see also H^+
provoked lower oesophageal contractions
    (PLOC) 866–7
proximal tubule, renal 363, 371–7
    bicarbonate re-absorption 373, 375–6,
        389–90
    cell morphology 371
    chloride re-absorption 372–3
    lateral intercellular spaces (LIS) 371,
        376, 377, 384
    pars convoluta 371
    pars recta 371
    peritubular capillaries 377
    re-absorption of other solutes 374–6
    secretion 376–7
    sodium re-absorption 371–2
    water re-absorption 376
PRST (Evan's) score 866
pruritus, opioid-induced 625
'pseudo-coarctation', in aortic rupture
    181

pseudocholinesterase *see* cholinesterase, plasma
psychological methods, labour analgesia 83
pudendal nerve 143
pulmonary arterial pressure (PAP) 414
  in functional zones of lung 415–16
  mean (MPAP) 325
pulmonary artery 413–14
  partial pressure of volatile agent in 590
pulmonary artery catheter (PAC) 322, 324, 325
pulmonary artery diastolic pressure (PADP) 324
pulmonary blood flow 413
  distribution 415–16
  volatile agent uptake and 590
pulmonary capillaries 414
pulmonary capillary wedge pressure (PCWP) 324, 325
pulmonary circulation 333, 413–18
  physiological shunt 417–18
  in pregnancy 517–18
  pressures 414
pulmonary embolism (PE)
  intra-operative 55
  post operative 69, 70
pulmonary function testing
  in asthma 8
  devices 846–7
  pre-operative 9, 10
  see also lung volumes
pulmonary hypertension 415
  of the newborn, persistent (PPHN) 531
pulmonary oedema, post operative 65
pulmonary valve 201, 316
  lesions 16
  sounds 317
pulmonary vascular resistance (PVR) 325, 336
  factors affecting 414
  in newborn infant 531
  in pregnancy 517
pulmonary vasculature 413–14
  blood filtration 422
  innervation 414
  transmural pressure 414, 415
pulse oximeters 861–2
  calibration 862
  prolonged response times 862
pulse oximetry 50, 860–3
  principles 860–1
  sources of error 862–3
pulse pressure 337
pulseless electrical activity (PEA) 153, 154
  in paediatric patients 166
  in pregnancy 164
pumping effect, vaporisers 887
purinergic receptors 449
purines 486
Purkinje fibres 201–2, 307
putamen 439
pyeloplasty 113
pyloric glands 462
pylorus 458–9

pyramidal tract
  corticospinal tract 203, 204, 435
  direct 203
pyrazinamide 765–6
pyrexia *see* fever
pyridoxine deficiency 476
pyrimidines 486
pyruvate 480, 481, 484
  in fatty acid metabolism 487
  oxidation 482
pyruvate dehydrogenase 482

Q–T interval 309
Q wave, in pulmonary embolism 70
QRS complex 308–9
quadratic functions 775–6
quadrupole method, mass spectrometry 852
quartiles 917, 918
Quetelet's test 475
quinidine 701–2
Quinke needle 128
quinolone antibiotics 763–4

R–R interval 308, 310
racemic mixture 546–7
racoon eyes 179
radial artery 216
radial nerve 215, 216
  injury 79
radiation 826–9
  biological effect 829
  dose 829
  exposure 828–9
  from radioactive isotopes 828
  heat 493, 796
  sickness 828–9
radicular arteries 435
radio-allergosorbent test (RAST) 29
radio-iodine 725
radio-opaque drugs 551
radioactive isotopes (radio-isotopes) 539, 826–9
  applications 828
  decay 828
  decay half life 828
  radiation emitted 828
radioactivity, units 828
radiographs, plain *see* X rays
radionucleotide scanning 13, 356, 358
RAE (Ring, Adair, Elwyn) endotracheal tube 895
Raman light scattering 854
ramipril 707
randomisation 771
randomised controlled trial (RCT) 769
ranitidine 39, 731, 735–6
rapacuronium 648–9
Rapaport–Leubering shunt 260
rapid eye movement (REM) sleep 432
rapid sequence induction (RSI) 40–1, 90
RAST testing 29
Rayleigh Refractometer 854
re-absorption, renal tubular 370
reactance 805
reboxetine 677
receptor occupancy (r) 562

agonists 563–4
  irreversible competitive antagonists 567, 568
  partial agonists 565
  response inconsistencies 568
  reversible competitive antagonists 566
receptor-operated (ligand-gated) ion channels 230, 236, 552
  anaesthetic agent actions 555–6
receptors 234, 235–6, 547
  binding site modulation 236
  downregulation 497
  drug actions via 552–3
  hormone actions 497
  intracellular 237
  properties 235–6
  upregulation 497
  see also drug–receptor interactions
Recklinghausen's oscillotonometer 843
record keeping 80
recovery, post operative 61
recovery room 61
  criteria for discharge to ward 61
  management 61
rectal administration 574
rectal temperature 869
rectum, surgery to 111
rectus abdominis muscle 214
rectus muscles, extraocular 217
rectus sheath 214
recurrent laryngeal nerve 143, 197
red blood cells 259–64
  antigens 265
  carbon dioxide transport 412, 413
  streaming 336–7
red cell volume 244
  measurement 244
  in pregnancy 515
'red man syndrome' 760
reflection 820–1
  total internal 821
reflex arc 435–9
  monosynaptic 436, 437
  polysynaptic 436, 437, 439
refraction 820
refractive index 820
  gas analysis based on 854
refractoriness, cardiac action potentials 304–5
refractory period, neuronal action potentials 428
refusal, epidural analgesia in labour 84
regional anaesthesia/analgesia 123–45
  contra-indications 125
  for day case surgery 98
  equipment 907
  intravenous (IVRA) 144–5, 659
  in major trauma 184
  for obstetric surgery 89
  paediatric patients 92
  patient preparation 125
  peri-operative management 125–6
  practical requirements 125
  see also central neural blockade; local anaesthesia; peripheral nerve blocks
Regnault's hygrometer 871

regression, linear 923–4
regression coefficient 923, 924
regurgitation 38–40
    causes 38
    prevention 39–40
relative risk 770
relatives
    withholding resuscitation and 168
    witnessing resuscitation 169
relaxin 520–1
remifentanil 627
    pharmacokinetics 623, 627
    pharmacology 636–7
renal artery 363–4
renal blood flow (RBF) 363, 367
    calculation 369
    regulation 369–70
renal clearance see clearance, renal
renal disease 20, 101–2
renal failure 20, 21, 101–2
    acute 21
    antimicrobial therapy 755
    chronic 20, 21, 101
renal function
    in foetus/newborn 534
    NSAIDs and 631
    in pregnancy 520, 521
renal physiology 361–94
renal plasma flow (RPF) 367
    effective 369
    measurement 368–9
renal stones 113
renal tubules see tubules, renal
renin 383
renin–angiotensin system 383–4, 503
    in haemorrhage 352–3
    pharmacological antagonism 707–8,
        727
repaglinide 725
rescue breathing 151
reserpine 691
reservoir bags 889
    'feel' 37
    oxygen 894
residual volume (RV) 399
resistance 805, 806–7
    parallel 806, 807
    series 806
resistance vessels 345
resistor 806
resonancies 837
respiration
    CNS chemoreceptor control 254–5
    expired air (EAR) see expired air
        respiration
    mechanics 402–8
        in pregnancy 516–17, 518
    periodic, in newborn infants 534
    see also breathing; ventilation
respiratory acidosis 387, 392
respiratory alkalosis 387, 392–3
respiratory arrest 149
    in paediatric patients 164
respiratory centre stimulants 717–18
respiratory centres, brain stem 419
respiratory chain 482–3

respiratory complications, post operative
    62–7
respiratory depression
    opioid-induced 66, 74, 75, 623–4
    post operative 66
    volatile agent-induced 593, 595
respiratory disease
    gas analysis errors 854
    hypoxic ventilatory drive 8, 73, 421
    post operative complications 67
    pre-operative assessment 7–9
    pulmonary vascular resistance 414
respiratory distress syndrome (RDS),
    neonatal 533–4
respiratory failure, chronic 8, 73
respiratory muscles 402–3
    accessory 402–3
    inadequate post operative function
        66–7
respiratory quotient (RQ) 409
respiratory system 395–424
    ageing 239
    anatomy 191–9, 397–8
    barbiturate effects 606
    benzodiazepine effects 613
    compliance 403–6
        dynamic 404
        factors decreasing 404
        measurement 404
        mechanical ventilation and 406,
            899, 900, 901
        in spontaneous ventilation 405–6
        static 404
    conducting airways 397
    ketamine effects 609
    local anaesthetic effects 658
    newborn infant 533–4
    NSAID effects 630–1
    opioid effects 623–4
    patient positioning and 45
    pharmacology 713–20
    in pregnancy 516–18
    pressure–volume loop 405
    propofol effects 611
    reflexes 419–20
    in spinal anaesthesia 128
    volatile agent effects 593, 595
    see also airway(s); lung
respiratory tract infection, upper (URTI)
    7
response time 835, 851
resting membrane potential (RMP) 293,
    303–4, 427
resuscitation 147–69
    abandoning 169
    breathing systems 153, 893–4
    in burns 184–5
    cannulation of major vessels 186–7
    cardiopulmonary see cardiopulmonary
        resuscitation
    ethical aspects 168–9
    indications 168–9
    in major trauma 174–8
    withholding 168
    witnessing by relatives 169
retching 471
reteplase 750

reticular-activating system (RAS) 432
reticular formation 433
retina 443
retinal surgery 119
reversible inhibitors of monoamine
        oxidase A (RIMAs) 677
Reye's syndrome 75, 632
Reynold's number (Re) 406, 800
Rhesus (Rh) system 264–5
    blood grouping and screening 266
    D antigens 264–5
    haplotype frequencies 265
rheumatoid arthritis 19–20
rhodonase 692
ribavirin 766
riboflavin deficiency 476
ribonuclease 464
ribonucleic acid (RNA) 232, 233
ribose 5-phosphate 481, 482
ribosomes 224, 233
ribs
    first 212–13, 214
    flaring, in pregnancy 516
    fractures 187
rifampicin 764–5
rifamycins 764–5
right atrium (RA) 201
    pressure 315
right coronary artery 202
right ventricle (RV) 201, 313
    LV interactions 329
    pressure 314
righting reflexes 440
rigidity, decerebrate 440
rimantadine 766
rimiterol 716
rise time 835, 851
Ritchie whistle 881, 882
Riva-Rocci cuff 843
RNA 232, 233
road traffic accidents 184
rocuronium 644, 646
    in ophthalmic surgery 119
    pharmacology 649, 651
röntgen 829
root mean square (RMS) value 805
ropivacaine 656, 662, 665
    epidural anaesthesia 87, 133
    hyperbaric, for spinal anaesthesia 89
    maximum dose 658
    peripheral nerve blocks 138
    structure 663
rosiglitazone 725
rotameter 847–8
    block, features 848, 849
    gas flow pattern 848
routes of drug administration 573, 574
rRNA 233
Rubens non-rebreathing valve 893–4
ruby laser 825, 826
'rule of nines' 184, 185
ryanodine receptors 287, 289
    defects 56, 492

S cells 464
S wave, in pulmonary embolism 70

SA (sinoatrial) node 201–2, 305, 307
sacral plexus 205, 209
sacrum, anatomy 135, 213
salbutamol 687, 688, 715–16, 719
salicylism 632
saline, normal (0.9%) 78, 79, 739, 740
saliva 250, 461, 462
salivary glands 462
saltatory conduction 427
sample size 770
Sanders injector 117, 802
saphenous nerve 141, 206
    block 142
    injury 79
saphenous vein cut down 186
sarcolemma 285, 301
sarcomere 285, 301, 302
sarcoplasmic reticulum (SR)
    cardiac muscle 301, 302
    skeletal muscle 286, 287
sarcotubular system 286, 287
satiety centre, hypothalamic 448
saturated vapour pressure (SVP) 792, 794
    and temperature 794
scalars 783–4
Scarpa's fascia 215
scavenging systems 895–6
    absorbers 896
    active 896, 897
    passive 896, 897
Schlemm, canal of 255, 442
Schrader probe 877
Schrader sockets 877
Schwann cells 427
sciatic nerve 205
scintillography (radionuclide scanning)
    13, 356, 358
scleral haemorrhage 179
screen pneumotachograph 849, 850
second gas effect 590
second messengers 237–8
    anaesthetic agent actions via 556
    drug actions via 552
    enzymes 226, 228
secondary pressure regulators 881
secondary survey 179–83
secretin 457, 464, 466
secretion, renal tubular 370
sedatives, anti-emetic 672
'Seebeck effect' 870
seizures
    drug treatment 674–5
    volatile agent-induced 595, 596
Seldinger technique 906
selectins 227
selective imidazoline receptor agonists
    (SIRA) 707
selective norepinephrine reuptake
    inhibitors 677
selective serotonin re-uptake inhibitors
    (SSRI) 677
selegiline 676, 679
self-inflating bag 153, 893, 894
semilunar valves see aortic valve;
    pulmonary valve
semipermeable membranes 245–9, 544–5
senses, special 442–5

sensitivity 834
sensory receptors 430, 431
sensory testing, in spinal anaesthesia 129
sepsis, epidural analgesia 86
septic shock, transfusion-related 266
sequential analysis 924–5
serotonin (5-hydroxytryptamine) 429
serotonin/norepinephrine reuptake
        inhibitors 677
sevoflurane 597–8
    blood/gas partition coefficient 544
    chemical structure 593
    clinical properties 592–4, 595, 597–8
    for induction 41
    physical properties 592, 597, 883
sex differences, total body water 243
sharps disposal 106
shear rate 798, 799
shear stress 798, 799
shivering 492
    post anaesthetic 70–1
shock
    anaphylactic 28, 29, 30
    haemorrhagic 177–8
    septic 266
shunt, physiological 417–18
shunt equation 418
shunt fraction 417–18
SI system 784, 785
Sibson's fascia 213
sick sinus syndrome 308
sickle cell disease 18, 260, 261–3
    clinical features 262
    diagnosis 262
    geography 261–2
    management 262–3
    pathophysiology 261
    vaso-occlusive crises 262–3
sickle cell trait 262
Sickledex test 18
sickling disorders 262
sievert (Sv) 829
Siggard–Andersen diagram 857
signal-to-noise (S/N) ratio 839
signal processing 839–40
signal transduction 236–7
    intracellular 237
    membrane 236
silver/silver chloride electrode 860
sine–cosine pairs 838
sine functions 778
    in electrical signals 779
sine wave 838
single twitch
    in neuromuscular monitoring 642, 864
    physiology 289, 290
sinoatrial (SA) node 201–2, 305, 307
sinus arrhythmia 312
sinus rhythm 312
sinuses of Valsalva 202
sinusoids, hepatic 489–90
sitting position, for spinal anaesthesia 129
skewed data distribution 917, 918
skin blood flow, in thermoregulation 492
skin damage, post operative 80
skull base
    anatomy 218

fractures 179
sleep
    effect on ventilation 421
    non-rapid eye movement (NREM)
        432
    rapid eye movement (REM) 432
sleep apnoea 62
small bowel
    motility 460–1
    secretion 461
smoking 7
smooth muscle 295–6
    contraction 295–6, 455
    extrinsic control 296
    gastro-intestinal 455
    membrane potential 296, 455
    multi-unit 295, 296
    plasticity 296
    properties 296
    single-unit 295, 296
    structure 295
    tone 296
    vascular 346
    vs skeletal and cardiac muscle 296–7
smooth muscle relaxants, direct-acting
        734
sneeze reflex 422
Snell's law 820
Snow, John 865–6
soda lime 594, 891
    'channelling' 891
    humidifying effect 905
    sevoflurane degradation 598
sodium (Na$^+$)
    anti-port carriers 231, 372
    balance
        disorders 250–2
        role of aldosterone 503–4
    bicarbonate re-absorption and 389–90
    in body fluids 249–50
    in cardiac action potentials 304, 305
    glucose co-transport 375
    intestinal re-absorption 467
    in intravenous fluids 740
    in neuromuscular transmission 292,
        293
    in neuronal action potentials 428
    renal re-absorption
        in loop of Henle 378, 379
        in proximal tubule 371–2, 373, 374,
            377
        regulation 382–7
    symport carriers 231, 372
    transmembrane gradient 248–9, 303,
        427
sodium bicarbonate
    8.4% solution 739, 740
    in anaphylaxis 30
    as antacid 733
    in CPR 154, 156, 168
sodium channels
    cardiac 304, 306
        anti-arrhythmic drug actions 701–2
    fast voltage-gated neuronal 430
        local anaesthetic actions 655, 656
        phenytoin actions 674
    kidney 371

sodium chloride (NaCl) 540, 544
  0.9% solution 78, 79, 739, 740
  bicarbonate re-absorption and 389–90
sodium citrate 39, 90, 733
sodium nitroprusside 691, 692, 697
sodium pump *see* Na⁺K⁺ ATPase
solids 791
solubility 543–4
solubility coefficient 544
solute 544–5
solutions 245–9
  concentration 245
  intravenous 740
  osmolality and osmolarity 246–7
  tonicity 229, 247–8
solvent 544
somatomedins 499
somatostatin 457, 510
somatosympathetic reflex 351
sore throat, post operative 79
sotalol 701, 703
sound, velocity in gas 854
Spearman correlation coefficient 923
specific heat capacity 791
specific latent heat of fusion 795
specific latent heat of vaporisation 795
SPECT scanning 358
spectral analysis 840
sphenoid sinus 192, 194
sphincter of Oddi 466
spina bifida 85
spinal anaesthesia 126–30
  accidental 88, 137
  anatomy 126–7
  complications 130
  drug doses and volumes 130
  equipment 128, 907
  in femoral neck fractures 114–16
  indications 126
  for obstetric surgery 89
  physiology 127–8
  technique 128–30
  for transurethral resection of prostate
    112
  vs epidural anaesthesia 131
  see also combined spinal–epidural
    (CSE) anaesthesia
spinal cord 203, 433–5
  ascending tracts 203, 204, 434, 436
  blood supply 203, 435
  complete transection 434
  descending tracts 203, 204, 434, 435
  dorsal horn 449, 450, 451
  hemisection 434–5
  injury 183, 434–5
  intermediolateral (IML) grey columns
    349
  meninges 127, 204, 433
  opioid receptors 622
  postural reflexes 440
  structure 433–4
spinal needles 128, 907
spinal nerves 127, 205, 433
spinal shock 434
spine *see* vertebral column
spinocerebellar tracts 203, 204, 436
spinocerebellum 439

spinotectal tract 436
spinothalamic tract 203, 204, 436, 449
spiral arteries, uterine 521
spirometry 398–9
  device 846
  pre-operative tests 9, 10
spironolactone 709–10
splanchnic nerves 218
Sprotte needle 89, 128, 907
squint surgery 93, 118–19
St. John's Wort 23
ST segment 309
'stacking' (of breaths) 903
staircase effect 327–8
standard deviation (SD) 916–17
standard error of the mean (SEM) 917
Starling curve 320
Starling forces 343–4
  proximal tubular Na⁺ re-absorption
    and 384–5
  renal peritubular capillaries 377
starvation 489
  pre-operative 4, 39
statistical analysis 772
statistical significance 771, 919
statistical tests 918–25
  comparing more than two groups 921
  one– and two-tailed 924
  paired data 921
  qualitative data 919–20
  quantitative data 920–1
  selection 919
  sequential analysis 924–5
statistics 913–26
  descriptive 915–17
status epilepticus 675
stavudine 766
step response 835
  gas analysers 850–1
stereoisomerism 546–7
stereoisomers 546–7
sterilisation (equipment) 908
  labels used after 909
  methods 908
sterilisation, laparoscopic 116
sterno-hyoid muscle 196
steroid anaesthetic agents 607–8
steroids *see* corticosteroids
Steward–Hamilton equation 322
stimulant laxatives 735
stimulated emission 824, 825
stockings, thrombo-embolic deterrent 70
stoichiometric concentrations 817
stomach
  full, induction of anaesthesia 40–1
  mucus 462–3
  see also gastric
streptokinase 750
streptomycin 760, 761
stress incontinence 113
stress response 446, 447
  catecholamine secretion 506
  glucocorticoid secretion 504
  see also sympathetic activation
stretch reflex 436, 437, 438
  in control of posture 440
  inverse 438

striatum 439
stridor, post operative 62
stroke, in sickle cell disease 262
stroke index (SI) 321
stroke volume (SV) 321
  control 323–6
  measurement 321
  in pregnancy 513
stroke volume work index (SVWI) 326
stroke work (SW) 318, 326, 790
stroma-free haemoglobin (SFH) 742–3
Student's t-test 919, 920
  more than two groups 921
  paired 919, 921
study power 770, 921–2
stylet, to aid tracheal intubation 32
styloglossus muscle 191
stylomastoid foramen 218
sub-acute combined degeneration of the
  cord 599
subarachnoid anaesthesia *see* spinal
  anaesthesia
subarachnoid space 433
  in pregnancy 520
subclavian artery 216
subclavian brachial plexus block 138–9
subclavian vein 216
  cannulation 186–7
subcostal nerve 214
subdural haematoma 94
subdural space 433
subhyaloid haemorrhage 179
sublimation 794
substance P 348, 451, 635
substrates, false 553, 570
sucralfate 733–4
sucrase 475
suction termination of pregnancy
  (STOP) 116–17
sufentanil 627
sugar, blood *see* glucose, blood
sulci 431
sulphasalazine 19
sulphonamides 765
sulphonylureas 22, 724
sulpiride 678
superficial peroneal nerve 141
  block 142
superior alveolar nerves 191
superior epigastric vessels 214
superior laryngeal nerve 143, 197
  block 144
superior oblique muscle 217
superior thyroid artery 197
supine hypotension syndrome 514
supine position 46
supplementary motor area 439
supraclavicular block 137, 138–9
supraorbital nerve palsy 79–80
supraspinous ligament 87, 126
supraventricular tachycardia (SVT)
  paroxysmal 53, 158
  peri-arrest 157–8
  post operative 69
sural nerve 141, 205
  block 142
surfactant 198, 405

foetal production 533–4
  treatment 718
surgery 109–21
  day case 97–9
  patient positioning 45
  see also specific types
surgical disease, concurrent 23–4
suxamethonium 642
  apnoea 57–8, 66–7
  chemical structure 652
  clinical features 642–3
  in head injury 95–6
  mechanism of action 642, 645
  metabolism 643
  muscle pains 79, 643
  pharmacology 650
  phase I blockade 644
  phase II blockade 644
  in upper airway obstruction 62, 63
swallowing 458
sweat 244, 250
sweating 492, 493
swimmers view, cervical spine 180
Sylvian fissure 431
symbols, medical devices 909
sympathetic activation 446, 447
  during awareness 48
  during exercise 353–4, 355
  in haemorrhage 352
  renal response 369–70, 383, 386
  see also stress response
sympathetic blockade, post operative 68
sympathetic nervous system 206, 445,
      446
  catecholamine secretion 506–7
  coronary blood flow regulation 356–7
  effects of stimulation *see* sympathetic
      activation
  gut innervation 456
  heart rate control 326–7
  kidney 386
  lungs 414
  in neuropathic pain 451
  neurotransmitters and receptors 445–6
  in pregnancy 520
  vascular control 346, 348
sympathetic tone 445
symport carriers 230, 231, 372
synapses 428–30
  mechanism of transmission 429–30
  structure 429
synaptic cleft 429
synchronised intermittent mandatory
      ventilation (SIMV) 901, 903
syncytiotrophoblast 521–3
syncytium 301
synergism, drug 556
syringe
  force required to inject with 788
  loss of resistance 132
systemic circulation 333
  flow 335–6
systemic inflammatory response
      syndrome (SIRS) 173–4
systemic vascular impedance 325
systemic vascular resistance (SVR) 325,
      336

effect on arterial pressures 339–40
  in pregnancy 514
  volatile agent effects 593
systole 313, 314–15

T-cell receptor (TCR) 274, 276
T-cells *see* T-lymphocytes
T-helper cells (T_H) 274, 275, 276
  in hypersensitivity reactions 282
  memory cells 275
T-lymphocytes 279
  antigen presentation to 274–5
  B cell interactions 275
  in cell-mediated immunity 276
  cytotoxic (T_C) 276
  pulmonary 422
t test *see* Student's t-test
T tubules 286, 287, 301, 302
T wave 308, 309
T_3 *see* tri-iodothyronine
T_4 (thyroxine) 501, 502, 725
tachycardia
  broad complex 157–8, 159, 163
  cardiac output 327–8
  intra-operative 53
  narrow complex 158, 160, 163
  peri-arrest 157–8, 162
  post operative 69
  sinus 312
  see also supraventricular tachycardia;
      ventricular tachycardia
tachykinins 635
tare weight, gas cylinders 879
target concentration 586
target controlled infusion 47
taste 444–5
taste buds 444
tautomer 545
tautomerism 545
technetium scan 13, 356
teeth 191
  broken 79
  extraction 92–3, 119–20
  wisdom, removal 120
teicoplanin 759, 760
temazepam 611, 613, 614
temperature
  body *see* body temperature
  critical (T_C) 792, 793
  latent heat and 794
  measurement 868–70
  physical state and 792, 793
  relative humidity and 795, 871
  saturated vapour pressure and 794
  scales 791, 868–9
    interconversions 869
  vaporiser performance and 886
  viscosity and 798
temporal lobe 431
terbutaline 715–16
terlipressin 727
termination of pregnancy, suction
      (STOP) 116–17
tetanic fade 642, 644, 865
tetanic stimulation 289, 290, 642, 865
tetracyclines 761–2

Δ^9-tetrahydrocannabinol (Δ^9-THC) 634,
      672
thalamus 449–50
thalassaemia 260, 263–4
  α 263
    homozygous 263
    trait 263
  β 263–4
    homozygous (major) 263
    trait 264
thallium scan 13, 356
theophylline 716, 717
therapeutic index 569
thermal conductivity, gases 853
thermistors 870
thermocouple 870
thermodilution, cardiac output
      measurement 322
thermodynamic theory 554
thermogenesis, non shivering 492, 534
thermometers 869–70
  chemical 869
  dial 870
  direct-reading 869–70
  liquid expansion 869
  remote-reading 869, 870
  resistance 870
  wet and dry bulb 871, 872
thermoregulation 492–3
  disturbances 492–3
  in newborn infants 534
  physiological mechanisms 492
  responses 492
  see also body temperature
θ rhythm 432, 867
thiamine
  absorption 467
  deficiency 476
thiamine pyrophosphate 479
thiazide diuretics 10, 709
thiazolidinediones 725
thiobarbiturates 604
thiols 691
thiopentone 604, 605–7, 618
  adverse reactions 603
  clinical effects 606, 618
  complications 605, 607
  isomerism 545
  maintenance of anaesthesia 47
  metabolism 606
  pharmacokinetics 603, 618
  physical properties 605–6
thioridazine 678
thioureylenes 725
thioxanthines 678
third space
  concept 50–2
  fluid losses 77
thirst 448
thoracic cage *see* chest wall
thoracic impedance 321
thoracic inlet 212–13
thoracic pump 341–2
thoracic sympathetic chain 198, 202
thoracic vertebrae 212
thorax *see* chest
Thorel bundle 307

three-compartment model 579
'3 in 1' block 140
threshold potential (TP) 304, 305, 307
thrombin 269–70, 271
thrombin time (TT) 270
thrombo-embolism
    intra-operative 55
    post operative 69–70
    risk group classification 70
thrombocytopenia 19, 267
    in pregnancy 515
thrombocytopenic purpura, thrombotic
        268
thrombomodulin 271
thromboplastin 269
thromboprophylaxis 70
    central nerve blocks and 134
thrombotic thrombocytopenic purpura
        268
thromboxane A$_2$ 273, 346, 630
    aspirin actions 750
    kidney 386
thromboxanes 629
thymol 887
thyro-arytenoid muscle 196
thyro-hyoid membrane 195, 196
thyro-hyoid muscle 196
thyroid cartilage 194, 195, 196
thyroid gland 500–2
    in pregnancy 520
thyroid hormones 221, 501–2
    abnormalities of secretion 502
    metabolism 502
    pharmacology 725
    physiological effects 502
    secretion and transport 501–2
    synthesis 501
thyroid-stimulating hormone (TSH)
        498, 500, 502
thyroid surgery 111
thyrotrophin-releasing hormone (TRH)
        498, 502
thyroxine binding globulin (TBG) 502
thyroxine (T$_4$) 501, 502, 725
tibial nerve 141, 205
    block 142
tidal volume (V$_T$) 50, 399
    calculation 782
    mechanical ventilators 898, 899
    paediatric patients 91
    in pregnancy 516
    preset 899, 900, 901
tight junctions 225
time 786
time constants 581–5, 776
'time-variant' signals 837–8
tissue
    blood flow to 576–7
    compartments, drug distribution 576,
        577
    distribution of volatile agents 591
    drug uptake 576
tissue factor 268, 271
tissue factor pathway inhibitor 271
tissue-type plasminogen activator (t-PA)
        272, 750
T$_m$-limited transport 374–5, 376

tolerance
    acute, to thiopentone 606
    opioid 624
tongue 191–2
tonic labyrinthine reflex 440
tonic neck reflex 440
tonicity 229, 247–8
tonsillectomy 93, 117–18
    haemorrhage after 117–18
tonsils
    nasopharyngeal 194
    palatine 194
topical administration 574
topical anaesthesia, mouth and
        oropharynx 144
Toronto frame 114, 115
torsade-de-pointes 158
total body water (TBW) 77, 243
    disturbances 251
    measurement 244
    see also fluid(s); water
total intravenous anaesthesia (TIVA) 47,
        586
total lung capacity (TLC) 399
total lung volume (TLV) 45
touch, neuromuscular monitoring 863
tourniquets 144
trabeculae carnae 201
trace elements 475
    deficiencies 476
trachea 197–8, 397
    intubation see endotracheal intubation
tracheobronchial injury 183
tracheostomy 118
    emergency 153
    in major trauma 183
    percutaneous dilatational 153
trachlight 32
train of four (TOF) stimulation 642,
        864–5, 866
tramadol 633–4
tranexamic acid 750
transaminases 100
transamination 484
transcellular fluids 243, 244
    composition 250
transcellular movement, renal tubules
        370, 371
transcervical resection of endometrium
        (TCRE) 116
transcription 233, 234
transcription factors 234
transcutaneous CO$_2$ electrodes 858
transcutaneous electrical nerve
        stimulation (TENS), in labour
        83
transcutaneous oxygen electrodes 856
transcytosis 248
transdermal administration 575
transducer 833
    signal-conditioning unit 833–4
    transmission path 833, 841
transfer
    in head injury 96–7
    to recovery room 61
transferrin 469
transformer 806, 810, 811

isolating 814
transfusion 264–7
    in emergencies 266
    infective risks 105
    intra-operative 52, 55
    in major trauma 178
    massive 55, 267, 268
    post operative 79
    pre-operative 17–18
    reactions 266–7
        delayed 267
        with dyspnoea 266
        febrile non haemolytic (FNHTR)
            266–7
        immediate haemolytic 266
        incompatibility 55, 266
    in renal failure 101
    in sickle cell disease 18, 263
    in thalassaemia 263
transfusion-associated acute lung injury
        (TRALI) 266
transient tachypnoea of the newborn
        (TTN) 533
transistor 806, 811
translation 234
transmembrane transport systems 553
transmission path 833, 841
transport
    active see active transport
    mechanisms 228–31, 248
    membrane 228–31
    renal tubular 370–1
    T$_m$-limited 374–5, 376
transport carriers 226, 230–1
transpulmonary pressure 403
transthyretin 501–2
transtracheal block 144
transurethral resection of bladder tumour
        (TURBT) 112
transurethral resection of the prostate
        (TURP) 112
transurethral (TUR) syndrome 6, 112–13
transvaginal tension-free tape (TVT) 113
transverse crico-arytenoid muscle 196
transverse waves 818, 819
trauma 171–87
    anaesthesia 185–6
    analgesia 184
    assessment and management 174–84
    cannulation of major vessels 186–7
    chest drain insertion 187
    medical history 184
    in paediatric patients 92
    pathophysiology 173–4
    prehospital management 174
    preparation for resuscitation 174
    primary survey and resuscitation
        (ABCDE) 174–8
    secondary survey 179–83
    team 174
    see also burns; head injury
Trendelenburg position 45
Treppe effect 327–8
tri-fluoroacetyl halide (of halothane) 101
tri-iodothyronine (T$_3$) 501, 502, 725
    reverse (RT$_3$) 501, 502
triad, sarcotubular 286, 287

triamcinolone 725
trichloroethylene 592, 600
triclofos 615
tricuspid valve 201, 315–16
  lesions 16
  sounds 317
tricyclic antidepressants 23, 676
trigeminal nerve (V) 143, 208–10
triglycerides 486, 487
trigonometric functions 777–9
trimetaphan 685
  tachyphylaxis 685
trimethoprim 765
triple response 346
trismus 121
trk receptors 449, 451
tRNA 233
trochlear nerve (IV) 208, 217
troglitazone 725
trophoblast 521, 522
tropomyosin 285–6, 287, 301
troponin 286, 301
  C 286, 288–9
  I 181, 286, 287
  T 286, 287
trypsin(ogen) 464, 466
tryptase 281, 629
  serum 29
D-tubocurarine 646, 649–50, 651
tubular maximum (T_m)-limited transport
    374–5, 376
tubules, renal 363, 370–81
  blood supply 363, 364
  transport mechanisms 370–1
  see also collecting tubules, renal; distal
      tubule, renal; loop of Henle;
      proximal tubule, renal
tubulo-glomerular feedback 367, 370
Tuffier's line 129
tumour necrosis factor (TNF) 276, 277,
    279, 629
tumour necrosis factor α (TNF-α) 629
Tunstall's 'isolated arm' technique 866
Tuohy needle 132, 133, 907
turbulent flow 801
  blood 335
  gas in airway 406–7, 801
TVT (transvaginal tension-free tape) 113
two-compartment model 579
tympanic membrane, temperature 869
type I error 919, 921
type II error 770, 921–2
tyrosine kinase 509, 723
  receptors (trkB and trkC) 449

ulnar artery 216
ulnar nerve injury 79
ultra violet (UV) absorption gas analyser
    852–3
ultrasound
  in abdominal trauma 183
  see also Doppler ultrasound;
      echocardiography
umbilical arteries 359, 523, 531
umbilical vein 359, 523
unconscious patient

airway management 62, 63
  basic life support 150, 151, 164
  in head injury 94, 95
  post operative care 61
  see also consciousness
underdamping 836
uniport carriers 230, 231
units 784–6
  derived 785
  fundamental 784
  multiplication factors 785
  named derived 785
Universal Gas Constant 797
upper airway
  functional anatomy 397
  local anaesthesia 143–4
  nerve anatomy 143
  obstruction see airway obstruction,
      upper
upper respiratory tract infection (URTI)
    7
uranium series 828, 829
urea
  in countercurrent mechanism 380–1
  cycle 485, 486
  formation 491
  pharmacology 710
  re-absorption in proximal tubule
      375–6
uric acid 486
uridine triphosphate (UTP) 486
urinary catheterisation, in trauma 178
urine
  buffering 390
  concentration mechanism 380–1
  titratable acidity 391
urokinase 750
urological surgery 112–13
  day case 97
  paediatric patients 92
urticarial transfusion reactions 267
uterine blood flow (UBF), in pregnancy
    514, 523
uvula 191

'v' wave 315, 317, 340
V₂ receptors 382
vacuum, medical 878
vacuum insulated evaporator (VIE) 877
vagus nerve (X) 210–11
  airway innervation 143, 198
  dorsal nucleus 210, 211
  gut innervation 456
  heart rate control 327
  pharyngeal branches 194
  in vomiting 471
valency 539–40
valproate 675
Valsalva, A.M. 353
Valsalva, sinuses of 202
Valsalva manoeuvre 342, 353
valsartan 708
valves
  adjustable pressure limiting (APL)
      expiratory 888
  non-rebreathing 893–4
  one way 88

valvular heart disease 316
  murmurs 317
  pre-operative assessment 15–16
van der Waals forces 541, 543
  in protein binding 548
van Slyke apparatus 850
vancomycin 759–60
vancomycin resistant enterococci (VRE)
    759
vanilloid receptors 449
van't Hoff equation 246
Vaporiser Inside Circle (VIC) 891
Vaporiser Outside Circle (VOC) 891
vaporisers 883–7
  backbar connections 882
  carrier gas composition 887
  checklist 910
  design 883, 887
  draw over 883, 885
  flow splitting ratio 884
  functions 883
  maintenance 887
  measured flow 883, 884, 885
  mechanical stability 887
  overfilling 887
  performance 886–7
  plenum 883, 884
  safety interlock system 882
  variable bypass 883, 884–5
vapours 792–4
  anaesthetic see anaesthetic gases and
      vapours
  analysis methods 850–4
  in cylinders 879
variability 770
variance 916, 917
variation, general 568–9
vasa recta 363, 364, 381
vascular function curve 351, 352
vascular resistance 336
  see also pulmonary vascular resistance;
      systemic vascular resistance
vascular smooth muscle 346
  local control mechanisms 346
  neurological control 348
vascular system 333–7
  control 345–51
  pressure and flow 333–6
  see also blood vessels; circulation
vasoactive intestinal peptide (VIP) 348,
    446
vasoconstriction
  mechanisms 346–51
  in thermoregulation 492
  ventricular contractility and 329
vasoconstrictors, in local anaesthetic
      solutions 662–3
vasodilatation
  mechanisms 346–51
  post operative peripheral 69
  in thermoregulation 492
  ventricular contractility and 329
vasodilating agents, direct-acting 691–2
vasomotor centres 348–9
vasopressin see anti-diuretic hormone
vasopressor drugs
  in CPR 156